Pediatric Nutrition

7TH EDITION

Ronald E. Kleinman, MD, FAAP
Editor

Frank R. Greer, MD, FAAP
Associate Editor

Suggested Citation:
American Academy of Pediatrics
Committee on Nutrition.
[chapter title]. In: Kleinman RE,
Greer FR, eds. *Pediatric Nutrition*.
7th ed. Elk Grove Village, IL:
American Academy of Pediatrics;
2014:[page number]

D1713563

Policy of the American Academy of Pediatrics

American Academy of Pediatrics
141 Northwest Point Blvd
Elk Grove Village, IL 60007-1098

Library of Congress Control Number: 2013951100
ISBN: 978-1-58110 816-3
eISBN: 978-1-58110-819-4
MA0676

The recommendations in this publication do not indicate an exclusive course of treatment or serve as a standard of care. Variations, taking into account individual circumstances, may be appropriate.

This book has been developed by the American Academy of Pediatrics. The authors, editors, and contributors are expert authorities in the field of pediatrics. No commercial involvement of any kind has been solicited or accepted in the development of the content of this publication.

Products are mentioned for informational purposes only. Inclusion in the publication does not imply endorsement by the American Academy of Pediatrics.

The publishers have made every effort to trace the copyright holders for borrowed material. If they have inadvertently overlooked any, they will be pleased to make the necessary arrangements at first opportunity.

Cover photo credits: (breastfeeding) © Goldmund Photography/iStockphoto; (vegetables) © Jasmina/iStockphoto; (fruits) © Picture Partners/iStockphoto; (family cooking) © Chinaview/Shutterstock; (milk) © Getty Images

3-239/1013

2 3 4 5 6 7 8 9 10

Committee on Nutrition
2012-2013

Jatinder J.S. Bhatia, MD, FAAP, Chairperson
Steven A. Abrams, MD, FAAP
Mark R. Corkins, MD, FAAP
Sarah D. de Ferranti, MD, FAAP
Neville H. Golden, MD, FAAP
Sheela N. Magge, MD, FAAP
Sarah Jane Schwarzenberg, MD, FAAP

Former Committee Members

Frank R. Greer, MD, FAAP, Former Chairperson
Stephen R. Daniels, MD, PhD, FAAP
Marcie B. Schneider, MD, FAAP
Janet Silverstein, MD, FAAP
Nicolas Stettler, MD, MSCE, FAAP
Dan W. Thomas, MD, FAAP

Liaisons

Laurence Grummer-Strawn, PhD, *Centers for Disease Control and Prevention*
Jeff Critch, MD, *Canadian Paediatric Society*
Van S. Hubbard, MD, PhD, FAAP, *National Institutes of Health*
Benson M. Silverman, MD, *US Food and Drug Administration*
Valery Soto, MS, RD, LD, *US Department of Food and Agriculture*

Staff

Debra L. Burrowes, MHA

Preface

Malnutrition and overweight and their consequences remain pervasive public health issues for infants and children across the globe. The recent Joint Child Malnutrition Estimates from the United Nations Children's Fund, the World Health Organization, and The World Bank[1] reported that in Africa and Asia in 2011, 36% and 27% of children, respectively, younger than 5 years are stunted. At the same time, overweight affects a third of the children in many resource-rich countries and, in some communities, as many as 60% of school-aged children. An increasing trend for overweight is occurring even in developing countries. Poor nutrition in infants and children has immediate consequences for health and well-being, growth, and development and can lead to long-term and intergenerational effects on health, reproduction, cognition, and chronic disease. This 7th edition of *Pediatric Nutrition* is meant to serve as a current resource for the practicing clinician to provide an understanding of the role of nutrients in human metabolism, the role of nutrition in the prevention and treatment of acute and chronic illnesses and the interaction between nutrients and gene function. Every attempt has been made to provide additional resources within each of the chapters that include references to printed materials, listings of Web-based resources and tools, as well as contacts for both government and private organizations that will be useful for both clinicians and patients. This edition of the handbook is the work of more than 100 authors and editors, all of whom are recognized experts for the topics on which they have written. All chapters are intended to reflect the current position statements and guidelines of the American Academy of Pediatrics Committee on Nutrition. Our most sincere thanks go to the members of the Committee on Nutrition, chaired by Dr. Jatinder Bhatia during the preparation of this latest edition of *Pediatric Nutrition*.

Ronald E. Kleinman, MD, FAAP, and Frank R. Greer, MD, FAAP, Editors

1. United Nations Children's Fund, World Health Organization, The World Bank. *UNICEF-WHO-The World Bank. Joint Child Malnutrition Estimates.* New York, NY: UNICEF; Geneva, Switzerland: World Health Organization; Washington, DC: The World Bank; 2012

Contributors

The American Academy of Pediatrics gratefully acknowledges the invaluable assistance provided by the following individuals who contributed to the preparation of this edition of *Pediatric Nutrition*. Every attempt has been made to recognize all who have contributed; we regret any omissions that may have occurred.

Steve Abrams, MD, FAAP

Jean Ashland, PhD, CCC-SLP

Robert Baker, MD, PhD, FAAP

Susan Baker, MD, PhD, FAAP

Jatinder Bhatia, MD, FAAP

Helen Binns, MD, MPH, FAAP

Margaux E. Black, BA

Christopher R. Braden, MD

Carol Brunzell, RD, LD, CDE

Nancy F. Butte, PhD

Ben Caballero, MD, PhD

Jong Chung, MD

Stephanie Cooks, MA, RD

Stephen Daniels, MD, PhD, MPH, FAAP

Ronald W. Day, MD, FAAP

Christopher Duggan, MD

Kamryn T. Eddy, PhD

Richard A. Ehrenkranz, MD, FAAP

Nancy Emenaker, PhD, MEd, RD

Phil Farrell, MD, PhD, FAAP

Drew Feranchak, MD

Eileen Ferruggiaro, RD, PhD

Marta Fiorotta, PhD

Jennifer Fisher, PhD

Deborah Frank, MD

Ellen Fung, PhD, RD, CCD

Amy Gates, RD, CSP, LD

Paulette Gaynor, PhD

Mark A. Goldstein, MD, FAAP

Rose C. Graham, MD, MSCE

Frank R. Greer, MD, FAAP

Ian Griffin, MD

Cary Harding, MD

Sandra G. Hassink, MD, FAAP

Katherine Hebel, RD, LDN

William C. Heird, MD

David Herzog, MD

Melvin B. Heyman, MD, MPH, FAAP

Kathleen Huntington, MS, RD, LD

Esther Israel, MD

W. Daniel Jackson, MD, FAAP

Susan L. Johnson, PhD

Katherine M. Joyce, MPH

Doron Kahana, MD

Bittoo Kanwar, MD

Martha Ann Keels, DDS, PhD, FAAP

Jae Kim, MD, PhD, FAAP

Ronald E. Kleinman, MD, FAAP

Pamela Kling, MD, FAAP
Nancy Krebs, MD, MS, FAAP
Michele LaBotz, MD, FAAP
HuiChuan Lai, PhD, RD
Melissa N. Laska, PhD, RD
Michele Lawler, MS, RD
Lynne Levitsky, MD, FAAP
Ximena Lopez, MD
David A. Lyczkowski, MD, FAAP
Martha Lynch, MS, RD, LDN, CNSC
William MacLean, Jr, MD, CM, FAAP
Laurie D. Manzo, MEd, RD
Valérie Marchand, MD
Martin G. Martin, MD, MPP
Antonia Mattia, PhD
Shilpa McManus, MD, MPH, FAAP
Nilesh Mehta, MD
Robert Merker, PhD
Tracie L. Miller, MD
John Milner, PhD
Robert D. Murray, MD
Brandon Nathan, MD
Anjali Nayak, MD
Karen Neil, MD, MSPH, FAAP
Daniella Neri, MS, RD, LD
Josef Neu, MD, FAAP
Kenneth Ng, DO

Theresa Nicklas, DrPH
Kate E. Nyquist, MD
Irene Olsen, PhD, RD
Carol O'Neil, PhD, MPH, RD
Lois Parker, RPh
Heidi H. Pfeifer, RD, LDN
Moraima Ramos-Valle, MS
Sue J. Rhee, MD
Michael J. Rock, MD
Phil Rosenthal, MD, FAAP
Stephanie Lynn Ross
Alanna E. F. Rudzik, MSc, PhD
Gary Russell, MD
Daniel W. Sellen, PhD
Robert Shulman, MD, FAAP
Scott Sicherer, MD, FAAP
John Snyder, MD, FAAP
Denise Sofka, MPH, RD
Valery Soto, MS, RD
Jamie Stang, PhD, MPH, RD
Elizabeth A. Thiele, MD, PhD
Vasu Tolia, MD
Steven J. Wassner, MD, FAAP
Jaime Liou Wolfe, MD
Garrett Zella, MD
Babette Zemel, PhD

Table of Contents

IV Micronutrients and Macronutrients

VII   Nutrition and Public Health

Appendices

Chapter 1

Nutrient-Gene Interactions

Introduction

Revolutionary developments in genome sequencing, evaluation of polymorphisms, gene product analysis, epigenetics, analytic software, and bioinformatics can now be used to fine-tune nutritional regimens to individuals rather than populations. Information based on epidemiologic studies of populations in the absence of specific knowledge of the individual's genetics and metabolic response to nutrients may result in erroneous nutritional recommendations. One interesting example is the "milk, it does the body good" concept, which applies quite well to half the world's population, but after infancy in the other half, symptoms of lactose intolerance may preclude ingesting this food in significant quantities.

Prior to the complete sequencing of genomes, the research community was unable to take an integrative approach to explore the role of diet on disease onset. The majority of experimental designs, including epidemiologic studies, used common and well-characterized but relatively uninformative biomarkers to advance our understanding of various disease states. For example, studies aimed at elucidating the molecular mechanisms promoting cardiovascular diseases have primarily used classical biomarkers, such as plasma cholesterol, triglycerides, or C-reactive protein, rather than ones that may provide better clues to an individual's gene response to a nutrient.[1]

The paradigm that has been based on epidemiologic studies, family history, and previous and current environment is shifting to an approach that takes into account an "n=1" (one's self).[2] Individual nutrient-gene interactions have become critical in this regard so that a proper diet can be selected for the individual rather than as a "pyramid" or "My Plate" approach aimed at an entire population. Nutrients contribute to phenotypic changes through various molecular targets, including DNA, RNA, proteins, and metabolites. These are based on the individual's genotype and environmental interactions, including epigenetic alterations (Fig 1.1).[3] This schema leads to the obvious conclusion that gene-nutrient interactions can follow different pathways and lead to different phenotypes on the basis of individual variations and environmental stimuli. Accordingly, 2 new fields—nutrigenomics and nutrigenetics—have a common goal to elucidate the interaction between diet and genes with a common ultimate goal to optimize health through the personalization of diet.[4] Nutrigenomics and nutrigenetics attempt to unravel the complex relationship between nutritional molecules, genetic polymorphisms, and the biological system as a whole—ushering in the era of so-called "personalized medicine."[5]

Fig 1.1.
Nutrients contribute to phenotypic changes through various molecular targets, including DNA, RNA, proteins, and metabolites. These are based on the individual's genotype and environmental interactions, including epigenetic alterations. Adapted with permission from Costa et al.[3]

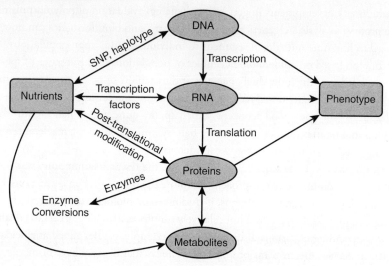

Nutrigenetics (Also Called Nutrigenics)

Human beings are not genetically identical and live in different environments. Thus, each person's response to diet would not be expected to be equivalent. Nutrigenetics refers to gene-nutrient interactions and how an individual responds to a certain diet on the basis of one's genome and, thus, considers underlying genetic polymorphisms.[6]

The following are examples of nutrigenetics:

1. For decades, dietary interventions have been required of individuals with phenylketonuria[7] or galactosemia.[8] These "inborn errors of metabolism" are caused by a single-gene defect that responds to dietary treatment with a low-phenylalanine or low-galactose diet. Galactosemia is caused by a rare recessive trait in galactose-1-phosphate uridyltransferase (GALT), leading to the accumulation of galactose in the blood and increasing the risk of mental retardation.[8] Phenylketonuria is characterized by the defective phenylalanine hydroxylase (PAH) enzyme, resulting in the accumulation of phenylalanine in

the blood, which drastically increases the risk of neurologic damage.[7] Galactose-free and phenylalanine-restricted tyrosine-supplemented diets are a means to treat these monogenic diseases nutritionally, respectively.

2. Individuals with 5,10-methylenetetrahydrofolate reductase (MHTFR) mutation might respond idiosyncratically to folate intakes with established dietary references. A specific thermolabile variant of this enzyme has been described in 5% to 15% of the "normal" population. This variant is associated with coronary heart disease and an increased risk of neural tube defects. Using red cell and plasma folate concentrations, it has been found that folate concentrations were lower in nonpregnant women and even lower still in pregnant women with a TT variant of this gene.[9] Dietary intervention or closer observation of pregnant women with this variant is warranted.

3. Intestinal fatty acid binding protein (IFABP) is exclusively expressed in the small intestine. IFABP is believed to bind and transport long-chain fatty acids (LCFAs) in the cytoplasm of columnar absorptive epithelial cells of the small intestine.[10,11] A polymorphism at codon 54 of the IFABP gene (Ala54Thr), resulting in a change from alanine to threonine, has been associated with a heightened affinity to bind LCFAs and increase TG secretion. The Thr54 allele has been associated with impaired insulin action and increased fat oxidation in several populations.[11,12] Healthy Pima Indian people homozygous for the Thr54 form have higher plasma concentrations of nonesterified fatty acids (NEFAs) and an increased insulin response after the consumption of a meal with high fat content.[12] This suggests that the effects of IFABP polymorphisms on LCFA transport may compromise health by modulating the bioavailability of dietary components.

These single-gene disorders tend to be relatively rare, with incidence less than 1 in 1000 births. On the other hand, much more common genomic variants with multigenic and multifactorial pathogenesis are being discovered using genome-wide association studies (GWAS). Examples include coronary heart disease, diabetes mellitus, various cancers, folate metabolism variants, and autoimmune diseases. The high prevalence of these common genetic variants underline that there is no such thing as a normal population with respect to nutrient requirements and that established dietary references for these individuals may be much less than optimal. These diseases have reached epidemic proportions in the Western world and most often arise from dysfunctional biological networks and not a single mutated gene (ie, polygenic diseases). Dietary intervention to prevent the onset of such diseases is complex and will require not only knowledge of how a single nutrient may affect a biological system but also how a complex mixture (ie, diet) of nutrients will interact to modulate biological functions.[13]

Nutrigenomics

Nutrigenomics refers to how an individual's environment may alter his or her response to a diet. Nutrigenomics aims to determine the influence of common dietary ingredients on the genome and attempts to relate the resulting different phenotypes to differences in the cellular and/or genetic response of the biological system.[14] Nutrigenomics uses functional genomic tools to probe a biological system following a nutritional stimulus that will permit an increased understanding of how nutritional molecules affect metabolic pathways and homeostatic control.[15] High-throughput tools are being used in nutrigenomics that enable millions of genetic screening tests to be conducted at a single time. This allows the examination of how nutrients affect the thousands of genes present in the human genome. Nutrigenomics involves the characterization of gene products that are affected by nutrients and the physiological function and interactions of these products, which include RNA and proteins. Examples include: (1) how an individual will adapt to increased dietary cholesterol intake by increasing 3-hydroxy-3-methylglutaryl coenzyme A (HMG-CoA) reductase concentrations; (2) how different carbohydrate intakes in early life will predispose an individual to metabolic syndrome in adulthood; and (3) how caloric restriction might result in an increased lifespan. As previously mentioned, nutrigenomics offers a powerful and exciting approach to unravel the effects of diet on health.

Epigenetics

Although much emphasis is being placed directly on nutrient-gene interactions, epigenetic relationships are also likely to play an important role. Dietary exposures can have consequences for health years or decades later, as seen in various epidemiologic studies. Epigenetics has raised questions about the mechanisms through which such exposures are "remembered" as pathogenic factors for common complex and chronic diseases not only in the individual but also for subsequent generations. Epigenetics encompasses changes that may alter gene expression but that do not involve changes in the primary DNA sequence. These include 3 distinct but closely interacting mechanisms—DNA methylation, histone modifications, and noncoding microRNAs (miRNA) (Fig 1.2).[16,17]

Epigenetic mechanisms have been implicated in early nutritional programming in utero or by early life environmental stimuli that cause adaptations, such as a "thrifty phenotype" as a response to nutritional deprivation, which may persist into adult life when this adaptation is no longer needed (eg, when there is an abundance of food). The persistence of this adaptation then contributes to the development of the metabolic syndrome.

There is growing evidence that numerous dietary factors, including micronutrients and nonnutrient dietary components, can modify epigenetic marks. In some cases, for

Fig 1.2.
Epigenetic mechanisms: 3 major mechanisms for epigenetic alterations in gene expression have been described. Reproduced with permission from Zaidi SK, Young DW, Montecino MA, et al. Mitotic bookmarking of genes: a novel dimension to epigenetic control. *Nature Rev Genet.* 2010;11(8):583-589.[17]

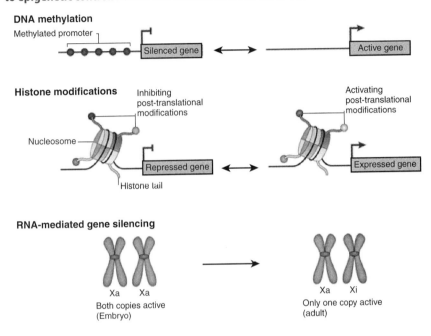

example, the effects of altered dietary supply of methyl donors on DNA methylation, there are plausible explanations for the observed epigenetic changes, but to a large extent, the mechanisms responsible for diet-epigenome-health relationships remain to be discovered. Fig 1.3 illustrates interactions between genetics, environment, epigenetics, and the subsequent development of the metabolic syndrome.[16]

Systems Biology

Along with nutrigenetics, nutrigenomics, and epigenetics, another new paradigm—the "systems" approach to biological phenomenon—is being utilized to evaluate complete sets of circumstances rather than the classic approach. In the classic or reductionist approach, as many variables as possible are controlled, altering one stimulus and determining its effect on a dependent variable. This provides limited information as to how complex systems relate to one another.

Fig 1.3.

Interaction of genetic and epigenetic background with environmental factors that can directly alter gene expression and development of the metabolic syndrome.

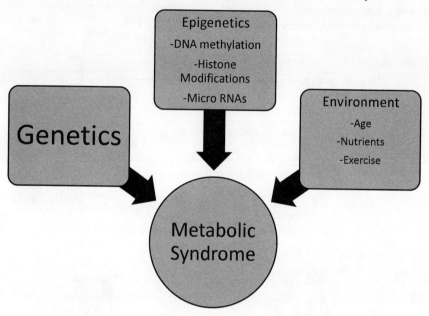

An important challenge in the development of functional foods for the prevention of complex (multifactorial) diseases and enhancement of health through personalized nutrition is to obtain a better and improved overview of the metabolic process a nutritional intervention mitigates. Thus, integration of all information at the different levels of genomic expression (mRNA, protein, metabolite) provides the capacity to measure perturbations of the pathway resulting from nutritional influences. Systems approaches accomplish this in that they model, analyze, and attempt to relate complex biological and chemical systems at multiple levels.[6] They integrate data from a variety of experimental platforms to provide insight into the molecular and chemical interactions and cellular phenotypes and disease processes. This incorporates the ability to obtain, integrate, and analyze complex data from multiple experimental sources using interdisciplinary tools. The experimental techniques that most suit systems biology are those that are system wide and attempt to be as complete as possible. Therefore, transcriptomics, metabolomics, proteomics, and high-throughput techniques are used to collect quantitative data for the construction and validation of models. These technologies are still emerging, and many face the problem in that the larger the quantity of data produced, the lower the quality.

Computational biologists, statisticians, mathematicians, computer scientists, engineers, and physicists are working to improve the quality of these approaches.[6]

The Future

The prevalences of food-related diseases, such as obesity, type 2 diabetes mellitus, and coronary heart disease, are on the rise in Westernized nations. A primary reason for the increase in these diseases is thought be changes in our lifestyle—an abundance of food coupled with low levels of physical activity. However, it is commonly observed that 2 individuals with an equivalent level of physical activity eat an identical diet, and only 1 person gains weight. The different responses between individuals to a given diet clearly highlight the limitations of population-based nutritional recommendations and suggest that our understanding of the mechanisms responsible for interindividual differences are far from being understood.

The observed differences in an individual's response to diet have been attributed to differences in the underlying generic makeup, prompting exploration into the role of nutrient-gene interactions in the determination of a healthy phenotype. Thus, in contrast to pharmaceutical agents that treat a particular disease, nutrition involves a myriad of agents that drastically increase the number of molecular endpoints that are capable of influencing phenotype and, thereby, places the field of nutrition in a prime position to benefit from the technologic innovations brought forth by the postgenomic era. Understanding nutrient-gene interactions will benefit from the concept of systems biology (or integrative metabolism), which aims to understand physiology and disease by integrating and considering molecular pathways, regulatory networks, cells, tissues, organs, and ultimately, the whole organism[18,19]; however, such an approach is not routinely used in nutrition and is conceptually challenging because of the large quantities of data generated. If the goal of a personalized nutrition is to be realized, we must begin to think of the biological system as a physiological network that is intricately connected rather than composed of individual and unrelated elements.

A goal for the future is that a biological sample (blood, urine, buccal swab, saliva) could be rapidly analyzed for its comprehensive metabolite profile, the information could be uploaded into software capable of comparing this profile with those present in a massive database, and then the information procured from the analysis could enable the physician to make dietary recommendations to optimize health. The technical and ethical[20] challenges of this goal remain daunting. Even more difficult will be the storage, management, and interpretation of the vast quantity of data. Nutrition in this century will be an exciting field as we get closer to achieving the goal of highly personalized nutrition.

References

1. Willerson JT, Ridker PM. Inflammation as a cardiovascular risk factor. *Circulation.* 2004;109(21 Suppl 1):II2-II10

2. van der Greef J, Hankemeier T, McBurney RN. Metabolomics-based systems biology and personalized medicine: moving towards n = 1 clinical trials? *Pharmacogenomics.* 2006;7(7):1087-1094

3. Costa V, Casamassimi A, Ciccodicola A. Nutritional genomics era: opportunities toward a genome-tailored nutritional regimen. *J Nutr Biochem.* 2010;21(6):457-467

4. Simopoulos AP. Nutrigenetics/nutrigenomics. *Annu Rev Public Health.* 2010;31:53-68

5. Kaput J. Nutrigenomics research for personalized nutrition and medicine. *Curr Opin Biotechnol.* 2008;19:110-120

6. Panagiotou G, Nielsen J. Nutritional systems biology: definitions and approaches. *Annu Rev Nutr.* 2009;29:329-339

7. Folling A. Ueber Ausscheidung von Phenylbrenztraubensaeure in den Harn als Stoffwechselanomalie in Verbindung mit Imbezillitaet. *Ztschr Physiol Chem.* 1934;227:169-176

8. Goppert F. Galaktosurie nach Milchzuckergabe bei angeborenem, familiaerem chronischem Leberleiden. *Klin Wschr.* 1917;54:473-477

9. Lucock MD. Synergy of genes and nutrients: the case of homocysteine. *Curr Opin Clin Nutr Metab Care.* 2006;9:748-756

10. Pratley RE, Baier L, Pan DA, et al. Effects of an Ala54Thr polymorphism in the intestinal fatty acid-binding protein on responses to dietary fat in humans. *J Lipid Res.* 200;41(12):2002-2008

11. Baier LJ, Sacchettini JC, Knowler WC, et al. An amino acid substitution in the human intestinal fatty acid binding protein is associated with increased fatty acid binding, increased fat oxidation, and insulin resistance. *J Clin Invest.* 1995;95(3):1281-1287

12. Agren JJ, Vidgren HM, Valve RS, Laakso M, Uusitupa MI. Postprandial responses of individual fatty acids in subjects homozygous for the threonine- or alanine-encoding allele in codon 54 of the intestinal fatty acid binding protein 2 gene. *Am J Clin Nutr.* 2001;73(1):31-35

13. Arab L. Individualized nutritional recommendations: do we have the measurements needed to assess risk and make dietary recommendations? *Proc Nutr Soc.* 2004;63(1):167-172

14. Ordovas JM, Mooser V. Nutrigenomics and nutrigenetics. *Curr Opin Lipidol.* 2004;15(2):101-108

15. Muller M, Kersten S. Nutrigenomics: goals and strategies. *Nat Rev Genet.* 2003;4(4):315-322

16. McKay JA, Mathers JC. Diet induced epigenetic changes and their implications for health. *Acta Physiol (Oxf).* 2011;202(2):103-118

17. Zaidi SK, Young DW, Montecino MA, et al. Mitotic bookmarking of genes: a novel dimension to epigenetic control. *Nature Rev Genet.* 2010;11(8):583-589

18. Butcher EC, Berg EL, Kunkel EJ. Systems biology in drug discovery. *Nat Biotechnol.* 2004;22(10):1253-1259

19. Desiere F. Towards a systems biology understanding of human health: interplay between genotype, environment and nutrition. *Biotechnol Annu Rev.* 2004;10:51-84

20. Lévesque L, Ozdemir V, Gremmen B, Godard B. Integrating anticipated nutrigenomics bioscience applications with ethical aspects. *OMICS.* 2008;12(1):1-16

Feeding the Infant

II

Chapter 2

Development of Gastrointestinal Function

Development of Gastrointestinal Function

The design of the gastrointestinal tract allows for the assimilation of environmental nutrients for the purposes of growth, maintenance, and reproduction. The gut has an incredibly intricate physiological and mechanical design, with a large yet limited capacity for nutrient assimilation.[1] The absorptive *capacity* of the gut is a function of multiple variables, including surface area, digestion, facilitative and active transport, motility, perfusion, microflora, and metabolism. Ultimately, capacity of the gut is designed to assimilate the dietary *load* to meet energy requirements for growth and metabolism.[2] The study of the development of gastrointestinal function reveals strong evolutionary concepts and triumphant adaptations for the purposes served.[3]

Development of the Gastrointestinal Tract

The embryonic period is the time of organogenesis. It begins in the third week with gastrulation, the process that establishes the 3 germ layers—*ectoderm, mesoderm,* and *endoderm.* The mammalian digestive tract begins to form soon after the embryo begins to undergo cephalocaudal and lateral folding, resulting in the incorporation of a portion of the endoderm-lined yolk sac cavity into the embryo. This forms the *primitive gut* that is differentiated into 3 parts: *foregut, midgut,* and *hindgut.*[4] Throughout embryogenesis, the gut lumen seals and recanalizes several times for the purpose of elongation. Most of the gut and visceral organs are derived from the *endodermal* cell layer; however, the interaction of *ectodermal* and *mesodermal* tissues is crucial, and several structures contain a mixture of primordial cells.

The lining of the digestive tube and its glands are generated by endodermal cells.[5] Endodermal cells also derive the parenchyma of the liver, gallbladder, and pancreas, and mesodermal tissue surrounds the tube and forms the smooth muscle necessary for intestinal peristalsis. Regional patterning sets the stage for the differential development of primary organs. Anterior (cranial) and posterior (caudal) patterning of the gut tube occurs through the expression of several genes (eg, *sonic hedgehog* [SHH]) that regulate gut development.[6,7] And as primary organs emerge, endodermal and mesodermal layers coordinate their differentiation via direct signaling between adjacent tissues and cells.[8] Investigators have recently succeeded in recapitulating the patterning of human gut in a 3-dimensional organ culture derived from pluripotent stem cells.[9] Specifically, sequential development of definitive and posterior endoderm and hindgut specification were promoted by activin (TGF-β protein superfamily) and subsequent FGF4 and Wnt3A signals.

The foregut differentiates into the pharynx, esophagus, and stomach, up to the second part of the duodenum, and gives rise to the liver and pancreas. Organs of the foregut ingest food and initiate digestion. The midgut is largely responsible for nutrient absorption and gives rise to the structures from the third part of the duodenum to the first two thirds of the large intestine. The hindgut gives rise to the structures from the remaining large intestine through to the rectum and is responsible for the resorption of water and ions, as well as fermentation and expulsion of digestive waste.

The glandular epithelium of the liver and the biliary drainage system, including the gallbladder, are all formed from the *hepatic diverticulum*, a tube of endoderm that extends out from the foregut into the surrounding mesenchyme. The pancreas develops from the fusion of 2 distinct *dorsal* and *ventral diverticula*, both derived of endodermal cells immediately caudal to the stomach. Portions of the gut tube and its derivatives are designated *intraperitoneal* if they are suspended from the dorsal and ventral body wall by a double layer of peritoneum that enclose and connect them to the body wall. Organs and portions of the intestinal tube that lie up against the posterior body-wall, covered by peritoneum on their anterior surface only are called *retroperitoneal*. Most of the gut lies intraperitoneally and is free floating, the exceptions being the majority of the duodenum and parts of the colon. The duodenum turns and exits into the retroperitoneal space just past the bulb and re-enters the peritoneum at the location of its fixation to the left crus of the diaphragm by the *ligament of Treitz*, which also marks the beginning of the jejunum. In most individuals, the left colon and right colon also lay retroperitoneally.[5]

Developmental Disorders

Several well-known complications of embryogenesis constitute a significant portion of the abnormalities seen in neonates and infants, yet their molecular basis has only been defined in a few incidences. Esophageal abnormalities include esophageal *atresia, stenosis*, and tracheoesophageal *fistula*. Esophageal *stenosis* can be the result of a vascular abnormality. Stomach malformations include *duplication* and prepyloric *septum*. Duodenal *atresia* and *stenosis* are believed to be the result of incomplete recanalization of the intestinal lumen. Midgut atresias are often considered to be secondary to a vascular accident caused by intestinal *malrotation*. Normally, the primary intestinal loop rotates 270° counterclockwise during embryogenesis. Failure of the gut to rotate fully, or its reverse rotation, results in malrotation and predisposes the child to abnormal movement of the gut and *volvulus*. *Gastroschisis* (ie, the herniation of abdominal contents through the body wall directly into the amniotic cavity) and *omphalocele* (ie, the herniation of abdominal contents through an enlarged umbilical ring) can also result in loss of viable intestines, leading to *short gut syndrome*. Rectoanal *atresias* and congenital *fistulas* are caused by abnormalities in formation of the cloaca and ectopic positioning of the anal opening. *Imperforate anus* occurs as a result of improper recanalization of the lower portion of the anal canal. *Hirschsprung disease* is caused by the absence of parasympathetic ganglia in the bowel wall. These ganglia are neural crest derived and normally migrate from the neural folds down to the wall of the bowel.[10]

Variation in liver architecture and lobulation is most often asymptomatic. Extrahepatic ducts can fail to recanalize, resulting in extrahepatic *biliary atresia*. *Intrahepatic biliary duct hypoplasia* is often caused by fetal infections (eg, cytomegalovirus infection), or Alagille syndrome, an autosomal-dominant disorder that is secondary to mutations in Jagged-1 (JAG1) and associated with complex congenital heart disease, and other anomalies.[11] Mild pancreatic abnormalities are relatively common, are often asymptomatic, and are usually the result of poor migration of the pancreatic buds. The lack of fusion of the 2 pancreatic ducts is called pancreatic *divisum* and may be associated with an increased risk of pancreatitis in children. A serious malformation is when an annular pancreas surrounds the duodenum, which can constrict the duodenum and present with intestinal obstructive symptoms.

Development of the Intestinal Epithelium

The rapid epithelial cell turnover of the gastrointestinal tract continues throughout life. This process is maintained and regulated by populations of *stem cells* that generate both absorptive and secretory epithelial cell lineages.[12] These cells form a clonal population called a *niche* toward the base of crypts, and their activity is regulated by paracrine secretion of growth factors and cytokines from surrounding mesenchymal cells. Stem cell division is usually asymmetric, with the identical daughter cell becoming a committed progenitor cell and retaining the ability to continue dividing until terminally differentiated. Symmetric division may result in either 2 daughter cells, with loss of stem cell function, or formation of 2 stem cells and eventual clone dominance. The apparent stochastic extinction of some stem cell lines with eventual dominance of a single cell line is called *niche succession*.[13]

Active and quiescent stem cell populations have recently been identified and reside in specific locations within crypts and are marked by specific molecular signatures, including LGR5 and OLFM4, which have been primarily established in mice.[14,15] Specifically, active stem cells are located in the crypt base columnar cells (CBCs) nested between Paneth cells that secrete luminal beta-defensins that probably protect the CBCs from a slew of microbes and pathogens and presumably secrete Wnt signals to support the proliferation of the active stem cell population.[16] In contrast, quiescent stem cells are believed to reside primarily in position +4 in the crypt and appear to proliferate following destruction of the active CBC population of cells during various types of injury like radiation. Whether the various markers such as BMI1, HOPX, and others define distinct quiescent stem cell populations that respond differently during injury/repair has not been established.[17] However, radiation injury obliterates the active cells, resulting in the subsequent induction of cell cycle proliferation of BMI1+ quiescent stem cells and the repopulation of the LGR5+ active stem cells.[18]

The active stem cells produce proliferating transit-amplifying (TA) progenitor cells of the epithelium that become increasingly differentiated along the *crypt-villus axis*, undergo spontaneous apoptosis within 4 to 5 days, and are shed into the lumen where they are digested and phagocytosed.[19] Five main epithelial cell lineages are derived from this active LGR5+ stem cells: *columnar* cells are the most abundant and are specialized for absorption and secretion by the presence of apical microvilli; *goblet* cells are named for their swollen shape, a consequence of mucin granule production; *enteroendocrine* cells secrete peptide hormones in an endo- and paracrine fashion, influencing gastrointestinal function in a variety of ways; *Paneth* cells are large cells that migrate down to the crypt base, where they express and secrete several proteins, including lysozyme, tumor necrosis factor alpha, and antibacterial *defensins*, all of which help keep the crypt sterile[20,21]; and the rarer *tuft cells* are distinguished by long microvilli.[22] M (*membranous* or *microfold*) cells are a sixth type of epithelial cell found near *Peyer patches* and are involved in antigen transport.[23]

The *lamina propria* forms the *basement membrane*, providing a supporting network for the epithelium and regulating epithelial cell function. It contains numerous kinds of cells, including *fibroblasts, myofibroblasts, fibrocytes, vascular endothelial* and *smooth muscle* cells, and various blood lineages. Some of these cells secrete growth factors, such as R-spondin, Wnt, and *transforming growth factor-beta 2*, essential for stem cell proliferation and epithelial cell differentiation.[24]

Infant Nutrient Assimilation

The neonatal gut has several major functions. It is obviously an organ of nutrition, with digestive, absorptive, secretory, and motile functions adapted to a milk diet. However, it is also part of the immune system, containing both humoral and cellular elements of the gut-associated lymphoid tissue (GALT). It is a large and diffuse endocrine organ that secretes locally acting gut hormones and paracrine factors that help regulate intestinal and metabolic adaptation to extrauterine life.[25] It plays a role in water conservation and electrolyte homeostasis and maintains a symbiotic relationship with a microbial flora, which assists in the digestion and absorption of certain nutrients. The intestinal *microbiota* also plays a vital role in health and disease.[26]

The neonatal intestine replaces the role of the placenta quite abruptly at birth, with most intestinal nutrient transport mechanisms intact well before birth.

The neonatal intestine is uniquely capable of absorbing intact macromolecules via *endocytosis*, a function utilized for the transport for various maternal growth factors imperative for intestinal development.[27,28] Yet, the overall absorptive and digestive capacity of the gut is impaired in the neonatal period, and early infant growth requires a special nutrient environment.[29] The degree to which alterations in digestive and absorptive capacity seen during and after infancy are genetically determined has yet to be established. For example, although the decline in lactase activity seen with weaning occurs despite an ongoing lactose load, the upregulation of fructose transporters in response to increased fructose consumption is altered by load.[30] Thus, there is evidence of both genetic hard-wired preprogramming and an adaptation mechanism responsive to nutrient load.

Dietary Fats

Fat, or *lipid*, is defined as a class of compounds insoluble in water but soluble in organic solvents, such as alcohol. Lipids contain carbon, hydrogen, and oxygen but have far less oxygen proportionally than do carbohydrates. Lipids vary considerably in size and polarity, ranging from hydrophobic triglycerides and sterol esters to the more water-soluble phospholipids and cardiolipins. Dietary lipids also include cholesterol and phytosterols. These compounds are distinguished from other dietary macronutrients in that they must undergo specialized processing during digestion, absorption, transport, storage, and utilization.[31]

Triglycerides (TGs) make up the largest proportion of dietary lipids. TGs are composed of 3 *fatty acids* (FAs) esterified onto a glycerol molecule. These FAs are generally nonbranched and have an even number of carbons, from 4 to 26, although *very long-chain fatty acids* (VLCFAs) are found in the brain and specialized tissue, such as retina and spermatozoa.[32] Double bonds are identified relative to the methyl end by the designation "n" or "ω" to indicate the distance from the first bond. For example, ω-6 indicates that the initial double bond is situated between the sixth and seventh carbon atom from the methyl group end. Because the biosynthetic process can only insert double bonds at the ω-9 position or higher, *essential FAs* are considered those with double bonds at the ω-6 and ω-3 positions. Most food contains double bonds in the *cis* configuration, whereas bonds that are *trans* result from hydrogenation, an industrial process used to increase the viscosity of oils. Trans-FAs have reduced internal rotation, which makes them more resistant to electrophilic additions, such as hydration, and increases their melting point. Trans-fats are heavily implicated in obesity and may contribute to development of obesity-related heart disease, diabetes, and atherosclerosis.[33]

Phospholipids are distinct from TGs in that they contain polar head groups that make them amphipathic and, therefore, capable of forming micelles in water. They include glycerol, choline, serine, inositol, and ethanolamine. Sterols, such as *cholesterol*, are also amphipathic molecules made up of a steroid nucleus and a branched hydrocarbon tail. Although cholesterol is found only in food of animal origin, plants do contain phytosterols, which are chemically related to cholesterol.

Fat Digestion

Digestion of dietary fat requires a series of processes that enable absorption through the aqueous milieu of the epithelium of the gut. Digestion begins in the oral cavity as salivation, mastication, and *lingual lipase* begin to release largely short-chain fatty acids (SCFAs) from TGs. Lingual lipase is produced by *von Ebner* serous glands located on the proximal, dorsal tongue,[34] and *gastric lipase* is produced by stomach *chief cells*.[35] Both lipases have been shown to remain largely active in the gastric milieu.[36] Both lingual and gastric (ie, preduodenal) lipases preferentially hydrolyze SCFAs and *medium-chain triglycerides* (MCTs), which can be absorbed directly from the stomach.[37,38,39] Thus, monoglycerides are poorly hydrolyzed in the stomach, and the release of *long-chain fatty acids* (LCFAs) and VLCFAs requires the presence of bile and pancreatic lipases.

Pancreatic lipase requires the presence of colipase to remove the inhibitory effect of bile salts. It is more active against insoluble, emulsified substrates. A second pancreatic lipase, *carboxylase esterase*, is more active against micellar (ie, soluble) substrates and is strongly stimulated by bile salts.

Bile is composed of bile salts, phospholipids, and sterols. It emulsifies the hydrophobic groups of dietary lipids and allows pancreatic lipases to hydrolyze the ester bonds of the glycerol moiety. Bile also increases the surface area available to enzymes and protects enzymes from proteolysis themselves. The bile of infants has a lower concentration of bile acids than does the bile of older children and adults, with a higher relative ratio of *cholic acid* to *chenodeoxycholic acid*.[40] This is believed to be secondary to a slower synthetic rate of bile acids in neonates than in adults.[41] Moreover, neonatal bile acids are conjugated primarily with taurine, whereas in older infants they are conjugated primarily with glycine.[42] The ileal mechanism for transport of *cholyltaurine* (ie, the expression of the *apical sodium-dependent bile acid transporter* [ASBT]) is not well developed in the newborn infant, resulting in poor recycling of bile acids.[43,44]

Fat Absorption

The absorption of lipids is through both active transport and passive diffusion of micellar products and free FAs across the brush-border membrane (BBM). *Fatty acid binding proteins* (FABPs) assist in the transmucosal shunting of free FAs, monoglycerides, and bile salts.[45] Both increased FA saturation and chain length correlate negatively with absorptive efficiency across the BBM.[46]

Fat Assimilation in the Newborn Infant

Human milk consists of approximately 4% fat, mostly in the form of MCTs and long-chain triglycerides (LCTs).[47] Because almost half of the total calories in an infant's diet are derived from fat, the digestion and absorption of fat must be very efficient in infancy.[48,49] Both salivary and gastric lipases are produced early in fetal development (gastric lipase is detectable in the developing fetus as early as 10 weeks' gestation and reaches adult levels by early infancy),[50] yet neonatal pancreatic and biliary excretion is generally low in early infancy.[51,52,53] Therefore, it is likely that certain evolutionary measures were preferentially selected for, such as the greater capacity for absorption of intact macromolecules by receptor-mediated endocytosis in the neonatal intestine as well as the production of various lipases and proteolytic inhibitors in the maternal mammary glands. The importance of human milk factors to infant fat digestion is well-documented, as hydrolysis of fat has been shown to be more than twice as efficient in breastfed infants compared with formula-fed infants.[54]

Human milk lipases include *bile salt-stimulated lipase* (BSSL), which is made in the mammary glands and remains inactive until coming into contact with bile salts in the infant's duodenum.[55,56] BSSL survives the stomach milieu and is activated in the duodenum by bile acids to convert monoglycerides to glycerol and free FAs.[57,58] Without BSSL, the monoglyceride load would likely exceed neonatal absorptive capacity and much would escape unabsorbed. BSSL performs other functions, such as the hydrolysis of retinol esters allowing for retinol absorption[59] as well as hydrolysis of *ceramide*, the main sphingomyelin (a phospholipid) in human milk.[60] The importance of BSSL is supported by a study of low birth weight preterm infants (3 to 6 weeks old) who were fed raw versus heat-treated (ie, pasteurized or boiled) human milk. Fat absorption was significantly higher in the former group (74%) compared with the latter (54% and 46%, respectively).[61] Other lipases, such as *lipoprotein lipase,* are also present in human milk (see Human Milk, p 25).[62]

Dietary Carbohydrates

Carbohydrates are a class of substances with a molar ratio of carbon to hydrogen to oxygen of 1:2:1, $C_n(H_2O)_n$, plus oligosaccharides, polysaccharides, and the sugar alcohols (sorbitol, maltitol, mannitol, galactitol, and lactitol). *Complex* carbohydrates are mainly plant starch and animal glycogen but include also pectin, cellulose, and gum. *Simple* carbohydrates include the hexose *monosaccharides* glucose, galactose, and fructose, the *disaccharides* maltose (glucose-glucose), sucrose (glucose-fructose), and lactose (glucose-galactose), as well as sporadic trioses, tetroses, and pentoses. Pentoses (ie, ribose, $C_5H_{10}O_5$) are important constituents of nucleic acids.[63]

Oligosaccharides are generally defined as yielding 3 to 10 monosaccharides on hydrolysis (eg, maltose, isomaltose, maltotriose, maltodextrin), whereas *polysaccharides* yield more than 10.[64] *Starch*, by far the most common dietary polysaccharide, consists of only glucose units and is, thus, designated a *glucosan*. Starch is composed of 2 homopolymers of glucose: *amylose* (linear 1-4 linkages) and *amylopectin* (branched 1-6 and 1-4 linkages).

Carbohydrate Digestion

The digestion of carbohydrates requires complete hydrolysis of poly-, oligo-, and disaccharides, because absorption of dietary carbohydrates in the intestine is limited to the monosaccharides glucose, galactose, and fructose. Digestion begins with salivary *amylase,* which acts only on the interior (1-4) linkages of polysaccharides, not the outer (1-6) linkages, releasing α-disaccharides (eg, maltose) and *trisaccharides* (eg, maltotriose) and creating large oligosaccharides (eg, dextrins). *Dextrins* are sugar molecules containing an average of 8 glucose units with 1 or more outer links, requiring further digestion by *glucoamylase. Pancreatic amylase*, similar to salivary amylase, cleaves only interior links. The *disaccharidases* (eg, lactase, fructose, and sucrase-isomaltase) are necessary to ultimately yield free monosaccharide molecules.

Carbohydrate Absorption

Glucose is the major source of metabolic energy. As a hydrophilic polar molecule, it relies on transport across the relatively impermeable hydrophobic intestinal brush-border membrane. Transport occurs via both a family of facilitative *glucose transporters* (GLUTs) as well as active symporters, such as the *sodium-glucose cotransporters* (SGLTs).[65,66,67] GLUTs are membrane integral proteins found on the surface of all cells. They transport glucose down its concentration gradient, and the energy for the transfer comes from dissipation of the concentration difference. SGLTs allow for glucose transport against the concentration gradient and are expressed mostly in enterocytes of the small intestine and epithelial cells of the kidney's proximal tubule.[68] The transport of glucose up its concentration gradient occurs in the presence of sodium and results in the passive resorption of water.[69] This concept explains the rationale behind oral rehydration solutions.

Galactose shares the same transport mechanisms as glucose in the enterocytes, namely apical SGLT cotransporters and the basolateral GLUT2. Once it enters the portal blood circulation, it is practically cleared in its first passage through the liver, where it is converted by *galactokinase* into galactose-1-phosphate. The latter is then transformed enzymatically into glucose-1-phosphate and converted into glycogen. Lactose is the sole dietary source of galactose in humans, although glucose can be converted into galactose for supply of cellular needs (eg, glycoproteins and mucopolysaccharides).

Fructose is transported across the BBM by the facilitated transporter GLUT5. Fructose malabsorption is well documented in infants and toddlers and is associated with diarrhea and abdominal pain.[70] GLUT5 is believed to undergo upregulation with increased dietary intake of fructose. Once absorbed, fructose is metabolized by the abundant enzyme *fructokinase* and then cleaved by *aldolase* to produce glyceraldehyde and dihydroxyacetone phosphate. The metabolites ultimately enter the glycolytic pathway and produce glycogen. Small amounts of fructose act catalytically to enhance glucose metabolism, perhaps via activation of *glucokinase*.[71] However, large amounts of fructose may saturate the glycolytic pathway with intermediate metabolites that may be used for triglyceride synthesis.

Carbohydrate Assimilation in the Newborn Infant

The concentration of salivary and pancreatic *amylase*, as well as brush-border glucoamylase and disaccharidases (eg, lactase) are low in the neonatal period but increase to mature concentrations quite rapidly in the postnatal period.[72,73,74] Approximately 25% of 1-week-old term infants exhibit some lactose malabsorption, and lactase activity in the neonatal period appears to be inducible by lactose intake.[75,76,77,78] Lactose malabsorption in the neonate is generally mild and asymptomatic, with malabsorbed lactose salvaged in the colon with bacterial fermentation and production of SCFAs. Thus, the finite capacity of the neonatal intestine to absorb lactose may serve to promote healthy intestinal microflora and provide colonocytes with an important nutrient (ie, butyric acid).[79]

Starch digestion is limited in newborn infants, and pancreatic secretion of α-amylase may remain insufficient for several months.[80] Thus, carbohydrate needs in infancy are met largely via the digestion of lactose into glucose and galactose, and the need for α-amylase digestion is minimal until weaning. Weaning is also the time at which all studied nonhuman mammals and most humans begin to experience a decline in lactase concentrations.[81] Individuals who are *lactase persistent* are generally of Western European descent, a product of natural selection in areas where animal farming and milking have occurred for centuries. *Hypolactasia* occurs in most other individuals, as early as 2 years of age in children from Thailand and Bangladesh and 10 years of age for other Asians, African-American, and Latin-American children. For many white children (eg Finnish, Irish), it is a steady and slow decrease.[82,83]

The molecular basis of hypolactasia is hard wired and has recently been elucidated. Specifically, 2 single nucleotide polymorphisms, C/T_{-13910} and G/A_{-22018}, located in regulatory control regions upstream of the transcriptional start site of the *lactase-phlorizin hydrolase (LPH)* gene, have been associated with adult-onset hypolactasia.[84] At position 13 910, the T polymorphism is associated with lactase persistence in the European population and is associated with enhanced binding by the Oct-1 transcription factor.[85] Therefore, these single nucleotide polymorphisms are believed to modulate binding of other transcription proteins that mediate lactase expression.

Dietary Protein

Made of *amino acids*, proteins direct and facilitate the biochemical reactions of life. Proteins include enzymes, transporters, signaling peptides, and muscle fiber. Its requirement diminishes greatly after infancy, as the rate of accretion of new protein is reduced; although during accelerated growth phases, as seen in early childhood and adolescence, as well as in athletes, protein requirement is increased to near-infant levels. The metabolic rate of conversion and utilization of individual amino acids differs in the body depending on age, gender, nutrient exposure, and level of activity.[86]

Indispensable amino acids make up about a third of the protein requirement in infancy but only about a fifth later in childhood and a tenth in adulthood.[87] The need for high-quality protein, defined by the protein's ability to support growth, also decreases with age.[88] High-quality proteins characteristically have an abundance of indispensable amino acids, are easily digestible, and lack contaminating molecules, such as inhibitors of digestive enzymes (eg, trypsin inhibitors) or antigens that may trigger allergic stimuli.

Protein differs from carbohydrates and fat in that it contains nitrogen, on average about 16% by weight. When amino acids are oxidized in the citric acid (ie, Krebs or TCA) cycle to carbon dioxide and water to produce energy, nitrogen is produced as a waste product and must be expelled from the body. The body can utilize dietary protein for energy, muscle incorporation, or incorporation into other nitrogen-containing compounds.

Amino acids can be converted to glucose via gluconeogenesis to provide a continuous supply of glucose after glycogen stores are consumed. Similar to carbohydrates, degradation of amino acids by oxidation produces approximately 4 kcal/g of protein. The carbon skeletons may also be used for formation of fat via elongation of acetyl units and carbohydrates through the conversion of alanine into pyruvate. Amino acids are also incorporated into various products, such as creatine, nitric oxide, purines and pyrimidines, glutathione, porphyrins (hemoglobin and cytochromes), histamine, serotonin, nicotinic acid, thyroid hormone, catecholamines, and carnitine, among many others.

Protein Digestion

Digestion of protein begins in the stomach with *pepsin* secretion in gastric juice. Pepsin cleaves the C-terminus of tyrosine, phenylalanine, and tryptophan. Pepsin output and *parietal* cell activity are believed to be lower in the neonate than in older infants.[89] The buffering of gastric acidity following milk feeds may also result in suboptimal pepsin activity in early infancy.[90,91] Yet, it is important to note that secretion of gastric acid, *intrinsic factor*, and *gastrin* is noted as early as the middle of the second gestational trimester,[92] and infants are able to maintain a gastric pH well below 4 from the first day of life.[93,94] Indeed, infants have been shown to be capable of hydrogen ion secretion,[95] with the level of gastric H^+/K^+-*adenosine triphosphatase* (H^+/K^+-ATPase) *proton pump* increasing significantly with advanced gestational age and during the first 3 months of life.[96] Pepsin activity is shown to increase soon after initiating feeding.[97]

Proteolytic enzymes secreted from the pancreas and intestinal mucosa break down proteins into smaller peptides. Their activity is largely dependent on the amino acid residue composition of the protein ingested. Pancreatic secretion begins in utero at about the fifth month of gestation.[98] Although trypsin values may be lower in the preterm infant,[99] a substantial difference in trypsin concentration in duodenal fluid between 2 days and 7 weeks of age is not observed,[100] and mature trypsin concentration is reached by as early as 1 to 3 months of age. *Chymotrypsin* activity may also be low in the newborn infant but increases rapidly, approaching the levels of older children at about 6 months of age and adult levels by 3 years of age.[101] Nonetheless, adults can digest protein at about a 60% faster rate than children can.[102]

Pancreatic digestive enzymes are secreted in the form of *zymogens*, precursors that are converted into active proteolytic enzymes in the intestinal lumen. *Trypsin* is activated from *trypsinogen* by *enterokinase*, a brush-border enzyme. Trypsin cleaves the C-terminal of positively charged amino acids, such as lysine and arginine, and activates *chymotrypsin* from *chymotrypsinogen*. Chymotrypsin attacks the same bonds cleaved by pepsin, which is inactivated by the increased pH of duodenal content. *Carboxypeptidase* cleaves the amide bond at the C-terminus of aromatic and branched-chain amino acids, such as tyrosine, tryptophan, and phenylalanine. *Elastase* preferentially cleaves peptide bonds at the C-terminal of small, hydrophobic amino acids, such as glycine, alanine, serine, and valine. Elastase is highly active against *elastin*, a component of connective tissue. *Nucleases* hydrolyze ingested nucleic acids (RNA and DNA) into their component nucleotides.

The oligopeptide products of gastric and pancreatic proteolysis undergo further hydrolysis in the BBM of the small intestine by *carboxypeptidase* and *aminopeptidase*. These 2 enzymes hydrolyze the carboxyl and amino terminals of oligopeptides, respectively, releasing tripeptides, dipeptides, and individual amino acids. Tri- and dipeptides can cross the BBM to be hydrolyzed intracellularly by *tri-* and *dipeptidases*. Activity of carboxypeptidase, aminopeptidase, tripeptidase, and dipeptidase is detectable in the intestines of fetuses as early as in the second trimester of gestation.[76,103]

Protein Absorption

Free amino acids are absorbed by active and specific transporters into the mucosa. Several transport systems are ubiquitously expressed and exhibit preference for certain amino acids. Systems *A* and *ASC*, for example, prefer amino acids with small side chains (eg, glycine, alanine, serine). System *L* transports amino acids with bulky side chains (eg, tyrosine, arginine, valine, asparagine, glutamine). The *B* system (eg, $B^{O,+}$, b^+), which has broad specificity for neutral amino acids, is produced largely in the small intestine.[104] Other specific amino acid transport systems in the intestine include *IMINO* (proline and glycine) and *rBAT* (cystine and dibasic amino acids). The transport of amino acids across the mucosa of the small intestine has been shown in fetuses as young as 12 weeks' gestational age.[105]

Protein Assimilation in the Newborn Infant

Larger peptides and proteins can enter the gut intact. Although the adult intestine absorbs about a quarter of its dietary protein as *dipeptides* and *tripeptides*, utilizing intracellular *hydrolases* to free amino acids into the portal blood, the neonate relies on the transfer of macromolecules to a much greater extent. Macromolecules from maternal milk include enzymes, growth factors, and immunoglobulins, which help shape the neonate's digestive, barrier, and immunologic function. Macromolecules can cross the intestinal epithelium either *transcellularly* (ie, through cells) or *paracellularly* (ie, between cells). *Endocytosis*, a transcellular pathway, is the major pathway for macromolecules to cross the mucosal brush border.[106] The paracellular passage of macromolecules across "leaks" between epithelial cell junctions (ie, *tight junctions*) remains controversial.

The uptake of macromolecules by the neonatal gut may represent the persistence of intrauterine absorptive processes, because amniotic fluid is known to contain a range of protein macromolecules, including immunoglobulins, hormones, enzymes, and growth factors.[107] The small intestine is noted to be more permeable to intact proteins in the neonatal period, and infant serum often contains higher titers of antibodies to food antigens than does the serum of adults.[108-110] It is not fully understood how protein antigens escape luminal digestion and cross the brush-border membrane in sufficient amount to trigger an immune response, but the transport of maternal biological compounds intact may have served an evolutionary advantage.[111] Recent data suggest that the epithelial immunoglobulin G (IgG) receptor (FcRn) facilitates the recycling of IgG between the intestinal lumen and systemic circulatory compartments, including antigen-immunoglobulin complexes.[112]

Vitamins and Minerals

Fat-soluble micronutrients, such as prostaglandins and vitamins A, D, E, and K, are emulsified within lipid and cross the mucosal BBM as lipophilic molecules. Water-soluble vitamins cross the intestinal BBM by the action of specific carrier-mediated transport. These include the *Na$^+$-dependent multivitamin transporter* (SMVT), which is produced by enterocytes and transports vitamins such as B complex and pantothenate.[113] Vitamin C (L-ascorbic acid) transport occurs via the recently identified mammalian family of a *Na$^+$-dependent L-ascorbic acid transporter* (SVCT1). Thought to be essential in diminishing oxidant injury in rapidly growing tissue, vitamin C serum concentrations decline rapidly postpartum. Thus, SVCT1 expression in neonates may be of vital importance for vitamin C regulation.[114,115]

Most mineral absorption depends on specific carrier-mediated transport as well. Mineral accretion in the fetus occurs only during the last trimester of gestation, increasing the risk of mineral deficiencies in the preterm infant. The transport of calcium is sensitive to the presence and abundance of other nutrients, such as lactose and fatty acids.[116-118] The impact of calcium on newborn bone mineral content (BMC) depends on several factors, including maternal vitamin D concentrations, gestational age, fetal size, and maternal glucose homeostasis.[119] Infants of diabetic mothers have low BMC at birth, implying that factors in pregnancy have an effect on fetal BMC or that decreased transplacental mineral transfer may occur, because otherwise, BMC is consistently increased with increased newborn weight and length. Moreover, although race and gender differences in BMC appear early in life, they do not appear to exist at birth.

Young animals absorb iron, lead, calcium, and strontium much better than do adult animals.[120,121] A divalent cation transporter named DCT1 is the main iron carrier in the small intestine.[122] The specificity of this transporter is limited to the reduced or ferrous form of iron. However, it can transport other divalent cationic minerals, such as zinc, copper, manganese, nickel, lead, cobalt, and cadmium. Its affinity to lead makes human infants at greater risk than adults for lead toxicity.[123]

Human Milk

The relationship between lactating mammary function and neonatal gastrointestinal function is an example of the parallel evolution of 2 organs that, after birth, together undertake functions previously performed by the placenta.[111] Human milk contains both nutrients required by the newborn infant for energy and metabolism and nonnutritional components that promote infant health, growth, and development. Nonnutritional components include antimicrobial factors, digestive enzymes, hormones, trophic factors, and growth modulators. Energy nutrients include metabolic fuel (ie, fat, protein, carbohydrates), free water, and raw material necessary for tissue growth and development, such as long-chain fatty acids, essential amino acids, minerals, vitamins, and trace elements. For most infants, nutrient intake from human milk becomes increasingly insufficient after 4 to 6 months of age, and other foods need to be added to the diet.

More than 98% of the fat in human milk is in the form of triglycerides, made within the mammary glands from medium- and long-chain fatty acids. *Oleic acid* (18:1) and *palmitic acid* (16:0) are the most abundant fatty acids, with palmitic acid occupying the central position of the glycerol molecule in most human milk triglycerides, a property that increases its overall digestibility.[124] Similarly high proportions of the essential fatty acids *linoleic acid* (18:2 ω-6) and *linolenic acid* (18:3 ω-3) and of other long-chain polyunsaturated fatty acids, such as *arachidonic acid* (20:4 ω-6, ARA) and *docosahexaenoic acid* (22:6 ω-3, DHA), are also present.[125] These long-chain polyunsaturated fatty acids (LCPUFAs) are constituents of brain and neural tissue and are needed in early life for mental and visual development.[126] Studies have established that plasma and red blood cell LCPUFA concentrations of infants fed formulas supplemented with both ω-6 and ω-3 LCPUFAs were closer to those of breastfed infants than to those of infants fed formulas containing no LCPUFAs.[127] Still, infants fed formulas supplemented with LCPUFAs did not match the status of breastfed infants.[128] Although fewer than half of all studies report beneficial effects of LCPUFAs on visual, mental, and/or psychomotor function, the body of literature suggests that LCPUFAs are important to the growth and development of infants.[129]

Proteins account for approximately 75% of the nitrogen-containing compounds in human milk. Nonprotein nitrogen substances include urea, nucleotides, peptides, free amino acids, and DNA. The proteins of human milk can be divided into 2 categories: micellar caseins and aqueous whey proteins, present in the ratio of about 40:60.[130] The predominant casein of human milk is β-*casein*, which forms micelles of relatively small volume and produces a soft, flocculent curd in the infant's stomach. Certain human milk proteases, such as *plasmin*, which is highly active against *casein*, increase infant capacity for protein digestion.

The major proteins found in human milk are α-*lactalbumin*, *lactoferrin*, *secretory IgA*, and *serum albumin*, with a large number of other proteins present in smaller amounts. Secretory IgA is the principal immunoglobulin of human milk and, together with lactoferrin, represents about 30% of all milk protein.[131] It is synthesized in the mammary epithelial cell when 2 IgA molecules, produced locally by lymphocytes resident in the breast tissue, are coupled with 2 proteins, a J-chain and a secretory component produced from the polymeric IgA receptor, pIgR. The specificity of human milk secretory IgA antibodies reflects the mother's exposure to various antigens and is independent of the specificity profile of bloodborne IgA.[132,133] *Lactoferrin*, which transports and promotes the absorption of iron, is also a bacteriostatic agent to a range of organisms. Ultimately, once digested into amino acids, it can be absorbed and used by the body for energy requirement.[131]

The principal carbohydrate of human milk is *lactose*, a β-disaccharide manufactured in the mammary epithelial cell from glucose by a reaction involving α-lactalbumin.[134] In addition, human milk contains significant quantities of oligosaccharides, predominantly lactose-N-tetraose and its monofucosylated derivatives, representing about 10% of total milk carbohydrate. Oligosaccharides can escape luminal digestion and are believed to serve as growth factors for intestinal microflora (eg, *Bifidobacterium bifidum*).[135] They are also suspected of altering bacterial adhesion to intestinal epithelial cells.[136]

In addition to energy nutrients, human milk contains a wealth of bioactive components that have beneficial yet nonnutritional functions.[137,138] Nonnutrient factors compensate for the neonate's immature digestive and barrier functions and modulate the transition from intrauterine to extrauterine life. These factors include a wide range of specific and nonspecific antimicrobial factors, cytokines, and anti-inflammatory substances, as well as hormones, growth modulators, and digestive enzymes. These components may be of particular importance for young infants, because their digestive systems and host defenses are still immature, making them susceptible to infection. The physiological significance of many of these substances is not fully determined, and some may represent merely a "spillover" of excretory products from metabolic processes occurring within the mammary epithelial cell. For those with established significance, the site of action may be within the mother's breast, within the infant's alimentary canal, or within the infant's body.

Of the trophic factors active in the newborn infant, *epidermal growth factor* (EGF) is the best studied. A small polypeptide with mitogenic, antisecretory, and cytoprotective properties, EGF is present in amniotic fluid and colostrum, suggesting that it plays an important role in perinatal adaptation to extrauterine nutrition and gut function.[139] Its roles in activating mucosal function, diminishing gastric hydrolysis of potentially useful milk macromolecules, and protecting the gut epithelium from autodigestion are well described.[140,141] EGF has also been implicated in the induction of lactase secretion and the repression of sucrase activity.[142]

Pancreatic lipase secretion in the preterm infant is only about 10% of an adult's, and the bile-salt pool is only about 50% of that found in the mature neonate.[143] The depressed pancreatic function ensures that the immature microvillus membrane is spared digestion by pancreatic proteolytic enzymes, and permits prolonged activity of essential brush border enzymes and mammary gland factors. The evolutionary advantage of maintaining certain maternal human milk proteins intact is clear. Such infants are able to maintain the function of immunoglobulins and other biologically important peptides, including enzymes such as salivary and human milk amylases and lipases, which are able to continue their activity in the neutral environment of the duodenum even after temporary inactivation in gastric pH. A sufficient proportion of antimicrobial proteins is known to escape digestion altogether and emerge in the feces, suggesting that antimicrobial activity continues throughout the length of the infant's gastrointestinal tract.

Some antimicrobial components are active both within the breast, minimizing the risk of breast infection and mastitis,[144] and within the infant's gastrointestinal and respiratory tracts, protecting the mucosal surfaces from infection by bacteria, viruses, and parasites.[130] The site of action of the peptide *feedback inhibitor of lactation* (FIL), for example, is within the breast itself, its function being the autocrine regulation of milk production.[145] Many bioactive substances also become valuable nutrient sources once they are digested and absorbed.

Intestinal Microbiota in the Infant

The gastrointestinal tract is sterile at birth and is subsequently colonized by microbes acquired from the mother and the surrounding environment.[146] The colonization of the neonate is known to be influenced by the mode of delivery, the type of feeding, and age.[147-149] Bacteria are predominant, but a variety of protozoa, bacteriophages, and aerobic and anaerobic fungi are present.[150,151] It is estimated that the human colon contains more than 10^{11} bacterial cells/g of mucosa, outnumbering host cells by a factor of 10 and belonging to as many as 400 different species.[152] Anaerobic bacteria predominate, and >99% of the bacteria isolated from human fecal specimens will not grow in the presence of atmospheric oxygen.[153] The vital role of the gastrointestinal tract *microbiota* and its profound influence on our immunologic, nutritional, physiologic, and protective processes make some consider it the largest metabolically adaptable and rapidly renewable organ of the body.[154]

The gut is initially colonized by lactic acid bacteria (eg, lactobacillus, bifidobacteria), enterobacteria, and streptococci. Recent studies using multiplexed 16S rRNA gene pyrosequencing has confirmed that the bacterial communities of vaginally delivered neonates resembles the mother's vaginal microbiota (*Lactobacillus, Prevotella,* or *Sneathia* species); similarly, neonates delivered by Cesarean section have a microbiota similar to the maternal skin flora (*Staphylococcus, Corynebacterium,* and *Propionibacterium* species).[147] The gastric microbiota of newborn infants is similar to that of their mothers' cervix,[155] and the colonization of the nasopharynx of most neonates is consistent with those of their mothers' vaginas immediately before delivery.[156] Enterobacteria and streptococci are the first groups to colonize the intestines, and all infants are colonized with *Escherichia coli* within a few days.[157] The intestinal microflora differs between breastfed and formula-fed infants, with the predominant species in breastfed infants being *Lactobacillus* and *Bifidobacterium* and the predominant species in formula-fed infants being *Bacteroides* and *Enterobacter*.[158,159] However, the predominance of bifidobacteria within the microbiota of young infants has recently been challenged, because they were only detected after several months of age, and thereafter persisted only as a minor population.[148] Human milk contains up to 10^9 microbes/L, the most frequent groups being staphylococci, streptococci, corynebacteria, lactobacilli, micrococci, propionibacteria, and bifidobacteria.[160,161] After the introduction of solid foods, obligate anaerobes increase in number and diversity until a pattern similar to that seen in adults is achieved, normally by the age of 2 to 3 years. Lactobacilli and most gram-negative bacteria, such as *E coli* and other members of the Enterobacteriaceae family, can adhere to enterocytes.[162] The study of the molecular basis for bacterial adhesion to enterocytes may help elucidate some of the mechanisms by which indigenous bacteria stimulate the development of host immunity in the intestinal tract. This may lead to insights into a variety of pediatric conditions, including food allergies, inflammatory bowel disease, and autoimmune conditions, including eczema.[163]

References

1. Steyermark AC, Lam MM, Diamond J. Quantitative evolutionary design of nutrient processing: glucose. *Proc Natl Acad Sci U S A*. 2002;99(13):8754-8759
2. O'Connor TP, Lam MM, Diamond J. Magnitude of functional adaptation after intestinal resection. *Am J Physiol*. 1999;76(5 Pt 2):R1265-R1275
3. Tracy CR, Diamond J. Regulation of gut function varies with life-history traits in chuckwallas (Sauromalus obesus: Iguanidae). *Physiol Biochem Zool*. 2005;78(4):469-481
4. Sadler TW. Third to eighth week: the embryonic period. In: Sadler TW, ed. *Langman's Medical Embryology*. 9th ed. Philadelphia, PA: Lippincott Williams & Wilkins; 2004:87-115
5. Sadler TW. Digestive system. In *Langman's Medical Embryology*, 9th ed. Lippincott Williams & Wilkins 2004. 285-319.
6. Apelqvist A, Ahlgreen U, Edlund H. Sonic hedgehog directs specialized mesoderm differentiation in the intestines and pancreas. *Curr Biol*. 1997;7(10):801-804
7. Moore-Scott BA, Manley NR. Differential expression of Sonic hedgehog along the anterior-posterior axis regulates patterning of pharyngeal pouch endoderm and pharyngeal endoderm-derived organs. *Dev Biol*. 2005;278(2):323-335
8. Kiefer JC. Molecular mechanisms of early gut organogenesis: a primer on development of the digestive tract. *Dev Dynamics*. 2003;228:287-291

9. Spence JR, Mayhew CN, Rankin SA, Kuhar MF, Vallance JE, Tolle K, Hoskins EE, Kalinichenko VV, Wells SI, Zorn AM, Shroyer NF, Wells JM. Directed differentiation of human pluripotent stem cells into intestinal tissue in vitro. *Nature.* 2011;470(7332): 105-109

10. Amiel J, Lyonnet S. Hirschsprung disease, associated syndromes, and genetics: a review. *J Med Genet* 2001;38:729-739

11. Li L, Krantz ID, Deng Y, et al. Alagille syndrome is caused by mutations in human Jagged1, which encodes a ligand for Notch1. *Nature Genet.* 1997;16:243-251

12. Bjerknes M, Cheng H. Gastrointestinal stem cells. II. Intestinal stem cells. *Am J Physiol Gastrointest Liver Physiol.* 2005;289:G381-G387

13. Leedham SJ, Brittan M, McDonald SAC, Wright NA. Intestinal stem cells. *J Cell Mol Med.* 2005;9:1:11-24

14. Sato T, Vries RG, Snippert HJ, et al. Single Lgr5 stem cells build crypt-villus structures in vitro without a mesenchymal niche. *Nature.*

15. van der Flier LG, Haegebarth A, Stange DE, van de Wetering M, Clevers H. OLFM4 is a robust marker for stem cells in human intestine and marks a subset of colorectal cancer cells. *Gastroenterology.* 2009;137(1):15-17

16. Sato T, van Es JH, Snippert HJ, Stange DE, Vries RG, van den Born M, Barker N, Shroyer NF, van de Wetering M, Clevers H. Paneth cells constitute the niche for Lgr5 stem cells in intestinal crypts. *Nature.* 2011;469(7330):415-418

17. Takeda N, Jain R, LeBoeuf MR, Wang Q, Lu MM, Epstein JA. Interconversion between intestinal stem cell populations in distinct niches. *Science.* 2011;334(6061):1420-1424

18. Li L, Clevers H. Coexistence of quiescent and active adult stem cells in mammals. *Science.* 2010;327(5965):542-545

19. Hall PA, Coates PJ, Ansari B, Hopwood D. Regulation of cell number in the mammalian gastrointestinal tract: the importance of apoptosis. *J Cell Sci.* 1994;107(Pt 12):3569-3577

20. Bjerknes M, Cheng H. The stem-cell zone of the small intestinal epithelium. I. Evidence from Paneth cells in the adult mouse. *Am J Anat.* 1981;160(1):51-63

21. Ouellette AJ. Defensin-mediated innate immunity in the small intestine. *Best Pract Res Clin Gastroenterol.* 2004;18(2):405-419

22. Bjerknes M, Khandanpour C, Möröy T, et al. Origin of the brush cell lineage in the mouse intestinal epithelium. *Dev Biol.* 2012;362(2):194-218

23. Gebert A. The role of M cells in the protection of mucosal membranes. *Histochem Cell Biol.* 1997;108(6):455-470

24. Powell DW, Mifflin RC, Valentich JD, Crowe SE, Saada JL, West AB. Myofibroblasts. II. Intestinal subepithelial myofibroblasts. *Am J Physiol.* 1999;277(2 Pt 1):C183-C201

25. Aynsley-Green A. Metabolic and endocrine interrelations in the human fetus and neonate. *Am J Clin Nutr.* 1985;41(2 Suppl):339-417

26. Salminen S, Isolauri E. Intestinal colonization, microbiota, and probiotics. *J Pediatr.* 2006;149(3 Suppl):S115-S120

27. Menard D. Growth-promoting factors and the development of the human gut. In: Lebenthal E, ed. *Human Gastrointestinal Development.* New York, NY: Raven Press: 1989:123-150

28. Weaver LT, Laker MF, Nelson R. Intestinal permeability in the newborn. *Arch Dis Child.* 1984;59:236-241

29. Lebenthal E. Concepts in gastrointestinal development. Lebenthal E, ed. *Human Gastrointestinal Development.* New York, NY: Raven Press; 1989:3-18

30. Ferraris RP, Diamond JM. Specific regulation of intestinal nutrient transporters by their dietary substrates. *Annu Rev Physiol.* 1989;51:125

31. Jones PJH, Kubow S. Lipids, sterols, and their metabolites. In: Shils ME, Shike M, Ross AC, Caballero B, Cousins RJ, eds. *Modern Nutrition in Health and Disease.* 10th ed. Philadelphia, PA: Lippincott Williams & Wilkins; 2006:92-122

32. Poulos A, Beckman K, Johnson DW, et al. Very long-chain fatty acids in peroxisomal disease. *Adv Exp Med Biol.* 1992;318:331-340

33. Hu FB, van Dam RM, Liu S. Diet and risk of type II diabetes: the role of types of fat and carbohydrate. *Diabetologia.* 2001;44(7):805-817

34. von Ebner K. Die acinosen drusen der zunge und ihre beziehungen zu den geschmacksorganen. In: Hoelliker V, ed. *Handbook der Geweblehre des Menschen.* Graz, Austria: Leuschner and Lubensky; 1899:18-38

35. Menard D, Monfils S, Tremblay E. Ontogeny of human gastric lipase and pepsin activities. *Gastroenterology.* 1995;154(6):362-364

36. Fink CS, Hamosh P, Hamosh M. Fat digestion in the stomach: stability of lingual lipase in the gastric environment. *Pediatr Res.* 1984;18(3):248-254

37. Jensen RG, DeJong FA, Clark RM, Palmgren LG, Liao TH, Hamosh M. Stereospecificity of premature human infant lingual lipase. *Lipids* 1982;17(8):570-572

38. Gargouri Y, Pieroni G, Riviere C, et al. Kinetic assay of human gastric lipase on short- and long-chain triacylglycerol emulsions. *Gastroenterology.* 1986;91(3):919-925

39. Faber J, Goldstein R, Blondheim O, et al. Absorption of medium chain triglycerides in the stomach of the human infant. *J Pediatr Gastroenterol Nutr.* 1988;7(2):189-195

40. Encrantz J-C, Sjovall J. On the bile acids in duodenal contents of infants and children. *Clin Chim Acta.* 1959;4:793-799

41. Heubi JE, Balistreri WF, Suchy FJ. Bile salt metabolism in the first year of life. *J Lab Clin Med.* 1982;100(1):127-136

42. Boehm G, Bierbach U, Senger H, et al. Activities of lipase and trypsin in duodenal juice of infants small for gestational age. *J Pediatr Gastroenterol Nutr.* 1991;12(3):324-327

43. de Belle RC, Vaupshas V, Vitullo BB, et al. Intestinal absorption of bile salts: immature development in the neonate. *J Pediatr.* 1979;94(3):472-476

44. Wong MH, Oelkers P, Craddock AL, Dawson PA. Expression cloning and characterization of the hamster ileal sodium-dependent bile acid transporter. *J Biol Chem.* 1994;269(2):1340-1347

45. Reinhart GA, Mahan DC, Lepine AJ, Simmen FA, Moore BE. Dietary clofibric acid increases intestinal fatty acid binding protein activity and apparent lipid digestibility in weanling swine. *J Anim Sci.* 1993;71(10):2693-2699

46. Liao TH, Hamosh M, Scanlon JW, Hamosh P. Preduodenal fat digestion in the newborn infant: effect of fatty acid chain length on triglyceride hydrolysis. *Clin Res.* 1980;28:820

47. Bitman J, Wood L, Hamosh M, Hamosh P, Mehta N. Comparison of the lipid composition of breast milk from mothers of term and preterm infants. *J Clin Nutr.* 1983;38(2):300-312

48. Roy CC, Ste-Marie M, Chartrand L, Weber A, Bard H, Doray B. Correction of the malabsorption of the preterm infant with a medium-chain triglyceride formula. *J Pediatr.* 1975;29(3):546-551

49. Tantibhedhyangkul P, Hashim SA. Medium-chain triglyceride feeding in premature infants: effects on fat and nitrogen absorption. *Pediatrics.* 1975;55(3):359-370

50. Sarles J, Moreau H, Verger R. Human gastric lipase: ontogeny and variations in children. *Acta Paediatr.* 1992;81(6-7):511-513

51. Zoppi G, Andreotti G, Pajno-Ferrara F, Njai DM, Gaburro D. Exocrine pancreas function in premature and full term neonates. *Pediatr Res.* 1972;6(12):880-886

52. Boehm G, Bierbach U, DelSanto A, Moro G, Minoli I. Activities of trypsin and lipase in duodenal aspirates of healthy preterm infants: effects of gestational and postnatal age. *Biol Neonate.* 1995;67(4):248-253

53. Brueton MJ, Berger HM, Brown GA, Ablitt L, Iyngkaran N, Wharton BA. Duodenal bile acid conjugation patterns and dietary sulphur amino acids in the newborn. *Gut.* 1978;19(2):95-98

54. Armand M, Hamosh M, Mehta NR, et al. Effect of human milk or formula on gastric function and fat digestion in the premature infant. *Pediatr Res.* 1996;40(3):429-437

55. Mehta NR, Jones JB, Hamosh M. Lipases in preterm human milk: ontogeny and physiologic significance. *J Pediatr Gastroenterol Nutr.* 1982;1(3):317-326

56. Blackberg L, Hernell O. The bile-salt stimulated lipase in human milk: purification and characterization. *Eur J Biochem.* 1981;116(2):221-225

57. Hernell O, Blackberg L. Digestion of human milk lipids: physiologic significance of sn-2 monoglycerol hydrolysis by bile salt-stimulated lipase. *Pediatr Res.* 1982;16(10):882-885

58. Hernell O. Human milk lipases. III. Physiological implications of the bile salt-stimulated lipase. *Eur J Clin Invest.* 1975;5(3):267-272

59. Fredrikzon B, Olivecrona T. Decrease of lipase and esterase activities in intestinal contents of newborn infants during test meals. *Pediatr Res.* 1978;12(5):631-634

60. Nyberg L, Farooqi A, Blackberg L, Duan RD, Nilsson A, Hernell O. Digestion of ceramide by human mild bile salt-stimulated lipase. *J Pediatr Gastroenterol Nutr.* 1998;27(5):560-567

61. Williamson S, Finucane E, Ellis H, Gamsu HR. Effect of heat treatment of human milk on absorption of nitrogen, fat, sodium, calcium, and phosphorus by preterm infants. *Arch Dis Child.* 1978;53(7):555-563

62. Wang CS, Kuksis A, Manganaro F. Studies on the substrate specificity of purified human milk lipoprotein lipase. *Lipids.* 1982;17(4):278-284

63. Keim NL, Levin RJ, Havel PJ. Carbohydrates. In: Shils ME, Shike M, Ross AC, Caballero B, Cousins RJ, eds. *Modern Nutrition in Health and Disease.* 10th ed. Philadelphia, PA: Lippincott Williams & Wilkins; 2006:62-82

64. Eggermont E. The hydrolysis of the naturally occurring alpha-glucosides by the human intestinal mucosa. *Eur J Biochem.* 1969;9(4):483-487

65. Wright EM, Loo DD. Coupling between Na$^+$, sugar, and water transport across the intestine. *Ann N Y Acad Sci*. 2000;915:54-66

66. Koldovsky O, Heringova A, Jirsova V, Jirasek JE, Uher J. Transport of glucose against a concentration gradient in everted sacs of jejunum and ileum of human fetuses. *Gastroenterology*. 1965;48:185-187

67. Malo C. Separation of two distinct Na$^+$/D-glucose cotransport systems in the human fetal jejunum by means of their differential specificity for 3-O-methylglucose. *Biochim Biophys Acta*. 1990;1022(1):8-16

68. Lee W-S, Kanal Y, Wells RG, et al. *J Biol Chem*. 1994;269(16):12032-12039

69. Loo DD, Hirayama BA, Meinild AK, Chandy G, Zeuthen T, Wright EM. Passive water and ion transport by cotransporters. *J Physiol*. 1999;518(Pt 1):195-202

70. Hoekstra JH. Fructose breath hydrogen tests in infants with chronic non-specific diarrhoea. *Eur J Pediatr*. 1995;154(5):362-364

71. Moore MC, Charrington AD, Mann SL, et al. Acute fructose administration decreases the glycemic response to an oral glucose tolerance test in normal adults. *J Clin Endocrinol Metab*. 2000;85(12):4515-4519

72. Rossiter MA, Barrowman JA, Dand A, Wharton BA. Amylase content of mixed saliva in children. *Acta Paediatr Scand*. 1974;63(3):389-392

73. Delachaume-Salem E, Sarles H. Normal human pancreatic secretion in relation to age [French]. *Biol Gastroenterol (Paris)*. 1970;2:135-146

74. Lebenthal E, Lee PC. Development of functional responses in human exocrine pancreas. *Pediatrics*. 1980;66(4):556-560

75. Antonowicz I, Chang SK, Grand RJ. Development and distribution of lysosomal enzymes and disaccharides in human fetal intestine. *Gastroenterology*. 1974;67(1):51-58

76. Raul F, Lacroix B, Aprahamian M. Longitudinal distribution of brush border hydrolases and morphological maturation in the intestine of the preterm infant. *Early Hum Dev*. 1986;13(2):225-234

77. Shulman RJ, Schanler RJ, Lau C, Heitkemper M, Ou CN, Smith EO. Early feeding, feeding intolerance, and lactase activity in preterm infants. *J Pediatr*. 1998;133(5):645-649

78. Douwes AC, Oosterkamp RF, Fernandes J, Los T, Jongbloed AA. Sugar malabsorption in healthy neonates estimated by breath hydrogen. *Arch Dis Child*. 1980;55(7):512-515

79. Topping DL, Clifton PM. Short-chain fatty acids and human colonic function: roles of resistant starch and nonstarch polysaccharides. *Physiol Rev*. 2001;81(3):1031-1064

80. Gray GM. Starch digestion and absorption in nonruminants. *J Nutr*. 1992;122:172-177

81. Rings EH, Grand RJ, Buller HA. Lactose intolerance and lactase deficiency in children. *Curr Opin Pediatr*. 1994;6(5):562-567

82. Northrop-Clewes CA, Lunn PG, Downes RM. Lactose maldigestion in breast-feeding Gambian infants. *J Pediatr Gastroenterol Nutr*. 1997;24(3):257-263

83. Koldovsky O. Digestive-absorptive functions in fetuses, infants, and children. In: Polin RA, Fox WW, eds. *Fetal and Neonatal Physiology*. Philadelphia, PA: WB Saunders Co; 1992:1060-1077

84. Enattah NS, Sahi T, Savilahti E, Terwilliger JD, Peltonen L, Järvelä I. Identification of a variant associated with adult-type hypolactasia. *Nat Genet*. 2002;30(2):233-237

85. Jensen TG, Liebert A, Lewinsky R, Swallow DM, Olsen J, Troelsen JT. The -14010*C variant associated with lactase persistence is located between an Oct-1 and HNF1α binding site and increases lactase promoter activity. *Hum Genet.* 2011;130(4):483-493

86. Matthews DE. Proteins and amino acids. In: Shils ME, Shike M, Ross AC, Caballero B, Cousins RJ, eds. *Modern Nutrition in Health and Disease.* 10th ed. Philadelphia, PA: Lippincott Williams & Wilkins; 2006:23-61

87. Young VR. Adult amino acid requirements: the case for major revision in current recommendations. *J Nutr.* 1994;124(8 Suppl):1517S-1523S

88. Bjelton L, Sandberg G, Wennberg A et al. Assessment of biological quality of amino acid solutions for intravenous nutrition. In: Kinney JM, Borum PR, eds. *Perspectives in Clinical Nutrition.* Baltimore, MD: Urban & Schwarzenberg; 1989:31-41

89. Mouterde O, Dacher JN, Basuyau JP, Mallet E. Gastric secretion in infants: application to the study of sudden infant death syndrome and apparently life-threatening events. *Biol Neonate.* 1992;62(1):15-22

90. Mitchell DJ, McClure BG, Tubman TR. Simultaneous monitoring of gastric and oesophageal pH reveals limitations of conventional oesophageal pH monitoring in milk fed infants. *Arch Dis Child.* 2001;84(3):273-276

91. Omari TI, Davidson GP. Multipoint measurement of intragastric pH in healthy preterm infants. *Arch Dis Child Fetal Neonatal Ed.* 2003;88(6):F517-F520

92. Kelly EJ, Brownlee KG. When is the fetus first capable of gastric acid, intrinsic factor and gastrin secretion? *Biol Neonate.* 1993;63(3):153-156

93. Kelly EJ, Brownlee KG, Newell SJ. Gastric secretory function in the developing human stomach. *Early Hum Dev.* 1992;31(2):163-166

94. Hyman PE, Clarke DD, Everett SL, et al. Gastric acid secretory function in preterm infants. *J Pediatr.* 1985;106(3):467-471

95. Kelly EJ, Newell SJ, Brownlee KG, Primrose JN, Dear PR. Gastric acid secretion in preterm infants. *Early Hum Dev.* 1993;35(3):215-220

96. Grahnquist L, Ruuska T, Finkel Y. Early development of human gastric H,K-adenosine triphosphatase. *J Pediatr Gastroenterol Nutr.* 2000;30(5):533-537

97. Yahav J, Carrion V, Lee PC, Lebenthal E. Meal-stimulated pepsinogen secretion in premature infants. *J Pediatr.* 1987;110(6):949-951

98. Lieberman J. Proteolytic enzyme activity in fetal pancreas and meconium: demonstration of plasminogen and trypsinogen activators in pancreatic tissue. *Gastroenterology.* 1966;50:183-190

99. Borgstrom B, Lindquist B, Lundh G. Enzyme concentration and absorption of protein and glucose in duodenum of premature infants. *Am J Dis Child.* 1960;99:338-343

100. Madey S, Dancis J. Proteolytic enzymes of the premature infant: with special reference to his ability to digest unsplit protein food. *Pediatrics.* 1949;4(2):177-182

101. Bujanover Y, Harel A, Geter R, Blau H, Yahav J, Spirer Z. The development of the chymotrypsin activity during postnatal life using the bentiromide test. *Int J Pancreatol.* 1988;3(1):53-58

102. Lindberg T. Proteolytic activity in duodenal juice in infants, children, and adults. *Acta Paediatr Scand.* 1974;63(6):805-808

II

103. Kushak RI, Winter HS. Regulation of intestinal peptidases by nutrients in human fetuses and children. *Comp Biochem Physiol A Mol Integr Physiol.* 1999;124(2):191-198

104. Palacin M, Estevez R, Bertran J, Zorzano A. Molecular biology of mammalian plasma membrane amino acid transporters. *Physiol Rev.* 1998;78(4):969-1054

105. Malo C. Multiple pathways for amino acid transport in brush border membrane vesicles isolated from the human fetal small intestine. *Gastroenterology.* 1991;100(6):1644-1652

106. Weaver LT, Walker WA. Uptake of macromolecules in the neonate. In: Lebenthal E, ed. *Human Gastrointestinal Development.* New York, NY: Raven Press; 1989:731-748

107. Lind T. Amniotic fluid. In: Lentner C, ed. *Geigy Scientific Tables.* 8th ed. Basel, Switzerland: Ciba-Geigy Pharmaceutical; 1981:197-212

108. Roberton DM, Paganelli R, Dinwiddie R, Levinsky RJ. Milk antigen absorption in the preterm and term neonate. *Arch Dis Child.* 1982;57(5):369-372

109. Walker WA. Absorption of protein and protein fragments in the developing intestine: role in immunologic/allergic reactions. *Pediatrics.* 1985;75(1 Pt 2):167-171

110. Gruskay FL, Cooke RE. The gastrointestinal absorption of unaltered protein in normal infants and in infants recovering from diarrhea. *Pediatrics.* 1955;16:763-768

111. Weaver LT. Breast and gut: the relationship between lactating mammary function and neonatal gastrointestinal function. *Proc Nutrition Soc.* 1992;51(2):155-163

112. Yoshida M, Kobayashi K, Kuo TT, et al. Neonatal Fc receptor for IgG regulates mucosal immune responses to luminal bacteria. *J Clin Invest.* 2006;116(8):2142–2151

113. Prasad PD, Wang H, Huang W, Fei YJ, Leibach FH, Devoe LD, Ganapathy V. Molecular and functional characterization of the intestinal Na^+-dependent multivitamin transporter. *Arch Biochem Biophys.* 1999;366(1):95-106

114. Bass WT, Malati N, Castle MC, White LE. Evidence for the safety of ascorbic acid administration to the premature infant. *Am J Perinatol.* 1998;15(2):133-140

115. Tsukaguchi H, Tokui T, Mackenzie B, et al. A family of mammalian Na^+-dependent L-ascorbic acid transporters. *Nature.* 1999;399(6731):70-75

116. Ziegler EE, Fomon SJ. Lactose enhances mineral absorption in infancy. *J Pediatr Gastroenterol Nutr.* 1983;2(2):288-294

117. Ghishan FK, Stroop S, Meneely R. The effect of lactose on the intestinal absorption of calcium and zinc in the rat during maturation. *Pediatr Res.* 1982;16(7):566-568

118. Barnes LA, Morrow G III, Silverio J, Finnegan LP, Heitman SE. Calcium and fat absorption from infant formulas with different fat blends. *Pediatrics.* 1974;54(2):217-221

119. Namgung R, Tsang RC. Factors affecting newborn bone mineral content: in utero effects on newborn bone mineralization. *Proc Nutr Soc.* 2000;59(1):55-63

120. Ghishan FK, Parker P, Nichols S, Hoyumpa A. Kinetics of intestinal calcium transport during maturation in rats. *Pediatr Res.* 1984;18(3):235-239

121. Forbes GB, Reina JC. Effect of age on gastrointestinal absorption (Fe, Sr, Pb) in the rat. *J Nutr.* 1972;102(5):647-652

122. Gunshin H, Mackenzie B, Berger UV, et al. Cloning and characterization of a mammalian proton-coupled metal-ion transporter. *Nature.* 1997;388(6641):482-488

123. Ziegler EE, Edwards BB, Jensen RL, Mahaffey KR, Fomon SJ. Absorption and retention of lead by infants. *Pediatr Res.* 1978;12(1):29-34

124. Carnielli VP, Luijendijk IHT, van Goudoever JB, Sulkers EJ, Boerlage AA, Degenhart HJ, Sauer PJJ. Feeding premature newborn infants palmitic acid in amounts and stereoisomeric position similar to that of human milk: effects on fat and mineral balance. *Am J Clin Nutr.* 1995;61(5):1037-1042

125. Jensen RG. Lipids in human milk-composition and fat soluble vitamins. In: Lebenthals E, ed. *Textbook of Gastroenterology and Nutrition in Infancy.* New York, NY: Raven Press; 1989:157-208

126. Ballabriga A. Essential fatty acids and human tissue composition. An overview. *Acta Paediatr.* 1994;402:63-68

127. Clandinin MT. Brain development and assessing the supply of polyunsaturated fatty acids. *Lipids.* 1999;34(2):131-137

128. Sala-Vila A, Castellote AI, Campoy C, Rivero M, Rodriquez-Palmero M, Lopez-Sabater MC. The source of long-chain PUFA in formula supplements does not affect the fatty acid composition of plasma lipids in full-term infants. *J Nutr.* 2004;134(4):868-873

129. Fleith M, Clandinin MT. Dietary PUFA for preterm and term infants: review of clinical studies. *Crit Rev Food Sci Nutr.* 2005;45(3):205-229

130. Lonnerdal B. Biochemistry and physiological functions of human milk proteins. *Am J Clin Nutr.* 1985;42(6):1299-1317

131. Prentice A, Ewing G, Roberts SB, Lucas A, MacCarthy A, Jarjou LM, Whitehead RG. The nutritional role of breast milk IgA and lactoferrin. *Acta Paediatr Scand.* 1987;76(4): 592-598

132. Kleinman RE, Walker WA. The enteromammary immune system. *Digestive Dis Sci.* 1979;24(4):876-882

133. Mata L. Breastfeeding and host defense. *Front Gastrointest Res.* 1986;13:119-133

134. Mepham TB. *Physiology of Lactation.* Milton Keynes, UK: Open University Press; 1987

135. Kunz C, Rudloff S. Biological functions of oligosaccharides in human milk. *Acta Paediatr.* 1993;82(11):903-912

136. Gnoth MJ, Rudloff S, Kunz C, Kinne RK. Investigations on the in vitro transport of human milk oligosaccharides by a Caco-2 monolayer using a novel high performance liquid chromatography-mass spectrometry technique. *J Biol Chem.* 2001;276(37):34363-34370

137. Koldovsky O. Hormonally active peptides in human milk. *Acta Pediatr (Suppl).* 1994;402:89-93

138. Goldman AS, Goldblum RM. Defense agents in human milk. In: Jensens RG, ed. *Handbook of Milk Composition.* New York, NY: Academic Press; 1995:727-745

139. Weaver LT, Walker WA. Epidermal growth factor and the developing human gut. *Gastroenterology.* 1988;94(3):845-847

140. Weaver LT, Freiberg E, Israel EJ, Walker WA. Epidermal growth factor in human amniotic fluid. *Gastroenterology.* 1989;95(5):1346

141. Weaver LT, Gonnella PA, Israel EJ, Walker WA. Uptake and transport of epidermal growth factor (EGF) by the small intestinal epithelium of the fetal rat. *Gastroenterology.* 1990;96(4):828-837

142. Menard D, Arsenault P, Pothier P. Biologic effects of epidermal growth factor in human fetal jejunum. *Gastroenterology.* 1988;94(3):656-663

143. Watkins JB, Szczepanik P, Gould JP, Klein P, Lester R. Bile salt metabolism in the human premature infant. Preliminary observations of pool size and synthesis rate following prenatal administration of dexamethasone and phenobarbital. *Gastroenterology*. 1975;69(3):706-713

144. Prentice A, Prentice AM, Lamb WH. Mastitis in rural Gambian mothers and the protection of the breast by milk antimicrobial factors. *Trans R Soc Trop Med Hyg*. 1985;79(1):90-95

145. Wilde CJ, Prentice A, Peaker M. Breastfeeding: matching supply with demand in human lactation. *Proc Nutr Soc*. 1995;54(2):401-406

146. Mackie RI, Sghir A, Gaskins HR. Developmental microbial ecology of the neonatal gastrointestinal tract. *Am J Clin Nutr*. 1999;69(Suppl):1035S-1045S

147. Dominguez-Bello MG, Costello EK, Contreras M, et al. Delivery mode shapes the acquisition and structure of the initial microbiota across multiple body habitats in newborns. *Proc Natl Acad Sci U S A*. 2010;107(26):11971-11975

148. Palmer C, Bik EM, DiGiulio DB, Relman DA, Brown PO. Development of the human infant intestinal microbiota. *PLoS Biol*. 2007;5(7):e177

149. Turroni F, Peano C, Pass DA, Foroni E, Severgnini M, et al. Diversity of bifidobacteria within the infant gut microbiota. *PLoS ONE*. 2012;7(5):e36957

150. Clarke RTJ. The gut and its micro-organisms. In: Clarke RTJ, Bauchop T, eds. *Microbial Ecology of the Gut*. New York, NY: Academic Press; 1977:35-71

151. Hespell RB, Akin DE, Dehority BA. Bacteria, fungi and protozoa of the rumen. In: Mackie RI, White BA, Isaacson RE, eds. *Gastrointestinal Microbiology*. Vol 2. New York, NY: Chapman and Hall; 1997:59-141

152. Conway PL. Microbial ecology of the human large intestine. In: Gibson GR, Macfarlane GT, eds. *Human Colonic Bacteria*. Boca Raton, FL: CRC Press; 1995:1-24

153. Savage DS. Microbial ecology of the gastrointestinal tract. *Annu Rev Microbiol*. 1977;31:107-133

154. Berg RD. The indigenous gastrointestinal microflora. *Trends Microbiol*. 1996;4(11): 430-435

155. Brook I, Barett C, Brinkman C, Martin W, Finegold S. Aerobic and anaerobic bacterial flora of the maternal cervix and newborn gastric fluid and conjunctiva: a prospective study. *Pediatrics*. 1979;63(3):451-455

156. MacGregor RR, Tunnessen WW. The incidence of pathogenic organisms in the normal flora of the neonates external ear and nasopharynx. *Clin Pediatr (Phila)*. 1973;12(12): 697-700

157. Adlerberth I, Carlsson B, de Man P, et al. Intestinal colonization with Enterobacteriaceae in Pakistan and Swedish hospital delivered infants. *Acta Paediatr Scand*. 1991;80(6-7):602-610

158. Parrett AM, Edwards CA. In vitro fermentation of carbohydrate by breast fed and formula fed infants. *Arch Dis Child*. 1997;76(3):249-253

159. Mata LJ, Urrutia JJ. Intestinal colonization of breast-fed children in a rural area of low socioeconomic level. *Ann N Y Acad Sci*. 1971;176(2):93-108

160. Asquith MT, Harrod JR. Reduction in bacterial contamination in banked human milk. *J Pediatr.* 1979;95(6):993-994

161. West PA, Hewitt JH, Murphy OM. The influence of methods of collection and storage on the bacteriology of human milk. *J Appl Bacteriol.* 1979;46(2):269-277

162. Duguid JP, Old DC. Adhesive properties of Enterobacteriaceae. In: Beachey EH, ed. *Bacterial Adherence, Receptors and Recognition.* Vol 6. London, England: Chapman and Hall; 1980:185-217

163. Kalliomäki M, Salminen S, Arvilommi H, Kero P, Koskinen P, Isolauri E. Probiotics in primary prevention of atopic disease: a randomised placebo-controlled trial. *Lancet.* 2001;357(9262):1076-1079

Chapter 3

Breastfeeding

Introduction

The American Academy of Pediatrics (AAP) recommends human milk as the sole nutrient for healthy, term infants for approximately the first 6 months of life and supports continued breastfeeding for at least 12 months.[1] It also recommends human milk as the preferred source of enteral nutrition for the preterm infant. Human milk offers specific advantages, and lack of access is associated with disadvantages. This chapter discusses the recent epidemiology of breastfeeding, composition of human milk, duration of breastfeeding, contraindications to breastfeeding, and how to support breastfeeding, especially for infants who do not thrive.

Recent Epidemiology

In the early part of the 20th century, breastfeeding was the norm in the United States, but by the early 1970s, breastfeeding rates had decreased to 24.7%. Since that time, they have steadily increased.[2] The 2011 Breastfeeding Report Card from the Centers for Disease Control and Prevention (CDC) found that 75% of mothers initiate breastfeeding, 44% are breastfeeding at 6 months, and 24% are breastfeeding at 12 months. Rates of exclusive breastfeeding are 35% and 15% at 3 and 6 months, respectively.[3] The achievement of a 75% initiation rate and an increase in the rates of exclusive breastfeeding at 3 and 6 months by 4% to 5% since the first Breastfeeding Report Card in 2007 is not attributable to any one factor. Surprisingly, fewer than 5% of US infants are born in certified Baby-Friendly Hospitals (see How to Support Breastfeeding). Nevertheless, the ability of hospitals to participate in the Maternity Practices in Infant Nutrition and Care (mPINC) survey undoubtedly has led to improved maternity care practices supportive of breastfeeding initiation and encouraged hospitals to adopt practices consistent with the Baby-Friendly Hospital initiative. In addition, breastfeeding is receiving more support from state governments, communities, employers, and the health care system.[3] Healthy People 2020 aims for 82% of mothers to breastfeed in the early postpartum period, 60% of mothers to be breastfeeding at 6 months, and 34% of mothers to be breastfeeding at 1 year, with additional goals of 46% and 25% for exclusive breastfeeding at 3 and 6 months, respectively. Additional objectives include increasing the proportion of employers that have worksite lactation support, reducing the proportion of breastfed newborn infants who receive formula supplementation within the first 2 days of life, and increasing the proportion of live births that occur in facilities that provide recommended care for lactating mothers and their newborn infants.[4]

On average, mothers who breastfeed have higher educational levels, are older, are more likely to be white, have a middle-level income, and have a higher employment rate than the overall US female population.[5] Despite the gains made in breastfeeding rates, racial, ethnic, socioeconomic, and geographic disparities exist. For example, breastfeeding rates for black infants are approximately 50% lower than those for white infants, rates among mothers receiving Special Supplemental Nutrition Program for Women, Infants, and Children (WIC) benefits are 25% lower than those among mothers who are WIC ineligible, and rates among mothers who graduated from college are 31% higher than those among mothers who did not graduate from high school.[6] Geographic disparities are prominent. Fewer than 55% of mothers initiate breastfeeding in Mississippi, and in general, fewer mothers have ever breastfed in the southern United States compared with other US regions, whereas more than 75% of children were ever breastfed in the west, central, and northeast United States.[7] Women living in rural areas are more likely never to have breastfed than are those living in urban areas.[8,9] Groups with low breastfeeding rates merit special attention to help mothers understand the benefits of breastfeeding and learn how to breastfeed and to make available the necessary support systems to ensure success. Guidance for cultural- and ethnic-based approaches to breastfeeding in the United States is available.[10]

Milk

Human milk is a complex fluid that consists of various compartments, including a true solution, colloidal dispersions of casein molecules, emulsions of fat globules, fat globule membranes, and live cells. Table 3.1 gives the approximate concentrations of some of the constituents of human milk, and Table 3.2 provides a list of important bioactive factors. The concentration of milk constituents varies over the course of lactation, during a single feed, over a 24-hour period, and among women. The first milk, colostrum, is ingested in very small amounts (15 ± 11 g in the first 24 hours of life)[11] and has high concentrations of proteins, fat-soluble vitamins, minerals, electrolytes, and antibodies. Colostrum contains 70% to 80% whey and 20% to 30% casein, and this ratio decreases over time to approximately 55% whey and 44% casein in mature milk. Transition milk, milk from about 7 to 14 days postpartum, is characterized by a decrease in the concentration of immunoglobulins and total proteins and an increase in lactose, fat, and total calories. Mature milk, milk produced after about 2 weeks postpartum, is the fully developed milk that supports healthy term infants exclusively for the first months of life. The milk produced by mothers who continue to lactate beyond 6 to 7 months, extended lactation milk, is characterized by declining concentrations of vitamins and minerals.[12]

Table 3.1.
Representative Values for Constituents of Human Milk

Constituent (per Liter)	Mature Milk (After 2 Weeks' Lactation)
Energy (kcal)	650-700
Macronutrients	
Lactose (g)	67-70
Oligosaccharides (g)	12-14
Total nitrogen (g)	1.9
Nonprotein nitrogen (% total nitrogen)	23
Protein nitrogen (% total nitrogen)	77
Total protein (g)	9
Total lipids (g)	35
Triglyceride (% total lipids)	97-98
Cholesterol (% total lipids)	0.4-0.5
Phospholipids (% total lipids)	0.6-0.8
Water-Soluble Vitamins	
Ascorbic acid (mg)	100
Thiamin (μg)	200
Riboflavin (μg)	400-600
Niacin (mg)	1.8-6.0
Vitamin B_6 (μg)	0.09-0.31
Folate (μg)	80-140
Vitamin B_{12} (μg)	0.5-1.0
Pantothenic acid (mg)	2.0-2.5
Biotin (μg)	5-9
Fat-Soluble Vitamins	
Retinol (mg)	0.3-0.6
Carotenoids (mg)	0.2-0.6
Vitamin K (μg)	2-3
Vitamin D (μg)	0.33
Vitamin E (mg)	3-8
Minerals	
Calcium (mg)	200-250
Magnesium (mg)	30-35

II

Table 3.1. *(continued)*
Representative Values for Constituents of Human Milk

Constituent (per Liter)	Mature Milk (After 2 Weeks' Lactation)
Phosphorus (mg)	120-140
Sodium (mg)	120-250
Potassium (mg)	400-550
Chloride (mg)	400-450
Trace Elements	
Iron (mg)	0.3-0.9
Zinc (mg)	1-3
Copper (mg)	0.2-0.4
Manganese (μg)	3
Selenium (μg)	7-33
Iodine (μg)	150
Fluoride (μg)	4-15

Reproduced with permission from Schanler RJ, Dooley S, Gartner LM, Krebs NF, Mass SB, eds. *Breastfeeding Handbook for Physicians*. Elk Grove Village, IL: American Academy of Pediatrics; 2006.

The volume and content of major nutrients in mature milk from individual mothers is highly variable, as shown in Tables 3.3 and 3.4. Most mothers are able to breastfeed successfully, and this may be because infants can adapt to achieve normal growth despite variability of nutrient intake and differences in the utilization of dietary nitrogen and energy.[13] However, the concentrations of some nutrients, such as iron, vitamin K, and vitamin D, are low in human milk, and deficiency in the infant can occur. Therefore, the AAP recommends supplementation of breastfed infants with these nutrients. For vitamin D, supplementation should begin with 400 IU/day in the first few days of life and continue until the infant is weaned to at least 1 L/day or 1 quart/day of vitamin D-fortified formula or whole milk.[14] Iron supplementation should start at 4 months of age with 1 mg/kg/day oral iron and continue until the infant consumes adequate oral iron from foods.[15] One way to ensure adequate iron intake during weaning is to introduce meats as the first complementary food (see chapter 6). Meats provide a highly bioavailable source of iron and zinc.

Fetuses receive immunoglobulin (Ig) G through the placenta. IgA is the predominant antibody isotype in human milk and provides passive protection against enteric pathogens to which the infant is exposed.[16-19] Colostrum also contains viable cells and other bioactive proteins, such as lysozyme, lactoferrin, haptocorrin,

Table 3.2.
Selected Bioactive Factors in Human Milk

Substance	Function
Secretory IgA	Specific antigen-targeted anti-infection action
Lactoferrin	Immunomodulation, iron chelation, anti-adhesive, trophic for intestinal growth
Lysozyme	Bacterial lysis, immunomodulation
κ-Casein	Anti-adhesive, bacterial flora
Oligosaccharides (prebiotics)	Block bacterial attachment
Cytokines	Anti-inflammatory, epithelial barrier function
Nucleotides	Enhance antibody responses, bacterial flora
Vitamins A, E, C	Antioxidants
Amino acids (including glutamine)	Intestinal cell fuel, immune responses
Lipids	Anti-infective properties
Growth Factors	
Epidermal growth factor	Luminal surveillance, repair of intestines
Transforming growth factor	Promotes lymphocyte function
Nerve growth factor	Growth
Enzymes	
PAF-acetylhydrolase	Blocks action of platelet-activating factor
Glutathione peroxidase	Prevents lipid oxidation

Reproduced with permission from Schanler RJ, Dooley S, Gartner LM, Krebs NF, Mass SB, eds. *Breastfeeding Handbook for Physicians*. Elk Grove Village, IL: American Academy of Pediatrics; 2006.

alpha-1 antitrypsin, transforming growth factor-beta,[18] and various cytokines.[20-22] Thus, human milk offers many advantages for the healthy term infant, including a clean, safe source of nutrition. A review performed by the Agency for Healthcare Research and Quality (AHRQ) found that in the industrialized world, a history of breastfeeding is associated with a reduced risk of acute otitis media, nonspecific gastroenteritis, severe lower respiratory tract infections, atopic dermatitis, asthma in young children, obesity, type 1 and 2 diabetes, childhood leukemia, sudden infant death, and necrotizing enterocolitis. No relationship was found between cognitive performance and a history of breastfeeding, and the relationship between breastfeeding and cardiovascular diseases and infant mortality were unclear.[23] The AHRQ cautions, however, that almost all the available data were from observational studies, and there was a wide range of quality among the data. Thus, causality between breastfeeding and these outcomes cannot be inferred.

Table 3.3.
Variation in Human Milk Volume and Content of Macronutrients

Volume (mL)	Protein g/100mL	Fat g/100 mL	NPN mg/100 mL	Energy Kcal/day	Comments	Reference
308-957	0.79-1.33	1.45-4.70	34-90	NG	Human milk for analysis obtained at second week of infant life	Hytten[a]
	1.12-1.82					
425->1000	NG	NG	NG	NG		Michaelsen[b]
800-1800	1.8	1.9-3.0	NG	NG		Saint[c]
Pooled Observations						
337-637					Volumes obtained by weighing infants at second week of life	Wallgren[d]
364-1096	1.44 ± 0.2	4.92 ± 1.05	NG	273-752	Volume obtained by infant and mother weighing at ~1 mo of age	Dewey[e]
NG	0.4-4.6	NG	10-110	38-80	Range is over time of the 4 lowest and four highest pooled	Hibberd[f]
780	1.17	4.0	NG	500		Institute of Medicine[g]

NPN = nonprotein nitrogen, NG = not given

[a] Hytten FE. Clinical and chemical studies in human lactation. *Br Med J*. 1954;1(4856):249-255
[b] Michaelsen KF, Larsen PS, Thomsen BL, Samuelson G. The Copenhagen Cohort Study on Infant Nutrition and Growth: breast-milk intake, human milk macronutrient content, and influencing factors. *Am J Clin Nutr*. 1994;59(3):600-611
[c] Saint L, Smith M, Hartmann PE. The yield and nutrient content of colostrum and milk of women from giving birth to 1 month post-partum. *Br J Nutr*. 1984;52(1):87-95
[d] Wallgren A. Breast-milk consumption of healthy full-term infants. *Acta Paediatr*. 1945;32(3-4):778-790
[e] Dewey KG, Lonnerdal B. Milk and nutrient intake of breast-fed infants from 1 to 6 months: relation to growth and fatness. *J Pediatr Gastroenterol Nutr*. 1983;2(3):497-506
[f] Hibberd CM, Brooke OG, Carter ND, Haug M, Harzer G. Variation in the composition of breast milk during the first 5 weeks of lactation: implications for the feeding of preterm infants. *Arch Dis Child*. 1982;57(9):658-662
[g] Institute of Medicine, Food and Nutrition Board. *Dietary Reference intakes for Energy, Carbohydrate, Fiber, Fat, Fatty Acids, Cholesterol, Protein and Amino Acids*. Washington, DC: National Academies Press; 2005

Table 3.4.
Variation in Human Milk Minerals and Trace Elements

Na (mg/100 mL)	K (mg/100 mL)	P (mg/100 mL)	Ca (mg/100 mL)	Mg (mg/100 mL)	Cu (µg/100 mL)	Zn (µg/100 mL)	Iron (mg/100 mL)	References
10.8–126.1	45.7–80.6		12.2–32.7	1.85–6.43	14.3–68.5	45.1–935.1		Hibberd[a]
14.3 ± 2.5	46.4 ± 9.3	15.5 ± 2.6	29.6 ± 6.1	2.8 ± 0.6	21.3 ± 68	221 ± 129	32.8 ± 11.7	Picciano[b]
16	50	12.4	26.4	3.4	25	40–120	35	Institute of Medicine[c-g]

[a] Hibberd CM, Brooke OG, Carter ND, Haug M, Harzer G. Variation in the composition of breast milk during the first 5 weeks of lactation: implications for the feeding of preterm infants. *Arch Dis Child.* 1982;57(9):658-662

[b] Picciano MF, Calkins EJ, Garrick JR, Deering RH. Milk and mineral intakes of breastfed infants. *Acta Paediatr Scand.* 1981;70(2):189-194

[c] Institute of Medicine, Food and Nutrition Board. *Dietary Reference Intakes for Vitamin C, Vitamin E, Selenium and Carotenoids.* Washington, DC: National Academies Press; 2000

[d] Institute of Medicine, Food and Nutrition Board. *Dietary Reference Intakes for Water, Potassium, Sodium, Chloride, and Sulfate.* Washington, DC: National Academies Press; 2005

[e] Institute of Medicine, Food and Nutrition Board. *Dietary Reference Intakes for Vitamin A, Vitamin K, Arsenic, Boron, Chromium, Copper, Iodine, Iron, Manganese, Molybdenum, Nickel, Silicon, Vanadium, and Zinc.* Washington, DC: National Academies Press; 2002

[f] Institute of Medicine, Food and Nutrition Board. *Dietary Reference Intakes for Calcium, Phosphorus, Magnesium, Vitamin D, and Fluoride.* Washington, DC: National Academies Press; 1997

[g] Institute of Medicine, Food and Nutrition Board. *Dietary Reference Intakes for Calcium and Vitamin D.* Washington, DC: National Academies Press; 2010

Duration of Breastfeeding

For approximately the past decade, there has been an effort to increase the prevalence and duration of time that infants are exclusively breastfed. Table 3.5 lists definitions for breastfeeding. Of note, the definition of exclusive breastfeeding encompasses the administration of supplements, such as vitamins. The AAP recommends exclusive breastfeeding for approximately the first 6 months of life and continuation after complementary foods have been introduced for at least the first year of life and beyond, as long as mutually desired by mother and child.[1] This approach acknowledges the need for flexibility in that mothers may introduce complementary foods for personal, social, and economic reasons. In addition, a flexible approach also acknowledges the variations in human development that occur. Nevertheless, 2 recent publications raised concern about extended periods of exclusive breastfeeding. The first report[24] addressed the doubling of the prevalence of peanut allergy in the past 10 years in England and compared it with

Table 3.5.
Definitions of Breastfeeding

Type	Description
Exclusive	Human milk is the only food provided. Medicines, minerals, and vitamins may also be given under this definition but no water, juice, or other preparations. Infants fed expressed human milk from their own mothers or from a milk bank by gavage tube, cup, or bottle also can be included in this definition if they have had no nonhuman milk or foods.
Almost exclusive	Human milk is the predominant food provided with very rare feedings of other milk or food. The infant may have been given 1 or 2 formula bottles during the first few days of life but none after that.
Partial or mixed	This may vary from mostly human milk with small amounts of infrequent feedings of nonhuman milk or food *(high partial),* to infants receiving significant amounts of nonhuman milk or food as well as human milk *(medium partial),* to infants receiving predominantly nonhuman milk or food with some human milk *(low partial).*
Token	The infant is fed almost entirely with nonhuman milk and food but either had some human milk shortly after birth or continues to have occasional human milk. This type of breastfeeding may be seen late in the weaning process.
Any breastfeeding	This definition includes all of the above.
Never breastfed	This infant has *never* received *any* human milk, either by direct breastfeeding or expressed milk with artificial means of delivery.

Reproduced with permission from Schanler RJ, Dooley S, Gartner LM, Krebs NF, Mass SB, eds. *Breastfeeding Handbook for Physicians.* Elk Grove Village, IL: American Academy of Pediatrics; 2006 the prevalence in Israel, where it was 10 times lower. The significant differences in feeding during the first year of life between the 2 populations included longer exclusive breastfeeding and lack of introduction of peanuts in the diet of British infants and children. In Israel, a common food for weaning infants contains peanuts. The investigators suggested that early introduction of the peanut protein could allow tolerance to develop and, hence, explained the difference in the prevalence of peanut allergy between the 2 countries.

The second report by Fewtrell[25] et al sought to assess the 2003 change in breast-feeding policy in the United Kingdom, announced by the Health Minister without input from the British Department of Health's Scientific Advisory Committee on Nutrition. The 2003 United Kingdom policy, which was based on a World Health Organization (WHO) systematic review of the literature,[26] recommended that infants be breastfed exclusively for 6 months, in concert with WHO recommendations. The policy noted that the definition of exclusive breastfeeding varied among the studies in the WHO review, but exclusive breastfeeding to 6 months was not associated with growth failure and was associated with a reduction in diarrhea and respiratory infections. The authors of the systematic review noted that there were few advantages for exclusive breastfeeding beyond 4 months from a disease standpoint, including the risk of atopic disease or asthma, but cautioned that some exclusively breastfed infants are at risk of developing iron deficiency.[26] Because of the quality of the studies, causality, again, could not be inferred. Fewtrell et al raised concerns that prolonged exclusive breastfeeding is associated with a higher risk of iron deficiency anemia, with a higher incidence of food allergies and a higher risk of celiac disease.[25] The AAP is also concerned with the development of iron deficiency in infants for whom exclusive breastfeeding is prolonged and, therefore, recommends iron supplementation after 4 months of age for exclusively breastfed infants.[15]

Contraindications to Breastfeeding

Most women can successfully breastfeed their infants, but some should not and some cannot. In the United States, women who are infected with human immuno-deficiency virus (HIV) or human T-cell lymphotropic virus (HTLV type 1 and 2) or active pulmonary tuberculosis who have not completed 2 weeks of treatment should not breastfeed.[27] Infants with inborn errors of metabolism, such as galactosemia, should not be breastfed.

Because of concern for the effect of maternal drugs on nursing infants, pediatricians often recommend cessation of breastfeeding to mothers who require medications. Perhaps most problematic is the increasing usage of a wide variety of maternal psychotropic agents, including selective serotonin-reuptake inhibitors, by lactating mothers. In general, there are inadequate pharmacologic data and little information on short- and long-term neurobehavioral effects from infant exposure to these psychotropic agents. Many medications taken by lactating women are safe for their infants, however. Before advising a mother to discontinue breastfeeding, the medication can be reviewed on the Drugs and Lactation Database (LactMed). LactMed is supported by the US National Library of Medicine and has up-to-date, peer-reviewed information for pediatricians and mothers on prescribed medications and recreational drugs. This information can be accessed at http://toxnet.nlm.nih.gov and is the preferred source for information on medications for nursing mothers.

How to Support Breastfeeding

To begin to meet the goals of Healthy People 2020, families require support to initiate and continue breastfeeding. For initiation, it is helpful to have the physician acknowledge support for breastfeeding early in the pregnancy so families can begin to consider the concept and put into place support systems. Unless there is a medical condition that prevents early initiation of breastfeeding, the infant should be placed at the mother's breast within 1 hour of delivery and should remain with the mother. Most infants will find the nipple, but some may need assistance by labor and delivery nurses or lactation consultants. Although breastfeeding is natural, it is a learned skill, and mothers benefit from bedside teaching of positioning, latching on, and sucking. Follow-up with committed personnel while mother and infant are in the hospital is essential to provide answers to questions, offer suggestions, and support and problem solve. During this time, the hospital is very important in terms of attitudes, support systems, and policies. All hospitals are encouraged to adopt the Ten Steps for successful breastfeeding recommended by the WHO and endorsed by the AAP.[1,28] These are listed in Table 3.6 and are an important part of being certified as a Baby-Friendly Hospital and have been shown to improve the duration of successful breastfeeding.[29,30] Currently, fewer than 5% of US infants are born in US hospitals that are certified as Baby-Friendly Hospitals.[3] The CDC mPINC survey has assessed the lactation practices in more than 80% of US hospitals and noted that the mean score for implementation was only 6.3 for the Ten Steps[9]; 65% of hospitals erroneously advised mothers to limit the duration of breastfeeding, and 45% of hospitals presented pacifiers to more than half of infants.[9]

Table 3.6.
Ten Steps to Successful Breastfeeding

Step	Activity
Step 1	Have a written breastfeeding policy that is routinely communicated to all health care staff.
Step 2	Train all health care staff in skills necessary to implement this policy.
Step 3	Inform all pregnant women about the benefits and management of breastfeeding.
Step 4	Help mothers initiate breastfeeding within 1 hour of birth.
Step 5	Show mothers how to breastfeed and how to maintain lactation, even if they should be separated from their infants.
Step 6	Give breastfeeding newborn infants no food or drink other than human milk, unless medically indicated.
Step 7	Rooming-in—all mothers and infants to remain together 24 hours a day.
Step 8	Encourage breastfeeding on demand.
Step 9	Give no artificial teats or pacifiers to breastfeeding infants.[a]
Step 10	Foster the establishment of breastfeeding support groups and refer mothers to them on discharge from the hospital.

Reproduced with permission from Schanler RJ, Dooley S, Gartner LM, Krebs NF, Mass SB, eds. *Breastfeeding Handbook for Physicians.* Elk Grove Village, IL: American Academy of Pediatrics; 2006

[a] The AAP does not support a categorical ban on pacifiers because of their role in SIDS risk reduction and their analgesic benefit during painful procedures when breastfeeding cannot provide the analgesia. Pacifier use in the hospital in the neonatal periods should be limited to specific medical indications, including pain reduction, calming in a drug-exposed infant, nonnutritive sucking in preterm infants, etc. Mothers of healthy term infants should be instructed to delay pacifier use until breastfeeding is well established, usually about 3 to 4 weeks after birth.

Maintenance of breastfeeding involves issues for the infant and mother. Most importantly, a supportive family and access to good information are needed for new mothers. Women often have concerns about their ability to produce adequate milk. There are many possible and manageable causes for inadequate milk intake and, hence, failure to thrive in breastfed infants. These include preterm birth, illness in the mother or child, mother-baby separation, cessation of lactation for a period of time, and anxiety, fatigue, and emotional stress. Most often, milk production can be increased by increasing the frequency of breastfeeding, using relaxation techniques, having psychological support, and having an experienced lactation expert, such as a certified lactation consultant, to help with the mechanics of breastfeeding.

If an infant is receiving insufficient milk, the infant will have delayed bowel movements, decreased urinary output, early jaundice, hunger, and lethargy and will lose more than 7% of his or her birth weight. Serial weights will identify whether the infant is getting adequate milk volume. If the infant fails to grow, the infant most likely is receiving insufficient milk. At times, this can be overcome by increasing the frequency of feedings. For example, an infant who sleeps through the night can be awakened and breastfed. If maternal anxiety or exhaustion are contributing, then support for the mother can be sought. Schanler et al suggest an organized approach to assessment of inadequate human milk intake that considers infant and maternal factors.[27] However, if objective measures, such as inadequate weight gain, persist despite all efforts, the mother most likely has insufficient milk syndrome, the most common cause of breastfeeding failure.[31] Insufficient milk syndrome occurs in approximately 5% of women. Maternal history can suggest insufficient milk syndrome. Lack of breast enlargement during pregnancy, lack of breast fullness by 5 days after birth, or a history of breast reduction surgery are predictive of insufficient milk syndrome. Women with poor milk production may request galactogogues, substances that induce, maintain, and increase human milk production. The currently available galactogogues were recently reviewed[32]; however, the authors cautioned that the use of substances to enhance milk production should be limited to those women who have no treatable cause for the reduced milk production. Supplementation is often necessary for infants receiving insufficient human milk. Appropriate supplementation includes stored human milk or infant formula. The recommendation that donor's milk be used must be approached with caution to be sure that the milk comes from a bank that abides by the protocols of the Human Milk Banking Association of North America (HMBANA)[33] and voluntarily follows the recommendations of the Food and Drug Administration and CDC. These banks follow standards for cleanliness and storage of human milk. The milk from these banks is tested for HIV-1 and HIV-2, hepatitis B and C, and syphilis, and donors must state that they are healthy, that their infants are thriving, and that they are taking no medications. In addition, there are many Web sites that offer human milk that may or may not follow the protocols of the HMBANA, and the use of milk from these sources should be approached with great caution. There is no government oversight or standards for donor milk including nutrient content, whether offered online or via established human milk banks.

Regular concerns of mothers with regard to breastfeeding include nipple pain, engorgement, and mastitis. Nipple pain is common in the first week or so of breastfeeding. If it persists, the breast and feeding technique should be observed by a lactation expert. Poor positioning and improper latching on are common, as is trauma caused by vigorous sucking that results in nipple cracking. Fungal infections are rare. Application of human milk to the nipple after a feed may be helpful, or manual expression for a day or 2 to allow the cracks to heal may ease the pain. Engorgement is usually caused by infrequent or ineffective milk removal. Engorgement is treated by increasing the frequency of breastfeeding. A clogged duct occurs when the breast is incompletely emptied, milk remains in the duct, and inflammation develops. It is diagnosed by palpating a lump in the breast. Treatment is increased nursing to drain the breast.

Mastitis presents as a localized area of warmth, tenderness, edema, and erythema in a breast more than 10 days after delivery. It may also present with systemic signs such as fever, malaise, and intense breast pain. Mastitis is treated with antibiotics and by increasing the frequency of breastfeeding to drain the breast.

Jaundice associated with breastfeeding has been divided into 2 distinct entities: breast milk jaundice and breastfeeding jaundice. Breast milk jaundice occurs in many breastfed infants and is characterized by a high unconjugated bilirubin concentration that may remain elevated for 6 to 12 weeks. Infants with breast milk jaundice are generally healthy, and in most circumstances, the family can be reassured. The factor in human milk that is responsible for prolonged unconjugated hyperbilirubinemia has not been identified. The infant should be assessed to be sure there is no other cause for the unconjugated hyperbilirubinemia, such as inadequate milk intake, galactosemia, hypothyroidism, urinary tract infection, or hemolysis. If the conjugated bilirubin concentration is greater than 1.5 mg/dL, an evaluation for liver disease must be performed.

Severe jaundice may occur with the second entity, breastfeeding jaundice. Severe jaundice is the most common reason for readmission for term or near-term infants to the hospital after delivery, and in one very large study, almost all the infants admitted for severe jaundice were breastfed.[34] Thus, poor breastfeeding management is often a contributing factor. Jaundice occurs in the first week of life and can be associated with inadequate milk intake and dehydration, leading some authorities to refer to this as "non-breastfeeding jaundice." Other medical factors, such as ABO incompatibility or urinary tract infection, may contribute to the severity of the jaundice. Generally, concentrations of total bilirubin in severe jaundice are 25 mg/dL or greater. These infants should be managed according the AAP policy on neonatal jaundice.[35] In addition, insufficient milk syndrome must be ruled out, and evaluation of breastfeeding technique should occur.

Nutrition of the Lactating Mother

Dietary reference intakes for breastfeeding mothers are similar to or greater than those during pregnancy. The lactating mother has an increased daily energy need of 450 to 500 kcal/day that can be met by modest increases in a normally balanced diet. Although most clinicians recommend the continued use of prenatal vitamins during lactation, there is no routine recommendation for these supplements.[36] The recommended dietary allowance for vitamin D in lactating women is 600 IU per day, with an upper limit of 4000 IU per day.[37] An intake of 4000 IU per day in lactating women has been demonstrated to significantly increased the vitamin D content of maternal milk and to increase serum vitamin D concentrations in breast-feeding infants, although more studies are needed to determine what is an appropriate level of supplementation of vitamin D for lactating women.[38]

Consumption of 1 to 2 servings of ocean-going fish per week is recommended to meet the need for an average daily intake of 200 to 300 mg of ω-3 long-chain fatty acids (docosahexaenoic acid [DHA]). Although there is concern for the risk of intake of excessive mercury or other contaminants, the risk is offset by the neurobehavioral benefits of adequate DHA intake.[39]

Growth of the Breastfed Infant

Until the 2006 publication of the World Health Organization (WHO) growth charts,[40] the CDC growth charts from 2000 for infants and children were used by most pediatric health care providers in the United States.[41] The CDC charts are a growth reference and describe how US children grow across a wide range of social, ethnic, and economic conditions (see chapter 25 and Appendix A). These charts included data from more than 82 million US birth certificates as well as various cross-sectional databases, which included 4697 infants 2 to 24 months of age with healthy as well as unhealthy growth.[41] However, the data points were sparse in the first few months of life, and there were no data points between birth and 2 months of age. The CDC charts used data from infants that approximated the mix of feedings that infants received in the 1970s and 1980s. During this period, one third of US infants were breastfed up to 3 months of age, and the other two thirds were predominantly formula fed. However, as noted previously, the feeding pattern in the United States has changed, and as of 2011, 75% of US mothers initiate breastfeeding, and 44% of infants are still receiving some human milk at 6 months of age.[3]

In contrast, the 2006 WHO charts demonstrate how infants "should" grow under ideal conditions not subject to economic restraints and, thus, are considered a growth "standard." The charts from birth to 2 years of age are based on 903 infants who were exclusively/predominantly breastfed for 4 to 6 months and who continued breastfeeding for at least 12 months. The median duration of breastfeeding was 17.8 months, and complementary foods were introduced at a mean age of 5.1 months.[42] The data were largely longitudinal, and infants were weighed and measured 21 times in 24 months.[43] After comparison of growth curves, in 2010 the CDC published a report detailing new recommendations for the use of the WHO Multicenter Growth Reference Study growth charts for children younger than 24 months (regardless of diet) in place of the 2000 CDC growth charts[44] (see Chapter 25 and Appendix A). These charts include weight for age, length for age, head circumference for age, weight for length, and body mass index for age.

Comparing the 2006 WHO and 2000 CDC growth curves will reveal the differences in growth between breastfed and formula-fed infants. The WHO curves have a steeper increase in weight from 0 to 3 months of age than the CDC curves do, so more infants are identified as having low weight for age using the WHO curves. After 3 months of age, however, the WHO curves have a slower increase in weight and length for age than the CDC charts do, so fewer 6- to 23-month-old children are identified as low weight for age and low weight for length.[44] If using the 2006 WHO curves, the CDC and the AAP recommend using the 2.3[rd] and 97.7[th] percentiles (labeled as 2nd and 98th percentiles on the curves, or 2 standard deviations above and below the mean) to identify infants and young children with potentially suboptimal growth in the first 24 months after birth. The differences in the prevalence of overweight and shortness between the 2 sets of curves are minimized if the recommended CDC and WHO cut point for overweight (>95th percentile for CDC 2000, >97.7[th] percentile for WHO 2006) and short stature (<5th percentile for CDC 2000, <2.3 percentile for WHO 2006) are used on their respective growth charts.[45]

Expressing and Storing Milk

At times, mothers cannot breastfeed, and having a supply of milk available to the infant is desirable. There are many manuals and online resources on the expression of milk. How a particular mother expresses her milk is a matter of choice. Milk can be hand expressed or expressed using any one of a variety of pumps. Before expressing milk, the mother should wash her hands and breasts with warm, soapy water. If using a pump, she should wash all components of the pump with warm, soapy water. The expressed milk should be placed in a glass or hard plastic container and frozen if not used within 72 hours. Milk should be stored as individual feedings so the same milk is not frozen and thawed numerous times. The milk should be labeled with the date it was collected. Milk can be kept frozen for 3 to 6 months. When needed, it can be thawed rapidly by holding the container under running tepid water. New data suggest that human milk can be stored at refrigerator temperature (4°C) in a neonatal intensive care unit for as long as 96 hours after thawing.[46] Human milk should never be refrozen.

Special Situations

Infants who are ill, have developmental delays, or are born preterm present special challenges for breastfeeding. Depending on the illness, an infant may or may not be able to feed for a period of time. If possible, mothers can express and store milk for the time when the infant is able to take nutrients via the gastrointestinal tract. If an infant cannot physically breastfeed, the mother's milk can be expressed and provided through tube feedings to the infant. This is often the case for infants who have significant developmental delays or are born preterm. However, these infants must be carefully followed by an experienced nutrition team, because the fat in human milk adheres to tubing and the infant may not receive adequate fat, fat-soluble vitamins, and calories.

Human milk is the preferred feeding for preterm infants (see Chapter 5). Mothers can express milk for ill or very small preterm infants, and if maternal milk is not available, pasteurized donor milk can be used. Preterm infants who weigh less than 1500 g at birth require a human milk fortifier to provide adequate nutrients to support growth. The fortifier should continue until the infant successfully breastfeeds or reaches a weight of at least 2000 g or is near the time of discharge. Subsequently, depending on the status of the infant, unfortified human milk may be appropriate.

Conclusion

Breastfeeding is a natural extension of pregnancy and the early life of the infant. If positive attitudes exist in the family, community, workplace, and the health care system, 95% of mothers can breastfeed successfully. Breastfeeding confers benefits on the infant, and lack of access to human milk can be disadvantageous for the infant. The duration of breastfeeding depends on the desires of the mother and the needs of her infant and her family, especially if she is working. Exclusively breastfed infants must be supplemented with iron and vitamin D, and complementary foods can be introduced at about 6 months of age.

References

1. American Academy of Pediatrics, Section on Breastfeeding. Breastfeeding and the use of human milk. *Pediatrics*. 2012;129(3):e827-e841

2. American Academy of Pediatrics, Committee on Nutrition. *Pediatric Nutrition Handbook*. Kleinman RE, ed. 6th ed. Elk Grove Village, IL: American Academy of Pediatrics; 2009

3. Center for Disease Control and Prevention. Breastfeeding Report 2010, United States: Outcome Indicators. Available at: http://www.cdc.gov/breastfeeding/data/reportcard2. htm. Accessed September 6, 2012

4. Center for Disease Control and Prevention. Healthy People 2020 Breastfeeding Objectives. Available at: http://www.cdc.gov/breastfeeding/policy/hp2010.htm. Accessed September 6, 2012

5. Fein SB, Labiner-Wolfe J, Shealy KR, Li R, Chen J, Grummer-Strawn LM. Infant Feeding Practices Study II: study methods. *Pediatrics*. 2008;122(Suppl 2):S28-S35

6. Ryan AS, Wenjun Z, Acosta A. Breastfeeding continues to increase into the new millennium. *Pediatrics*. 2002;110(6):1103-1109

7. US Department of Health and Human Services. The Surgeon General's Call to Action to Support Breastfeeding. Washington, DC: US Department of Health and Human Services, Office of the Surgeon General; 2011

8. Centers for Disease Control and Prevention. Breastfeeding trends and updated national health objectives for exclusive breastfeeding—United States, birth years 2000–2004. *MMWR Morb Mortal Wkly Rep.* 2007;56(30):760-763

9. Centers for Disease Control and Prevention. Breastfeeding-related maternity practices at hospitals and birth centers—United States, 2007. *MMWR Morb Mortal Wkly Rep.* 2008;57(23):621-625

10. Pak-Gorstein S, Haq A, Graham EA. Cultural influences on infant feeding practices. *Pediatr Rev.* 2009;30(3):e11-e21

11. Santoro W Jr, Martinez FE, Ricco RG, Jorge SM. Colostrum ingested during the first day of life by exclusively breastfed healthy newborn infants. *J Pediatr.* 2010;156(1):29-32

12. Karra MV, Udipi SA, Kirksey A, Roepke JL. Changes in specific nutrients in breast milk during extended lactation. *Am J Clin Nutr.* 1986;43(4):495-503

13. Motil KJ, Sheng HP, Montandon CM, Wong WW. Human milk protein does not limit growth of breast-fed infants. *J Pediatr Gastroenterol Nutr.* 1997;24(1):10-17

14. Wagner CL; Greer FR, American Academy of Pediatrics, Section on Breastfeeding, Committee on Nutrition. Prevention of rickets and vitamin D deficiency in infants, children, and adolescents. *Pediatrics.* 2008;122(5):1142-1152

15. Baker RD; Greer FR; American Academy of Pediatrics, Committee on Nutrition. Diagnosis and prevention of iron deficiency and iron-deficiency anemia in infants and young children (0-3 years of age). *Pediatrics.* 2010;126(5):1040-1050

16. Hanson LA, Ahlstedt S, Andersson B, et al. Protective factors in milk and the development of the immune system. *Pediatrics.* 1985;75(1 Pt 2):172-176

17. Brandtzaeg P. The mucosal immune system and its integration with the mammary glands. *J Pediatr.* 2010;156(2 Suppl):S8-S15

18. Manjarrez-Hernandez HA, Gavilanes-Parra S, Chavez-Berrocal E, Navarro-Ocana A, Cravioto A. Antigen detection in enteropathogenic *Escherichia coli* using secretory immunoglobulin A antibodies isolated from human breast milk. *Infect Immunol.* 2000;68(9):5030-5036

19. Parissi-Crivelli A, Parissi-Crivelli JM, Giron JA. Recognition of enteropathogenic Escherichia coli virulence determinants by human colostrum and serum antibodies. *J Clin Microbiol.* 2000;38(7):2696-2700

20. Sanches MI, Keller R, Hartland EL, et al. Human colostrum and serum contain antibodies reactive to the intimin-binding region of the enteropathogenic Escherichia coli translocated intimin receptor. *J Pediatr Gastroenterol Nutr.* 2000;30(1):73-77

21. Lonnerdal B. Bioactive proteins in human milk: mechanisms of action. *J Pediatr.* 2010;156(2 Suppl):S26-S30

22. Garofalo R. Cytokines in human milk. *J Pediatr.* 2010;156(2 Suppl):S36-S40

23. Ip S, Chung M, Raman G, Chew P, Magula N, De Vine D, Trikalinos T, Lau J. *Breastfeeding and Maternal and Infant Health Outcomes in Developed Countries.* Rockvill, MD: Agency for Healthcare Research and Quality; 2007. AHRQ Publication No. 07-E007

24. Du Toit G, Katz Y, Sasieni P, et al. Early consumption of peanuts in infancy is associated with a low prevalence of peanut allergy. *J Allergy Clin Immunol.* 2008;122(5):984-991

25. Fewtrell M, Wilson DC, Booth I, Lucas A. Six months of exclusive breastfeeding: how good is the evidence? *BMJ*. 2010;324:c5955

26. Kramer MS, Kakuma R. *The Optimum Duration of Breastfeeding: A Systematic Review*. Geneva, Switzerland: World Health Organization; 2002

27. Schanler RJ, Dooley S, Gartner LM, Krebs NF, Mass SB, eds. *Breastfeeding Handbook for Physicians*. Elk Grove Village, IL: American Academy of Pediatrics; 2006

28. UNICEF. *Ten Steps to Successful Breastfeeding*. Geneva, Switzerland: World Health Organization; 1991

29. Step 10: Strives to Achieve the WHO/UNICEF Ten Steps of the Baby-Friendly Hospital Initiative to Promote Successful Breastfeeding: The Coalition for Improving Maternity Services. *J Perinat Educ*. 2007;16(Suppl 1):79S-80S

30. Kramer MS, Chalmers B, Hodnett ED, et al. PROBIT Study Group. Promotion of Breastfeeding Intervention Trial (PROBIT): a randomized trial in the Republic of Balarus. *JAMA*. 2001;285(4):413-420

31. Sjolin S, Hofvander Y, Hillervik C. Factors related to early termination of breastfeeding. A retrospective study in Sweden. *Acta Paediatr Scand*. 1977;66(4):505-511

32. Zuppa AA, Sindico P, Orchi C, Carducci C, Cardiello V, Romagnoli C. Safety and efficacy of galactogogues: substances that induce, maintain and increase breast milk production. *J Pharm Pharm Sci*. 2010;13(2):162-174

33. Human Milk Banking Association of North America. *Guidelines for the Establishment and Operation of a Donor Human Milk Bank*. Fort Worth, TX: Human Milk Banking Association of North America; 1994

34. Newman TB, Liljestrand P, Escobar GJ. Infants with bilirubin levels of 30 mg/dL or more in a large managed care organization. *Pediatrics*. 2003;111(6 Pt 1):1303-1311

35. Maisels MJ, Bhutani VK, Bogen D, Newman TB, Stark AR, Watchko JF. Hyperbilirubinemia in the newborn infant > or =35 weeks' gestation: an update with clarifications. *Pediatrics*. 2009;124(4):1193-1198

36. Picciano MF, McGuire MK. Use of dietary supplements by pregnant and lactating women in North America. *Am J Clin Nutr*. 2009;89(2):663S-667S

37. Institute of Medicine. *Dietary Reference Intakes for Calcium and Vitamin D*. Washington, DC: National Academies Press; 2011

38. Hollis BW, Wagner CL. Vitamin D requirements during lactation: high dose maternal supplementation as therapy to prevent hypovitaminosis D for both the mother and the nursing infant. *Am J Clin Nutr*. 2004;80(6 Suppl):1752S-1758S

39. Carlson SE. Docosahexenoic acid supplementation in pregancy and lactation. *Am J Clin Nutr*. 2009;89(2):678S-684S

40. World Health Organization Multicenter Growth Reference Study. Enrollment and baseline characteristics in the WHO Multicenter Growth Reference Study. *Acta Paediatr Suppl*. 2006;450:7-15

41. Ogden CL, Kuczmarski RJ, Flegal KM, et al. Centers for Disease Control and Prevention 2000 growth charts for the United States: improvement to the 1977 National Center for Health Statistics version. *Pediatrics*. 2002;109(1):45-60

42. World Health Organization Multicenter Growth Reference Study. Breastfeeding in the WHO Multicenter Growth Reference Study. *Acta Paediatr Suppl*. 2006;450:16-26

43. World Health Organization Multicenter Growth Reference Study. Assessment of differences in linear growth among populations in the WHO Multicenter Growth Reference Study. *Acta Paediatr Suppl*. 2006;450:56-65

44. Centers for Disease Control and Prevention. Use of World Health Organization and CDC growth charts for children aged 0-59 months in the United States. *MMWR Recomm Rep*. 2010;59(RR-9):1-15

45. Mei Z, Ogden CL, Flegal KM, Grummer-Strawn LM. Comparison of the prevalence of shortness, underweight, and overweight among US children aged 0-59 months by using the CDC 2000 and the WHO 2006 growth charts. *J Pediatr*. 2008;153(5):622-628

46. Slutzah M, Codipilly C, Potak D, Clark RM, Shanler RJ. Refrigerator storage of expressed human milk in the neonatal intensive care unit. *J Pediatr*. 2010;156(1):26-28

II

Chapter 4

Formula Feeding of Term Infants

General Considerations

In the absence of human milk, iron-fortified infant formulas are the most appropriate substitutes for feeding healthy, full-term infants during the first year of life. Although infant formulas do not duplicate the composition of human milk, formulas are continuously being modified as new nutritional information, ingredients, and technology become available. All currently available formulas meet all of the energy and nutrient requirements for healthy term infants during the first 4 to 6 months of life. After 6 months of age, formulas complement the increasing variety of solid foods in the diet and continue to supply a significant part of the infant's nutritional requirements.[1] The practice of delaying the introduction of complementary foods until approximately 6 months of age has accentuated the importance of the liquid part of the diet throughout the first year of life.[2]

Rates of Breastfeeding and Formula Feeding

The Centers for Disease Control and Prevention (CDC)'s Breastfeeding Report Card in 2010 revealed that 75% of US infants initially were breastfed.[3] Breastfeeding initiation rates and breastfeeding continuation rates at 6 months of age are highest among women who are 20 years or older; are white, Hispanic, or Asian American; have had at least some college education; are relatively affluent; and live in the western or northeastern United States. The lowest rates of breastfeeding are observed among black mothers who are younger than 20 years and mothers who have lower incomes or live in the southeastern United States.[3-5] The CDC study did not address employment status of women, but an earlier study found that breastfeeding initiation rates did not differ between women who were employed (full- or part-time) and those who were unemployed, although employment status did affect length of breastfeeding, as might be expected since this study was performed before legislation requiring workplace support for breastfeeding (Patient Protection and Affordable Care Act [Pub L No. 111-148]) and before guidelines for supporting breastfeeding in child care centers were published.[4] The CDC Report Card showed that the percentage of infants who were still at least partially breastfed at 6 and 12 months of age was approximately 42% and 21%, respectively.

Approximately 80% of infants are fed an infant formula or some form of whole cow milk by 1 year of age.[2] Commercial infant formulas are widely available and play a substantial role in meeting the nutritional needs of infants in the United States. Because of concern that mothers may choose not to initiate breastfeeding or may stop prematurely, the American Academy of Pediatrics (AAP) and other organizations have expressed disapproval of direct advertising of infant formula to the general public. Such advertising runs counter to the World Health Organization's "International Code of Marketing of Breastmilk Substitutes," to which the United States is not a signatory.

Indications for the Use of Infant Formula

There are 3 indications for the use of infant formulas: (1) as a substitute (or supplement) for human milk in infants whose mothers choose not to breastfeed (or not to do so exclusively); (2) as a substitute for human milk in infants for whom breastfeeding is medically contraindicated (eg, some inborn errors of metabolism); and (3) as a supplement for breastfed infants whose intake of human milk is inadequate to support adequate weight gain. In the latter case, supplementation should be instituted only after attempts to increase milk supply have proven ineffective, because the introduction of formula may lead to a decrease in milk supply. Because of the beneficial properties of human milk, mothers should be encouraged to continue breastfeeding even if formula is used as a supplement.

History of Infant Formula Development

Alternatives for feeding the infant something other than human milk have been a problem for centuries, and often, "wet nurses" or the unaltered milks of cows and other animals were used. The first scientific comparison of the composition of human milk and cow milk was published in 1838. After that study was published, several often complicated systems of altering cow milk to make it more suitable for infant feeding were developed. In 1919, Gerstenberger published a report on his 3-year experience with a cow milk formula, "synthetic milk adapted," which had concentrations of protein, fat, and carbohydrate similar to those of human milk. Commercially produced formulas soon followed.[6,7] Nevertheless, for many years, infant formulas were predominantly prepared in the home using whole or evaporated cow milk, corn syrup, and water. The protein content of these formulas was much higher than that found in human milk or currently available commercial formulas. The fat largely comprised saturated fatty acids, which are poorly absorbed by young infants, and small amounts of the essential fatty acids. The carbohydrate content was a mixture of lactose and added corn syrup (dextrins, glucose polymers). Vitamins needed to be supplemented separately. The composition of infant formulas has evolved considerably over the ensuing years. Each of the macronutrients (protein, fat, and carbohydrate) has been modified in currently available preparations to approximate more closely the macronutrient composition of human milk. Ongoing research has led to continued modification of infant formula through the present day.

Rationale for Development of Current Infant Formulas

Although the composition of human milk provides a basis for the composition of infant formulas, formulas do not duplicate the composition of human milk, for several reasons. First, human milk contains a number of components, such as hormones, growth factors, antibodies, immune-modulatory factors, enzymes, and live cells, that are difficult, if not impossible, to add to infant formula. Second, infant formulas are made from cow milk and other ingredients, which often provide nutrients that are dissimilar in chemical form and composition to the corresponding nutrients in human milk. For example, although the whey-to-casein ratio of cow milk-based infant formulas can be adjusted to approximate that of human milk, the types of whey and casein proteins in cow milk and their amino acid compositions are not the same as those found in human milk. Third, whereas human milk is usually consumed within hours of being produced, infant formulas are heat-treated and must have long shelf lives, generally at least 1 year. All of these factors make it impossible to duplicate the composition of human milk. Additionally, the bioavailability of some nutrients in infant formula may be lower than that of the same nutrients in human milk. Increasingly in recent years, because of the inability to match the composition of human milk per se, the development of infant formulas has focused on trying to duplicate the growth, physiology, and developmental outcomes of the breastfed infant through formula feeding. This requires a different approach to infant formula research and development and increases the reliance on the results of randomized clinical trials rather than on compositional similarity.[8]

Regulatory agencies have implicitly recognized that infant formulas should not be identical in composition to human milk. In the United States, for example, the standards for nutrient concentrations in infant formulas (see Appendix B) are specified by the Infant Formula Act of 1980 (Pub L No. 96-359), which was amended in 1986 (Pub L No. 99-570).[9] This act established the minimum levels of 29 nutrients and the maximum levels of 9 nutrients. In the case of 19 nutrients, the *minimum* amount required in infant formula is above the *average* level found in human milk. The same is true when one examines the minimums in the 2007 revision of the Codex infant formula standard, which is used in many countries around the world.[10] Although all formulas sold in the US must meet the requirements set forth in the Infant Formula Act, the compositions of both branded and generic formulas may differ qualitatively and quantitatively within the ranges allowed by the law.

Available Forms of Infant Formula

Infant formulas are available in 3 forms: ready-to-feed, concentrated liquid, and powder. The different forms of a given product are nearly identical in nutrient composition, but small differences may exist for technical reasons. Ready-to-feed formulas for healthy, full-term infants are available principally in 32-fl oz containers and also in smaller volume containers (2, 3, 6, and 8 fl oz), depending on the product and manufacturer. Concentrated liquid products are available in 13-fl oz and 1-quart containers. When diluted with equal amounts of water, concentrated liquids yield formula with nutrient levels that are the same as the corresponding ready-to-feed product. Powder products are available in a number of different sizes of containers that have anywhere from the amount needed to prepare a single serving to 2.2 lb of powder. Depending on the manufacturer, when prepared according to instructions, a 12.4- to 12.5-oz container yields approximately 90 fl oz of standard formula, and larger cans yield proportionally more.

Infant Formula Labels

The Infant Formula Act requires the manufacturer to ensure by analysis the amount of all 29 essential nutrients in each batch of formula and to make a quantitative declaration for each nutrient on the label. In the United States, this "label claim" for the amount of each nutrient is the *minimum* amount of the nutrient that will be present in the formula at the end of shelf life.[a] It is not the average amount of the nutrient in the formula, as is commonly thought and is the case in many other countries. Thus, the actual content of a given nutrient in a formula will always be higher than the level declared on the label. A survey of *actual* nutrient levels in infant formulas produced between 2000 and 2005 and sold in the United States and other countries revealed that although all formulas met label claim requirements, there was wide variability of actual levels of many nutrients from batch to batch.[11] Consequently, health care professionals who need to prescribe carefully defined diets based on infant formulas are advised to contact manufacturers to obtain the average or typical amounts of the nutrient(s) of interest in the formula being used. Among other requirements of the Infant Formula Act, all labels must have detailed mixing instructions, which may differ among manufacturers' products and should be followed for the specific formula being used.

---

[a] This is especially important for some vitamins. Although some vitamins degrade very little over shelf life (eg, vitamin K), others, such as riboflavin, vitamin B_{12}, and vitamin C, are subject to considerable loss. This means that early in shelf life, the levels of those vitamins that degrade are higher than at the end of shelf life, although in all cases, the final actual levels will be above the amount claimed on the label.

Safe Preparation of Infant Formula

All infant formulas must be manufactured in adherence to Good Manufacturing Practices, and all production facilities are inspected at least annually by the US Food and Drug Administration (FDA). Ready-to-feed and concentrated liquid products are commercially sterile—that is, they contain no pathogenic organisms. (Liquid products may contain small numbers of nonpathogenic organisms that are capable of growing only at very high temperatures—so-called thermophiles; these organisms may spoil the formula if it has not been stored properly.) Although powder products are heat-treated during manufacture and must meet strict standards regarding the allowable amounts and types of bacteria they may contain, they are not completely sterile and, in rare cases, may contain pathogenic organisms. Of recent concern has been the occasional presence of *Cronobacter sakazakii* (formerly *Enterobacter sakazakii*) in some powder infant formulas. This opportunistic organism has been the sporadic cause of severe infections in preterm infants in the early months of life and in other immunocompromised infants. For this reason, powder infant formulas generally are not recommended for these infants.

Careful preparation and handling of infant formulas are important to ensure their safety. Ready-to-feed formula should be shaken before being poured into the bottle to resuspend any mineral sediment that may have settled during storage. The normal preparation of formula from concentrated liquid products requires dilution with an equal volume of water; concentrated liquids also should be shaken before being poured for mixing. In preparing formula from powder products, it is important to adhere closely to the manufacturers' instructions on the label; most powders of standard formulas are mixed using 1 level, unpacked scoop of powder per 2 fl oz of water (for infants younger than 3 months of age, the US Department of Agriculture recommends using boiled water [see later discussion]). It is important to use the scoop provided by the manufacturer with the specific product and not to rely on standard measuring spoons or scoops from other products, because powders from different manufacturers provide slightly different amounts of nutrients per unit of volume, and scoop sizes will vary accordingly.

For special feeding situations, both powders and concentrated liquids can be reconstituted to provide formulas with more than the standard energy (calorie) concentration, which normally varies from about 19 kcal/fl oz to 20 kcal/fl oz. Most concentrated liquid products contain 40 kcal/fl oz; consequently, the same instructions for preparation of more-concentrated formula from concentrated liquid can be used for all of those products. These mixing instructions are shown in Appendix C. The table also shows how to mix more-concentrated formulas from concentrated liquids that contain 38 kcal/oz. As mentioned previously, because powders differ among manufacturers, a single approach cannot safely be used for all powder products. Instructions for preparation of more-concentrated formulas from powder should be obtained from the manufacturer for the specific product in question. In some instances, instructions may be available on the manufacturers' Web sites.

All formulas need to be prepared in clean containers and fed from clean bottles with clean nipples. In most cases, it is not necessary to sterilize bottles (or nipples) before mixing formula in them, especially if they have been washed in a dishwasher. Ready-to-feed formula can be poured into the bottle and fed immediately. Formula from concentrated liquid or powder can be prepared in individual bottles just before each feeding or in larger quantities in a clean container before transferring the desired amounts to individual bottles. In the latter case, use of a blender is specifically advised against. In all cases, safe, potable water needs to be used (see next paragraph). Although there are few recent data, terminal sterilization of formulas in the home seems to be performed far less frequently than in the past, possibly because of the improved level of hygiene in most homes and the practice of preparing single bottles just before feeding. The apparent abandonment of terminal sterilization increases the importance of cleanliness during preparation.

"Safe, potable water" implies that the water is both free of microorganisms capable of causing disease and low in minerals and other contaminants that may be detrimental. Municipal water supplies are generally free of pathogenic microorganisms. Well water needs to be tested regularly. In some cases, the use of bottled water may be the best alternative. If there is any doubt about bacterial contamination, water to be used for preparation should be brought to a rolling boil for 1 minute; longer boiling may concentrate minerals to an undesirable degree. Instructions from most manufacturers suggest allowing the water to cool to at least 38°C (approximately 100°F) and using this lukewarm water to prepare formula. Several years ago, after a 2004 meeting of an expert group, the Food and Agriculture Organization of the United Nations and the World Health Organization (FAO/WHO) recommended that powder formula be prepared with water that is at least 70°C (approx 158°F) to decrease the risk of infection with *C sakazakii*. Their data suggested that this approach could result in as much as a 4-log decrease in the concentrations of *C sakazakii*.[12] This recommendation has since been adopted and promulgated by other groups. A temperature of 70°C implies that after boiling, water is cooled at room temperature for no more than 30 minutes before it is used. It should be noted, however, that use of water at this temperature can cause substantial decreases in the concentrations of certain heat-labile nutrients, notably vitamin C; the concentrations of heat-labile nutrients in current powder formulas were formulated on the assumption of using cooler water for preparation, before the FAO/WHO recommendations were made. Parents may also complain that the use of excessively hot water causes clumping of the formula. There is no reason not to allow water to cool fully after boiling when reconstituting concentrated liquid.

Municipal water supplies may contain variable concentrations of minerals, including fluoride, depending on the source; well water may contain high concentrations of fluoride as well as other minerals, such as copper. (Formulas prepared with well water with very high concentrations of copper have been reported to cause hepatotoxicity.) Infant formulas are produced with defluoridated water. Fluoride is not specifically added during production, but some of the other ingredients used naturally contain fluoride. It has been recommended that the concentration of fluoride in formula be less than 60 to 100 µg/100 kcal (400–670 µg/L).

AAP

Formula Preparation

Water used for mixing infant formula must be from a safe water source, as defined by the state or local health department. If you are concerned or uncertain about the safety of the tap water, you may use bottled water or bring cold tap water to a rolling boil for 1 minute (no longer), then cool the water to room temperature for no more than 30 minutes before it is used.

Warmed water should be tested in advance to make sure it is not too hot for the infant. The easiest way to test the temperature is to shake a few drops on the inside of your wrist. Otherwise, a bottle can be prepared by adding powdered formula and room temperature water from the tap just before feeding. Bottles made in this way from powdered formula can be ready for feeding, as no additional refrigeration or warming would be required.

Prepared formula must be discarded within 1 hour after serving an infant. Prepared formula that has not been given to an infant may be stored in the refrigerator for 24 hours to prevent bacterial contamination. An open container of ready-to-feed formula, concentrated formula, or formula prepared from concentrated formula, should be covered, refrigerated, and discarded after 48 hours if not used.

There is no need to supplement the diet of the formula-fed infant with fluoride during the first 6 months of life. Health care professionals should ascertain the fluoride concentrations in the local water supplies of the communities in which their patients live. If the fluoride content of the municipal or well water used to prepare infant formula is high, bottled water that has been defluoridated should be used. After 6 months of age, the need for additional fluoride will depend principally on the fluoride content of the water (for recommendations, see Chapter 50: Nutrition and Oral Health).

Safe Handling and Storage of Infant Formula

Parents should be instructed to use proper hand-washing techniques whenever preparing infant formula or feeding their infant. They also should be given guidance on (1) proper storage of formula product remaining in the original container that will be used or mixed later; and (2) proper storage of formula that has been prepared, if it is not to be fed immediately. Once opened, cans of ready-to-feed and concentrated liquid product can generally be stored covered (with a plastic overcap or aluminum foil) in the refrigerator for no longer than 48 hours. Powder formula (both unopened and opened cans) should be stored in a cool, dry place, not in the refrigerator. Once opened, cans of powder should be covered with the overcap; opened product can be used for up to 4 weeks with no loss of quality if proper precautions are taken to avoid microbiologic contamination.

Prepared formula should not be left out of the refrigerator. If more than 1 bottle is prepared at a time, bottles for later use should be refrigerated immediately. This is especially important for powder products prepared with hot water, because they require longer to cool to reach a safe storage temperature. Regardless, all bottles should be used within 24 hours. "Unopened" bottles of prepared formula should be taken out of the refrigerator no more than 2 hours before being fed. Once the feeding has begun, the contents should be fed within an hour or discarded.

In the early months of life especially, infants prefer warm infant formula. This warming can be accomplished by putting the unopened bottle in a bowl of warm water for 5 to 10 minutes prior to feeding. Bottles of infant formula should not be warmed in a microwave oven. Microwave ovens can create "hot spots" in the formula in the bottle, and burns to the infant's mouth can occur despite the formula seeming to be at the right temperature when tested by the mother before feeding.

Guidelines for Length of Exclusive Formula Feeding and Supplementation With Solid Foods

Formula should be offered ad libitum, the goal being to allow the infant to regulate intake to meet his or her energy needs. The usual intake will be 140 to 200 mL/kg per day for the first 3 months of life. This intake provides approximately 90 to 135 kcal/kg of body weight per day and should result in an initial weight gain of 25 to 30 g/day. Between 3 and 6 months of age, weight gain decreases to 15 to 20 g/day, and between 6 and 12 months of age, weight gain decreases to 10 to 15 g/day. If human milk or formula intake is adequate, healthy infants do not need additional water, except when the environmental temperature is extremely high.

Although most infants thrive on formulas derived from cow milk, some infants may exhibit intolerance to these formulas. Vomiting or spitting up is common for the first few months of life and usually requires no change in the feeding regimen if weight gain is adequate. Constipation coupled with slow weight gain may indicate inadequate intake of formula. When a transition from one formula to another is undertaken because of tolerance, cost, availability, or a specific desire to alter the nutrient composition of the diet, the change from one formula to another can almost always be made abruptly.

Complementary foods may be introduced at approximately 6 months of age on the basis of developmental readiness (eg, oro-motor coordination, head control) and nutritional needs of the growing infant. With regard to complementary feeding and breastfeeding, the AAP supports exclusive breastfeeding (in which all fluid, energy, and nutrients come from human milk, with the possible exception of small amounts of medicinal/nutrient supplements) for approximately 6 months. After 6 months, in addition to solid foods, either breastfeeding or iron-fortified infant formula should be used for the remainder of first year of life, rather than feeding any form of cow milk. This reduces the risk of inadequate intakes of nutrients such as zinc, the essential fatty acids, and other important long-chain, polyunsaturated fatty acids. These practices also help prevent excessive intakes of certain nutrients, such as protein and sodium, during this time.

Intact Cow Milk Protein-Based Formulas

Composition

Commercial, intact cow milk protein-based formulas have many similarities but also differ substantially from one another in sources and quantities of nutrients. Although the different manufacturers provide a rationale for formula composition, physiologically significant differences have not always been clearly demonstrated among the various products. The composition of formulas may change over time and is reflected on the formula label. In attempting to differentiate among different formulas, health care professionals should rely on the results of clinical studies rather than on composition alone whenever possible.

Because the composition of available formulas for healthy, full-term infants evolves constantly and at different rates for different products, published nutrient composition tables go out of date quickly. Consequently, in lieu of product composition tables in appendices, this handbook provides links to manufacturers' Web sites (found at the end of this chapter) so that health care professionals and their patients will have access to the most up-to-date information.

Energy (Calories)

The energy (calorie) content of human milk varies, and although the US Infant Formula Act specifies minimum and maximum levels of protein and fat, it does not specify minimum and maximum energy levels. An expert panel convened at the request of the FDA recommended in 1998 that energy levels in standard formulas should fall between 63 and 71 kcal/dL (18.6–21 kcal/fl oz).[13] In 2003, the European Scientific Committee on Food suggested a similar range, 60 to 70 kcal/dL (17.8–20.7 kcal/fl oz).[14] Standard formulas currently available in the United States range from about 640 to 670 kcal/dL (18.9–20 kcal/fl oz).

Protein

Cow milk-based formulas in the United States contain protein at concentrations varying from approximately 1.4 to 1.8 g/dL. These concentrations represent almost 50% more protein than the average amount found in human milk (0.9-1.0 g/dL). The ratio between the predominant types of cow milk proteins (ie, whey proteins and casein proteins) varies considerably among these formulas. Some formulas contain cow milk protein with its unaltered whey-to-casein ratio of 18:82. Other formulas contain added cow milk whey protein in an effort to approach the whey-to-casein ratio of human milk; these have whey-to-casein ratios of between 48:52 and 60:40. One "standard" infant formula containing 100% partially hydrolyzed whey protein also is available.

The whey-to-casein ratio of human milk is variable and changes throughout early lactation.[15] Additionally, as stated previously, there are compositional and functional differences between the principal whey and casein proteins in cow milk and in human milk.[16] The predominant whey protein in cow milk is β-lactoglobulin, whereas the predominant whey protein in human milk is α-lactalbumin. Similarly, there are differences in the amounts of alpha, beta, and kappa caseins of human milk and cow milk. Because of these and other differences in the amino acid composition of these proteins, compared with breastfed infants, formula-fed infants have increased serum concentrations of several amino acids, and each type of formula results in a characteristic amino acid pattern. The clinical importance of these various patterns has not been demonstrated.

Fat

Fat provides 40% to 50% of the energy in cow milk-based formulas and is provided principally by mixtures of vegetable oils. These blends are better absorbed than the butterfat of cow milk and provide more appropriate amounts of the essential fatty acids. Fat blends are selected to provide a balance of saturated, monounsaturated, and polyunsaturated fatty acids. Commonly used oils include coconut oil (a good source of short-, medium- and long-chain saturated fatty acids), palm and palm olein oils (a source of long-chain, saturated fatty acids), and soy, corn, and safflower or sunflower oils (rich sources of polyunsaturated fatty acids). Some manufacturers use high-oleic variants of safflower or sunflower oils to increase monounsaturated fatty acids in the fat blend. The concentrations and ratio of the 2 essential fatty acids (linoleic acid, 18:2 omega-6; and alpha-linolenic acid, 18:3 omega-3) meet current guidelines. In contrast to human milk, which is high in cholesterol, commercially available infant formulas contain little or no cholesterol; the value of adding cholesterol to infant formulas has not been demonstrated.

Determination of the ideal fatty acid composition for infant formulas has been an area of intense research, particularly with regard to the omega-6 and omega-3 essential fatty acids and their very long-chain, polyunsaturated derivatives arachidonic acid (ARA) and docosahexaenoic acid (DHA). ARA and DHA are found in a wide range of concentrations in human milk, depending on maternal diet. They also can be synthesized from their precursor essential fatty acids by both preterm and term infants. Some, but not all, clinical studies have found improved short-term and long-term performance in tests of visual and cognitive functions both in preterm and in term infants fed formulas supplemented with ARA and DHA (see Chapter 17: Fats and Fatty Acids). ARA and DHA derived from single-cell microfungi and microalgae, respectively, have been classified as "generally recognized as safe" (GRAS) for use in infant formula when added at approved concentrations and ratios. Although there is no regulatory requirement for the inclusion of ARA and DHA in infant formulas, with the exception of a few "specialty products," standard formulas for term infants in the United States now contained added ARA and DHA.

Carbohydrate

Lactose is the major carbohydrate in human milk and in most standard cow milk-based infant formulas. Lactose is hydrolyzed in the small intestine by the action of lactase, which is located on the brush border of the intestinal villus epithelial cell. Lactase appears later than other brush-border disaccharidases in the developing fetal intestine but is present in maximal amounts in full-term infants. Nevertheless, even in full-term infants, some lactose enters the large intestine, where it is fermented. The end products of fermentation are short-chain fatty acids and several gases, among them carbon dioxide and hydrogen. This fermentation helps to maintain an acidic environment in the colon, which in turn fosters an acidophilic bacterial flora that includes lactobacilli and other organisms that suppress the growth of more pathogenic organisms. In addition to lactose, some formulas for term infants also contain modified starch or other complex carbohydrates, such as maltodextrins.

Iron

All routinely used cow milk-based formulas in the United States are now available only in "iron-fortified" versions. By law, a formula with an iron concentration ≥ 6.7 mg/L (≥ 1 mg/100 kcal) is considered iron-fortified and must be labeled as such.[9] Commercially available infant formulas originally were low in iron. During the 1950s, in response to a high prevalence of iron deficiency among infants in the

United States and to link iron with a major source of dietary energy, iron was added to infant formulas at a concentration of 12 mg/L. This amount was determined by the amount of iron needed in the first year of life, using estimates of iron absorption and formula intake. However, low-iron versions of milk-based formulas also continued to be available, principally because iron was perceived by some parents and physicians to cause constipation and other feeding problems. Well-controlled studies consistently failed to show any increase in prevalence of fussiness, cramping, colic, gastroesophageal reflux, constipation, or flatulence with the use of iron-fortified formulas. From the late 1990s onward, the AAP consistently stated that there was no role for low-iron formulas in the feeding of healthy term infants.[17,18] Low-iron formulas were gradually removed from the market over the ensuing decade. Although the relatively large amount of iron in infant formula has been controversial, this degree of fortification is required by the Special Supplemental Nutrition Program for Women, Infants, and Children (WIC) and supported by the AAP.[19]

Other Nutrients

The other required nutrients in infant formula (mostly vitamins and trace minerals) are inherent in the ingredients used to supply the macronutrients and/or are specifically added during manufacture. A number of micronutrients may come from more than one ingredient. All the ingredients used to produce formulas are regulated by the FDA and must be generally recognized as safe for use in infant formula.

Since the early 1980s, other nutrients not required by the Infant Formula Act have been added to infant formulas, and this will undoubtedly continue. The products to which these optional nutrients have been added vary by manufacturer and product. The additions have been made after preclinical and clinical studies of safety and possible efficacy, and all cases of new or modified infant formula notifications were filed with the FDA. Examples of these additions are the following:

- *Taurine*, an amino acid found in high concentrations in the brain and retina (see Chapter 15 – Protein);
- *Nucleotides*, semi-essential nutrients that have been added to many formulas and that may enhance development of immune function and promote the development of a less pathogenic intestinal flora (see Chapter 36 – Nutrition and Immunity);
- *Prebiotics and probiotics,* which are discussed briefly below (see also Chapters 36 – Nutrition and Immunity and 28 – Chronic Diarrheal Disease).

Prebiotics. In addition to lactose, human milk contains more complex carbohydrates, oligosaccharides, which account for approximately 10% of the carbohydrate. These oligosaccharides are not digestible in the small intestine but are fermentable in the large intestine and help maintain an acidic environment in the colon, which favors growth of nonpathogenic, acidophilic flora. The majority of US formula manufacturers now offer at least 1 formula with added indigestible, complex carbohydrates that, like the oligosaccharides in human milk, can be fermented in the colon. These carbohydrates are referred to a prebiotics. The commonly used prebiotics are galacto-oligosaccharides, fructo-oligosaccharides, and polydextrose. The goal of such additions is to foster the growth of those bacteria that are part of a healthy colonic mircroflora more typical of a healthy breastfed infant.[20] However, the AAP does not believe that the available evidence supports any benefit to adding prebiotics to infant formula at the present time.[20]

Probiotics. Although not nutrients, probiotics—nonpathogenic microorganisms, especially strains of some bacteria that ferment lactose, oligosaccharides, and other prebiotics and that may affect the colonic microflora and immune system—have also been added to some infant formulas. Because these are viable organisms, their addition has been limited to powder products, which do not undergo the stringent heat treatment involved in sterilization of liquid products. The AAP believes that although the addition of probiotics to infant formulas appears at this time to be safe for healthy infants, such formulas should not be fed to children who are immunocompromised or seriously ill. Furthermore, the evidence of clinical efficacy for probiotics "is insufficient to recommend the routine use of these formulas."[20]

Soy Formulas

Although soy formulas date back to the 1920s, during the 1960s and 1970s, improved, better-tolerated formulas were developed that were based on more refined soy protein isolates. Soy formulas are lactose free and have been used to feed infants who cannot tolerate milk protein or lactose. Soy formulas currently constitute approximately 13% of all formula sold, a decrease from approximately 20% several years ago.[21] The cause of this decline in usage could relate to the increased array of formulas marketed as "problem solvers," with various structure-function claims on the labels (ie, for "fussiness"), a common reason for switching to soy, as well as concerns about phytoestrogens in soy (see below).

Soy formulas support growth equivalent to that of breastfed and cow milk-based formula-fed infants.[22] Bone mineralization is similar in full-term infants fed soy and cow milk-based formulas.[23-25] Earlier formulations of currently available soy formulas were associated with an increased incidence of osteopenia in preterm infants. Data on the effects of newer formulations of soy formulas on bone mineralization in preterm infants are scarce, and consequently, the use of soy formulas in these infants should be avoided if possible. Special formulas with higher nutrient concentrations than standard milk-based or soy formulas for term infants have been developed for feeding preterm infants after discharge, and their use is preferred whenever possible.

Uses

There are several indications for the use of soy formulas. Infants for whom soy formula is indicated include those with primary (very rare) and secondary intolerance to lactose, those with intolerance to milk protein (in many instances), those with galactosemia, and those whose parents are vegetarian and wish for their infant's diet to be vegetarian.

All soy formulas in the United States are lactose free and are recommended for infants with clinically significant lactose intolerance or galactosemia.[19] Lactose intolerance occurs in some infants as a result of acute gastroenteritis; soy formulas are recommended for postdiarrheal refeeding only in patients who have signs and symptoms of clinically significant lactose intolerance.[26] Those who do require a lactose-free formula generally can be rechallenged with a lactose-containing formula after 1 month. Other symptoms of intolerance to cow milk-based formulas, such as colic, loose stools, spitting up, or vomiting, sometimes prompt a switch to soy formula. Most of these problems are unrelated to the formula being fed; occasionally, however, some infants respond positively to soy formulas for reasons not totally understood. Finally, infants in whom sucrase-isomaltase deficiency or hereditary fructose intolerance is suspected or diagnosed should not be fed soy formulas that contain sucrose as part of the carbohydrate.

Most infants who have an immunoglobulin E-associated reaction to cow milk proteins do well when fed soy formulas (up to 85% in one prospective study).[27,28] These formulas taste better and cost less than formulas based on extensively hydrolyzed protein. Nevertheless, although soy protein does not cross-react with cow milk protein, 10% to 14% of infants who are allergic to cow milk protein will develop an allergy to soy protein as well.[25,27,28] Soy formulas should specifically be avoided in those infants with milk protein-induced enterocolitis or intestinal blood loss. There is no indication for use of soy formula for the prevention of food allergy in general or atopic disease[19,29] (see Chapter 35 – Food Sensitivity).

Composition

Protein concentrations in soy infant formulas are slightly higher than those in cow milk-based formulas. In addition, methionine is added to compensate for the low concentration of this essential amino acid in soy protein. The fat blends in soy formulas are similar to those found in cow milk-based formulas. Lactose, the major carbohydrate of human milk and most cow milk-based formulas, is not used in soy formulas to avoid contamination with milk proteins. Carbohydrate in various soy formulas is supplied by sucrose and/or corn syrup solids and corn maltodextrins. The required concentrations of minerals and vitamins in soy formulas do not differ from those required in milk-based formulas. The concentrations of a number of nutrients differ in soy compared with cow milk-based formulas, as much because of the concentrations inherent in the ingredients used in their manufacture as because of any specific addition. Phytates present in soy protein isolates may affect the absorption of some minerals, and there are increased concentrations of minerals in some soy formulas to compensate for this lower bioavailability (eg, calcium). Soy formulas were the first to be available only in iron-fortified versions. This fact is of particular interest because of the belief by many health care professionals and parents that soy formulas are useful in the management of infants with feeding intolerance, and it belies the belief that iron is a cause of such intolerance. Carnitine, which is involved in intracellular fatty acid transport, is inherently low in soy formulas and, thus, is added to them.

Soy formulas contain phytoestrogens, which have been demonstrated to have physiological activity in rodent models. To address the possible long-term effects relating to the presence of phytoestrogens in soy formulas, a long-term follow-up study in 2001 compared early and later growth, pubertal development, and reproductive outcomes in 20- to 34-year-olds who, as infants, had been fed cow milk-based or soy formulas in studies at the University of Iowa. There were no significant differences in the outcomes of these 2 groups related to the type of formula that had been fed in infancy.[30] In 2008, the AAP stated: "there is no conclusive evidence from animal, adult human, or infant populations that dietary soy isoflavones may adversely affect human development, reproduction, or endocrine function."[19] In 2010, the National Toxicology Program of the National Institute of Health's Institute of Environmental Health Sciences concluded there was *"minimal concern for adverse effects on development in infants who consume soy infant formula."*[21]

AAP

The American Academy of Pediatrics finds that isolated soy protein-based formulas are a safe and nutritionally equivalent alternative to cow milk-based formula for term infants whose nutritional needs are not met from human milk.

The AAP specifically recommends the use of soy formulas for the following:

1. Term infants with galactosemia or hereditary lactase deficiency.
2. Term infants with documented transient lactase deficiency.
3. Infants with documented immunoglobulin E-associated allergy to cow milk who are not also allergic to soy protein.
4. Patients seeking a vegetarian-based diet for a term infant.

The use of soy protein-based formula is not recommended for the following:

1. Preterm infants with birth weights less than 1800 g.
2. Prevention of colic or allergy.
3. Infants with cow milk protein-induced enterocolitis or enteropathy.

Bhatia J; Greer FR; American Academy of Pediatrics, Committee on Nutrition. The use of soy protein-based formulas in infant feeding. *Pediatrics.* 2008;121(5):1062-1068

Protein Hydrolysate Formulas

Protein hydrolysate formulas may contain either partially hydrolyzed protein or extensively hydrolyzed protein. The indications for use of these 2 types of formula are distinctly different.

Infant Formula With Partially Hydrolyzed Protein

There are several infant formulas with partially hydrolyzed protein available in the US market. They have fat blends similar to those found in other standard infant formulas. Carbohydrate is supplied by corn maltodextrins or corn syrup solids and, in some cases, lactose. These formulas are used in the United States for routine feeding of healthy term infants and some are marketed as "problem solvers," depending on the overall composition. Formulas with partially hydrolyzed protein may be useful as part of a dietary regimen during infancy aimed at preventing atopic dermatitis, but on the basis of clinical studies, these results are not consistent for all products, and the effects are modest[29] (see Chapter 35). Because the protein in these formulas is not extensively hydrolyzed, these hydrolysates contain peptides that, to some degree, retain their antigenic nature; thus, these formulas are contraindicated in the management of infants with documented cow milk protein allergy.

Infant Formulas With Extensively Hydrolyzed Protein

Uses

Formulas based on hydrolyzed casein were originally developed for infants who could not digest or were severely intolerant to intact cow milk protein. The protein in these hydrolysate formulas is extensively hydrolyzed to produce a mixture of free amino acids and di-, tri-, and short-chain peptides that are incapable of eliciting an immunologic response in most infants. Formulas containing protein hydrolysates of this type are the preferred formulas for infants allergic to cow milk proteins and soy proteins. They also may be helpful as part of a dietary regimen during infancy aimed at preventing atopic disease, but as with the partially hydrolyzed products, the results are not consistent[29] (see Chapter 35). Because these formulas are lactose free and, in some cases, include substantial amounts of medium-chain triglycerides, they are also often useful in infants with significant malabsorption caused by gastrointestinal or hepatobiliary disease (eg, cystic fibrosis, short gut syndrome, biliary atresia, cholestasis, and protracted diarrhea). In such cases, protein hydrolysate formulas can be lifesaving and are preferable to the alternative of total parenteral nutrition. Disadvantages of protein hydrolysate formulas include their poor taste (because of the presence of specific amino acids and some peptides with bitter tastes), greater cost, and in some cases, higher osmolalities. It should be noted that despite their taste, these formulas are generally well accepted when introduced in the early months of life, before the infant's sense of bitter taste is well developed.

Composition

The unique compositions of the different protein hydrolysate formulas are available on manufacturers' Web sites. In contrast to the partially hydrolyzed protein formulas discussed previously, all infant formulas with extensively hydrolyzed protein are based on casein that has been heat-treated and enzymatically hydrolyzed. The resulting hydrolysate, consisting of free amino acids and short-chain peptides of varying lengths, is then fortified with selected amino acids to compensate for amino acids that are lost in the manufacturing process. Although in vitro tests and animal immunization studies have proven useful in the preclinical evaluation of extensively hydrolyzed proteins, the assurance of the hypoallergenicity of infant formulas containing these protein sources relies on carefully conducted clinical trials that document their efficacy in highly allergic infants and children. All infant formulas based on extensively hydrolyzed protein are lactose free. Manufacturers use sucrose, tapioca starch, corn syrup solids, and modified starches in various mixtures as sources of carbohydrate. Fat in some of these formulas contains varying amounts of medium-chain triglycerides to facilitate absorption of fat. Other polyunsaturated vegetable oils are used to supply essential fatty acids. Products differ significantly from each other; the manufacturers' Web sites should be consulted for explanations of the differences.

Other Formulas

Other special formulas are available for infants with low birth weight (see Chapter 5: Nutritional Needs of the Preterm Infant) and for infants with inborn errors of metabolism (see Chapter 30: Inborn Errors of Metabolism).

Amino Acid-Based Formulas

Amino acid-based formulas specifically designed for infants are indicated for extreme protein hypersensitivity—when symptoms persist even when extensively hydrolyzed protein formulas are used.[31,32] These formulas are more costly than cow milk protein- and soy protein-based formulas.

Follow-up Formulas

Referred to variously as "follow-up" or "follow-on formulas," these formulas are directed at infants older than 6 months who are taking solid food and, in many countries, are seen as a normal step in the progression of an infant's diet. This concept and these products have never gained the same popularity in the United States. Follow-up formulas and formulas for older babies, which are directed at children at the end of the first and into the second year of life and "sometimes referred to as growing up milks," are available in the United States in milk-based and soy-based forms. Their compositions, by convention, differ from those of standard formulas (increased protein and minerals, among other differences), but unlike other countries, the United States does not have separate regulatory requirements for their nutrient levels. They are nutritionally adequate. They offer no clear advantage over standard infant formula during the first year of life, although the iron fortification and balance of nutrients they contain may be an advantage for toddlers receiving inadequate amounts in their solid feedings.

Cow Milk

Full-fat cow milk, 1% to 2% fat cow milk, "skim" or fat-free cow milk, goat milk, evaporated milk, and other "milks" have levels of nutrients, both excesses and deficiencies, that are not well suited for meeting the infant's nutritional requirements, and they are not recommended for use during the first 12 months of life.[18] The Centers for Disease Control and Prevention previously reported that the use of cow milk during the first year of life, or an intake of more than 750 mL (approx 25 fl oz) per day in the second year of life, was associated with iron deficiency.[33] Infants fed cow milk in the first 12 months of life are at risk of depleting their iron stores and ultimately developing iron-deficiency anemia because of the low concentration and bioavailability of iron in cow milk and possible intestinal blood loss. The higher intakes of protein, sodium, potassium, and chloride associated with the use of cow milk inappropriately increase the renal solute load.[34] The limited amounts of essential fatty acids as well as vitamin E, zinc, and perhaps other micronutrients may not be adequate to prevent deficiencies. Skim milks may cause the infant to consume excessive amounts of protein, because large volumes of these hypocaloric milks will be ingested as the infant tries to satisfy his or her caloric needs.[35]

Web Links to Manufacturers for Product Composition and Other Information

Abbott Nutrition - http://abbottnutrition.com/

Earth's Best - http://www.earthsbest.com/node/12

Gerber (Nestlé) Infant Formulas - http://medical.gerber.com/products/Default.aspx

Mead Johnson Nutritionals - http://www.meadjohnson.com/Brands/Pages/Products-by-Need.aspx

Nutricia - http://www.nutricia-na.com/

Perrigo Nutritionals (many store brands) - http://www.pbmproducts.com/products.aspx

References

1. Heinig MJ, Nommsen LA, Peerson JM, Lonnerdal B, Dewey KG. Energy and protein intakes of breast-fed and formula-fed infants during the first year of life and their association with growth velocity: the DARLING Study. *Am J Clin Nutr*. 1993;58(2): 152-161

2. Siega-Riz AM, Deming DM, Reidy KC, Fox MK, Condon E, Briefel RR. Food consumption patterns of infants and toddlers: where are we now? *J Am Diet Assoc*. 2010;110(12 Suppl):S38-S51

3. Centers for Disease Control and Prevention. Breastfeeding Report Card – 2010, United States. Available at: http://www.cdc.gov/breastfeeding/pdf/ BreastfeedingReportCard2010.pdf. Accessed September 11, 2012

4. Ryan AS, Zhou W. Lower breastfeeding rates persist among the Special Supplemental Nutrition Program for Women, Infants, and Children participants, 1978-2003. *Pediatrics*. 2006;117(4):1136-1146

5. Centers for Disease Control and Prevention. Progress in increasing breastfeeding and reducing racial/ethnic differences—United States, 2000-2008 births. *MMWR Morb Mortal Wkly Rep*. 2013;62(5):77-80

6. Cone TE Jr. Infant feeding of paramount concern. In: Cone TE Jr, ed. *History of American Pediatrics*. Boston, MA: Little, Brown & Co; 1979:131-148

7. Schuman AJ. A concise history of infant formula (twists and turns included). *Contemp Pediatr*. 2003;20(2):91-103

8. European Society of Paediatric Gastroenterology, Hepatology and Nutrition, Committee on Nutrition. The nutritional and safety assessment of breast milk substitutes and other dietary products for infants: a commentary by the ESPGHAN Committee on Nutrition. *J Pediatr Gastroenterol Nutr*. 2001;32(3):256-258

9. Food and Drugs. 21 CFR 107. Available at: http://www.access.gpo.gov/nara/cfr/ waisidx_09/21cfr107_09.html. Accessed September 11, 2012

10. Codex Alimentarius Commission, 2007a. Standards for Infant Formulas and Formulas for Special Medical Purposes Intended for Infants (Codex Stan 72-1981) (Revised 2007). www.codexalimentarius.net/ownload/standards/288/CXS_072e.pdf10. Accessed May 18, 2011

11. MacLean WC Jr, Van Dael P, Clemens R, et al. Upper levels of nutrients in infant formulas: comparison of analytical data with the revised Codex infant formula standard. *J Food Comp Analysis*. 2010;23(1):44-53

12. Food and Agriculture Organization of the United Nations, World Health Organization. *Enterobacter sakazakii* and other microorganisms in powdered infant formula: meeting report. Microbiological Risk Assessment Series 10. Geneva, Switzerland: World Health Organization and Food and Agriculture Organization of the United Nations; 2004. Available at: ftp://ftp.fao.org/docrep/fao/007/y5502e/y5502e00.pdf. Accessed September 11, 2012

13. Life Sciences Research Office. *Life Sciences Research Office Report: Executive Summary for the Report: Assessment of Nutrient Requirements for Infant Formulas.* Washington, DC: Center for Food Safety and Applied Nutrition, Food and Drug Administration, Department of Health and Human Services; 1998. Available at: http://jn.nutrition.org/content/128/11/suppl/DC1. Accessed September 11, 2012

14. Scientific Committee on Food. Report on the Revision of Essential Requirements of Infant Formulae and Follow-on Formulae. SCF/CS/NUT/IF/65. Brussels, Belgium: European Commission; 2003. Available at: http://ec.europa.eu/food/fs/sc/scf/out199_en.pdf. Accessed September 11, 2012

15. Kunz C, Lonnerdal B. Re-evaluation of the whey protein/casein ratio of human milk. *Acta Paediatr.* 1992;81(2):107-112

16. Heine WE, Klein PD, Reeds PJ. The importance of alpha-lactalbumin in infant nutrition. *J Nutr.* 1991;121(2):277-283

17. American Academy of Pediatrics, Committee on Nutrition. Iron fortification of infant formulas. *Pediatrics.* 1999;104(5):119-123

18. Baker RD; Greer FR; American Academy of Pediatrics, Committee on Nutrition. Diagnosis and prevention of iron deficiency and iron-deficiency anemia in infants and young children (0–3 years of age). *Pediatrics.* 2010;126(5):1040-1050

19. Bhatia J; Greer FR; American Academy of Pediatrics, Committee on Nutrition. The use of soy protein-based formulas in infant feeding. *Pediatrics.* 2008;121(5):1062-1068

20. Thomas DW; Greer FR; American Academy of Pediatrics, Committee on Nutrition, Section on Gastroenterology, Hepatology, and Nutrition. Probiotics and prebiotics in pediatrics. *Pediatrics.* 2010;126(6):1217-1231

21. National Toxicology Program, Center for the Evaluation of Risks to Human Reproduction. NTP Brief on Soy Formula. Washington, DC: National Institute of Environmental Health Sciences, National Institutes of Health, US Department of Health and Human Services; September 2010. Available at: http://ntp.niehs.nih.gov/NTP/ohat/genistein-soy/SoyFormulaUpdt/FinalNTPBriefSoyFormula_9_20_2010.pdf. Accessed September 11, 2012

22. Lasekan JB, Ostrom KM, Jacobs JR, et al. Growth of newborn, term infants fed soy formulas for 1 year. *Clin Pediatr (Phila).* 1999;38(10):563-571

23. Mimouni F, Campaigne B, Neylan M, Tsang RC. Bone mineralization in the first year of life in infants fed human milk, cow-milk formula, or soy-based formula. *J Pediatr.* 1993;122(3):348-354

24. Hillman LS, Chow W, Salmons SS, Weaver E, Erickson M, Hansen J. Vitamin D metabolism, mineral homeostasis, and bone mineralization in term infants fed human milk, cow milk-based formula, or soy-based formula. *J Pediatr.* 1988;112(6):864-874

25. Venkataraman PS, Luhar H, Neylan MJ. Bone mineral metabolism in full-term infants fed human milk, cow milk-based, and soy-based formulas. *Am J Dis Child.* 1992;146(6):1302-1305

26. Brown KH, Peerson JM, Fontaine O. Use of nonhuman milks in the dietary management of young children with acute diarrhea: a meta-analysis of clinical trials. *Pediatrics.* 1994;93(1):17-27

27. Zeiger RS, Sampson HA, Bock SA, et al. Soy allergy in infants and children with IgE-associated cow's milk allergy. *J Pediatr.* 1999;134(5):614-622

28. Cordle CT. Soy protein allergy: incidence and relative severity. *J Nutr.* 2004;134(5):1213S-1219S

29. Greer FR; Sicherer SH; Burks AW; American Academy of Pediatrics, Committee on Nutrition, Section on Allergy and Immunology. The effects of early nutritional interventions on the development of atopic disease in infants and children: the role of maternal dietary restriction, breastfeeding, timing of introduction of complementary foods, and hydrolyzed formulas. *Pediatrics.* 2008;121(1):183-191

30. Strom BL, Schinnar R, Ziegler EE, et al. Exposure to soy-based formula in infancy and endocrinological and reproductive outcomes in young adulthood. *JAMA.* 2001;286(7):807-814

31. Sampson HA, James JM, Bernhisel-Broadbent J. Safety of an amino acid-derived infant formula in children allergic to cow milk. *Pediatrics.* 1992;90(3):463-465

32. Kelso JM, Sampson HA. Food protein-induced enterocolitis to casein hydrolysate formulas. *J Allergy Clin Immunol.* 1993;92(6):909-910

33. Centers for Disease Control and Prevention. Recommendations to prevent and control iron deficiency in the United States. *MMWR Recomm Rep.* 1998;47(RR-3):1-29

34. Ziegler EE, Fomon SJ. Potential renal solute load of infant formulas. *J Nutr.* 1989;119(12 Suppl):1785-1788

35. Ryan AS, Martinez GA, Krieger FW. Feeding low-fat milk during infancy. *Am J Phys Anthropol.* 1987;73(4):539-548

Chapter 5

Nutritional Needs of the Preterm Infant

II

Introduction

Although optimal nutrition is critical in the management of small preterm infants, no standard has been set for the precise nutritional needs of infants born prematurely. Current recommendations for parenteral (Table 5.1) and enteral (Table 5.2) nutrition are designed to provide nutrients to approximate the rate of growth and composition of weight gain for a normal fetus of the same postmenstrual age and to maintain normal concentrations of blood and tissue nutrients.[1-3] Nearly all extremely low birth weight infants (<1000 g birth weight) experience significant growth restriction during their stay in the neonatal intensive care unit (NICU), and the intrauterine growth rate is typically not obtained until well after term equivalent gestational age is achieved.[4,5] Growth restriction among preterm infants is largely attributable to the interaction of acute neonatal illnesses and nutritional practices in which inadequate parenteral and enteral support facilitate the development of energy, protein, and mineral deficits. However, the implementation of practices in which parenteral nutrition is initiated within hours of birth and enteral nutrition is initiated within several days of birth has begun to reduce the risk of extrauterine growth restriction.[6]

Table 5.1

Comparison of Parenteral Intake Recommendations for Growing Preterm Infants in Stable Clinical Condition

| | Consensus Recommendations | | | |
| | Weight <1000 g | | Weight 1000-1500 g | |
	g/kg/day	g/100 kcal	g/kg/day	g/100 kcal
Water/fluids, mL	140-180	122-171	120-160	120-178
Energy, kcal	105-115	100	90-100	100
Protein, g	3.5-4.0	3.0-3.8	3.2-3.8	3.2-4.2
Carbohydrate, g	13-17	11.3-16.2	9.7-15	9.7-16.7
Fat, g	3-4	2.6-3.8	3-4	3.0-4.4
Linoleic acid, mg	340-800	296-762	340-800	340-889
Linoleate:linolenate = C18:2/C18:3	5-15	5-15	5-15	5-15
Vitamin A, IU	700-1500	609-1429	700-1500	700-1667
Vitamin D, IU	40-160	35-152	40-160	40-178

Table 5.1 *(continued)*
Comparison of Parenteral Intake Recommendations for Growing Preterm Infants in Stable Clinical Condition

	Consensus Recommendations			
	Weight <1000 g		Weight 1000-1500 g	
	g/kg/day	g/100 kcal	g/kg/day	g/100 kcal
Vitamin E, IU	2.8-3.5	2.4-3.3	2.8-3.5	2.8-3.9
Vitamin K$_1$ µg	10	8.7-9.5	10	10.0-11.1
Ascorbate, mg	15-25	13.0-23.8	15-25	15.0-27.8
Thiamine, µg	200-350	174-333	200-350	200-389
Riboflavin, µg	150-200	130-190	150-200	150-222
Pyridoxine, µg	150-200	130-190	150-200	150-222
Niacin, mg	4-6.8	3.5-6.5	4-6.8	4.0-7.6
Pantothenate, mg	1-2	0.9-1.9	1.2	1.0-2.2
Biotin, µg	5-8	1.3-7.6	5-8	5.0-8.9
Folate, µg	56	49-53	56	56-62
Vitamin B$_{12}$, µg	0.3	0.26-0.29	0.3	0.30-0.33
Sodium, mg	69-115	60-110	69-115	69-128
Potassium, mg	78-117	68-111	78-117	78-130
Chloride, mg	107-249	93-237	107-249	107-277
Calcium, mg	60-80	52-76	60-80	60-89
Phosphorus, mg	45-60	39-57	45-60	45-67
Magnesium, mg	4.3-7.2	3.7-6.9	4.3-7.2	4.3-8.0
Iron, µg	100-200	87-190	100-200	100-222
Zinc, µg	400	348-381	400	400-444
Copper, µg	20	17-19	20	20-22
Selenium, µg	1.5-4.5	1.3-4.3	1.5-4.5	1.5-5.0
Chromium, µg	0.05-0.3	0.04-0.29	0.05-0.3	0.05-0.33
Manganese, µg	1	0.87-0.95	1	1.00-1.11
Molybdenum, µg	0.25	0.22-0.24	0.25	0.25-0.28
Iodine, µg	1	0.87-0.95	1	1.00-1.11
Taurine, mg	1.88-3.75	1.6-3.6	1.88-3.75	1.9-4.2
Carnitine, mg	≈2.9	≈2.5-2.8	≈2.9	≈2.9-3.2
Inositol, mg	54	47-51	54	54-60
Choline, mg	14.4-28	12.5-26.7	14.4-28	14.4-31.1

Table 5.2.
Comparison of Enteral Intake Recommendations for Growing Preterm Infants in Stable Clinical Condition[3]

	Consensus Recommendations			
	Weight <1000 g		Weight 1000-1500 g	
	g/kg/day	g/100 kcal	g/kg/day	g/100 kcal
Energy, kcal	130-150	100	110-130	100
Protein, g	3.8-4.4	2.5-3.4	3.4-4.2	2.6-3.8
Carbohydrate, g	9-20	6.0-15.4	7-17	5.4-15.5
Fat, g	6.2-8.4	4.1-6.5	5.3-7.2	4.1-6.5
Linoleic acid, mg	700-1680	467-1292	600-1440	462-1309
Linoleate:linolenate = C18:2/C18:3	5-15	5-15	5-15	5-15
Docosahexaenoic acid, mg	≥21	≥16	>18	≥16
Arachidonic acid, mg	≥28	≥22	≥24	≥22
Vitamin A, IU	700-1500	467-1154	700-1500	538-1364
Vitamin D, IU	150-400	100 308	150-400	115-364
Vitamin E, IU	6-12	4.0-9.2	6-12	4.6-10.9
Vitamin K_1, μg	8-10	5.3-7.7	8-10	6.2-9.1
Ascorbate, mg	18-24	12.0-18.5	18-24	13.8-21.8
Thiamine, μg	180-240	120-185	180-240	138-218
Riboflavin, μg	250-360	167-277	250-360	192-327
Pyridoxine, μg	150-210	100-162	150-210	115-191
Niacin, mg	3.6-4.8	2.4-3.7	3.6-4.8	2.8-4.4
Pantothenate, mg	1.2-1.7	0.8-1.3	1.2-1.7	0.9-1.5
Biotin, μg	3.6-6	2.4-4.6	3.6-6	2.8-5.5
Folate, μg	25-50	17-38	25-50	19-45
Vitamin B_{12}, μg	0.3	0.2-0.23	0.3	0.23-0.27
Sodium, mg	69-115	46-88	69-115	53-105
Potassium, mg	78-117	52-90	78-117	60-106
Chloride, mg	107-249	71-192	107-249	82-226
Calcium, mg	100-220	67-169	100-220	77-200
Phosphorus, mg	60-140	40-108	60-140	46-127
Magnesium, mg	7.9-15	5.3-11.5	7.9-15	6.1-13.6

II

Table 5.2. (continued)
Comparison of Enteral Intake Recommendations for Growing Preterm Infants in Stable Clinical Condition

	Consensus Recommendations			
	Weight <1000 g		Weight 1000-1500 g	
	g/kg/day	g/100 kcal	g/kg/day	g/100 kcal
Iron, mg	2-4	1.33-3.08	2-4	1.54-3.64
Zinc, µg	1000-3000	337-2308	1000-3000	769-2727
Copper, µg	120-150	80-115	120-150	92-136
Selenium, µg	1.3-4.5	0.9-3.5	1.3-4.5	1.0-4.1
Chromium, µg	0.1-2.25	0.07-1.73	0.1-2.25	0.08-2.05
Manganese, µg	0.7-7.75	0.5-5.8	0.7-7.75	0.5-6.8
Molybdenum, µg	0.3	0.20-0.23	0.3	0.23-0.27
Iodine, µg	10-60	6.7-46.2	10-60	7.7-54.5
Taurine, mg	4.5-9.0	3.0-6.9	4.5-9.0	3.5-8.2
Carnitine, mg	≈2.9	≈1.9-2.2	≈2.9	≈2.2-2.6
Inositol, mg	32-81	21-62	32-81	25-74
Choline, mg	14.4-28	9.6-21.5	14.4-28	11.1-25.2

Parenteral Nutrition

Parenteral administration of glucose, fat, and amino acids is an important aspect of the nutritional care of preterm infants, particularly those who weigh less than 1500 g (Table 5.1). Feeding intolerance is a common problem as a result of limited gastric capacity, intestinal hypomotility, and complicating illnesses in small preterm infants. These factors dictate the slow advancement of the volume of enteral feeding and delays in achieving full enteral feeding. Parenteral nutrition is, thus, an essential supplement to enteral feedings so that total daily intake by both means of support meets the infant's nutritional needs. When necessary, basic nutritional needs can be met for considerable periods by the parenteral route alone.

Parenteral nutrition for preterm infants weighing greater than 1500 g and for late preterm infants (≥34 weeks' gestation) has not been well studied, despite the needs for increased nutritional support compared with those of term infants.[7,8] Decisions to start parenteral nutrition in these infants are best made on a case-by-case basis. On the other hand, infants with intrauterine growth restriction require special nutritional considerations at any gestational age.

Fluid therapy is designed to avoid dehydration or overhydration, to provide stable electrolyte and glucose concentrations, and to avoid abnormal acid-base balance. Because insensible water losses occurring primarily through the skin vary tremendously depending on gestational age and birth weight, emphasis is placed on individualized fluid management. For preterm infants with birth weights ≥1000 g, fluid requirements approximate 60 to 80 mL/kg on the first day, increasing by 20 mL/kg/day, to a total of 120 to 140 mL/kg/day by day 4 of life. Parenteral sodium intake is restricted until the physiological postnatal loss of extracellular fluid is underway.[9] Sodium should be added after serum sodium concentration decreases below 140 mg/dL with up to 3 to 4 mEq/kg/day of sodium as an appropriate mixture of chloride and acetate to correct both sodium losses and metabolic acidosis.[9,10]

For infants weighing less than 1000 g at birth, generally higher fluid intakes are necessary in the first 5 days of life, depending on urine output and insensible water losses, which may be 5 to 7 mL/kg/hour in extreme cases.[9,11] Eventually, if total parenteral nutrition is used exclusively for nutritional support, fluid rates of up to 140 to 160 mL/kg/day will be needed for most infants to achieve a weight gain of 15 to 20 g/kg/day. The addition of 2 to 4 mEq/kg/day of sodium and chloride and 1.5 to 2 mEq/kg/day of potassium will be needed for this period of active growth.[10,11] Higher intakes of sodium and chloride may be required in extremely preterm infants with the inability to conserve sodium and prevent the high urinary excretion of electrolytes.

Protein

Glucose infusions without amino acids increases the loss of body protein in preterm infants, because they require a minimum of 1.2 g/kg/day of amino acids to match protein breakdown and urinary losses.[12-15] Very low birth weight (VLBW) infants should be provided a minimum of 2 to 3 g/kg/day of amino acids within the first few hours of life to preserve body protein stores and maximize plasma concentrations.[16] This can be achieved through the provision of intravenous amino acids using preprepared (stock) amino acid solutions (2%-4%) before full parenteral nutrition is instituted.[12-17] Studies have documented no significant increases in metabolic acidosis, blood urea nitrogen concentration, or serum ammonia concentration with early amino acid administration.[18,19]

Positive nitrogen balance and an anabolic state can occur with parenteral lipid and glucose energy intakes of 60 kcal/kg/day and amino acid intakes of 2.5 to 3.0 g/kg/day.[20] With nonprotein energy intakes of 80 to 85 kcal/kg per day and amino acid intakes of 2.7 to 4 g/kg per day, nitrogen retention may occur at the fetal rate.[21,22] Growth generally requires a minimum parenteral nonprotein energy intake of 70 kcal/kg/day.

Glucose

Use of glucose as the sole nonprotein energy source presents several problems. Concentrations of glucose higher than 12.5 g/dL cause local irritation of peripheral veins. In addition, VLBW preterm infants with ongoing gluconeogenesis despite glucose intake develop hyperglycemia (serum glucose concentration >150 mg/dL), occurring frequently when glucose infusion rates exceed 6 mg/kg/minute.[23] To avoid the potentially adverse effects of widely varying serum osmolality and a potential osmotic diuresis from glycosuria, glucose infusion rates should start at less than 6 mg/kg/minute (8.6 g/kg/day). Usually, a steady increase of the glucose infusion rate stimulates endogenous insulin secretion, and an infusion rate of 11 to 12 mg/kg/minute (130–140 mL/kg/day of a 13-g/dL solution) is tolerated after 5 to 7 days of parenteral nutrition. In addition, early initiation and advancement of protein infusions has resulted in less hyperglycemia and hyperkalemia.[24] In the past, intravenous insulin has been administered to increase glucose tolerance and improve energy uptake, but this should be avoided because of issues with adherence to intravenous tubing resulting in fluctuations in insulin delivery and serum glucose concentrations, which have resulted in higher complications and mortality rates.[25-29]

Intravenous Lipids

The availability of intravenous lipid preparations has allowed the provision of a dense energy source adequate for growth via peripheral veins. These lipids have a high concentration of calories (2 kcal/mL in the 20% preparation) but have the same osmolality as plasma and, thus, do not irritate the veins. Lipid tolerance is optimal with a 20% phospholipid preparation and is preferred in neonates.[30] A minimum provision of 0.5 g/kg/day protects against essential fatty acid deficiency.[31] The tolerance for parenteral lipid is less in newborn infants than in older children and is even further decreased in the smallest preterm infants.[32,33] In addition, infants with restricted intrauterine growth have less parenteral fat tolerance than would be predicted from their gestational ages. Unlike amino acid delivery, the benefits of very early lipid administration are less clear, but lipid should be administered continuously over 24 hours/day at an initial dose of 1.0 to 2.0 g/kg/day. This should be increased to a maximum of 3.0 g/kg/day during the first few days of life. Fat tolerance can be assessed indirectly by measuring serum triglyceride concentrations, which should be kept less than 200 mg/dL by convention. Lipid intake should usually provide 25% to 40% of nonprotein calories in fully parenterally fed patients.[34]

Carnitine is an important amino acid that assists in the metabolism of fat. Blood and tissue carnitine concentrations are low in preterm infants.[35] Intravenous carnitine may enhance the preterm infant's ability to use exogenous fat for energy, although clinical studies are contradictory in demonstrating metabolic or physiologic benefit in preterm infants following addition of carnitine to parenteral nutrition solutions.[36,37] If carnitine is added to parenteral solutions, it should be provided up to 10 mg/kg/day.

Intravenous lipids increase serum free fatty acid concentrations that can displace bilirubin from albumin binding sites. However, studies have demonstrated that if parenteral lipids are provided up to 3 to 3.5 g/kg/day continuously over a 24-hour period, free bilirubin is unaffected, and intravenous lipids do not need to be discontinued in jaundiced infants.[30,38]

The primary soybean sources of intravenous lipid emulsions that are currently approved in the United States (Intralipid [Sigma Aldrich, St Louis, MO] or Liposyn [Hospira, Lake Forest, IL]) have been considered not well suited for prolonged (>2 weeks) parenteral nutrition administration as they may hasten the development of cholestasis and liver dysfunction.[39,40] Alternative lipid emulsions are not yet available in North America. Cycling of lipids alone has not been shown to reduce parenteral nutrition-associated liver disease, although for those that are already cholestatic, decreasing the rate of lipid infusion to as low as 1 mg/kg/day may impede the progression of cholestasis.[40] Another consideration is that lipids are a source of oxidants that may stimulate inflammation.[41] The clinical implications of the oxidative products generated when lipids or multivitamins are exposed to light are not well understood. All-in-one parenteral nutrition solutions are used for providing single solution administration, but the addition of vitamins and trace elements may increase oxidation in the presence of light.[42] Iron, in particular, should not be added to the admixture. Light protection of parenteral nutrition solutions is not currently recommended but has been promoted by some investigators.[42]

Calcium, Phosphorus, and Trace Minerals

Levels of fetal calcium and phosphorus accretion cannot generally be met with parenteral nutrition, but severe metabolic bone disease in preterm infants can be minimized by adding calcium and phosphorous to parenteral amino acid solutions containing at least 2.5 g/dL amino acids and by administering calcium- and phosphorous-containing solution at 120 to 150 mL/kg per day.[43] Each institution should establish calcium and phosphorous solubility curves for their parenteral nutrition solutions. The provision of calcium and phosphorus intravenously is optimized by the addition of cysteine to amino acid mixtures, because cysteine lowers the pH, permitting a higher amount of calcium and phosphorus to solubilize in the parenteral nutrition solution. Additional strategies to maximize mineral delivery include the use of calcium glycerophosphate in parenteral solutions, but this remains unavailable in North America.[44] Goals for calcium intake are 60 to 80 mg/kg/day, and goals for phosphorous intake are 39 to 67 mg/kg/day.[43]

When parenteral nutrition supplements enteral feedings or is limited to 1 to 2 weeks, zinc is the only trace mineral that needs to be added. If total parenteral nutrition is required for a longer period, the other trace minerals may be added; however, manganese should be omitted in patients with cholestatic jaundice, and selenium and chromium should be omitted in patients with renal dysfunction.[45] Removal of copper will depend on copper concentrations, because copper is necessary for antioxidant synthesis and is variably accumulated in the presence of cholestasis secondary to prolonged parenteral nutrition therapy.[46]

Multivitamins

Several parenteral vitamin solutions are available for use in preterm infants in the United States. The recommended daily dose of parenteral vitamins for preterm infants is 40% of the currently available reconstituted single dose (5 mL) of the multivitamin mixture (Table 5.3).[47,48] Vitamin mixtures given at this dosage provide the recommended amounts of vitamins E and K, low levels of vitamin A and D, and excess levels of most B vitamins. However, a more appropriate mixture is not available, and individual vitamins are not available for parenteral use. A practical problem in providing fat-soluble vitamins parenterally is adherence to the plastic tubing in intravenous administration sets, especially for vitamin A. This can be overcome, in part, by administering the multivitamin mixture in the lipid emulsion used for parenteral nutrition.[49] However, the addition of multivitamin to lipid solutions is associated with lipid peroxidation, particularly when combined with ambient light exposure.[42]

Parenteral to Enteral Transition

The transition from parenteral nutrition to complete enteral nutrition is a critical period when total nutrient requirements may fluctuate as parenteral nutrition is weaned and enteral intake is insufficient. Care must be taken in calculating concentrations of each nutrient in parenteral nutrition to minimize avoidable reductions in nutrient delivery during this period. This is particularly important for protein. For most infants, parenteral nutrition can generally be discontinued when enteral feeds are at least 120 mL/kg/day, because basic fluid requirements will be met.

Enteral Feeding

The quality of postnatal growth depends on the type, quantity, and quality of feedings consumed. Preterm infants fed standard infant formulas gain a higher percentage of their weight as fat when compared with a fetus of the same maturity.[50] The use of specially formulated preterm infant formulas and preterm human milk fortifiers results in a composition of weight gain and bone mineralization closer to that of the reference fetus, as compared with infants fed standard formulas for term infants or unfortified human milk.

Table 5.3.
Vitamins Provided with PN Solutions[a]

Vitamin	Amount Provided Per 5 mL
Ascorbic acid (vitamin C)	80 mg
Vitamin A (retinol)[b]	2300 USP units
Vitamin D[b]	400 USP units
Thiamine (vitamin B$_1$) (as the hydrochloride)	1.20 mg
Riboflavin (vitamin B$_2$) (as riboflavin-5-phosphate sodium)	1.4 mg
Pyridoxine (vitamin B$_6$) (as the hydrochloride)	1.0 mg
Niacinamide	17.0 mg
Dexpanthenol (pantothenyl alcohol)	5 mg
Vitamin E (d-α-tocopheryl acetate)	7.0 USP units
Biotin	20 μg
Folic acid	140 μg
Vitamin B$_{12}$ (cyanocobalamine)	1.0 μg
Vitamin K$_1$ (phylloquinone)[b]	200 μg

[a] MVI Pediatric is a lyophilized, sterile powder intended for reconstitution and dilution in intravenous infusions. INFUVITE Pediatric is provided as a 4-mL and 1-mL vial that can be combined for administration. For each vitamin mixture, 5 mL of reconstituted product provides the indicated amounts of the vitamins. The recommended dose is 40% (2 mL) of the currently available reconstituted single dose (5 mL) of the MVI mixture.

[b] Fat-soluble vitamins solubilized with polysorbate 80.

Randomized prospective trials of specially formulated formulas for preterm infants have shown significant improvements in growth and cognitive development compared with standard formulas for term infants.[51] These findings underscore the need for the health care professional to carefully plan and monitor the nutritional care of preterm infants during hospitalization and after discharge, especially for the preterm infant maintained on unfortified human milk after discharge.

A consensus recommendation of nutrition experts on specific nutrient requirements in preterm infants summarizes available data and recommendations and should be referred to for more detailed information.[3]

General Energy Requirements

Energy is required for body maintenance and growth. VLBW infants are particularly sensitive to energy fluctuations because of their exceptionally high growth demands. The estimated resting metabolic rate of preterm infants, with minimal physical activity, is lower during the first week after birth. In a thermoneutral environment, the resting metabolic rate is approximately 40 kcal/kg/day when the infant is parenterally fed and 50 kcal/kg/day by 2 to 3 weeks of age when the infant is fed orally.[52] By 6 weeks, most preterm infants have a baseline energy expenditure of 80 kcal/kg/day.[53] Each gram of weight gain, including the stored energy and the energy cost of synthesis, requires between 3 and 4.5 kcal.[52] Thus, a daily weight gain of 15 g/kg requires a caloric expenditure of 45 to 67 kcal/kg above the 50 kcal/kg/day for the resting metabolic rate. Estimated average energy requirements of preterm infants during the neonatal period are shown in Table 5.4.[54] It must be noted, however, that these energy requirements have largely been determined in healthy growing preterm infants at 3 to 4 weeks of age.

Table 5.4.
Estimation of the Energy Requirement of the Low-Birth-Weight Infant[a]

	Average Estimation, kcal/kg per day
Energy expended	40-60
Resting metabolic rate	40-50[b]
Activity	0-5[b]
Thermoregulation	0-5[b]
Synthesis	15[c]
Energy stored	20-30[c]
Energy excreted	15
Energy intake	90-120

[a] Adapted from the Committee on Nutrition of the Preterm Infant, European Society of Paediatric Gastroenterology and Nutrition.[9]

[b] Energy for maintenance.

[c] Energy cost of growth.

The energy needs for activity, basal energy expenditure at thermoneutrality, nutrient absorption, and new tissue synthesis (growth) vary among infants. These variations may be more pronounced in growth-restricted or small-for-gestational-age infants. In practice, energy intake by the enteral route of 105 to 130 kcal/kg/day enables most preterm infants to achieve satisfactory rates of growth. More calories may be given if growth is unsatisfactory at these intakes, particularly with the increased energy requirements of chronic lung disease.

Protein

Enteral protein intakes between 3.0 and 4.0 g/kg per day are adequate and non-toxic. The estimated requirements on the basis of the fetal accretion rate of protein are 3.5 to 4 g/kg per day, with higher protein intakes correlating with lower gestational ages. One study suggests that in very low birth weight infants, a higher protein content of 3.6 g/100 kcal versus a standard 3.0 g/100 kcal formula results in increased protein accretion and weight gain without evidence of metabolic stress.[55] This finding was supported by a Cochrane review.[56]

The type and quantity of protein in infant formulas most suitable for preterm infants has been examined in multiple studies.[57] In general, term infants fed whey-predominant formulas had metabolic indices and plasma amino acid concentrations closer to those of infants fed pooled, mature human milk. Partially hydrolyzed formula versus intact bovine formula use in term infants have been shown to reduce the incidence of atopic dermatitis.[58] However, no data are available for preterm infants. Soy-based formulas, as presently constituted, are not recommended for preterm infants, because optimal carbohydrate, protein, and mineral absorption and utilization are not well documented for soy-based formulas.[59]

Fat

Fat provides a major source of energy for growing preterm infants. In human milk, approximately 50% of the energy is from fat; in commercial formulas, fat provides 40% to 50% of the energy. These feedings provide 5 to 7 g/kg of fat per day. The saturated fat of human milk is well absorbed by the preterm infant, in part because of the distribution pattern of fatty acids on the triglyceride molecule. Palmitic acid is present in the beta position in human milk fat and is more easily absorbed than palmitic acid in the alpha position, which occurs in cow milk, most other animal fats, and vegetable oils. Gastric lipase, pancreatic lipase-related protein 2, and bile salt-stimulated lipase facilitate the digestion of triglycerides into fatty acids and glycerol digestion in the gastrointestinal tract.[60] These lipase activities substitute for the low pancreatic lipase of preterm infants and low intraluminal bile salt concentration of preterm infants. In formula-fed preterm infants, fat absorption is increased when human milk is mixed with the formula, presumably because of the lipases in human milk.[61] Human milk, therefore, has decided advantages to formula in digestibility of fats.

Preterm infant formulas contain a mixture of medium-chain triglycerides (MCTs) and vegetable oils rich in polyunsaturated, long-chain triglycerides, both of which are well absorbed by preterm infants.[3,57] This fat blend meets the estimated essential fatty acid requirement of at least 3% of energy in the form of linoleic acid with additional small amounts of alpha-linolenic acid. Formulas designed for preterm infants contain a much higher amount of MCTs than does human milk, with no observed differences in weight gain or fat deposition.[62]

Human milk contains small amounts of the fatty acids docosahexaenoic acid (DHA) and arachidonic acid (ARA). Although endogenous synthesis of these fatty acids is observed from stable isotope studies in both term and preterm infants, demonstrating their capacity to synthesize DHA and ARA, it is not sufficient in the preterm infant.[63,64] Preterm infants fed formula void of DHA or ARA show decreasing concentrations of these lipids in their tissue compared with those that are supplemented or fed human milk. Relatively short-term visual and cognitive improvements were observed with formula supplemented with DHA and ARA to concentrations similar to human milk.[65,66] Because DHA concentrations in human milk vary tremendously on the basis of maternal diet, additional DHA supplementation with fish oil may provide further neurodevelopmental benefits in the long-term to the preterm infant fed human milk, although this is not recommended, because additional studies with longer-term follow-up are needed.[67]

Carbohydrates

Carbohydrates contribute a readily usable energy source and protect against tissue catabolism. Once the infant's condition is stabilized, the requirement for carbo-hydrate is estimated at 40% to 50% of calories, or approximately 10 to 14 g/kg per day. By 34 weeks' postconceptional age, preterm infants have intestinal lactase activities that are only 30% of term infants.[68] However, in clinical settings, lactose intolerance is rarely a problem with formula and human milk, which may be attributable to the fact that preterm infants acquire a relatively efficient capacity to hydrolyze lactose in the small intestine at an earlier developmental stage than do infants in utero.[69] Glycosidase enzymes for glucose polymers are active in small preterm infants, and these polymers are well tolerated by preterm infants. Because glucose polymers add fewer osmotic particles to the formula per unit weight than does lactose, they permit the use of a high-carbohydrate formula with an osmolal-ity below 300 mOsm/kg of water. Lactose enhances calcium absorption. Formulas designed for preterm infants contain approximately 40% to 50% lactose and 50% to 60% glucose polymers, a ratio that does not impair mineral absorption.[70]

Oligosaccharides (Prebiotics)

Human milk oligosaccharides protect the infant by stimulating the growth of components of a healthy microflora (such as bifidobacteria and lactobacilli) in the colon.[71-73] Oligosaccharides are carbohydrate substances that are composed of between 3 and 10 monosaccharide units. The concentration of oligosaccharides in human milk varies from 20 g/L in colostrum to 5 to 14 g/L in mature human milk.[74] Oligosaccharides are the third-most abundant component of human milk, following lactose and lipids. Oligosaccharides are only partially digested in the small intestine; therefore, they reach the colon, where they are able to selectively stimulate the growth and development of probiotic flora.[75] Approximately 90% of oligosaccharides are found in the infant's feces, acting as dietary fibers.[76] Oligosaccharides are determined genetically but the biochemistry is still very poorly understood. Over 200 different oligosaccharides have been identified in human milk. The structural diversity and abundance of oligosaccharides in human milk distinguishes human milk from cow milk-based infant formulas, as there are only trace amounts of oligosaccharides present in mature cow milk.[75-77] Although there is no natural alternative to the oligosaccharides found in human milk, there is insufficient evidence to add oligosaccharides to formulas for preterm infants. Current efforts to synthesize oligosaccharides found in human milk may enable future studies in this area. Some formulas for term infants are supplemented with oligosaccharides not generally found in human milk, including galacto- and fructo-oligosaccharides.[75]

Minerals

Sodium, Potassium, and Chloride

Preterm infants, particularly VLBW infants, have high fractional excretion rates of sodium for at least the first 10 to 14 days after birth, although urinary loss of sodium is also related to total fluid intake. The low sodium concentrations of human milk, formulas for term infants, or human milk fortifiers designed for the feeding of preterm infants, may lead to hyponatremia. Special formulas for preterm infants provide 1.7 to 2.2 mEq/kg per day of sodium at full feeding levels (Appendix D).[11] During the stable and growing period, sodium requirements are usually met with a daily intake of 2 to 3 mEq/kg per day. The potassium requirement of preterm infants seems to be similar to that of term infants, 2 to 3 mEq/kg per day.

Calcium, Phosphorus, and Magnesium

During the last trimester of pregnancy, the human fetus accrues approximately 80% of the calcium, phosphorus, and magnesium present at term. To achieve similar rates of accretion for normal growth and bone mineralization, small preterm infants require higher intakes of these minerals per kilogram of body weight than do term infants.[43,78] Current recommendations (Tables 5.1 and 5.2) reflect the high daily intake requirements for these minerals. However, providing adequate amounts of these nutrients, particularly calcium and phosphorus, to VLBW infants during the first few weeks of life is not always possible. As a result, osteopenia is common in these infants, and fractures develop in some. The American Academy of Pediatrics (AAP) has recently made recommendations to maximize calcium, phosphorus, and vitamin D intakes in enterally fed preterm infants to prevent osteopenia.[79]

Cow milk-based formulas used for term infants contain 53 to 76 mg of calcium per 100 kcal and 42 to 57 mg of phosphorus per 100 kcal. Bone mineral content (BMC) in preterm infants consuming these formulas, as determined by photon absorptiometry, is less than normal fetal values.[79] However, the use of formulas specially designed for preterm infants (Appendix D) that contain 165 to 180 mg of calcium per 100 kcal and 82 to 100 mg of phosphorus per 100 kcal may improve the mineral balance and BMC to levels similar to fetal values.[80,81] Preterm human milk contains approximately 40 mg of calcium per 100 kcal and 20 mg of phosphorus per 100 kcal. It has been associated with impaired bone mineralization and rickets. The addition of powdered or liquid human milk fortifiers has improved mineral balance and bone mineralization.[81-83]

Iron

Most of the iron accumulation in the human fetus also occurs during the last trimester of pregnancy. On a weight basis, the iron content of preterm infants at birth is lower than the iron content of term infants (75 mg/kg).[84] Most of the iron is in the circulating hemoglobin, and the frequent blood sampling that occurs with some preterm infants further depletes the amount of iron available for erythropoiesis. However, blood transfusions with packed red blood cells supply 1 mg/mL of elemental iron, and these transfusions may be given frequently to VLBW infants.

During the first 2 weeks of life, no clear indication exists for iron supplementation, as the early physiologic anemia of prematurity is not ameliorated by iron therapy. However, after 2 weeks of age, 2 to 4 mg/kg day of iron should be provided to growing preterm infants.[84] Preterm infants on iron fortified formulas for preterm infants do not need additional iron. However, all preterm infants (even those who are breastfed) should receive at least 2 mg/kg/day of iron until 12 months of age. There is no role for the use of low-iron formulas in these infants. Iron-fortified formulas can be used from the first feeding in formula-fed preterm infants.

Many controversial questions remain regarding the practice of neonatal red blood cell transfusions versus the use of recombinant human erythropoietin in the treatment of the anemia of prematurity.[85] On the basis of a large number of clinical trials and a meta-analysis of these trials, it is impossible to clearly recommend one treatment strategy over the other. Clearly, recombinant human erythropoietin has efficacy in stimulating erythropoiesis in preterm infants, but success in the elimination or marked reduction in the need for red blood cell transfusions has not been definitively demonstrated, especially if care is taken to minimize the number of blood draws for laboratory testing.[86] Thus, the use of recombinant erythropoietin to prevent or treat anemia of prematurity is probably not indicated in most preterm infants, including the smallest preterm infants (birth weight <1000 g).[87,88] If erythropoietin is used, iron supplementation up to 6 mg/kg/day is needed, because active erythropoiesis requires additional iron as a substrate.[89]

Trace Minerals

Zinc (Zn)

During the last trimester of pregnancy, the estimated fetal accretion rate for zinc is 850 μg/day.[90] Although the zinc concentration of colostrum is high, its concentration in human milk rapidly declines to concentrations of 2.5 mg/L by 1 month and 1.1 mg/L by 3 months postpartum. These concentrations of zinc are inadequate to meet the requirements of the stable growing preterm infant, as demonstrated by reports of clinical zinc deficiency among human milk-fed preterm infants.[91] Current enteral recommendations for zinc are 1 to 3 mg/kg/day (Table 5.2). Currently marketed formulas for preterm and term infants as well as human milk fortifiers provide sufficient zinc to meet these recommendations (see Appendix D).

Copper (Cu)

Copper retention by the fetus has been estimated to be 56 μg/kg per day. Human milk from mothers of preterm infants contains 58 to 72 μg/dL during the first month after birth. Preterm infants absorb copper at rates of 57% from fortified human milk to 27% from standard cow milk-based formula.[92] Copper absorption is affected by the concentration of dietary zinc. Copper deficiency has been identified among infants primarily fed cow milk or given prolonged copper-free parenteral nutrition. The recommended daily intake (Table 5.2) can be met by using human milk or preterm infant formula.[45]

Iodine (I)

The iodine content of human milk varies depending on the mother's intake, which is related to the geographic location of her food sources. Transient hypothyroidism has been reported among preterm infants receiving 10 to 30 μg/kg per day of iodine, though the recommended iodine intake is 10 to 60 μg/kg/day.[45,93] All formulas for preterm infants will supply this amount. Currently available powdered human milk fortifiers do not contain added iodine. Human milk may not supply enough iodine by itself if the preterm infant is maintained for extended periods on human milk, although the needs for supplementation in this population have not been definitely established.

Other trace elements

Deficiency of selenium, chromium, molybdenum, or manganese has not been reported for healthy preterm infants fed human milk.[45] Current minimum recommendations for these microminerals are based on the concentration in human milk. (see Table 5.2 and Chapter 3).

Water-Soluble Vitamins

The recommended intake of water-soluble vitamins is based on the estimated amount provided by human milk and current feeding regimens, an understanding of their physiologic functions and excretion, stability during storage, and a very limited amount of research data on the water-soluble vitamin needs of preterm infants (Table 5.2).[48] As a group, the body's reserves of water-soluble vitamins are limited, and a continuing supply of these nutrients is essential for normal metabolism. The higher recommended intakes for preterm infants compared with those for term infants is based on their higher protein requirements and reduced vitamin reserves associated with shortened gestation. The recommended enteral intakes of water-soluble vitamins for preterm infants fed human milk may be achieved by using a vitamin-containing human milk fortifier. Relatively few of these vitamins are provided by standard, oral multivitamin supplements. In formula-fed preterm infants, recommendations may be met by feeding formulas designed for preterm infants that contain higher levels of water-soluble vitamins than standard formulas for term infants. There are no guidelines for supplementing preterm infants with water-soluble vitamins after hospital discharge, and no published studies are available.

The ascorbic acid (vitamin C) content of human milk is approximately 8 mg/100 kcal, and that of formulas for preterm infants ranges from 20 to 40 mg/100 kcal. Although no reports of deficiency among preterm infants receiving these feedings have occurred, no published studies have assessed the ascorbic acid status of enterally fed preterm infants. Because ascorbic acid is essential for the metabolism of several amino acids, its requirement may be increased because of the high level of protein metabolism in the growing preterm infant. Enteral supplementation of ascorbic acid has not shown net benefit for any neonatal morbidity, including bronchopulmonary dysplasia.[94] Loss of ascorbic acid can occur during handling and storage of human milk, but ascorbic acid supplementation of human milk with a human milk fortifier or multivitamins can offset this. Current guidelines for ascorbic acid intake are 18 to 24 mg/kg/day[48] (Table 5.2).

Thiamine (vitamin B_1) is a cofactor for 3 enzyme complexes required for carbohydrate metabolism as well as for the decarboxylation of branched-chain amino acids. The thiamine content of human milk is 29 μg/100 kcal, and thiamine content of formulas for preterm infants is 200 to 250 μg/100 kcal (Appendix D). Commercially available human milk fortifiers provide an equivalent amount of thiamine when used to fortify human milk to 24 kcal/oz. Recommendations for thiamine intake range from 180 to 240 μg/kg/day.[48]

Riboflavin (vitamin B_2) is a primary component of flavoproteins that serve as hydrogen carriers in numerous oxidation-reduction reactions. Infants with a negative nitrogen balance may have increased urinary losses of riboflavin, and those requiring phototherapy may use their reserves of riboflavin in the photocatabolism of bilirubin. The riboflavin content is 49 μg/100 kcal in human milk and 150 to 620 μg/100 kcal in formulas for preterm infants (Appendix D). Commercially available human milk fortifiers provide 250 to 500 μg/100 kcal when used to fortify human milk to 24 kcal/oz. Because of the photosensitivity of riboflavin, its content in human milk decreases during storage and handling. Guidelines for riboflavin intake range from 250 to 360 μg/kg/day.[48] The higher intake allows for increased losses of riboflavin associated with medical problems commonly found among preterm infants.

Pyridoxine (vitamin B_6) is a cofactor for numerous reactions involved in amino acid synthesis and catabolism. The requirement for pyridoxine is directly related to protein intake. The pyridoxine content of human milk is 28 μg/100 kcal, and pyridoxine content of formula for preterm infants is 150 to 250 μg/100 kcal (Appendix D). Human milk fortifiers contain the equivalent amount when used as directed. Current recommendations for pyridoxine intake range from 150 to 210 μg/kg/day.[48]

Niacin (vitamin B_3) is a primary component of cofactors that function in numerous oxidation-reduction reactions, including glycolysis, electron transport, and fatty acid synthesis. Human milk contains 210 μg of niacin/100 kcal, and formulas for preterm infants contain 3900 to 5000 μg of niacin/100 kcal (Appendix D). Human milk fortifiers contain the equivalent amount when used as directed. No cases of niacin deficiency have been reported among healthy preterm infants using current feeding regimens; however, no studies of niacin status among enterally fed infants are available. Recommended intake ranges from 3.6 to 4.8 mg/kg/day.[48]

Biotin is a cofactor for 4 carboxylation reactions and is active in folate metabolism. The only reports of biotin deficiency have occurred among infants supported on biotin-free parenteral nutrition for several weeks.[95] The biotin content of human milk is 0.56 μg/100 kcal, and the content of formulas for preterm infants is 3.9 to 37 μg/100 kcal (Appendix D). Powdered human milk fortifiers contain the equivalent amount when used as directed. The recommended daily intake ranges from 3.6 to 6 μg/kg/day.[48]

Pantothenic acid (vitamin B_5) is a component of the acyl transfer group coenzyme A that is essential for fat, carbohydrate, and protein metabolism. Human milk provides 250 μg of pantothenic acid/100 kcal, and formulas for preterm infants contain from 1200 to 1900 μg of pantothenic acid/100 kcal (Appendix D), which will easily provide the recommended daily intake of 1.2 to 1.7 mg/kg/day.[48] Powdered human milk fortifiers contain the equivalent amount when used as directed.

Folic acid (vitamin B_9) is a cofactor that serves as an acceptor and donor of one-carbon units in amino acid and nucleotide metabolism. Deficiency alters cell division, particularly in tissues with rapid cell turnover, such as the intestine and bone marrow. Preterm infants are at increased risk of folate deficiency because of limited hepatic stores and rapid postnatal growth. Studies of preterm infants have shown improved folate status, assessed by red blood cell folate concentrations, among those provided supplemental folic acid.[96,97] On the basis of these studies, recommendations for folic acid intake range from 25 to 50 µg/kg.[48] Human milk provides approximately 7 µg/100 kcal of folic acid. Formulas for preterm infants contain 20 to 37 µg folic acid/100 kcal (Appendix D). Powdered human milk fortifiers will supply up to 30 µg folic acid/100 kcal when used as directed.

Vitamin B_{12} (cobalamine) is a cofactor involved in the synthesis of DNA and the transfer of methyl groups. Clinical symptoms of deficiency have been reported among infants who were exclusively breastfed by vegetarian mothers.[98] Deficiency has not been reported among term or preterm infants born to well-nourished mothers. Vitamin B_{12} is well absorbed from human milk and infant formula. Human milk provides 0.07 µg of vitamin B_{12}/100 kcal and preterm infant formulas provide 0.25 to 0.55 µg of vitamin B_{12}/100 kcal (Appendix D). Powdered human milk fortifiers will provide 0.22 to 0.79 µg of vitamin B_{12}/100 kcal when used as directed. The recommended intake is 0.3 µg/kg/day.[48]

Fat-Soluble Vitamins

Fat-soluble vitamins are provided in both parenteral and enteral nutrition to the preterm infant. There is little information regarding supplementation of fat-soluble vitamins after hospital discharge. For infants fed human milk, supplements of A, D, and E are readily available as oral solutions. None of these contain vitamin K. Supplementing formula-fed infants is more problematic, but in general, if preterm infants are discharged on standard term infant formulas, they may not receive the recommended amounts of these vitamins, as discussed previously, until they reach a weight of 3 kg. Thus in the "healthy" preterm infant, it is probably not necessary to supplement with fat-soluble vitamins after attaining a weight of 3 kg, except for vitamin D. On the other hand, formulas designed for preterm infants postdischarge from the NICU should supply adequate amounts of fat-soluble vitamins (Appendix D).

Vitamin A is a fat-soluble vitamin that promotes normal growth and differentiation of epithelial tissues. The liver is the primary storage site for vitamin A. At birth, the hepatic vitamin A content of preterm infants is low.[99] Measured concentrations have indicated limited reserves and, in some cases, depletion. In addition, the plasma retinol, retinol binding protein (RBP), and retinol-to-RBP molar ratios of preterm infants are less than those of infants born at term.[100] The low vitamin

A reserves in conjunction with impaired absorption, attributable to reduced hydrolysis of fats and low levels of intestinal carrier proteins for retinol, place the preterm infant at risk of vitamin A deficiency. The preterm infant's vitamin A status may affect the maintenance and development of pulmonary epithelial tissue. The recommendations for vitamin A intake range from 700 to 1500 IU/kg/day.[47] Supplementation of preterm infants with 1500 IU/kg/day results in normalization of serum retinol and RBP concentrations.[101] Given their high vitamin A content (10 150 IU/L [1250 IU/100 kcal], Appendix D), special formulas for preterm infants will supply this amount. Human milk, with a vitamin A concentration of 2230 IU/L (338 IU/100 kcal), will not supply the recommended intake. Human milk fortifiers, when used as directed, will provide an additional 6200 to 9500 IU/L. Several studies have indicated that normal vitamin A status reduces the incidence and severity of lung disease in the preterm infant.[102] The largest study to date demonstrated a reduction in bronchopulmonary dysplasia, defined as the need for oxygen treatment among survivors at 36 weeks' postmenstrual age.[103] Although additional supplementation may be beneficial for preterm infants at risk of lung disease, clinicians must weigh the modest benefits against necessity for repeated intramuscular injections.[102] Postdischarge blood concentrations of vitamin A in preterm infants do not reach those of term infants and may not be sufficient with current supplemental approaches using supplemental vitamins.[104]

Vitamin E is an antioxidant that actively inhibits fatty acid peroxidation in cell membranes. The vitamin E requirement increases with the amount of polyunsaturated fatty acids (PUFAs) in the diet. Vitamin E deficiency-induced hemolytic anemia has been reported among preterm infants.[105,106] This syndrome has been associated with the use of formulas that contain high amounts of PUFAs with inadequate vitamin E while providing supplemental iron, which functions as an oxidant.[107,108] Current formulas have been designed to provide a ratio of vitamin E to PUFAs that prevents this problem. The enteral intake should provide a minimum of 0.7 IU of vitamin E/100 kcal and at least 1 IU/g of linoleic acid. Pharmacologic doses of vitamin E for the prevention or treatment of retinopathy of prematurity, bronchopulmonary dysplasia, and intraventricular hemorrhage are not recommended.[109] There is a general consensus in the United States that the VLBW infant should receive 6 to 12 IU/kg/day enterally (Table 5.2).[47] Preterm infant formulas supply 4 to 6 IU of vitamin E/100 kcal/day. Because the vitamin E content of mature human milk is quite variable and generally low, powdered human milk fortifiers supply the equivalent amount per 100 kcal/day.

Vitamin D is a pluripotent steroid hormone that, in addition to having a pivotal role in maintaining bone health, may be increasingly important in numerous health conditions.[110] Most tissues and cells in the body have a vitamin D receptor.

Vitamin D has been associated with improved cardiovascular health, stimulation of the immune system, and cancer prevention as well as prevention of other chronic diseases. Vitamin D deficiency can cause growth restriction and skeletal deformities and increases the risk of hip fracture later in life. Maternal vitamin D status is highly variable, and many mothers may be silently insufficient or deficient in vitamin D stores and, therefore, may put their fetus at risk of having low vitamin D concentrations.[111]

Osteopenia of prematurity is primarily caused by insufficient calcium and phosphorus intake, but low vitamin D status may contribute as well.[112] The importance of exercise in improving bone mineral density remains controversial in preterm infants.[113] The recommended enteral intake of vitamin D is between 150 and 400 IU/kg/day (Table 5.2).[43,114] Preterm infants with birth weight <1250 g and gestational age <32 weeks who receive a high mineral-containing cow milk-based formula and a daily vitamin D intake of approximately 400 IU maintain normal serum 25-hydroxyvitamin D and appropriately elevated 1,25-dihydroxyvitamin D for many months,[115] although 200 IU per day is acceptable.[114] There is no compelling evidence to give the preterm infant any more than 400 IU/day of vitamin D, and the AAP recommends an enteral intake of 200-400 IU/day of vitamin D for preterm infants.[79] Both the AAP and the Institute of Medicine have also determined an adequate intake of 400 IU for healthy term infants 0 to 6 months of age.[116,117] Current liquid and powdered human milk fortifiers and special formulas for preterm infants supply between 200 and 400 IU per day when fed in the usual amounts; thus, additional vitamin D supplements may be needed for these infants.

Vitamin K is poorly stored, and therefore, daily intake is important. Hemorrhagic disease of the newborn infant, most commonly seen in exclusively breastfed infants, results from vitamin K deficiency.[118] As a preventive measure, an intramuscular injection of vitamin K is routinely provided after birth. In preterm infants who weigh more than 1 kg at birth, the standard prophylactic dose of 1 mg of phylloquinone is appropriate. For infants weighing less than 1 kg, a dose of 0.3 mg/kg of phylloquinone is recommended. Formulas for preterm infants provide sufficient vitamin K to meet daily needs thereafter. Human milk has a low vitamin K content. The use of human milk fortifiers that contain supplemental vitamins will provide the additional vitamin K needed to meet the recommended intake of 8 to 10 µg/kg per day (Table 5.2).[47]

Energy Density and Water Requirements

The energy density of preterm and term human milk is approximately 67 kcal/dL (20 kcal/oz) at 21 days of lactation. Energy density in human milk varies largely between mothers, by time of day, and by fraction of milk pumped (foremilk vs hind milk, the latter containing more fat).[119,120] Formulas of this energy density (67 kcal/

dL) may be used for feeding preterm infants, but more concentrated formulas (ie, 81 kcal/dL [24 kcal/oz]) are often preferred. The increased caloric density allows smaller feeding volumes, an advantage when the gastric capacity is limited or fluid restriction is necessary. Formulas of this concentration provide most preterm infants with sufficient water for the excretion of protein metabolic products and electrolytes derived from the formula.

Human Milk

Human milk from the preterm infant's mother is the enteral feeding of choice. Human milk is generally well tolerated by preterm infants and has been reported to promote earlier achievement of full enteral feeding compared with infant formula. In addition to its nutritional value, human milk provides immunologic and antimicrobial components, hormones, and enzymes that may contribute positively to the infant's health and development.[121] The presence of milk enzymes, such as bile salt-stimulated lipase and lipoprotein lipase, may facilitate nutrient bioavailability. Nevertheless, once growth is established, the nutritional needs of the preterm infant exceed those amounts in human milk for protein, calcium, phosphorus, magnesium, sodium, copper, zinc, folic acid, and vitamins B_2 (riboflavin), B_6 (pyridoxine), C, D, E, and K.[121,122]

Unlike infant formula, the composition of human milk varies within a single feeding (or expression), diurnally, and throughout the course of lactation. Milk from mothers of preterm infants, especially during the first 2 weeks after delivery, contains higher levels of energy and higher concentrations of fat, protein, and sodium but slightly lower concentrations of lactose, calcium, and phosphorus compared with milk from mothers of term infants.[123] The higher fat content accounts for the higher energy density of preterm milk. The higher protein content of preterm milk expressed during the first 2 to 3 weeks of lactation may be sufficient to match the fetal growth requirement for nitrogen when consumed at very high volumes (180–200 mL/kg per day). However, by the end of the first month of lactation, the protein content of milk from a mother of a preterm infant is inadequate to meet the needs of most preterm infants.[124] Metabolic complications associated with the long-term use of unsupplemented human milk in preterm infants include hyponatremia at 4 to 5 weeks,[125] hypoproteinemia at 8 to 12 weeks,[121,126] osteopenia at 4 to 5 months,[127] and zinc deficiency at 2 to 6 months.[45]

To correct the nutritional inadequacies of human milk for preterm infants, human milk fortifiers are available and provide additional protein, minerals, and vitamins (Appendix D). When these supplements are added to human milk in the first month postpartum, the resultant nutrient, mineral, and vitamin concentrations are similar to those of formulas developed for feeding preterm infants. Clinical studies of human milk fortified with commercially available powdered mixtures show metabolic and growth effects approaching those of formulas designed for infants with low birth weight.[81,82]

Human milk intake is associated with a reduction in the incidence necrotizing enterocolitis (NEC), likely because of immunologic and antimicrobial components in human milk.[128-130] A dose-dependent effect of human milk on survival without NEC has been observed in a retrospective analysis of a national neonatal database.[131] The use of an exclusive human milk feeding regimen that includes human milk and human milk-derived milk fortifier has been shown to decrease NEC and surgical NEC in infants born weighing less than 1250 g.[132] However, the control group was fed mother's own milk fortified with bovine human milk fortifier as well as formula for preterm infants when mother's milk was not available. VLBW infants should be encouraged to consume as much human milk (mother's own or donor milk) within the period when NEC occurs most often—before 34 weeks' postconceptional age. In addition, pasteurized donor milk with the addition of human milk fortifier is likely advantageous for the prevention of NEC when the mother's milk is not available.

In addition, the use of human milk from a preterm infant's own mother may promote neurologic development. A nonrandomized study reported higher developmental scores at 18 months and 7.5 to 8 years of age among former preterm infants fed their mother's milk than among those fed formula for term infants.[51] There were many confounding variables in this study, however. A dose-dependent effect of mother's own milk intake was observed with neurodevelopmental outcomes at 30 months, with an increase in the Mental Developmental Index by 0.59 for every 10 mL/kg/day.[133]

Facilitating Lactation and Human Milk Handling

Mothers of preterm infants should be encouraged to provide their milk for feeding their infants. Even mothers who plan to feed infant formula at discharge are often willing to express their milk for a few weeks after delivery. This milk can then be used to establish enteral feeding during the early critical weeks of life when the infant's medical condition is less stable.

Mothers should begin expressing their milk within the first 24 hours after delivery. They should be given verbal and written instructions about appropriate methods for collection, storage, and handling of their milk and assisted in locating a supplier for breast pumping equipment needed to establish and maintain a milk supply.[134] Individual counseling about lactation management issues, such as pumping frequency, methods to facilitate milk letdown, and breast and nipple care, should be readily available.

Fresh milk from an infant's mother may be fed immediately or refrigerated at approximately 4° C. Refrigerated milk can be safely fed within 96 hours of expression.[135] Any milk that will not be fed within 48 to 96 hours should be frozen at −20° C immediately after it has been expressed. Freezing and heat treatment of human milk alter such labile factors as cellular elements, IgA, IgM, lactoferrin, lysozyme, and C3 complement. However, freezing generally preserves these factors better than heat treatment. Human milk that has been frozen retains most of its immunologic properties (except for cellular elements) and vitamin content, when fed within 3 months of expression. Routine bacteriologic testing and pasteurization of human milk is not necessary when it is fed to the mother's own infant.[134]

Frozen milk should be thawed gradually in the refrigerator or in lukewarm water (running tap water or standing basin). Commercial milk warmers are also available to thaw milk and warm up milk to body temperature at steady rates. Care should be taken to avoid contaminating the lids of the milk containers by placing them in plastic bags before warming or contact with water. Thawing in a microwave oven is not recommended, because it reduces the levels of immunoglobulin A and lysozyme activity and may produce hot spots in the milk.[136,137] Thawed human milk should be stored in a refrigerator and used within 24 hours.

Donor Human Milk

The use of donor human milk has become an established practice in North America over the past century. Donor human milk was used frequently for term and preterm infants until there were concerns for HIV transmission in the 1980s, at which time the use of donor milk banking decreased in medical practice. With appropriate screening and preparations standards, the use of donor milk has increased significantly over the past decade, and donor human milk is especially targeted for use in the preterm infant. The dozen or more North American nonprofit milk banks are all members of the Human Milk Banking Association of North America (HMBANA), which has established practice and safety guidelines. Each bank follows specific procedures set by HMBANA for screening potential donors for infectious diseases, medical history, and lifestyle behaviors that could affect the quality of donated milk. Commercial human milk banking is also available in the United States. Pooled donor human milk is made available to hospitals through physician prescription. Although there are no federal regulations or guidelines for banking human milk, the FDA has endorsed the use of human milk banking and deemed informal sharing of human milk to be unsafe. Donor milk is pooled, pasteurized, tested for bacteria and HIV, and frozen for storage.[a] Donor milk consists

---

[a] Information about donor human milk banks in the United States and Canada is available from the Human Milk Banking Association of North America Web site (www.hmbana.org).

primarily of human milk from mothers of term infants, with some donations coming from mothers of preterm infants. Like mother's milk, donor milk requires fortification when used as a feeding for preterm infants.

Human Milk Fortification

As described previously, powdered and liquid milk fortifiers are available for supplementing human milk for the preterm infant (Appendix D). These fortifiers are well balanced and contain similar amounts of protein, minerals, and vitamins and can be used to supplement human milk for the preterm infant up to 24 kcal/oz. The human milk based liquid fortifiers do require vitamin supplementation, especially vitamin D. They are designed for mixing with human milk at the bedside.

Commercial Formulas for Preterm Infants

Commercial formulas for preterm infants (Appendix D) have been developed to meet the unique nutritional needs of the growing preterm infant. Characteristics of this group of formulas include increased amounts of protein and minerals compared with standard formulas for term infants, carbohydrate blends of lactose and glucose polymers, and fat blends containing a portion of the fat as MCTs. The vitamin contents of these formulas are sufficient that, in general, no additional multivitamin supplementation is necessary. Formulas for preterm infants are whey-predominant, cow milk-based formulas. One formula provides partially hydrolyzed whey protein as its primary source of protein. Formulas for preterm infants provide 2.7 to 3.5 g of protein per 100 kcal, which promotes a rate of weight gain and body composition similar to that of the reference fetus.[138-140]

The higher intake of calcium and phosphorus provided by formulas for preterm infants increases net mineral retention and improves bone mineral content compared with standard formulas for term infants.[80,81] No additional supplements of vitamin D are needed.

The fat blends of formulas for preterm infants have been designed to optimize absorption. Of the fat, 40% to 50% is provided as MCTs. These fats help reduce losses attributable to low intestinal lipase or bile salt levels. The amount of MCTs in formula for preterm infants may lead to increased plasma ketones and urinary dicarboxylic acid excretion in preterm infants, but this has not been shown to be detrimental to date.[141,142]

In 2002, the FDA alerted the pediatric medical community about reports of serious infections in infants caused by *Cronobacter sakazakii* (reclassified from *Enterobacter sakazakii*) that were traced to milk-based powdered infant formulas that were contaminated with the organism.[143] Powdered infants formulas are not commercially sterile products. Preterm infants and those with underlying medical conditions may be at the highest risk of developing infection[144]; therefore, the FDA recommended that powdered infant formulas not be used in preterm or immuno-compromised infants and that only commercially sterile liquid formulas designed specifically for preterm infants be used. Preterm infants who are not being fed human milk are generally on sterile liquid formula for preterm infants, but most human milk-fed infants continue to receive nonsterile powdered milk fortifiers. The World Health Organization and the Food and Agriculture Organization of the United Nations made further recommendations, including the encouragement of industry partners to develop an affordable range of sterile formula options.[145] New liquid alternatives to current powdered human milk fortifiers are now emerging that will permit further reduction in the use of powdered milk products for the preterm infant. Infant formula preparation guidelines established by the Academy of Nutrition and Dietetics are a practical resource to minimize contamination risks during the preparation and delivery of enteral nutrition in preterm infants (http://www.eatright.org).

Significant data have accumulated outside of North America suggesting protec-tive effects of probiotics against NEC and all-cause mortality.[146] Probiotics have been introduced into some formulas for term infants but not those for preterm infants. Further research is warranted before specific probiotics are included in the diet of preterm infants.

Methods of Enteral Feeding

The method of enteral feeding chosen for each infant should be based on gesta-tional age, birth weight, clinical condition, and experience of the hospital nursing personnel. Specific feeding decisions that must be made by the clinician include age to initiate feeding, type of feeding (formula, human milk), method of delivery, feeding frequency, and rate of advancement. Implementation of feeding protocols for preterm infants results in earlier full enteral feeding along with a reduction in neonatal morbidities, such as NEC.[147-149]

Trophic Feeding

Although there is no uniform definition of so-called "trophic," "priming," or "minimal enteral" feedings, these terms have been used in the literature to describe nonnutritive intakes ranging from 1 to 25 mL/kg/day. Some clinicians recom-mend that trophic feedings, especially of human milk, be started as soon as possible after birth. Among the benefits reported for early enteral nutrition are a decreased incidence of indirect hyperbilirubinemia, cholestatic jaundice, and metabolic bone disease; increased levels of gastrin and other enteric hormones; fewer days to achieve full enteral feeding; and increased weight gain. Studies have not found an increased incidence of NEC among preterm infants receiving early, minimal enteral feedings.[150,151] Therefore, on the basis of available evidence, the institution of early enteral feedings should be considered for all VLBW infants, even when infants are critically ill or labile following birth.[150,151]

Route of Feeding

The route for enteral feeding is determined by the infant's ability to coordinate sucking, swallowing, and breathing, which appear at approximately 32 to 34 weeks of gestation. Preterm infants of this postconceptional age who are alert and vigorous may be fed by nipple or offered the breast. Infants who are more premature or critically ill require feeding by tube. Nasogastric and orogastric tube feedings are the most commonly used tube feedings. Use of the stomach maximizes the digestive capability of the gastrointestinal tract. With formula feeding, studies demonstrated increased feeding intolerance and decreased growth in preterm infants fed continuously compared with those fed by bolus, whereas with early human milk feeding, the opposite effects have been demonstrated, with early achievement of full feeds and faster growth rates.[151] Transpyloric feedings provide no improvement in energy intake or growth and may be associated with significant risks.[152] This method of feeding should be undertaken only in rare instances (ie, prolonged gastroparesis or severe gastroesophageal reflux) and gastric feedings resumed as soon as possible. Gastrostomy tube feeding should be considered for infants who will be unable to nipple feed for long periods of time to decrease negative oral stimulation associated with feeding tubes and other complications, such as aspiration.

Infants who receive nasogastric, orogastric, or gastrostomy tube feedings may be fed on an intermittent bolus or continuous schedule. Because of the significant differences in the criteria used to define feeding intolerance in existing studies, it is difficult to compare the effect of these 2 feeding methods on feeding tolerance. Bolus feedings have been associated with cyclical hormone release that is commonly thought to be more physiologic.[153] On the other hand, in a study of the duodenal motor response to feeding in preterm infants, full-strength formula given continuously over 2 hours produced a normal duodenal motility pattern, whereas the same volume administered as a 15-minute bolus feeding actually inhibited motor activity.[154] On the basis of these findings, a "slow bolus" technique (ie, intermittent feedings lasting from 30 minutes to 1-2 hours) may be the best tolerated feeding method. In a small study of infants born at less than 29 weeks' gestational age and with birth weight less than 1200 g, those receiving continuous drip feedings achieved full enteral feedings an average of 1 week earlier than controls ($P < .027$). However, there were no differences in feeding tolerance or in the incidence of NEC between feeding groups.[155] Reduced nutrient absorption is also a problem associated with continuous drip feeding.[156] Fat from human milk and MCT additives tends to adhere to the feeding tube surfaces and reduce energy density.[157,158] Likewise, the loss of nutrients from fortifiers used to supplement human milk is increased when given in a continuous feeding.[159] The ideal initial feeding is full-strength human milk, with full-strength formula used only when human milk is not available. There is no evidence to support use of diluted human milk or formula as the initial feeding, a strategy that only serves to decrease nutrient intake.

A randomized control trial has demonstrated that early, aggressive enteral and parenteral nutrition in sick VLBW infants can improve growth outcomes without increasing the risk of all measured clinical and metabolic sequelae.[160]

Feeding the Preterm Infant After Discharge

With infants now being discharged home from the NICU weighing as little as 1500 g and/or receiving human milk, the nutrition of preterm infants has assumed new importance and is of growing concern. The VLBW infant is at highest risk of accumulating significant nutritional deficits by the time of hospital discharge. Even though the rate of intrauterine weight gain may be achieved prior to discharge with intensive dietary management, catch-up growth itself does not occur until well after discharge.[4,5]

In general, there is a paucity of data on what to feed the preterm infant after hospital discharge, especially if the goal is to achieve "catch-up" growth. How fast these preterm infants (and especially those born growth restricted) should demonstrate catch-up growth after hospital discharge is an area of critical research need, given the increased risk of these infants developing metabolic syndrome later in life.[161-163]

The preferred milk feeding at discharge is human milk, but in the Vermont Oxford Network, fewer than half of all VLBW infants are receiving any human milk by the time of discharge.[164] The high variability in nutrient content of human milk as well as the gradual decline in its protein content over time place exclusively human milk-fed infants at higher risk of nutritional deficiencies.[165] Human milk feeding alone at discharge may not be sufficient to provide an adequate amount of calories, protein, minerals, and vitamins without additional supplementation. The existing data on the need for postdischarge fortification for human milk-fed preterm infants are conflicting and limited.[166,167] In the study by Aimone et al, in infants weighing less than 1800 g, human milk was fortified to 22 kcal/oz with human milk fortifier powder after discharge. These infants had better growth and bone mineral density at 1 year follow-up than did controls.[167] No data thus far have demonstrated that postdischarge human milk fortification improves short-term neurodevelopmental outcomes, however. Therefore, decisions to fortify human milk should be individualized to optimize the growth trajectory of the infant over the first year of life. Strong consideration should be given to fortification of human milk for a minimum of 12 weeks for those infants who weigh less than 1250 g at birth and/or have incurred intrauterine or extrauterine growth restriction, because they represent the highest nutritional risk categories. Current practical strategies include additional human milk fortification with the addition of powdered post-discharge formula (22 kcal/oz), the use of several bottle feedings per day of postdis-charge formula, or liquid fortification with high-calorie formula for preterm infants (30 kcal/oz). Powder options are concerning given the inability to sterilize these products. These infants also require supplements of vitamins and iron.

For formula-fed infants, the change from formulas for preterm infants to special postdischarge formulas may occur as weight approaches 2000 g and the time of hospital discharge nears.[168-176] These formulas may be mixed to 22 or 24 kcal/oz (see Appendix C). Because the vitamin content of postdischarge formulas is higher than those of standard infant formulas, supplemental vitamins are not required. A meta-analysis of randomized controlled trials concluded that postdischarge formulas with higher calorie and protein content had limited benefits, at best, for growth and development up to 18 months post-term compared with standard infant formulas.[177] In some of the randomized trials, infants on standard formulas simply increased their volume of intake compared with infants on the special discharge formulas, thus largely compensating for any additional nutrients from the special discharge formulas.[169,171,173] In infants who are maintained on standard formulas after discharge, supplemental vitamins should also be given, and any formula used should be iron fortified. However, there is no information that indicates how long after discharge these supplements should be continued. Similar to human milk fortification, decisions to provide postdischarge formula should be individualized to optimize the growth trajectory of the infant over the first year of life.

Infants being discharged home need to be followed closely, with nutritional assessment of growth, iron, vitamin, and mineral status by their primary care physician. This can be facilitated with the primary care physician receiving an inpatient growth chart and nutritional recommendations as part of the medical discharge summary. Monitoring growth, including matching body composition with the term infant, may produce better neurodevelopmental outcomes. However, reliable, cost-effective measures of body composition and bone mineral density are still not readily available. For infants receiving any human milk at discharge, appropriate lactation support should be provided to the mother to promote breastfeeding and/or pumping for the first 6 months of adjusted age to be consistent with the benefits recommended to the term infant for exclusive breastfeeding.

Conclusion

Nutrition plays a critical role in the optimal health and developmental outcomes of the increasing number of surviving VLBW preterm infants. Because of the potential effects of inadequate nutrition during the early neonatal period, the goal of feeding the preterm infant is to provide nutritional support to ensure optimal growth and development and to prevent nutrition-related morbidity and mortality. The implementation of early, aggressive nutrition is targeted at reducing postnatal growth delays seen in many preterm infants, even at the time of discharge. Determining the optimal postdischarge nutritional strategy for the VLBW preterm infant with further research is of paramount importance.

References

1. American Academy of Pediatrics, Committee on Nutrition. Nutritional needs of low-birth-weight infants. *Pediatrics*. 1985;75(5):976-986

2. Agostoni C, Buonocore G, Carnielli VP, et al. Enteral nutrient supply for preterm infants: commentary from the European Society for Pediatric Gastroenterology Hepatology, and Nutrition, Committee on Nutrition. *J Pediatr Gastroenterol Nutr*. 2010;50(1):85-91

3. Tsang RC. *Nutrition of the Preterm Infant: Scientific Basis and Practice Guidelines*. 2nd ed. Cincinnati, OH: Digital Educational Publishing Inc; 2005

4. Ehrenkranz RA, Younes N, Lemons JA, et al. Longitudinal growth of hospitalized very low birth weight infants. *Pediatrics*. 1999;104(2 Pt 1):280-289

5. Lemons JA, Bauer CR, Oh W, et al. Very low birth weight outcomes of the National Institute of Child Health and Human Development Neonatal Research Network, January 1995 through December 1996. NICHD Neonatal Research Network. *Pediatrics*. 2001;107(1):e1

6. Dusick AM, Poindexter BB, Ehrenkranz RA, et al. Growth failure in the preterm infant: can we catch up? *Seminars in Perinatology*. 2003;27(4):302-310

7. Fenton TR. A new growth chart for preterm babies: Babson and Benda's chart updated with recent data and a new format. *BMC Pediatr*. 2003;3:13

8. Olsen IE, Groveman SA, Lawson ML, et al. New intrauterine growth curves based on United States data. *Pediatrics*. 2010;125(2):e214-e224

9. Modi N. Management of fluid balance in the very immature neonate. *Arch Dis Child Fetal Neonatal Ed*. 2004;89(2):F108-F111

10. Ekblad H, Kero P, Takala J, et al. Water, sodium and acid-base balance in premature infants: therapeutical aspects. *Acta Paediatr Scan*.1987;76(1):47-53

11. Fusch CH, Jochum F. Water, sodium, potassium and chloride. In: Tsang RC, Uauy R, Koletzko B, Zlotkin SH, eds. *Nutrition of the Preterm Infant: Scientific Basis and Practical Guidelines*. Cincinnati, OH: Digital Educational Publishing; 2005:201-244

12. Denne SC, Karn CA, Ahlrichs JA, et al. Proteolysis and phenylalanine hydroxylation in response to parenteral nutrition in extremely premature and normal newborns. *J Clin Invest*. 1996;97(3):746-754

13. Hay WW, Thureen P. Protein for preterm infants: how much is needed? How much is enough? How much is too much? *Pediatr Neonatol*. 2010;51(4):198-207

14. Mitton SG, Calder AG, Garlick PJ. Protein turnover rates in sick, premature neonates during the first few days of life. *Pediatr Res*. 1991;30(5):418-422

15. Rivera A Jr, Bell EF, Bier DM. Effect of intravenous amino acids on protein metabolism of preterm infants during the first three days of life. *Pediatr Res.* 1992;33(2):106-111

16. Blanco CL, Gong AK, Green BK, et al. Early changes in plasma amino acid concentrations during aggressive nutritional therapy in extremely low birth weight infants. *J Pediatr.* 2010;158(4):543-548

17. Van Goudoever JB, Colen T, Wattimena JL, et al. Immediate commencement of amino acid supplementation in preterm infants: effect on serum amino acid concentrations and protein kinetics on the first day of life. *J Pediatr.* 1995;127(3):458-465

18. Ridout E, Melara D, Rottinghaus S, et al. Blood urea nitrogen concentration as a marker of amino-acid intolerance in neonates with birthweight less than 1250 g. *J Perinatol.* 2005;25(2):130-133

19. Thureen PJ., Melara D, Fennessey PV, et al. Effect of low versus high intravenous amino acid intake on very low birth weight infants in the early neonatal period. *Pediatr Res.* 2003;53(1):24-32

20. Anderson TL, Muttart CR, Bieber MA, et al. A controlled trial of glucose versus glucose and amino acids in premature infants. *J Pediatr.* 1979;94(6):947-951

21. Duffy B, Gunn T, Collinge J, et al. The effect of varying protein quality and energy intake on the nitrogen metabolism of parenterally fed very low birthweight (less than 1600 g) infants. *Pediatric Res.* 1981;15(7):1040-1044

22. Zlotkin SH, Bryan MH, Anderson GH. Intravenous nitrogen and energy intakes required to duplicate in utero nitrogen accretion in prematurely born human infants. *J Pediatr.* 1981;99(1):115-120

23. Dweck HS, Cassady G. Glucose intolerance in infants of very low birth weight. I. Incidence of hyperglycemia in infants of birth weights 1,100 grams or less. *Pediatrics.* 1974;53(2):189-195

24. Blanco CL, Falck A, Green BK, et al. Metabolic responses to early and high protein supplementation in a randomized trial evaluating the prevention of hyperkalemia in extremely low birth weight infants. *J Pediatr.* 2008;153(4):535-540

25. Beardsall K, Vanhaesebrouck S, Ogilvy-Stuart AL, et al. Early insulin therapy in very-low-birth-weight infants. *N Engl J Med.* 2008;359(18):1873-1884

26. Binder ND, Raschko PK, Benda GI, et al. Insulin infusion with parenteral nutrition in extremely low birth weight infants with hyperglycemia. *J Pediatr.* 1989;114(2):273-280

27. Collins JW Jr, Hoppe M, Brown K, et al. A controlled trial of insulin infusion and parenteral nutrition in extremely low birth weight infants with glucose intolerance. *J Pediatr.* 1991;118(6):921-927

28. Kanarek KS, Santeiro ML, Malone JI. Continuous infusion of insulin in hyperglycemic low-birth weight infants receiving parenteral nutrition with and without lipid emulsion. *JPEN J Parenter Enteral Nutr.* 1991;15(4):417-420

29. Poindexter BB, Karn CA, Denne SC. Exogenous insulin reduces proteolysis and protein synthesis in extremely low birth weight infants. *J Pediatr.* 1988;132(6):948-953

30. Putet G. Lipid metabolism of the micropremie. *Clin Perinatol.* 2000;27(1):57-69

31. Hay WW Jr. Strategies for feeding the preterm infant. *Neonatology.* 2008;94(4):245-254

32. Andrew G, Chan G, Schiff D. Lipid metabolism in the neonate. I. The effects of Intralipid infusion on plasma triglyceride and free fatty acid concentrations in the neonate. *J Pediatr.* 1976;88(2):273-278

33. Shennan AT, Bryan MH, Angel A. The effect of gestational age on intralipid tolerance in newborn infants. *J Pediatr.* 1997;91(1):134-137

34. Koletzko B, Goulet O, Hunt J, et al. 1. Guidelines on Paediatric Parenteral Nutrition of the European Society of Paediatric Gastroenterology, Hepatology and Nutrition (ESPGHAN) and the European Society for Clinical Nutrition and Metabolism (ESPEN), Supported by the European Society of Paediatric Research (ESPR). *J Pediatr Gastroenterol Nutr.* 2005;41(Suppl 2):S1-S87

35. Penn D, Schmidt-Sommerfeld E, Pascu F. Decreased tissue carnitine concentrations in newborn infants receiving total parenteral nutrition. *J Pediatr.* 1981;98(6):976-978

36. Larsson LE, Olegard R, Ljung BM, et al. Parenteral nutrition in preterm neonates with and without carnitine supplementation. *Acta Anaesthesiol Scand.* 1990;34(6):501-505

37. Schmidt-Sommerfeld E, Penn D. Carnitine and total parenteral nutrition of the neonate. *Biol Neonate.* 1990;58(Suppl 1):81-88

38. Brans YW, Ritter DA, Kenny JD, et al. Influence of intravenous fat emulsion on serum bilirubin in very low birthweight neonates. *Arch Dis Child.* 1987;62(2):156-160

39. Carter BA, Shulman RJ. Mechanisms of disease: update on the molecular etiology and fundamentals of parenteral nutrition associated cholestasis. *Nat Clin Pract Gastroenterol Hepatol.* 2007;4(5):277-287

40. Colomb V, Jobert-Giraud A, Lacaille F, at al. Role of lipid emulsions in cholestasis associated with long-term parenteral nutrition in children. *JPEN J Parenter Enteral Nutr.* 2000;24(6):345-350

41. Lavoie PM, Lavoie JC, Watson C, et al. Inflammatory response in preterm infants is induced early in life by oxygen and modulated by total parenteral nutrition. *Pediatr Res.* 2010;68(3):248-251

42. Grand A, Jalabert A, Mercier G, et al. Influence of vitamins, trace elements, and iron on lipid peroxidation reactions in all-in-one admixtures for neonatal parenteral nutrition. *JPEN J Parenter Enteral Nutr.* 2011;35(4):505-510

43. Atkinson S, Tsang RC. Calcium, magnesium, phosphorus, and vitamin D. In: Tsang RC, Uauy R, Koletzko B, Zlotkin SH, eds. *Nutrition of the Preterm Infant: Scientific Basis and Practical Guidelines.* Cincinnati, OH: Digital Educational Publishing Inc; 2005:135-155

44. Hanning RM, Atkinson SA, Whyte RK. Efficacy of calcium glycerophosphate vs conventional mineral salts for total parenteral nutrition in low-birth-weight infants: a randomized clinical trial. *Am J Clin Nutr.* 1991;54(5):903-908

45. Rao R, Georgieff MK. Microminerals. In: Tsang RC, Uauy R, Koletzko B, Zlotkin SH, eds. *Nutrition of the Preterm Infant: Scientific Basis and Practical Guidelines.* Cincinnati, OH: Digital Educational Publishing; 2005:277-310

46. Zambrano E, El-Hennawy M, Ehrenkranz RA, et al. Total parenteral nutrition induced liver pathology: an autopsy series of 24 newborn cases. *Pediatr Dev Pathol.* 2004;7(5):425-432

47. Greer FR. Vitamins A, E, and K. In: Tsang RC, Uauy R, Koletzko B, Zlotkin SH, eds. *Nutrition of the Preterm Infant: Scientific Basis and Practical Guidelines*. Cincinnati, OH: Digital Educational Publishing; 2005:141-172

48. Schanler R. Water soluble vitamins. In: Tsang RC, Uauy R, Koletzko B, Zlotkin SH, eds. *Nutrition of the Preterm Infant: Scientific Basis and Practical Guidelines*. Cincinnati, OH: Digital Educational Publishing; 2005:173-200

49. Baeckert PA, Greene HL, Fritz I, et al. Vitamin concentrations in very low birth weight infants given vitamins intravenously in a lipid emulsion: measurement of vitamins A, D, and E and riboflavin. *J Pediatr*. 1988;113(6):1057-1065

50. Reichman B, Chessex P, Putet G, et al. Diet, fat accretion, and growth in premature infants. *N Engl J Med*. 1981;305(25):1495-1500

51. Morley R, Lucas A. Influence of early diet on outcome in preterm infants. *Acta Paediatr Suppl*. 1994;405:123-126

52. Roberts SB, Young VR. Energy costs of fat and protein deposition in the human infant. *Am J Clin Nutr*. 1988;48(4):951-955

53. Bauer J, Werner C, Gerss J. Metabolic rate analysis of healthy preterm and full-term infants during the first weeks of life. *Am J Clin Nutr*. 2009;90(6):1517-1524

54. European Society for Paediatric Gastroenterology, Hepatology and Nutrition, Committee on Nutrition. *Nutrition and Feeding of Preterm Infants*. Oxford, England: Blackwell Scientific Publications; 1987

55. Cooke R, Embleton N, Rigo J, et al. High protein pre-term infant formula: effect on nutrient balance, metabolic status and growth. *Pediatr Res*. 2006;59(2):265-270

56. Premji S, Fenton T, Sauve R. Does amount of protein in formula matter for low-birthweight infants? A Cochrane systematic review. *JPEN J Parenter Enteral Nutr*. 2006;30(6):507-514

57. Klein CJ. Nutrient requirements for preterm infant formulas. *J Nutr*. 2002;132(6 Suppl 1):1395S-1577S

58. Alexander DD, Cabana MD. Partially hydrolyzed 100% whey protein infant formula and reduced risk of atopic dermatitis: a meta-analysis. *J Pediatr Gastroenterol Nutr*. 2010;50(4):422-430

59. Shenai JP, Jhaveri BM, Reynolds JW, et al. Nutritional balance studies in very-low-birth-weight infants: role of soy formula. *Pediatrics*. 1981;67(5):631-637

60. Lindquist S, Hernell O. Lipid digestion and absorption in early life: an update. *Curr Opin Clin Nutr Metab Care*. 2010;13(3):314-320

61. Alemi B, Hamosh M, Scanlon JW, et al. Fat digestion in very-low-birth-weight infants: effect of addition of human milk to low-birth-weight formula. *Pediatrics*. 1981;68(4):484-489

62. Bustamante SA, Fiello A, Pollack PF. Growth of premature infants fed formulas with 10%, 30%, or 50% medium-chain triglycerides. *Am J Dis Child*. 1987;141(5):516-519

63. Carnielli VP, Wattimena DJ, Luijendijk IH, et al. The very low birth weight premature infant is capable of synthesizing arachidonic and docosahexaenoic acids from linoleic and linolenic acids. *Pediatr Res*. 1996;40(1):169-174

64. Sauerwald TU, Hachey DL, Jensen CL, et al. Intermediates in endogenous synthesis of C22:6 omega 3 and C20:4 omega 6 by term and preterm infants. *Pediatr Res.* 1997;41(2):183-187

65. O'Connor DL, Hall R, Adamkin D, et al. Growth and development in preterm infants fed long-chain polyunsaturated fatty acids: a prospective, randomized controlled trial. *Pediatrics.* 2001;108(2):359-371

66. Fleith M, Clandinin MT. Dietary PUFA for preterm and term infants: review of clinical studies. *Crit Rev Food Sci Nutr.* 2005;45(3):205-229

67. Makrides M, Gibson RA, McPhee AJ, et al. Neurodevelopmental outcomes of preterm infants fed high-dose docosahexaenoic acid: a randomized controlled trial. *JAMA.* 2009;301(2):175-182

68. Kien CL, Heitlinger LA, Li BU, et al. Digestion, absorption, and fermentation of carbohydrates. *Semin Perinatol.* 1989;13(2):78-87

69. Parimi P, Kalhan S. Carbohydrates including oligosaccharides and inositol. In: Tsang RC, Uauy R, Koletzko B, Zlotkin SH, eds. *Nutrition of the Preterm Infant: Scientific Basis and Practical Guidelines.* Cincinnati, OH: Digital Educational Publishing; 2005:81-96

70. Wirth FH Jr, Numerof B, Pleban P, et al. Effect of lactose on mineral absorption in preterm infants. *J Pediatr.* 1990;117(2 Pt 1):283-287

71. Coppa G, Pierani P, Zampini L, et al. Characterization of oligosaccharides in milk and faeces of breast-fed infants by high-perfromance anion-exchange chromatography. *Adv Exp Med Biol.* 2001;501:307-314

72. Engfer M, Stahl B, Finke B, et al. Human milk oligosaccharides are resistant to enzymatic hydrolysis in the upper gastrointestinal tract. *Am J Clin Nutr.* 2000;71(6):1589-1596

73. German JB, Freeman SL, Lebrilla CB, et al. Human milk oligosaccharides: evolution, structures and bioselectivity as substrates for intestinal bacteria. Presented at: *62nd Nestle Nutrition Institute Workshop Series: Pediatric Program.* Basel, Switzerland; Karger: 2008

74. Donovan SM. Human milk oligosaccharides—the plot thickens. *Br J Nutr.* 2008;101(9):1267-1269

75. Coppa GV, Zampini L, Galeazzi T, Gabrielli O. Prebiotics in human milk: a review. *Dig Liver Dis.* 2006;38(2):S291-S294

76. Bode L. Human milk oligosaccharides: prebiotics and beyond. *Nutr Rev.* 2009;67(2):S183-S191

77. Boehm G, Stahl B, Jelinek J, et al. Prebiotic carbohydrates in human milk and formula. *Acta Paediatricia.* 2005;94(10 Suppl 449):18-21

78. Rigo J, Pieltain C, Salle B, et al. Enteral calcium, phosphate and vitamin D requirements and bone mineralization in preterm infants. *Acta Paediatr.* 2007;96(7):969-974

79. Abrams SA; American Academy of Pediatrics, Committee on Nutrition. Clinical report: calcium and vitamin D requirements of enterally fed preterm infants. *Pediatrics.* 2013;131(5):e1676-e1683

80. Chan GM, Mileur L, Hansen JW. Effects of increased calcium and phosphorous formulas and human milk on bone mineralization in preterm infants. *J Pediatr Gastroenterol Nutr.* 1986;5(3):444-449

II

81. Ehrenkranz RA, Gettner PA, Nelli CM. Nutrient balance studies in premature infants fed premature formula or fortified preterm human milk. *J Pediatr Gastroenterol Nutr.* 1989;8(1):58-67

82. Greer FR, McCormick A. Improved bone mineralization and growth in premature infants fed fortified own mother's milk. *J Pediatr.* 1988;112(6):961-969

83. Schanler RJ, Garza C. Improved mineral balance in very low birth weight infants fed fortified human milk. *J Pediatr.* 1988;112(3):452-456

84. Rao R, Georgieff MK. Iron in fetal and neonatal nutrition. *Semin Fetal Neonatal Med.* 2007;12(1):54-63

85. Von Kohorn I, Ehrenkranz RA. Anemia in the preterm infant: erythropoietin versus erythrocyte transfusion—it's not that simple. *Clin Perinatol.* 2009;36(1):111-123

86. Strauss RG. Controversies in the management of the anemia of prematurity using single-donor red blood cell transfusions and/or recombinant human erythropoietin. *Transfus Med Rev.* 2006;20(1):34-44

87. Ohls RK. Erythropoietin treatment in extremely low birth weight infants: blood in versus blood out. *J Pediatr.* 2002;141(1):3-6

88. Zipursky A. Erythropoietin therapy for premature infants: cost without benefit? *Pediatr Res.* 2000;48(2):136

89. Franz AR, Mihatsch WA, Sander S, et al. Prospective randomized trial of early versus late enteral iron supplementation in infants with a birth weight of less than 1301 grams. *Pediatrics.* 2000;106(4):700-706

90. Widdowson EM, Southgate DAT, Hey E. Fetal growth and body composition. In: Lindblad B, ed. *Perinatal Nutrition.* New York, NY: Academic Press; 1998:3-14

91. Zlotkin SH. Assessment of trace element requirements (zinc) in newborns and young infants, including the infant born prematurely. In: Chandra RK, ed. *Trace Elements in Nutrition of Children II.* Vol. 23. New York, NY: Raven Press; 1991:49-64

92. Ehrenkranz RA, Gettner PA, Nelli CM, et al. Zinc and copper nutritional studies in very low birth weight infants: comparison of stable isotopic extrinsic tag and chemical balance methods. *Pediatr Res.* 1989;26(4):298-307

93. Delange F, Dalhem A, Bourdoux P, et al. Increased risk of primary hypothyroidism in preterm infants. *J Pediatr.* 1984;105(3):462-469

94. Darlow BA, Buss H, McGill F, et al. Vitamin C supplementation in very preterm infants: a randomised controlled trial. *Arch Dis Child Fetal Neonatal Ed.* 2005;90(2):F117-F122

95. Mock DM, deLorimer AA, Liebman WM, et al. Biotin deficiency: an unusual complication of parenteral alimentation. *N Engl J Med.* 1981;304(14):820-823

96. Stevens D, Burman D, Strelling MK, et al. Folic acid supplementation in low birth weight infants. *Pediatrics.* 1979;64(3):333-335

97. Kendall AC, Jones EE, Wilson CI, et al. Folic acid in low birthweight infants. *Arch Dis Child.* 1974;49(9):736-738

98. Higginbottom MC, Sweetman L, Nyhan WL. A syndrome of methylmalonic aciduria, homocystinuria, megaloblastic anemia and neurologic abnormalities in a vitamin B12-deficient breast-fed infant of a strict vegetarian. *N Engl J Med.* 1978;299(7):317-323

99. Shenai JP, Chytil F, & Stahlman MT. Liver vitamin A reserves of very low birth weight neonates. *Pediatr Res.* 1985;19(9):892-893

100. Shenai JP, Chytil F, Jhaveri A, et al. Plasma vitamin A and retinol-binding protein in premature and term neonates. *J Pediatr.* 1981;99(2):302-305

101. Shenai JP, Rush MG, Stahlman MT, et al. Plasma retinol-binding protein response to vitamin A administration in infants susceptible to bronchopulmonary dysplasia. *J Pediatr.* 1990;116(4):607-614

102. Darlow BA, Graham PJ. Vitamin A supplementation to prevent mortality and short and long-term morbidity in very low birthweight infants. *Cochrane Database Syst Rev.* 2007;(4):CD000501

103. Tyson JE, Wright LL, Oh W, et al. Vitamin A supplementation for extremely-low-birth-weight infants. National Institute of Child Health and Human Development Neonatal Research Network. *N Engl J Med.* 1999;340(25):1962-1968

104. Salle BL, Delvin E, Claris O, et al. Is it justifiable to administrate vitamin A, E and D for 6 months in the premature infants? *Arch Pediatr.* 2007;14(12):1408-1412

105. Oski FA, Barness LA. Vitamin E deficiency: a previously unrecognized cause of hemolytic anemia in the premature infant. *J Pediatr.* 1967;70(2):211-220

106. Ritchie JH, Fish MB, McMasters V, et al. Edema and hemolytic anemia in premature infants. A vitamin E deficiency syndrome. *N Engl J Med.* 1968;279(22):1185-1190

107. Gross S, Melhorn DK. Vitamin E-dependent anemia in the premature infant. *J Pediatr.* 1974;85(6):753-759

108. Williams ML, Shoot RJ, O'Neal PL, et al. Role of dietary iron and fat on vitamin E deficiency anemia of infancy. *N Engl J Med.* 1975;292(17):887-890

109. Brion LP, Bell EF, Raghuveer TS. Vitamin E supplementation for prevention of morbidity and mortality in preterm infants. *Cochrane Database Syst Rev.* 2003;(4):CD003665

110. Holick MF. Vitamin D deficiency. *N Eng J Med.* 2007;357(3):266-281

111. Hollis BW, Wagner CL. Assessment of dietary vitamin D requirements during pregnancy and lactation. *Am J Clin Nutr.* 2004;79(5):717-726

112. Rigo, J, De Curtis M, Pieltain C, et al. Bone mineral metabolism in the micropremie. *Clin Perinatol.* 2000;27(1):147-170

113. Schulzke SM, Trachsel D, Patole SK. Physical activity programs for promoting bone mineralization and growth in preterm infants. *Cochrane Database Syst Rev.* 2007;(2):CD005387

114. Abrams SA; American Academy of Pediatrics, Committee on Nutrition. Calcium and vitamin D requirements of enterally fed preterm infants. *Pediatrics.* 2013;131(5):e1676-e1683

115. Cooke R, Hollis B, Conner C, et al. Vitamin D and mineral metabolism in the very low birth weight infant receiving 400 IU of vitamin D. *J Pediatr.* 1990;116(3):423-428

116. Institute of Medicine, Food and Nutrition Board. *Dietary Reference Intakes for Calcium and Vitamin D.* Washington, DC: National Academies Press; 2011

117. Wagner CL, Greer FR. Prevention of rickets and vitamin d deficiency in infants, children, and adolescents. *Pediatrics.* 2008;122(5):1142-1152

118. Greer FR. Vitamin K the basics—what's new? *Early Hum Dev.* 2010;86(Suppl 1):43-47

119. Daly SE, Di Rosso A, Owens RA, et al. Degree of breast emptying explains changes in the fat content, but not fatty acid composition, of human milk. *Exp Physiol.* 1993;78(6): 741-755

120. Lubetzky R, Littner Y, Mimouni FB, et al. Circadian variations in fat content of expressed breast milk from mothers of preterm infants. *J Am Coll Nutr.* 2006;25(2):151-154

121. Schanler RJ, Lau C, Hurst NM, et al. Randomized trial of donor human milk versus preterm formula as substitutes for mothers' own milk in the feeding of extremely premature infants. *Pediatrics.* 2005;116(2):400-406

122. Victor YH, Simmer K. Enteral nutrition: practical aspects, strategy, and management. In: Tsang RC, Uauy R, Koletzko B, Zlotkin SH, eds. *Nutrition of the Preterm Infant: Scientific Basis and Practical Guidelines.* Cincinnati, OH: Digital Educational Publishing; 2005: 311-333

123. Atkinson SA. Effects of gestational age at delivery on human milk components. In: Jensen RG, ed. *Handbook of Milk Composition.* San Diego, CA: Academic Press; 1995:2 22-237

124. Lucas A, Hudson GJ. Preterm milk as a source of protein for low birthweight infants. *Arch Dis Child.* 1984;59(9):831-836

125. Engelke SC, Shah BL, Vasan U, et al. Sodium balance in very low-birth-weight infants. *J Pediatr.* 1978;93(5):837-841

126. Ronnholm KA, Sipila I, Siimes MA. Human milk protein supplementation for the prevention of hypoproteinemia without metabolic imbalance in breast milk-fed, very low-birth-weight infants. *J Pediatr.* 1982;101(2):243-247

127. Greer FR., Steichen JJ, Tsang RC. Calcium and phosphate supplements in breast milk-related rickets. Results in a very-low-birth-weight infant. *Am J Dis Child.* 1982;136(7):581-583

128. Lucas A, Cole TJ. Breast milk and neonatal necrotising enterocolitis. *Lancet.* 1990;336(8730):1519-1523

129. Schanler RJ. Human milk. In: Tsang RC, Uauy R, Koletzko B, Zlotkin SH, eds. *Nutrition of the Preterm Infant: Scientific Basis and Practical Guidelines.* Cincinnati, OH: Digital Educational Publishing; 2005:333-356

130. Schanler RJ, Shulman RJ, Lau C. Feeding strategies for premature infants: beneficial outcomes of feeding fortified human milk versus preterm formula. *Pediatrics.* 1999;103(6 Pt 1):1150-1157

131. Meinzen-Derr J, Poindexter B, Wrage L, et al. Role of human milk in extremely low birth weight infants' risk of necrotizing enterocolitis or death. *J Perinatol.* 2009;29(1):57-62

132. Sullivan S, Schanler RJ, Kim JH et al. An exclusively human milk-based diet is associated with a lower rate of necrotizing enterocolitis than a diet of human milk and bovine milk-based products. *J Pediatr.* 2010;156(4):562-567

133. Vohr BR, Poindexter BB, Dusick AM, et al. Persistent beneficial effects of breast milk ingested in the neonatal intensive care unit on outcomes of extremely low birth weight infants at 30 months of age. *Pediatrics.* 2007;120(4):e953-e959

134. Jones F. *Best Practice for Expressing, Storing and Handling Human Milk in Hospitals, Homes and Child Care Settings.* 3rd ed. Fort Worth, TX: Human Milk Banking Association of North America Inc; 2011

135. Slutzah M, Codipilly CN, Potak D, et al. Refrigerator storage of expressed human milk in the neonatal intensive care unit. *J Pediatr.* 2010;156(1):26-28

136. Quan R, Yang C, Rubinstein S, et al. Effects of microwave radiation on anti-infective factors in human milk. *Pediatrics.* 1992;89(4 Pt 1):667-669

137. Sigman M, Burke KI, Swarner OW, et al. Effects of microwaving human milk: changes in IgA content and bacterial count. *J Am Diet Assoc.* 1989;89(5):690-692

138. Gross SJ. Growth and biochemical response of preterm infants fed human milk or modified infant formula. *N Engl J Med.* 1983;308(5):237-241

139. Putet G, Senterre J, Rigo J, et al. Nutrient balance, energy utilization, and composition of weight gain in very-low-birth-weight infants fed pooled human milk or a preterm formula. *J Pediatr.* 1984;105(1):79-85

140. Schulze KF, Stefanski M, Masterson J, et al. Energy expenditure, energy balance, and composition of weight gain in low birth weight infants fed diets of different protein and energy content. *J Pediatr.* 1987;110(5):753-759

141. Odle J. New insights into the utilization of medium-chain triglycerides by the neonate: observations from a piglet model. *J Nutr.* 1997;127(6):1061-1067

142. Sulkers EJ, Lafeber HN, Sauer PJ. Quantitation of oxidation of medium-chain triglycerides in preterm infants. *Pediatr Res.* 1989;26(4):294-297

143. Taylor C. Health professionals letter on *Enterobacter sakazakii* infections associated with the use of powdered (dry) infant formulas in neonatal intensive care units. Silver Spring, MD: US Food and Drug Administration, Center for Food Safety and Applied Nutrition, Office of Nutritional Products, Labeling and Dietary Supplements; 2002

144. Bowen AB, Braden CR. Invasive *Enterobacter sakazakii* disease in infants. *Emerg Infect Dis.* 2006;12(8):1185-1189

145. World Health Organization. *Enterobacter sakazakii* and other microorganisms in powdered infant formula. Meeting report. *Microbiol Risk Assess Series.* Vol 6. Geneva, Switzerland: World Health Organization; 2004

146. Alfaleh K, Anabrees J, Bassler D, et al. Probiotics for prevention of necrotizing enterocolitis in preterm infants. *Cochrane Database Syst Rev.* 2011;(3):CD005496

147. McCallie KR, Lee HC, Mayer O, et al. Improved outcomes with a standardized feeding protocol for very low birth weight infants. *J Perinatol.* 2011;31(Suppl 1):S61-S67

148. Patole SK, de Klerk N. Impact of standardised feeding regimens on incidence of neonatal necrotising enterocolitis: a systematic review and meta-analysis of observational studies. *Arch Dis Child Fetal Neonatal Ed.* 2005;90(2):F147-F151

149. Wiedmeier SE, Henry E, Baer VL, et al. Center differences in NEC within one health-care system may depend on feeding protocol. *Am J Perinatol.* 2008;25(1):5-11

150. McClure RJ, Newell SJ. Randomised controlled trial of trophic feeding and gut motility. *Arch Dis Child Fetal Neonatal Ed.* 1999;80(1):F54-F58

151. Schanler RJ, Shulman RJ, Lau C, Smith EO, Heitkemper MM. Feeding strategies for premature infants: randomized trial of gastrointestinal priming and tube-feeding methods. *Pediatrics.* 1999;103(2):434-439

152. McGuire W, McEwan P. Transpyloric versus gastric tube feeding for preterm infants. *Cochrane Database Syst Rev.* 2007;(3):CD003487

153. Aynsley-Green A, Adrian TE, et al. Feeding and the development of enteroinsular hormone secretion in the preterm infant: effects of continuous gastric infusions of human milk compared with intermittent boluses. *Acta Paediatr Scand.* 1982;71(3): 379-383

154. Baker JH., Berseth CL. Duodenal motor responses in preterm infants fed formula with varying concentrations and rates of infusion. *Pediatr Res.* 1997;42(5):618-622

155. Dsilna A, Christensson K, Alfredsson L, et al. Continuous feeding promotes gastrointestinal tolerance and growth in very low birth weight infants. *J Pediatr.* 2005;147(1):43-49

156. Roy RN, Pollnitz RB, Hamilton JR, et al. Impaired assimilation of nasojejunal feeds in healthy low-birth-weight newborn infants. *J Pediatr.* 1977;90(3):431-434

157. Greer FR, McCormick A, Loker J. Changes in fat concentration of human milk during delivery by intermittent bolus and continuous mechanical pump infusion. *J Pediatr.* 1984;105(5):745-749

158. Mehta NR, Hamosh M, Bitman J, et al. Adherence of medium-chain fatty acids to feeding tubes during gavage feeding of human milk fortified with medium-chain triglycerides. *J Pediatr.* 1988;112(3):474-476

159. Bhatia J, Rassin DK. Human milk supplementation. Delivery of energy, calcium, phosphorus, magnesium, copper, and zinc. *Am J Dis Child.* 1988;142(4):445-447

160. Wilson DC, Cairns P, Halliday HL, et al. Randomised controlled trial of an aggressive nutritional regimen in sick very low birthweight infants. *Arch Dis Child Fetal Neonatal Ed.* 1997;77(1):F4-F11

161. Euser AM, Finken MJ, Keijzer-Veen MG, et al. Associations between prenatal and infancy weight gain and BMI, fat mass, and fat distribution in young adulthood: a prospective cohort study in males and females born very preterm. *Am J Clin Nutr.* 2005;81(2): 480-487

162. Singhal A, Fewtrell M, Cole TJ, et al. Low nutrient intake and early growth for later insulin resistance in adolescents born preterm. *Lancet.* 2003;361(9363):1089-1097

163. Singhal A, Lucas A. Early origins of cardiovascular disease: is there a unifying hypothesis? *Lancet.* 2004;363(9421):1642-1645

164. Vermont Oxford Network. Available at: http://www.vtoxford.org/. Accessed September 18, 2012

165. Saarela T, Kokkonen J, Koivisto M. Macronutrient and energy contents of human milk fractions during the first six months of lactation. *Acta Paediatrica.* 2005;94(9):1176-1181

166. Aimone A, Rovet J, Ward W. Growth and body composition of human milk-fed premature infants provided with extra energy and nutrients early after hospital discharge: 1-year follow-up. *J Pediatr Gastroenterol Nutr.* 2009;49(4):456-466

167. Zachariassen G, Faerk J, Grytter C, et al. Nutrient enrichment of mother's milk and growth of very preterm infants after hospital discharge. *Pediatrics.* 2011;127(4):e995-e1003

168. Bishop NJ, King FJ, Lucas A. Increased bone mineral content of preterm infants fed with a nutrient enriched formula after discharge from hospital. *Arch Dis Child.* 1993;68(5 Spec No):573-578

169. Carver JD, Wu PY, Hall RT, et al. Growth of preterm infants fed nutrient-enriched or term formula after hospital discharge. *Pediatrics.* 2001;107(4):683-689

170. Chan GM. Growth and bone mineral status of discharged very low birth weight infants fed different formulas or human milk. *J Pediatr.* 1993;123(3):439-443

171. Cooke RJ, Embleton ND, Griffin IJ, et al. Feeding preterm infants after hospital discharge: growth and development at 18 months of age. *Pediatr Res.* 2001;49(5):719-722

172. Cooke RJ, Griffin IJ, McCormick K,et al. Feeding preterm infants after hospital discharge: effect of dietary manipulation on nutrient intake and growth. *Pediatr Res.* 1998;43(3):355-360

173. Koo WW, Hockman EM. Posthospital discharge feeding for preterm infants: effects of standard compared with enriched milk formula on growth, bone mass, and body composition. *Am J Clin Nutr.* 2006;84(6):1357-1364

174. Lapillonne A, Salle BL, Glorieux FH, et al. Bone mineralization and growth are enhanced in preterm infants fed an isocaloric, nutrient-enriched preterm formula through term. *Am J Clin Nutr.* 2004;80(6):1595-1603

175. Lucas A, Bishop NJ, King FJ, et al. Randomised trial of nutrition for preterm infants after discharge. *Arch Dis Child.* 1992;67(3):324-327

176. Wheeler RE, Hall RT. Feeding of premature infant formula after hospital discharge of infants weighing less than 1800 grams at birth. *J Perinatol.* 1996;16(2 Pt 1):111-116

177. Henderson G, Fahey T, McGuire W. Calorie and protein-enriched formula versus standard term formula for improving growth and development in preterm or low birth weight infants following hospital discharge. *Cochrane Database Syst Rev.* 2005;(2):CD004696

II

Chapter 6

Complementary Feeding

Introduction

The importance of complementary feeding has received tremendous recognition in international nutrition circles because of the well-established risk of infectious diseases and malnutrition with premature introduction of complementary food and nonexclusive breastfeeding during early infancy. For older infants, inadequate complementary feeding, either because of delayed introduction and/or reliance on poor-quality foods, is cited as a major cause of preventable mortality in young children.[1]

In industrialized nations, however, the high prevalence of nonexclusive breastfeeding and formula feeding as well as the availability of relatively inexpensive, hygienically prepared commercial foods in a bewildering array of choices designed specifically for infants, has largely mitigated concerns about micronutrient deficiencies, with the possible exception of iron. Rather, the increasing prevalence of overweight and obesity in young children has directed attention to the potential for excessive caloric intake from complementary foods. Such a narrow focus, however, belies the complexity of the nutritional and developmental progression that underlies the complementary feeding process. Despite this importance, remarkably limited data are available for determining "best practices." Rather, much of the advice provided on complementary feeding is based on traditions rather than evidence. This chapter will briefly review biological, nutritional, developmental, and behavioral issues related to successful complementary feeding for the normal, healthy infant and toddler.

Definitions

Complementary foods refer to nutrient- and energy-containing solid or semi-solid foods (or liquids) fed to infants in addition to human milk or formula. Importantly, the choice of complementary foods ideally "complements" the nutritional gaps that develop as a result of the dynamic nutritional composition of human milk and the dynamic nutritional needs of the infant. Generally, the progression from the fully liquid diet of the young infant to the mixed diet of "family foods" occurs from mid-way through the first year of life through the second year—that is, approximately 6 to 24 months of age.

Nutritional Considerations

The most important factor affecting an infant's dependence on complementary food choices to meet nutritional requirements is whether he or she has been exclusively breastfed or formula fed (or if mixed, the balance between human milk and formula). For simplicity, the following discussion, after first addressing energy and macronutrient needs, will address human milk compared with formula feeding but will not specifically address so-called "mixed feeding," which is very common[2,3] and clearly influences nutritional intake and nutrient utilization. The following subsections discuss general considerations for energy and nutritional requirements of older infants and toddlers up to 24 months of age.

Energy Requirements

Over the first year of life, energy requirements relative to body weight gradually decrease, whereas total calorie needs increase as physical activity increases. The proportion of energy required to support growth also steadily decreases, from 25% to 30% between birth and 4 months of age to approximately 5% by the end of the first year (Fig 6.1).[4]

Fig 6.1.
Allocation of energy expenditure during the first year of life.[4]

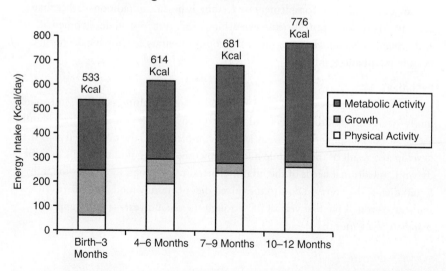

Figure drawn from data presented in *Arch Dis Child* 1998;78:131–136 and *Am J Clin Nutr* 2000;72:1558–1569.

Estimated daily energy requirements for infants and toddlers are presented in Table 6.1.[4]

Table 6.1.
Total Energy Requirements in Infants and Toddlers

Age	Energy Requirement (kcal/day) for Boys	Energy Requirement (kcal/day) for Girls
3 mo	535 ± 105	530 ± 100
6 mo	630 ± 110	615 ± 110
9 mo	750 ± 110	680 ± 100
12 mo	830 ± 170	775 ± 125
18 mo	950 ± 115	855 ± 170
24 mo	1000 ± 150	990 ± 170

Adapted with permission from Butte et al[4]; figures rounded to nearest 5 kcal.

For breastfed infants, the volume of milk intake typically decreases over the first year of life, in both developing and industrialized countries, with the extent being influenced by the availability and intake of calories from other sources. Ideally, the total caloric intake to support normal growth will reflect a decrease in the milk/formula component as intake of complementary foods increases. According to estimates derived from direct measurements of energy expenditure along with careful growth and body composition measurements, the average total energy requirements for the intervals 6 through 8, 9 through 11, and 12 to 24 months of age are approximately 615, 685, and 895 kcal/day, respectively.[4] Considering the average energy transferred from human milk at each of these age intervals, the average energy intake required from complementary foods is approximately 200, 300, and 550 kcal/day, respectively.[4]

For bottle-fed infants, typically receiving infant formula, for whom there is more propensity to overfeed, the volume of formula should, likewise, decrease as intake of complementary foods increases.[5,6] The revised food packages for the Special Supplemental Nutrition Program for Women, Infants, and Children (WIC) reflect this decreased need, as the amount of formula provided between 6 to 12 months of age is less than that provided for younger infants.[7]

Although estimates of caloric needs of infants and young children are useful for programmatic planning and for feeding under controlled conditions (eg, in the hospital or with nutrition support), for a healthy individual child, energy requirements are impossible to gauge precisely. This is because of the impossibility of accurately estimating caloric requirements for physical activity and for basal metabolic activity, which is influenced by body composition. The daily energy requirements noted previously are, thus, best considered "first approximation" estimates. Therefore, recommendations for specific caloric goals to parents or care providers can be misleading and may result in undue focus on a "number" instead of on healthy/appropriate eating patterns. More appropriately, an infant or toddler's growth should guide energy intake recommendations. For infants gaining weight too rapidly, an emphasis on foods with low caloric density, such as selected vegetables and fruits, is appropriate. For infants with evidence of faltering weight gain, foods with higher caloric density, such as those with higher fat and protein content, should be encouraged.[8,9] Careful investigations of the effect of energy density and frequency of feeding have demonstrated that for any frequency of feeding, a higher energy density of complementary foods results in higher total energy intake.[8] Inappropriately rapid or slow weight gain should be explored and addressed in the context of food choices and feeding behaviors, not by specific calorie intake goals.

Macronutrient Recommendations

Protein

As with energy, protein requirements relative to body weight decrease with age but increase in absolute amounts. By 6 months of age, the average requirement for protein per kg is about two thirds that for a newborn infant, and by 2 years of age, protein requirement decreases further to about 50% of that for a newborn infant.[10] The quantity of protein in human milk, although of high quality, decreases modestly over the course of lactation. By late infancy, typical protein intakes from human milk alone will be marginally adequate and reflect a moderate dependence on complementary foods to meet the total requirement. For example, an average weight, 8-month-old breastfed infant weighing 8 kg and consuming 700 mL of human milk (a generous estimate providing ~ 60 kcal/kg) would receive approximately 6.3 g or 0.8 g of protein/kg/day. The quality of protein in human milk is maintained independently of maternal diet. In contrast to breastfed infants, an 8-kg formula-fed infant consuming a similar amount of formula would receive approximately 1.3 g of protein/kg/day.[6]

Fat

Lipids contribute approximately 45% to 50% of the calories in human milk, infant formulas, and whole cow milk. Notably, plant-based so-called "milks" (eg, soy, almond, rice, etc) tend to be lower in fat and, hence, in calories compared with animal milks and formulas. In contrast to protein, the fatty acid composition of human milk does reflect maternal intake (see Chapter 3, Breastfeeding). Fats from "milk" products are an important source of concentrated calories to maintain normal growth in older infants and young children. As complementary foods gradually provide a larger percentage of energy intake, they should ideally include sources of "healthy" mono- and polyunsaturated fatty acids, including the long-chain polyunsaturated fatty acids. Recommendations for fat intake for young children are approximately 30% to 40% of daily energy.[11] As noted later in this chapter, the traditional and current emphasis on cereals, vegetables, and fruits results in fat intakes that may be unnecessarily and potentially undesirably low. Recent data from a survey of US infants and children reported that approximately 23% of 12- through 23-month-olds have fat intakes less than recommended.[12] However, diets containing less than 30% of calories from fat for older infants and toddlers have been shown to be safe in terms of growth and development,[13] unless total energy intake is suboptimal reflected by underweight and growth faltering, in which case increasing the fat intake of the diet is an efficient and effective intervention.

Carbohydrate

As complementary foods provide increasing amounts of calories and nutrients in the diet, carbohydrates become the major source of energy, providing 55% to 60% of total calorie intake. This is in contrast to the young infant's diet, in which approximately 40% of calories in human milk (or formula) are provided by carbohydrate as lactose. Similar to recommendations for older children and adults, the recommendations for type of carbohydrate in complementary foods emphasize complex, unrefined sources over simple, added sugars.

Micronutrient Requirements

Because of the fortification of all standard infant formulas with generous levels of virtually all essential micronutrients, the risk of micronutrient deficiencies in formula-fed infants is very low. After 12 months of age, when most healthy infants are no longer consuming formula, the risk of certain micronutrient deficiencies gradually increases if the diet is restricted to a few foods. However, data from the Feeding Infants and Toddlers Study (FITS) indicated that the average intakes of most micronutrients, including antioxidants, B vitamins, and other micronutrients, were adequate.[12]

For breastfed infants, assuming maternal diet is adequate and unrestricted, the gap between typical intake from human milk and the micronutrient requirement is highest for the micronutrients iron and zinc.[9] In practice, iron and zinc are defined as "problem nutrients" because of the great discrepancy between their content in human milk and traditional complementary foods and the estimated daily requirements.[9] These gaps in intakes must be made up from complementary foods (or dietary supplements). As for vitamin D, because human milk, like most complementary foods, contains small amounts, vitamin D supplements are the principal means to meet requirements (see Chapter 21).

Iron

As noted, infant formula is fortified with iron (12 mg/L in the United States). However, human milk is distinctly low in iron. Although the relatively favorable bioavailability enhances its absorption, the low iron concentration means that the contribution of human milk to infants' iron needs is very modest. Maternal iron status has no effect on milk iron concentrations, although it affects fetal iron accretion. In general, healthy term infants are born with 75 mg/kg of total body iron. As discussed in Chapter 19, the breastfed infant's need for iron from complementary foods is dictated by gestational age (iron stores are acquired during the third trimester), complications of pregnancy (ie, infants of mothers with diabetes and infants who are small for gestational age or have intrauterine growth restriction have decreased iron stores), whether or not there is late umbilical cord clamping, postnatal growth rate, and duration of exclusive breastfeeding. The healthy term infant who is exclusively breastfed will need to begin either consuming iron-rich complementary foods or receiving iron supplements to support erythropoiesis and normal brain development between 4 and 6 months of age. The risk of iron deficiency and iron-deficiency anemia increases progressively the longer complementary foods (or other sources of iron, such as dietary supplements) are delayed beyond 6 months.[14]

The common practice of introducing infant cereals as a first complementary food is based on the recognized need for iron; essentially all commercial infant cereals in the United States are iron fortified. Accounting for the low bioavailability of the electrolytic iron fortificant, 1 to 2 servings per day are recommended to meet iron requirements. Indeed, the Recommended Dietary Allowance of 11 mg/day for infants 7 to 12 months of age is based on the assumption that most iron consumed by the older infant will be from cereal and, thus, will be poorly absorbed.[11] Plant foods, including whole grains, legumes, and most vegetables, are naturally low in iron and may contain inhibitors of iron absorption, such as phytate, tannins, or polyphenols. Flesh foods, especially red meats, are naturally rich in heme iron, which has a much more favorable bioavailability (20%-35% absorption rate).[14]

Zinc

The older exclusively breastfed infant also is strongly dependent on complementary foods to provide adequate zinc intake, unlike the formula-fed infant. In contrast to iron, human milk initially contains high concentrations of zinc, but a sharp physiologic decrease in human milk zinc content over the first several months postpartum (independent of maternal zinc status) results in inadequate intake if other dietary sources are not consumed. As with iron, high absorption efficiency of zinc in human milk does not compensate for the low concentrations and intakes by approximately 5 to 6 months of age.[15] Zinc fortification of infant cereals is not routine in the United States, and the zinc content of plant foods, including cereal grains and legumes, tends to be low and/or poorly absorbed. Red meats (and liver) are the best source of zinc in the diet, with pork and poultry being medium rich and fish and eggs being lowest in zinc content of animal products. Dairy foods, such as cow milk, yogurt, and cheese, are only moderately rich sources of zinc.

Fruits and vegetables are low in zinc; whole grains and legumes have moderately high concentrations, but absorption is inhibited by intrinsic compounds in the plants (eg, phytate). Commercially available mixed dinners, which combine a vegetable or starch with a meat source, contain much lower amounts of zinc and iron than "single-ingredient" pureed meats.[15]

Vitamin D

The content of vitamin D in human milk is quite low relative to requirements, even with adequate maternal vitamin D status. With the exception of fatty fish, fortified cow milk, some other dairy products, and selected calcium/vitamin D-fortified juices, complementary foods are not good sources of vitamin D. Sunlight provides the ultraviolet light to convert the precursor in skin to active vitamin, but sunscreen, when applied appropriately, blocks this conversion. Thus, the American Academy of Pediatrics (AAP) has recommended routine vitamin D supplements of 400 IU/day for breastfed infants to avoid development of deficiency[16] (see Chapter 21).

Other Vitamins

For well-nourished mothers, the human milk content of vitamins will generally be adequate to meet breastfed infants' nutritional requirements; thus, complementary food choices are less critical to meet requirements for these micronutrients. An important exception to this generalization is vitamin B_{12} for vegan mothers. (see Chapter 11). If the mother has not taken supplements during pregnancy and lactation, her milk may be low in vitamin B_{12}, and the breastfed infant will be at risk of deficiency. Case reports of vitamin B_{12} deficiency in breastfed infants of vegan mothers are readily found in the literature.[17] Furthermore, if parents wish to provide a vegan diet for the weanling infant and toddler, the risk of vitamin B_{12} is moderately high (especially if mother has not used supplements), as are the risks of iron and zinc deficiencies.

Physiologic and Developmental Considerations

The normal progression of physiologic and motor maturation aligns typically midway through the first year of life. The infant gastrointestinal tract is able to digest and efficiently absorb virtually all nutrients by 2 to 3 months of age. Therefore, it follows that by the time complementary feeding is recommended, no foods need to be avoided on the basis of gastrointestinal tract immaturity. Developmentally, an infant should have truncal strength and stability to allow sitting in an upright position with little or no support, skills typically present between 4 and 7 months of age. The sucking, rooting, and extrusion primitive reflexes will normally have diminished by this time, and oral motor skills to handle nonliquid foods should be emerging. The gag reflex also gradually declines during this period and the infant is able to handle more complex textures.

Oral motor skills needed for greater manipulation of food within the mouth and for handling of more complex textures like thicker purees, appear at approximately 6 months of age and include up-down jaw movements, tongue lateralization, and rotary motion of jaws. By the end of the first year, relatively refined chewing jaw motions and incisor teeth allow controlled bites of soft solids.[18]

The ability to transfer objects to and across the midline, exploration of objects and food by bringing them to the mouth, and refinement of pincer grasp all develop progressively after 6 months and support self-feeding skills.[18] Finger-feeding skills and desire are often particularly strong after 9 months of age, and preference to this over being spoon fed by an adult may be quite firm. Because effective handling of a spoon, however, does not typically develop until after 12 months of age, parents may be encouraged to offer as many "finger foods" as possible, to encourage self-feeding and to support the child's emerging autonomy. Cup skills, with assistance, progressively improve between 7 and 8 months of age, and by 12 months of age, most infants are able to hold a cup with 2 hands and take several swallows without choking.[18] The ubiquitous use of "sippy cups" facilitates cup-drinking skills while minimizing spillage, but the spill-proof designs may also encourage grazing behavior for toddlers allowed to have continuous access to them.

The pace at which infants obtain oral motor skills and accept new tastes and textures varies as widely as any other aspect of human development. Parents should be encouraged to respect the pace their infant dictates, and they should be reassured that infants who are otherwise developmentally normal will eventually be able and willing to handle a wide variety of textures and tastes. One study found that infantile "feeding disorders" followed a final common pathway, linking an interaction between food refusal and intrusive feeding by care providers. A bidirectional pattern leading to disrupted feeding behaviors was described: either intrusive feeding by parents led to food refusal, or an episode of infant feeding refusal was followed by an inappropriate parental response, which then was associated with persistent disordered feeding[19] (see Chapter 26).

The period from 6 to 8 months of age is often referred to as a critical window for initiating complementary feeding because of the developmental processes that are occurring at this time. As the infant's own desire for autonomy progresses toward the end of the first year and through the second year, the potential for conflict around "being fed" versus self-feeding increases.

When to Initiate Complementary Feeding
Several organizations, including the World Health Organization (WHO), have recommended exclusive breastfeeding through 6 months of age. The AAP supports

this recommendation, stipulating introduction of complementary foods at approximately 6 months of age (see Chapter 3). The most recent systematic review on the optimal duration of exclusive breastfeeding concluded that exclusive breastfeeding for 6 months is associated with less morbidity from nonhospitalized gastrointestinal tract disease, and possibly respiratory disease, compared with mixed feeding by 3 to 4 months of age. Growth deficits were not identified with exclusive breastfeeding for 6 months or longer, although sample sizes were rarely adequate to rule out small effects on growth.[20] The review concluded that the evidence demonstrated no apparent risks, as a general recommendation, for exclusive breastfeeding for 6 months in both industrialized and developing nations. Of note, however, the report also emphasized the distinction between recommendations for populations and those for individual infants. All individual infants should be monitored for growth faltering or other adverse effects, and appropriate interventions should be undertaken when indicated. Similarly, caregivers should take into consideration the wide variations in the attainment of oral motor skills in infants when deciding when to initiate complementary feeding, as noted previously.

The data supporting an effect of timing of complementary feeding on later obesity are limited, and findings from studies have provided mixed results.[21] Introduction of complementary foods prior to 4 months of age is most consistently identified as contributing to later overweight.[22-24] Such feeding practices may contribute to higher early rates of weight gain, which have been associated with later overweight and obesity.[25]

Timing of complementary feeding has also been examined in relation to prevention of atopic disease. One evidence review comparing introduction of complementary foods at 3 to 4 months of age versus 6 months of age found no protective effect of the later introduction.[20] A large study from Finland reported neither protection from exclusive breastfeeding nor late introduction of complementary foods to be protective against allergic sensitization at 5 years of age.[26] The AAP has, likewise, concluded that evidence does not support a strong relationship between timing of complementary feeding and development of atopic disease.[27] A systematic review by the Cochrane group also found no significant reduction in atopic outcomes associated with exclusive breastfeeding for 6 months.[20]

For reasons described previously, iron and zinc deficiencies are not uncommon in older breastfed infants, with the risk progressively increasing after 6 months if nutrient-rich complementary foods or supplements are not consumed. One study in the United States specifically examined the risk of iron deficiency in toddlers associated with full breastfeeding for 6 versus 4 months by analyzing data from the National Health and Nutrition Examination Survey (NHANES) III (1988-1994) and from the 1999-2002 NHANES data set. A significantly lower risk of iron deficiency (low ferritin) without anemia was found in those who were exclusively breastfed for 4 to 5 months versus those who were exclusively breastfed for 6 months or longer without any dietary supplements of iron.[28] National surveillance data are not available in the United States for infants younger than 12 months. In a small study of exclusively breastfed infants who started complementary foods between 5 and 6 months of age, 36% of the infants had iron deficiency (ferritin <12 µg/L), and 20% were anemic at 9 months of age.[29] Although plasma zinc is not a very sensitive biomarker of zinc status, 36% of the infants also had zinc concentrations below the suggested cutoff of 65 µg/dL, suggesting at least mild zinc deficiency in these 9-month-olds.[29]

Current Practice for Complementary Feedings

Introduction of solid foods prior to 4 months of age in the United States has reportedly decreased over the past decade from 26% to 10%.[30,31] Longitudinal data of US infants reported by the Infant Feeding Practices Study II, conducted by the Centers for Disease Control and Prevention and the Food and Drug Administration, indicated that by 4 months of age, 40% of infants had consumed cereal, and 17% had consumed fruits or vegetables. By 5 months' completed age, the majority (approximately 80%) were receiving solid foods. Compared with those not fed solids at 4 months of age, infants with such early introduction of complementary foods were more likely to have discontinued breastfeeding by 6 months of age and to have reported intakes of sugary or fatty foods at the 12-month data point.[1]

Which Complementary Foods to Feed

In its guidelines for complementary feeding, with an emphasis on resource-limited settings and populations with generally high rates of breastfeeding, the WHO emphasizes the importance of variety in food choices. Specifically, the WHO recommends that flesh foods, including meats, poultry, and fish, as well as eggs, be eaten daily or as often as possible. Diets with adequate fat content are recommended. Vegetarian diets are noted to be unlikely to meet nutrient needs at this age unless nutrient supplements or fortified products are used. Recommendations also include avoidance of low-nutrient drinks, such as teas, coffee, and sugary drinks such as soda; limits on juice are also recommended to avoid displacement of more nutritious foods.[32]

In contrast, in industrialized nations such as the United States, emphasis has been on iron-fortified cereals, followed by fruits or vegetables, with later introduction of meats. The ready availability and common use of infant formulas reduces the reliance on specific choices of complementary foods. As more infants are breastfed in the United States, however, the importance of complementary feeding patterns has gained more attention. Data from the Infant Feeding Practices Study II indicate that nearly 20% of 6-month-old breastfed or mixed-fed (human milk and formula fed) infants had received neither iron-fortified cereals nor meat in the past week, and 15% had never received cereal, meat, or supplements. Despite being at the highest risk of iron deficiency, exclusively breastfed infants at 6 months of age had the highest rates of noncompliance with recommendations for iron intake, with 70% having less than 2 servings of infant cereal, meat, or formula and receiving iron supplements less than daily. Compliance with recommendations for iron intake was even lower for preterm breastfed and mixed-fed infants.[33]

Although at the 9-month data collection point for the Infant Feeding Practices Study II, more than 80% of all infants received "baby cereal" (presumed to be iron fortified); this decreased to less than 50% by 12 months. Additionally, at 9 months, approximately 70% received "other" cereals and starches, which would not necessarily be fortified with iron (or zinc) to levels recommended for infants. By 1 year, this category had increased to more than 90%.[2] Consistent with these observations were the findings from the Feeding Infants and Toddlers Study (FITS), a cross-sectional survey of a random sample of US children from birth to 4 years of age. Compared with data obtained in the 2002 Feeding Infants and Toddlers Study, in 2008 significantly fewer 9- to 11.9-month-old infants were consuming iron-fortified infant cereals, but more than 40% were consuming noninfant cereals.[31] At the same time, meat consumption decreased by nearly 80% between the 2 survey periods, while yogurt consumption (a poor source of iron) increased significantly.[31] Thus, common complementary feeding practices in the United States often are not consistent with the distinctly different risk profiles for micronutrient deficiencies in breastfed infants, compared with formula–fed infants.

With the recognition of the potential value of meats as a source of heme iron with enhanced iron absorption and as a source of bioavailable zinc, the AAP encourages consumption of meats, vegetables with higher iron content, and iron-fortified cereals for infants and toddlers between 6 and 24 months of age.[14] Data are lacking to determine actual amounts of foods needed to achieve absorption to meet iron or zinc physiologic requirements.[34] The complexity of iron absorption, in particular, and the dependence of iron requirements on such factors as iron stores at birth, growth rate, gender, iron status, and the adverse effects of infection on absorption emphasize the challenge of determining adequacy of iron status by dietary intake alone (see Chapter 19 for recommendations for screening iron status). For zinc, limited absorption data suggest that intakes approximating the estimated average requirement of 2.5 mg/day for populations or Recommended Dietary Allowance of 3 mg/day for individuals will result in adequate absorbed zinc for healthy infants and toddlers.[34]

A good variety of healthy foods generally promotes good nutritional status for infants and toddlers. Because the digestive and absorptive functions are mature well before 6 months of age, there is no reason to introduce whole food groups sequentially. Rather, considering the dynamic changes in infants' nutritional needs in the second half of the first year of life, gradual introduction of foods from all groups may be a better paradigm. To identify adverse reactions, new foods should be introduced singly every 3 to 5 days. Beyond that, however, introduction of new foods from different food groups should proceed once complementary feeding is initiated. For example, an infant cereal may be the first food, followed by meats, fruits, and vegetables. Progression to foods from 4 food groups (cereals, meats, fruits, and vegetables) could reasonably be achieved within the first month of complementary feeding. Amounts of each food and variety are expected to gradually increase with the infant's age. Infants have been demonstrated to accept cereals and meats equally well after 6 months of age.[29]

Food choices to be encouraged, whether home or commercially prepared, are those with no added salt or sugar. Fats, particularly healthy fats, such as those containing mono- and polyunsaturated fatty acids, should not be discouraged. The findings of the 2008 Feeding Infants and Toddlers Study suggest that nearly one quarter of toddlers had intakes of fat below recommended levels.[12] Energy intakes of older infants and toddlers are notoriously difficult to measure, and energy requirements are difficult to estimate. Reported energy intakes may have exceeded the estimated requirements for 20% to 30% of infants and toddlers in the Feeding Infants and Toddlers Study, but these figures must be interpreted cautiously.[12] Appropriateness of energy intake for an individual child is best judged by appropriateness of growth.

How to Guide Complementary Feeding

The following guiding principles are provided for introduction of complementary foods and for the progression through the second year of life.

1. **Choose first foods that provide key nutrients and help meet energy needs.**
   As discussed in the preceding sections, iron and zinc are the micronutrients that become limiting for primarily breastfed infants, and they are also the most likely to be low in the diets of older infants. To provide these nutrients, iron- and zinc-fortified infant cereals and meats are excellent first foods and are equally well accepted by infants.[29] The suggested intake is approximately 2 servings/day for cereal (2 tablespoons/serving) or meat (1-2 oz/day meat or 1-2 small jars of commercially prepared meat/day).

2. **Introduce one "single-ingredient" new food at a time**, from any food group. Do not introduce other new foods for 3 to 5 days to observe for possible allergic reactions or intolerance. Foods most commonly associated with infant allergies are cow milk, eggs, soy, peanuts, tree nuts (and seeds), wheat, fish, and shell fish. Although solid foods should not be introduced before approximately 6 months of age, there is no current convincing evidence that delaying the introduction of those foods most associated with allergy beyond this period has a significant protective effect on the development of atopic disease. For some food allergies, there may be a window of time after which introduction of the food actually increases the risk of allergy (see Chapter 35).

3. **Introduce a variety of foods.** By 7 to 8 months of age, infants should be consuming foods from all food groups. The food variety should progressively increase over next several months. Parents should be encouraged to offer foods multiple times ($\geq$10 exposures) for infants and toddlers to become accepting.[35]

4. **Withhold cow milk (and other "milks" not formulated for infants) during the first year of life.** Fresh cow milk has been associated with low-grade intestinal blood loss in infants and, thus, is not recommended. Liquids, so-called "milks," based on plant foods (eg, soy, rice, almond, or hemp) should not be used as a human milk or infant formula substitute (ie, when human milk or infant formula provides a significant portion of daily energy intake). The caloric density of these products is typically lower than that of human milk or infant formula; protein quality is low; products are not fortified with micronutrients to levels recommended for infants and young children; and some contain high levels of phytate, which bind iron, zinc, and calcium. Use of such alternative fluids as major component of the diet at these ages has been associated with protein energy malnutrition and with growth faltering.[36]

5. **During the second year of life, low-fat milk may be considered** if growth and weight gain are appropriate or especially if weight gain is excessive or family history is positive for obesity, dyslipidemia, or cardiovascular disease[37] (see Chapter 33). Total daily milk intake of 16 to 24 oz is appropriate to meet calcium needs. Intakes above 32 oz/day predispose to iron deficiency.

6. **Juice consumption should be limited.** No juice should be offered before 6 months of age, and it should not be served in a nursing bottle. Total daily volume should not exceed 4 to 6 oz/day for children younger than 6 years.[38] Juice drinks, which typically contain added sweeteners, should be discouraged. Dilution of juice with water may encourage excessive fluid consumption and grazing behaviors.

7. **Ensure that homemade complementary foods are prepared in a safe manner.** Home preparation of pureed or mashed table foods is practical for many families. Practices to encourage include:
   a. Matching texture and consistency to infant's oral motor skills;
   b. Use thickened purees to enhance caloric density;
   c. Provide healthy "single ingredient" foods, especially while total variety is still limited;
   d. Avoid added sugar or salt;
   e. Avoid foods that could be choking or aspiration risks (hot dogs, nuts, grapes, raisins, raw carrots, popcorn, hard candies);
   f. Use caution when using microwave to warm foods; check temperature prior to feeding to infants.
8. **Encourage infant's involvement in feeding process.** By 9 months of age, infants should be presented with finger foods, and a cup may be introduced. Effective use of utensils develops progressively after approximately 12 months of age.
9. **Encourage "responsive feeding," watching for and responding to infant's hunger and satiety cues.** General feeding practices to encourage:
   a. Avoid intrusive behaviors (eg, or force feeding) by care providers;
   b. Establish routines for meals and snacks in a predictable schedule, typically allowing 2 to 3 hours between eating and drinking opportunities, resulting in eating 5 to 6 times per day (eg, 3 meals, 2-3 snacks);
   c. Avoid "grazing" behaviors with snacks or liquids by allowing constant access to foods and drinks; eat only in high chair, at table, or at other designated areas;
   d. Limit meals to 15 to 20 minutes, as appropriate for infants' or toddlers' attention spans;
   e. Praise eating but resist attention for not eating; withholding or rewarding with food as means of punishment or rewards is not appropriate;
   f. Minimize distractions during meal times (TV, videos, pets, etc).
10. **Monitor appropriateness of growth as a guide to adequacy of complementary feeding practices.** Avoid giving calorie goals to parents, which encourages overemphasis on numbers and may lead to intrusive feeding behaviors. The focus should be on the quality of the feeding environment, feeding routines, and behaviors and food choices.

References

1. Black RE, Allen LH, Bhutta ZA, et al. Maternal and child undernutrition: global and regional exposures and health consequences. *Lancet*. 2008;371(9608):243-260

2. Grummer-Strawn LM, Scanlon KS, Fein SB. Infant feeding and feeding transitions during the first year of life. *Pediatrics*. 2008;122(Suppl 2):S36-S42

3. Shealy KR, Scanlon KS, Labiner-Wolfe J, Fein SB, Grummer-Strawn LM. Characteristics of breastfeeding practices among US mothers. *Pediatrics*. 2008;122(Suppl 2):S50-S5

4. Butte NF, Wong WW, Hopkinson JM, Heinz CJ, Mehta NR, Smith EO. Energy requirements derived from total energy expenditure and energy deposition during the first 2 y of life. *Am J Clin Nutr*. 2000;72(6):1558-1569

5. Li R, Fein SB, Grummer-Strawn LM. Do infants fed from bottles lack self-regulation of milk intake compared with directly breastfed infants? *Pediatrics*. 2010;125(6):e1386-e1393

6. Heinig MJ, Nommsen LA, Peerson JM, Lonnerdal B, Dewey KG. Energy and protein intakes of breast-fed and formula-fed infants during the first year of life and their association with growth velocity: the DARLING Study. *Am J Clin Nutr*. 1993;58(2):152-161

7. Institute of Medicine. *WIC Food Packages: Time for a Change*. Washington, DC: National Academies Press; 2005

8. Brown KH, Sanchez-Grinan M, Perez F, Peerson JM, Ganoza L, Stern JS. Effects of dietary energy density and feeding frequency on total daily energy intakes of recovering malnourished children. *Am J Clin Nutr*. 1995;62(1):13-18

9. Dewey KG, Brown KH. Update on technical issues concerning complementary feeding of young children in developing countries and implications for intervention programs. *Food Nutr Bull*. 2003;24(1):5-28

10. Fomon SJ. Requirements and recommended dietary intakes of protein during infancy. *Pediatr Res*. 1991;30:391-395.

11. Institute of Medicine. *Dietary Reference Intakes: The Essential Guide to Nutrient Requirements*. Washington, DC: National Academies Press; 2006

12. Butte NF, Fox MK, Briefel RR, et al. Nutrient intakes of US infants, toddlers, and preschoolers meet or exceed dietary reference intakes. *J Am Diet Assoc*. 2010;110(12 Suppl):S27-S37

13. Simell O, Niinikoski H, Ronnemaa T, et al. Cohort Profile: the STRIP Study (Special Turku Coronary Risk Factor Intervention Project), an Infancy-onset Dietary and Life-style Intervention Trial. *Int J Epidemiol*. 2009;38(3):650-655

14. Baker RD; Greer FR; American Academy of Pediatrics, Committee on Nutrition. Clinical report: diagnosis and prevention of iron deficiency and iron-deficiency anemia in infants and young children (0-3 years of age). *Pediatrics*. 2010;126(5):1040-1050

15. Krebs NF, Hambidge KM. Complementary feeding: clinically relevant factors affecting timing and composition. *Am J Clin Nutr*. 2007;85(Suppl):639S-645S

16. Wagner CL, Greer FR. Prevention of rickets and vitamin D deficiency in infants, children, and adolescents. *Pediatrics*. 2008;122:1142-1152

II

17. Chalouhi C, Faesch S, Anthoine-Milhomme MC, Fulla Y, Dulac O, Cheron G. Neurological consequences of vitamin B12 deficiency and its treatment. *Pediatr Emerg Care*. 2008;24(8):538-541

18. Pridham KF. Feeding behavior of 6- to 12-month-old infants: assessment and sources of parental information. *J Pediatr*. 1990;117(2 Pt 2):S174-S180

19. Levine A, Bachar L, Tsangen Z, et al. Screening criteria for diagnosis of infantile feeding disorders as a cause of poor feeding or food refusal. *J Pediatr Gastroenterol Nutr*. 2011;52(5):563-568

20. Kramer MS, Kakuma R. Optimal duration of exclusive breastfeeding. *Cochrane Database Syst Rev*. 2012;(8):CD003517

21. Burdette HL, Whitaker RC, Hall WC, Daniels SR. Breastfeeding, introduction of complementary foods, and adiposity at 5 y of age. *Am J Clin Nutr*. 2006;83(3):550-558

22. Taveras EM, Gillman MW, Kleinman K, Rich-Edwards JW, Rifas-Shiman SL. Racial/ethnic differences in early-life risk factors for childhood obesity. *Pediatrics*. 2010;125(4):686-695

23. Huh SY, Rifas-Shiman SL, Taveras EM, Oken E, Gillman MW. Timing of solid food introduction and risk of obesity in preschool-aged children. *Pediatrics*. 2011;127(3):e544-e551

24. Baker JL, Michaelsen KF, Rasmussen KM, Sorensen TI. Maternal prepregnant body mass index, duration of breastfeeding, and timing of complementary food introduction are associated with infant weight gain. *Am J Clin Nutr*. 2004;80(6):1579-1588

25. Stettler N, Iotova V. Early growth patterns and long-term obesity risk. *Curr Opin Clin Nutr Metab Care*. 2010;13(3):294-299

26. Nwaru BI, Erkkola M, Ahonen S, et al. Age at the introduction of solid foods during the first year and allergic sensitization at age 5 years. *Pediatrics*. 2010;125(1):50-59

27. Greer FR, Sicherer SH, Burks AW. Effects of early nutritional interventions on the development of atopic disease in infants and children: the role of maternal dietary restriction, breastfeeding, timing of introduction of complementary foods, and hydrolyzed formulas. *Pediatrics*. 2008;121(1):183-191

28. Chantry CJ, Howard CR, Auinger P. Full breastfeeding duration and risk for iron deficiency in U.S. infants. *Breastfeed Med*. 2007;2(2):63-73

29. Krebs NF, Westcott JE, Butler N, Robinson C, Bell M, Hambidge KM. Meat as a first complementary food for breastfed infants: feasibility and impact on zinc intake and status. *J Pediatr Gastroenterol Nutr*. 2006;42(2):207-214

30. Hendricks K, Briefel R, Novak T, Ziegler P. Maternal and child characteristics associated with infant and toddler feeding practices. *J Am Diet Assoc*. 2006;106(1 Suppl):S135-S148

31. Siega-Riz AM, Deming DM, Reidy KC, Fox MK, Condon E, Briefel RR. Food consumption patterns of infants and toddlers: where are we now? *J Am Diet Assoc*. 2010;110(12 Suppl):S38-S51

32. Pan American Health Organization/World Health Organization. *Guiding Principles for Complementary Feeding of the Breastfed Child*. Washington, DC: Pan American Health Organization; 2003

33. Dee DL, Sharma AJ, Cogswell ME, Grummer-Strawn LM, Fein SB, Scanlon KS. Sources of supplemental iron among breastfed infants during the first year of life. *Pediatrics.* 2008;122(Suppl 2):S98-S104

34. Institute of Medicine, Food and Nutrition Board. *Dietary Reference Intakes for Vitamin A, Vitamin K, Boron, Chromium, Copper, Iodine, Iron, Manganese, Molybdenum, Nickel, Silicon, Vanadium and Zinc.* Washington, DC: National Academies Press; 2001

35. Sullivan SA, Birch LL. Infant dietary experience and acceptance of solid foods. *Pediatrics.* 1994;93(2):271-277

36. Liu T, Howard RM, Mancini AJ, et al. Kwashiorkor in the United States: fad diets, perceived and true milk allergy, and nutritional ignorance. *Arch Dermatol.* 2001;137(5):630-636

37. National Heart, Lung, and Blood Institute. *Expert Panel on Integrated Guidelines for Cardiovascular Health and Risk Reduction in Children and Adolescents.* November 2011. Available at: www.nhlbi.nih.gov/guidelines/cvd_ped/. Accessed October 31, 2012

38. American Academy of Pediatrics. The use and misuse of fruit juice in pediatrics. *Pediatrics.* 2001;107(5):1210-1213. Reaffirmed October 2006

Feeding the Child and Adolescent

III

Chapter 7

Feeling the Child

Introduction

Following infancy, children experience developmental progress that is fundamentally tied to the evolution and establishment of eating behavior. In contrast to infancy, however, the period from 1 year of age to puberty is a slower period of physical growth. Birth weight is tripled during the first year of life but is not quadrupled until 2 years of age; birth length is increased by 50% during the first year but is not doubled until 4 years of age. Although growth patterns vary in individual children, children from 2 years of age to puberty gain an average of 2 to 3 kg (4.5–6.5 lb) and grow 5 to 8 cm (2.5–3.5 in) in height per year.[1,2] As growth rates decline during the preschool years, appetites often decrease, and food intake may appear erratic and unpredictable. Parental confusion and concern are not uncommon. Frequently expressed concerns include the limited variety of foods ingested, dawdling and distractibility, limited consumption of vegetables and meats, and a desire for too many sweets. Parental concern regarding children's eating behaviors, whether warranted or unfounded, should be addressed with developmentally appropriate nutrition information. Anticipatory guidance for parents and caregivers is key to preventing many feeding problems.

An important goal of early childhood nutrition is to ensure children's present and future health by fostering the development of healthy eating behaviors. Parents and caregivers are called on to offer foods at developmentally appropriate moments—matching the child's age and stage of development with his or her nutrition needs. Appropriate limits for children's eating are set by adhering to a division of responsibility in child feeding.[3] Parents and caregivers are responsible for providing a variety of nutritious foods, defining the structure and timing of meals, and creating a developmentally appropriate mealtime environment that facilitates eating and social exchange. Children are responsible for participating in choices about food selection and should take primary responsibility for determining how much is consumed at each eating occasion.

Toddlerhood

Toddler eating patterns are characterized by independence both in terms of the physical skills that facilitate mobility and self-feeding and the acquisition of language skills that enable the toddler to verbally express eating preferences and needs. Between 7 and 12 months of age, most infants become capable of grasping food with their hands, removing food from the spoon with their lips, and making the transition to eating soft foods or those with tiny lumps without gagging.[3,4] By 15 months of age, the toddler is generally capable of self-feeding firmer table foods and drinking from a "sippy" cup without help.[5] Weaning from the bottle should occur during the transition from infancy to toddlerhood. Bottle use beyond 12 to 15 months of age should be discouraged, given the associated risks of iron deficiency,[5,6] obesity,[7,8] and dental caries. Avoiding the use of juice in bottles and bottles during sleeping, in particular, reduces exposure to sugars and risk of caries[9] (see Chapter 50: Nutrition and Oral Health). Between the first and second year, infants move from gross motor skills required for holding a spoon to developing fine motor skills needed to scoop food, dip food, and bring the spoon to the mouth with limited spilling.[3,4] These skills allow children to begin to participate in family meals, including serving themselves with assistance. Supporting self-feeding is thought to encourage the maintenance of self-regulation of energy intake, the mastery of feeding skills, and the socialization of eating behaviors. Given earlier opportunities for mastery of self-feeding skills, the older toddler (2 years) is ready to consume most of the same foods offered to the rest of the family, with some extra preparation to prevent choking and gagging.

Toddlers continually explore cause-and-effect relationships. In the eating domain, this translates into using utensils to move foods and using food and eating to elicit responses from the parent. These interactions are part of children's learning about the family's and the culture's standards for behavior; children as young as 2 years have demonstrated the ability to evaluate their actions according to its badness or goodness in relation to parental standards for behavior.[10] An example of this type of learning is the toddler's response of "uh-oh" to dropping food or drink on the floor. Toddlers seek attention and will find ways, positive or negative, to engage the notice of parents. Helping parents focus on children's positive eating behaviors, rather than on food refusals or negative conduct, will keep mealtimes pleasant and productive.

Preventing Choking

Gagging and choking are realistic concerns for infants and young children,[11] with 69% of food-related choking injuries and 79% of choking fatalities occurring in US children younger than 3 years.[12] Incomplete dentition, small airway diameter, immature swallowing coordination, and high activity levels during eating (eg, running) make young children particularly vulnerable to choking. Foods that are small and cylindrical as well as hard, highly elastic, slippery, or crunchy present the greatest risk.[13] Analysis of US choking-related injuries and fatalities among young children identified hot dogs, peanuts/nuts, seeds, hard candy/chewing gum, carrots, popcorn, and apples as the highest-risk foods.[11,12] Anticipatory guidance for caregivers should include selecting appropriate foods, adequately processing foods offered, and supervising children during eating.[13] Toddlers should be given foods that gradually build self-feeding skills—starting with soft, mashed, or ground foods and building to prepared table foods by 12 to 18 months. Soft, round foods, such as hot dogs, grapes, and string cheese, must be cut into very small pieces or avoided entirely.

AAP

More than 10 000 emergency department visits annually are attributable to food-related choking for children younger than 14 years.

Risk factors for choking include age younger than 4 years, swallowing and neuromuscular disorders, developmental delay, and traumatic brain injury. Behavioral risk factors, such as walking or running while eating, laughing and talking with food in the mouth, and eating quickly, may also increase risk of choking.

High-risk foods for choking in all young children include: hot dogs, hard candy, peanuts/nuts, seeds, whole grapes, raw carrots, apples, popcorn, chunks of peanut butter, marshmallows, chewing gum, and sausages.

American Academy of Pediatrics, Committee on Injury, Violence, and Poison Prevention. Prevention of choking among children. *Pediatrics.* 2010;125(3):601-607

Parents or caregivers should always be present during feeding, and children should be seated in a high chair during mealtimes. The mealtime environment should ideally be free of distractions like television, loud music, and activities. Eating in the car should be discouraged, because (1) aiding the child quickly is difficult; and (2) with obesity prevention in mind, eating should not be encouraged in environments that are not related to mealtime (ie, in cars, in front of television/computers, etc). Finally, analgesics used to numb the gums during teething may anesthetize the posterior pharynx. Children who receive such medications should be carefully observed during feeding.

Food Acceptance

Preferences for the taste of sweet have been observed shortly after birth,[14] and young children show the capacity to readily form preferences for the flavors of energy-rich foods.[15] Early experiences in utero and early infant feeding, via transmission of aromatic compounds from the maternal diet into amniotic fluid and human milk,[16] also strongly influence flavor and food acceptance. These experiences are believed to set the stage for later food choices and may be important in establishing lifelong food habits. Acceptance of some foods, like vegetables, is not immediate and may only occur after 8 to 10 exposures to those foods in a noncoercive manner.[17-19] Many parents are not aware of the lengthy but normal course of food acceptance in young children; approximately 25% of mothers with toddlers reported offering new foods only 1 or 2 times before deciding whether the child liked it, and approximately half made similar judgments after serving new foods 3 to 5 times.[20] Touching, smelling, and playing with new foods as well as putting them in the mouth and spitting them back out are normal exploratory behaviors that precede acceptance and even willingness to taste and swallow foods.[17] Beginning around 2 years of age, children become characteristically resistant to consuming new foods— and sometimes dietary variety seemingly diminishes to a handful well-accepted favorites. In a study of 3022 infants and toddlers ranging from 6 to 24 months, half of mothers with 19- to 24-month-old toddlers reported picky eating, whereas only 19% reported picky eating among 4- to 6-month-old infants.[20] It should be stressed to families that children's failure to immediately accept new foods is a normal stage of child development that, although potentially frustrating, can be dealt with effectively with knowledge, consistency, and patience. Recent studies have shown that acceptance can be promoted by offering children very small tastes of new and previously disliked vegetables.[21,22] Further, whereas pressuring children to eat can produce dislike,[23] noncoercive strategies that emphasize "liking" over "eating" appear to promote food acceptance, include enthusiastic modeling,[24-27] praising children for trying new foods, providing small token rewards (eg, stickers),[28-30] reading books with food-related characters and themes,[31,32] and offering foods with "dips" or other preferred accompaniments.[33] There is some suggestion that exposure to a variety of healthful foods and textures during weaning and toddlerhood acts to promote acceptance into childhood.[34-36]

Although toddlers are in a generally explorative phase, they can go on food "jags," during which certain foods are preferentially consumed to the exclusion of others.[37] Parents who become concerned when a "good eater" in infancy becomes a "fair to poor" or "picky" eater as a toddler should be reassured that this change in acceptance is developmentally normative and, in most cases, lasts for a relatively short duration (<2 years).[38]

Preschool-Aged Children

The preschool-aged child has more fully developed motor skills, handles utensils and cups efficiently, and can sit at the table for meals. Because growth has slowed, their interest in eating may be unpredictable, with characteristic periods of disinterest in food. Their attention span may limit the amount of time that they can spend in the mealtime setting; however, they should be encouraged to attend and partake in family meals for reasonable periods of time (15–20 minutes)—whether they choose to eat or not.

As children move from toddlerhood to the preschool years, they become increasingly aware of the environment in which eating occurs, particularly the social aspects of eating. By interacting with and observing other children and adults, preschool-aged children become more aware of when and where eating takes place, what types of foods are consumed at specific eating occasions (ie, ice cream is a dessert food), and how much of those foods are consumed at each eating occasion (ie, "finish your vegetables"). Consequently, children's food selection and intake patterns are influenced by a variety of environmental cues, including the time of day[39]; energy-dense foods (defined as high amounts of energy per volume of food and drink in grams)[40-42] and large portion sizes[43-45] of foods; parental feeding styles and controlling child feeding practices, including restriction and pressure to eat[46,47]; and the preferences and eating behaviors of importance to others.[26,48,49]

During the preschool period, most children have moved from eating on demand to a more adult-like eating pattern, consuming 3 meals each day as well as several smaller snacks. Although children's intake from meal-to-meal may appear to be erratic, children show the capacity to adjust food intake such that total daily energy intake remains fairly constant.[50] Children show the ability to respond to the energy content of foods by adjusting their intake to reflect the energy density of the diet.[51-54] It is important to note, however, that this ability can be diminished when large food portion sizes of energy dense foods are frequently offered. In contrast to their skills in regulation of food intake, young children do not appear to have the innate ability to choose a well-balanced diet.[37,55] Rather, they depend on adults to offer them a variety of nutritious and developmentally appropriate foods and to model the consumption of those foods.

School-Aged Children

During the school years, increases in memory and logic abilities are accompanied by reading, writing, and math skills. This developmental period is one in which basic nutrition education concepts can be successfully introduced. Emphasis should be placed on enjoying the taste of fruits and vegetables rather than to focus exclusively on their healthfulness, because young children tend to think of taste and healthfulness as mutually exclusive.[56] Socially, children are learning rules and conventions and also begin to develop friendships. During the period between 8 and 11 years of age, children begin making more peer comparisons, including those pertaining to weight and body shape. An awareness of the physical self begins to emerge, and comparisons with social norms for weight and weight status begin to occur. During this period, children vary greatly in weight, body shape, and growth rate, and teasing of those who fall outside the perceived norms for weight status frequently occurs. Friends and those outside the family can alter food attitudes and choices, which may have either a beneficial or a negative effect on the nutritional status of a given child.

School-aged children have increased freedom over their food choices and, during the school year, eat at least 1 meal per day away from the home. These choices, such as the decision to consume school lunch or a snack bar meal, may affect dietary quality.[57]

Eating Patterns and Nutrient Needs

Toddlers

Toddlers eat, on average, 7 times each day, with snacks representing approximately one quarter of daily energy intake. Between 15 and 24 months of age, approximately 59% of energy comes from table foods.[58] Milk constitutes the leading source of daily energy (approx 25%), macronutrients, and many vitamins and minerals, including vitamins A and D, calcium, and zinc.[59] Recent data indicate that a majority of US toddlers' diets contain adequate amounts of protein, carbohydrate, and fat.[60] Alternatively, fruit and vegetable intake are notably low or absent among some toddlers. Approximately one third of 2-year-olds do not consume vegetables or fruit (other than fruit juice) on a given day.[61] French fries remain the most commonly consumed vegetable among 2-year-olds.[61] Finally, close to one quarter of 2-year-olds consume salty snacks daily and nearly half consume higher-than-recommended levels of sodium.[60,61] Micronutrient-rich animal-source proteins should be encouraged in light of a recent focus on iron deficiency (ID) and iron deficiency anemia (IDA) in young children, which remains relatively common in toddlers (6.6%–15.2%), depending on race/ethnicity and socioeconomic status, according to a recent clinical report from the American Academy of Pediatrics (AAP).[62] These findings collectively suggest that anticipatory guidance should focus on encouraging intake of whole fruits and vegetables as well as lower-sodium foods at snacks and meals and should further stress that young children have high nutrient needs and relatively low energy requirements, leaving little room for sugar- and fat-dense foods (Table 7.1).[60]

Table 7.1.
Key Eating and Activity Concerns

Toddlers and Preschoolers	School-Aged Children
• Choosing appropriate weaning foods • Perceived decreases in appetite • Avoiding juice, sugar-sweetened beverage consumption • Avoiding energy-dense, nutrient-poor snack consumption • Encouraging fruit and vegetable acceptance • Maintaining appropriate routines for eating and physical activity • Limiting television and screen time	• Avoiding beverages and foods with added sugar • Limiting high-energy, nutrient-poor snacks • Increasing fruit and vegetable intakes • Increasing fiber intake • Increasing milk consumption • Limiting television and screen time • Preoccupation with dieting and body image

Preschool- and School-Aged Children

Fruit and vegetable intake among children is also well below current recommendations.[63,64] As such, a majority of preschool-aged children consume less than the recommended amounts of fiber and potassium,[60] with low-fiber fruits, such as applesauce and fruit cocktail, having the greatest contributions to daily fiber intake.[65] Alternatively, children's intakes of "extra" or "empty" calories from solid fats and added sugars are notably high,[60,63,64,66] representing nearly 40% of daily energy consumed by US children 2 to 18 years of age.[67] On a given day, approximately half of US 3-year-olds consume sweetened beverages, and three quarters consume desserts or candies,[61] which are top sources of added sugars. This results in higher energy intakes in preschool- and school-aged children.[40-42,68] Young children who consume high levels of added sugar (>25% of daily energy) have lower micronutrient intakes and may be at greater risk of inadequate intakes of number of micronutrients, particularly vitamins A and E, calcium, and potassium.[69] Greater intake of energy-rich, nutrient-poor foods accompanies an increase in the frequency of snacking. A shift to foods prepared and consumed away from home results in increasing food portion sizes.[70-73]

Energy Needs

Dietary Reference Intakes (DRIs) are a set of nutrient-based reference values that can be used for planning and assessing diets of individuals and groups[74] (see Appendix E). The DRIs also include data on safety and efficacy, reduction of chronic degenerative disease (in addition to the avoidance of nutritional deficiency), and data on upper levels of intake (where available). The Estimated Average Requirement (EAR) refers to the median usual intake value that is estimated to meet the requirements of one half of apparently healthy individuals of a given age and sex over time. The Recommended Dietary Allowance (RDA) refers to the level of intake that is adequate for nearly all healthy individuals of a given sex and age (97%–98%). When the EAR or RDA has not been established, an Adequate Intake (AI) is provided and is based on average intake of a nutrient based on intakes of healthy people. The Tolerable Upper Intake Level (UL) is the highest level of continuing daily nutrient intake that is likely to pose no risk of adverse health effects in almost all individuals. The UL, however, is *not* intended to be a recommended level of intake. Using the age- and sex-specific EAR, it is possible to make a quantitative statistical assessment of the adequacy of an individual's usual intake of a nutrient and to assess the safety of an individual's usual intake by comparison with the UL.

Energy needs are highly variable in children and depend on basal metabolism, rate of growth, physical activity, body size, sex, and onset of puberty (see also Chapter 14: Energy). Many nutrient requirements depend on energy needs and intake. Micronutrients that are most likely to be low or deficient in the diets of

III

young children are iron, zinc, vitamin E, and potassium.[60,75-77] Of note, intakes of synthetic folate, preformed vitamin A, zinc, and sodium are reported as increasingly exceeding ULs for a significant proportion of toddlers and preschool-aged children. This is likely related to high intakes of fortified foods and use of supplements. Although the ULs for nutrients are not meant to be used as rigid cutoffs or standards for ingestion, nutrients that are consumed in amounts over the ULs merit consideration regarding source (food-based vs supplement sources) and for potential adverse effects resulting from excessive consumption.[77]

Supplements

Parents frequently ask health care professionals whether their children need vitamin supplements, and many routinely give supplements to their children, with recent estimates suggesting that approximately 25% of toddlers and 40% preschool-aged children are given a vitamin/mineral supplement daily.[60] The children who receive the supplements are not necessarily the children who need them most, however, and, in some cases, adequate or bioavailable amounts of marginal nutrients in their diets, such as calcium and zinc, are not included in the supplement. Routine supplementation is not necessary for healthy growing children who consume a varied diet. For children and adolescents who cannot or will not consume adequate amounts of micronutrients from any dietary sources, the use of mineral supplements should be considered. Children at nutritional risk who may benefit from supplementation include those:

1. with anorexia or an inadequate appetite or who have extremely selective diets;
2. with chronic disease (eg, cystic fibrosis, inflammatory bowel disease, or hepatic disease;
3. from food-deprived families or who suffer parental neglect or abuse;
4. who participate in a dietary program for managing obesity;
5. who consume a vegetarian diet without adequate dairy products;
6. with growth faltering (failure to thrive); or
7. with developmental disabilities.

Evaluation of the dietary intake should be included in any assessment of the need for supplementation. If parents wish to give their children supplements, a standard pediatric vitamin-mineral product containing nutrients in amounts no larger than the DRI (EAR or RDA) poses little risk. Levels higher than the DRI should be discouraged and counseling provided about the potential adverse effects, especially of fat-soluble vitamins and synthetic folate. Because the taste, shape, and color of most pediatric preparations are as attractive as candy, parents should be cautioned to keep them out of reach of children (refer to Chapters 18-21 for more information on vitamins and minerals).

Dietary Fat

In recent decades, emphasis and educational efforts supporting low-fat, low-cholesterol diets for the general population have increased. A variety of health organizations, including the AAP, recommend against fat or cholesterol restriction for infants younger than 2 years, when rapid growth and development require high energy intakes.[78] For this reason, nonfat and low-fat milks are not recommended for use during the first 2 years of life. Subsequently, fat intake should be gradually decreased during the toddler years so that fat intake, averaged across several days, should provide approximately 30% of total energy.[78-81] Parents should be reassured that this level of intake is sufficient for adequate growth[82,83] and does not place children at increased risk of nutritional inadequacy.[66] Concerns have been expressed that some parents and their children may overinterpret the need to restrict their fat intakes. Indeed, 23% of toddlers 12 to 23 months of age and 47% of preschool-aged children 24 to 47 months of age consume less fat than recommended.[60] At the same time, as many as 76% of preschool-aged children consume higher levels of saturated fats than recommended. Whole milk is a primary source of solid fats in young children's diets,[67] and recent data suggest that one third of 2-year-olds and one quarter of 3-year-olds consume whole milk at least once in a day.[61] Transitioning children's diets to provide 30% energy from fat can be achieved by substituting low-fat milk products and dairy products, fruits, vegetables, beans, lean meat, poultry, fish, and whole-grain foods for those higher in fat and saturated fats.[78]

Dietary Guidelines and ChooseMyPlate

The US Department of Agriculture has developed 2 main nutritional guides that can be used in feeding children. Dietary Guidelines for Americans 2010 is intended for children 2 years and older to encourage 2 main concepts: (1) balancing calories to achieve and manage weight over time; (2) focus on consuming nutrient-dense foods and beverages.[84] A significant shift in the 2010 Dietary Guidelines was toward the adoption of the ChooseMyPlate concept, which recommends: (1) "building a healthy plate" with a focus on increasing fruit, vegetable, and whole grain consumption; and 2) choosing appropriate portion sizes. These 2 strategies are aimed at increasing nutrient density and balancing energy intakes with energy expenditure. On the whole, the Dietary Guidelines urge adults and children to eat fewer calories, be active, and make wise food choices. Parents are encouraged to: (1) help children to maintain appropriate calorie balance during childhood and adolescence and to consume adequate amounts of fruits, vegetables, and whole-grain products; (2) reduce intake of sugar-sweetened beverages; (3) monitor intakes of 100% fruit juice, especially for children who are overweight; (4) enable children to achieve at least 60 minutes of physical activity on most, if not all, days of the week and to reduce sedentary pastimes by limiting screen time; (5) reduce intakes of sodium, calories from solid fats and added sugars, and refined grain products and limit intakes of *trans* fatty acids.

ChooseMyPlate[85] (see Appendix F) translates the Dietary Guidelines into food group-based recommendations for a healthful diet for young children. In addition to helping parents understand the amounts that children need from each food group, this tool can be used to convey basic nutrition concepts for feeding young children, such as variety, moderation, the allowance for all types of foods in the diet, and appropriate portion sizes. MyPyramid, a tool previously used to translate the Dietary Guidelines for Americans into actionable steps for the consumer, continues to be available and utilized by health care and nutrition education professionals in tandem with ChooseMyPlate (see Appendix F).

Recognition that appropriate child portions are considerably smaller than those for adults is important in light of increases in standard marketplace food portions that have occurred in recent decades.[86,87] Nationally representative survey data show that daily energy intake among infants[88,89] and children[90] increases as the average food portion size consumed increases. Further, laboratory studies confirm that serving entrée portions in excess of age-appropriate norms increases energy intake at meals among children as young as 2 years.[43,44] Table 7.2 gives examples of how appropriate portion sizes differ by age across food groups. One standard for portions that may be followed for young children (2-6 years of age) is to initially offer 1 tablespoon of foods (fruits, vegetables, and protein/main course foods) for every year of age, with more provided according to appetite.[91,92]

In all settings where children are offered food and beverage, attention to food safety is paramount. Observance of good food safety protocols includes the steps in Table 7.3 (see also Chapter 53: Food Safety: Infectious Disease).

Parenting and the Feeding Relationship

Feeding can be challenging, particularly during the toddler and preschool years. Satter's division of responsibility—in which parents provide structure in mealtime, a healthy variety of foods, and opportunities for learning and the child ultimately decides how much and whether they will eat on a given eating occasion—represents a theoretical basis for implementing appropriate child-feeding practices (Table 7.4).[91]

Table 7.2.
Feeding Guide for Children

Food	Age, y 2 to 3 (1000–1400 kcal) Portion Size	Daily Amounts	4 to 6 (1200–1800 kcal) Portion Size	Daily Amounts	7 to 12 (1400–2000 kcal) Portion Size	Daily Amounts	Comments
Low-fat milk and dairy	½ cup (4 oz)	2½ cups	½–¾ cup (4–6 oz)	2½–3 cups	½–1 cup (4–8 oz)	2½–3 cups	The following may be substituted for ½ cup fluid milk: ½ oz natural cheese, 1 oz processed cheese, ½ cup low-fat yogurt, 2½ T nonfat dry milk.
Meat, fish, poultry or equivalent	1–2 oz (2–3 T)	2–4 oz	1–2 oz (4–6 T)	3–5 oz	2 oz	4–5½ oz	The following may be substituted for 1 oz meat, fish, or poultry: 1 egg, 1 T peanut butter, ¼ cup cooked beans or peas.
Vegetables and fruit							
Vegetables Cooked, Raw^a	2–3 T / Few pieces	1½ cup	4–6 T / Few pieces	1½–2½ cups	¼–½ cup / Several pieces	1½–2½ cups	Include dark green (1 cup per week) and orange vegetables (3 cups per week) for vitamin A, such as carrots, spinach, broccoli, winter squash, or greens. Limit starchy vegetables (potatoes) to 3½ cups weekly.
Fruit Raw, Canned, Juice	½–1 small / 2–3 T / 3–4 oz	1½ cup	½–1 small / 4–6 T / 4 oz	1–1½ cups	1 medium / ¼–½ cup / 4 oz	1½–2 cups	Include one vitamin C-rich fruit, vegetable, or juice, such as citrus juices, orange, grapefruit, strawberries, melon, tomato, or broccoli.
Grain products Whole grain or enriched bread / Cooked cereal / Dry cereal	½–1 slice / ¼–½ cup / ½–1 cup	3–5 oz 1½–2½ oz whole grain	1 slice / ½ cup / 1 cup	4–6 oz	1 slice / ½–1cup / 1 cup	5–6 oz	The following may be substituted for 1 slice of bread: ½ cup spaghetti, macaroni, noodles, or rice; 5 saltines; ½ English muffin or bagel; 1 tortilla; corn grits; or posole. Make ½ of grain intake *whole grains*.
Oils		4 tsp		4–5 tsp		4–6 tsp	Choose soft margarines. Avoid *trans* fats. Use liquid vegetable oils rather than solid fats.

Adapted from ChooseMyPlate at http://www.choosemyplate.gov/ and the 2010 Dietary Guidelines for Americans.

^a Do not give to young children until they can chew well.

Table 7.3
Appropriate Food Safety Protocols

- **Clean** hands, food-contact surfaces, and vegetables and fruits.
- **Separate** raw, cooked, and ready-to-eat foods while shopping, storing, and preparing foods.
- **Cook** foods to a safe temperature.
- **Chill** (refrigerate) perishable foods promptly.
- Some foods pose high risk of foodborne illness. These include raw (unpasteurized) milk, cheeses, and juices; raw or undercooked animal foods, such as seafood, meat, poultry, and eggs; and raw sprouts.

Federal Food Safety Gateway: www.foodsafety.gov and http://www.fightbac.org

Table 7.4
Feeding Guidance for Parents

Parents' responsibilities include:
- Choosing food.
- Setting mealtime routines.
- Creating positive mealtime environments with appropriate physical components (chairs, tables, utensils, cups, etc) that are free of distractions (television, loud music).
- Learning how to offer developmentally appropriate portion sizes to children.
- Modeling behaviors that they desire their children learn, like consuming a varied and healthy diet.
- Regarding mealtime as a time of learning and mastery with respect to eating and social skills, and with respect to family and community time.

Children decide which of the foods (that are selected by parents) that they will consume. They also decide how much to eat.

Parents can be reminded that:
- Foods should be offered repeatedly (up to 8-10 times) and patiently to establish children's acceptance of the food. Building food acceptance requires experience with trying (new) foods that may fall short of parental expectations for quantities to be consumed.
- Children need a routine of 3 meals and 2 snacks per day.
- Appropriate demands for mastery (like using a spoon, drinking from a cup, helping prepare meals when they are able) facilitate children's learning and sense of accomplishment.
- Pressure and coercion may have short-term benefits but will ultimately make feeding more difficult and eating less rewarding and pleasurable.

Structure and routine for eating occasions is particularly important for the young child. During the preschool years, young children begin to transition to adult-like eating patterns in which opportunities for consumption should center on the provision of routinely scheduled meals and snacks (4-6 eating occasions per day) and limited grazing. The physical environment should also be structured to promote healthy eating with distractions from television or other activities avoided. Ideally, eating should occur in a designated area of the home with a developmentally appropriate chair for the child. Family meals, with adults present and eating at least some of the same foods as children, provide occasions to learn and model healthful eating habits as well as opportunities to include the social aspects of eating.

The "job" of early childhood is to learn about the self and the external environment. Young children respond well when appropriate maturity demands are made. Children *want* to learn and *want* to eat. They also desire to participate in decisions about their own eating. To facilitate learning in the eating domain, parents should provide repeated opportunities for learning about new foods. Research suggests that it may take many exposures (up to 8-10) to help a child accept a novel food. Therefore, patience and consistency are required to facilitate children's acceptance of some foods, particularly vegetables, which are neither energy-rich nor appreciably sweet and are sometimes bitter.[18] However, parental responsibility falls short of "getting" children to eat or like particular foods. Pressuring children to consume foods or rewarding them for consuming specific foods is counterproductive in the long run, because it is likely to build resistance and food dislikes rather than acceptance. Instead, considering mealtime from the child's perspective—where everything is new and different—and recognizing that "finicky eating" is a normal stage of development that children outgrow—is a more productive outlook.

Experience is the only established positive predictor of acceptance and liking. Therefore, encouraging learning—using all senses and various modes for learning (eg, food shopping and preparation; reading to children about food, eating, and cultures)—can promote more enthusiasm for trying new foods and ultimately more healthful eating. Allowing children the opportunities for mastery of eating, even when it translates into extra time, work, and cleanup for adults, ultimately promotes self-regulation and autonomy building, not to mention more pleasant mealtimes for and feeding interactions with children. This can be a challenging message for parents who are stressed because of lack of time, money, or knowledge.

Parents' concerns can be diminished if the focus becomes the adequacy of children's growth rather than children's behavior at individual eating occasions. Encouraging parents to gather information about what their child eats from other settings in which children consume meals and snacks (eg, child care) may also alleviate parental concern.

The manner in which parents approach feeding has important implications for child behavioral, dietary, and weight outcomes.[93-96] Authoritative approaches to feeding, characterized by adults encouraging children to eat healthy foods and allowing the child to have limited choices but stopping short of pressuring or forcing, has been associated with increased availability and intake of fruits, vegetables, and dairy and lower intake of "less nutritious" foods.[93,97] In contrast, authoritarian approaches to feeding, characterized by attempts to control children's eating, have been associated with lower intakes of fruit, juices, and vegetables. Highly controlling feeding practices, including the use of bribes, threats, and food restriction, have negative effects on eating behaviors in young children and have been related to the inability to regulate energy intake and weight status in some studies.[52,98]

III

Alternatively, some parents have difficulty saying "no" to their toddlers' demands and indulge children's wishes rather than establish limits. Indulgent approaches to feeding, characterized by little structure or limit-setting in feeding, has been associated with greater intake of fat and sweet foods, more snacks, fewer healthy food choices, and overweight among preschool-aged children.[47,94,99]

Special Topics

Feeding During Illness

A common treatment for acute diarrhea has been a clear liquid diet until symptoms improve. The AAP clinical practice guideline on the management of acute gastroenteritis in young children recommends that only oral electrolyte solutions be used to rehydrate infants and young children and that a normal diet be continued throughout an episode of gastroenteritis[100,101] (see also Chapter 29: Oral Rehydration Therapy). Infants and young children can experience a decrease in nutritional status and the illness can be prolonged with a clear liquid diet, especially when it is extended beyond a few days.[102] Continuous or early refeeding has been shown to shorten the duration of the diarrhea. Recommendations for toddlers and preschool-aged children include reintroduction of solid foods shortly after rehydration. Foods that are usually well tolerated include rice cereals, bananas, potatoes, eggs, rice, plain pasta, and other similar foods. Dairy products, in recommended amounts, can also be included. During viral illnesses, colds, and other acute childhood illnesses, a variety of foods should be offered according to the child's appetite and tolerance, with extra fluids provided when fever, diarrhea, or vomiting is present.

AAP

The American Academy of Pediatrics endorsed guidelines from the Centers for Disease Control and Prevention on nutritional therapy for acute gastroenteritis.

Recommendations depend on the age and diet history of the child. Breastfed infants should continue feeding on demand, and formula-fed infants should continue with usual formula feeding after rehydration to meet energy and nutrient needs.

Children consuming pureed or solid foods should continue to consume their regular diet. Foods high in simple sugars (eg, soft drinks, gelatin, juice) should be avoided to avoid increases in osmotic load.

Early feeding reduces illness duration and improves nutrition outcome. Recommended foods include age-appropriate diets including complex carbohydrates, meats, yogurt, fruits and vegetables.

Pediatrics. 2004;114(2):507
MMWR. 2003;52(RR-16):1-16

Breakfast

Children and adolescents skip breakfast more than any other meal. Nationally representative data indicate that 20% of children skip breakfast on any given day, with the numbers growing to nearly a third of children by adolescence.[103,104] Among school-aged children, common barriers to eating breakfast include lack of time and not being hungry in the morning.[103] Children who frequently consume breakfast have superior nutritional profiles compared with those children who do not.[105] School breakfast programs, which heavily serve children from low-income families,[103] decrease breakfast skipping[106] and are associated with improvements in children's nutrient intake and overall diet quality.[107] Although one study reported that children who frequently skip breakfast may make up for missed energy by consuming greater energy from snacks in the afternoon and evening,[108] other research has found that skipping breakfast leads to lower daily energy and nutrient intakes.[109] Children and adolescents who eat regularly eat breakfast show better cognitive performance, particularly memory,[110,111] at school, with benefits most pronounced among children at nutritional risk.[112,113] School breakfast participation has also been associated with increases in attendance and academic performance, with benefits again most pronounced among children at nutritional risk.[114,115] An increasing number of studies indicate that some types of breakfast may offer more benefits to children than others. Breakfasts with lower levels of rapidly absorbing carbohydrates are associated with better cognitive performance in some, but not all studies.[116] Ready-to-eat cereal consumption has also been associated with better dietary quality among children and represents a major source of fiber, folate, vitamin C, iron, and zinc in young children's diets.[117-119] An increasing number of studies, several of which were prospective, have reported a protective association of breakfast consumption on body mass index (BMI) in children and adolescents,[103,120-122] particularly for ready-to-eat breakfast cereal.[117,119,123] Anticipatory guidance should encourage parents and caregivers to provide breakfast regularly to young children—either at home or school—that includes low-sugar, ready-to-eat cereals[124] and other foods with low levels of rapidly absorbing carbohydrates,[125] whole grains, and low-fat dairy.[126] Encouragement by pediatricians to have eligible children partake in school breakfast and to support efforts at improving the quality of school breakfast will both improve children's nutrient intakes and support chronic disease-prevention efforts.[127]

Obesity

The prevalence of overweight among children has increased drastically over the past 3 decades and is alarmingly high; currently, 31.8% of children 2 to 19 years of age are overweight or obese (see also Chapter 34: Obesity).[128,129] In 2009–2010, the prevalence of obesity reached 12.1% for children 2 to 5 years of age,

18% for children 6 to 11 years of age, and 18.4% for adolescents 12 to 19 years of age.[128] Overweight children are at increased risk of social stigmatization, hyperlipidemia, abnormal glucose tolerance, noninsulin-dependent diabetes mellitus, and hypertension.[130] Environmental influences that promote problematic eating have been given attention in light of the fact that secular increases in overweight have occurred too rapidly to be explained by genetic influences alone.[131,132] It must be acknowledged that the food supply has also changed drastically in recent decades. The number of foods available has increased in all major food categories, and average daily calories available per person increased approximately 600 kcal, with the greatest increases in the availability of added fats and oils, grains, milk and milk products, and caloric sweeteners. Parents have an important role in the etiology of childhood overweight, because they provide children with both genes and the environment in which eating and physical activity take place.[133] Evidence of this point is found in the fact that the tracking of childhood overweight into adulthood is particularly strong among children who have one or more overweight parents.[134]

It is recommended that children 3 years or older with BMI ≥85th percentile and with complications of obesity or with a BMI ≥95th percentile with or without medical complications undergo evaluation and possible treatment.[135] A longitudinal developmental approach by pediatricians is encouraged to help identify children early in the excess weight gain trajectory. Prevention efforts, at a minimum, should include adherence to recommendations to plot and track BMI on growth charts and to discuss obesity-related topics frequently (see Chapter 34: Obesity). When possible, guidance to promote healthful eating patterns in the overweight child should be directed toward modifying the dietary intake patterns and behaviors of the family as a whole rather than targeting only the overweight child.[136] Referring the family for nutrition and physical activity education and counseling may be useful to help parents discuss behavioral issues involved in child feeding. These discussions should focus on the types of foods that are available in the home, identifying appropriate portion sizes, and incorporating low-energy, nutrient-rich foods into the child's and family's diet, advocating the concept of energy balance, for example, as referenced earlier in the discussion of ChooseMyPlate.gov. Helping parents and caregivers to assess their home food and physical activity environments, including foods that should be limited (such as sweetened beverages, high-calorie snacks, and processed foods), and to determine what changes can be made to the environment may be helpful. Parents should also be made aware that highly restrictive approaches to child feeding are not effective but rather appear to promote the intake of restricted foods[137-139] and contribute to low self-appraisal.[140] Further, parents should be encouraged to exhibit the eating behaviors they would like their children to adopt, because children learn to model their parents' eating and behaviors.[57,141]

Increased physical activity is a critical component of childhood obesity prevention, because sedentary behavior has been associated with overweight among children[142,143]; health care professionals should inquire about the child's amount of screen time and whether there is a television in the child's bedroom.[144,145] Parents should be encouraged to limit screen time to 2 hours or less per day and to avoid media exposure for children younger than 2 years. Parents and caregivers have a central responsibility in this area, because they serve as role models for active lifestyles and are children's gatekeepers to opportunities to be physically active. Play and adequate sleep time are essential to children's healthy development and well-being.[146] Health care professionals should convey the importance of encouraging activity in the entire family as well as among individuals within the family. Children should be encouraged to participate in discussions of modifications of diet and physical activity. Taking into account their preferences will allow them a sense of responsibility for decisions about their behavior.

Beverage Consumption

Fruit juices, fruit-flavored juices, and soft drinks are increasingly common beverages consumed by young children at home and in group settings.[147] Between 1977 and 2001, soft drink intake among children 2 to 18 years of age more than doubled, largely because of increases in the average portion size consumed.[148] On any given day, 60% of toddlers consumed 100% fruit juice, with 1 in 10 children consuming more than 14 oz of 100% fruit juice daily.[149] Further, sweetened beverages are one of the top 3 contributors (4.7%) to daily energy intake in this age group, with 40% of toddlers consuming fruit drinks and 11% consumed carbonated beverages on any given day.[59] Among older children, these types of beverages provide roughly 10% of energy in the diets of 2- to 19-year-olds, with soft drinks providing as much as 8% of total daily energy for adolescents.[150] Children's soft drink consumption exceeds that of 100% fruit juice by 5 years of age and that of milk by 13 years of age.[151] Soft drinks, a main source of added sugar in young children's diets,[152] have been shown to replace milk in the diet and are associated with lower intakes of key nutrients, particularly calcium.[153-156]

> **AAP**
>
> ### AAP Recommendations for Fruit Juice Consumption
>
> - Intake of fruit juice should be limited to 4 to 6 oz per day for children 1 through 6 years old. For children 7 through 17 years old, juice intake should be limited to 8 to 12 oz or 2 servings per day.
> - Children should be encouraged to eat whole fruits to meet their recommended daily fruit intake.
> - Children should not consume unpasteurized juice.
> - Health care professionals should determine the amount of juice consumed by children being evaluated for malnutrition (overnutrition and undernutrition), chronic diarrhea, excessive flatulence, abdominal pain and bloating, and dental caries.
> - Pediatricians should routinely discuss fruit juice, fruit drinks, and the difference between the 2 with parents.
>
> American Academy of Pediatrics, Committee on Nutrition. The use and misuse of fruit juice in pediatrics. *Pediatrics.* 2001;107(5):1210-1213

According to ChooseMyPlate, caregivers should look for and choose fruit options, including 100% fruit juice, in fast food restaurants.[85] Fresh, frozen, canned, and dried fruits provide more fiber than juice. Preschool-aged children may be offered up to ½ cup to ¾ cup (4-6 oz) of 100% fruit juice (http://www.choosemyplate.gov/preschoolers/daily-food-plans/about-fruit.html) per day.[157] Fruit punch and fruit drinks contain little or no fruit. These drinks, as well as some flavored waters, sweetened teas, and sports drinks, provide calories, but few or no nutrients.[3]

Perhaps the most significant increase of late in caloric beverage consumption comes from sports and energy drinks being marketed to children and adolescents.[158] Although both contain significant calories, a primary distinction between sports and energy drinks is the caffeine content of energy drinks. Energy drinks contain large and varied amounts of caffeine, with the total amount of caffeine in some energy drinks exceeding 500 mg (equivalent to 14 cans of caffeinated soft drinks).[159] A lethal dose of caffeine is considered to be 200 to 400 mg/kg.[160] Because of the potential adverse effects, the AAP recommends that children do not consume caffeine.[158] Pediatricians should inquire about the use of sports and energy drinks during routine health visits (see side bar).

Growth faltering (failure to thrive) has been associated anecdotally with excessive intake of fruit juice,[161] and at least one study found carbohydrate malabsorption following consumption of large amounts of fruit juices in healthy children with chronic nonspecific diarrhea.[162] In addition, weight gain and adiposity have been linked to excess energy-containing beverage consumption.[163,164] For all young children, consumption of sweetened beverages should be monitored.[165] For those with either chronic diarrhea or excessive weight gain, obtaining a diet history, including the volume of fruit juice and soft drinks consumed, is useful for anticipatory guidance (see side bar). Intake of fruit juice should be limited. Parents should be encouraged to routinely offer plain, unflavored water to children, particularly for fluids consumed outside of meals and snacks.[166]

Snacking

Because of smaller capacities and fluctuating appetites, most young children fare best when fed 4 to 6 times a day. Nationally representative data, however, indicate that young children snack more frequently and consume more energy at each snack and a greater proportion of their daily energy intakes from snacks than in previous decades.[167] Children younger than 2 years consume as much as 15% to 25% of their daily energy intake from snacks,[168] and preschool-aged children consume approximately 27% of their daily energy from snacks.[167] Half of all snacking calories consumed by US children 2 to 18 years of age come from foods known to be high in solid fats and added sugars,[167] with desserts and salty snacks representing the greater sources of snacks in children's diets. A recent observational study found that school-aged children living in low-income urban neighborhoods purchased, on average, more than 350 kcal of energy-rich, nutrient-poor foods and beverages per convenience store trip and for only a little more than $1 per purchase.[169] Although frequent snacking has been suggested to contribute to obesity, the available evidence supports an inverse relationship between eating frequency and weight[170-172] or no relationship.[173] Anticipatory guidance should encourage parents and caregivers to think of snacks as "mini-meals" and planned so they contribute to the total day's nutrient intake. Healthful snacks accepted by many children include fresh fruit, cheese, whole-grain crackers, bread products (eg, bagels, pita, tortillas, and rice crackers), milk, raw vegetables, 100% fruit juices, sandwiches, peanut butter, and yogurt.

Media Influences on Children's Eating

Among US children 2 to 15 years of age, 47% watch television, play video games, or sit in front of computer screens for 2 or more hours daily.[174] One study showed that even preschool-aged children spend an average of 4 hours each day watching television and videos.[175] Children watch more television than any other type of media. The more time children spend watching television, the more likely they are to have higher energy intakes and to be overweight compared with children who watch less television. Exposure to advertisements for foods high in solid fats, added salt, and sugar, including fast foods and carbonated beverages, may contribute to this relationship.[173] In 2006, companies spent $1.6 billion in targeted food marketing to children 2 to 17 years of age.[176] Analysis of television advertisements on popular children's television in 11 countries showed that 53% to 87% of foods advertised were high in undesirable nutrients, including added sugars and fats. Children who are exposed to food advertisements are more likely to recall and prefer advertised foods and brands and to request[177] and consume advertised brands.[178] In fact, young children prefer[179] and choose[179,180] foods that have been associated with popular food brands and cartoon characters. Anticipatory guidance should strongly encourage parents and caregivers to limit screen time for toddlers and young children.

The Role of Anticipatory Guidance in Promoting Healthy Eating Behaviors

Appropriate feeding behavior is vital in promoting healthy growth and development but also in engendering healthy behaviors and habits that can prevent the advent of chronic disease. The feeding relationship is critical for establishing a healthy parent-child relationship. Feeding provides opportunities for pleasure, for self-discovery, for learning self-control, and ultimately for helping children to establish the internal motivation to consume a healthy diet and maintain healthy weight.

For the parent, a healthy feeding environment requires knowledge structure, limit-setting, an appreciation of children's developing capabilities, and perhaps most of all, patience and endurance. The pediatrician's role includes the timely delivery of information. Each well-child visit can be structured to include short, targeted nutrition guidance that is relevant to the child's development and growth. Information regarding a child's growth and weight status (by use of BMI curves adjusted for sex and age) and interpretation of the child's growth tracking, over time, is both critical and enlightening for parents. Further, anticipating and addressing problematic childhood behaviors (eg, resistance to unfamiliar foods, preferences for sweet-tasting and energy-dense foods, how to handle diminishing appetites and food refusal) and framing them in a developmental light often alleviates parental overconcern. Guiding parents to identify and define their goals for family eating patterns and then to establish and adopt routines for eating and physical activity from infancy through adolescence will greatly assist parents to prioritize healthy eating and activity patterns. Pediatricians can support families by offering continued encouragement and direction regarding the benefits of a varied diet, appropriate expectations for growth and development, and the importance of physical activity.

References

1. World Health Organization, Multicentre Growth Reference Study Group. Length/height-for-age, weight-for-age, weight-for-length, weight-for-height and body mass index-for-age: Methods and development. Geneva, Switzerland: World Health Organization; 2006. Available at: http://www.who.int/childgrowth/standards/technical_report/en/index.html. Accessed September 25, 2012

2. Dibley MJ, Goldsby JB, Staehling NW, Trowbridge FL. Development of normalized curves for the international growth reference: historical and technical considerations. *Am J Clin Nutr*. 1987;46(5):736-748

3. Carruth BR, Skinner JD. Feeding behaviors and other motor development in healthy children (2-24 months). *J Am Coll Nutr*. 2002;21(2):88-96

4. Carruth BR, Ziegler PJ, Gordon A, Hendricks K. Developmental milestones and self-feeding behaviors in infants and toddlers. *J Am Diet Assoc*. 2004;104(1 Suppl 1):S51-S56

5. Brotanek JM, Halterman JS, Auinger P, Flores G, Weitzman M. Iron deficiency, prolonged bottle-feeding, and racial/ethnic disparities in young children. *Arch Pediatr Adolesc Med*. 2005;159(11):1038-1042

6. Brotanek JM, Schroer D, Valentyn L, Tomany-Korman S, Flores G. Reasons for prolonged bottle-feeding and iron deficiency among Mexican-American toddlers: an ethnographic study. *Acad Pediatr*. 2009;9(1):17-25

7. Kimbro RT, Brooks-Gunn J, McLanahan S. Racial and ethnic differentials in overweight and obesity among 3-year-old children. *Am J Public Health*. 2007;97(2):298-305

8. Gooze RA, Anderson SE, Whitaker RC. Prolonged bottle use and obesity at 5.5 years of age in US children. *J Pediatr*. 2011;159(3):431-436

9. American Academy of Pediatrics, Section on Pediatric Dentistry and Oral Health. Preventive oral health intervention for pediatricians. *Pediatrics*. 2008;122(6):1387–1394

10. Burhans KK, Dweck CS. Helplessness in early childhood: the role of contingent worth. *Child Dev*. 1995;66(6):1719-1738

11. Centers for Disease Control and Prevention. Nonfatal choking-related episodes among children—United States, 2001. *MMWR Morb Mortal Wkly Rep*. 2002;51(42):945-948

12. Altkorn R, Chen X, Milkovich S, Stool D, Rider G, Bailey CM, et al. Fatal and non-fatal food injuries among children (aged 0-14 years). *Int J Pediatr Otorhinolaryngol*. 2008;72(7):1041-1046

13. American Academy of Pediatrics, Committee on Injury, Violence, and Poison Prevention. Policy Statement: prevention of choking among children. *Pediatrics*. 2010;125(3): 601-607

14. Desor JA, Maller O, Turner RE. Taste in acceptance of sugars by human infants. *J Comp Physiol Psychol*. 1973;84(3):496-501

15. Kern DL, McPhee L, Fisher J, Johnson S, Birch LL. The postingestive consequences of fat condition preferences for flavors associated with high dietary fat. *Physiol Behav*. 1993;54(1):71-76

16. Beauchamp GK, Mennella JA. Early flavor learning and its impact on later feeding behavior. *J Pediatr Gastroenterol Nutr*. 2009;48(Suppl 1):S25-S30

17. Johnson SL, Bellows L, Beckstrom L, Anderson J. Evaluation of a social marketing campaign targeting preschool children. *Am J Health Behav*. 2007;31(1):44-55

18. Sullivan S, Birch LL. Pass the sugar; pass the salt; experience dictates preference. *Dev Psychol*. 1990;26(4):546-551

19. Wardle J, Cooke LJ, Gibson EL, Sapochnik M, Sheiham A, Lawson M. Increasing children's acceptance of vegetables; a randomized trial of parent-led exposure. *Appetite*. 2003;40(2):155-162

20. Carruth BR, Ziegler PJ, Gordon A, Barr SI. Prevalence of picky eaters among infants and toddlers and their caregivers' decisions about offering a new food. *J Am Diet Assoc*. 2004;104(1 Suppl 1):S57-S64

21. Lakkakula A, Geaghan JP, Wong WP, Zanovec M, Pierce SH, Tuuri G. A cafeteria-based tasting program increased liking of fruits and vegetables by lower, middle and upper elementary school-age children. *Appetite*. 2011;57(1):299-302

22. Lakkakula A, Geaghan J, Zanovec M, Pierce S, Tuuri G. Repeated taste exposure increases liking for vegetables by low-income elementary school children. *Appetite*. 2010;55(2):226-231

23. Birch LL, Birch D, Marlin DW, Kramer L. Effects of instrumental consumption on children's food preference. *Appetite*. 1982;3(2):125-134

24. Hendy HM. Comparison of five teacher actions to encourage children's new food acceptance. *Ann Behav Med*. 1999;21(1):20-26

25. Hendy HM. Effectiveness of trained peer models to encourage food acceptance in preschool children. *Appetite*. 2002;39(3):217-225

26. Hendy HM, Raudenbush B. Effectiveness of teacher modeling to encourage food acceptance in preschool children. *Appetite*. 2000;34(1):61-76

27. Addessi E, Galloway AT, Visalberghi E, Birch LL. Specific social influences on the acceptance of novel foods in 2-5-year-old children. *Appetite*. 2005;45(3):264-271

28. Cooke LJ, Chambers LC, Anez EV, Croker HA, Boniface D, Yeomans MR, et al. Eating for pleasure or profit: the effect of incentives on children's enjoyment of vegetables. *Psychol Sci*. 2011;22(2):190-196

29. Horne PJ, Greenhalgh J, Erjavec M, Lowe CF, Viktor S, Whitaker CJ. Increasing pre-school children's consumption of fruit and vegetables. A modelling and rewards intervention. *Appetite*. 2011;56(2):375-385

30. Corsini N, Slater A, Harrison A, Cooke L, Cox DN. Rewards can be used effectively with repeated exposure to increase liking of vegetables in 4-6-year-old children. *Public Health Nutr.* 2011;7:1-10

31. Houston-Price C, Butler L, Shiba P. Visual exposure impacts on toddlers' willingness to taste fruits and vegetables. *Appetite.* 2009;53(3):450-453

32. Heath PM, Houston-Price C, Kennedy OB. Can visual exposure impact on children's visual preferences for fruit and vegetables? *Proc Nutr Soc.* 2010;69(OCE6):e422

33. Fisher JO, Mennella JA, Hughes SO, Liu Y, Mendoza P, Patrick H. Offering "dip" promotes intake of a moderately-liked raw vegetable among preschoolers with genetic sensitivity to bitterness. *J Am Diet Assoc.* 2012;112(2):235-245

34. Cooke LJ, Wardle J, Gibson EL, Sapochnik M, Sheiham A, Lawson M. Demographic, familial and trait predictors of fruit and vegetable consumption by pre-school children. *Public Health Nutr.* 2004;7(2):295-302

35. Northstone K, Emmett P, Nethersole F. The effect of age of introduction to lumpy solids on foods eaten and reported feeding difficulties at 6 and 15 months. *J Hum Nutr Diet.* 2001;14(1):43-54

36. Skinner JD, Carruth BR, Bounds W, Ziegler P, Reidy K. Do food-related experiences in the first 2 years of life predict dietary variety in school-aged children? *J Nutr Educ Behav.* 2002;34(6):310-315

37. Nutrition classics. American Journal of Diseases of Children, Volume 36 October, 1928: Number 4. Self selection of diet by newly weaned infants: an experimental study. By Clara M. Davis. *Nutr Rev.* 1986;44(3):114-116

38. Mascola AJ, Bryson SW, Agras WS. Picky eating during childhood: a longitudinal study to age 11 years. *Eat Behav.* 2010;11(4):253-257

39. Birch LL, Billman J, Richards SS. Time of day influences food acceptability. *Appetite.* 1984;5(2):109-116

40. Leahy KE, Birch LL, Rolls BJ. Reducing the energy density of multiple meals decreases the energy intake of preschool-age children. *Am J Clin Nutr.* 2008;88(6):1459-1468

41. Leahy KE, Birch LL, Fisher JO, Rolls BJ. Reductions in entree energy density increase children's vegetable intake and reduce energy intake. *Obesity (Silver Spring).* 2008;16(7):1559-1565

42. Leahy KE, Birch LL, Rolls BJ. Reducing the energy density of an entree decreases children's energy intake at lunch. *J Am Diet Assoc.* 2008;108(1):41-48

43. Fisher JO. Effects of age on children's intake of large and self-selected food portions. *Obesity (Silver Spring).* 2007;15(2):403-412

44. Fisher JO, Rolls BJ, Birch LL. Children's bite size and intake of an entree are greater with large portions than with age-appropriate or self-selected portions. *Am J Clin Nutr.* 2003;77(5):1164-1170

45. Rolls BJ, Engell D, Birch LL. Serving portion size influences 5-year-old but not 3-year-old children's food intakes. *J Am Diet Assoc.* 2000;100(2):232-234

46. Ventura AK, Birch LL. Does parenting affect children's eating and weight status? *Int J Behav Nutr Phys Act.* 2008;5:15

III

47. Hurley KM, Cross MB, Hughes SO. A systematic review of responsive feeding and child obesity in high-income countries. *J Nutr*. 2011;141(3):495-501

48. Birch LL. Effects of peer models' food choices and eating behaviors on preschoolers' food preferences. *Child Dev*. 1980;51:489-96

49. Salvy SJ, Kieffer E, Epstein LH. Effects of social context on overweight and normal-weight children's food selection. *Eat Behav*. 2008;9(2):190-196

50. Birch LL, Johnson SL, Andresen G, Peters JC, Schulte MC. The variability of young children's energy intake. *N Engl J Med*. 1991;324(4):232-235

51. Birch LL, Deysher M. Conditioned and unconditioned caloric compensation: evidence for self-regulation of food intake by young children. *Learn Motiv*. 1985;16:341-355

52. Johnson SL, Birch LL. Parents' and children's adiposity and eating style. *Pediatrics*. 1994;94(5):653-661

53. Savage JS, Fisher JO, Marini M, Birch LL. Serving smaller age-appropriate entree portions to children aged 3-5 y increases fruit and vegetable intake and reduces energy density and energy intake at lunch. *Am J Clin Nutr*. 2012;95(2):335-341

54. Faith MS, Pietrobelli A, Heo M, et al. A twin study of self-regulatory eating in early childhood: estimates of genetic and environmental influence, and measurement considerations. *Int J Obes (Lond)*. 2012;36(7):931-937

55. Davis CM. Results of the self-selection of diets by young children. *Can Med Assoc J*. 1939;41(3):257-261

56. Wardle J, Huon G. An experimental investigation of the influence of health information on children's taste preferences. *Health Educ Res*. 2000;15(1):39-44

57. Cullen KW, Eagan J, Baranowski T, Owens E, de Moor C. Effect of a la carte and snack bar foods at school on children's lunchtime intake of fruits and vegetables. *J Am Diet Assoc*. 2000;100(12):1482-1486

58. Briefel RR, Reidy K, Karwe V, Jankowski L, Hendricks K. Toddlers' transition to table foods: Impact on nutrient intakes and food patterns. *J Am Diet Assoc*. 2004;104(1 Suppl 1):S38-S44

59. Fox MK, Reidy K, Novak T, Ziegler P. Sources of energy and nutrients in the diets of infants and toddlers. *J Am Diet Assoc*. 2006;106(1 Suppl 1):S28-S42

60. Butte NF, Fox MK, Briefel RR, et al. Nutrient intakes of US infants, toddlers, and preschoolers meet or exceed dietary reference intakes. *J Am Diet Assoc*. 2010;110(12 Suppl):S27-S37

61. Fox MK, Condon E, Briefel RR, Reidy KC, Deming DM. Food consumption patterns of young preschoolers: are they starting off on the right path? *J Am Diet Assoc*. 2010;110(12 Suppl):S52-S9

62. Baker RD, Greer FR. Diagnosis and prevention of iron deficiency and iron-deficiency anemia in infants and young children (0-3 years of age). *Pediatrics*. 2010;126(5):1040-1050

63. Krebs-Smith SM, Cook A, Subar AF, Cleveland L, Friday J, Kahle LL. Fruit and vegetable intakes of children and adolescents in the United States. *Arch Pediatr Adolesc Med*. 1996;150(1):81-86

64. Munoz KA, Krebs-Smith SM, Ballard-Barbash R, Cleveland LE. Food intakes of US children and adolescents compared with recommendations. *Pediatrics*. 1997;100(3 Pt 1):323-329

65. Kranz S, Mitchell DC, Siega-Riz AM, Smiciklas-Wright H. Dietary fiber intake by American preschoolers is associated with more nutrient-dense diets. *J Am Diet Assoc*. 2005;105(2):221-225

66. Ballew C, Kuester S, Serdula M, Bowman B, Dietz W. Nutrient intakes and dietary patterns of young children by dietary fat intakes. *J Pediatr*. 2000;136(2):181-187

67. Reedy J, Krebs-Smith SM. Dietary sources of energy, solid fats, and added sugars among children and adolescents in the United States. *J Am Diet Assoc*. 2010;110(10):1477-1484

68. Mendoza JA, Drewnowski A, Cheadle A, Christakis DA. Dietary energy density is associated with selected predictors of obesity in U.S. children. *J Nutr*. 2006;136(5):370-378

69. Marriott BP, Olsho L, Hadden L, Connor P. Intake of added sugars and selected nutrients in the United States, National Health and Nutrition Examination Survey (NHANES) 2003-2006. *Crit Rev Food Sci Nutr*. 2010;50(3):228-258

70. Poti JM, Popkin BM. Trends in energy intake among US children by eating location and food source, 1977-2006. *J Am Diet Assoc*. 2011;111(8):1156-1164

71. Bowman SA, Gortmaker SL, Ebbeling CB, Pereira MA, Ludwig DS. Effects of fast-food consumption on energy intake and diet quality among children in a national household survey. *Pediatrics*. 2004;113(1 Pt 1):112-118

72. Jahns L, Siega-Riz AM, Popkin BM. The increasing prevalence of snacking among US children from 1977-1996. *J Pediatr*. 2001;138(4):493-498

73. Nielsen SJ, Siega-Riz AM, Popkin BM. Trends in energy intake in U.S. between 1977-1996: Similar shifts seen across age groups. *Obes Res*. 2002;5:370-378

74. Wiecha JL, Peterson KE, Ludwig DS, Kim J, Sobol A, Gortmaker SL. When children eat what they watch: Impact of television viewing on dietary intake in youth. *Arch Pediatr Adolesc Med*. 2006;160(4):436-442

75. Alaimo K, McDowell MA, Briefel RR, et al. Dietary intake of vitamins, minerals, and fiber of persons ages 2 months and over in the United States: Third National Health and Nutrition Examination Survey, Phase 1, 1988-91. *Adv Data*. 1994;Nov 14(258):1-28

76. Federation of American Societies for Experimental Biology, Life Sciences Research Office. *Third Report on Nutrition Monitoring in the United States*. Washington, DC: US Government Printing Office; 1995:365

77. Fulgoni VL, 3rd, Keast DR, Bailey RL, Dwyer J. Foods, fortificants, and supplements: Where do Americans get their nutrients? *J Nutr*. 2011;141(10):1847-1854

78. Daniels SR, Greer FR. Lipid screening and cardiovascular health in childhood. *Pediatrics*. 2008;122(1):198-208

79. American Academy of Pediatrics, Committee on Nutrition. Statement on cholesterol. *Pediatrics*. 1998;101(1):141-147

80. US Department of Agriculture. Food Guide Pyramid for Kids. MyPyramid.gov Web site. Available at: http://www.cnpp.usda.gov/FGP4Children.htm. Accessed September 25, 2012

81. Grundy SM, Cleeman JI, Daniels SR, et al. Diagnosis and management of the metabolic syndrome: an American Heart Association/National Heart, Lung, and Blood Institute Scientific Statement. *Circulation*. 2005;112(17):2735-2752

82. Butte NF. Fat intake of children in relation to energy requirements. *Am J Clin Nutr*. 2000;72(5 Suppl):1246S-1252S

83. Obarzanek E, Hunsberger SA, Van Horn L, et al. Safety of a fat-reduced diet: the Dietary Intervention Study in Children (DISC). *Pediatrics*. 1997;100(1):51-59

84. US Department of Agriculture. *Dietary Guidelines for Americans*. Washington, DC: US Government Printing Office; 2005

85. US Department of Agriculture. ChooseMyPlate.gov Web site. Available at: http://www .choosemyplate.gov/food-groups/fruits-tips.html. Accessed September 25, 2012

86. Nielsen SJ, Popkin BM. Patterns and trends in food portion sizes, 1977-1998. *JAMA*. 2003;289(4):450-453

87. Young LR, Nestle MS. Portion sizes in dietary assessment: issues and policy implications. *Nutr Rev*. 1995;53(6):149-158

88. Fox MK, Devaney B, Reidy K, Razafindrakoto C, Ziegler P. Relationship between portion size and energy intake among infants and toddlers: evidence of self-regulation. *J Am Diet Assoc*. 2006;106(1 Suppl):77-83

89. McConahy KL, Smiciklas-Wright H, Birch LL, Mitchell DC, Picciano MF. Food portions are positively related to energy intake and body weight in early childhood. *J Pediatr*. 2002;140(3):340-347

90. McConahy KL, Smiciklas-Wright H, Mitchell DC, Picciano MF. Portion size of common foods predicts energy intake among preschool-aged children. *J Am Diet Assoc*. 2004;104(6):975-979

91. Satter E. *How to Get Your Kid to Eat...but Not Too Much*. Palo Alto, CA: Bull Publishing Company; 1987

92. Ramsay SA, Branen LJ, Johnson SL. How much is enough? Tablespoon per year of age approach meets nutrient needs for children. *Appetite*. 2012;58(1):163-167

93. Gable S, Lutz S. Household, parent, and child contributions to childhood obesity. *Fam Relat*. 2000;49:293-300

94. De Bourdeaudhuij I. Family food rules and healthy eating in adolescents. *J Health Psychol*. 1997;2(1):45-56

95. Fisher JO, Birch LL. Restricting access to palatable foods affects children's behavioral response, food selection, and intake. *Am J Clin Nutr*. 1999;69(6):1264-1272

96. Rhee KE, Lumeng JC, Appugliese DP, Kaciroti N, Bradley RH. Parenting styles and overweight status in first grade. *Pediatrics*. 2006 ;117(6):2047-2054

97. Patrick H, Nicklas TA, Hughes SO, Morales M. The benefits of authoritative feeding style: caregiver feeding styles and children's food consumption patterns. *Appetite*. 2005;44(2):243-249

98. Faith MS, Berkowitz RI, Stallings VA, Kerns J, Storey M, Stunkard AJ. Parental feeding attitudes and styles and child body mass index: prospective analysis of a gene-environment interaction. *Pediatrics*. 2004;114(4):e429-e436

99. Olvera N, Power TG. Brief report: parenting styles and obesity in Mexican American children: a longitudinal study. *J Pediatr Psychol*. 2010;35(3):243-249

100. King CK, Glass R, Bresee JS, Duggan C. Managing acute gastroenteritis among children: oral rehydration, maintenance, and nutritional therapy. *MMWR Recomm Rep*. 2003;52(RR-16):1-16

101. American Academy of Pediatrics. Statement of endorsement: managing acute gastroenteritis among children: oral rehydration, maintenance, and nutritional therapy. *Pediatrics*. 2004;114(2):507

102. Brown KH. Dietary management of acute childhood diarrhea: optimal timing of feeding and appropriate use of milks and mixed diets. *J Pediatr*. 1991;118(4 Pt 2):S92-S98

103. Deshmukh-Taskar PR, Nicklas TA, O'Neil CE, Keast DR, Radcliffe JD, Cho S. The relationship of breakfast skipping and type of breakfast consumption with nutrient intake and weight status in children and adolescents: the National Health and Nutrition Examination Survey 1999-2006. *J Am Diet Assoc*. 2010;110(6):869-878

104. Siega-Riz AM, Popkin BM, Carson T. Trends in breakfast consumption for children in the United States from 1965-1991. *Am J Clin Nutr*. 1998;67(4):748S-756S

105. Rampersaud GC, Pereira MA, Girard BL, Adams J, Metzl JD. Breakfast habits, nutritional status, body weight, and academic performance in children and adolescents. *J Am Diet Assoc*. 2005;105(5):743-760

106. Morris CT, Courtney A, Bryant CA, McDermott RJ. Grab N' Go breakfast at school: observations from a pilot program. *J Nutr Educ Behav*. 2010;42(3):208-209

107. Bhattacharya J, Currie J, Haider SJ. Evaluating the impact of school nutrition programs: final report. Washington, DC: US Department of Agriculture, Food Assistance and Nutrition Research Program; 2004:48

108. Dubois L, Girard M, Potvin Kent M, Farmer A, Tatone-Tokuda F. Breakfast skipping is associated with differences in meal patterns, macronutrient intakes and overweight among pre-school children. *Public Health Nutr*. 2009;12(1):19-28

109. Berkey CS, Rockett HR, Gillman MW, Field AE, Colditz GA. Longitudinal study of skipping breakfast and weight change in adolescents. *Int J Obes Relat Metab Disord*. 2003;27(10):1258-1266

110. Mahoney CR, Taylor HA, Kanarek RB, Samuel P. Effect of breakfast composition on cognitive processes in elementary school children. *Physiol Behav*. 2005;85(5):635-645

111. Wesnes KA, Pincock C, Richardson D, Helm G, Hails S. Breakfast reduces declines in attention and memory over the morning in schoolchildren. *Appetite*. 2003;41(3):329-331

112. Cooper SB, Bandelow S, Nevill ME. Breakfast consumption and cognitive function in adolescent schoolchildren. *Physiol Behav*. 2011;103(5):431-439

113. Cueto S, Jacoby E, Pollitt E. Breakfast prevents delays on attention and memory functions among nutritionally at-risk boys. *J Appl Dev Psychol*. 1998;19:219-233

114. Kleinman RE, Hall S, Green H, Korzec-Ramirez D, Patton K, Pagano ME, et al. Diet, breakfast, and academic performance in children. *Ann Nutr Metab*. 2002;46(Suppl 1):24-30

115. Murphy JM, Pagano ME, Nachmani J, Sperling P, Kane S, Kleinman RE. The relationship of school breakfast to psychosocial and academic functioning: cross-sectional and longitudinal observations in an inner-city school sample. *Arch Pediatr Adolesc Med.* 1998;152(9):899-907

116. Micha R, Rogers PJ, Nelson M. The glycaemic potency of breakfast and cognitive function in school children. *Eur J Clin Nutr.* 2010;64(9):948-957

117. Barton BA, Eldridge AL, Thompson D, et al. The relationship of breakfast and cereal consumption to nutrient intake and body mass index: the National Heart, Lung, and Blood Institute Growth and Health Study. *J Am Diet Assoc.* 2005;105(9):1383-1389

118. Subar AF, Krebs-Smith SM, Cook A, Kahle LL. Dietary sources of nutrients among US children, 1989-1991. *Pediatrics.* 1998;102(4 Pt 1):913-923

119. Williams BM, O'Neil CE, Keast DR, Cho S, Nicklas TA. Are breakfast consumption patterns associated with weight status and nutrient adequacy in African-American children? *Public Health Nutr.* 2009;12(4):489-496

120. Sandercock GR, Voss C, Dye L. Associations between habitual school-day breakfast consumption, body mass index, physical activity and cardiorespiratory fitness in English schoolchildren. *Eur J Clin Nutr.* 2010;64(10):1086-1092

121. Szajewska H, Ruszczynski M. Systematic review demonstrating that breakfast consumption influences body weight outcomes in children and adolescents in Europe. *Crit Rev Food Sci Nutr.* 2010;50(2):113-119

122. Tin SP, Ho SY, Mak KH, Wan KL, Lam TH. Breakfast skipping and change in body mass index in young children. *Int J Obes (Lond).* 2011;35(7):899-906

123. Albertson AM, Anderson GH, Crockett SJ, Goebel MT. Ready-to-eat cereal consumption: its relationship with BMI and nutrient intake of children aged 4 to 12 years. *J Am Diet Assoc.* 2003;103(12):1613-1619

124. Harris JL, Schwartz MB, Ustjanauskas A, Ohri-Vachaspati P, Brownell KD. Effects of serving high-sugar cereals on children's breakfast-eating behavior. *Pediatrics.* 2011;127(1):71-76

125. Agostoni C, Brighenti F. Dietary choices for breakfast in children and adolescents. *Crit Rev Food Sci Nutr.* 2010;50(2):120-128

126. Pereira MA, Erickson E, McKee P, et al. Breakfast frequency and quality may affect glycemia and appetite in adults and children. *J Nutr.* 2011;141(1):163-168

127. Crawford PB, Gosliner W, Kayman H. The ethical basis for promoting nutritional health in public schools in the United States. *Prev Chronic Dis.* 2011;8(5):A98

128. Ogden CL, Carroll MD, Kit BK, Flegal KM. Prevalence of obesity and trends in body mass index among US children and adolescents, 1999-2010. *JAMA.* 2012;307(5):483-490

129. Ogden CL, Flegal KM, Carroll MD, Johnson CL. Prevalence and trends in overweight among US children and adolescents. *JAMA.* 2002;288(14):1728-1732

130. Dietz WH. Health consequences of obesity in youth: childhood predictors of adult disease. *Pediatrics.* 1998;101(3 Pt 2):518-525

131. Hill JO, Peters JC. Environmental contributions to the obesity epidemic. *Science.* 1998;280(5368):1371-1374

132. Poston WS, 2nd, Foreyt JP. Obesity is an environmental issue. *Atherosclerosis*. 1999;146(2):201-209

133. US Department of Agriculture. ERS Food Availability (per Capita). 2011. Available at: http://www.ers.usda.gov/Data/FoodConsumption/. Accessed September 25, 2012

134. Whitaker RC, Wright JA, Pepe MS, Seidel KD, Dietz WH. Predicting obesity in young adulthood from childhood and parental obesity. *N Engl J Med*. 1997;337(13):869-873

135. Barlow SE, Dietz WH. Obesity evaluation and treatment: expert Committee recommendations. The Maternal and Child Health Bureau, Health Resources and Services Administration, and the Department of Health and Human Services. *Pediatrics*. 1998;102(3):e29

136. Krebs NF, Himes JH, Jacobson D, Nicklas TA, Guilday P, Styne D. Assessment of child and adolescent overweight and obesity. *Pediatrics*. 2007;120(Suppl 4):S193-S228

137. Birch LL, Fisher JO. Mothers' child-feeding practices influence daughters' eating and weight. *Am J Clin Nutr*. 2000;71(5):1054-1061

138. Fisher JO, Birch LL. Restricting access to foods and children's eating. *Appetite*. 1999;32(3):405-419

139. Boles RE, Scharf C, Stark LJ. Developing a treatment program for obesity in preschool age children: preliminary data. *Child Health Care*. 2010;39(1):34

140. Davison KK, Birch LL. Weight status, parent reaction, and self-concept in five-year-old girls. *Pediatrics*. 2001;107(1):46-53

141. Cutting TM, Fisher JO, Grimm-Thomas K, Birch LL. Like mother, like daughter: familial patterns of overweight are mediated by mothers' dietary disinhibition. *Am J Clin Nutr*. 1999;69(4):608-613

142. Crespo CJ, Smit E, Troiano RP, Bartlett SJ, Macera CA, Andersen RE. Television watching, energy intake, and obesity in US children: results from the third National Health and Nutrition Examination Survey, 1988-1994. *Arch Pediatr Adolesc Med*. 2001;155(3):360-365

143. American Academy of Pediatrics, Committee on Public Education. Children, adolescents, and television. *Pediatrics*. 2001;107(2):423-426

144. American Academy of Pediatrics, Council on Communications and Media. Media use by children younger than 2 years. *Pediatrics*. 2011;128(5):1040–1045

145. Strasburger VC; American Academy of Pediatrics, Council on Communications and Media. Children, adolescents, obesity, and the media. *Pediatrics*. 2011;128(1):201-208

146. Milteer RM; Ginsburg; Kenneth R; American Academy of Pediatrics, Council on Communications and Media, Committee on Psychosocial Aspects of Child and Family Health. The importance of play in promoting healthy child development and maintaining strong parent-child bond: focus on children in poverty. *Pediatrics*. 2012;129(1):e204-e213

147. Briefel RR, Johnson CL. Secular trends in dietary intake in the United States. *Annu Rev Nutr*. 2004;24:401-431

148. Nielsen SJ, Popkin BM. Changes in beverage intake between 1977 and 2001. *Am J Prev Med*. 2004;27(2):205-210

149. Skinner JD, Ziegler P, Ponza M. Transitions in infants' and toddlers' beverage patterns. *J Am Diet Assoc*. 2004;104(1 Suppl 1):S45-S50

150. Troiano RP, Briefel RR, Carroll MD, Bialostosky K. Energy and fat intakes of children and adolescents in the united states: data from the national health and nutrition examination surveys. *Am J Clin Nutr*. 2000;72(5 Suppl):1343S-1353S

151. Rampersaud GC, Bailey LB, Kauwell GP. National survey beverage consumption data for children and adolescents indicate the need to encourage a shift toward more nutritive beverages. *J Am Diet Assoc*. 2003;103(1):97-100

152. Kranz S, Smiciklas-Wright H, Siega-Riz AM, Mitchell D. Adverse effect of high added sugar consumption on dietary intake in American preschoolers. *J Pediatr*. 2005;146(1):105-111

153. Fisher JO, Mitchell DC, Smiciklas-Wright H, Birch LL. Maternal milk consumption predicts the trade-off between milk and soft drinks in young girls' diets. *J Nutr*. 2001;131:246-250

154. Frary CD, Johnson RK, Wang MQ. Children and adolescents' choices of foods and beverages high in added sugars are associated with intakes of key nutrients and food groups. *J Adolesc Health*. 2004;34(1):56-63

155. Marshall TA, Eichenberger Gilmore JM, Broffitt B, Stumbo PJ, Levy SM. Diet quality in young children is influenced by beverage consumption. *J Am Coll Nutr*. 2005;24(1):65-75

156. Striegel-Moore RH, Thompson D, Affenito SG, Franko DL, Obarzanek E, Barton BA, et al. Correlates of beverage intake in adolescent girls: the National Heart, Lung, and Blood Institute Growth and Health Study. *J Pediatr*. 2006;148(2):183-187

157. American Academy of Pediatrics, Committee on Nutrition. The use and misuse of fruit juice in pediatrics. *Pediatrics*. 2001;107(5):1210-1213

158. American Academy of Pediatrics, Committee on Nutrition and Council on Sports Medicine and Fitness. Sports drinks and energy drinks for children and adolescents: are they appropriate? *Pediatrics*. 2011;127(6):1182-1189

159. Reissig CJ, Strain EC, Griffiths RR. Caffeinated energy drinks—a growing problem. *Drug Alcohol Depend*. 2009;99(1-3):1-10

160. Berger AJ, Alford K. Cardiac arrest in a young man following excess consumption of caffeinated "energy drinks." *Med J Aust*. 2009;190(1):41-43

161. Smith MM, Lifshitz F. Excess fruit juice consumption as a contributing factor in nonorganic failure to thrive. *Pediatrics*. 1994;93(3):438-443

162. Lifshitz F, Ament ME, Kleinman RE, et al. Role of juice carbohydrate malabsorption in chronic nonspecific diarrhea in children. *J Pediatr*. 1992;120(5):825-829

163. Ludwig DS, Peterson KE, Gortmaker SL. Relation between consumption of sugar-sweetened drinks and childhood obesity: a prospective, observational analysis. *Lancet*. 2001;357(9255):505-508

164. Welsh JA, Cogswell ME, Rogers S, Rockett H, Mei Z, Grummer-Strawn LM. Overweight among low-income preschool children associated with the consumption of sweet drinks: Missouri, 1999-2002. *Pediatrics*. 2005;115(2):e223-e229

165. Dietz WH. Sugar-sweetened beverages, milk intake, and obesity in children and adolescents. *J Pediatr*. 2006;148(2):152-154

166. American Academy of Pediatrics, Committee on Sports Medicine and Fitness. Climatic heat stress and the exercising child and adolescent. *Pediatrics*. 2000;106(1 Pt 1):158-159

167. Piernas C, Popkin BM. Trends in snacking among U.S. children. *Health Aff (Millwood)*. 2010;29(3):398-404

168. Skinner JD, Ziegler P, Pac S, Devaney B. Meal and snack patterns of infants and toddlers. *J Am Diet Assoc*. 2004;104(1 Suppl 1):S65-S70

169. Borradaile KE, Sherman S, Vander Veur SS, McCoy T, Sandoval B, Nachmani J, et al. Snacking in children: the role of urban corner stores. *Pediatrics*. 2009;124(5):1293-1298

170. Vader AM, Walters ST, Harris TR, Hoelscher DM. Television viewing and snacking behaviors of fourth- and eighth-grade schoolchildren in Texas. *Prev Chronic Dis*. 2009;6(3):A89

171. Keast DR, Nicklas TA, O'Neil CE. Snacking is associated with reduced risk of overweight and reduced abdominal obesity in adolescents: National Health and Nutrition Examination Survey (NHANES) 1999-2004. *Am J Clin Nutr*. 2010;92(2):428-435

172. Lioret S, Touvier M, Lafay L, Volatier JL, Maire B. Are eating occasions and their energy content related to child overweight and socioeconomic status? *Obesity (Silver Spring)*. 2008;16(11):2518-2523

173. Maffeis C, Grezzani A, Perrone L, Del Giudice EM, Saggese G, Tato L. Could the savory taste of snacks be a further risk factor for overweight in children? *J Pediatr Gastroenterol Nutr*. 2008;46(4):429-437

174. Sisson SB, Broyles ST, Baker BL, Katzmarzyk PI. Screen time, physical activity, and overweight in U.S. youth: national survey of children's health 2003. *J Adolesc Health*. 2010;47(3):309-311

175. Tandon PS, Zhou C, Lozano P, Christakis DA. Preschoolers' total daily screen time at home and by type of child care. *J Pediatr*. 2011;158(2):297-300

176. Marketing Food to Children and Adolescents: A Review of Industry Expenditures, Activities, and Self-Regulation. Federal Trade Commission Report to Congress. 2008. Available at: http://www.ftc.gov/os/2008/07/P064504foodmktingreport.pdf. Accessed September 25, 2012

177. Chamberlain LJ, Wang Y, Robinson TN. Does children's screen time predict requests for advertised products? Cross-sectional and prospective analyses. *Arch Pediatr Adolesc Med*. 2006;160(4):363-368

178. Institute of Medicine. *Food Marketing to Children and Youth: Threat or Opportunity?* Washington, DC: National Academies Press; 2006

179. Robinson TN, Borzekowski DL, Matheson DM, Kraemer HC. Effects of fast food branding on young children's taste preferences. *Arch Pediatr Adolesc Med*. 2007;161(8):792-797

180. Roberto CA, Baik J, Harris JL, Brownell KD. Influence of licensed characters on children's taste and snack preferences. *Pediatrics*. 2010;126(1):88-93

III

Chapter 8

Adolescent Nutrition

Introduction

Approximately 40 million people in the United States, or 14% of the population, are 10 to 19 years old.[1] For this age group, there is a dramatic increase in physical growth and development that requires the adolescent to adjust to a new body size with new physiological requirements. Although the requirements for all major nutrients are increased, many adolescents consume inadequate amounts of vitamins and minerals (including folic acid; vitamins A, D, E, and B_6; calcium; iron; zinc; magnesium; and fiber), as well as several important food groups, such as fruits, vegetables, and whole grains.[2-4] Adolescent diets also frequently exceed recommendations for fat, saturated fat, sodium, and cholesterol. Furthermore, a substantial number of teenagers experience excess weight gain, frequently eat energy-dense foods (such as fast food and sugar-sweetened beverages), and are physically inactive.[4,5] Special situations, such as pregnancy, chronic disease, and physical conditioning, increase nutritional requirements of the adolescent. Some disorders observed during adolescence, such as anorexia nervosa, bulimia nervosa, and obesity, are associated with insufficient or excessive nutrient intake.

Factors Influencing Nutritional Needs of Adolescents

In comparison to other age groups, the nutritional needs of the adolescent are determined by the degree of sexual maturation and biological maturity rather than chronological age.[6] The onset of puberty, with its associated increased growth rate, changes in body composition, physical activity, and onset of menstruation in girls, affects normal nutritional needs during adolescence. Increased growth rates occur in girls between 10 and 12 years of age and in boys about 2 years later, although substantial individual variability occurs. Growth in girls is accompanied by a greater increase in the proportion of body fat than in boys, and growth in boys is accompanied by a greater increase in the proportion of lean body mass and blood volume than in girls. Health care professionals should use the sexual maturation rating or Tanner stages to assess the degree of pubertal maturation in the adolescent at each office visit (see Table 8.1). Of the 5 Tanner stages, stage 1 corresponds with prepubertal growth and development, and stages 2 through 5 denote the period of puberty. In adolescent females, menarche occurs 2 to 3 years after the development of breast buds and pubic hair, most commonly during the sexual maturation rating breast stage 4 (average age, 12.4 years). There are racial differences in the development of secondary sexual characteristics in females, with non-Hispanic black females developing pubic hair at an average of 9.4 years of age, compared with 10.4 years of age for Mexican American and 10.5 years for non-Hispanic white females. The average age of onset of menarche is 12.06 years for non-Hispanic black females, 12.25 years for Hispanic females, and 12.55 for non-Hispanic white females. However, completion of sexual secondary maturation occurs at approximately the same time for all racial groups.[7]

Table 8.1.
Sexual Maturity Rating for Girls and Boys

Girls Stage	Breast Development	Pubic Hair Growth
1	Prepubertal; nipple elevation only	Prepubertal; no pubic hair
2	Small, raised breast bud	Sparse growth of hair along labia
3	General enlargement of breast extending beyond areola	Pigmentation, coarsening, and curling, with an increase in amount
4	Further enlargement with projection of areola and nipple as secondary mound	Hair resembles adult type, but not spread to medial thighs
5	Mature, adult contour, with areola in same contour as breast, and only nipple projecting	Adult type and quantity, spread to medial thighs
Boys Stage	**Genital Development**	**Pubic Hair Growth**
1	Prepubertal; no change in size or proportion of testes, scrotum, and penis from early childhood	Prepubertal; no pubic hair
2	Enlargement of scrotum and testes; reddening and change in texture in skin of scrotum; little or no penis enlargement	Sparse growth of hair at base of penis
3	Increase first in length, then width of penis; growth of testes and scrotum	Darkening, coarsening, and curling; increase in amount
4	Enlargement of penis with growth in breadth and development of glands; further growth of testes and scrotum, darkening of scrotal skin	Hair resembles adult type, but not spread to medial thighs
5	Adult size and shape genitalia	Adult type and quantity, spread to medial thighs

Dietary Reference Intakes

The Dietary Reference Intakes (DRIs) provide guidelines for normal nutrition for adolescent males and females in 2 age categories, 9 to 13 years and 14 to 18 years (Appendix E) and include Recommended Dietary Allowances (RDAs) for many nutrients, which provide an estimate of the minimum daily average dietary level that meets the nutrient requirements for 97% to 98% of healthy individuals. Although there are no RDAs established for energy intake, Estimated Energy Requirements

(EERs) provide guidance on the calorie intakes needed to maintain energy balance on the basis of age, gender, weight, height, and physical activity. Among adolescents, individual variability occurs in the rates of physical growth, timing of growth spurts, and physiologic maturation, all of which may affect energy needs. In addition, individual physical activity patterns vary widely. For these reasons, assessment of energy needs of adolescents should include consideration of appetite, growth, activity, and weight gain in relation to deposition of subcutaneous fat. Restricted food intake in the physically active adolescent results in diminished growth and a drop in the basal metabolic rate and, in girls, amenorrhea. The RDAs for micronutrients, including vitamins and minerals, are designed to meet the needs of almost all healthy adolescents; therefore, they exceed the requirements for the average person. A healthy diet for the whole population, including adolescents, should provide approximately 25% to 35% of calories from fat, 45% to 65% of calories from carbohydrate, and 10% to 30% of calories from dietary protein.[8] Average caloric intake for moderately active adolescents is approximately 2700 kcal for males and 2300 kcal for females.[6]

During adolescence, increases in requirements for energy and such nutrients as calcium, nitrogen, and iron are determined by increases in lean body mass rather than an increase in body weight, with its variable fat content. Assuming that the lean body contents of calcium, iron, nitrogen, zinc, and magnesium of adolescents are the same as those of adults, the daily increments of body nutrients for the growing adolescent can be estimated (Table 8.2).[9] The incremental increases of these nutrients and the increased nutrient needs are not constant throughout adolescence and are more closely associated with the degree of sexual maturation and growth rate rather than the chronological age, as noted previously.

Table 8.2.
Daily Increments in Body Content of Minerals and Nitrogen During Adolescent Growth[a]

Mineral	Sex	Average for 10-20 y, mg	Average at Peak of Growth Spurt, m
Calcium	M	210	400
	F	110	240
Iron	M	0.57	1.1
	F	0.23	0.9
Nitrogen*	M	320	610
	F	160	360
Zinc	M	0.27	0.50
	F	0.18	0.31
Magnesium	M	4.4	8.4
	F	2.3	5.0

Adapted with permission from Forbes.[9]

[a] Multiply by 0.00625 to obtain g of protein.

Nutrition Concerns During Adolescence

Many teenagers in the United States, particularly females, consume inadequate amounts of numerous vitamins and minerals, including folic acid; vitamins A, D, E, and B_6; calcium; iron; zinc; magnesium; and fiber. In addition, adolescent diets also frequently exceed recommendations for fat, saturated fat, sodium, and cholesterol. Moreover, adolescents 9 to 18 years of age consume inadequate amounts of several important food groups, including fruits, vegetables, and whole grains.[4,10] For example, among adolescents 14 to 18 years of age, males consume an average of 1 cup of fruit/day, and females consume 0.8 cups/day, approximately half of recommended levels (2 cups for males of this age, 1.5 cups for females). Vegetables are also frequently underconsumed; males 14 to 18 years of age consume an average of 1.5 cups/day, and females consume 1.2 cups/day, far less than the 3 cups recommended for males and 2.5 cups for females. Furthermore, few adolescents are consuming nutrient-dense vegetables, highlighted by the fact that more than 95% of 9- to 18-year-olds consumed fewer than 0.2 cups of dark-green vegetables daily. In addition, a vast majority (>95%) of adolescents consume an insufficient level of whole grains and a substantial amount of added sugar in their diets.[10]

Food habits of adolescents are characterized by: (1) an increased tendency to skip meals, especially breakfast and lunch; (2) eating more meals outside the home; (3) snacking, especially energy-dense foods and beverages; (4) consumption of fast foods; and (5) dieting.[6] Some adhere to vegetarian diets or to more restrictive dietary regimens, such as Zen macrobiotic diets (see Chapter 11). Although it is very possible for young people to maintain healthy dietary intakes when consuming a vegetarian diet, some adolescents may use vegetarian diets as a means of controlling their intake in unhealthy ways; thus, such diets at this age may be associated with some disordered eating behaviors[6] (see Chapter 39). Overall, many adolescents may attempt to follow fad diets and may change their eating habits frequently. These behavioral patterns are explained by the adolescents' independence and busy schedule, difficulty in accepting existing values, dissatisfaction with body image, search for self-identification, desire for peer acceptance, and need to conform to the adolescent lifestyle.

The following describe specific nutrient needs and concerns associated with the intake of nutrients during adolescence:

1. **Energy:** Results from the 2007-2008 National Health and Nutrition Examination Survey (NHANES) revealed that 34.2% of individuals between 12 and 19 years of age were overweight and an additional 18.1% were obese. This had leveled off and slightly decreased by 2009-2010, with 32.6% of adolescents overweight and 17.1% obese,[11] although the prevalence remained alarmingly high (see Chapter 34: Obesity).

2. **Protein:** During adolescence, protein needs, like those for energy, correlate more closely with growth pattern than with chronologic age.

3. **Iron:** The need for iron for males and females is increased during adolescence to sustain the rapidly enlarging lean body mass and hemoglobin mass; in females, it is needed to offset menstrual losses as well.

4. **Zinc:** Zinc is essential for growth and sexual maturation. Growth retardation and hypogonadism have been reported in adolescent males with zinc deficiency.

5. **Vegan diets:** Adolescents who consume no animal products may be vulnerable to deficiencies of several nutrients, particularly vitamins D and B_{12}, riboflavin, protein, calcium, iron, zinc, and perhaps other trace elements (see Chapter 11).

6. **Dental caries:** Although dental caries begin in early childhood, they are a highly prevalent nutrition-related problem of adolescence. Caries are associated with low fluoride intake in childhood and frequent consumption of foods containing carbohydrates (see Chapter 50).

7. **Conditioned deficiencies:** A number of drug-nutrient interactions have been described[12] (Appendix G). Anticonvulsant drugs, especially phenytoin and phenobarbital, interfere with the metabolism of vitamin D and can lead to rickets and/or osteomalacia; therefore, supplementation with vitamin D may be desirable. Isoniazid interferes with pyridoxine metabolism. Oral contraceptives increase serum lipid concentrations, an effect that may have some clinical significance.[13]

8. **Chronic disease:** Adolescents may have inflammatory bowel disease, diabetes mellitus, juvenile rheumatoid arthritis, or sickle cell disease, among others. These chronic diseases can profoundly affect nutritional status (see appropriate chapters).

9. **Adolescent bone health:** see next section.

10. **Pregnancy:** see later section.

Nutritional Concerns for Adolescent Bone Health
(Also See Chapter 18: Calcium, Phosphorus, and Magnesium)

By the time the adolescent growth spurt occurs, the bones of the extremities have largely completed their growth. The main bone growth associated with adolescence occurs in the axial bones and is accompanied by a large increase in bone mineral density.[14,15] Peak bone mineral accretion rates occur at an average of 12.5 years of age for girls and 14.0 years for boys. Bone mineral density reaches its peak between the ages of 20 and 30 years and declines thereafter.[14,15] Adolescence is of utmost importance with regard to long-term bone health, because fully half of adult bone calcium is accreted during that time.[15] Factors that influence bone growth and mineral accretion during adolescence include genetics, hormonal status, exercise, adequacy of dietary calcium and vitamin D, general nutrition, and health. Although genetic factors account for more than half of the variance in final bone mineral density, the remaining factors are amenable to manipulation.[15]

There are a number of impediments to the teenager attaining optimal bone health. Most teenagers in the United States do not ingest the recommended daily amount of calcium of 1300 mg/day.[16] One of the principal causes is the general decline in dairy intake during these years and the inadequate consumption of calcium-rich dairy alternatives. The AAP recommends that teenagers consume 3 cups of dairy or the equivalent per day.[15] Teenagers decrease their milk consumption for various reasons. Some are truly lactose intolerant, some do not like the taste, and others consider milk to be a "child's drink." A substantial number of adolescents also may substitute sugar-sweetened beverages (such as soda) for plain milk in their diet, perhaps partly in response to the substantial advertising and marketing efforts of the manufacturers of these products that specifically target adolescents. Whatever the reason, if a teenager is not consuming dairy products, alternative sources of calcium and vitamin D need to be identified. Juices and ready-to-eat cereals fortified with calcium and vitamin D are commercially available. Other nondairy sources of calcium include some types of fish (such as sardines, canned with bones) and fortified soy products. Green, leafy vegetables that are not high in oxalates, such as broccoli, have bioavailable calcium; spinach, because of its high oxalate level, is not an optimal source of calcium. Finally, to promote optimal bone health, weight-bearing physical activity should be encouraged.[15] As adolescents age, routine daily physical activity tends to decline and sedentary behaviors (such as "screen time") increase substantially. These trends can be detrimental to good bone health as well as many other health outcomes.

Nutritional Considerations During Pregnancy

The rate of pregnancy among US adolescent females was estimated at 39.1/1000 teenagers 15 to 19 years of age in 2009.[17] Pregnancy is much more common among adolescent females 18 to 19 years of age than among younger adolescent females. Nutrient needs are higher during adolescence than at any other time in a female's life, and the additional nutrient needs of pregnancy can make it difficult for teenagers to obtain adequate nutrient intakes. Iron deficiency is particularly common among pregnant adolescents, with rates of 29% found in a national sample of low-income women during their third trimester of pregnancy.[18] As with iron, calcium intakes are low and requirements are high among adolescents. However, the recent revision of the RDA of 1300 mg of calcium for pregnant and lactating adolescents is the same for nonpregnant and nonlactating adolescents.[16]

Weight gain during pregnancy is an important issue to be addressed by health care professionals and was the subject of a recent Institute of Medicine report.[19] Obesity prior to pregnancy is an increasingly common issue that places both the mother and fetus at risk of poor pregnancy outcomes.[12] Higher rates of gestational diabetes, birth defects, preeclampsia, cesarean delivery, postpartum weight retention, large- and small-for-gestational-age infants, and preterm birth have been associated with females who enter pregnancy obese. However, the recent IOM report did not find enough evidence to support the idea that weight gain itself during pregnancy was associated with gestational diabetes and preeclampsia. Prepregnancy obesity status and excessive gestational weight gain have been found to be predictive of the development of obesity within 1 to 9 years postpartum among primiparous adolescent mothers.[20,21]

A review of nutrition interventions among pregnant adolescents found that prenatal care enhanced with intensive nutrition counseling and supplemental foods has been shown to improve rates of low birth weight, very low birth weight, and preterm birth.[22] School-based nutrition education and nursing home-visit programs have been shown to lead to modest improvements in dietary intake but no improvements in birth outcomes.[22] A comprehensive health care program for the pregnant adolescent should include proper prenatal care; monitoring of weight gain; nutritional assessment, counseling, and support; and family planning. Whenever possible, the parents or other caregiver should be included in counseling sessions.

Assessing and Maintaining Adequate Nutrition in Adolescents

Health guidance for adolescents should begin with an annual screening for indicators of nutritional risk (see Table 8.3). These include overweight and underweight, eating disorders, hyperlipidemia, hypertension, and iron-deficiency anemia. Unhealthy eating practices for which the adolescent should be screened include frequent dieting, meal skipping, food fads, and increased consumption of foods and beverages high in fat and sugar, such as fast foods and soft drinks. Nutrition screening should include a physical examination with measurement of blood pressure, an assessment of sexual maturity rating (Table 8.1), an accurate measurement of height and weight, and a calculation of body mass index (BMI). Nutrition screening should also include a broader dietary assessment of adolescents who are at increased nutritional risk (see Table 8.3) with a food frequency questionnaire, 24-hour dietary recall, or a food diary to further define nutritional problems.

Table 8.3
Tools for Practice—Adolescent Nutrition

Tool	Description	Reference
CDC Growth Curves 2000	For children 2 to 20 years; includes BMI, height, weight, and head circumference	www.cdc.gov/growthcharts/whocharts.htm
Adolescent Nutritional Questionnaire	Assesses dietary intake with selective questions about nutritional status to be completed prior to the office visit; includes interpretive notes	Tool C: Nutrition Questionnaire for Adolescents. In : American Academy of Pediatrics. *Bright Futures Nutrition*. 3rd ed. Elk Grove Village, IL: American Academy of Pediatrics; 2011:233-238
Assessing Nutrition Risk	Includes screening for food intakes, meeting dietary guidelines, excessive intakes of fats and sweets, poor dietary practices (fast foods, meal skipping, dieting, food fads, eating disorders), obesity, iron deficiency, dental caries, alcohol and tobacco use; includes criteria for further screening and assessment	Tool D: Key Indicators of Nutritional Risk for Children and Adolescents. In: American Academy of Pediatrics. *Bright Futures Nutrition*. 3rd ed. Elk Grove Village, IL: American Academy of Pediatrics; 2011:239-243
Nutrition Counseling	A simplified approach to behavior modification and nutrition counseling for children and adolescents—could be used for obesity and eating disorders	Tool F: Stages of Change—A Model for Nutrition Counseling. In : American Academy of Pediatrics. *Bright Futures Nutrition*. 3rd ed. Elk Grove Village, IL: American Academy of Pediatrics; 2011:249-250
Promotion of Healthy Eating Behavior	Tips for promoting healthy eating behavior at the office visit for adolescents	Tool G: Strategies of Health Professionals to Promote Healthy Eating Behaviors. In : American Academy of Pediatrics. *Bright Futures Nutrition*. 3rd ed. Elk Grove Village, IL: American Academy of Pediatrics; 2011:251-253
Promoting Positive Body Image	Useful for counseling adolescents with a distorted body image	Tool I: Tips for Fostering a Positive Body Image Among Children and Adolescents. In : American Academy of Pediatrics. *Bright Futures Nutrition*. 3rd ed. Elk Grove Village, IL: American Academy of Pediatrics; 2011:257-258
Scoff Questionnaire for Identifying Eating Disorders	Although only validated in adults, provides useful screening questions about eating and body image that should be asked of adolescents	See reference 23
Dietary Guidelines for Americans 2010 and My Plate	Contains specific and detailed information about specific nutrient requirements for adolescents and food based guidelines for a healthy diet	See references 24 and 25

CDC indicates Centers for Disease Control and Prevention.

Anthropometric measures should be plotted on the National Center for Health Statistics 2000 growth charts (www.cdc.gov/growthcharts/whocharts.htm). Adolescents with weight or BMI less than the 5th percentile are underweight and should undergo additional evaluation. Those with a BMI greater than the 85th percentile but less than the 95th percentile are considered overweight and should also undergo additional evaluation. Adolescents with a BMI greater than or equal to the 95th percentile are obese and should be referred for a full-scale medical evaluation as well as to a weight management program designed to meet the needs of adolescents and their families.

As noted previously, obesity prevention in adolescents is a real concern for the health care professional, and obese adolescents are at risk of becoming obese adults with the metabolic syndrome.[25] Adolescents are very concerned about physical appearance and maintaining a healthy weight. Those engaged in competitive sports can be encouraged to maintain a healthy energy intake as a competitive advantage. The AAP has recently endorsed the report from the Expert Panel on Integrated Guidelines for Cardiovascular Health and Risk Reduction in Children and Adolescents sponsored by the National Heart, Lung, and Blood Institute of the National Institutes of Health.[26] This report recommended a universal lipid screening between 9 and 11 years of age and again between 18 and 21 years of age with a nonfasting non-high-density lipoprotein (HDL) or fasting lipid panel.[26] Adolescents between 12 and 17 years of age may need additional fasting lipid panels to be performed if significant risk factors for cardiovascular disease develop, such as obesity. Dietary intervention should include avoiding high intakes of saturated fats and trans fats as well as cholesterol. For adolescents, the Expert Panel recommended that energy from fat not exceed 25% to 35% of total energy intake. If lipid screening reveals an abnormality, adolescents will need close follow-up and ongoing dietary management.[26] These adolescents are also at risk of the metabolic syndrome, including type 2 diabetes mellitus, although no acceptable definition of this syndrome exists for children or adolescents.[26]

As noted previously, relatively few adolescents meet the dietary guidelines for intakes of fruits, vegetables, whole grains, and dairy products, although they often exceed their daily energy requirement—males more so than females.[27] Fast food snacks account for 25% to 33% of daily energy intake and tend to be energy dense and nutrient poor. Directing food choices toward nutritionally dense foods, especially for foods eaten outside of the home, is very important advice to give to the adolescent by both physician and parents.

Parents are still the gatekeepers of foods and again serve as important role models for eating behavior. They should be advised to keep a variety of healthy foods in the home, provide fruits and vegetables at every meal, and use whole-grain breads and cereals. Adolescents require 3 servings a day of low-fat (1%) or non-fat milk or other low-fat dairy products to provide adequate amounts of calcium and vitamin D for strong bones.[16] Lean meats, including chicken and fish, should be served. High-fat foods, sweetened beverages, and fast foods low in nutrient density should be avoided. Eating meals as a family has been shown to improve dietary intake, with higher intakes of essential nutrient such as calcium, iron, and vitamins. The intake of fruits and vegetables is also increased with family meals.[28] The tendency for meal skipping also increases, with breakfast being the most frequently skipped meal but one that has been shown to have a positive effect on school performance.[29] Skipping breakfast also adversely affects dietary intake, as this promotes snacking on less healthy food throughout the day to make up for the loss in energy intake.[30]

Adolescents engage in significant amounts of screen time, and the influence of the media and the Internet have an increasingly negative effect on dietary intake, with their emphasis on foods with low nutrient density and increased amounts of fat, sugar, and salt.[28] Parents should be encouraged to keep healthy snacks around the home and to encourage adolescents to take breakfast bars or fruit with them to school rather than skipping breakfast.

Encouraging participation in both organized and unorganized physical activity is crucial, as there is often a significant drop in physical activity at adolescence, especially among females.[31] It is recommended that adolescents engage in 60 minutes or more of physical activity per day, the energy and nutrient needs of these activities varying widely.[27] Electronic social networking is greatly increased in adolescence, and parents should be encouraged to limit screen time (TV, video, computer) to 2 hours per day and never allow television watching in the bedroom.[28] This intervention is important in obesity prevention as well.[32]

Average caloric intake for moderately active adolescents is approximately 2700 kcal for males and 2300 kcal for females.[27] Individual energy needs will vary greatly depending on age, gender, body size, degree of physical maturation, rate of growth, and level of physical activity (Table 8.4). The assessment of growth rate is key to determining adequate energy intake. Adolescents also need large amounts of protein, up to 0.5 g/lb of body weight per day. Thus, a 124-lb adolescent will need approximately 60 g of daily protein intake.[27] The RDA for iron is 15 mg/day for females and 12 mg/day for males, the difference being menstrual losses of blood in females.[33] Heme iron from meat (including shell fish) is the best source of iron, given its relatively high absorption rate. Adolescents should be screened for iron deficiency if, by history, they are at risk of iron deficiency.[33]

Table 8.4.
Estimated Calorie Needs per Day by Age, Gender, and Physical Activity Level

Males			
	Activity Level		
	Sedentary	**Moderately Active**	**Active**
Age (y)			
12	1800	2200	2400
13	2000	2200	2600
14	2000	2400	2800
15	2200	2600	3000
16	2400	2800	3200
17	2400	2800	3200
19-20	2600	2800	3000
Females			
	Activity Level		
	Sedentary	**Moderately Active**	**Active**
Age (y)			
12	1600	2000	2200
13	1600	2000	2200
14	1800	2000	2400
15	1800	2000	2400
16	1800	2000	2400
17	1800	2000	2400
19-20	2000	2200	2400

Adapted from the US Department of Agriculture and the US Department of Health and Human Services. *Dietary Guidelines for Americans, 2010.*[27]

Other key nutrients for adolescents include adequate calcium and vitamin D for bone growth. The RDA for calcium, according to the IOM, is 1300 mg for adolescents.[16] This can be achieved with 3 to 4 servings of dairy products a day. Fortified milk will also supply the daily 600 IU of vitamin D recommended for adolescents.[16] Weight-conscious adolescents should be assured that reduced-fat or skim milk contains just as much calcium and vitamin D as does whole milk. Alternative sources of calcium are tofu, fortified soy milk, and dark green, leafy vegetables, although very large quantities of vegetables will have to be consumed to match the iron intake from meat. As noted previously, many adolescents fail to achieve the required intakes of vitamins and minerals because of their food choices.[16,33]

References

1. US Census Bureau. Age and Sex Composition: 2010. 2010 Census Briefs. Available at: http://www.census.gov/prod/cen2010/briefs/c2010br-03.pdf. Accessed September 26, 2012

2. Stang J, Story MT, Harnack L, Neumark-Stzainer D. Relationship between vitamin and mineral supplement use, dietary intake, and dietary adequacy among adolescents. *J Am Diet Assoc*. 2000;100(8):905-910

3. US Department of Agriculture, Agricultural Research Service. What we eat in America. 2002-2008. Available at: http://www.ars.usda.gov/Services/docs.htm?docid=18349. Accessed September 26, 2012

4. Centers for Disease Control and Prevention. Fruit and vegetable consumption among high school students—United States, 2010. *MMWR Morb Mortal Wkly Rep*. 2012;307(2):135-137

5. Centers for Disease Control and Prevention. Youth risk behavior surveillance—United States, 2005. *MMWR Surveill Summ*. 2006;55(SS-5):1-108

6. Kliegman RM, Berhman RE, Jenson HB, Stanton BF. *Nelson Textbook of Pediatrics*. 18th ed. Philadelphia, PA: Saunders Elsevier; 2007

7. American Academy of Pediatrics, Committee on Adolescence; American College of Obstetricians and Gynecologists, Committee on Adolescent Health Care. Menstruation in girls and adolescents: using the menstrual cycle as a vital sign. *Pediatrics*. 2006;118(5):2245-2250

8. Institute of Medicine, Food and Nutrition Board. *Dietary Reference Intakes: The Essential Guide to Nutrient Requirements*. JJ Otten, JP Hellwig, LD Meyers, eds. Washington DC: National Academies Press; 2006

9. Forbes GB. Nutritional requirements in adolescence. In: Suskind RM, ed. *Textbook of Pediatric Nutrition*. New York, NY: Raven Press; 1981:381-391

10. US National Institutes of Health, National Cancer Institute. Usual Dietary Intakes: Food Intakes, US Food Population, 2001-04. Risk Factor Monitoring and Methods, Cancer Control and Population Sciences. Available at: http://riskfactor.cancer.gov/diet/usualintakes/pop/. Accessed September 26, 2012

11. Ogden CL, Carroll MD, Kit BK, Flegal KM. Prevalence of obesity and trends in body mass index among US children and adolescents, 1999-2010. *JAMA*. 2012;307(5):483-490

12. Roe DA. Diet-drug interactions and incompatibilities. In: Hathcock JN, Coon J, eds. *Nutrition and Drug Interrelations*. New York, NY: Academic Press; 1978:319-345

13. Webber LS, Hunter SM, Johnson CC, Srinivasan SR, Berenson GS. Smoking, alcohol, and oral contraceptives: effect on lipids during adolescence and young adulthood: Bogalusa Heart Study. *Ann N Y Acad Sci*. 1991;623:135-154

14. Steelman J, Zeitler P. Osteoporosis in pediatrics. *Pediatr Rev*. 2001;22(2):56-65

15. Greer FR, Krebs NF. Committee on Nutrition. Optimizing bone health and calcium intakes of infants, children, and adolescents. *Pediatrics*. 2006;117(2):578-585

16. Institute of Medicine, Food and Nutrition Board. *Dietary Reference Intakes for Calcium and Vitamin D*. Washington, DC: National Academies Press; 2011

17. Centers for Disease Control and Prevention. Vital signs: teen pregnancy—United States, 1991-2009. *MMWR Morb Mort Wkly Rep.* 2011;60(13):414-420

18. Centers for Disease Control and Prevention. Recommendations to prevention and control iron deficiency in the United States. *MMWR Recomm Rep.* 1998;47(RR-3):1-29

19. Institute of Medicine. *Weight Gain During Pregnancy: Reexamining the Guidelines.* Washington, DC: National Academies Press; 2009

20. Groth SW. The long-term impact of adolescent gestational weight gain. *Res Nurs Health.* 2008;31(2):108–118

21. Nielsen JN, Gittelsohn J, Anliker J, O'Brien K. Interventions to improve diet and weight gain among pregnant adolescents and recommendations for future research. *J Am Diet Assoc.* 2006;106(11):1825-1840

22. Joseph NP, Hunkali KB, Wilson B, Morgan E, Cross M, Freund KM. Pre-pregnancy body mass index among pregnant adolescents: gestational weight gain and long-term post partum weight retention. *J Pediatr Adolesc Gynecol.* 2008;21(4):195-200

23. Rosen DS. Identification and management of eating disorders in children and adolescents. *Pediatrics.* 2010;126(5):1240-1253

24. US Department of Agriculture. MyPlate. Available at: http://www.choosemyplate.gov/food-groups/. Accessed September 26, 2012

25. Ogden CL, Lamb MM, Carroll MD, Flegal KM. Obesity and socioeconomic status in children and adolescents: United States, 2005-2008. *NCHS Data Brief.* 2010 Dec;(51):1-8

26. Expert Panel on Integrated Guidelines for Cardiovascular Health and Risk Reduction in Children and Adolescents: Summary Report. National Heart, Lung, and Blood Institute, National Institutes of Health. *Pediatrics.* 2011;128(Suppl 5):S213-S256

27. US Department of Health and Human Services. Dietary Guidelines for Americans. Available at: http://www.health.gov/dietaryguidelines/. Accessed September 26, 2012

28. Liang T, Kuhle S. Veugelers PJ. Nutrition and body weights of Canadian children watching television and eating while watching television. *Public Health Nutr.* 2009;12(12):2457-2463

29. Hoyland A, Dye L, Lawton CL. A systematic review of the effect of breakfast on the cognitive performance of children and adolescents. *Nutr Res Rev.* 2009;22(2):220-243

30. Szajewska H, Ruszczynski M. Systematic review demonstrating that breakfast consumption influences body weight in outcomes in children and adolescents in Europe. *Crit Rev Food Sci Nutr.* 2010;50(2):113-119

31. Kimm SY, Glynn NW, Kriska AM, et al. Decline in physical activity in black girls and white girls during adolescence. *N Engl J Med.* 2002;347(10):709-715

32. Robinson TN. Reducing children's television viewing to prevent obesity: a randomized controlled trial. *JAMA.* 1999;282(16):1561-1567

33. Institute of Medicine, Food and Nutrition Board. *Dietary Reference Intakes for Vitamin A, Vitamin K, Arsenic, Boron, Chromium, Copper, Iodine, Iron, Manganese, Molybdenum, Nickel, Silicon, Vanadium, and Zinc.* Washington, DC: National Academies Press; 2005

III

CHAPTER 9

Nutrition in School, Preschool, and Child Care

Introduction

The sudden doubling of obesity rates among children in the 1980s and 1990s left nearly 1 of every 3 children overweight and 1 of every 6 obese. This has heightened concerns about the quality of foods and beverages provided in the school setting, not only in school meal programs but also in vending machines, school stores, cafeterias, school fundraisers, and special occasions in the classroom. A series of strong policies and practices have been introduced to ensure more nutritious school meals and improve the school food environment as one important measure to help address childhood obesity, ushering in yet another phase in the evolution of the national school meal programs.[1]

School food is complex. Besides the programs supported by the US Department of Agriculture (USDA) in schools, such as the School Breakfast Program, the National School Lunch Program, the After-School Food Program, and the Child and Adult Food Program, there are many other entry points for food in schools (see Chapter 51). Although the school environment has been described as a contributor to, as well as a potential solution for, overweight, its role is much broader. It should be recognized that the primary intent of school meals is to support the needs of children who come from families with food insufficiency and hunger (food insecurity). In 2011, more than 95% of American children, 55 million, attended public or private schools.[2] A typical child spends as much as 6 hours per day in school and consumes 35% of their daily energy at school, compared with 56% at home.[3] School nutrition should underscore the concept that a healthy child is a better student, particularly children and adolescents with economic or social disadvantages.[4]

The US Nutritional Safety Net

The USDA Food and Nutrition Service oversees a series of federal programs that form a nutritional safety net for vulnerable populations, including children and adolescents during and after school hours as well as during the summer[5] (see Chapter 51). These programs have a profound effect on the diet quality of US children at highest risk.[6] Assistance programs from the Food and Nutrition Service that directly affect children and adolescents in school represent an investment of $13.7 billion in cash reimbursement and commodity costs annually (estimated fiscal year 2010 expenses) to fund a series of specialized offerings intended to address specific problem areas or populations, including:

- The National School Lunch Program
- The School Breakfast Program
- After School Snacks
- The Special Milk Program
- The Fresh Fruit and Vegetable Program
- The Child and Adult Care Food Program
- The Seamless Summer Program
- Team Nutrition

The History of School Meals

In 1946, even before Congress passed and President Harry Truman signed the National School Lunch Act (Pub L No. 79-396), it was recognized that children in poverty needed school meals both for nutritional stability and for academic productivity. Early models of school meals began in the late 1800s. The National School Lunch Program was created in response to the recognition that physical inadequacies were linked with poor nutrition among young men rejected for the armed services in World War II. The intent of the National School Lunch Program was to provide children with at least 1 nutritious meal every day at school. The type A lunch was designed to provide one third to one half of the daily requirements for a 10- to 12-year-old child, a benchmark that was sustained for 3 decades. Over time, growth and development as well as provision of balanced macronutrients and targeted recommended daily amounts (RDAs) of micronutrients served as the scientific foundation for the program. The most recent reauthorizations of the Child Nutrition Act (the Healthy, Hunger-Free Kids Act of 2010 [Pub L No. 111-196]) have tailored the National School Lunch Program to match the Dietary Guidelines for Americans. Since its inception, the number of children participating in the National School Lunch Program has increased from 7.1 million in 1946-1947 to 29.5 million 60 years later in more than 100 000 schools both public and nonprofit private as well as residential child care institutions. The Child Nutrition Act of 1966 established the School Breakfast Program as a pilot for low-income children, especially those traveling long distances to school. In 1975, the School Breakfast Program became a permanent entitlement program alongside the National School Lunch Program, administered by the USDA Food and Nutrition Service.

Approximately half of National School Lunch Program participants and three quarters of School Breakfast Program participants fit the criteria for eligibility on the basis of low family income, indicating that the original mission of the school food programs is being met. Newman and Ralston,[7] using data from the National

Health and Nutrition Examination Survey as well as the Survey of Income and Program Participation Survey, found that by 2006, free lunches were being served to white, African-American, and Hispanic participants almost evenly, with the highest proportion among 8- to 13-year-old children. Further, two thirds of children and teenagers from female-headed households were benefiting from free lunch.

New Nutrition Standards for School Meals

Optimal nutrition for children older than 2 years is described by the Dietary Guidelines for Americans.[8] The most recent guidelines (2010) were released in January 2011, on the basis of recommendations from the Dietary Guidelines for Americans Advisory Committee. The report of the committee reviewed current issues related to child and adolescent nutrition. The Dietary Guidelines for Americans Committee set goals for children's diets, including consumption of a nutrient-rich diet pattern based on 5 food groups: vegetables, fruits, grains and whole grains, low-fat or no-fat milk and dairy, and quality protein sources. Dietary attributes of the nutrient rich concept have been discussed in a clinical practice paper of the American Dietetic Association (now the Academy of Nutrition and Dietetics).[9]

The new Dietary Guidelines for Americans stress limiting the intake of solid fats, added sugars, and sodium. For children and adolescents 2 to 18 years of age, the most common sources of daily energy vary with age but collectively are grain-based desserts, pizza, sweetened soft drinks, yeast breads, and chicken or "dishes," that is, combination items. The leading sources of solid fats are pizza, grain desserts, whole milk, regular cheese, and fatty meats; leading sources of added sugars are sweetened soft drinks, fruit drinks, grain desserts, dairy desserts, and candy.[10] The Dietary Guidelines for Americans stressed the need for greater physical activity at all ages with an emphasis on achieving energy balance, matching caloric intake with routine activity levels. The Dietary Guidelines for Americans also identified 4 nutrients that, because of low consumption, put Americans at a high level of health risk: potassium, fiber, vitamin D, and calcium.

The Child Nutrition Reauthorization, termed *The Healthy, Hunger-Free Kids Act of 2010* (Pub L No. 111-296), passed the most significant changes for school food in more than 3 decades. Providing funding of $4.5 billion over 10 years, the bill included several new provisions to shape foods offered in school:

- Provides 0.06 cents additional funding to schools per reimbursed meal to improve nutritional quality;
- Helps communities establish local farm-to-school networks;
- Augments USDA efforts to improve the nutritional quality of commodity foods for school meal programs;

- Expands access to drinking water in schools, particularly during meal times;

- Gives the USDA the authority to set nutritional standards for all foods regularly sold during the school day, including vended and a la carte items and those sold in school stores;

- Sets basic standards for school wellness policies, including goals for nutrition, education, and physical activity;

- Promotes nutrition and wellness in child-care settings through the Child and Adult Care Food Program;

- Improves access to food by increasing eligibility and simplifying the process by which a child can meet requirements while allowing for more universal access in high-poverty communities through eligibility based on census data;

- Enhances food safety and nutritional standards by mandating school audits every 3 years;

- Gives the USDA the authority to support more meals for high-risk children through after-school programs; and

- Provides more training for school nutrition staff to support these provisions.

The Institute of Medicine (IOM) provided new recommendations for school meals based on the 2005 Dietary Guidelines for Americans.[11] This report and the subsequent proposed Food and Nutrition Service rule in 2011 recommended school meals based on the 5 basic food groups and established food frequency and serving size as well as minimum and maximum caloric intake targets by age and grade (Table 9.1). This approach reflects the emphasis of the Dietary Guidelines for Americans on overall dietary patterns of food intake for healthy eating rather than intake of specific nutrients.

Table 9.1.
Proposed Minimum and Maximum Calorie Intakes[11]

Grades	Breakfast Program	Lunch Program
K-5	350-500 kcal	550-650 kcal
6-8	400-550 kcal	600-700 kcal
9-12	450-600 kcal	750-850 kcal

School breakfast aims to provide 25% of a student's average nutrient needs, and school lunch aims to provide 33% of a student's average nutrient needs spread over the course of a week. An example school breakfast pattern is presented in Table 9.2. The recommended food patterns provide more fruit at breakfast, more vegetables at lunch, and more whole grains at both meals.

Table 9.2.
The Proposed School Breakfast Meal Pattern[11]

Average Total Amount of Food Per Week			
	Grades K-5	**Grades 6-8**	**Grades 9-12**
Fruits (cups)	5 At least 1/day	5 At least 1/day	5 At least 1/day
Vegetables (cups)	0	0	0
Grains (ounces)	7-10 At least 1/day	8-10 At least 1/day	9-10 At least 1/day
Meats/Meat Alternatives (ounces)	5 At least 1/day	5 At least 1/day	7-10 At least 1/day
Fluid milk (cups)	5 At least 1/day	5 At least 1/day	5 At least 1/day
Daily Amount Based on the Average for a 5-Day Week			
Calorie range	350-500	400-550	450-600
Saturated Fat (% of total calories)	<10	<10	<10
Sodium (mg)	<430	<470	<500
Trans Fat	0	0	0

Within the meal patterns, trans fats are stringently curtailed and sodium is reduced by 25% for school breakfasts and 50% for school lunches over a 10-year period. The IOM report also proposed the new category of "starchy vegetable" (potatoes, corn, lima beans, and green peas) and recommended that it be limited to 1 cup (2 servings) per week to ensure that a variety of other vegetables were offered to students. Subsequently, Congress overturned this proposed restriction on potatoes. Using the suggested approach, it was determined that students could meet the Daily Recommended Intakes (DRIs) for 24 nutrients.

Adherence to these guidelines, with their emphasis on whole-grain foods, fruits, and vegetables, naturally limits discretionary solid fats and added sugars in school meals. The minimum and maximum calorie recommendations are intended to represent the average daily amount for a 5-day school week and not a per-meal or per-day basis. For certain age groups, such as adolescent males, the minimum daily calories may be high enough to be a challenge for school food service to achieve consistently. To address this, discretionary sources of calories (solid fats and added sugars) may be added to the meal pattern, provided that they are within the specifications for calories, saturated fat, trans fat, and sodium.

Alternatives for meat servings may include other protein sources, such as nuts, seeds, or nut butters or flours; yogurt products; and enriched macaroni. Forms of meats or meat alternatives may not be repeated more than 3 times weekly. Similarly, fluid milk substitutes may be used if warranted for students with medical, dietary, or cultural needs. However, nondairy substitutes must follow fortification guidelines of the Food and Drug Administration (Table 9.3).

Table 9.3.
Nondairy Alternative Fortification Requirements

Nutrient	Per cup (8 fl oz)
Calcium	276 mg
Protein	8 g
Vitamin A	500 IU
Vitamin D	100 IU
Magnesium	24 mg
Phosphorus	222 mg
Potassium	349 mg
Riboflavin	0.44 mg
Vitamin B_{12}	1.1 μg

The Infrastructure of School Food Service

The USDA Food and Nutrition Service policies direct how the menu should be designed and provided to students. The school food service staff is responsible for producing meals that are palatable and economical and can be delivered within a strict time frame set aside in the school day. The school nutrition supervisor completes core training in nutrition, menu planning, quantity food preparation, purchasing, personnel, and organization management. Supervisors also must continue their training on a prescribed basis. School nutrition staff members receive training and staff development as dictated by their school district. One of the greatest challenges for improving school nutrition services is increasing the professional qualifications of the individuals who manage them. A majority of districts require only a high school diploma or general educational development (GED) credential as the minimum educational requirement.[12] On a voluntary basis, the School Nutrition Association provides credentialing, certification, resources for helping programs to produce and improve their meal programs, and continuing education opportunities and national advocacy for those in the field.[13] Over the past 2 decades, data from the 3 School Nutrition Dietary Assessment (SNDA) studies have shown a rapid improvement in the nutritional quality of school meals.[14-16]

The Economics of the School Meal

School meal programs aim to provide nutritious food for disadvantaged children. To accomplish this, the USDA provides subsidies to schools to allow them to provide meals at no cost or low cost to children meeting specified household financial criteria. The income and eligibility requirements are based on the federal poverty guidelines published by the US Department of Health and Human Services. The income cutoff for those eligible for free school meals is 130% of the defined poverty cut-point and for reduced-price meals is 185% of the poverty cut-point. During periods of economic downturn, many more children rely on school meal subsidies. One measure of successful outreach is the ratio of school breakfast compared with school lunch participation. Of the 29 largest urban school districts, only 2 exceeded 70%, whereas many enrolled as few as 30% to 40%.[17]

Perhaps the most difficult responsibility for food service managers is balancing the dual challenges of operating costs versus federal nutrition requirements. Generally, the school food service director is responsible to the district's chief financial officer to maintain a cost-neutral program, at minimum. Revenue is tied to federal reimbursement rates, outlined in Table 9.4.

Table 9.4.
Government Per Meal Reimbursement Rates for School Meal Programs in the Contiguous 48 States[23,a]

Student's Status	Breakfast	Lunch/Supper	Snack
Free meal	$1.51	$2.79	$0.76
Reduced price meal	$1.21	$2.39	$0.38
Full price meal	$0.27	$0.28	$0.007

[a] Reimbursement is higher for Alaska and Hawaii.[23]

Rising food and transportation costs, as well as ever-increasing expenses related to personnel for health care and other benefits, are not fully offset by the annual cost-of-living adjustments that are built into the Child Nutrition Reauthorizations. Labor accounts for nearly half of all expenses, whereas the USDA subsidies account for only half of all food service revenue (student payments = 24%, competitive food sales = 16%, and state and local funding = 9%).[18] Additional noncommodity funds to improve the quality of school meals have remained relatively flat over the past 20 years.[19] According to the School Lunch and Breakfast Cost Study II,[20] in 2004-2005, school food service authorities reported that the cost of producing the National School Lunch Program reimbursable lunch averaged $2.28 and the

School Breakfast Program reimbursable breakfast averaged $1.92, below the lunch reimbursement of $2.51 but well above the breakfast reimbursement of $1.27. But these costs do not reflect the full costs carried by the school district. Meal time supervision, administrative labor, payroll and accounting, and indirect costs, such as equipment and utility charges, are not reflected in the food service budget. When estimates for total costs are included, the real cost of a school lunch is approximately $2.91 per meal, well above the reimbursement rate. Further, these numbers are skewed by larger school districts that are able to maintain relatively low costs per meal by a high volume of meals and by efficiencies in production.[18]

Many districts use lucrative a la carte and vended foods to provide added revenues.[18] The Government Accounting Office in 2005 reported that revenues to middle and high schools from competitive foods generated nearly $125 000 per school, funds that typically are used to offset food service expenses.[21,22] In the 2010 Child Nutrition Reauthorization, a supplementary 0.6 cents per meal was included to aid schools in supplying the additional fruits, vegetables, whole grains, and water that were mandated in the new rule from the Food and Nutrition Service, although it is unlikely to fully address the additional funds needed.[23] The most effective strategy for school food services to increase revenue is to have higher student participation in school meals.[18]

The Commodity School Program

Even at the inception of the school lunch program in 1946, Congress recognized the need to augment the meal reimbursement to schools with food stocks from the nation's agricultural surplus. The Commodity School Program is a critical supplement to help schools meet nutritional guidelines and maintain a reasonable cost.[24] Commodities provide approximately 15% to 20% of the food items served. More than 180 products are available to schools that cover all 5 food groups, including sauces, meats, canned and frozen vegetables, fruits, juices, and grains. Foods purchasing agents, the American Marketing Service and Farm Service Agency, must meet the USDA's strict food safety guidelines. Each commodity is accompanied by a food fact sheet for use by the school nutrition staff that lists the food item, the amount, a description of the product, its nutrition fact label, and storage information and tips for preparation. Fruits are packed in extra light sucrose syrup or remain unsweetened, such as applesauce. Vegetable products are limited to 140 mg of sodium per serving or less, many as no-salt varieties. Meats are offered as lean, low-fat servings. Lard and butter have been eliminated altogether as commodity products. In this way, the USDA contributes to the provisions of the 2010 Dietary Guidelines for Americans as it helps the nation's 100 000 schools meet the directives of the Food and Nutrition Service. In fiscal year 2010, the commodity food service was estimated to have delivered to schools agricultural products valued at more than $1.12 billion dollars.

The Nutritional Effectiveness of the School Meal Programs

The first national study of school meal programs, the School Nutrition Dietary Assessment Study,[14] found that most programs met a variety of important nutrition goals but fell well short of achieving the Dietary Guidelines for Americans recommendations for children, particularly in terms of fat and saturated fat intake. In that same year, the USDA introduced the School Meals Initiative for Healthy Children to improve nutritional quality through closer adherence to the Dietary Guidelines. Subsequent SNDA studies II and III showed rapid progress after introduction of a defined process for meal planning.[15,16] Prior to the 2011 Food and Nutrition Service proposed rule changes for school nutrition, school meals were designed to be balanced in terms of macronutrients and selected micronutrients in a specified manner using software to aid menu planning (at least one third the RDA for protein, calcium, iron, vitamin A, and vitamin C at lunch and one quarter the RDA for each at breakfast). Two approaches were offered to the schools: the nutrient analysis method (Nutrient Standard Menu Planning and Assisted Nutrient Standard menu planning for nutrients and energy) or the food-based menu method (Traditional or Enhanced menu planning for specific meal patterns). Previous standards did not specify levels of cholesterol, sodium, carbohydrate, or dietary fiber, although over the past decade, school food services have addressed these nutrients. Guidelines set an age-appropriate minimum but not a maximum limit of calories. In addition, the percentage calories from fat could not exceed 30% of the total, and those of saturated fat could not exceed 10% of the total. The nutrient balance was not required by USDA standards to be averaged daily but rather over the course of a school week. This methodology proved effective in ensuring the nutritional quality of school meals.

Nutrition Goals and the National School Lunch Program

The National School Lunch Program is one of the nation's most powerful nutrition programs. Nearly every public school (99%) in the country participates. Of the 30 million lunches served daily, 49% are provided free and another 10% provided at reduced cost to low-income children.[25] Not only is the planned or offered meal of high quality, but also, the meal actually selected by students meets the USDA benchmark, the School Meals Initiative for Healthy Children (SMI).[26] Comparisons between the 3 SNDA studies—I in 1995, II in 2000, and III in 2007—show impressive improvements in nutritional quality over a short period.[14-16] Intake of protein, vitamins A and B_{12}, riboflavin, calcium, phosphorus, potassium, and zinc were higher among participants than nonparticipants in the National School Lunch Program.

Still, the most recent School Health Policies and Programs Study (SHPPS) and the SNDA III study revealed several potential areas for improvement.[12,26] Only 9 of 22 specific food-preparation practices recommended by nutritionists as strategies for reducing the total fat, saturated fat, sodium, and added sugar content of school meals were implemented "almost always" or "always" by more than half of districts and schools.[12] Only 6% of schools offered lunches that met all of the SMI standards. Approximately 60% met the fat standard of 25% to 35% of total calories, but only 30% kept saturated fat under 10% of calories. Saturated fats in schools, such as fatty meats, cheeses, and high-fat milks, were still prevalent in school meals in SNDA III. In addition, almost no school met the goals for sodium on the basis of current recommendations.[26] Raw or fresh vegetables and fresh fruits were found to be unavailable in 42% and 50% of schools, respectively. Only 5% of the breads or rolls offered were whole grain. On the other hand, the SHPPS survey showed that approximately two thirds of schools offered students a choice each day for lunch between 2 or more types of fruit or 100% fruit juice, between 2 or more entrees or main courses, and between 2 or more vegetables. Most schools offered either low-fat milk or skim milk; less than half of milk offered was whole or 2% milk. Removal of fryers from school kitchens has been one recent, highly successful campaign of the School Nutrition Association.[12,13]

The Nutrition Potential of the School Breakfast Program

Over 10 million children per day, nearly one-quarter of all students, participated in the School Breakfast Program in 2007. This represents only one-third of those participating in the National School Lunch Program, presenting a potentially powerful opportunity to improve the nutritional status of American children.[27,28] More than 70% of breakfasts are provided free, and another 10% are provided at a reduced price.[26] Skipping breakfast becomes increasingly common as children age.[29] The nutritional quality of breakfast has improved progressively over the past decade, on the basis of comparison of data from the SNDA II and SNDA III.[30] Children who consume school breakfast show a greater intake of selected micronutrients than those who do not participate.[28-30] Recommendations for improving school breakfasts include decreasing the reliance on 100% fruit juice and increasing whole fruits; limiting high-fat meats, such as sausage; offering only nonfat or 1% milk; and substituting more unsweetened whole grain products for the current sweet pastries and breads. The IOM report[11] reflected these changes, and they have been incorporated into the provisional 2011 USDA rule for the School Breakfast Program.

In the United States in 2007, nearly 70% of schools offered some form of breakfast to students. Two thirds of schools participated in the USDA reimbursable School Breakfast Program, and 11.9% offered other breakfast options to students.[12]

Many schools are starting to offer universal breakfast to take advantage of this important first meal. According to the SHPPS nationwide survey in 2007, 18.0% of states had adopted a policy offering breakfast to all students.[12] An additional 44.0% of states had adopted a policy stating that some categories of schools, such as those with a certain percentage of students eligible for free or reduced-price meals, now must offer universal breakfast. But according to the Food Research and Action Center, no states serve breakfast to more than 61% of those children eligible for free or reduced price lunches.[17] If just the 29 largest urban districts in the United States had achieved a 70% rate, an additional 595 000 children would have been fed daily, and schools would have collected an additional $151 million in available federal dollars. For these districts, universal breakfast eliminates much of the challenge of verification while offering students and schools a tremendous benefit.[17]

Several national organizations, including the School Nutrition Association, Food Research and Action Center, and others, are promoting breakfast in the classroom as a simple means to achieve highest participation rates.[17,31] Although school administrators often voice worries over problems with transportation timing, personnel needs, children consuming double meals, supervision during breakfast, and even infestations of the school, all these issues have been overcome successfully in both large urban and rural schools using the breakfast-in-the-classroom strategy.[29] Especially for children with chronic food insecurity, daily classroom breakfast offer substantial benefits, not only for diet quality but also for many measures of psychosocial functioning, in addition to decreasing tardiness or absenteeism and improving classroom behavior.[4,27,32,33] Of course, merely serving a breakfast will not necessarily improve a student's overall diet quality. Crepinsek et al[34] stressed that a quality breakfast is required to improve overall nutrition and maximize breakfast's benefits.

Special Challenges for School Food Service

As specified in the Individuals with Disabilities Education Act (IDEA), children with disabilities are to be provided with a free and appropriate public education to prepare them for future employment and independent living. As a result, schools, school nurses, and the school food service have developed policies and practices to address a variety of nutritional challenges, such as food allergy, celiac disease, lactose intolerance, special diets for genetic or medical conditions, and religious and lifestyle preferences or vegetarian or vegan diets. Such accommodations can be costly for schools, not only in terms of supplying and preparing unique menus for a variety of different children, but also in personnel, quality control, and monitoring.

The most prevalent of the specific dietary adjustments is for food allergies. CDC data show that food allergies, especially more severe cases, are on the rise.[35,36] The largest and most recent study of allergic children found that 8% (5.9 million) have food allergies, and of that group, 30% have allergies to multiple foods and 39% had severe forms of the reaction.[37] In 90% of the nation's schools, more than one child in attendance has a food allergy. Half of these schools have experienced an allergic reaction.[38] Because food allergies are the most common cause of anaphylaxis, representing a sudden, potentially fatal, reaction, parents of children with severe food allergies have concerns about the potential for contact with allergic trigger foods both in the school meals and in packed meals of other students. Although the food service staff is trained to deal with allergy by careful food handling techniques, packed lunches, food trading, and contaminated surfaces make the cafeteria environment difficult to control. Misconceptions about food allergy prevalence, definition, and triggers are common. Among physicians, strategies for approaching food allergies differ widely, making uniform dietary approaches difficult.[37]

Although any food can elicit a reaction, there are 8 foods that account for 90% of all food allergies in children: egg, milk, soy, wheat, peanuts, tree nuts, fish, and shellfish. The most frequent reactions occur in young children but generally are milder. Severe anaphylactic or fatal reactions in children usually are attributable to peanut and tree nuts (eg, walnuts, cashews, etc), milk, and seafood. Anaphylaxis is often associated with adolescence and underlying asthma. In 25% of cases involving anaphylaxis in schools, no prior diagnosis of food allergy existed.[39]

The management of proven food allergy relies on 3 components: strict avoidance of the food, recognition of symptoms (intestinal, respiratory, and neurologic), and the administration of epinephrine as soon as possible. In schools, treatment is more challenging, although the 3 pillars of management remain the same. The most important approach for schools is to have available the student's Individualized Health Care Plan (IHCP) as a management strategy. To write the IHCP, the school nurse will require documentation of the food allergy from the primary care physician along with a description of the food allergy, triggers, warning signals noted, and a history of past reactions, including anaphylactic reactions.

Avoidance is the front-line strategy for food allergies. Little is published in the way of controlled studies on approaches to avoidance in schools and child-care centers, but best practice guidelines are available.[40-42] Some basic principles can be applied. Skin contact and routine inhalation, which might occur routinely without heat vaporization, do not induce systemic reactions.[43] Cleaning of hands and surfaces with soap and water or commercial wipes are effective; antibacterial gels alone are not. Although the concept of an "allergen-safe table" in the cafeteria may be important for some hypersensitive children, they need not be physically separated from their friends or other children, provided that the others at the table are eating safe foods. Within the classroom environment, blanket bans of offending allergens may be warranted, particularly for younger children with a higher likelihood of incidental spread and ingestion of the allergen. Eating bans on field trips and school buses also are important means of control. Education is the most effective way to prevent an unforeseen allergic reaction.[39]

The school food service is responsible for the cleanliness of surfaces in food preparation areas as well as in the cafeteria. Menu ingredients, food preparation, and handling require knowledge of ingredient labels, including any manufacturer modifications to food products that may have introduced an offending allergen. Cross-contamination of equipment or storage containers is another common route for exposure. The routine of maintaining food ingredient lists for a few days allows the school food service director to help identify new food allergies as they are identified in the student population.

Food Safety

To protect the safety of school meals, several safety measures are written into the law. The USDA Food and Nutrition Service rule requires that schools participating in the federal school breakfast and lunch programs must obtain 2 inspections yearly, post the inspection report, and release a copy to the public on request. The protocols examine such issues as food handling, hand washing, equipment, food temperature, storage, and environment. Although this rule has been in effect since 2004 and was reiterated in the 2010 Child Nutrition Reauthorization, fiscal pressures and the lack of tangible punitive measures at the state level may have limited compliance. A report in 2010 showed that of the 100 000 schools, one quarter had 1 or 0 inspections. Nevertheless, despite a remarkable 38 million meals served daily in US schools, reports of foodborne illnesses are extremely rare, probably as a result of careful training, increased requirements for written school policies, better continuing-education programs for food service personnel, and the commitment of the food service staff to protect the children in their care.

A school foodborne infection outbreak is an significant event for the dietary staff and costly for school districts, resulting in disruption of food service, loss of participation in the school meal programs, and potential liability for medical expenses, attorney fees, increased insurance rates, and additional training or equipment to rectify food safety practices. In the decade between 1990 and 1999, there were only 292 outbreaks in schools, involving 16 232 children and teenagers.[44,45] This can be compared with the national statistics at the same time, which showed that the 7 most serious food pathogens caused 325 000 hospitalizations and 5000 deaths and cost as much as $34.9 billion annual in medical costs and lost productivity.[46]

Competitive Foods in Schools

Competitive foods are widely available in the nation's schools.[47] They represent a double-edged sword for the food service. On the one hand, a la carte and vending machine purchases during school meal times subtract consumers from the School Breakfast Program and National School Lunch Program rolls, robbing the school of USDA subsidies. Fixed costs, such as equipment and personnel, remain unchanged, so this loss of revenue is a double hardship. Additionally, consumption of a poor-quality diet is especially detrimental for impoverished children. On the other hand, a la carte and vending sales are attractive to students and can be lucrative for schools, although some recent evidence suggests that, in many cases, the revenues from competitive food sales do not make up for the nonreimbursed income from missed school meals.[48,49] A recent literature review found that schools that substitute foods of higher nutritional quality to replace energy-dense, nutrient-poor foods do not report subsequent losses in total revenues from the competitive food sales.[50,51] Emphasizing taste, value, and convenience within food choices can ensure stable revenue.

Despite variations in the definition of an "empty calorie," studies in recent years have shown a consistency in their influence on the overall diet quality of youth. Typically, the energy density of a food is the amount of energy consumed per gram weight of the product. Using NHANES data from 2003-2004, researchers showed that approximately 30% to 40% of daily energy consumed by 2- to 18-year-olds were in the form of empty calories—that is, energy-dense, nutrient-poor items.[52] Of these calories, 433 kcal came from solid fats and 365 kcal came from added sugars. Half of the empty calories could be attributed to just 6 foods: sweetened soft drinks, fruit drinks, dairy desserts, grain desserts, pizza, and full-fat milk (as opposed to low- or nonfat milks, which are supported by the Dietary Guidelines for Americans). Briefel et al[53] reported that most of these calories were consumed away from school and that more stringent school policy provisions lessened the likelihood of high consumption.

The taste appeal of processed snack foods is a result of the interaction of fats, sugar, and salt in the foods, a triad that holds powerful appeal even for very young children.[54-56] The attributes of taste, convenience, and value are readily apparent in the school environment. School food policies affect children's access to snack foods and drinks.[57] Often, in higher grades, snack foods serve as alternatives to eating a balanced school meal. Access to "empty calories" at school has been related to increased daily energy intake and higher body mass index (BMI) among children in middle school.[53,58] Equally important, energy-dense nutrient-poor products displace more healthful alternatives that contain essential nutrients.

Snacking is nearly ubiquitous among American children, having increased steadily over the course of the obesity epidemic. The number of eating occasions per day has been positively correlated with energy intake and obesity.[59] Nearly 40% reported snacking at school, the frequency of which was tied directly to the number of snack machines and the school's policy affording easy availability.[60,61] Sources of snack-type foods and beverages included snack bars, school stores, bake sales or fundraisers outside the cafeteria, class parties, or foods offered as rewards for classroom performance. Further, a school district's participation in a "pouring rights" contract from a beverage business has been tied with increased sales and consumption of sweetened beverages in the school,[61] a practice of great concern to the AAP.[62] Such contracts have become increasingly rare since 2005, when the Alliance for a Healthier Generation, in conjunction with the beverage industry, published national guidelines curtailing contracts that included sweetened, high-calorie beverages in schools.[63]

National Standards for Competitive Foods in Schools

At the request of the USDA, a committee of the IOM was formed to review all available research and present recommendations for school nutrition standards for foods sold outside the federally reimbursable school meal program (competitive foods). The IOM report concluded that to achieve dietary stability for children and at the same time maintain a financial footing for the food service, competitive foods should be curtailed significantly.[64] They cited the Dietary Guidelines for Americans as the most comprehensive science-based benchmark.

In the IOM report, recommendations were presented in 2 tiers. Tier 1 foods and beverages were appropriate for all students. This class of foods contained no more than 200 kcal per portion as packaged and had no more than 35% of calories from fat, less than 10% from saturated fats, minimal trans fats (<0.5% g/serving), 35% or less from total sugars (excepting yogurt), and 200 mg or less of sodium per portion, as packaged. For beverages, the report recommended water, low-fat and nonfat milk in 8-oz portions (including lactose-free and soy as well as flavored milk with no more than 22 g of total sugars/8-oz portion), and 100% fruit juice in 4-oz portions for elementary schools and 8-oz portions for high school. The IOM also urged that all products be caffeine free. A la carte entrees should meet the same standards and calorie limits as the National School Lunch Program while not exceeding 480 g/serving of sodium. Finally, combination products must contain a total of 1 or more servings of fruit, vegetables, or whole-grain products per portion. Tier 2 products were intended for high school students after school. They mirror the Tier 1 recommendations but allow for vending noncaffeinated, nonfortified beverages with less than 5 kcal per portion, with or without nonnutritive sweeteners, carbonation, or flavorings. Primarily, this includes water and diet drinks sweetened with nonnutritive sweeteners.

Wellness Advisory Committees and School Nutrition Policies

In retrospect, one of the most important clauses in the Child Nutrition and WIC Reauthorization Act of 2004 (Pub L No. 108-265 §204) was a simple directive that all school districts participating in the National School Lunch Program adopt and implement a local wellness policy by the 2006-2007 school year. The legislation required that:

- Goals be established for nutrition education, physical activity, and other school activities;
- Nutrition guidelines be established for all foods available on school campus;
- Nutrition standards for school meals be at least as restrictive as existing federal guidelines;
- Schools design a plan for measuring implementation of the local wellness policy, including designation of a person or people with operational responsibility; and
- The wellness advisory council writing the policy include parents and students, school nutrition leaders, school administrators, and other members of the public.

Local school wellness policies have provided an unprecedented opportunity to mold the school environment in terms of nutrition and physical activity. A recent comprehensive study showed that nearly all students in the United States were under a district wellness policy.[65] However, examination of individual school policies revealed a range from strong and specific to ineffective and vague. Strengthening school wellness policies and helping to design evaluations and plans for continuous quality improvement is a primary target of the 2010 Child Nutrition Reauthorization.[66] Pediatricians, particularly those looking for a way to be involved in their own child's school, should consider participating in the school and district wellness councils. An influential national organization with chapters in every state, Action for Healthy Kids, has many resources to assist physicians and others in the public who participate on councils.[67]

Controversies Surrounding School Nutrition

Obesity and School Food

Concerns about school food as a cause of obesity are commonly expressed. In their analysis of federal food policy and childhood obesity, Kimbro and Rigby[68] found that school meal participation was beneficial for child weight status, not detrimental to it. Similarly, using SNDA III data, Gleason and Dodd[27] carefully controlled for both student-level and school-level confounders. Their study found no evidence that National School Lunch Program participation was associated with a student's BMI or risk of overweight. Additionally, they found a diminished risk of overweight for those students consuming school breakfast regularly. Fox et al[58] cited a few school food factors that could be associated with higher BMI, however. Potato products and desserts served more than once a week in elementary school and energy-dense vended foods and a la carte foods in middle and high schools correlated with higher BMI. Their study, among others, showed that sound school food policies had a positive effect on prevention of excess weight gain by students.[58,69,70]

School Lunch Versus Packed Lunch
Despite commonly expressed misgivings about the nutritional quality of school food, it has been shown repeatedly in the 3 SNDA studies that the National School Lunch Program is superior nutritionally compared with alternatives brought from home, purchased from vending or a la carte lines, or obtained off campus during "open" lunch periods.[71,72] The impact of a la carte and vended food on diet quality can be either negative or positive, depending on the school's oversight.[57]

Soft Drinks, Rehydration Drinks, Energy Drinks, and the Beverage Industry
In 2004, the AAP Council on School Health published its policy statement, "Soft Drinks in Schools" to alert pediatricians, the public, and school administrators about the burgeoning availability of soft drinks in schools.[62] Consistently, high intake of sweetened drinks has been associated with greater energy and lower nutrient consumption.[73] Further, studies of the effects of more restrictive school beverage policies on exposure and consumption showed significant improvements.[74] Recently, several positive developments have occurred.

The Alliance for a Healthier Generation was formed by the William J. Clinton Foundation, in collaboration with the American Heart Association, and aimed to combat childhood obesity. The Alliance's initial efforts involved publication of the "School Beverage Guidelines" in 2007.[63] In it, the beverage industry committed to altering the availability and mix of beverages in schools, removing full-calorie soft drinks, and replacing them with lower-calorie, higher nutrient products of a smaller portion size. The final progress report by the industry was published in 2010, reporting an 88% decrease in calories shipped to schools, a 95% decrease (ounces) in shipment of full-calorie carbonated soft drinks and an increase in alternatives, such as water, 100% fruit juice, and rehydration drinks in smaller portion sizes.[63] However, studies still record widespread availability of sweetened beverages in US schools, at least partly because of use of vendors outside of exclusive or formal contracts in half the schools surveyed.[75] Decreasing carbonated soft drinks has opened the way for other beverages in schools: some beneficial, such as water and milk, and some less so, such as rehydration and energy drinks. Recently, a clinical report

III

from the AAP Committee on Nutrition and Council on Sports Medicine clarified the role of sport drinks and energy drinks consumed by children and adolescents, warning that their use outside of moderate to vigorous physical activity involving fluid and electrolyte depletion is an unwarranted source of energy, added sugar, and in many cases, caffeine and other additives[76] (see Chapter 12). Along with other sweetened drinks, these products represent a substantial source of added sugars and empty calories for sale in schools. Public health and beverage industry efforts, grassroots advocacy, local school wellness committees, and school policy improvements have combined to lower the availability of high-energy drinks in schools, although continued progress will require ongoing surveillance and reevaluation.

Obesity, Added Sugars, Flavored Milk, and School Policy

Many have a strong conviction that added sugars are a primary cause of obesity. Nicklas et al,[77] examining added sugars and weight change in children, did not find a connection. Similarly, the Dietary Guideline Advisory committee[78] did not identify a direct correlation between consumption of sugars and obesity, type 2 diabetes mellitus, heart disease, or behavioral disorders. Only when its consumption begins to limit recommended intakes of other nutrients does added sugar cause nutritional harm. The IOM suggested that this occurs when added sugars approach 25% of daily energy.[79] Others argue that the issue is complex enough that no such threshold truly exists.[80,81]

A recent, rigorous evaluation, which used the new National Cancer Institute's usual intake estimation model, determined that only 13% of the population had added sugar intake above 25% of energy; the majority ranged from 5% to 20% of energy as added sugars, the equivalent of roughly 10 to 23 teaspoons of sucrose per day.[82] The study found that irrespective of added sugar consumption, the dietary patterns for all ages were low in many micronutrients relative to DRI recommendations. When the effect of added sugar intake was included in the analysis, non-Hispanic black people and people in poverty were found to have the highest added sugar consumption. But surprisingly, obese individuals consumed only an average amount of energy as added sugars.[82] This data is consistent with other studies that have shown an inverse relationship between carbohydrate intake and BMI rather than the positive relationship that is commonly assumed.[83]

Still, a panel of the American Heart Association that examined dietary sugars and cardiovascular health recommended that Americans strictly limit their added sugars.[84] The "prudent upper limit" recommended was one half of the total discretionary calories. For most, the sucrose equivalent would range from 4 to 18 teaspoons per day, depending on age, gender, and activity level. For most females, 5 teaspoons or 100 kcal per day would be the recommended limit, and for most males, 9 teaspoons or 144 kcal per day would be the recommended limit.

But the AHA panel recognized differences in the form in which added sugars are consumed. Soft drinks, sugar, and sweets were identified as more likely to have a negative impact on diet quality than were dairy foods, milk drinks, or presweetened cereals, which were not correlated with obesity or diminished diet quality.[84,85]

A controversy over flavored milk in school has arisen from the tension between those advocating cutting unnecessary fats and added sugars to reduce the risk of obesity and those promoting the use of acceptable amounts of fats and sugars to increase consumption of foods with high nutritional value. Advocates of removal suggest that there is no need for sweetened milk in schools and that it represents the type of excess calories that the Dietary Guidelines have stressed removing from a child's diet. Proponents of removal believe that in the absence of sweetened milk, children will switch to white milk. Those promoting flavored milk in schools emphasize that studies have not shown a link between flavored milk consumption and obesity,[85] that when flavored milk is removed from school, consumption of milk falls by one third and does not rebound with time,[86] and that milk within the school meal provides many nutrients in support of the overall diet quality at a low cost-per-nutrient for the school food service.[87]

To date, through its policy statements and clinical reports, the AAP has supported the use of flavored milk for children as one means to achieve nutrition goals, particularly of vitamin D and calcium.[62,88,89] The IOM also included flavored milk in its recommendations to the USDA for nutrition standards in schools, albeit only in nonfat form.[64] Because of concerns about cardiovascular disease, type 2 diabetes mellitus, cancer, and metabolic syndrome as well as bone health and related diseases, the 2010 Dietary Guidelines for Americans emphasized 4 nutrients of highest public health concern: fiber, calcium, vitamin D, and potassium.[8] Presently, fluid milk is the primary source in the American supply for the latter 3 nutrients.

The milk consumed in school does not reflect that consumed when out of school in several ways. The Centers for Disease Control and Prevention reported that for children and adolescents 2 to 19 years of age, milk consumed in the United States comprised 32.4% as full-fat milk, 45.4% as 2% reduced-fat milk, and only 20.2% as low-fat milk (1% or nonfat types).[90] But in schools, the low-fat category accounts for 78% of consumption, and among flavored milks, the low-fat and nonfat varieties account for nearly 90% (51% as 1% reduced-fat and 38.5% as nonfat skim milk).[91] At the same time, according to dairy industry surveys, sugar content of chocolate milk in school has been reduced by 30% nationwide in 5 years, from 16.7 g to 11.8 g per serving.[92] Further reduction or elimination of added sugars have been achieved when noncaloric sweeteners are used. Typically, the flavored milks available in schools are not the same formulations as those sold at retail stores.

The Dairy Research Institute, in an analysis of the NHANES 2003-2006 data from children 2 to 19 years of age, found that flavored milk accounted for less than 5% of the total dietary added sugars at any age.[93] Frary and Johnson[94] stressed that all added sugars are not alike. Sweetened dairy products and presweetened cereals made positive contributions to the child's diet. It is the soft drinks, fruit drinks, energy and sports drinks, grain desserts, and candy that account for three quarters of the added sugars in children's diets, according to the Dietary Guidelines Advisory Committee.[78] Unfortunately, many of these still can be found in schools. A school wellness committee seeking to cut excess added sugars and fats will have the greatest effect, with the least risk of nutritional harm, by targeting the many foods and drinks of low nutritional value consumed outside the school meal programs.

Food Marketing in Schools

Repeatedly, leaders in pediatric health care have called attention to the link between public health problems, particularly obesity and poor nutrition, and the marketing food products to children.[95,96] Calls to restrict the type and timing of advertising to children have been made by the World Health Organization.[97] Some have suggested that the same methodology used by marketing firms be used to promote consumption of nutritious foods in children.[98] Clearly, one part of the solution will be to incorporate media training in school-based health education curricula to sharpen the consumer skills of children and adolescents.[98] New guidelines are due to be proposed by the Food and Drug Administration in conjunction with other federal agencies. In response to this development, a coalition of leading food industries, responsible for 70% to 80% of food advertising to children, has proposed its own voluntary guidelines titled the Children's Food and Beverages Advertising Initiative (CFBAI).[99]

Activity, Recess, and Structured Versus Unstructured Play

Nutrition and daily activity are complementary components of the Dietary Guidelines for Americans 2010. A trend toward reallocating time in school to accentuate academics has threatened recess as integral part of a child's school day.[100] Ironically, minimizing or eliminating recess may be counterproductive to academic achievement.[101] Recess offers cognitive, social, emotional, and physical benefits that may not be fully appreciated when a decision is made to diminish it. Recess is unique from, and a complement to, physical education—not a substitute for it. The AAP has supported recess as a necessary break in the child's day, emphasizing that it should not be withheld for punitive or academic reasons.[101] Concerns about obesity have led to calls for a more active, structured form of recess. Although this approach ensures activity for all students, it sacrifices the role of recess as a personal, free time that encourages creativity and exploration.[100,101] But whether structured or unstructured, recess should be safe and well supervised.

Several national programs have been developed to emphasize the link between nutrition and daily activity. For instance, the USDA Food and Nutrition Service created Team Nutrition to help schools improve their curricula and policies, including the school wellness policy.[102] Recognition for excellence is offered through the HealthierUS School Challenge. Another national program offering resources for schools is Fuel Up to Play 60, a collaboration between the National Football League and the National Dairy Council,[103] which is unique in being student designed and directed. Adult mentors and professional football players join to help the students engage their whole school in projects to improve nutrition and increase regular physical activity.

Nutrition Standards in Preschool and Child Care

Child care may offer one of the best opportunities for laying a foundation of quality nutrition and routine physical activity in early life.[104] Experiences in various child-care settings offer the potential for optimal, balanced nutrition that could help to shape a child's preferences and habits. Conversely, poor policies and practices could result in detrimental feeding practices, greater energy intake, and weight gain. More than 60% of women with children younger than 6 years are employed, the majority full time. As a result, more than 75% of children younger than 6 years spend some time in organized care settings, with many additional children in unregulated and unregistered informal care.[105] Working mothers use many different types of care, including center-based care (45%), child care in another family's home (14%), or leaving the child with the other parent (18%) or relative (17%) or with a nanny/babysitter (6%).[105] Currently, there are approximately 120 000 child-care centers but an estimated additional 2.5-fold more informal sites, which are far less easily influenced by national or state policies.[106]

State-by-state regulations for nutrition and activity are variable, becoming less strict as the setting diminishes in structure, from organized care centers, to modest less-formal sites, to small family homes, respectively. Guidelines to shape the quality of child care in all types of sites are available, however. Recently, a self-assessment tool was developed and tested in child care settings to improve the standards for nutrition and physical activities.[107] In a position statement on nutrition in child care settings, the Academy of Nutrition and Dietetics encouraged all child care providers to align their food offerings with the Dietary Guidelines for Americans 2010 recommendations and the USDA Child and Adult Care Food Programs (CACFP) meal patterns and portion sizes.[108] State requirements for nutrition in child-care settings most commonly follow the CACFP meal plans.[104] The CACFP, like the school meal programs for older children, reimburses free or reduced price meals for very young children on the basis of financial need in child care centers, group homes, and in-home care settings for 3 age categories: 1 through 2 years, 3 through 5 years, and 6 through 12 years. The CACFP designates nutrition quality on the basis of a meal pattern approach, offering portion size guidance and nutrition education. Head Start, the preschool program for low-income or high-risk children, participates in CACFP. Individual states often augment these basic standards with provisions that further limit foods of low nutritional value in child care settings.[108]

The AAP has published comprehensive standards for nutrition and physical activity in child care.[109] These standards suggest 3 eating occasions (meals and snacks) for children in child care for 8 hours and 4 eating occasions for those staying longer, essentially offering energy every 2 to 3 hours. The Feeding Infants and Toddlers Study (FITS) revealed that total energy intake at lunch was highest in child care (332 kcal) or away-from-home (308 kcal), compared with home (281 kcal), so special attention toward age-appropriate portion sizes is warranted.[110] Some centers allow or require parents to send in lunches in place of the center-prepared food. Parental sack lunches usually fail to conform to CACFP portion and servings standards, but food choices can be influenced by education offered through the child care center.[111]

The IOM recently published guidelines for child care settings that specifically targeted the issue of obesity prevention in the young child.[112] For physical activity, the committee recommended a variety of activities, indoor and outside, that blend developmentally appropriate moderate and vigorous activities throughout the day. The chapter on nutrition directs child care providers to align with national policy, such as the CACFP and the Dietary Guidelines for Americans 2010. A variety of foods from the 5 food groups in age-appropriate portions should form the basis of school policy. Training of staff in food planning skills was strongly recommended, as well.

The quality of child care experiences varies widely in the United States. Falbe et al[113] recently published a 65-point tool to assess the quality of a child care center's policies. National guidelines have advocated facilitated structured play that promotes fundamental motor skill development, such as running, jumping, throwing, and kicking, as the foundation for more sophisticated physical activity.[114,115] More than three quarters of disadvantaged preschool-aged children showed deficits in these skills, particularly females, which hampered engagement in activity and directly correlated with preschool obesity rates.[116] The IOM report not only made recommendations to support nutrition and activity policies but also included guidance on sleep and sedentary screen time, emerging issues for mitigating the risk of obesity in child care settings.[112]

Summary

The obesity epidemic has focused the concern of health care and public health professionals on the link between the American diet and future health. In the first years of life, child care policies offer our best opportunity to help shape the child and family's food preferences, sense of portion size, and understanding of proper proportionality of food servings. With 55 million children and adolescents in child care and school, food policies can directly affect not only the student's daily well-being but also his or her ability to function academically. School nutrition is a complex mix of federally subsidized meals, vended options, and a host of other sources in which foods and beverages reach children. New guidelines for school meal programs, along with new national nutrition standards for foods sold in competition with school meal programs, should result in a significant improvement in diet quality. School wellness policies, an excellent opportunity for input from health care professionals, can make a substantial contribution toward nutrition and physical activity. The well-informed pediatrician is in a unique position to contribute his or her perspective to the policies of local schools, preschools, and child care centers.

References

1. Story M, Kaphingst KM, French S. The role of schools in obesity prevention. *Future Child.* 2006;16(1):109-142

2. US Department of Education, National Center for Education Statistics. Back to School Statistics. Available at: http://nces.ed.gov/fastfacts/display.asp?id=372. Accessed October 31, 2012

3. Breifel RR, Wilson A, Gleason PM. consumption of low-nutrient, energy-dense foods and beverages at school, home and other locations among school lunch participants and nonparticipants. *J Am Diet Assoc.* 2009;109(Suppl 1):S79-S90

4. Basch C. *Healthier Students Are Better Learners: A Missing Link in Efforts to Close the Achievement Gap.* Equity Matters Research Review No. 6 March 2010. Available at: http://www.equitycampaign.org/i/a/document/12558_EquityMattersVol6_WebFINAL.pdf. Accessed October 31, 2012

5. US Department of Agriculture, Food and Nutrition Service. Nutrition Assistance Programs. Available at: http://www.fns.usda.gov/fns/. Accessed October 31, 2012

6. Linz P, Lee M, Bell L. *Obesity, Poverty, and Participation in Nutrition Assistance Programs.* Alexandria, VA: US Department of Agriculture, Food and Nutrition Service, Office of Analysis, Nutrition and Evaluation; 2005

7. Newman C, Ralston K. *Profiles of Participants in the National School Lunch Program: Data from Two National Surveys.* Washington, DC: US Department of Agriculture, Economic Research Service; 2006

8. US Department of Agriculture. Dietary Guidelines for Americans. Washington, DC: US Department of Agriculture, Center for Nutrition Policy and Promotion; 2010. Available at: http://www.cnpp.usda.gov/dietaryguidelines.htm. Accessed October 31, 2012

9. Practice paper of the American Dietetic Association: nutrient density: meeting nutrient goals within calorie needs. *J Am Diet Assoc.* 2007;107(5):860-868

10. Reedy J, Krebs-Smith SM. Dietary sources of energy, solid fats and added sugars among children and adolescents in the United States. *J Am Diet Assoc.* 2010;110(10):1477-1484

11. Institute of Medicine, Food and Nutrition Board. *School Meals: Building Blocks for Health Children.* Washington, DC: National Academies Press; 2009

12. O'Toole TP, Anderson S, Miller C, Guthrie J. Nutrition services and foods and beverages available at school: results from the School Health Policies and Programs Study 2006. *J School Health.* 2007;77(Suppl):500-521

13. School Nutrition Association. Available at: http://www.schoolnutrition.org. Accessed October 31, 2012

14. Burghardt JA, Devaney BL, Gordon AR. The School Nutrition Dietary Assessment Study: summary and discussion. *Am J Clin Nutr.* 1995;61(1 Suppl):252S-257S

15. Fox MK, Crepinsek MK, Connor P, Battaglia M. *School Nutrition Dietary Assessment Study II: Summary of Findings.* Alexandria, VA: US Department of Agriculture, Food and Nutrition Service, Office of Research, Nutrition, and Analysis; 2001. Available at: http://www.fns.usda.gov/ora/menu/published/CNP/FILES/SNDAIIfind.pdf. Accessed October 31, 2012

16. Gordon AR, Fox MK. *School Nutrition Dietary Assessment Study III: Summary of Findings.* Alexandria, VA: US Department of Agriculture, Food and Nutrition Service, Office of Research, Nutrition, and Analysis; 2007. Available at: http://www.fns.usda.gov/ora/menu/published/CNP/FILES/SNDAIII-SummaryofFindings.pdf. Accessed October 31, 2012

17. Food Research and Action Center. Record Demand for School Meals, But Breakfast Participation Still Falling Short. Washington, DC: Food Research and Action Center; 2011. Available at: http://frac.org/2010-school-breakfast-report/. Accessed October 31, 2012

18. Newman C, Ralston K, Clauson A. Balancing nutrition, participation and cost in the National School Lunch Program. *Amber Waves.* 2008;6(4)

19. Weber JA. Increasing food costs for consumers and food programs straining pocketbooks. *J Am Diet Assoc.* 2008;108(4):615-617

20. Bartlett S, Glanz F, Logan C. School Lunch and Breakfast Cost Study II. Available at: http://www.fns.usda.gov/Ora/menu/Published/CNP/FILES/MealCostStudy.pdf. Accessed October 31, 2012

21. Government Accounting Office. *Report to Congress: School Meal Programs: Competitive Foods Are Widely Available and Generate Substantial Revenue for Schools.* Washington, DC: Government Accounting Office; 2005

22. Government Accounting Office. *National School Lunch Program: School Food Service Account Revenue Amendments Related to the Healthy, Hunger-Free Kids Act of 2010.* Available at: http://www.gao.gov/decisions/majrule/d11792r.pdf. Accessed October 31, 2012

23. US Department of Agriculture, Food and Nutrition Service. National School Lunch, Special Milk, and School Breakfast Programs, National Average Payments/Maximum Reimbursement Rates. *Fed Regist.* 2011;76(139):43256-43259

24. USDA School Commodities Program. Available at: http://www.fns.usda.gov/fdd/foods/healthy/USDAFoods_FactSheet_FINAL.pdf. Accessed October 31, 2012

25. US Department of Agriculture, Economic Research Service. *The Food Assistance Landscape: FY 2007 Annual Report.* Washington, DC: US Department of Agriculture; 2008. Economic Information Bulletin No. 6-5

26. Crepinsek MK, Gordon AR, McKinney PM, Condon EM, Wilson A. Meals offered and served in US public schools: do they meet nutrient standards? *J Am Diet Assoc.* 2009;109(Suppl 1):S31-S43

27. Gleason PM, Dodd AH. School breakfast program but not school lunch program participation is associated with lower body mass index. *J Am Diet Assoc.* 2009;109: (Suppl 1):S118-S126

28. Rampersaud GC, Pereira MA, Girard BL, Adams J, Metzl JD. Breakfast habits, nutritional status, body weight, and academic performance in children and adolescents. *J Am Diet Assoc.* 2005;105(5):743-760

29. Briefel RR, Crepinsek MK, Cabili C, Wilson A, Gleason PM. School food environments and practices affect dietary behaviors of US public school children. *J Am Diet Assoc.* 2009;109(Suppl 1):S91-S107

30. Story M, Brown JL, Beardslee WH, Prothrow-Stith D. *Impact of School Breakfast on Children's Health and Learning: An Analysis of the Scientific Research.* Gaithersburg, MD: Sodexo Foundation; 2008. Available at: http://www.sodexofoundation.org/hunger_us/Images/Impact%20of%20School%20Breakfast%20Study_tcm150-212606.pdf. Accessed October 31, 2012

31. School Nutrition Association. School Nutrition Foundation provides breakfast in the classroom [press release]. Alexandria, VA: School Nutrition Association; January, 2011

32. Hoyland A, Dye L, Lawton CL. A systematic review of the effect of breakfast on cognitive performance of children and adolescents. *Nutr Res Rev.* 2009;22(2):220-243

33. Grantham-McGregor S. Can the provision of breakfast benefit school performance? *Food Nutr Bull.* 2005;26(Suppl 2):S144-S158

34. Crepinsek MK, Singh A, Bernstein LS, McLaughlin JE. Dietary effects of universal-free school breakfast: findings from the evaluation of the school breakfast program pilot project. *J Am Diet Assoc.* 2006;106(11):1796-1803

35. Centers for Disease Control and Prevention, National Center for Health Statistics. Food allergies in children. *NCHS Data Brief.* 2008;10. Available at: http://www.cdc.gov/nchs/data/databriefs/db10.pdf. Accessed October 31, 2012

36. Branum AM, Lukacs SL. Food allergies among U.S. children: Trends in prevalence and hospitalizations. *NCHS Data Brief.* 2008;10. Available at: http://www.cdc.gov/nchs/data/databriefs/db10.pdf. Accessed October 31, 2012

37. Gupta RS, Springston EE, Warrier MR, Smith B, Kumar R, Pongracic J, Holl JL. The prevalence, severity and distribution of childhood food allergy in the United States. *Pediatrics.* 2011;128(1):e9-e17

38. Nowak-Wegrzyn A, Conover-Walker MK, Wood RA. Food-allergic reactions in schools and preschools. *Arch Pediatr Adolesc Med.* 2001;155(7):790-795

39. Sicherer SH; Mahr TA; American Academy of Pediatrics, Section on Allergy and Immunology. Management of food allergy in the school setting. *Pediatrics.* 2010;126(6):1232-1239

40. American College of Allergy, Asthma, and Immunology. Food allergy: a practice parameter. *Ann Allergy Asthma Immunol.* 2006;96(3 Suppl 2):S1-S68

41. Sicherer SH, Sampson HA. Peanut allergy: emerging concepts and approaches for an apparent epidemic. *J Allergy Clin Immunol.* 2007;120(3):491-503

42. Baumgart K, Brown S, Gold M, et al. ASCIA guidelines for prevention of food anaphylactic reactions in schools, preschools and child-care centres. *J Paediatr Child Health.* 2004;40(12):669-671

43. Wainstein BK, Kashef S, Ziegler M, Jelley D, Ziegler JB. Frequency and significance of immediate contact reactions to peanut in peanut-sensitive children. *Clin Exp Allergy.* 2007;37(6):211-215

44. Government Accounting Office. School Meal Programs: Few Outbreaks of Food Borne Illness Reported. Washington, DC: Government Accounting Office; 2000. Available at: http://www.gao.gov/new.items/rc00053.pdf. Accessed October 31, 2012

45. Government Accounting Office. *Continued Vigilance Needed to Ensure Safety of School Meals.* Washington, DC: Government Accounting Office; 2002. Available at: http://www.gao.gov/new.items/d02669t.pdf. Accessed July 22, 2011

46. Partnership for Food Safety Education. *The Costs of Food Borne Illness.* Available at: http://www.fightbac.org/about-foodborne-illness/costs-to-society. Accessed October 31, 2012

47. Fox MK, Gordon A, Nogales R, Wilson A. Availability and consumption of competitive foods in US public schools. *J Am Diet Assoc.* 2009;109(Suppl 1): S57-S66

48. General Accounting Office. School Meals Programs: Competitive Foods Are Widely Available and Generate Substantial Revenue for Schools. Washington, DC: General Accounting Office; 2005. Available at: http://www.gao.gov/new.items/d05563.pdf. Accessed October 31, 2012

49. Food Research and Action Center. How competitive foods in schools impact student health, school meal programs, and students from low-income families. Food Research and Action Center Issue Briefs for Child Nutrition Reauthorization. June 2010;5. Available at: http://www.frac.org/pdf/CNR05_competitivefoods.pdf. Accessed October 31, 2012

50. Wharton CM, Long M, Schwartz MB. Changing nutrition standards in schools: the emerging impact on school revenue. *J Sch Health.* 2008;78(5):245-251

51. Schwartz MB, Novak SA, Fiore SS. The impact of removing snacks of low nutritional value from middle schools. *Health Educ Behav.* 2009;36(6):999-1011

52. Reedy J, Krebs-Smith SM. Dietary sources of energy, solid fats, and added sugars among children and adolescents in the United States. *J Am Diet Assoc.* 2010;110(10):1477-1484

53. Briefel RR, Wilson A, Gleason PM. Consumption of low-nutrient energy-dense foods and beverages at school, home and other locations among school lunch participants and nonparticipants. *J Am Diet Assoc.* 2009;109(Suppl 1):S79-S90

54. Drewnowski A, Bellisle F. Liquid calories, sugar, and body weight. *Am J Clin Nutr.* 2007;85(3):651-661

55. Drewnowski A. the real contribution of added sugars and fats to obesity. *Epidemiol Rev.* 2007;29:160-171

56. Kessler DA. *The End of Overeating: Taking control of the insatiable American appetite.* New York, NY: Rodale Press; 2009

57. Story M, Kaphingest KM, Robinson-O'Brien R, Glanz K. Creating healthy food and eating environments: policy and environmental approaches. *Annu Rev Public Health.* 2008;29:253-272

58. Fox MK, Dodd AH, Wilson A, Gleason PM. Association between school food environment and practices and body mass index of US public school children. *J Am Diet Assoc.* 2009;109(Suppl 1):S108-S117

59. Franko DL, Streigel-Moore RH, Thompson D, Affenito SG, Daniels SR, Crawford PB. The relationship between meal frequency and body mass index in black and white adolescent girls: more is less. *Int J Obes (Lond).* 2008;32(1):23-29

60. Park S, Sappenfield WM, Huang Y, Sherry B, Bensyl DM. The impact of the availability of school vending machines on eating behavior during lunch: The Youth Physical Activity and Nutrition Survey. *J Am Diet Assoc.* 2010;110(10):1532-1536

61. Briefel RR, Crepinsek MK, Cabili C, Wilson A, Gleason PM. School food environments and practices affect dietary behaviors of US public school children. *J Am Diet Assoc.* 2009;109(2 suppl 1):S91-S107

62. American Academy of Pediatrics, Council on School Health. Soft drinks in schools. *Pediatrics.* 2004;113(1):152-154

63. American Beverage Association. Alliance School Beverage Guidelines: Final Progress Report. March 8, 2010. Available at: http://www.healthiergeneration.org/uploadedFiles/About_The_Alliance/SBG%20FINAL%20PROGRESS%20REPORT%20(March%202010).pdf. Accessed October 31, 2012

64. Institute of Medicine, Food and Nutrition Board. *Nutrition Standards for Foods in Schools: Leading the Way Toward Healthier Youth.* Washington, DC: National Academies Press; 2007. Available at: http://www.nap.edu/catalog/11899.html. Accessed October 31, 2012

65. Bridging the Gap. *School District Wellness Policies: Evaluating Progress and Potential for Improving Children's Health Three Years After the Federal Mandate.* August 2010. Available at: http://www.bridgingthegapresearch.org/_asset/r08bgt/WP_2010_report.pdf. Accessed October 31, 2012

66. US Department of Agriculture. Local School Wellness Policy. Available at: http://teamnutrition.usda.gov/healthy/wellnesspolicy.html. Accessed October 31, 2012

67. Action for Healthy Kids. Wellness Policy Toolkit. Available at: http://www.actionforhealthykids.org/school-programs/our-programs/wellness-policy-tool/. Accessed October 31, 2012

68. Kimbro RT, Rigby E. Federal food policy and childhood obesity: a solution or part of the problem? *Health Affairs.* 2011;29(3):411-418

69. Kubik MY, Lytle LA, Story M. Schoolwide food practices are associated with body mass index in middle school students. *Arch Pediatr Adolesc Med.* 2005;159(12):1111-1114

70. Terry-McElrath YM, O'Malley PM, Delva J, Johnston LD. The school food environment and student body mass index and food consumption: 2004 to 2007 national data. *J Adolesc Health.* 2009;45:S45-S56

71. Clark MA, Fox MK. Nutritional quality of the diets of US public school children and the role of the school meal programs. *J Am Diet Assoc.* 2009;109(Suppl 1):S44-S56

72. Rovner AJ, Nansel TR, Wang J, Lannotti RJ. Food sold in school vending machines is associated with overall student dietary intake. *J Adolesc Health.* 2011;48(1):13-19

73. Vartanian LR, Schwartz MB, Brownell KD. Effects of soft drink consumption on nutrition and health: a systematic review and meta-analysis. *Am J Public Health.* 2007;97(4):667-675

74. Johnson DB, Bruemmer B, Lund AE, Evens CC, Mar CM. Impact of school district sugar-sweetened beverage policies on student beverage exposure and consumption in middle schools. *J Adolesc Health.* 2009;45(3 Suppl):S30-S37

75. Turner L, Chaloupka FJ. Wide availability of high-calorie beverages in US elementary schools. *Arch Pediatr Adolesc Med.* 2011;165(3):223-228

76. Schneider M; Benjamin H; American Academy of Pediatrics, Committee on Nutrition and Council on Sports Medicine and Fitness. Sports drinks and energy drinks for children and adolescents: are they appropriate? *Pediatrics.* 2011;127(6):1182-1189

77. Nicklas TA, O'Neil CE, Liu Y. Intake of added sugars is not associated with weight measures in children 6 to 18 years: National Health and Nutrition Examination Surveys 2003-2006. *Nutr Res.* 2011;31(5):338-346

78. US Department of Agriculture, Center for Nutrition Policy and Promotion. Report of the Dietary Guidelines Advisory Committee on the Dietary Guidelines for Americans, 2010. Available at: http://www.cnpp.usda.gov/dgas2010-dgacreport.htm. Accessed October 31, 2012

79. Institute of Medicine, Food and Nutrition Board. *Dietary Reference Intakes for Energy, Carbohydrate, Fiber, Fat, Fatty Acids, Cholesterol, Protein and Amino Acids.* Washington, DC: National Academies Press, 2002

80. Gibson S, Boyd A. Associations between added sugars and micronutrient intakes and status: further analysis of data from the National Diet and Nutrition Survey of Young People aged 4 to 18 years. *Br J Nutr.* 2009;101(1):100-107

81. Rennie KL, Livingstone MB. Associations between dietary added sugar intake and micronutrient intake: a systematic review. *Br J Nutr.* 2007;97(5):832-841

82. Marriott BP, Olsho L, Hadden L, Connor P. Intake of added sugars and selected nutrients in the United States, National Health and Nutrition Examination Survey (NHANES) 2003-2006. *Crit Rev Food Sci Nutr.* 2010;50(3):228-258

83. Gaesser GA. Carbohydrate quantity and quality in relation to body mass index. *J Am Diet Assoc.* 2007;107(10):1768-1780

84. Johnson RK, Appel LJ, Brands M, Howard BV, Lefevre M, Lustig RH, Sacks F, Steffen LM, Wylie-Rosett J. Dietary Sugars Intake and cardiovascular health: A scientific statement from the American Heart Association. *Circulation.* 2009;120(11):1011-1020

85. Murphy MM, Douglass JS, Johnson RK, Spence LA. Drinking flavored or plain milk is positively associated with nutrient intake and is not associated with adverse effects on weight status in US children and adolescents. *J Am Diet Assoc.* 2008;108(4):631-639

86. Adams D, Fahey N, Pryslak J, Wilhelm B. Changes in school children's milk consumption and nutrient intake as a result of changing the availability of flavored milk in schools. Prime Consulting Group; March, 2010. Available at: http://www.midwestdairy.com/download_file.cfm?FILE_ID=603. Accessed October 31, 2012

87. Fulgoni VL, Keast DR, Auestad N, Quann EE. Nutrients from dairy foods are difficult to replace in diets of Americans: food pattern modeling and an analyses of the National Health and Nutrition Examination Survey 2003-2006. *Nutr Res*. 2011;31(10):759-765

88. Wagner CL; Greer FR; American Academy of Pediatrics, Section on Breastfeeding and Committee on Nutrition. Prevention of rickets and vitamin D deficiency in infants, children and adolescents. *Pediatrics*. 2008;122(5):1142-1152

89. Heyman MB; American Academy of Pediatrics, Committee on Nutrition. Clinical report: lactose intolerance in infants, children and adolescents. *Pediatrics*. 2006;118(3): 1279-1286

90. Kit BK, Carroll MD, Ogden CL. Low-fat milk consumption among children and adolescents in the United States, 2007-2008. US Department of Health and Human Services. *NCHS Data Brief*. 2011 Sep;(75):1-8

91. School Nutrition Association, Children's Nutrition Foundation, National Dairy Council Survey Report: *Availability of Flavored Milks in Schools*. 2006. http://www.schoolnutrition.org/uploadedFiles_old/ASFSA/newsroom/bookstore/availabillityofflavoredmilk.pdf. Accessed October 31, 2012

92. Prime Consulting Group. 2011-2012 Projected School Milk Product Profile. Available at: http://www.nationaldairycouncil.org/flavoredmilk. Accessed October 31, 2012

93. Dairy Research Institute. Proprietary NHANES 2003-2006 Analyses, Ages 2+ Years. Data Source: Centers for Disease Control and Prevention, National Center for Health Statistics, National Health and Nutrition Examination Survey. Hyattsville, MD: US Department of Health and Human Services, Centers for Disease Control and Prevention, 2003-2006. Available at: www.cdc/nchs/nhanes.htm. Accessed October 31, 2012

94. Frary CD, Johnson RK, Wang MQ. Children and adolescents' choice of foods and beverages high in added sugars are associated with intakes of key nutrients and food groups. *J Adolesc Health*. 2004;34(1):56-63

95. Powell LM, Szczypka G, Chaloupka FJ. Trends in exposure to television food advertisements among children and adolescents in the United States. *Arch Pediatr Adolesc Med*. 2010;164(9):794-802

96. Strasburger VC; American Academy of Pediatrics, Council on Communications and Media. Children, adolescents, obesity and the media. *Pediatrics*. 2011;128(1):201-208

97. Zarocostas J. WHO calls for action to restrict marketing of unhealthy foods and drinks to children. *BMJ*. 2011 Jan 25;342:d503

98. Strasburger VC, Jordan AB, Donnerstein E. Health effects of media on children and adolescents. *Pediatrics*. 2010;125(4):756-767

99. Better Business Bureau. Children's Food and Beverage Advertising Initiative. Available at: http://www.bbb.org/us/children-food-beverage-advertising-initiative/. Accessed October 31, 2012

100. Ramstetter CL, Murray R, Garner AS. The crucial role of recess. *J Sch Health*. 2010;80: 517-552

101. American Academy of Pediatrics, Council on School HealthPolicy statement: the crucial role of recess in school. *Pediatrics*. 2013; in press

102. US Department of Agriculture, Food and Nutrition Service. Team Nutrition. Available at: http://www.fns.usda.gov/tn/. Accessed October 31, 2012

103. Fuel Up to Play 60. Available at: http://www.fueluptoplay60.com/. Accessed October 31, 2012

104. Kaphingst KM, Story M. Child care as an untapped setting for obesity prevention: State child care licensing regulations related to nutrition, physical activity and media use for preschool-aged children in the United States. *Prev Chronic Dis.* 2009;6(1):A11

105. National Association of Child Care Resource and Referral Agencies. *Child Care in America. 2008 State Fact Sheets.* Available at: http://www.naccrra.org/. Accessed October 31, 2012

106. Survey of Income and Program Participation, 2010. US Census Bureau. http://www.census.gov/hhes/childcare/. Accessed October 31, 2012

107. Benjamin SE, Ammerman A, Sommers J, Dodds J, Neelon B, Ward DS. Nutrition and Physical Activity Self-assessment for Child Care (NAP SACC): results from a pilot intervention. *J Nutr Educ Behav.* 2007;39(3):142-149

108. Position Statement of the American Dietetic Association: benchmarks for nutrition in child care. *J Am Diet Assoc.* 2011;111(4):607-615

109. American Academy of Pediatrics, American Public Health Association, National Resource Center for Health and Safety in Child Care and Early Education. *Preventing Childhood Obesity in Early Care and Education: Selected Nutrition and Physical Activity Standards from the Third Edition of Caring for Our Children.* Aurora, CO: National Resource Center for Health and Safety in Child Care and Early Education; 2010

110. Ziegler P, Briefel R, Ponza M, Novak T, Hendricks K. Nutrient intakes of food patterns of toddlers' lunches and snacks: influence of location. *J Am Diet Assoc.* 2006;106(1 Suppl 1):S124-S134

111. Sweitzer SJ, Briley ME, Roberts-Gray C, Hoelscher DM, Harrist RB, Staskel DM, Almansour FD. Lunch is in the bag: increasing fruits, vegetables and whole grains in sack lunches of preschool-aged children. *J Am Diet Assoc.* 2010;110(7):1058-1064

112. Institute of Medicine. *Early Childhood Obesity Prevention Policies.* Washington, DC: National Academies Press; 2011. Available at: http://www.nap.edu/catalog.php?record_id=13124. Accessed October 31, 2012

113. Falbe J, Kenney EL, Henderson KE, Schwartz MB. The Wellness Childcare Assessment Tool: a measure to assess the quality of written nutrition and physical activity policies. *J Am Diet Assoc.* 2011;111(12):1852-1860

114. Crowe H, Goodway JD, Robinson LE. Gender differences in fundamental motor skill development in disadvantaged preschoolers from two geographical regions. *Res Q Exerc Sport.* 2010;81(1):17-24

115. National Association for Sport and Physical Education. Active Start: A Statement of Physical Activity Guidelines for Children Birth to Five Years. Reston, VA: National Association for Sport and Physical Education; 2002. Available at: http://www.aahperd.org/naspe/standards/nationalGuidelines/ActiveStart.cfm. Accessed October 31, 2012

116. Logan SW, Modlesky C, Scarabis-Fletcher K, Getchell N. The relationship between motor skill proficiency and body mass index in preschool children. *Res Q Exerc Sport.* 2011;82(3):442-444

CHAPTER 10

Cultural Considerations in Feeding Infants and Young Children

Importance of Addressing Cultural Influence on Feeding Practices

Infants and young children need physiologically and psychosocially adequate care and feeding to survive, develop to their full potential, and achieve and maintain adult health.[1,2] Parent and caregiver feeding practices that influence diet in the first 5 years of life, therefore, have significant and long-term effects on health for any child. However, ideas about "care," "nutrition," and "child needs" vary among cultural groups that self-identify on the basis of language, national heritage, religion, age, gender, and many other social and historical characteristics. Such cultural variation has the potential to influence the particular ways parents and other caregivers feed newborn infants, older infants, toddlers, and preschool-aged children or respond to health messages, advice, and guidelines and may contribute to a range of health disparities. Culturally competent advice on feeding and caregiving in family or other child-rearing contexts is, therefore, a key strategy to address diet- and nutrition-related health problems across ethnic groups.[3-6]

Challenges for Health Professionals

Most caregivers are aware of the importance of postnatal nutrition, but feeding newborn infants and older infants can seem like major a challenge. There may be gaps between "folk models" of how to meet infant and child feeding needs and current biomedical advice that must be bridged by effective knowledge translation. Culture may influence the gaps in how pediatricians and caregivers conceive and communicate about infant and child feeding. For example, although US pediatricians draw distinctions between infants and older children, many cultures frame the developmental cutoffs between "newborn infants," "babies" or "infants," "toddlers," and "preschoolers" in different ways. In some cases, specific cultural influences on infant and young child feeding practices may contribute to clinically relevant mismatch between everyday caregiver practices and evidence-based recommendations. Common examples worldwide include the very early introduction of nonnutritious liquids to newborn infants. Meeting the feeding needs of infants and young children, therefore, requires connecting clinical knowledge of the child's changing nutritional needs and requirements to caregiver expectations of infant and young child development. Health care professionals increasingly need new tools to protect, promote, and support healthier feeding practices in multicultural societies and to translate global and national recommendations and guidelines into culturally specific information.

In the United States, support for healthy infant and child feeding must be responsive to the historical and continuing diversification of American society and targeted to address the specific health needs of racial and ethnic minorities.[7-9] Three of the overarching goals of *Healthy People 2020,* the current set of national objectives for improving the health of all Americans, are to achieve health equity, eliminate disparities, and improve the health of all groups.[9] These objectives recognize that the United States is a culturally diverse nation[10] faced with a continuing challenge of reducing health disparities among population subgroups that vary in cultural heritage, income, education, economic empowerment, social history, and the politics of identity. Such disparities include higher proportions of low birth weight[11,12] and child overweight and obesity[13] among some minority, groups, principally non-white Hispanic and African American people. Improved neonatal, older infant, and preschool child feeding practices are recognized as a key component of strategies to reduce such disparities. For example, the Surgeon General's Call to Action to Support Breastfeeding[14] highlights the health and economic benefits of breastfeeding and some of the ethnic/racial disparities in breastfeeding rates. A useful fact sheet is available at: http://www.surgeongeneral.gov/library/calls/breastfeeding/factsheet.html.

Cultural Diversity in the United States

Officially recognized indicators of "cultural" difference in America include the socially constructed categories of race[15] and ethnicity. For example, recent US Census Bureau data captured information on "331 different race and ethnic groups."[16] Racial or ethnic groups are often considered to be distinct cultures within the United States, separated from the mainstream by traditions and practices even though many individuals born and raised in the United States may share ideas, behaviors, understandings, values, and attitudes embedded in the dominant culture.

Together, the officially recognized racial and ethnic minorities now represent roughly one third of the US population,[17] and foreign-born people represent more than 11%.[18] According to the US Census Bureau, "A minority is anyone who is not single-race white and not Hispanic."[19] However, current minorities will represent half of the US population by 2042,[17] and by 2023, half of all children will have a minority background. The proportion of non-Hispanic white births fell below that of all other groups for the first time in the year ending July 2011, during which minority groups such as black, Hispanic, Asian, and mixed-race accounted for 50.4% of 2.02 million births in the United States.[19] It is projected that the racial and ethnic diversity of the United States will continue to increase significantly in coming decades,[20] led by the child population.

How Is Culture Linked to Health?

Population differences in health are often attributed in part to complex effects of culture, but there are many difficulties in establishing causal links.[21] The concept of culture differs from the concept of race and ethnicity often used in health policy. Culture emerges from the dynamic expression in everyday life of socially learned understandings, values, attitudes, and behaviors that shape each person's experiences and interactions. The precise ways culture may influence health remain unclear, despite an apparent association with persistent disparities in health between racial and ethnic groups.[22,23] Genetic differences explain few of these health disparities; instead, evidence suggests that health has social determinants beginning in childhood[24] and that disparities in social conditions can contribute to poor health in "racialized" groups.[25] For example, in the United States, black and Hispanic children are more likely to be exposed to a suite of pre- and postnatal risk factors related to childhood obesity[26] for reasons more directly linked to economic and social historical factors than specifically cultural ones.

Recent advances in social science offer new ways to trace the mechanisms through which cultural factors modify health outcomes. One approach, cultural consensus modeling, views cultures as made up of overlapping shared "domains of significance" that structure understanding and transmit morals, values, traditions, behaviors, and practices.[27] Together, these domains form a cultural "model" with which an individual makes sense of how the world works, decides how to behave in any given situation, and interprets what the behavior of others means. This approach accommodates the fact that no 2 people share exactly the same mix of models, in part because of variation in social roles by age, gender, health, and economic status. Individuals often combine multiple models from different strands of their cultural heritage, and some individuals within cultural groups may hold more detailed knowledge and more "expertise" in certain cultural domains than others.

Cultural Influences on Feeding Practices

In looking at racial and ethnic variation in caregiver practices, it is critical to differentiate the variation attributable to disproportionate social and economic influences from variation attributable to cultural models. Everyday care practices within families and communities are strongly influenced by income, education, social autonomy, time demands, and health literacy of individual caregivers. Most people, whether parents, caregivers, or otherwise, hold cultural models of good, adequate caregiving and feeding practices. Such models usually combine several physical, psychosocial, and emotional dimensions. Diversity in infant and child feeding practices is linked to variation in such models. Sources of variation linked to social and cultural factors

III

include parental and other caregiver expectations and social roles, the processes of social learning of diverse cultural models of good feeding and healthy eating, and the symbolic meanings and social categories associated with food that strongly influence food choices, recipes, and diets. Food preferences, food preparation, and consumption practices and ideas about how healthy or appropriate specific foods or dishes may be begin in the childhood family or other caregiving context and are influenced throughout life by location, gender, social identity, ethnicity, income and class, commercial marketing, and social change. For example, feeding traditional and culturally meaningful foods may be important to caregivers, especially parents.

Early Infant Feeding

In 2010, US Secretary of State Hillary Clinton launched the international 1000 Days partnership[a] to focus international and national attention on the critical importance of good nutrition between conception and a child's second birthday. This developmental period offers a narrow window during which good nutrition has the most long-term effects and after which deficits attributable to undernutrition cannot be overcome. Specific feeding practices based on currently available clinical evidence are recommended to ensure optimal infant and child development and growth. The clearest recommendations relate to breastfeeding[28,29] and complementary feeding.[30,31] Other guidelines aim at building healthy dietary habits for preschool- and school-aged children[32] that reduce the risks of childhood overweight and obesity.[33]

Recommendations for Normal Breastfeeding and Complementary Feeding

The American Academy of Pediatrics (AAP) officially defines breastfeeding and human milk as "the normative standard for infant feeding and nutrition" and, in concert with the World Health Organization[29] and many other national authorities around the world, recommends "exclusive breastfeeding[1] for about 6 months."[28] The AAP also recommends babies sleep in the same room (but not in the same bed) as parents during the first 6 months of life,[34] which allows mothers to register subtle cues from a baby, encourages nursing through the night, and helps to maintain milk supply.[35] The AAP also recommends introducing appropriate complementary foods[b] at approximately 6 months of age and that breastfeeding should "continue for at least one year and thereafter for as long as mutually desired by mother and child."[28] This recommendation is in alignment with World Health Organization and UNICEF guidelines to continue breastfeeding to 2 years or longer,[29] feed complementary foods 2 to 3 times a day beginning at 6 months of age, and to feed 3 meals and 1 to 2 snacks a day to a breastfed child during the second year of life.[31]

[a] No other foods or liquids apart from medicines.

[b] Complementary foods are safe and nutritious foods fed to an older breastfed infant to promote health, growth, and development in the young child.

These recommendations apply to all ethnic and racial groups and are based on strong epidemiologic evidence that shows protection, promotion, and support of breastfeeding are among the most clinically and cost-effective global strategies for ensuring survival of healthy infants. Immediate postnatal initiation and exclusive breastfeeding for 6 months are a clear goal for global public nutrition because of the health benefits of breastfeeding. In industrialized countries, infants who are breastfed are healthier, and breastfeeding is associated with fewer respiratory infections; fewer episodes of diarrhea, pneumonia, and ear infections; and reduced risk of later asthma, obesity, and sudden infant death syndrome.[36-38] The timing of the introduction of complementary foods is somewhat controversial given the limited evidence linking infant age at introduction of foods to outcomes, such as iron deficiency, allergy, obesity, and later childhood eating habits[39,40] (also see Chapter 6: Complementary Feeding).

Current Practices

Recent data show that only 75% of American women initiate breastfeeding, less than half (43%) continue to breastfeed until at least 6 months, and only 13.3% continue to breastfeed exclusively until 6 months.[38] There is widespread introduction of foods or other substances before 6 months of age.[41]

Pediatricians should anticipate increasing momentum among policy makers, health care professionals, and employers toward increased support of breastfeeding across all sectors of the workforce and population subgroups. For example, the US Surgeon General recently released a Call to Action to Support Breastfeeding that explicitly recognizes a need for action across several societal domains to support mothers and other caregivers to meet current recommendations.[14] The Department of Health and Human Services has set Healthy People 2020 goals at 81.9% for the breastfeeding initiation, 60.6% breastfeeding at 6 months, and 25.5% exclusively breastfeeding at 6 months.[38] Globally, the economic value of increased breastfeeding both to families and nations may be high.[42] Evidence for reduced absenteeism among breastfeeding mothers suggests that supporting breastfeeding can benefit employers as well as the health of women and their children. In one study of breastfeeding and formula-feeding working mothers, three quarters of the one-day absences recorded over a year were among mothers of formula-fed infants, and 86% of infants who were never ill were breastfed.[43]

Cultural Influences on Breastfeeding Practices

Caregivers make decisions about infant feeding within an economic, social, and cultural context, and it is important to distinguish the relative influence of cultural history, social support (including family and health care professionals), income, and working conditions. These different factors change over time, and health care professionals should be aware of this wider context in advising caregivers. On one hand, historical declines in breastfeeding in America are partially reversing in response to ongoing social, business, and policy changes. On the other hand, a formidable range of barriers to breastfeeding is now deeply embedded within contemporary American culture. Health care professionals should be aware of some of the most widespread and powerful influences on parents and caregivers in their decision making regarding breastfeeding (see Table 10.1).

Table 10.1.
Selected Cultural Influences on Breastfeeding in Contemporary America

Type of Influence	Examples	Demonstrated Pathways (Effects on Breastfeeding: $+/-$)
Medical practices	Obstetric interventions	Elective Cesarian ($--$) Anaesthesia (-?) Doula care ($++$) Kangaroo care ($++$)
	Baby Friendly Hospitals	Institutionalized protection, promotion and support for breastfeeding in the peripartum ($++$)
	Infant sleep arrangements	Advice to separate from mother erodes breastfeeding ($--$)
	Scheduling feeds	Spacing breastfeeding bouts ($--$)
Public services	Provision of infant formula vs support for breastfeeding by WIC program	Large-scale provision of formula ($--$)
Business practices	Employment Maternity leave Breast-pumping facilities	Employment outside the home ($--$) ($++$) ($++$)
Legal frameworks	Legislation for protection of breastfeeding outside the home Maternity leave Breast pumping	Weak and inconsistent legal framework reflects a cultural discomfort with breastfeeding (-?) ($++$) Unknown: requires more study
Popular culture	Sexualization of the breast	Limited exposure to breastfeeding and reinforced negative concepts of breastfeeding ($--$)

Historical Changes

In America, some experts suggest culture (including gender relations), politics, and religion may have been as powerful as medicine, science, and the formula industry in shaping breastfeeding practices.[44] Infant feeding culture in colonial America mirrored European practices of the time, with breastfeeding the norm through the 17th and 18th centuries. For example, the Puritans promoted breastfeeding as a Christian duty, describing women who did not breastfeed as "criminal and blameworthy."[45] After independence, many women in the wealthier classes stopped breastfeeding their infants themselves, turning first to wet nurses (in some cases enslaved women of African descent) and eventually to patent infant foods.[46] Nevertheless, breastfeeding rates remained at 85% to 90% prior to and throughout the first third of the 20th century.

By mid-century, however, increased medicalization of childbirth and increased reliance on commercial formulas marketed as more "scientific" methods of infant feeding had significantly eroded rates of breastfeeding.[46] By 1971, only 3.2% of American infants were exclusively breastfed for 6 months.[47] Breastfeeding initiation rates have increased substantially over the most recent 4 decades, (from 26.5% in 1970 to 61.9% in 1982 and 75% in 2010[48]) as some of the many remaining gaps in protection, promotion, and support of continued breastfeeding have narrowed[48]), but the rate of exclusive breastfeeding at 6 months has lagged, increasing by only 10% since 1971, to 13.3% in 2010.[38]

Differences in Breastfeeding Rates Between Major Population Groups

Although the cultural factors discussed previously affect all women in the United States, large differences in breastfeeding rates exist between ethnic and racial groups. Within the last decade, breastfeeding initiation was rarer among non-Hispanic black mothers than among non-Hispanic white mothers in most states, whereas rates of initiation between Hispanic and non-Hispanic white mothers varied from east to west.[49] National breastfeeding indicators remain disproportionately low among groups self-identifying as non-Hispanic black or African American, American Indian, or Alaska Native (Table 10.2), and rates of initiation, exclusive breastfeeding, and continued breastfeeding will have to increase disproportionately across ethnic and racial groups to achieve Healthy People 2020 goals.

Table 10.2.

Maternal Breastfeeding Rates[a] for US Infants Born in 2009, by Census Ethnic and Racial Groups

Group	Any Breast-feeding	Breast-feeding at 6 mo	Breast-feeding at 12 mo	Exclusive Breast-feeding at 3 mo	Exclusive Breast-feeding at 6 mo
Asian	84.2	59.0	32.5	41.1	18.2
Hispanic or Latino	82.6	47.9	26.1	35.1	17.0
Native Hawaiian and other	61.6	33.0	19.3	33.0	17.2
Non-Hispanic white	78.4	50.4	27.1	35.9	17.4
American Indian or Alaska Native	71.5	33.1	19.3	27.8	8.0
Non-Hispanic black or African American	58.8	32.0	16.6	20.0	10.0
All women	76.9	47.2	25.5	33.0	16.3

Source: Centers for Disease Control and Prevention and Department of Health and Human Services. Breastfeeding among US children born 2000-2009, CDC National Immunization Survey. Available at: http://www.cdc.gov/breastfeeding/data/nis_data/.

[a] Percentage of births.

The underlying reasons for the persistent disparities in breastfeeding rates are not yet understood. It is clear that the most significant disparity is in breastfeeding initiation. Although Asian American women have the highest breastfeeding rates and non-Hispanic black women have the lowest rates for all breastfeeding measures, these differences are reduced when comparing only those women who initiated breastfeeding among population groups (Table 10.2). It is important to note that the differences attenuate as infant ages increase and also that the underlying factors associated with positive breastfeeding attitudes, intentions, and practices are similar across ethnic and racial groups and include various forms of support from partners and coparents, family members, community-based groups or services, and health care professionals. The following sections highlight findings from selected recent studies of the historical and cultural factors that underlie current observed differences among population subgroups distinguished by American definitions of race or ethnicity.

African American Women

Current breastfeeding rates are low among African American women compared with other racial and ethnic groups because of a mix of economic, cultural-historical, and political factors.[46] Again, generalization from a few focused studies is not advised because of large cultural diversity, even in single samples."[50] Inconsistent results are reported regarding the relative influence of knowledge on breastfeeding benefits, levels of social support, advice and encouragement, exposure to role models, past personal experience with breastfeeding, and self-efficacy in maternal decision-making.[51] Some studies suggest the prevalence of positive breastfeeding intentions may increase over time among some non-Hispanic black population subgroups because of increasing Afro-Caribbean immigration.[52]

Recent studies in selected African American communities suggest that generally high prenatal confidence in breastfeeding ability[51] is subsequently eroded among women with less self-efficacy by postpartum "ambivalence" toward breastfeeding, which is in turn linked to perceptions of the relative value of formula and the practical and social difficulties associated with breastfeeding.[51,53] Common challenges to breastfeeding in a southeastern sample included "perceived lack of information about benefits and management of breastfeeding, difficulties breastfeeding in public, and lack of a support system for continued breastfeeding."[50] Underlying factors included infrequent reports of health care professionals discussing breastfeeding during pregnancy. Specific beliefs also played a role, however. Beliefs among women in the study included that breastfeeding was an activity for white women only, that human milk is too sweet and rots the infant's teeth, and that breastfeeding "spoils" the child, and older men in their community believed that male children who were breastfed become "soft."[50]

Although the value of peer and other social supports for breastfeeding is often assumed, African American women interested in breastfeeding may feel isolated or out of place in support groups that tend to have more white members, such as La Leche League.[50] A socioecologic study that examined the effect of a variety of factors on rates of breastfeeding among an urban, northeastern sample of African American concluded that in specific situations "where breastfeeding role models are few, beliefs that discourage breastfeeding are many… [and]… where everyday life is full of danger and fear, it is understandable that breastfeeding is not considered practical."[54]

American Indian Women

As a group, American Indian women have the second-lowest breastfeeding rates in America (Table 10.2), but there have been few studies of the underlying reasons. In some American Indian communities in which consumption of local fish and game foods continues or is increasing because of health promotion and community decision making, women may be unwilling to breastfeed because of concerns about environmental pollutants in their milk. For example, in one such community, the Akwesasne Mohawk Nation, polychlorinated biphenyl levels in young adults were nearly twice as high as US national averages, and higher levels were associated with having been breastfed.[55] Another study found that almost all American

Indian women interviewed held positive breastfeeding attitudes prenatally and that those with a stronger sense of cultural identity or connection to their community were more likely to breastfeed exclusively to 6 months.[56] Although this suggests that factors other than traditional cultural practices underlie low rates of exclusive and continued breastfeeding, more studies across almost 600 federally recognized American Indian nations and many other communities are needed before general conclusions can be drawn.

Hispanic Women

The American context appears to exert a powerful influence that changes infant feeding decisions among both Hispanic and other women immigrating to the United States.[57] Compared with immigrant women from the same ethnic groups born outside the United States, groups of American-born Mexican Hispanic, non-Mexican Hispanic, and non-Hispanic women are all substantially less likely to initiate breastfeeding and to still be breastfeeding at 6 months (85% and 66% reduced likelihood, respectively[58]). Data from both the National Health and Nutrition Examination Survey (NHANES) and the National Survey of Children's Health show that, controlling for age, education, and poverty, more "acculturated" Hispanic women are less likely to breastfeed.[59,60] Studies of specific Latina groups show associations between less integration/acculturation and greater likelihood of continued breastfeeding.[61] Other studies have found that the odds of breastfeeding decreased by 4% for every year of residency in the United States among Hispanic immigrant couples[58] and in Mexican-origin women residing in the United States for more than 5 years.[4,62]

The clear conclusion for health care professionals is that strategies to support maintenance of cultural reinforcement for breastfeeding may be helpful. Hispanic immigrants often bring specific cultural models of appropriate infant feeding that support breastfeeding, such as the "cuarentena del bebe" (a 40-day postpartum period during which the mother focuses entirely on infant care, leaving housework and other responsibilities to family members, and infants are ideally breastfed exclusively).[57] Narrative data from qualitative studies indicate that Hispanic immigrants believe formula feeding is necessitated by the need to work and facilitated by the provision of free formula through the Special Supplemental Nutrition Program for Women, Infants, and Children (WIC).[57] Many Hispanic immigrant women come to believe that giving "los dos" (both human milk and formula) is a good option that combines the flexibility of bottle feeding with the benefits of breastfeeding.

Other Immigrant Populations

The strongest evidence of cultural influences on breastfeeding independent of other social and economic factors is found among newcomers. Foreign-born women from a range of ethnic backgrounds living in the United States are consistently reported to be at least as or more likely to initiate breastfeeding, to intend only to breastfeed, and to breastfeed exclusively as US-born women categorized in the same racial or ethnic group.[52,58,60] Several studies have found that rates of breastfeeding initiation and duration of breastfeeding also decrease among various ethnic groups of non-Hispanic immigrants with increased length of residence in the United States and reduced use of native language.[58] This suggests immigrant women's breastfeeding behaviors tend to converge with those of American-born women over time, presumably because of exposure to American cultural models. New studies among specific immigrant groups are beginning to trace the connections between infant feeding beliefs and practices and increased health risks, such as childhood overweight.[63]

Introduction of "First Foods" to Older Infants and Toddlers

Pediatric nutritional interest in the period from the beginning of complementary feeding of "first foods" through the preschool and kindergarten years has moved beyond characterizing nutrient requirements to investigation of the potential effects in later childhood and adulthood. Current guidelines in the United States and beyond provide advice based on fairly well-established evidence of the potential clinical importance of (1) the links between early exposure, later acceptance, and long-term benefits of early dietary variety; and (2) the influence of parenting and caregiving styles.[64] Recent research is refining the conceptual models for understanding the development of healthy and less healthy food habits[64] but is also highlighting problems in measuring caregiver practices through self-report and direct observation.[65]

Early Food Habit Formation

Exposure to varied foods early in life is key for acceptance and development of later food tastes.[66,67] Both breastfeeding and complementary feeding play a role.[68] Infants exposed to a flavor through their mother's amniotic fluid and human milk will enjoy the food more when first introduced to it as a complementary food. Accumulated evidence suggests that familiarity with foods underpins dietary preferences and that early experiences with diverse foods and flavors broaden future preferences.[70] Familiarity accounts for more than half the variance in children's food preferences, early exposure to foods improves subsequent food acceptance, and repeated exposure to foods reduces neophobia and increases both subjective ratings of liking and objective food consumption.[71]

Importance of Parent/Caregiver Practice

We can assume that parents and caregivers have a powerful gatekeeping influence on exposure to foods during infancy and early childhood. Giving infants and toddlers nutritious foods and finding strategies to ensure older children eat a balanced diet are probably goals shared by most mothers and other caregivers in all ethnic or racial groups. However, parent/caregiver perceptions and behavioral approaches to the challenge of introducing and subsequently feeding foods and helping younger children eat a healthy range of foods shows cultural variation.[65,72-74] Young children often show neophobia on exposure to new foods that must be resolved to ensure a varied and balanced diet and establish healthy dietary preferences and habits.[71] Successful introduction of complementary first foods often requires more perseverance, patience, and number of exposures than parents/caregivers expect. Culturally influenced variation in the timing of introduction, frequency of feeding, amounts fed, and types food eaten might affect child outcomes because of the potential effects on (1) meeting nutrient requirements (adequate or inadequate); (2) immune development (tolerance or allergy); (3) eating patterns (healthy or unhealthy); (4) child, adolescent, and adult nutritional status (normal range vs stunted, underweight, overweight, or obese); and (5) metabolic programming (appropriate vs increasing risk of development of insulin resistance, diabetes, or cardiovascular disease).

Parenting and Feeding Styles

Research to characterize and validate the existence of different "feeding styles" and their potential relationship to parenting styles, cultural and socioeconomic context and child nutrition outcomes has increased in recent years.[75] Recent reviews confirm the common assumption that parenting styles influence child body proportions, activity levels, diet quality, eating experiences, and behavior during meals.[76-78] Researchers have characterized parenting and feeding styles in a number of different ways that have changed over the years, but recent reviews of available data conclude that "authoritative" parenting and "responsive" feeding styles are more likely associated with healthy child weight and diet diversity at appropriate ages than either "authoritarian" (restrictive or controlling) or "laissez-faire" styles.[77] Caregivers show a responsive feeding style if they pay close attention to and interact with children, making sure foods are tried and consumed and tracking how much nutritious (eggs, lean meats, leafy greens, red/yellow vegetables, and fruits, etc) or unhealthy food (junk snacks, fast foods, high-fat and sweet foods) is eaten.[75] A more controlling style pressures the child to eat independently of child cues, and a more laissez-faire style provides little physical help or communication of encouragement to infants during feeding or children during meals.

Sources of Advice on First Foods

Today's parents and caregivers are exposed to a large and often bewildering number of nutrition recommendations for infants, older preschoolers, and school-aged children.[a] Social contacts of parents and caregivers commonly provide additional or alternative advice on infant feeding. Both maternal and paternal grandmothers are often reported as a major influence on maternal feeding decisions among Hispanic parents and other groups. Father or male partner involvement in infant feeding decisions is not well investigated but likely varies across cultural groups. Some evidence indicates interaction of gender and ethnicity in the interparental negotiation of advice on infant feeding. One study reported male partners as more likely to influence infant feeding in white couples and to encourage early introduction of complementary first foods across ethnic/racial groups.[79]

Ethnic/Racial Similarities and Differences

A nonsystematic review of findings from studies of differences in feeding practices among ethnic or racial groups indicates a mosaic of differences and similarities that is greatly complicated by noncultural factors as location, income, age, and education. Studies have looked for differences in key indicators of feeding practices among ethnic or racial groups, and recent years have seen publication of an increasing number of studies that test whether tools and constructs used to measure parenting styles, feeding styles, parental or caregiver self-efficacy, and other indicators can be used to make valid comparisons among ethnic, racial, and cultural groups. A major limitation of studies of feeding practices across groups is that, often because of the value of focused, qualitative research with relatively small samples of parents/caregivers, it is difficult to generalize the findings to all members of a particular ethnic/racial group. It is important to note that most of these studies have been conducted among low-income samples, many of which are drawn from participants in WIC, Head Start, and other such programs, and that they have highlighted important variation within the ethnic/racial groups studied as well as some between-group differences.

African American Practices

Specific studies of African American practices seem remarkably few, and general patterns are difficult to discern. Several studies have found that a high proportion of mothers of African American preschoolers adopt a restrictive feeding style[74] but that this is also associated with low income and high maternal weight.[65,80] Another study found that African American parents use food to calm their children more often than do English-speaking Hispanic parents.[81] One study found that lower

---

[a] At the time of writing, one Web site sponsored by the AAP (HealthyChildren.org) offered 36 articles with information on "nutrition and feeding" for the age range 0-12 months and another 15, 9, 17, and 21 articles for toddlers, preschoolers, grade-schoolers, and teenagers, respectively; http://www.healthychildren.org/english/ages-stages/baby/feeding-nutrition/Pages/default.aspx.

consumption of fruits and vegetables among African American toddlers from low-income families enrolled in Head Start programs was also associated with maternal perception of "picky" eating by toddlers and low maternal consumption of fruits and vegetables.[82]

Hispanic and Latina/Latino Practices

The heterogeneity of Hispanic and/or Latina mothers makes it particularly difficult to draw generalizations about Hispanic and Latino feeding beliefs, attitudes, and practices, but several patterns are reported are fairly consistently across studies. For example, compared with other populations in the United States, some groups of Hispanic and/or Latina mothers tend toward a more "indulgent" feeding style, use positive incentives to get the child to eat more,[83,84] and feed softer foods, such as purees and soups, more frequently to older infants.[85] Heterogeneity is consistently observed with respect to language (English or Spanish speaking), time of residence in the United States, and measures of acculturation.[83] Among a recent sample of Latina WIC participants, foreign-born and less-educated women were more likely to show a pressuring feeding style.[72] Less acculturated and/or Spanish-speaking Hispanic participants from the southwest were more likely than their English-speaking counterparts to employ a controlling style, and this is linked to greater concerns about childhood overweight or underweight.[83]

Asian and Asian American Practices

The heterogeneity represented among Asian American and Asian people living in the United States again suggests a need for caution in generalizing about feeding behaviors and style. This is supported by the diversity in study findings. In one study, Chinese-American parents of preschoolers scored higher than non-Hispanic white counterparts on monitoring, concern, and restrictive feeding behaviors.[73] In another study, Vietnamese and Cambodian parents were found to be more likely to have an "indulgent" feeding style compared with other ethnic/racial groups.[74] Once again, studies investigating level of acculturation suggest it can be an important modifying influence on feeding practices. In a recent study of Chinese and Korean immigrants, a history of parental material deprivation was associated with a laissez-faire parental feeding style, specifically with less monitoring, less concern about weight and diet, and lower perception of parental responsibility for the child's diet.[86] However, because the effect was not observed among more acculturated parents, increased time in the United States again appears to significantly alter parents' feeding behaviors.

Building Skills in Advising Parents and Caregivers

Cultural Self-Awareness

The majority of patients will not completely share the culture of the health care professional, whether because of socioeconomic background, age, gender, ethnicity, or other factors. To move beyond ethnocentrism, health care professionals must understand their own cultural models about how things are or should be. It is a worthwhile exercise to use "cultural competency" tools to understand the overlap between the culture of the health care professional and the culture of each patient, regardless of the level of similarity or difference that the health care professional perceives between the patient and himself or herself.

Cultural Competency

Cultural competency is a skill now widely advocated in the medical fields and increasingly incorporated into medical education curricula.[3] A central requirement of cultural competency is acknowledging that all individuals have culture. In fact, individuals who have successfully completed medical school have added a new cultural dimension to their identity, as they have taken on the beliefs, traditions, practices, and behaviors of medical science. It is important for health care professionals who interact with women who are pregnant or breastfeeding to understand their own cultural positioning, both as individuals and as part of the culture of medicine. It is important, because the relationship between health care professional and patient is an exchange that relies on views and values of each participant as well as (in some cases) others, such as the partner or family members.[87]

There are multiple approaches to cultural competency training, but in essence, skill in cultural competency involves learning from the patient about the ways in which their view of the world (and particularly of health-related issues) might differ from that of the health care professional. To avoid stereotyping, the focus should be kept on the individual rather than attempting to generate a list of characteristics of the group. Individual life history and experience is likely the dominant force in how patients view their health and care.[87] Cultural competency is framed as an ongoing process rather than an end-point that is reached once and remains thereafter.

Among several available tools for building cultural competency skills,[87] the Purnell model[88] highlights 12 cultural domains that may have relevance for health and health care and could be modified to increase cultural competency during counseling on breastfeeding and feeding of complementary first foods. Some domains of the Purnell model that might be especially important to investigate for health care professionals who are advising parents about the feeding of infants and young children are summarized in Table 10.3.

Table 10.3.
Domains of Cultural Importance in Breastfeeding Counselling, Adapted From the Purnell Model of Cultural Competence[88]

Gender roles	Who makes decisions in the patient's household? Is one partner or the other dominant in terms of decision making? Does breastfeeding fall into the same category as other decisions? Are gender roles likely to influence the woman's comfort level for breastfeeding whenever/wherever necessary?
Extended family	Does the patient's family have input into the mode of infant feeding? If the mother or mother-in-law is influential regarding infant feeding, is there a way to involve her in breastfeeding counselling or follow-up appointments? Conversely, is the patient far from her family or experiencing a lack of social support that can make breastfeeding more difficult to cope with?
Tobacco/alcohol/ drug use	How would you ask about the use of legal and illegal drugs? Perhaps offer advice about tobacco, alcohol and drug use to all patients, on the basis that often you can't tell whether someone uses or abuses these substances.
Autonomy	Is it culturally appropriate for the patient to make breastfeeding decisions for herself and her baby or is it expected that she will consult a partner, parent, or senior members of the community? Is the patient likely to view the health care professional as an authority figure and respond to questions in the way she perceives as most acceptable to the health care professional?
Dominant language/ language barriers	Does the patient prefer to use a language other than English? Are breastfeeding materials and classes available in the patient's preferred language? Written materials on breastfeeding are available in a wide variety of languages from sources such as WIC, Abbott Laboratories, and La Leche League International sites.
Postpartum traditions	Will the patient require home visits because of cultural practices that seclude the woman and baby for 40 days following the birth? Are there breastfeeding-related practices, such as expressing and disposing of the colostrum or using prelacteal feeds? Do women consume or avoid any particular foods to ensure human milk supply? Three questions to help determine an appropriate response to a traditional postpartum practice: Is it beneficial? Is it harmless? Is it harmful?
Meaning of foods	Does formula feeding signify something to the woman or her community? Many cultures have prescriptions and prohibitions regarding breastfeeding, so it is helpful to inquire about galactogogues, ritual foods, and prohibited foods for all women.

By using the Purnell model to investigate patient cultural models of domains related to breastfeeding, health care professionals can avoid reliance on generalizations or applying stereotypes to relate to patients. If applied to all patients, the framework has the potential to increase understanding of women's decisions about infant feeding and improve dialogue between health care professional and patient.

Summary

The United States is an increasingly culturally diverse country, and a wide variety of cultural factors contribute to infant and child feeding decisions by parents and other caregivers. Cultural considerations for health care professionals advising on infant and young child feeding include differences among ethnic and racial groups in the proportions of mothers initiating breastfeeding and adhering to recommendations on exclusive and continued breastfeeding and in the proportions of parents and other caregivers adopting different infant feeding styles for complementary feeding and feeding of toddlers and preschoolers up to the age of 5 years. Cultural factors also include more systemic influences beyond the level of individuals and families, such as government policy, legislative frameworks, the "medicalization" of birthing and management of newborn care, the influence of the formula industry and major public health programs in shaping perceptions and practices, expectations on working women and very limited support for breastfeeding in the workplace, popular culture, and historical loss of experiential knowledge across generations as a result of large-scale social change. Such factors may explain trends such as reduced breastfeeding and increased concordance with mainstream caregiver feeding styles with increased length of residence among recent immigrants and level of mainstream acculturation among ethnic groups.

Some cultural models influencing caregiver feeding practices in America's many and diverse ethnic and racial population subgroups may potentially differ from those of a particular health care professional. Health care professionals and service providers are, themselves, strongly influenced by the dominant "models" of care and feeding that pervade American society and include more than the evidence-based recommendations that represent the "gold standard" for feeding practices. Health care professionals counseling patients to improve the health of children can narrow the potential cultural gaps by training in cultural competency, increasing their knowledge about the potential different cultural models for feeding and care, and assessing caregivers to understand which models may be relevant to each pediatric case. Table 10.3 summarizes some cultural considerations to be taken into account in culturally aware counseling to support mothers and other caregivers to meet recommendations for breastfeeding and feeding of complementary first foods to infants and young children in different ethnic and racial groups in the United States.

III

References

1. One Thousand Days Web site. Available at: http://www.thousanddays.org/resource-slug/1000-days-infographic/. Accessed October 2, 2012

2. Ruel M, Hoddinott J. *Investing in Early Childhood Nutrition.* Washington, DC: International Food Policy Research Institute; 2008

3. Expert Panel on Cultural Competence Education for Students in Medicine and Public Health. *Cultural Competence Education for Students in Medicine and Public Health: Report of an Expert Panel.* Washington, DC: Association of American Medical Colleges and Association of Schools of Public Health; 2012

4. Crawford PB, Gosliner W, Anderson C, et al. Counseling Latina mothers of preschool children about weight issues: suggestions for a new framework. *J Am Diet Assoc.* 2004;104(3):387-394

5. Galvin S, Grossman X, Feldman-Winter L, Chaudhuri J, Merewood A. A practical intervention to increase breastfeeding initiation among Cambodian women in the US. *Matern Child Health J.* 2008;12(4):545-547

6. Noble LM, Noble A, Hand IL. Cultural competence of healthcare professionals caring for breastfeeding mothers in urban areas. *Breastfeed Med.* 2009;4(4):221-224

7. American Academy of Pediatrics, Committee on Pediatric Workforce. Culturally effective pediatric care: education and training issues. *Pediatrics.* 1999;103(1):167-170

8. Sidelinger DE, Meyer D, Blaschke GS, et al. Communities as teachers: learning to deliver culturally effective care in pediatrics. *Pediatrics.* 2005;115(Suppl 3):1160-1164

9. US Department of Health and Human Services. Healthy People 2020. Available at: http://healthypeople.gov/2020/TopicsObjectives2020/pdfs/HP2020_brochure_with_LHI_508.pdf. Accessed October 2, 2012

10. US Census Bureau. Minority Links. Available at: http://www.census.gov/newsroom/minority_links/minority_links.html. Accessed October 2, 2012

11. Bruckner TA, Saxton KB, Anderson E, Goldman S, Gould JB. From Paradox to disparity: trends in neonatal death in very low birth weight non-Hispanic black and white infants, 1989-2004. *J Pediatr.* 2009;155(4):482-487

12. Collins JW, David RJ. Racial disparity in low birth weight and infant mortality. *Clin Perinatol.* 2009;36(1):63-73

13. Long JM, Mareno N, Shabo R, Wilson AH. Overweight and obesity among white, black, and Mexican American children: implications for when to intervene. *J Spec Pediatr Nurs.* 2012;17(1):41-50

14. US Department of Health and Human Services. The Surgeon General's Call to Action to Support Breastfeeding. Washington, DC: US Public Health Service, Office of the Surgeon General; 2011

15. American Anthropological Association. Race: Are we so different? Available at: http://www.understandingrace.org/home.html. Accessed October 2, 2012

16. US Census Bureau. Census Bureau Releases New Race and Ethnic Demographic Information from the 2010 Census for Alaska, Louisiana, Michigan and New Jersey [press release]. Washington, DC: US Census Bureau; March 8, 2012. Available at: http://www.census.gov/newsroom/releases/archives/2010_census/cb12-cn16.html. Accessed October 2, 2012

17. US Census Bureau. National Population Projections. Available at: http://www.census.gov/population/www/projections/2008projections.html. Published 2008. Accessed October 2, 2012

18. US Census Bureau. The foreign-born population 2000. Census 2000 Brief. December 2003. Available at: http://www.census.gov/prod/2003pubs/c2kbr-34.pdf. Accessed October 2, 2012

19. US Census Bureau. Most Children Younger Than Age 1 are Minorities, Census Bureau Reports [press release]. Washington, DC: US Census Bureau; May 17, 2012. Available at: http://www.census.gov/newsroom/releases/archives/population/cb12-90.html. Accessed October 2, 2012

20. Ortman JM, Guarneri CE. *United States Population Projections: 2000 to 2050*. Washington, DC: US Census Bureau; 2012. Available at: http://www.census.gov/population/www/projections/analytical-document09.pdf. Accessed October 2, 2012

21. Hruschka DJ, Hadley C. A glossary of culture in epidemiology. *J Epidemiol Community Health*. 2008;62(11):947-951

22. Dressler WW. Culture and the risk of disease. *BMJ*. 2004;69(1):21-31

23. Hruschka DJ. Culture as an explanation in population health. *Ann Hum Biol*. 2009;36(3):235-247

24. Wilkinson R, Marmot M, eds. *Social Determinants of Health: The Solid Facts*. Copenhagen, Denmark: World Health Organization; 2003

25. Gravlee CC. How race becomes biology: embodiment of social inequality. *Am J Phys Anthropol*. 2009;139(1):47-57

26. Taveras EM, Gillman MW, Kleinman K, Rich-Edwards JW, Rifas-Shiman SL. Racial/ethnic differences in early-life risk factors for childhood obesity. *Pediatrics*. 2010;125(4):686-695

27. Dressler WW, Bindon JR. The health consequences of cultural consonance: cultural dimensions of lifestyle, social support, and arterial blood pressure in an African American community. *Am Anthropol*. 2000;102(2):244-260

28. American Academy of Pediatrics, Section on Breastfeeding. Policy statement: breastfeeding and the use of human milk. *Pediatrics*. 2012;129(3):e827-e841

29. World Health Organization, UNICEF. *Global Strategy for Infant and Young Child Feeding*. Geneva, Switzerland: World Health Organization; 2003

30. Dewey K. *Guiding Principles for Feeding Non-breastfed Children 6-24 Months of Age*. Geneva, Switzerland: World Health Organization; 2005

31. Dewey KG; Pan-American Health Organization. Guiding Principles for Complementary Feeding of the Breastfed Child. Washington, DC: Pan-American Health Organization; 2003

32. American Heart Association; Gidding SS, Dennison BA, Birch LL, et al. Dietary Recommendations for children and adolescents: a guide for practitioners. *Pediatrics*. 2006;117(2):544-559

33. American Academy of Pediatrics, Committee on Nutrition. Prevention of pediatric overweight and obesity. *Pediatrics*. 2003;112(2):424-430

34. American Academy of Pediatrics, Task Force on Sudden Infant Death Syndrome. SIDS and other sleep-related infant deaths: expansion of recommendations for a safe infant sleeping environment. *Pediatrics*. 2011;128(5):1030-1039

35. Ball HL. Breastfeeding, bed-sharing, and infant sleep. *Birth*. 2003;30(3):181-188

36. Ladomenou F, Moschandreas J, Kafatos A, Tselentis Y, Galanakis E. Protective effect of exclusive breastfeeding against infections during infancy: a prospective study. *Arch Dis Child*. 2010;95(12):1004-1008

37. Tarrant M, Kwok MK, Lam TH, Leung GM, Schooling CM. Breast-feeding and childhood hospitalizations for infections. *Epidemiology*. 2010;21(6):847-854

38. Centers for Disease Control and Prevention. Breastfeeding Report Card— United States, 2010. Available at: http://www.cdc.gov/breastfeeding/pdf/ BreastfeedingReportCard2010.pdf. Accessed October 2, 2012

39. Michaelsen KF, Larnkjaer A, Lauritzen L, Molgaard C. Science base of complementary feeding practice in infancy. *Curr Opin Clin Nutr Metab Care*. 2010;13(3):277-283

40. Moorcroft KE, Marshall JL, McCormick FM. Association between timing of introducing solid foods and obesity in infancy and childhood: a systematic review. *Matern Child Nutr*. 2011;7(1):3-26

41. Grummer-Strawn LM, Scanlon KS, Fein SB. Infant feeding and feeding transitions during the first year of life. *Pediatrics*. 2008;122(Suppl 2):S36-S42

42. Bartick M, Reinhold A. The burden of suboptimal breastfeeding in the United States: a pediatric cost analysis. *Pediatrics*. 2010;125(5):e1048-1056

43. Cohen R, Mrtek MB, Mrtek RG. Comparison of maternal absenteeism and infant illness rates among breast-feeding and formula-feeding women in two corporations. *Am J Health Promot*. 1995;10(2):148-153

44. Thulier D. Breastfeeding in America: a history of influencing factors. *J Hum Lact*. 2009;25(1):85-94

45. Blum LM. *At the Breast: Ideologies of Breastfeeding and Motherhood in the Contemporary United States*. Boston, MA: Beacon Press; 1999

46. Apple RD. Constructing mothers: scientific motherhood in the nineteenth and twentieth centuries. *Soc Hist Med*. 1995;8(2):161-178

47. Riordan J. *Breastfeeding and Human Lactation*. 3rd ed. Sudbury, MA: Jones and Bartlett; 2005

48. Sellen DW. Evolution of infant and young child feeding: implications for contemporary public health. *Annu Rev Nutr*. 2007;27:123-148

49. Centers for Disease C, Prevention. Racial and ethnic differences in breastfeeding initiation and duration, by state—National Immunization Survey, United States, 2004-2008. *MMWR Morb Mortal Wkly Rep*. 2010;59(11):327-334

50. Lewallen LP, Street DJ. Initiating and sustaining breastfeeding in African American women. *J Obstet Gynecol Neonatal Nurs*. 2010;39(6):667-674

51. Robinson KM, VandeVusse L. African American women's infant feeding choices prenatal breast-feeding self-efficacy and narratives from a black feminist perspective. *J Perinat Neonatal Nurs*. 2011;25(4):320-328

52. Bonuck KA, Freeman K, Trombley M. Country of origin and race/ethnicity: impact on breastfeeding intentions. *J Hum Lact*. 2005;21(3):320-326.

53. Kaufman L, Deenadayalan S, Karpati A. Breastfeeding ambivalence among low-income African American and Puerto Rican women in north and central Brooklyn. *Matern Child Health J*. 2010;14(5):696-704

54. Bentley ME, Dee DL, Jensen JL. Breastfeeding among low income, African-American women: power, beliefs and decision making. *J Nutr*. 2003;133(1 Suppl):305S-309S

55. Gallo MV, Schell LM, DeCaprio AP, Jacobs A. Levels of persistent organic pollutant and their predictors among young adults. *Chemosphere*. 2011;83(10):1374-1382

56. Rhodes KL, Hellerstedt WL, Davey CS, Pirie PL, Daly KA. American Indian breastfeeding attitudes and practices in Minnesota. *Matern Child Health J*. 2008;12(Suppl 1):46-54

57. Faraz A. Clinical recommendations for promoting breastfeeding among Hispanic women. *J Am Acad Nurse Pract*. 2010;22(6):292-299

58. Gibson-Davis CM, Brooks-Gunn J. Couples' immigration status and ethnicity as determinants of breastfeeding. *Am J Public Health*. 2006;96(4):641-646

59. Gibson MV, Diaz VA, Mainous AG, 3rd, Geesey ME. Prevalence of breastfeeding and acculturation in Hispanics: results from NHANES 1999-2000 study. *Birth*. 2005;32(2):93-98

60. Singh G, Kogan M, Dee D. Nativity/immigrant status, race/ethnicity, and socioeconomic determinants of breastfeeding initiation and duration in the United States, 2003. *Pediatrics*. 2007;119(1 Suppl):S38-S46

61. Chapman DJ, Perez-Escamilla R. Acculturative type is associated with breastfeeding duration among low-income Latinas. *Matern Child Nutr*. Epub ahead of print July 25, 2011. DOI: 10.1111/j.1740-8709.2011.00344.x

62. Harley K, Stamm N, Eskenazi B. The effect of time in the U.S. on the duration of breastfeeding in women of Mexican descent. *Matern Child Health J*. 2007;11(2):119-125

63. Steinman L, Doescher M, Keppel GA, et al. Understanding infant feeding beliefs, practices and preferred nutrition education and health provider approaches: an exploratory study with Somali mothers in the USA. *Matern Child Nutr*. 2010;6(1):67-88

64. Schwartz C, Scholtens PAMJ, Lalanne A, Weenen H, Nicklaus S. Development of healthy eating habits early in life. Review of recent evidence and selected guidelines. *Appetite*. 2011;57(3):796-807

65. Sacco LM, Bentley ME, Carby-Shields K, Borja JB, Goldman BD. Assessment of infant feeding styles among low-income African-American mothers: comparing reported and observed behaviors. *Appetite*. 2007;49(1):131-140

66. Hetherington MM, Cecil JE, Jackson DM, Schwartz C. Feeding infants and young children. From guidelines to practice. *Appetite*. 2011;57(3):791-795

67. Mennella JA, Trabulsi JC. Complementary foods and flavor experiences: setting the foundation. *Ann Nutr Metab*. 2012;60:40-50

68. Nicklaus S. Children's acceptance of new foods at weaning. Role of practices of weaning and of food sensory properties. *Appetite*. 2011;57(3):812-815

69. Mennella JA, Jagnow CP, Beauchamp GK. Prenatal and postnatal flavor learning by human infants. *Pediatrics*. 2001;107(6):e88

70. Cooke LJ, Wardle J, Gibson EL, Sapochnik M, Sheiham A, Lawson M. Demographic, familial and trait predictors of fruit and vegetable consumption by pre-school children. *Public Health Nutr*. 2004;7(2):295-302

71. Cooke L. The importance of exposure for healthy eating in childhood: a review. *J Hum Nutr Diet*. 2007;20(4):294-301

III

72. Gross RS, Fierman AH, Mendelsohn AL, et al. Maternal perceptions of infant hunger, satiety, and pressuring feeding styles in an urban Latina WIC population. *Acad Pediatr.* 2010;10(1):29-35

73. Huang SH, Parks EP, Kumanyika SK, et al. Child-feeding practices among Chinese-American and non-Hispanic white caregivers. *Appetite.* 2012;58(3):922-927

74. Ventura AK, Gromis JC, Lohse B. Feeding practices and styles used by a diverse sample of low-income parents of preschool-age children. *J Nutr Educ Behav.* 2010;42(4):242-249

75. Black MM, Aboud FE. Responsive feeding is embedded in a theoretical framework of responsive parenting. *J Nutr.* 2011;141(3):490-494

76. Hughes SO, Power TG, Papaioannou MA, et al. Emotional climate, feeding practices, and feeding styles: an observational analysis of the dinner meal in Head Start families. *Int J Behav Nutr Phys Act.* 2011;8:60

77. Hurley KM, Cross MB, Hughes SO. A systematic review of responsive feeding and child obesity in high-income countries. *J Nutr.* 2011;141(3):495-501

78. Sleddens EFC, Gerards SMPL, Thijs C, De Vries NK, Kremers SPJ. General parenting, childhood overweight and obesity-inducing behaviors: a review. *Int J Pediatr Obes.* 2011;6(2-2):e12-e27

79. McLorg PA, Bryant CA. Influence of social network members and health care professional on infant feeding practices of economically disadvantaged mothers. *Med Anthropol.* 1989;10(4):265-278

80. Powers SW, Chamberlin LA, van Schaick KB, Sherman SN, Whitaker RC. Maternal feeding strategies, child eating behaviors, and child BMI in low-income African-American preschoolers. *Obesity.* 2006;14(11):2026-2033

81. Evans A, Seth JG, Smith S, et al. Parental feeding practices and concerns related to child underweight, picky eating, and using food to calm differ according to ethnicity/race, acculturation, and income. *Matern Child Health J.* 2011;15(7):899-909

82. Horodynski MA, Stommel M, Brophy-Herb H, Xie Y, Weatherspoon L. Low-income African American and non-Hispanic white mothers' self-efficacy, "picky eater" perception, and toddler fruit and vegetable consumption. *Public Health Nurs.* 2010;27(5):408-417

83. Seth JG, Evans AE, Harris KK, et al. Preschooler feeding practices and beliefs: differences among Spanish- and English-speaking WIC clients. *Fam Community Health.* 2007;30(3):257-270

84. Chaidez V, Townsend M, Kaiser LL. Toddler-feeding practices among Mexican American mothers. A qualitative study. *Appetite.* 2011;56(3):629-632

85. Mennella JA, Ziegler P, Briefel R, Novak T. Feeding Infants and Toddlers Study: the types of foods fed to hispanic infants and toddlers. *J Am Diet Assoc.* 2006;106(1):S96-S106

86. Cheah CSL, Van Hook J. Chinese and Korean immigrants' early life deprivation: an important factor for child feeding practices and children's body weight in the United States. *Soc Sci Med.* 2012;74(5):744-752

87. Stein K. Moving cultural competency from abstract to act. *J Am Diet Assoc.* 2010;110(5 Suppl):S21-S27

88. Purnell L. The Purnell Model for Cultural Competence. *J Transcult Nurs.* 2002;13(3):193-196

Chapter 11

Nutritional Aspects of Vegetarian Diets

Vegetarian Diets

There are many variations of the vegetarian diet and the practice of vegetarianism. Vegetarianism, according to the Merriam–Webster dictionary, is defined as "the theory or practice of living on a diet made up of vegetables, fruits, grains, nuts, and sometimes eggs or dairy products." Vegetarianism is a way of life for many individuals for various reasons. However, there can be potentially serious implications for the growing pediatric and adolescent population as a result of self-imposed or misguided limitations of the vegetarian diet. Therefore, pediatricians should proactively ask and assess the nutritional status of their vegetarian patients to ensure optimal health and growth provide anticipatory guidance to prevent any potential deficits.

A true vegetarian is a person who does not eat meat, fish, or fowl or products containing these foods. Many so-called semivegetarians eat some meat, fish, or seafood products. Thus, vegetarians are a heterogenous group of individuals that may be categorized as shown in Table 11.1. A lacto-ovo-vegetarian eating pattern is based on grains, vegetables, fruits, legumes, seeds, nuts, dairy products, and eggs. The lacto-vegetarian excludes eggs but can consume milk products. The eating pattern of a vegan, or total vegetarian, is similar to the lacto-vegetarian diet, with the exclusion of dairy and all products of animal origin, including gelatin and honey. A macrobiotic diet is based largely on grains, legumes, and vegetables. Fruits, nuts, and seeds are consumed to a lesser extent.[1] However, some individuals on a macrobiotic diet also consume limited amounts of fish. A sproutarian eats primarily sprouted seeds (eg, bean, wheat, or broccoli sprouts) supplemented with other raw foods. Fruitarianism diets include fruits, berries, juices, grains, nuts, seeds, legumes, and a few vegetables. Raw foodism excludes anything cooked above 118°F; this is the temperature at which a number of enzymes present in foods begin to degrade.[2] People leading an anthroposophic lifestyle have a diet consisting of vegetables fermented by lactobacilli and a restriction on antibiotics, antipyretics, and immunizations.[3] A nutritarian diet has increased amounts of unrefined plant food with high amounts of micronutrients as well as avoidance or minimal intake of refined grain products.[4] Each of these eating styles has different implications for the nutrition and health of children and adolescents. Therefore, it is important for the nutrition counselor to determine which groups of foods are actually consumed and which are avoided and the degree of conviction and adherence to the dietary pattern, so as to provide appropriate recommendations.

Table 11.1.
Types of Vegetarians

Classic Vegetarians	New Vegetarians
Lacto-ovo-vegetarians	Low-meat vegetarians
Lacto-vegetarians	Almost vegetarians
Ovo-vegetarians	Semi-vegetarians
Vegans	Pesco-vegetarians
Raw food eaters	Pollo-vegetarians
Sproutarians	Pudding vegetarians
Fruitarians	
Nutritarians	
Macrobiotic vegetarians	
Anthroposophic vegetarians	

Adapted from Fuhrman and Ferreri[4] and Leitzmann.[30]

Some of the reasons that individuals give for following a vegetarian diet are listed in Table 11.2. Health considerations, concern for the environment, animal welfare activism, or economic considerations and religious beliefs, alone or in combination, are often cited to support a vegetarian diet pattern. In the United States, economic reasons alone are usually not prominent, because a wide variety of both plant and animal foods are widely available and inexpensive. Immigrants from developing countries (eg, mainland China, India, Pakistan, and Southeast Asia) may maintain vegetarian eating patterns from tradition, habit, and religious beliefs.[5] Other reasons for eating vegetarian diets include concerns about the risks of omnivorous diets and the negative publicity about bacterial foodborne disease from animal foods.[6] There is a group of moral vegetarians who avoid meat by linking it to cruelty, environmental degradation, or political reasons.[7] Ecologic reasons involving views that the environmental impact of meat and poultry production is an inefficient use of the planet's resources motivate others. Some have religious (eg, Seventh-Day Adventists, some Hindus, Jains, and Buddhists) or philosophical beliefs (macrobiotics, transcendental meditators, anthroposophists, some yogic groups) that encourage various types of vegetarian diets and/or other food avoidances in their followers. Among the health considerations that lead some to follow a vegetarian diet is the suggestion that children consuming a vegetarian diet have a higher IQ as young adults.[8] This, of course, remains highly speculative and poorly substantiated.

Table 11.2.
Reasons for Vegetarian Lifestyle

Health	Religion
Performance	Ethics
Economic reasons	Animal rights
Environmental concerns	Cosmetics
Hygiene	Social influence
Moral	New age

Adapted from Leitzmann.[30]

Trends

A survey conducted by the Vegetarian Resource Group in 2009 showed that approximately 3.4% of the US adult population consistently follows a vegetarian diet; 1% or approximately one third of that group were vegans.[9,10] Approximately 3% of 8- to 18-year-old children and adolescents in the United States are vegetarians, and around 0.5% of this age group is vegan.[11] In Europe, 0.3% to 4.2% of population is vegetarian, varying by country, and India has the highest proportion of vegetarians, at 40% of the population.[12]

As with any dietary pattern, the degree of adherence to vegetarian patterns varies, and thus, overall nutrient intake differs from one vegetarian to the next. Most dietary patterns can be accommodated while fulfilling nutrient needs with appropriate dietary planning based on scientific principles of sound nutrition. Most vegetarian parents welcome such advice. However, when goals are zealously pursued and nutrition principles are ignored, the health consequences can be unfortunate, especially for infants and young children. Overall, it is possible to provide a balanced diet to vegetarians and vegans.[13]

The extent and degree of animal food restriction does not always predict either the extent of other food avoidances or the divergences in lifestyle and philosophical beliefs from nonvegetarians, although there is some correspondence. Generally, vegetarians with the most restrictive diets have the largest number of reasons for their eating styles, and their dietary patterns are most closely interwoven into their philosophical and belief systems.

Position papers of the American Dietetic Association and Canadian Paediatric Society state that appropriately planned vegetarian diets are healthful and nutritionally adequate and provide health benefits in the prevention and treatment of certain diseases.[14,15] A vegetarian, including a vegan, diet can also meet current recommended daily requirements for protein, iron, zinc, calcium, vitamin D, riboflavin, vitamin B_{12}, vitamin A, omega-3 fatty acids, and iodine. In some cases, use of fortified foods or supplements can be helpful in meeting recommendations for individual nutrients. Well-planned vegan and other types of vegetarian diets are appropriate for all stages of the life cycle, including pregnancy, lactation, infancy, childhood, and adolescence. Vegetarian diets, in general, have lower levels of saturated fat and cholesterol and higher levels of complex carbohydrates, fiber, magnesium, vitamins C and E,[14] carotenoids, and phytochemicals.[16]

Although vegetarians also suffer from coronary artery disease, hypertension, type 2 diabetes mellitus, and prostate and colon cancer, the incidence of these diseases is lower than in omnivores.[17-20] There may be other advantages besides an improved lipid profile from vegetarian diets.[21] There is substantial epidemiologic evidence that a high consumption of fruit and vegetables is associated with reduced mortality from cardiovascular disease, stroke, cancer, and other causes.[22,23] In part, this may simply indicate that high fruit and vegetable consumption is a marker of a healthy lifestyle, but there is also strong evidence from in vitro studies and clinical trials that micronutrients and other components of fruit and vegetables have beneficial biological effects. A study evaluating circulating E-selectin levels, which include circulating intercellular adhesion molecule and circulating vascular adhesion molecule, in vegetarian and control adults showed that low circulating E-selectin levels of vegetarians may reflect the favorable cardiovascular risk profile of this group.[24] Most attention has focused on antioxidants, B group vitamins, minerals, and fiber, but several strands of evidence now indicate that increased intake of salicylates may be another benefit of fruit and vegetable consumption.[25,26] Urinary excretion of salicyluric acid and salicylic acid is significantly increased in vegetarians compared with nonvegetarians, but they excrete significantly less salicylic acid than do patients consuming 75 mg or 150 mg of aspirin per day.[27,28] The concentrations of salicylic acid in vegetarians have been shown to inhibit cyclooxygenase-2 (COX-2) in vitro.[29] Thus, it is plausible that dietary salicylates may contribute to the beneficial effects of a vegetarian diet.

Additional Implications of Vegetarianism

The lifestyle of vegetarians is different from omnivores in 3 major ways, which may have direct or indirect effects on children. First, they may practice abstinence or moderation in alcohol consumption, as well as other stimulating substances, including nicotine. Second, they tend to be engaged in increased physical activities as well. Third, overall, plant foods are less calorie dense and thus predispose to lower overall calorie intake. Thus, the overall benefit of a vegetarian diet may derive from a vegetarian lifestyle rather than diet alone.[30]

Families that follow an anthroposophic lifestyle often justify it by claiming overall health benefits for their children. Their diet is comprised of a high intake of organically produced food items, including spontaneously fermented vegetables, and foods containing live lactobacilli. In addition, these families restrict the use of antibiotics, antipyretics, and immunizations. A study evaluating gut flora in children younger than 2 years with this lifestyle in comparison with those with a traditional lifestyle reported that microflora associated characteristics were different between the 2 groups,[31] and it has been suggested that this provides a "probiotic" benefit.[32] Others have suggested that potential health benefits may be the result of restriction of antibiotics.[33] In an unmasked study in adults with refractory atopic dermatitis, alternative therapy with a low-energy, vegetarian diet caused a striking improvement in the severity of dermatitis as well as in lactate dehydrogenase-5 activity and in the number of circulating peripheral eosinophils.[34] Some have recently suggested that vegetarian diets have an effect on the development of allergy as a result of the fatty acid composition of the diet.[35]

There have been concerns that vegetarians, and in particular vegans, have lower-than-adequate intakes of vitamin B_{12}, vitamin D, calcium, zinc, and riboflavin.[36] A Polish study suggested that prepubertal vegetarian children had lower levels of leptin, a polypeptide that plays a role in bone growth, maturation, and weight regulation, in comparison with their omnivore counterparts,[37] which may contribute to reduced bone growth and development in childhood. A vegan diet may also put children at risk of vitamin A deficiency and subsequent keratomalacia, anemia, and protein and zinc deficiency if a proper evaluation of the diet is not performed and the family is not given appropriate information of the potential dietary deficiencies relevant to the vegetarian diet.[38] However, the overall belief that individuals following vegan or vegetarian diets suffer from nutritional deficiencies may be exaggerated, as reports of specific malnutrition in these populations are rare.[39,40]

Dietary practices among vegetarians are varied; hence, individual assessent of dietary intakes by a trained dietitian is important. Such assessments can be best made by using a 24- to 72-hour food recall and food frequency questionnaire.[41] Suggestions for balanced meal planning are shown in Table 11.3. A knowledgeable and skilled dietitian or physician can educate vegetarian patients about food sources of specific nutrients, food purchase and preparation, and any dietary modifications that may be necessary to meet individual needs. Menu planning for vegetarians can be simplified by use of a food guide that specifies food groups and serving sizes as shown in Fig 11.1 to 11.3. Such guidance is of particular importance in planning adequate meals for pediatric patients of all ages to ensure

III

proper growth and development.[42] A questionnaire to assess diet quality index with special reference to micronutrient adequacy for lacto-vegetarian adolescent girls was reported to be helpful as an assessment tool to suggest dietary intervention.[43]

Table 11.3.
Tips for Meal Planning

1. Encourage a variety of foods from Fig 11.1–11.3.
2. The number of servings in each group is for minimum daily intakes as shown in Fig 11.1 and 11.2. Choose more foods from any of the groups to meet energy needs.
3. A serving from the calcium-rich food group provides approximately 10% of adult daily requirements. Choose 8 or more servings a day. These also count towards servings from other food groups in the guide. For example, ½ cup (125 mL) of fortified fruit juice counts as a calcium-rich food and also counts toward servings from the fruit group.
4. Include 2 servings every day of foods that supply omega-3 fats. Foods rich in omega-3 fats are found in the legumes/nuts group and the fats group. A serving is 1 teaspoon (5 mL) of ground flaxseed oil, 3 teaspoons (15 mL) of canola or soybean oil, 1 tablespoon (15 mL) of ground flaxseed, or ¼ cup (60 mL) of walnuts. Olive and canola oil are the best choices for cooking.
5. Equivalent servings of nuts and seeds can replace servings from the fats group.
6. Vitamin D from daily sun exposure or through fortified foods or supplements. Cow milk and some brands of soy milk and breakfast cereals are fortified with vitamin D.
7. Include at least 3 good food sources of vitamin B_{12} in daily diet (eg, 1 tbsp (15 mL) of Red Star Vegetarian support formula nutritional yeast, 1 cup (250 mL) fortified soy milk, ½ cup (125 mL) cow milk, ¾ cup (185 mL) yogurt, 1 large egg, 1 oz of fortified breakfast cereal, 1 to 1½ oz of fortified meat analog. If these foods are not consumed regularly, (at least 3 servings per day) a daily vitamin B_{12} supplement of 5 to 10 µg or a weekly dose of 2000 µg is recommended.
8. Consume sweets or alcohol in moderation. Use foods in the Vegetarian Food Guide to get most of calories.

Adapted from Messina et al.[42]

Fig 11.1.
Vegan Pyramid

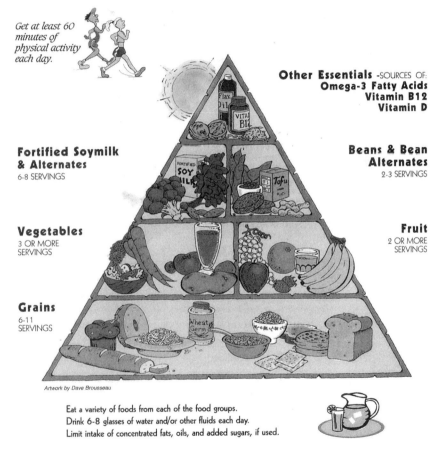

VEGAN FOOD GUIDE
DAILY PLAN FOR HEALTHY EATING

Get at least 60 minutes of physical activity each day.

Other Essentials -SOURCES OF:
Omega-3 Fatty Acids
Vitamin B12
Vitamin D

Fortified Soymilk & Alternates
6-8 SERVINGS

Beans & Bean Alternates
2-3 SERVINGS

Vegetables
3 OR MORE SERVINGS

Fruit
2 OR MORE SERVINGS

Grains
6-11 SERVINGS

Artwork by Dave Brousseau

Eat a variety of foods from each of the food groups.
Drink 6-8 glasses of water and/or other fluids each day.
Limit intake of concentrated fats, oils, and added sugars, if used.

Reproduced with permission from Messina et al.[42]

Fig 11.2.
Vegetarian Food Guide Pyramid

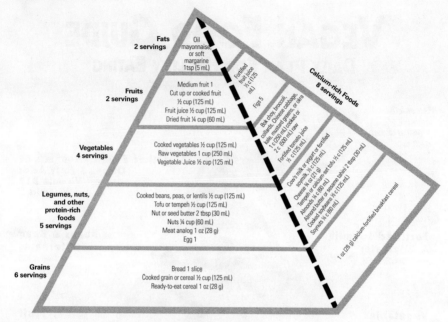

Reproduced with permission from Messina et al.[42]

Fig 11.3.
Vegetarian Food Guide Rainbow

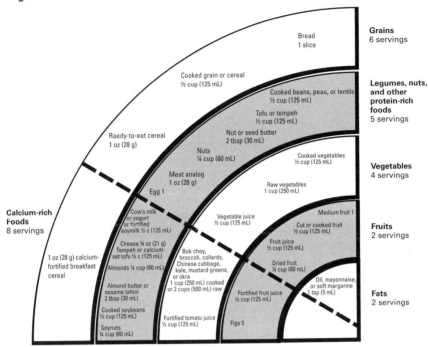

Reproduced with permission from Messina et al.[42]

Nutrient Intake Guidelines

Some basic guidelines are used to determine the daily nutrient requirements for healthy vegetarians. The recommendation for daily calorie intake is the same as for the general population. The recommendations for most other nutrient intakes are increased by 2 standard deviations above the Recommended Dietary Allowance to compensate for potential deficiencies or poor bioavailability of nutrients in the vegetarian diet and, thus, ensure adequacy of nutrient intke.[14,15,42]

Whole Foods Concept

The concept of whole foods as a principle of vegetarian diets relies on the fact that almost any kind of food processing, including freezing, heating, and cooking, can lead to loss of nutrients. Whole-grain products contain an excellent combination of nutrients to meet human needs, although they are deficient in calcium and vitamin C. Processing whole grains to white flour leads to a loss of minerals, vitamins, phytochemicals, and dietary fibers by 75% to 95%.[44] The changes that occur in freezing, baking, boiling, and frying may also be significant. However, the relevance of this concept to overall human nutrition is unclear, because processing has a number of functions, including increasing palatability and digestibility, food preservation, and safety and fortification. Thus, when an appropriate variety and amount of food is consumed over several days, both children and adults can meet their daily nutrient requirements.

Nutritional Considerations

Energy

Studies of vegan children have indicated that their energy intake is close to the recommended level for nonvegetarian controls.[39] During infancy and weaning, the amount of food needed to meet energy needs on vegan diets may exceed gastric capacity; hence, the child should be fed frequently.[45] Concentrated sources of calories that are acceptable for older infants and children include soy products, legumes, oils, nuts, nut butters, and fruit juices.[4,14]

Protein

Despite the low caloric density of strict vegetarian diets, food intakes are usually sufficient to support protein needs even for the weanling infant.[45,46] Plant protein can meet requirements when a variety of plant foods is consumed. Additional protein need not be consumed at the same meal, as long as the protein requirement is consumed over a period of 24 hours. Variations in plant protein quality, quantity, and digestibility are all of potential concern, especially when vegan-vegetarian diets are used during infancy. Compared with children fed a mixed diet, some studies suggest that the lower quality of protein sources in a vegan diet increases the protein requirements of infants by 30% to 35%, those of children 2 to 6 years of age by 20% to 30%, and those of children older than 6 years by 15% to 20%.[14,47]

The 5 major food sources of plant protein are legumes, cereals, nuts and seeds, fruits, and other vegetables. Each of these has nutritional advantages and disadvantages. For example, legumes and cereals provide relatively large amounts of high-quality protein, but they must be cooked or processed to enhance their palatability and to remove substances that decrease digestibility, such as tough skins, amylase inhibitors, lectins, and tannins.[42,46] A standard method for determining protein quality is the protein digestibility corrected amino acid score. Using this method, isolated soy protein is shown to meet protein needs as effectively as animal protein, unlike wheat protein, which is almost 50% less usable than animal protein.[48] Lysine is lower in all plant foods than in animal foods. The levels of the sulfur-containing amino acids, methionine and cysteine, are lower in legumes and fruits. The level of the essential amino acid, threonine, is lower in cereals, and tryptophan content tends to be lower in fruits than in most animal foods.[45] Therefore, if parents feed diets that are adequate in food energy and select a wide variety of plant foods with proteins that complement each other, vegetarian children should be able to receive an adequate amount of protein to grow and thrive.

Fat

Dietary fat intakes of vegetarian children older than 2 years are between 25% and 35% of total calories, which are a little lower than those of omnivores; effects on growth appear to be small.[49] However, when dietary fat falls below approximately 15% of calories, special care must be taken to ensure that recommended intakes of essential fatty acids are met. At least 3% of energy should be from linoleic acid (an omega-3 fatty acid), and 1% of energy should be from linolenic acid (an omega-6 fatty acid).[45] The recommended ratio of omega-6 fatty acids to omega-3 fatty acids is in the range of 2:1 to 4:1.[50,51] Linoleic acid is found in seeds, nuts, and grains. Alpha-linolenic acid is found in the green leaves of plants, in phytoplankton and algae, and in certain seeds, nuts, and legumes, such as flax seeds, canola seeds, walnuts, hazelnuts, and soybeans. These can be converted into more highly unsaturated fatty acids, including arachidonic acid, eicosapentaenoic acid (EPA) and docosahexaenoic acid (DHA).[52] Arachidonic acid (ARA) and EPA serve as precursors for the eicosanoids. Tentative recommended intakes for these polyunsaturated fatty acids range from 3% to 10% of total energy intakes.[51] ARA is found in animal foods such as meat, poultry, and eggs. EPA and DHA are largely found in fish and seafood. Vegan-vegetarians have no direct sources of these long-chain omega-3 fatty acids in their diets and, thus, must convert alpha-linolenic acid to them.[14] There is concern that pregnant women who are vegan or vegetarian or who follow a macrobiotic diet who consume little or no fish or other animal foods may not obtain enough of these fatty acids, especially during pregnancy and while breastfeeding.[14,15] Risks may be especially high if infants are preterm, because their capacity to desaturate alpha linolenic acid to DHA is limited.[14] Such individuals may need DHA supplements, either from fish oils, or from cultured micro algae.[53] Algae sources of DHA have been shown to positively affect blood levels of DHA and of EPA through retroconversion. However, such supplements for young infants should only be dispensed under a physician's direction, because they are also potent anticoagulants.

Fiber

Recommended daily fiber intake for 1- to 3-year-olds is 19 g/day, for 4 to 8-year-old children is 25 g/day, and for adolescents is up to 38 g/day.[52] In very small children, the sheer bulk and low energy density of such a high-fiber diet may make consumption of sufficient energy difficult for the child and may inhibit absorption of some minerals.[45] The sieving or mashing of cereals, pulses, and vegetables that are fed to infants can increase their digestibility, and partial replacement of whole-grain cereals with more highly refined cereals that are lower in fiber can further increase energy intakes and decrease bulk if this is a problem in small children. Lacto-ovo-vegetarian children usually consume adequate but not excessive amounts of dietary fiber.

Vitamins

Vitamin A/Beta Carotene

Because plant foods contain only dietary carotenoids, vitamin A requirements can be met by 3 servings a day of plant foods rich in beta carotene, such as leafy or deep yellow or orange vegetables and fruits. Absorption of beta carotene can be increased by cooking, chopping, or pureeing or addition of small amounts of fat.[14,15,54]

Riboflavin

Intakes of riboflavin appear to be similar in vegetarians and omnivores.[55] Riboflavin deficiency has occasionally occurred in people following severely restricted macrobiotic diets, but it is not a problem in other forms of vegetarianism. Good sources of riboflavin include yeast, wheat germ, soy, fortified cereals, and enriched grains.

Folic Acid

Usually, vegetarians who consume high amounts of vegetables and fruits as well as other plant foods have adequate intakes of folic acid. However, those who consume vegetables that are usually braised or fried at high temperature and who rarely drink fruit juices or eat grain products fortified with folic acid may be at risk. Additionally, postmenarchal adolescent girls who are capable of becoming pregnant should consume 400 µg of folic acid as a supplement or in fortified foods in addition to usual food sources of the nutrient.[14,55]

Vitamin B$_{12}$

No plant foods, except for certain sea vegetables, or plants foods that are fortified, contain vitamin B$_{12}$. Lacto-ovo-vegetarians get sufficient amounts of vitamin B$_{12}$ if dairy products are consumed on a regular basis.[56] Studies indicate that some strict vegans are deficient in vitamin B$_{12}$, and vegetarian diets typically high in folic acid mask hematologic symptoms of deficiency, sometimes leading to a delayed diagnosis.[57] In such situations, the presentation is often with neurologic symptoms.[58] Absorption is effective when small amounts of vitamin B$_{12}$ are consumed at regular intervals.[14,15] Regular intake of vitamin B$_{12}$-fortified foods or dairy products should be encouraged in vegetarians and especially in mothers of breastfed infants.

Vitamin D

Serum vitamin D levels are dependent on sunlight exposure and intake of vitamin D-rich foods or supplements. Infants and children synthesize vitamin D less efficiently than older individuals.[59] Foods such as cow milk, some types of soy milk and rice milk, and breakfast cereals that are enriched with vitamin D$_2$ (ergocalciferol) and/or vitamin D$_3$ (cholecalciferol, animal based) should be consumed. Intake of such fortified foods, wherever possible, should be encouraged. Vitamin D$_2$ may be less biologically active than vitamin D$_3$, thus raising the requirements for certain types of vegetarians.[60] A recent study reported that deficient consumption of vitamin D and calcium may reduce bone density in vegans by affecting bone turnover rate adversely; hence, vitamin D and calcium intakes should be monitored proactively in the pediatric vegetarian population.[61] If sunlight exposure and intake of fortified foods are insufficient or if sun-protective lotions are used, then supplements are recommended.[14,15,59]

Minerals

Iron

Iron is vital at all ages, and there is a risk of deficiency of this nutrient during infancy, the adolescent growth spurt, and pregnancy.[62-64] The iron status of vegetarian infants and children varies. Although iron deficiency is by far the most common of the micronutrient deficiencies exhibited by vegetarian children, the incidence of iron-deficiency anemia among vegetarians is similar to that among nonvegetarians.[65] Vegetarians have lower iron stores than do omnivores, but their serum ferritin levels are usually within the normal range.[14,15] Iron deficiency is particularly common in children consuming vegan diets, because plant foods contain non-heme iron as opposed to heme iron found in animal sources.[66] Non-heme iron is more sensitive to inhibitors of iron absorption, such as phytates, calcium, herbal teas, cocoa, some spices, and fiber.[66] Vitamin C and other organic acids in fruits and vegetables enhance the absorption of iron.[64] Recommended iron intakes for vegetarians are approximately 1.8 to 2 times those of omnivores because of the lower bioavailability of iron in a vegetarian diet.

Zinc

Approximately half of the zinc in the diet comes from meat, poultry, and fish.[62,67] The bioavailability of relatively rich plant sources of zinc, such as whole-grain cereals, soy, beans, lentils, peas, and nuts tends to be low, because most of them also contain large amounts of phytate and fiber, which inhibit zinc absorption.[68] In lacto-ovo-vegetarians, zinc absorption is approximately a third less than in omnivores.[69]

The requirement for zinc may be as much as 50% greater among strict vegetarians.[14,15] Vegetarian diets also tend to be lower in this mineral than are omnivorous diets.[70] When daily requirements for zinc are increased, as they are in infants and children, the risk of suboptimal zinc nutritional status is increased, because the ability to increase zinc absorption is limited. Because the presence of inhibitors is highest in vegan diets, vegans are at special risk. Despite this, zinc supplementation is not recommended, because clinical signs of deficiency are rare among vegetarians, even in children younger than 24 months.[71] Good plant sources of zinc are yeast-fermented whole-grain breads (the phytic acid content is reduced) and zinc-fortified infant and adult cereals.

Calcium

Calcium intakes of vegans tend to be lower than those of lacto-vegetarians and non-vegetarians.[59] Although oxalates, phytates, and fiber in plant foods decrease calcium availability, the bioavailability of calcium from plant foods and soy products can be higher than from milk,[72] although in general this is not the case. Calcium is present in a large number of plant and fortified foods, such as broccoli, Chinese cabbage, collards, kale, okra, and turnip greens. It has been suggested but not substantiated that soy products may have favorable effects on bone health apart from their calcium content.[73] If vegetarian children's diets do not contain adequate sources of dietary calcium, supplements may be advisable.

Iodine

Iodine deficiency is not commonly seen in vegetarian children when iodized salt is readily available. Vegans whose diets are restricted to kosher or sea salts, which are generally not iodized, or who also have a substantial intake of goitrogens, such as broccoli, mustard, kale, turnips, etc, are at risk of iodine deficiency. For these children, especially for those living in iodine-poor areas, iodine-fortified foods are recommended.[74]

Carnitine and Taurine

Serum carnitine and taurine levels are decreased in lacto-ovo-vegetarian and vegan diets; however, the functional significance of this is not apparent, and therefore, supplementation does not appear to be warranted.[75,76]

Vegetarian Diets for Special Populations

Infants

Exclusively breastfed infants of omnivorous mothers receive adequate amounts of energy and nutrients during the first 4 to 6 months of life.[77,78] The milk of vegetarian women is similar in nutrient composition to that of nonvegetarians. Vegetarian mothers should be encouraged to breastfeed. Soy formula is the only option for vegan infants who are not being breastfed. Soy and rice beverages and other homemade formulas should not be used to replace human milk or commercial formulas for those infants of vegan mothers who are not being breastfed.[15]

Guidelines for the introduction of complementary foods in infancy are similar for vegetarians and nonvegetarians.[77,78] Infants older than 6 months are potentially at the greatest risk of overt deficiency states related to inappropriate restrictions of the diet, although deficiencies of vitamins B_{12} and essential fatty acids may appear earlier.[78] They are particularly vulnerable during the weaning period if fed a macrobiotic diet and may experience psychomotor delay in some instances.[79] Anticipating these potential problems for vegetarian families by explaining the principles of providing calorie dense foods at the time of weaning is important so the increased bulk of vegetarian diets does not interfere with adequate consumption of energy, protein, and other nutrients.[14,15]

Children

Except for those on severely restricted diets, most vegetarian children exhibit growth comparable to their omnivore peers.[80] The average calorie and protein intake generally meets or exceeds recommendations. Vegan children may have slightly higher protein needs than nonvegan children because of differences in protein digestibility and amino acid profile of certain plant proteins, but this is usually met with an intake of a variety of plant foods. The importance of proper intake of calcium, zinc, and iron should be emphasized.[14,15]

Adolescents

Whether adolescents adopt a vegetarian diet at this age or have been vegetarians from infancy, nutritional imbalances in their diets may occur during this period of life. Vegetarianism may be adopted as a part of disordered eating attitudes and behaviors.[81,82] A vegetarian diet is practiced by some young women as a means of weight control.[83] Adolescent vegetarians were significantly more likely to exhibit bulimic behaviors in a Minnesota study.[84] Klopp et al reported that, although they found no differences in eating attitudes and behaviors between self-reported vegetarian and nonvegetarian college women, adolescent vegetarians were at greater risk than were omnivorous adolescents for unhealthy and extreme weight-control behaviors.[85] Vegetarian males also appear more vulnerable in this regard.[86] In a Turkish study to evaluate the prevalence of eating disorders associated with vegetarianism, abnormal eating habits, low self-esteem, high body image anxiety, and high trait anxiety were detected in Turkish vegetarian adolescents between 7 and 21 years of age.[87] Data from a study comparing fish-eating vegetarians with omnivores demonstrate that long-term adherence to a vegetarian diet is associated with maintained leanness and a lower body mass index (BMI).[88] Therefore, vegetarian practices may be a marker to help identify adolescents or young adults with eating disorder tendencies or weight obsession,[83] and adolescents who choose to become vegetarians may benefit significantly from dietary guidance (see Table 11.4).

Table 11.4.

Modifications to the Vegetarian Food Guide (Fig 11.2 and 11.3) for Children, Adolescents, and Pregnant and Lactating Women

| Stage | Food Group[a] | | |
	B$_{12}$-Rich Foods (Servings)	Beans/Nuts/ Seeds/Egg (Servings)	Calcium-Rich Foods (Servings)
Child, 4-8 y	2	5	6
Adolescent, 9-13 y	2	6	10
Adolescent, 14-18 y	3	6	10

[a] The number of servings in each group is the minimum amount needed. The minimum number of servings from other groups is not different from the vegetarian food guide (Fig 11.2 and 11.3). Additional foods can be chosen from any of the groups in the vegetarian food guide to meet energy needs.

Adapted from Messina et al.[42]

Athletes

With increasing interest in the potential health benefits of vegetarian diets, it is relevant to consider dietary practices that influence athletic performance. Athletes can meet their protein needs from a vegetarian diet.[4,89] Although long term-controlled studies are needed, a well-planned and appropriately supplemented vegetarian diet appears to effectively support the nutritional requirements of athletes.[4] Vegetarian female athletes should be informed of an increased risk of iron deficiency, which may limit endurance performance.[90] Vegetarian athletes have a lower mean muscle creatine concentration, and it has been suggested that they may experience greater performance increments after creatine loading in activities that rely on adenosine triphosphate/phosphocreatine systems,[91] although this requires substantiation. Training coaches need to be made aware of the use of a vegetarian diet as a form of weight control, and appropriate steps should be taken to determine that a balanced vegetarian diet is followed to ensure the good health of these athletes.

With Developmental and Neurological Delays

It is possible to provide oral and/or enteral feeding to pediatric patients with swallowing problems whose families elect to provide a vegetarian diet. A list of appropriate formulas for use by vegetarian and vegan diets at different ages is shown in Table 11.5.

Table 11.5.
Formulas for Gastrostomy Tube Feedings

Vegetarian		Vegan	
<1 y	>1 y	<1 y	>1 y
Alimentum	Kindercal	Isomil	Elecare
Enfamil	Next Step	Neocate	Isomil 2
Nutramigen	Nutren Jr/1.0/2.0	Prosobee	Neocate/Jr/One
Pregestamil	Pediasure	Carnation Soy	L-Emental
Similac	Peptamen/Jr	RCF (Ross)	Tolerex
Enfacare	Similac 2		Vivonex/Plus/Ten
Carnation	Ensure/Plus		Faa (Nestle)
	Jevity		Next Step Soy
	Isocal		

Vegetarian Diets in Management of the Metabolic Syndrome and Type 2 Diabetes Mellitus

Vegetarian diets present potential advantages for the management of type 2 diabetes mellitus.[92] Although most of the studies are in adults, the findings are applicable to children and adolescents. The increased intake of soluble and insoluble fiber in a vegetarian diet improves glucose metabolism in both diabetic and normal subjects, along with a reduced intake of saturated fats and high-glycemic-index foods.[93] Vegetarian diets have been shown to be efficacious, nutritionally complete under proper guidance, acceptable, and practical to follow.[94] The prevalence of type 2 diabetes mellitus in a large population of Adventists on different types of vegetarian diets was compared with that in omnivores using self-reported questionnaire.[95] Vegans had a 5-unit lower BMI than did nonvegetarians, even after adjustment for demographic and lifestyle factors, as well as a lower incidence of type 2 diabetes mellitus. This study provides further evidence of the advantage of a vegetarian lifestyle in protecting against obesity and reducing risk of type 2 diabetes mellitus. These observations were also noted in those following fish-vegetarian and semi-vegetarian diets. Reduced intramyocellular lipid concentrations and decreased iron stores may mediate the effects of plant-based diets on glycemia.[96] This, of course, is theoretical, and there is no direct evidence that iron requirements or stores should differ between vegetarians and nonvegetarians for health reasons.

Vegetarian Diets and Obesity

There is an increased prevalence of childhood overweight and obesity globally.[97,98] Evidence from epidemiologic studies suggests that children and adults on vegetarian diets have a lower BMI and a decreased prevalence of obesity.[99] Because vegetarian diets may reduce the risk of overweight and obesity, they should be considered a possible preventive measure against obesity in at risk pediatric patients, under supervision.[100] The low energy density of vegetarian foods, along with increased consumption of complex carbohydrates, fiber, and water, may increase satiety and metabolic rate. Most of these observations require further research, especially for the pediatric age group.

Conclusion

Vegetarian diets can meet the nutritional needs of children and adolescents if appropriately planned and monitored by a health care professional or dietitian. Table 11.6 lists a few useful Web sites for use by consumers and pediatricians. The current database of vegetarian studies convincingly indicate that plant based diets have health benefits as well. In addition to maintaining awareness of various relevant nutritional issues, health care professionals may also need to be familiar with the wide range of vegetarian diets and the social, cultural, and ideological systems present among vegetarians in their communities.

Table 11.6.
List of Useful Vegetarian Web sites

http://vegetariannutrition.net
http://www.kidshealth.org/parent/nutrition_fit/nutrition/vegetarianism.html
http://www.heart.org/HEARTORG/GettingHealthy/NutritionCenter/Vegetarian-Diets_UCM_306032_Article.jsp
http://www.nal.usda.gov/fnic/pubs/bibs/gen/vegetarian.pdf
http://www.vegansociety.com/food/nutrition/b12/
http://www.vrg.org
http://www.vegsoc.org/health

References

1. Kushi M, Jack A. *The Book of Macrobiotics: The Universal Way of Health, Happiness, and Peace*. Revised ed. Boston, MA: Japan Publications; 1987

2. Corliss R. Should we all be vegetarians? Would we be healthier? The risks and benefits of a meat free life. *Time*. 2002;160(3):48-56

3. Edmunds F. *An Introduction to Anthroposophy*. London, England: Rudolph Steiner Press; 2006

4. Fuhrman J, Ferreri DM. Fueling the vegetarian (vegan) athlete. *Curr Sports Med Rep*. 2010;9(4):233-241

5. Fox N, Ward K. Health, ethics and environment: a qualitative study of vegetarian motivations. *Appetite*. 2008;50(2-3):422-429

6. Fox N, Ward KJ. You are what you eat? Vegetarianism, health and identity. *Soc Sci Med*. 2008;66(12):2585-2595

7. Lea E, Worsley A. The cognitive contexts of beliefs about the healthiness of meat. *Public Health Nutr*. 2005(1):37-45

8. Gale CR, Deary IJ, Schoon I, Batty GD. IQ in childhood and vegetarianism in adulthood: 1970 British cohort study. *BMJ*. 2007;334(7587):245-248

9. The Vegetarian Resource Group. How Many Vegetarians Are There? Available at: http://www.vrg.org/press/2009poll.htm. Accessed October 2, 2012

10. Vegan Soapbox. How Many People Are Vegan? Available at: http://www.vegansoapbox.com/how-many-people-are-vegan/. Accessed October 2, 2012

11. Marcus MB. More young people go the vegetarian route. *USA Today*. October 15, 2007. Available at: http://www.usatoday.com/news/health/2007-10-14-veggie-kids_N.htm. Accessed October 2, 2012

12. Raw Food Health. The Number of Vegetarians in the World. Available at: http://www.raw-food-health.net/NumberOfVegetarians.html. Accessed October 2, 2012

13. Jacobs C, Dwyer JT. Vegetarian children: appropriate and inappropriate diets. *Am J Clin Nutr*. 1988;48(3 Suppl):811-818

14. Craig WJ; Mangels AR; American Dietetic Association. Position of the American Dietetic Association: vegetarian diets. *J Am Diet Assoc*. 2009;109(7):1266-1282

15. Amit M; Canadian Paediatric Society, Community Paediatrics Committee. Vegetarian diets in children and adolescents. *Paediatr Child Health*. 2010;15(5):303-314

16. Craig WJ. Nutrition concerns and health effects of vegetarian diets. *Nutr Clin Pract*. 2010;25(6):613-620

17. Joshipura KJ, Hu FB, Manson JE, et al. The effect of fruit and vegetable intake on risk for coronary heart disease. *Ann Intern Med*. 2001;134(12):1106-1114

18. Liu S, Manson JE, Lee I-M, et al. Fruit and vegetable intake and risk of cardiovascular disease: the women's health study. *Am J Clin Nutr*. 2000;72(4):922-928

19. Joshipura KJ, Ascherio A, Manson JE, et al. Fruit and vegetable intake in relation to risk of ischaemic stroke. *JAMA*. 1999;282(13):1233-1239

20. Key TJ, Allen NE, Spencer EA, et al. The effect of diet on risk of cancer. *Lancet*. 2002;360(9336):861-868

21. Richter V, Rassoul F, Hentschel B, et al. Age-dependence of lipid parameters in the general population and vegetarians. *Z Gerontol Geriatr.* 2004;37(3):207-213

22. Fraser GE. Vegetarian diets: what do we know of their effects on common chronic diseases? *Am J Clin Nutr.* 2009;89(Suppl):1607S-1612S

23. Key TJ, Fraser GE, Thorogood M, et al. Mortality in vegetarians and nonvegetarians: detailed findings from a collaborative analysis of 5 prospective studies. *Am J Clin Nutr.* 1999;70(3 Suppl):516S-524S

24. Purschwitz K, Rassoul F, Reuter W, Purschwitz R, Jahn N, Kellert D, Richter V. Soluble leukocyte adhesion molecules in vegetarians of various ages. *Z Gerontol Geriatr.* 2001;34(6):476-479

25. John JH, Ziebland S, Yudkin P, et al. Effects of fruit and vegetable consumption on plasma antioxidant concentrations and blood pressure: a randomized controlled trial. *Lancet.* 2002;359(9322):1969-1974

26. Hare LG, Woodside JV, Young IS. Dietary salicylates: another benefit of fruit and vegetable consumption? (Editorial). *J Clin Pathol.* 2003;56(9):649-650

27. Lawrence JR, Peter R, Baxter G, et al. Urinary excretion of salicyluric and salicylic acids by non-vegetarians, vegetarians and patients taking low-dose aspirin. *J Clin Pathol.* 2003;56(9):651-653

28. Blacklock CJ, Lawrence JR, Malcolm EA, et al. Salicylic acid in the serum of subjects not taking aspirin. Comparison of salicylic acid concentrations in the serum of vegetarians, non-vegetarians, and patients taking low-dose aspirin. *J Clin Pathol.* 2001;54(7):553-555

29. Xu XM, Sansores-Garcia L, Chen XM, et al. Suppression of inducible cyclo-oxygenase 2 gene transcription by aspirin and sodium salicylate. *Proc Natl Acad Sci.* 1999;96(9):5292-5297

30. Leitzmann C. Vegetarian diets: what are the advantages? *Forum Nutr.* 2005;57:147-156

31. Pershagen G, Reinders C, Wreiber K, Scheynius A. An anthroposophic lifestyle and intestinal microflora in infancy. *Pediatr Allergy Immunol.* 2002;13(6):402-411

32. Kalliomaki M, Salminen S, Arvilommi H, Kero P, Koskinen P, Isolauri E. Probiotics in primary prevention of atopic disease: a randomized placebo controlled trial. *Lancet.* 2001;357(9262):1076-1079

33. Matsuzaki T, Yamazaki R, Hashimoto S, Yokokura T. The effect of oral feeding of Lactobacilli casei strain Shirota on immunoglobulin E production in mice. *J Dairy Sci.* 1998;81(1):48-53

34. Tanaka T, Kouda K, Kotani M, et al. Vegetarian diet ameliorates symptoms of atopic dermatitis through reduction of the number of peripheral eosinophils and of PGE2 synthesis by monocytes. *J Physiol Anthropol.* 2001;20(6):353-361

35. Gorczyca D, Pasciak M, Szponar B, Gamian A, Jankowski A. An impact of the diet on serum fatty acid and lipid profiles in Polish vegetarian children and children with allergy. *Eur J Clin Nutr.* 2011;65(2):191-195

36. Craig WJ. Health effects of vegan diets. *Am J Clin Nutr.* 2009;89(Suppl):1627S-1633S

37. Ambroszkiewicz J, Laskowska-Klita T, Klemarczyk W. Low levels of osteocalcin and leptin in serum of vegetarian prepubertal children. *Med Wieku Rozwoj.* 2003;7(4 Pt 2):587-591

38. Colev M, Engel H, Mayers M, et al. Vegan diet and vitamin A deficiency. *Clin Pediatr (Phila)*. 2004;43(1):107-109

39. Moilanen BC. Vegan diets in infants, children and adolescents. *Pediatr Rev*. 2004;25(5):174-176

40. Dunham L, Kollar LM. Vegetarian eating for children and adolescents. *J Pediatr Health Care*. 2006;20(1):27-34

41. Sanders TA, Purves R. An anthropometric and dietary assessment of the nutritional status of vegan preschool children. *J Hum Nutr*. 1981;35(5):349-357

42. Messina V, Melina V, Mangels AR. A new food guide for North American vegetarians. *J Am Diet Assoc*. 2003;103(6):771-775

43. Chiplonkar SA, Tupe R. Development of a diet quality index with special reference to micronutrient adequacy for adolescent girls consuming a lacto-vegetarian diet. *J Am Diet Assoc*. 2010;110(6):926-931

44. Bishnoi S, Khetarpaul N. Protein digestability of vegetables and field peas (Pisum sativum). Varietal differences and effect of domestic processing and cooking methods. *Plant Foods Hum Nutr*. 1994;46(1):71-76

45. Institute of Medicine, Food and Nutrition Board. *Dietary Reference Intakes for Energy, Carbohydrate, Fiber, Fat, Fatty Acids, Cholesterol, Protein and Amino Acids*. Washington, DC: National Academies Press; 2005:386

46. Millward DJ. The nutritional value of plant based diets in relation to human amino acid and protein requirements. *Proc Nutr Soc*. 1999;58:249-260

47. Messina V, Mangels AR. Considerations in planning vegan diets: children. *J Am Diet Assoc*. 2001;101(6):661-669

48. Young VR, Fajardo L, Murray E, Rand WM, Scrimshaw NS. Protein requirements of man. Comparative nitrogen balance response within the submaintenance-to-maintenance range of intakes of wheat and beef proteins. *J Nutr*. 1975;105(5):534-542

49. Attwood CR. Low-fat diets for children: practicality and safety. *Am J Cardiol*. 1998;82(10B):77T-79T

50. World Health Organization, Food and Agriculture Organization of the United Nations. *Diet, Nutrition and the Prevention of Chronic Diseases*. Geneva, Switzerland: World Health Organization; 2003. Available at: http://whqlibdoc.who.int/trs/WHO_TRS_916.pdf. Accessed October 2, 2012

51. Kris-Etherton PM, Taylor DS, Yu-Poth S, et al. Polyunsaturated fatty acids in the food chain in the United States. *Am J Clin Nutr*. 2000;71(1 Suppl):179S-188S

52. Brenner RR, Peluffo RO. Regulation of unsaturated fatty acids biosynthesis. I. Effect of unsaturated fatty acid of 18 carbons of the microsomal desaturation of linoleic acid into gamma-linoleic acid. *Biochem Biophys Acta*. 1969;176(3):471-479

53. Conquer JA, Holub BJ. Supplementation with an algae source of docosahexanoic acid increases (n-3) fatty acid status and alters selected risk factors for heart disease in vegetarian subjects. *J Nutr*. 1996;126(12):3032-3039

54. Ribaya-Mercado JD. Influence of dietary fat on beta carotene absorption and bioconversion into vitamin A. *Nutr Rev*. 2002;60(4):104-110

55. Institute of Medicine. *Dietary Reference Intakes for Thiamin, Riboflavin, Niacin, Vitamin B 6, Folate, Vitamin B12, Pantothenic Acid, Biotin, and Choline.* Washington, DC: National Academies Press; 1998

56. Donaldson MS. Metabolic vitamin B12 status on a mostly raw vegan diet with follow up using tablets, nutritional yeast or probiotic supplements. *Ann Nutr Metab.* 2000;44(5-6):229-234

57. Weiss R, Fogelman Y, Bennett M. Severe vitamin B12 deficiency in an infant associated with a maternal deficiency and a strict vegetarian diet. *J Pediatr Hematol Oncol.* 2004;26(4):270-271

58. Gilois C, Wierzbicki AS, Hirani N, et al. The hematological and electrophysiological effects of cobalamin. Deficiency secondary to vegetarian diets. *Ann N Y Acad Sci.* 1992;669:345-8

59. Institute of Medicine. *Dietary Reference Intakes for Calcium, Phosphorous, Magnesium, Vitamin D, and Fluoride.* Washington, DC: National Academies Press; 1997

60. Trang HM, Cole DE, Rubin LA, Pierratos A, Siu S, Vieth R. Evidence that vitamin D3 increases serum 25 hydroxyvitamin D more efficiently than does Vitamin D2. *Am J Clin Nutr.* 1998;68(4):854-858

61. Ambroszkiewicz J, Klemarczyk W, Gajewska J, Chelchowska M, Franek E, Laskowska-Klita T. The influence of vegan diet on bone mineral density and biochemical bone turnover markers. *Pediatr Endocrinol Diabetes Metab.* 2010;16(3):201-204

62. Institute of Medicine. *Dietary Reference Intakes for Vitamin A, Vitamin K, Arsenic, Boron, Chromium, Copper, Iodine, Iron, Manganese, Molybdenum, Nickel, Silicon, Vanadium, and Zinc.* Washington, DC: National Academies Press; 2001

63. Hunt JR, Roughead ZK. Nonheme-iron absorption, fecal ferritin excretion and blood indexes of iron status in woman consuming controlled lactoovovegetarian diets for 8 weeks. *Am J Clin Nutr.* 1999;69(5):944-952

64. Donovan UM, Gibson R. Iron and zinc status of young women aged 14 to 19 years consuming vegetarian and omnivorous diets. *J Am Coll Nutr.* 1995;14:463-472

65. Haddad EH, Berk LS, Kettering JD, Gubbard RW, Peters RW. Dietary intake and biochemical, hematologic and immune status of vegans compared with nonvegetarians. *Am J Clin Nutr.* 1999;70(3 Suppl):586S-593S

66. Hunt JR, Roughead ZK. Adaptation of iron absorption in men consuming diets with high or low iron bioavailability. *Am J Clin Nutr.* 2000;71(1):94-102

67. Subar AF, Krebs-Smith SM, Cook A, Kahle LL. Dietary sources of nutrients among US adults, 1989 to 1991. *J Am Diet Assoc.* 1998;98(5):537-547

68. Harland BF, Oberleas D. Phytate in foods. *World Rev Nutr Diet.* 1987;52:235-259

69. Hunt JR, Matthys LA, Johnson LK. Zinc absorption, mineral balance and blood lipids in women consuming controlled lactoovovegetarian and omnivorous diets for 8 weeks. *Am J Clin Nutr.* 1998;67(3):421-430

70. Gibson RS. Content and bioavailability of trace elements in vegetarian diets. *Am J Clin Nutr.* 1994;59(5 Suppl):1223S-1232S

71. Taylor A, Redworth EW, Morgan JB. Influence of diet on iron, copper and zinc status in children under 24 months of age. *Biol Trace Element Res.* 2004;94(3):197-214

72. Heaney RP, Dowell MS, Rafferty K, Bierman J. Bioavailability of the calcium in fortified soy imitation milk, with some observations on method. *Am J Clin Nutr*. 2000;71(5): 1166-1169

73. Weaver C, Proulx W, Heaney R. Choices for achieving adequate dietary calcium with a vegetarian diet. *Am J Clin Nutr*. 1999;70(3 Suppl):543S-548S

74. Remer T, Neubert A, Manz F. Increased risk of iodine deficiency with vegetarian nutrition. *Br J Nutr*. 1999;81(1):45-49

75. Lombard KA, Olson AL, Nelson SE, Rebouche CJ. Carnitine status of lacto-ovo vegetarians and strict vegetarian adults and children. *Am J Clin Nutr*. 1989;50(2): 301-306

76. Laidlaw SA, Shultz TD, Cecchino JT, Kopple JD. Plasma and urine taurine levels in vegans. *Am J Clin Nutr*. 1988;47(4):660-663

77. Mangels AR, Messina V. Considerations in planning vegan diets: infants. *J Am Diet Assoc*. 2001;101(6):670-677

78. Sanders TA. Vegetarian diets and children. *Pediatr Clin North Am*. 1995;42(4):955-965

79. Sanders TA. Essential fatty acid requirements of vegetarians in pregnancy, lactation, and infancy. *Am J Clin Nutr*. 1999;70(3 Suppl):555S-559S

80. Hebbelinck M, Clarys P. Physical growth and development of vegetarian children and adolescents. In: Sabate J, ed. *Vegetarian Nutrition*. Boca Raton, FL: CRC Press Inc; 2001:173-193

81. Freeland-Graves JH, Greninger SA, Graves GR, Young RK. Health practices, attitudes and beliefs of vegetarians and nonvegetarians. *J Am Diet Assoc*. 1986;86(7):913-918

82. Worsley A, Skrzypiec G. Teenage vegetarianism: prevalence, social and cognitive contexts. *Appetite*. 1998;30(2):151-170

83. Gillbody SM, Kirk SFL, Hill AJ. Vegetarianism in young women: another means of weight control? *Int J Eat Disord*. 1999;26(1):87-90

84. Neumark-Sztainer D, Story M, Resnick MD, Blum RW. Adolescent vegetarians. A behavioral profile of a school based population in Minnesota. *Arch Pediatr Adolesc Med*. 1997;151(8):833-838

85. Klopp SA, Heiss CJ, Smith HS. Self-reported vegetarianism may be a marker for college women at risk for disordered eating. *J Am Diet Assoc*. 2003;103(6):745-747

86. Perry CL, Mcguire MT, Neumark-Sztainer D, Story M. Characteristics of vegetarian adolescents in a multi-ethnic urban population. *J Adolesc Health*. 2001;29(6):406-416

87. Bas M, Karabudak E, Kiziltan G. Vegetarianism and eating disorders: association between eating attitudes and other psychological factors among Turkish adolescents. *Appetite*. 2005;44(3):309-315

88. Phillips F, Hackett AF, Stratton G, Billington D. Effect of changing to a self-selected vegetarian diet on anthropometric measurements in UK adults. *J Hum Nutr Diet*. 2004;17(3):249-255

89. Nieman DC. Physical fitness and vegetarian diets. Is there a relation? *Am J Clin Nutr*. 1999;70(3 Suppl):570S-575S

90. Snyder AC, Dvorak LL, Roepke JB. Influence of dietary iron source on measures of iron status among female runners. *Med Sci Sports Exerc*. 1989;21(1):7-10

III

91. Burke DG, Chilibeck PD, Parise G, et al. Effect of creatine and weight training on muscle creatine and performance in vegetarians. *Med Sci Sports Exerc*. 2003;35(11):1946-1955

92. Barnard ND, Katcher HI, Jenkins DJ, Cohen J, Turner-McGrievy G. Vegetarian and vegan diets in type 2 diabetes management. *Nutr Rev*. 2009;67(5):255-263

93. Turner-McGrievy GM, Barnard ND, Cohen J, Jenkins DJ, Gloede L, Green AA. Changes in nutrient intake and dietary quality among participants with type 2 diabetes following a low-fat vegan diet or a conventional diabetes diet for 22 weeks. *J Am Diet Assoc*. 2008;108(10):1636-1645

94. Barnard ND, Gloede L, Cohen J, et al. A low-fat vegan diet elicits greater macronutrient changes, but is comparable in adherence and acceptability, compared with a more conventional diabetes diet among individuals with type 2 diabetes. *J Am Diet Assoc*. 2009;109(2):263-272

95. Tonstad S, Butler T, Yan R, Fraser GE. Type of vegetarian diet, body weight, and prevalence of type 2 diabetes. *Diabetes Care*. 2009;32(5):791-796

96. Trapp CB, Barnard ND. Usefulness of vegetarian and vegan diets for treating type 2 diabetes. *Curr Diab Rep*. 2010;10(2):152-158

97. Galson SK. Childhood overweight and obesity prevention. *Public Health Rep*. 2008;123(3):258-259

98. Azagury DE, Lautz DB. Obesity overview: epidemiology, health and financial impact, and guidelines for qualification for surgical therapy. *Gastrointest Endosc Clin North Am*. 2011;21(2):189-201

99. Sabate J, Ratzin-Turner RA, Brown JE. Vegetarian diets: description and trends. In: Sabate J, ed. *Vegetarian Nutrition*. Boca Raton, FL: CRC Press Inc; 2001:3-17

100. Sabate J, Wien M. Vegetarian diets and childhood obesity prevention. *Am J Clin Nutr*. 2010;91(5):1525S-1529S

Chapter 12

Sports Nutrition

Introduction

The majority of children and adolescents in the United States take part in sports. The 2009 Youth Risk Behavior Survey (YRBS) revealed that 64% of high school boys and 51% of high school girls participated on an organized sports team during the previous 12 months.[1] For boys, this rate of participation was not significantly different from that found in the 1999 YRBS; however, for girls, the rate of participation increased slightly. Over that time period, there was also a general increase in the intensity, volume, and specialization of training for young athletes. Many children are no longer encouraged to become "all around" scholastic athletes but rather will stick with a single, or several related, sports year-round and will often participate on multiple teams simultaneously.

When pediatricians are counseling patients and families on physical activity and sports, it is important to recognize that for the child younger than 8 or 9 years, diversity in physical activity is much more effective at enhancing motor development than repetition.[2] This is the rationale behind the endorsement of "free play" for younger children and for encouraging participation in a wide variety of sporting activity, particularly in younger children. Although varied activity and training remain important throughout an athletic career, as children move into early adolescence and beyond, repetition and practice become much more beneficial in terms of refining specific motor movement patterns and enhancing sports-specific skills.

In older children and adolescents, it is important to assess the volume and intensity of their training and ambition. Some of these athletes practice and play several hours daily on a year-round basis. The problem with this becomes evident with further consideration of some fundamental principles of sports training. Exercise creates a training stimulus or stress that affects not only musculoskeletal tissue but also multiple body systems. The body adapts to this stimulus in such a way that builds exercise capacity. The most successful training programs include:

1. A variety of training stimuli of sufficient intensity to create physiologic stress for the athlete.
2. Adequate recovery periods between training sessions to allow the body to rebuild and repair the microtrauma that occurs with sports training. This point is, unfortunately, lost on many young athletes and families who embrace the "more is better" philosophy. If athletes are not given adequate rest and recovery, they will not experience optimal performance improvements and markedly increase their risk of injury and burnout.

3. An appropriate nutritional base that provides fuel and fluid during periods of exercise, as well as readily available "building blocks" for postexercise recovery. This is the foundation for an effective sports nutrition philosophy and is the basis for this chapter.

Sports nutrition is a field rife with multiple claims of performance enhancement from a myriad of dietary and supplemental products and interests. This, combined with adolescents' (and often parents') goals for rapid gains and high levels of achievement, often leads to pursuit of nutritional "magic" that may be neither healthy nor effective. The goal of this chapter is to provide evidence-based information regarding the role of nutrition in young athletes. As much as possible, this information is based on results from studies performed in the pediatric population. The key points that will be covered in this chapter include:

- the use of appropriate fluids and macronutrients to provide fuel for, and to enhance recovery from, exercise and physical exertion;
- the role of select vitamins and minerals in the young athlete's diet;
- issues related to weight loss and weight gain in the athlete; and
- information regarding nutritional supplements in common use in youth sports.

Fuels for Activity

Overview of Exercise Metabolism

One of the basic tenets of sports nutrition is to ensure adequate fuel and fluid to optimize athletic efforts. The preferred fuel for physical activity depends on the intensity and duration of the physical effort as well as the nutritional and training status of the athlete. Fat is the primary fuel source at rest and during very low levels of activity, such as walking, but does not provide enough adenosine triphosphate (ATP) to fuel the level of physical activity required by most sports.

Higher-Intensity Activity

For intense physical exertion lasting less than 10 to 30 seconds, such as sprints or individual sets in weight training, the ATP/phosphocreatine system is the primary fuel substrate. As ATP is broken down to adenosine diphosphate (ADP) in the exercising muscle, phosphocreatine contained in muscle is used to regenerate ATP stores and provide additional energy. This appears to be the mechanism of action of the dietary supplement creatine, which will be discussed later in the chapter.

As intense activity continues beyond about 30 seconds, carbohydrates become the dominant fuel source. For the next several minutes of high-intensity activity, muscle glycogen becomes increasingly important and provides energy via the anaerobic glycolytic pathway. The resulting accumulation of lactic acid prohibits sustaining this level of effort beyond a brief period.

Lower-Intensity Activity

For lower-intensity efforts, once activity commences, carbohydrates begin to displace fatty acids as a fuel source, and as intensity and duration of training increase, carbohydrates become an increasingly dominant source. Aerobic metabolic pathways use glycogen initially as a carbohydrate energy source. However, as duration of exercise increases, blood glucose becomes a more important fuel source. This transition of fuel supply appears to be developmentally dependent. There is evidence that muscle glycogen stores may be 50% to 60% lower in children than in adults,[3,4] and this may contribute to several key differences between young and adult athletes and may have important nutrition ramifications:

1. Children and adolescents remain more reliant on lipids as an energy source for a given level of exercise compared with adults. This results in a relative sparing of muscle glycogen stores. This lipid reliance is further enhanced with endurance training.

2. Children and adolescents are more dependent on blood glucose, particularly exogenous/dietary sources, for their energy supply during physical activity compared with adults. Some studies comparing children with adults have found that ingested carbohydrates have a 50% greater contribution to energy supply during moderate and intense activity in children than in adults.[4] This may increase the significance of dietary choices before and during exercise in the young athlete.

Fueling the Workout: Carbohydrates

Carbohydrates, in the forms of muscle glycogen and blood glucose, are major sources of energy for most physical endeavors in the child and adolescent. Therefore, adequate carbohydrate intake and stores are keys to successful athletic pursuits. Although the current Recommended Dietary Allowance (RDA) for carbohydrates in children and adults is 130 g/day,[5] most young athletes require much higher intakes to support optimum training and participation. Maintenance of muscle glycogen requires intake of at least 4 to 5 g of carbohydrate/kg/day, with energy needs to support physical activity sometimes requiring intakes up to twice this amount.[6] Recommendations for adult athletes are 6 to 10 g of carbohydrate/kg/day.[6] This is likely an appropriate range for many adolescents as well and has significant overlap with the general recommendation in young athletes that at least 50% of caloric intake should be from carbohydrates. Carbohydrates should be ingested throughout the course of the day, but they are particularly important during the times surrounding athletic activity, as outlined below.

Before Exercise

Before working out, carbohydrates are important to bolster muscle glycogen and blood glucose. Muscle glycogen is best supported with a diet that is consistently high in carbohydrates throughout the athletic season. This is particularly important in the days leading up to endurance-type events, where glycogen is typically built up with consistent high carbohydrate intakes over multiple days. Studies in adults have shown marked increases in muscle glycogen after a single day of a diet high in carbohydrates with a high glycemic index (10 g of carbohydrate/kg/day).[7] More modest increases are noted approximately 4 hours after a single high-carbohydrate meal.[4] It is not known whether these same increases occur in the child and adolescent athlete.

There is a great deal of individual variability in the athlete's tolerance to preexercise food and fluid ingestion. The athlete's comfort should dictate the timing and content of any preexercise intake, but several general principles apply:

- Some trial and error is typical when determining an acceptable preexercise meal regimen. For the school-aged athlete, lunch typically occurs 3 to 4 hours before after-school training sessions. General recommendations would be for this meal to be in high in carbohydrates, which would allow for optimization of glycogen stores.[6] If a single larger meal creates gastric discomfort, smaller, more frequent snacks may need to be substituted.

- Select food and beverage that will empty from the stomach fairly quickly. Meals that are high in fat and protein tend to remain in the stomach for longer periods of time, which may cause gastric distress with exercise.

- It is generally recommended that blood glucose concentrations should be augmented with a small high-carbohydrate snack 30 to 60 minutes before beginning exercise.[8] Studies in adults have shown that, although this seems to enhance glucose availability and oxidation during subsequent exercise, results are mixed about direct effect on performance.[6,8] However, given young athletes' increased reliance on blood glucose as an energy source, this may be more important in the child athlete than in the adult.

- Although some studies have shown that ingestion of carbohydrates with high glycemic index are important in maximizing muscle glycogen stores,[9] and other reports encourage carbohydrates with low glycemic index shortly before exercise, the overall role of the glycemic index before exercise remains somewhat in doubt, with many studies and expert panels reporting inconclusive findings to date and deferring to individual preference.[6,9,10]

During Exercise

Intake of carbohydrates during activity appears to be beneficial as an ongoing fuel source and protects lean tissue from catabolism during and after exercise. This is best established for activity lasting greater than 1 hour[11] but may also be true for shorter activity.[6] Once again, gastric tolerance for ingested food and fluid during exercise will vary greatly. Gastric emptying significantly slows with higher-intensity exercise, and many athletes in running sports will need to experiment with different regimens before finding one that is effective and comfortable. The following general principles apply:

- Endurance athletes should consume 0.7 g of carbohydrate/kg/hour (30-60 g of carbohydrate/hour for full-grown individuals), divided into 15- to 20-minute intervals[6] (see Table 12.1 for sample carbohydrate content).

- The type and form of carbohydrate can be dictated by the athlete's preference and gastric tolerance. Hydration with recommended volumes of a 6% to 8% carbohydrate-containing sports drink during exercise also provides the recommended amount of carbohydrates (see Table 12.2 and fluid section below).

- Exogenous carbohydrate utilization during exercise appears to be limited by intestinal transport. Ingesting carbohydrates that utilize different transporters in the intestinal tract (ie, glucose and fructose) during exercise appears to increase available exogenous carbohydrate to fuel exercise in adults.[12] It is interesting to speculate how this may influence exercise performance in young athletes, who are already known to be more dependent on exogenous glucose, but no data are available to date.

- Many carbohydrate sources in common use by athletes contain fructose, which may cause gastric upset in some athletes. Sucrose- or glucose-based sources of carbohydrate may be better tolerated.

Table 12.1.

Carbohydrate Content of Sample Food and Products Commonly Ingested During Sports Activities

Food	Carbohydrate (g)
Apple, 1 medium	21
Banana, 1 medium	27
Clif Bar, 1 original	45
Clif Kid Z Bar, 1 original	25
Fig Newton, 2-oz single-serve packet	39
Fruit Roll Up, 1 roll	12
Gu Original Energy Gel, 1 packet	25
Jelly Belly Sport Beans, 1 packet	24
NutriGrain, 1 bar	24
Power Bar Iron Girl, 1 bar	28
Power Bar Performance, 1 bar	45
Pretzels, 1 oz (about 18 mini pretzels)	23
Raisins, 1.5-oz box	22

After Exercise

Many scholastic athletes train 1 to 2 hours/day at least 5 days/week, with some preseason training involving multiple sessions per day. For athletes training at this frequency, the postexercise meal becomes very important in replenishing diminished muscle glycogen, which becomes an important fuel source for the next workout. In addition, carbohydrate ingestion once again protects muscle in that the postexercise meal appears to have an important role in sparing muscle from postexercise catabolism. The following are guiding principles for postexercise meals:

- The postexercise meal is best ingested within 30 minutes of exercise, when muscles are most sensitive to the effects of insulin and when glycogen synthesis is maximized.[6] This is most important for athletes training multiple times per day or on multiple consecutive days. It is currently recommended that athletes ingest 1 to 1.5 g of carbohydrates/kg of body weight immediately after exercise and at 2-hour intervals, which can be repeated for up to 6 hours. However, some recent studies report optimal glycogen resynthesis when this amount is increased to 1.2 g of carbohydrate/kg per hour.[13]

- Glucose and sucrose appear to be more effective than fructose at restoring glycogen stores.[6]

- In adults, postexercise meals with a high glycemic index appear to be more effective than meals with a low glycemic index at restoring muscle glycogen stores.[6] However, it is not clear whether this is also true for the younger athlete. On the basis of current data, the quantity and timing of postexercise carbohydrates appear to be far more important determinants of glycogen replenishment than the glycemic index of the postexercise meal.

Despite the importance of carbohydrates in supporting optimal physical performance, multiple studies have shown that young and adolescent athletes often consume significantly less than recommended amounts. Convincing athletes to increase carbohydrate intake to cover the caloric demand of their activity can be a "hard sell" for some athletes, who are often used to functioning on far less. When carbohydrate intake is inadequate, the metabolic response is to catabolize muscle to provide needed fuel. In these cases, it is often helpful to inform athletes that the muscle and strength they are working so hard to gain is being broken down and used as an expendable fuel source.

III

Fluids for the Workout

Optimal physical performance relies on maintenance of adequate fluid volume, which is important for the delivery of oxygen and nutrients to exercising muscle and assisting with heat dissipation. This is particularly true for endurance, or aerobic, activities. Unfortunately, young athletes and their parents are often uncertain about the appropriate types and quantities of fluid needed to maintain hydration before, during, and after physical activity. A comparison of the carbohydrate, protein, and sodium content of various drinks is shown in Table 12.2.

Table 12.2.
Carbohydrate, Protein, and Sodium Content of Several Common Sports Drinks and Comparison Fluids

Product	% Carbohydrate	Carbohydrate (g/8-oz serving)	Protein (g/8-oz serving)	Sodium mEq/L
Gatorade	6	14	0	20
Powerade	8	19	0	10
Accelerade	6	15	4	21
Apple juice	16	38	0	4
Orange juice (from concentrate)	11	26	2	3
Cola	12	28	0	4
Milk	6	14	8	26
Milk, chocolate 2%	12	29	8	34

Before Exercise

Young athletes should be fully hydrated before beginning any training session and ideally should maintain euhydration throughout the day. This can be readily accomplished by having the athlete drink enough fluids to keep urine pale yellow or clear. In preparation for physical training, athletes should prehydrate 1 to 2 hours before training. This allows for gastric emptying and absorption into the vascular system before exertion begins.

Recommended prehydration fluid volumes are as follows:

Athletes <40 kg: 90-180 mL (3-6 oz)

Athletes >40 kg: 180-360 mL (6-12 oz)

Prehydration can be accomplished with water, milk, or other nutritive beverages. Sports drinks, which typically contain a low concentration of carbohydrates and a small amount of electrolytes, provide no advantage over other fluids for prehydration (see Appendix H).

During Exercise

Fluid requirements during exercise are highly variable, depending on intensity of training, climactic conditions, and the intrinsic sweat rate and acclimatization of the athlete. Sweat rates typically range from approximately 500 to 1300 mL/hour but can be much higher.[14,15,16] In the adolescent population, older or male athletes tend to have higher sweat rates than younger or female athletes. Although thirst is often recognized when dehydration approaches 3% to 5%, aerobic capacity, balance, and mental/cognitive performance appear to fall off at approximately 2% dehydration.[6,17] The goal for fluid intake during exercise is to keep fluid losses to less than 2% body weight. A good starting point for fluid recommendations for healthy adolescents is as follows:

Athletes ~40 kg: 150 mL (5 oz) every 20 min

Athletes ~60 kg: 240 mL (8 oz) every 20 min

For many physically active children and adolescents, water is the fluid of first choice, particularly for training sessions lasting less than an hour or of relatively low intensity.[18] For longer bouts of significant exertion, athletes may benefit from also ingesting a small amount of added carbohydrate and sodium.[6] Carbohydrate intake during exercise provides an ongoing source of blood glucose to fuel the working muscles. In addition, fluids containing carbohydrate concentrations of about 6% to 8% appear to empty from the stomach more quickly than plain water and may reduce stomach discomfort. For athletes who are not ingesting any solid food during exercise, sports drinks may be a convenient way to obtain this additional carbohydrate, but this same concentration can also be obtained by diluting many fruit juices by half with water.

Fluids with added sodium stimulate osmoreceptors and enhance additional intake. Many sports drinks contain 10 to 20 mmol of sodium/L, which appears sufficient to stimulate further drinking. However, contrary to common perception, this amount of sodium is not sufficient to significantly replace sweat-related sodium losses (sodium content in adolescent sweat is typically on the order of 40 to 70 mmol/L).

Some athletes will report gastric discomfort or nausea when attempting to drink recommended volumes of fluid. Gastric emptying of fluids in individuals participating in high-intensity intermittent running (such as seen in practices and games of many team sports) is reduced by 50% to 70% as compared with lower-intensity activity and may contribute to issues with gastric tolerance for recommended volumes of fluid.[19] For those athletes complaining of stomach discomfort when attempting appropriate volume intake, the following may be helpful:

- Temperate fluids empty quicker from the stomach than do cold fluids and may be better tolerated by some.
- Smaller, more frequent sips are generally better tolerated than less frequent, higher-volume intakes.
- Gastric tolerance can often be trained, so beginning with smaller volumes of fluid and then increasing gradually over several weeks to recommended amounts may help.
- It may take some experimenting with different fluid types to find what works for individual athletes.

The past decade has seen a marked increase in recognition of exertional hyponatremia in endurance activities. The mechanism of exertional hyponatremia is incompletely understood but appears to occur in athletes who have inappropriately reduced their excretion of free water.[20] It is mainly a phenomenon found in sustained endurance and ultra-endurance efforts of greater than 4 hours in duration, and as such, is not of significant concern for the majority of young athletes.

After Exercise

Given the variation in sweat losses, postexercise fluid recommendations should start by encouraging athletes to determine their individual fluid status. Athletes can be educated to weigh themselves before and after working out (making sure to remove sweat-soaked clothing) to calculate fluid losses during activity. Future intake can then be adjusted to avoid these losses in subsequent practice sessions. Adults are recommended to rehydrate with approximately 100% to 150% volume fluid lost, with some data suggesting improved fluid replacement at the higher levels.[6,21] This is likely appropriate for adolescents, but younger individuals may have difficulty with the higher volumes and should start with replacing on an ounce-per-ounce basis.

Recommended fluid replacement volumes are as follows:

Adolescents: 480-720 mL (16-24 oz) per pound of weight loss

Younger children: ~480 mL (16 oz) per pound of weight loss

For postexercise hydration, the volume of beverage is more important than the type of beverage used. Water, milk, or other nutritive beverages are all appropriate choices. Most young athletes will be also be ingesting solid food during this time period, which will provide the carbohydrate and sodium that appear to enhance fluid retention during rehydration. If food is not available, studies performed with hypertonic solutions containing 10% carbohydrate and 25 mmol of sodium/L appear more effective at restoring hydration than do hypotonic solutions.[22] One way to achieve this content is to add ¼ teaspoon of table salt to 1 L of orange or other fruit juice.

Several recent studies have found low-fat and chocolate milk to be effective recovery beverages. These milk products provide a combination of carbohydrate, sodium, potassium, and protein that not only enhances intra- and extracellular rehydration but also benefits restoration of glycogen stores and muscle recovery after exercise.[23,24]

Standard sports drinks provide insufficient carbohydrates to replenish glycogen and insufficient sodium to replace sweat losses and do not provide an advantage over other fluid selections for rehydration after exercise.[18]

Building Blocks for Recovery

The body repairs the microtrauma induced with a rigorous exercise session during the following 24 to 72 hours. This repair process results in hypertrophy and increased strength of skeletal muscle and other tissues and requires the following:

- Adequate protein intake to provide the "building blocks" for muscle synthesis and repair;
- Adequate carbohydrate intake to avoid excess muscle breakdown; and
- Adequate sleep and rest from additional physical stress.

Protein

Many adolescent athletes are highly interested in the role protein plays in building strength and muscle. RDAs for protein are 0.8 g/kg/day in adults, 0.85 g/kg/day in 14- to 18-year-olds, and 0.95 g/kg/day in 4- to 13-year-olds.[5] The higher values in children and adolescents accommodate the protein requirements for growth and development.

Research in adults has demonstrated that athletes have increased protein requirements relative to the sedentary population. These higher requirements are likely attributable, in part, to increased protein turnover with muscle breakdown and repair as well as utilization of some amino acids (especially the branched-chain amino acids) for fuel with activity. The following protein recommendations in adults are synthesized from several recently published position stands with the higher range appropriate for those training with a higher degree of intensity as well as for novice athletes who are just initiating a training regimen (for reference, the "average" US daily intake is 1.4 g/kg/day)[6,25]:

- Endurance-trained athletes: 1.0-1.7 g/kg/day
- Resistance-trained athletes: 1.2-2.0 g/kg/day
- Athletes in "intermittent" sports (most team sports): 1.4-1.7 g/kg/day
- General fitness training: 0.8-1.0 g/kg/day

Although there is a paucity of data on the pediatric athlete, the increased protein requirements for growth and athletic activity are probably cumulative but not necessarily additive. See Table 12.3 for protein content of some common foods and supplements.

Table 12.3.
Protein Content of Some Common Foods and Supplements Used by Athletes

Food	Protein (g)
Meats/eggs	
Hamburger (3 oz, extra-lean)	24
Chicken, roasted (3 oz)	21
Tuna (3 oz, water-packed)	20
Eggs (1 large)	6
Dairy	
Cottage cheese (1/2 cup, low-fat)	14
Yogurt (8 oz)	12
Milk (8 oz, whole or skim)	8
Non-fat dry milk (2 tablespoons)	3
Beans/legumes	
Tofu (1/2 cup)	10
Peanut butter (2 tablespoons)	10
Lentils (1/2 cup, cooked)	9
Black beans (1/2 cup)	8
Grains	
Pasta (1 cup, cooked)	7
Bread (whole wheat, 2 slices)	5
Other	
Protein supplements (per serving)	20-35
Promax bar	20
Clif bar (peanut butter flavor)	12
Carnation-brand instant breakfast (w/8 oz skim milk)	12
PowerBar	10
Ensure (8 oz.)	9
Snickers bar	4
Nutri-Grain bar	2

III

It has long been accepted that protein's main role in sports nutrition is to serve as building blocks for the repair and adaptation of muscle tissue after training. Traditionally, the goal has been to provide the body with a steady stream of amino acids throughout the 48 to 72 hours after working out for these repair efforts. However, more recent studies demonstrate that ingestion of protein, particularly the essential amino acids, appears not only to diminish the amount of muscle breakdown that occurs with exercise but also to augment muscle synthesis and promote a more anabolic hormonal profile.[26] This has been demonstrated consistently in adult studies when at least 20 g of protein is ingested in conjunction with adequate amounts of carbohydrate shortly after exercise.[9,13,27] Ratios of carbohydrate to protein in these studies are generally approximately 3:1.[26] This can be approximated with a peanut butter and jelly sandwich (2 tablespoons each of peanut butter and jelly on 2 slices of multigrain bread). It is important to emphasize that protein does not appear to enhance performance per se, but rather its addition around the time of exercise appears to optimize subsequent muscle recovery.

Some studies have examined the possibility that ingestion of a small amount of protein before and during exercise may decrease muscle breakdown, but findings are inconsistent.[26] Although there are a number of commercial products on the market promoting this practice, it is not yet supported by a significant body of evidence.

Micronutrients

Minerals

IRON

Iron has an important role in oxygen delivery and energy generation in the young athlete, and there are iron-related stressors that are unique to athletes and increase their need for iron and confound results for iron testing. These include:

- At the onset of aerobic training, athletes initially expand their plasma volume, which leads to a transient dilutional "pseudoanemia." As long as iron stores are sufficient, with continued training there is a subsequent increase in red blood cell mass, which normalizes hemoglobin and hematocrit concentrations for the majority of young athletes.[6,28]

- In endurance and ultra-endurance events, some athletes will lose small amounts of iron via sweat or through the gastrointestinal or genitourinary tracts. These losses are typically compensated by enhanced dietary absorption and are not likely clinically significant in the majority of young athletes.[28]

- In high-impact activity, especially running, hemolysis can occur with the forces generated during footstrike. The body is generally very good at recovering iron after hemolysis, but these athletes may have macrocytosis resulting from increased reticulocyte formation.

- Iron intake is often suboptimal in athletes who are in weight-controlled sports or are otherwise restricting dietary intake.

There is a high degree of interest among athletes and coaches regarding iron intake and iron status, and athletes presenting with fatigue or poor performance often question iron deficiency.

It is important to recognize that supplies of iron in the human body appear to exist on a functional continuum. Athletes with fully replete iron stores are capable of completely supporting the increases in red cell mass that occur with aerobic training. Athletes with mild depletion may develop a "relative anemia" in which hemoglobin concentrations are below optimal for the individual but still within population norms. Athletes with more significant decreases in iron stores may develop frank anemia.

Rates of iron-deficiency anemia are similar between athletes and nonathletes, and there is consensus that iron-deficiency anemia leads to significant decreases in athletic performance.[6] However, there is currently disagreement as to the definition and athletic impact of nonanemic iron-deficient states, and athletes do appear to be at greater risk of developing this condition.[28]

Ferritin is often used as a marker of iron stores, and there is disagreement over the lower concentration at which ferritin is still considered "normal." Many laboratories report the lower limit of normal ferritin concentrations at 12 ng/mL. However, iron absorption studies suggest that 35 ng/mL may be a more appropriate normal lower limit, and the up-regulation of iron absorption that is seen in deficient states has been demonstrated in some studies with ferritin concentrations as high 60 ng/mL.[28] Given the difficulties with the definition of "iron deficiency," it is not surprising that methodology and results of studies looking at the effects of nonanemic low iron stores on athletic performance have been inconsistent. Some studies have shown significant changes in maximal oxygen uptake and exercise performance in the nonanemic athlete with low ferritin, but others have not.[6,28]

There should be a low threshold for checking hemoglobin, hematocrit, and ferritin in athletes presenting with fatigue or decreases in performance. Although iron supplementation is common in young athletes, it is not without risk and should be reserved for those cases with documented iron deficiency in which symptoms, performance, and laboratory values are followed during treatment. Studies in nonanemic depleted athletes showed that doses of 50 mg of elemental iron/day have been sufficient at replenishing ferritin stores in an athletic population. A "relative anemia" can be detected by looking for a rebound in hemoglobin concentrations after supplementing for approximately 1 month.

III

CALCIUM

In childhood and adolescence, calcium intake and weight-bearing exercise are both important components in achieving peak bone mass. Increased calcium intake appears to protect against bone injuries in the athletic population, and there is evidence in younger adult female athletes that calcium intakes greater than 1500 mg/day reduces the risk of stress fractures.[29] This may be applicable for adolescents as well and is in stark contrast to current intakes in children and adolescents in the United States. Table 12.4 illustrates the discrepancy between RDAs and intake in children and adolescents in the United States and demonstrates that poor calcium intake is ubiquitous and not unique to the athletic population.

Table 12.4.

Calcium: Comparison of Recommended Daily Allowances and Calculated Daily Intakes

Athletes	RDA (mg/day)	Calcium intake (mg/day)		
		25th percentile	50th percentile	75th percentile
Males: 4-8 y	1000	855	1045	1207
Males: 9-13 y	1300	864	1055	1268
Males: 14-18 y	1300	884	1169	1565
Females: 4-8 y	1000	739	808	1106
Females: 9-13 y	1300	743	938	1162
Females: 14-18 y	1300	657	825	1048

Source: Institute of Medicine. *Dietary Reference Intakes for Calcium and Vitamin D*. Washington, DC: The National Academies Press; 2011 http://books.nap.edu/catalog.php?record_id=13050.

For a given level of calcium intake, most athletes, particularly those participating in high-impact activities, have higher bone density than their more sedentary peers. However, the athlete's demands for bone integrity are much greater than those of their peers, and athletes are at higher risk of developing stress fractures. This is particularly true for female athletes whose energy intake is too low to support their caloric requirements.[30] These girls will often suppress estrogen production, possibly resulting in pubertal delay or oligomenorrhea or amenorrhea. This combination of low caloric intake and decreased estrogen production results in diminished bone formation. This condition is known as "the female athlete triad," and these young athletes typically have bone density below average for their age group and are at markedly higher risk of developing bony stress injuries. There is good support in the athletic community for recommending minimum daily intakes of 1500 mg calcium/day for oligomenorrheic and amenorrheic female athletes.[6,30]

ZINC

Zinc plays a variety of roles in metabolism and growth, appears to be important in regulating concentrations of thyroid hormone, and also serves as an antioxidant.[31,32] Athletes who are vegetarian or restricting calories, particularly females, may be at increased risk of inadequate zinc intake. Zinc deficiency has been reported to have negative effects on strength and endurance performance[6]; however, athletic performance benefit with zinc supplementation has not been reliably demonstrated.[32] Many multivitamin and mineral supplements have zinc contents at or below the RDA of 15 mg/day, and supplementation at this level appears safe. However, higher doses (as often found in single-element zinc supplements) have been shown to interfere with iron absorption and markedly increase risk of iron deficiency.[32]

MAGNESIUM

Magnesium deficiency has been shown to contribute to suboptimal athletic performance in a variety of settings.[32] Athletes with restrictive eating patterns are at risk of inadequate magnesium intake, and in these athletes, supplementation may be beneficial. Although studies in older patients with coronary artery disease appear to show some increased exercise tolerance with magnesium, no benefit with supplementation has been found in younger athletes with adequate magnesium status.

Vitamins

B VITAMINS

The B vitamins are water-soluble coenzymes involved in energy production (thiamin, riboflavin, niacin, pyridoxine), DNA/red blood cell synthesis, and other tissue maintenance and repair (folate and vitamin B_{12}). There is some evidence in adults to suggest that athletes have increased turnover and utilization of B vitamins, possibly resulting in needs up twice those of current recommendations.[6] Although these increased needs are generally met with higher food intake in athletes, female diets, especially vegetarians and others with restrictive eating behaviors, often have low intakes of riboflavin, pyridoxine, folate, and vitamin B_{12}.[6] Athletic performance may be affected if folate or vitamin B_{12} deficiency results in anemia, but mild deficiencies of B vitamins do not appear to have a significant effect, and supplementation in nondeficient individuals does not appear to produce significant benefit to athletic performance.[6]

VITAMIN C

Much has been made of the potential benefit of vitamin C supplementation in the athletic population as a protectant against oxidative stress and protector of immune function. Studies examining oxidant stress and subsequent muscle damage and training adaptations as well as exercise performance do not appear to show significant difference between athletes supplemented with vitamin C or with placebo.[33,34] Adolescent and adult athletes already have enhanced antioxidant mechanisms, and exogenous supplementation does not seem to further augment these.[35,36]

Looking at immune function, a recent meta-analysis reports that vitamin C supplementation in endurance athletes (ie, marathoners and skiers) appears to reduce the risk of development of the common cold in half,[37] and vitamin C intakes of 100 to 1000 mg/day has been recommended in this population.[6] However, there does not appear to be significant immune benefit with vitamin C supplementation in studies performed in adolescents or at training intensities more typical of the young athlete.[38]

VITAMIN D

The roles of vitamin D particularly pertinent to the athletic population include attainment of optimal bone mass and support of muscle function. Vitamin D and physical activity appear to exert separate but complementary roles on bone development. A 2010 study in adolescents found that the positive correlation between exercise and bone density became stronger as vitamin D concentrations decreased, even as vitamin D concentrations decreased below 27.5 nmol/L.[39] This seems to indicate that exercise may provide increasing protection against bone loss with increasing vitamin D deficiency.

Stress fractures are more likely to occur in young athletes with decreased bone density. The interaction between physical activity, calcium, vitamin D, and the more recent recognition of the role of vitamin D receptor polymorphisms may explain the variable findings in some of the literature that has looked at the relationship between vitamin D and stress fracture development in athletes.[40] A military study showed that female Navy recruits with serum 25-hydroxyvitamin D (25-OH-D) concentrations <50 nmol/L were twice as likely to sustain stress fractures than those whose concentrations were >100 nmol/L.[41] Studies in young adults do appear to show that stress fractures are less frequent in subjects supplemented with calcium (2000 mg/day) and vitamin D (800 IU/day) compared with placebo[42] as well as in athletes with higher dairy intakes.[43] On the basis of these findings, many practitioners ascribe to a protective role for vitamin D in stress fracture development[44]; however, there remains a paucity of vigorous studies on this topic and essentially no published prospective studies performed with adolescent athletes.[29]

Vitamin D deficiency has long been associated with poor muscle function. Serum 25-OH-D concentrations <30 nmol/L have been associated with decreased muscle strength in adults.[45] The degree to which this holds true for adolescents and possibly affects athletic performance remains unclear. A 2009 study performed in asymptomatic 12- to 14-year-old British girls found a positive correlation between muscle power and serum 25-OH-D concentrations over a broad range.[46]

Recommendations regarding appropriate intake and optimal serum concentrations of vitamin D in the general pediatric population is a currently evolving topic (See Chapter 21.I). This is also true for the athletic population. Recent authors have proposed that young athletes benefit when serum 25-OH-D concentrations are above 70 to 100 nmol/L.[44,47] Particular attention should be paid to athletes who train indoors, because they appear to be at greater risk of deficiency.[48,49]

VITAMIN E

Vitamin E is similar to vitamin C in its role as an antioxidant. As with vitamin C, study results do not seem to support a role for supplemental vitamin E in terms of affecting exercise-associated oxidative damage and subsequent training adaptations and exercise performance.[34,35,36] Some concern exists that excess vitamin E may actually promote oxidative damage.[36]

Determination of Optimal Body Weight in Young Athletes

For a given athlete in a given sport, there is a range of body weights that support optimal performance. The specific weight range may change depending on choice of sport, developmental stage, body composition, and a variety of factors intrinsic to the individual. But this basic relationship holds: body weights at either extreme are associated with a drop in athletic performance and increase the potential for injury.[50]

Weight and body mass index (BMI) are 2 common measures in pediatric offices and, in that setting, are typically used to assess overall growth and development as well as possible health implications in over- or underweight individuals. Neither one is a good measure of body fat or athletic performance in athletes.[50,51] Further pursuit of weight and body composition assessments should be performed with caution and with an understanding of the rationale and implications for pursuing these measures.

Some sports (ie, wrestling and others with weight classifications) require calculations of body composition for weight class certification. Routine assessment of body composition in other athletes is not indicated and has the potential to be detrimental.[6,50] Body composition issues have an emotional overlay for many young athletes, and inappropriate use may trigger disordered eating patterns.[50] Sports performance measures (ie, speed, agility, jump height, etc) are far better gauges than body composition measures in determining optimal body weight for a given athlete.

If body composition assessment is pursued, skin-fold measurements and bioelectrical impedance in the euhydrated state usually give fairly accurate ranges of body fat in young athletes and are usually more readily accessible than other methods[51] (see Chapter 25). These calculations may then be used in conjunction with nutritional intervention to counsel young athletes regarding healthy dietary and activity choices. It is important to remember that optimal body composition parameters for athletic performance have not been determined, and specific goal setting for body composition should be avoided.[50] If body composition measures are clinically indicated, they should be obtained no more than twice per year.[50]

Principles of Weight Gain in Young Athletes

Despite the continuing epidemic of obesity in American youth, many adolescent males actively seek to gain weight. This is particularly true in American football, a sport in which players have much higher rates of overweight and obesity than population norms.[52,53] A 2005 study on community football players in Michigan demonstrated an upward drift in BMI starting at 11 years of age and median BMIs around the 90th percentile in boys 11 to 14 years of age.[52] Between 2001 and 2009, average weights for college-recruited high school offensive linemen and defensive tackles have been approximately 130 kg (286 lb).[54]

Unfortunately, this degree of obesity is also conferring significant increases in injury risk, heat illness, and early development of the metabolic syndrome.[55] Any performance benefit to weight gain needs to be tempered by concerns that excessive weight gain during childhood and adolescence often leads to a lifetime of issues with overweight and obesity, and athletic participation does not appear to protect these individuals from adverse health implications.

Adolescents who seek to gain weight should be advised to focus on gains in lean mass, while minimizing gains in fat mass. They should be aware that significant gains in lean body mass require:

1. Sufficient endogenous anabolic hormones to support hypertrophy of muscle and lean tissue.
2. Physical training (especially resistance training) sufficient to stimulate protein synthesis.
3. Sufficient carbohydrate intake to support training and minimize muscle catabolism.
4. Sufficient protein intake to support muscle repair and hypertrophy.
5. Appropriate recovery between training sessions.

A reasonable goal for most adolescents who are attempting to gain weight is approximately 1 lb of lean body mass/week. For athletes who are currently maintaining their weight, this requires an additional 300 to 400 kcal/day and maintenance of 1.5 to 1.8 g of protein/kg/day. Intakes higher than this or weight gains in excess of 1.5% of body weight/week will likely produce increased gains of fat mass.[56] See Table 12.5 for practical recommendations on weight gain in young athletes.

Table 12.5.
Strategies for Weight Gain in Young Athletes

Training:
Resistance training is a key aspect of making gains in lean mass:
   -For muscle hypertrophy: Multiple sets of 8-15 repetitions/set
   -For strength/power gain: Multiple sets of 4-6 repetitions/set
Appropriate rest:
   -Strength training for a given body part should be done on nonconsecutive days

Nutrition:
Calories:
   -Increase intake by 300-400 kcal/day over any increased expenditures
Protein:
   -Maintain 1.5-1.8 g/kg/day
Practical recommendations to attain above:
   -Increase frequency of meals/snacks
     -Do not skip breakfast
     -Aim to eat 5-9 times/day
   -Increase size of meals/portions
   -Change dietary composition to include foods with higher caloric density
Examples of ways to enhance calorie/protein content of foods in diet:
   -Enrich milk with nonfat dry milk, instant breakfast, other flavorings
   -Reconstitute canned soup with evaporated milk instead of water
   -Choose cranberry, grape, or pineapple juice instead of orange or grapefruit juice
   -Add dried fruits and/or nuts to hot cereal, sandwich fillings, etc
   -Create sandwiches with thick-sliced, dense bread instead of white
Fat: Consider increasing fat content of diet if:
   -Difficulty gaining weight or ingesting adequate calories, after implementing above recommendations
   -No contraindications/other risk factors for a higher-fat diet
Weight gain supplements (ie, "weight gainers"):
   -May provide between 500-2000 kcal/serving
     -If used as directed, will often result in excessive fat gains
   -Often with 20-35 g of protein/serving
   -Fat content variable
   -For young athletes, liquid food products (eg, Ensure, Carnation Instant Breakfast) are reasonable options
     -Regulated by Food and Drug Administration and widely available
     -2 servings/day often provide appropriate calories and protein to support lean tissue growth

III

Principles of Weight Loss in Young Athletes

Pursuit of weight loss is ubiquitous in American culture for both health and aesthetic reasons, and this can be particularly problematic for some females. Weight issues in athletes are often compounded by the perception in some sports that competing at the lowest possible weight is advantageous. This may be attributable to appearance concerns (particularly in aesthetic sports, such as gymnastics or figure skating), increased strength-to-mass ratio, or the desire to compete in a lower weight class. Weight loss practices of athletes can be generally divided into those techniques that produce rapid loss of fluid weight (ie, dehydration, also known as "cutting weight"), and those that result in more gradual reductions in lean tissue or fat mass.

Rapid loss of fluid weight is potentially life threatening and has been a particular problem in the sport of wrestling. In 1995, the National Federation of State High School Associations (NFHS) began a weight control program to minimize the weight loss fluctuations seen in many scholastic wrestlers and to certify an appropriate and healthy weight class for each wrestler. In 1998, the NFHS disallowed any means of achieving rapid weight loss. The current program for weight certification in high school wrestling varies from state to state, but several fundamentals are applicable nationwide:

1. Body composition (while appropriately hydrated) is obtained by an appropriately trained school or health professional before the beginning of the competitive season and is the foundation for calculating weight class and allowed rates of weight loss.
2. Weight class needs to accommodate a minimum of 7% body fat for high school males and 12% body fat for high school females.
3. Rate of weight loss may not exceed 1.5% of body weight/week.

A variety of weight-loss practices are used to produce longer term changes in body mass. Athletes who desire to lose weight should be instructed to avoid significant loss of lean mass, because this may lead to possible reductions in strength and performance as well as a reduction in caloric expenditure because of resulting decreases in resting metabolic rate. Protein intakes in the range of 2 g/kg/day appear more effective than lower levels of protein intake in helping maintain lean mass during periods of weight reduction.[57] In athletes who are currently maintaining their weight, weight loss should not exceed 1.5% of total body weight/week (usually 1-2 lb/week).[56] Weight loss of 1 lb/week requires a caloric deficit of 3500 kcal/week, which is best obtained by a combination of a reduction in caloric intake and an increase in caloric expenditure.

Once weight goals are met, weight maintenance should be emphasized. Cyclic fluctuations in weight should be strongly discouraged, because they tend to produce significant decreases in metabolic rate and lean body mass over time.

AAP

Promotion of Healthy Weight-Control Practices in Young Athletes

1. Physicians who care for young athletes should have knowledge of healthy weight-gain and weight-loss methods. They should understand minimal recommended weight, normal growth curves, and body composition measurements and be willing to educate athletes, families, coaches, athletic trainers, school administrators, and state and national organizations when appropriate. Physicians should understand that all athletes are unique and each athlete must be evaluated individually.

2. All physical examinations of young athletes should include a weight history and a history of eating patterns, hydration practices, eating disorders, heat illness, and other factors that may influence heat illness or weight control.

3. Physicians should be able to recognize early signs and symptoms of an eating disorder and obtain appropriate medical, psychological, and nutritional consultation for young athletes with these symptoms.

4. Nutritional needs for growth and development must be placed above athletic considerations. Fluid or food deprivation should never be allowed. There is no substitute for a healthy diet consisting of a variety of foods from all food groups with enough energy (calories) to support growth, daily physical activities, and sports activities. Daily caloric intake for most athletes should consist of a minimum of 8400 kJ (2000 kcal). Athletes need to consume enough fluids to maintain euhydration. Physicians should engage the services of a registered dietitian familiar with athletes to help with weight-control issues.

5. In sports for which weigh-ins are required, athletes' weight and body composition should be assessed once or twice per year. The most important assessment is obtained before the beginning of the sport season. This should include a determination of body fat and minimal allowable weight when the athlete is adequately hydrated (the National Wrestling Coaches' Association [NWCA] Internet Weight Classification Program is available at www.nwcaonline.com or by calling 717-653-8009). Weigh-ins for competition should be performed immediately before competition. Athletes should be permitted to compete in championship tournaments only at the weight class in which they have competed for most other athletic events that year.

6. Male high school athletes should not have less than 7% body fat. This minimal allowable body fat may be too low for some athletes and result in suboptimal performance. Female athletes should consume enough energy (calories) and nutrients to meet their energy requirements and experience normal menses. There are no recommendations on body-fat percentages in female athletes.

III

7. A program for the purpose of gaining or losing weight should (a) be started early to permit a gradual weight gain or loss over a realistic time period, (b) permit a change of 1.5% or less of one's body weight per week, (c) permit the loss of weight to be fat loss and the gain of weight to be muscle mass, (d) be coupled with an appropriate training program (both strength and conditioning), and (e) incorporate a well-balanced diet with adequate energy (calories), carbohydrates, protein, and fat. After athletes obtain their desired weight, they should be encouraged to maintain a constant weight and avoid fluctuations of weight. A weight-loss plan for athletic purposes should never be instituted before the 9th grade.

8. Any athlete who loses a significant amount of fluid during sports participation should weigh in before and after practices, games, meets, and competitions. Each pound of weight loss should be replaced with 1 pt of fluid containing carbohydrates and electrolytes before the next practice or competition. Fluids should be available, and the drinking of such should be encouraged at all practices and competitions.

9. Weight loss accomplished by overexercising; using rubber suits, steam baths, or saunas; prolonged fasting; fluid reduction; vomiting; or using anorexic drugs, laxatives, diuretics, diet pills, insulin, stimulants, nutritional supplements, or other legal or illegal drugs and/or nicotine should be prohibited at all ages.

10. Athletes who need to gain weight should consult their physician for resources on healthy weight gain and referral to a registered dietitian. They should be discouraged from gaining excessive weight, which may impair performance, increase the likelihood of heat illness, and increase the risk of developing complications from obesity.

11. Ergogenic aids and nontherapeutic use of supplements for weight management should be prohibited.

12. Young athletes should be involved in a total athletic program that includes acquisition of athletic skills and improvement in speed, flexibility, strength, and physical conditioning while maintaining good nutrition and normal hydration. This should be done under the supervision of a coach who stresses a positive attitude, character building, teamwork, and safety.

American Academy of Pediatrics, Committee on Sports Medicine and Fitness. Promotion of healthy weight-control practices in young athletes. *Pediatrics*. 2005;116(6):1557-1564

Vegetarian Athletes

In a 2005 nationwide survey, 3% of 8- to 18-year-olds were vegetarian, and almost 1% in this age group were vegan.[58] Although questions are often raised about athletic performance in vegetarians, limited studies show that vegetarian athletes who consume a well-planned diet demonstrate no difference in athletic performance compared with their omnivorous peers.[6] The challenge in a diet devoid of meat or animal products is the greater effort required to ensure daily intake of a full complement of essential amino acids and adequate amounts of vitamins B_{12} and D, riboflavin, zinc, and calcium.[6] Non-heme iron sources in the vegetarian diet are relatively poorly absorbed, and vegetarian athletes may be at higher risk of iron deficiency states. Some experts recommend routine monitoring of iron status in vegetarian athletes, particularly during periods of rapid growth.[6]

The amount of planning required to meet nutritional recommendations may be difficult for many vegetarian children and adolescents. However, as long as nutritional requirements are met, the dietary source does not seem to matter in terms of supporting athletic performance. Many vegetarian athletes, particularly at higher performance levels, may benefit from consultation with a sports nutritionist.[6] Registered sports nutritionists can be located at www.scandpg.org.

Dietary Supplements/Ergogenic Aids

Comparison and competition among peers is an inevitable part of youth and adolescence. This is especially true in the realm of sports and athletic participation, in which the desire for competitive advantage, or for rapid performance gains, may lead to experimentation with a variety of ergogenic aids. This often includes a number of dietary supplements. In a 2007 multistate survey, 71% of 8th through 12th grade students reported use of dietary supplements.[59] The most frequent supplements in use were multivitamins, reported by 59%, and energy drinks, reported by 32%. Supplement use increased significantly with grade, and with the exception of weight loss aids, boys used supplements more frequently than girls.

Despite the prevalence of supplement use, there is a paucity of data on the safety and efficacy of dietary supplements in young athletes. Knowledge of the effects of performance-enhancing aids is based almost solely on studies in adults, which may or may not be applicable to the pediatric population. The American Academy of Pediatrics (AAP) has taken a firm stand against the use of performance-enhancing substances in young athletes, citing both safety and ethical concerns.[60] The AAP states that pediatricians should directly ask their athletic patients about supplement use and should be prepared to provide unbiased information about risks and benefits.

> **AAP**
>
> # Use of Performance-Enhancing Substances
>
> 1. Use of performance-enhancing substances for athletic or other purposes should be strongly discouraged.
> 2. Parents should take a strong stand against the use of performance-enhancing substances and, whenever possible, demand that coaches be educated about the adverse health effects of performance-enhancing substances.
> 3. Schools and other sports organizations should be proactive in discouraging the use of performance-enhancing substances, incorporating this message into policy and educational materials for coaches, parents, and athletes.
> 4. Interventions for encouraging substance-free competition should be developed that are more positive than punitive, such as programs that teach sound nutrition and training practices along with skills to resist the social pressures to use performance-enhancing substances.
> 5. Colleges, schools, and sports clubs should make use of educational interventions that encourage open and frank discussion of issues related to the use of performance-enhancing substances, with the aim of promoting decisions about personal drug use based on principles of fair competition and character rather than on the fear of getting caught.
> 6. Coaches at all levels, including youth sports, should encourage wholesome and fair competition by emphasizing healthy nutrition and training practices, taking a strong stand against cheating, and avoiding the "win-at-all-costs" philosophy.
> 7. Inquiries about the use of performance-enhancing substances should be made in a manner similar to inquiries about use of tobacco, alcohol, or other substances of abuse. Guidelines for patient confidentiality should be followed and explained to the patient.
> 8. Athletes who admit using performance-enhancing substances should be provided unbiased medical information about benefits, known adverse effects, and other risks. When appropriate, additional testing may be necessary to investigate or rule out adverse medical effects.
> 9. The pediatric health care professional providing care for an athlete who admits to using a performance-enhancing substance should explore the athlete's motivations for using these substances, evaluate other associated high-risk behaviors, and provide counseling on safer, more appropriate alternatives for meeting fitness or sports-performance goals.
> 10. Nonusers of performance-enhancing substances should have their decisions reinforced while establishing an open channel of communication if questions about performance-enhancing substances arise in the future.
> 11. Pediatric health care professionals should promote safe physical activity and sports participation by providing or making available sound medical information on exercise physiology, conditioning, nutrition, weight management, and injury prevention and by helping to care for sports-related medical conditions and injuries.
>
> American Academy of Pediatrics, Committee on Sports Medicine and Fitness. Use of performance-enhancing substances. *Pediatrics*. 2005;115(4):1103-1106

Caffeine/Energy Drinks

Caffeine is arguably the most popular performance-enhancing agent in current use and is well known for its stimulant properties. In the United States, the average daily intake of caffeine is1 mg/kg/day in children and 3 mg/kg/day in adults, and in a 2004 study, 27% of adolescent athletes admitted to use of caffeine specifically for performance enhancement.[61] Previously, the dominant source of caffeine for children was soft drinks[18]; however, given the recent rapid growth of beverages in the "energy drink" category, it is unclear whether this is still the case. Although there is no formal definition for the term "energy drink," it is generally recognized as a flavored beverage containing relatively high amounts of caffeine, guarana, or other stimulants. See Table 12.6 for comparison of caffeine amounts found in common energy drinks and other beverages.

Table 12.6.
Comparison of Caffeine Contained in Energy Drinks With Amounts Found in Other Common Sources of Dietary Caffeine

Product	Caffeine Content (mg/"usual" serving size)
Coffee (drip)	100 mg/8oz
Starbucks Grande Mocha	175 mg/16 oz
Mountain Dew	46-55 mg/12 oz
Coca Cola	30-35 mg/12 oz
Diet Coke	38-47 mg/12 oz
Red Bull Energy Drink	80 mg/8 oz
Monster Energy Drink	140 mg/16 oz
SoBe No Fear Energy Drink	174 mg/16 oz
Jolt Energy	280 mg/23.5 oz
Energy "shots" (multiple brands)	200-350 mg/1-2oz

Energy drinks are now aggressively marketed to children and adolescents, and many companies are utilizing athletes in these marketing campaigns. Young athletes often do not recognize the difference between an energy drink, which is formulated for performance enhancement, versus a sports drink, which is formulated for rehydration; but it is an important distinction. The AAP states that energy drinks have no place in the diets of children and adolescents.[18] See the section on fluids for more information about sports drinks.

> ## AAP
>
> ### Sports Drinks and Energy Drinks for Children and Adolescents: Are They Appropriate?
>
> 1. Improve the education of children and adolescents and their parents in the area of sports and energy drinks. This education must highlight the difference between sports drinks and energy drinks and their associated potential health risks.
> 2. Understand that energy drinks pose potential health risks primarily because of stimulant content; therefore, they are not appropriate for children and adolescents and should never be consumed.
> 3. Counsel that routine ingestion of carbohydrate-containing sports drinks by children and adolescents should be avoided or restricted. Intake can lead to excessive caloric consumption and an increased risk of overweight and obesity as well as dental erosion.
> 4. Educate patients and families that sports drinks have a specific limited function for child and adolescent athletes. These drinks should be ingested when there is a need for more rapid replenishment of carbohydrates and/or electrolytes in combination with water during periods of prolonged, vigorous sports participation, or other intense physical activity.
> 5. Promote water, not sports or energy drinks, as the principal source of hydration for children and adolescents.
>
> American Academy of Pediatrics Committee on Nutrition and Council on Sports Medicine and Fitness. Sports drinks and energy drinks for children and adolescents: are they appropriate? *Pediatrics*. 2011; 127(6):1182-1189

One of the reasons caffeine is such a popular ergogenic aid is that it is effective. Caffeine has long been recognized as enhancing endurance performance by approximately 3% to 5%, but there is more recent work suggesting a possible benefit in shorter activities as well. A recent review reported performance gains with speed events lasting 60 to 180 seconds in duration as well as in studies that reproduced the short, intermittent bursts of activity that are typically seen in youth sports.[62] The performance benefit in these sprinting activities was less than 3%. Ergogenic doses of caffeine may be as low as 1 to 2 mg/kg, but more commonly studied doses are in the range of 3 to 6 mg/kg.[63]

Multiple adverse effects have been reported and studied with caffeine. Previous concerns about direct effects of caffeine on bone density and thermoregulation appear to be unfounded.[64,65] Although caffeine does induce a transient diuresis in individuals at rest, this does not persist for more than several hours and does not occur with exercise.[66] Although sinus tachycardia is common, ventricular arrhythmias do not appear to be significantly increased with moderate caffeine dosages.[67]

The most significant concerns regarding caffeine use in the young athlete appear to be issues of acute toxicity, chronic dependency, and possibly "gateway" concerns regarding future use of additional ergogenic aids or substances of abuse. Symptoms of toxicity typically include agitation, nausea/vomiting, dizziness, and tachycardia. In addition, case reports of caffeine toxicity include new onset seizures, acute mania, stroke, and death after excessive use of energy drinks.[68] Toxic doses appear to be highly variable and difficult to determine, because many products do not disclose caffeine content in their product. Children and adolescents who have not developed tolerance to caffeine's effects are particularly vulnerable.[68]

Dependency is a common problem, and withdrawal symptoms often start 12 to 24 hours after the last dose. Headache is the most common withdrawal symptom and is seen in approximately 50% of dependent users, but withdrawal can also include a variety of other generalized symptoms such as fatigue, dysphoria, and irritability. Symptoms can be severe enough to impair daily function in up to 13%.[68] Although causation is difficult to prove, there is an association between use of caffeine and subsequent use of tobacco products, alcohol, and anabolic agents.[68,69]

Protein and Amino Acid Supplements

Protein and amino acid supplementation is very common in young athletes. Complete protein supplements (ie, containing all of the essential amino acids) typically contain 20 to 40 g of protein/serving and are typically categorized by their food source. The most common include whey-, casein-, and soy-based products. Whey protein is typically marketed as being more rapidly metabolized and producing higher muscle synthetic rates. Although some studies have supported this assertion,[70] others have not.[71] Many experts currently believe that any complete, high-quality protein source will produce similar results and that there is no advantage to protein obtained from supplements over that obtained from whole food.[6,8,26]

Common amino acid supplements marketed to athletes are glutamine, arginine, and carnitine as well as mixtures of branched-chain and essential amino acids. Current evidence does not support use of individual amino acids as performance enhancers, and caution is warranted, because ingestion of an excess of one amino acid may impair the absorption of others. Amino acid mixtures have no advantage over equivalent protein amounts found in whole foods.[6]

Convenience is the primary advantage of protein supplements, although cost, taste, and potential issues of product quality and purity are the primary drawbacks. Athletes and parents typically perceive supplements as being very high in protein content; however, a serving of most supplements contains the same amount of protein as a 3- to 4-ounce serving of lean meat or poultry (see Table 12.3). One low-cost way to supplement protein for athletes who have difficulty achieving optimal intake is to enrich foods or beverages in the diet with nonfat powdered milk. This provides 3 g of protein per 2 tablespoons of powder, which may be added to milk, cereal, sandwiches, pasta sauce, etc.

"Weight Gainers"

These popular supplements are often higher-calorie versions of the protein supplements described previously, and their content is highly variable. Carbohydrates and/ or fats are added to increase the calorie count, with some preparations containing up to 2000 kcals/serving. They are often supplemented with significant amounts of vitamins and minerals and may contain additional herbal or other ingredients as well. The instructions for these products often direct the consumer to drink 1 to 2 servings/day in addition to regular meals. However, as described in the earlier section on weight gain, this caloric increase will typically result in significant increases in fat mass, which is often not the desired effect. See Table 12.5 for additional recommendations on weight gain.

Creatine

Creatine is a metabolite of arginine that has found widespread use among athletes as a dietary supplement. More than 90% of the body's store of creatine is found in skeletal muscle, where it serves as an energy source with initiation of high-intensity physical activity. Creatine is both ingested in the diet and also endogenously synthesized. Meat, fish, and poultry contain 2 to 5 g of creatine/lb, and the average US omnivorous diet contains approximately 1 g of creatine/day. Approximately 1 to 2 g of creatine/day are synthesized in the liver.

It is important to recognize that muscle has a finite carrying capacity for creatine and that any excess is excreted in the urine as creatinine. Several dosing patterns for maximizing muscle creatine have emerged, as follows:

Loading and maintenance:

Load: 20 g/day (5 g, 4 times/day) for 5 to 7 days

Maintenance: 2 g/day for 4 to 16 weeks

Low dose:

Daily: 2 to 3 g/day (demonstrated to increase intramuscular creatine over course of a month and maintain levels during supplementation)

It is important to note that some adolescents on an omnivorous diet may already be ingesting these maintenance doses of creatine in their daily diets and would not be expected to realize significant changes in creatine concentrations with additional supplementation.

Studies examining creatine use reveal much higher usage rates in boys than in girls, with increasing use throughout the high school years. A 2007 multistate survey revealed that 8% of 9th-grade boys reported creatine use, as compared with 22% of 12th-grade boys.[59] Prevalence of creatine use in 12th-grade girls was 1%.

Creatine is fairly unique among current "purported" ergogenic aids in that the body of evidence appears to favor some performance benefit but primarily in activities of <30 seconds' duration and with improvements typically on the order of 1% to 2%.[63] Creatine use is often accompanied by a 1.5-kg weight gain within the first 5 to 7 days of administration. Although this acute increase is primarily water, subsequent significant increases in lean tissue have often been seen in subjects who used creatine compared with placebo in conjunction with resistance training.[63] It is currently believed that this reflects the increased training capacity with creatine secondary to its effect in ATP regeneration. Although this fairly rapid increase in weight may be considered undesirable by many females and may be ergolytic in many sports, it is often very convincing to strength-trained young males that they are achieving their desired goals with creatine use and can make dissuasion of further use difficult.

Gastric upset is the most common adverse effect with creatine use and is reported in approximately 5% of users.[63] There have been published case reports linking creatine to cases of renal damage, elevated blood pressure, and possible deaths resulting from dehydration and heat illness. However, when reviewing the literature critically, many of these case reports have had other plausible and significant risk factors,[63] and a recent meta-analysis did not find evidence of creatine contributing significant risk to issues with heat or hydration.[72]

When discussing creatine use with young athletes and families, it is important to recognize the following:

- Benefit appears to occur only with repeat, anaerobic efforts.
- This benefit is only on the order of 1% to 2% (which will be undetectable by the vast majority of young athletes).
- Although creatine appears to be safe in studies of adults, there is no prospective literature evaluating safety data in children and adolescents.

Other Supplements

The evidence-based literature cannot keep up with the pace of development and the dissemination of information about dietary supplements and ergogenic aids. The Internet is a common source of nutritional information and misinformation for young athletes, and location of an appropriate Internet resource can be very helpful for the health care professional as well as for the athlete and his or her family. Two reputable Web sites include:

- www.nal.usda.gov/fnic. "Dietary supplements" and "ergogenic aids" serve as portals for a spectrum of information sources on dietary supplements and performance enhancing aids.

- www.thatsdope.org. A Web site designed by the United States Anti-Doping Agency (USADA) for adolescent and young adult athletes. USADA strongly opposes use of any ergogenic agents in sport. The Web site provides information and encourages critical thinking on issues related to sports nutrition and performance enhancement; www.usantidoping.org/education/youth is another USADA Web site with similar content but formatted for a preadolescent audience).

In young athletes, the most powerful combination for improving athletic performance includes: nutrition fundamentals, appropriate coaching and practice, and the onset of puberty. Although it is important to emphasize to athletes and their families that the vast majority of ergogenic claims by commercial products are unfounded, it is also important to acknowledge supplements that have been shown to be effective, such as caffeine and creatine. However, the 1% to 3% performance benefits that are reported in studies will not be detectable in the vast majority of adolescent athletes and will not likely translate to improved "on field" performance in the young athlete. The changes in strength, speed, endurance, and athletic proficiency that come with maturation and practice dwarfs even the most optimistic results of performance enhancement with any dietary supplement.

References

1. Eaton DK, Kann L, Kinchen S, et al. Youth Risk Behavior Surveillance—United States, 2009. *MMWR Surveill Summ.* 2010;59(SS-5):1-142
2. Stricker P. *Sports Success Rx! Your Child's Prescription for the Best Experience: How to Maximize Potential and Minimize Pressure.* Elk Grove Village, IL: American Academy of Pediatrics; 2006
3. Aucouturier J, Baker JS, Duche P. Fat and carbohydrate metabolism during submaximal exercise in children. *Sports Med.* 2008;38(3):213-238
4. Riddell MC. The endocrine response and substrate utilization during exercise in children and adolescents. *J Appl Physiol.* 2008;105(2):725-733
5. Institute of Medicine. *Dietary Reference Intakes for Energy, Carbohydrate, Fiber, Fat, Fatty Acids, Cholesterol, Protein and Amino Acids (Macronutrients).* Washington, DC: Then National Academies Press; 2005. Available at: http://www.nap.edu/catalog.php?record_id=10490. Accessed October 9, 2012
6. Position of the American Dietetic Association, Dietitians of Canada, and the American College of Sports Medicine. Nutrition and athletic performance. *J Am Diet Assoc.* 2009;109(3):509-527
7. Sedlock DA. The latest on carbohydrate loading: a practical approach. *Curr Sports Med Rep.* 2008;7(4):209-213
8. Kreider RB, Wilborn CD, Taylor L, et al. ISSN exercise and sport nutrition review: research and recommendations. *J Int Soc Sports Nutr.* 2010;7:7

9. Kerksick C, Harvey T, Stout J, et al. International Society of Sports Nutrition position stand: nutrient timing. *J Intl Soc Sports Nutr.* 2008;5:17

10. Donaldson CM, Perry TL, Rose MC. Glycemic index and endurance performance. *Int J Sport Nutr Exerc Metab.* 2010;20(2):154-165

11. Burke LM, Hawley JA, Wong SH, Jeukendrup AE. Carbohydrates for training and competition. *J Sports Sci.* 2011;29(Suppl 1):S17-S27

12. Currell K, Jeukendrup AE. Superior endurance performance with ingestion of multiple transportable carbohydrates. *Med Sci Sports Exerc.* 2008;40(2):275-281

13. Howarth KR, Moreau NA, Phillips SM, Gibala MJ. Coingestion of protein with carbohydrate during recovery from endurance exercise stimulates skeletal muscle protein synthesis in humans. *J Appl Physiol.* 2009;106(4):1394-1402

14. Bergeron MF, Laird MD, Marinik EL, et al. Repeated-bout exercise in the heat in young athletes: physiological strain and perceptual responses. *J Appl Physiol.* 2009;106(2): 476-485

15. Iuliano S, Naughton G, Collier G, Carlson J. Examination of the self-selected fluid intake practices by junior athletes during a simulated duathlon event. *Int J Sport Nutr.* 1998;8(1):10-23

16. Palmer MS, Logan HM, Spriet LL. On-ice sweat rate, voluntary fluid intake, and sodium balance during practice in male junior ice hockey players drinking water or a carbohydrate-electrolyte solution. *Appl Physiol Nutr Metab.* 2010;35(3):328-335

17. Montain SJ. Hydration recommendations for sport 2008. *Curr Sports Med Rep.* 2008;7(4):187-192

18. American Academy of Pediatrics, Committee on Nutrition and Council on Sports Medicine and Fitness. Clinical report-sports drinks and energy drinks for children and adolescents: are they appropriate? *Pediatrics.* 2011;127(6):1182-1189

19. Leiper JB, Nicholas CW, Ali A, Williams C, Maughan RJ. The effect of intermittent high-intensity running on gastric emptying of fluids in man. *Med Sci Sports Exerc.* 2005;37(2):240-247

20. Siegel AJ, d'Hemecourt P, Adner MM, et al. Exertional dysnatremia in collapsed marathon runners: a critical role for point-of-care testing to guide appropriate therapy. *Am J Clin Pathol.* 2009;132(3):336-340

21. Von Duvillard SP, Arciero PJ, Tietjen-Smith T, Alford K. Sports drinks, exercise training and competition. *Curr Sports Med Rep.* 2008;7(4):202-208

22. Evans GH, Shirreffs SM, Maughan RJ. Postexercise rehydration in man: the effects of osmolality and carbohydrate content of ingested drinks. *Nutrition.* 2009;25(9):905-913

23. Ferguson-Stegall L, McCleave EL, Ding Z, et al. Postexercise carbohydrate-protein supplementation improves subsequent exercise performance and intracellular signaling for protein synthesis. *J Strength Cond Res.* 2011;25(5):1210-1224

24. Roy BD. Milk: the new sports drink? A review. *J Int Soc Sports Nutr.* 2008;2:5-15

25. Campbell B, Kreider RB, Ziegenfuss T, et al. International Society of Sports Nutrition position stand: protein and exercise. *J Int Soc Sports Nutr.* 2007;4(8):5-17

26. Kumar V, Atherton P, Smith K, Rennie MJ. Human muscle protein synthesis and breakdown during and after exercise. *J Appl Physiol.* 2009;106(6):2026-2039

III

27. Miller BF. Human muscle protein synthesis after physical activity and feeding. *Exerc Sports Sci Rev*. 2007;35(22):50-55

28. Rodenberg RE, Gustafson S. Iron as en ergogenic aid: ironclad evidence? *Curr Sports Med Rep*. 2007;6(4):258-264

29. Tenforde AS, Sayres LC, Sainani KL, Fredericson M. Evaluating the relationship of calcium and vitamin D in the prevention of stress fracture injuries in the young athlete: a review of the literature. *PM R*. 2010;2(10):945-949

30. International Olympic Committee Position Stand: Female athlete triad. IOC Medical Commission Working Group Women in Sport. International Olympic Committee. Available at: http://www.olympic.org/Documents/Reports/EN/en_report_917.pdf. Accessed October 9, 2012

31. Kara E, Gunay M, Cicioglu I, et al. Effect of zinc supplementation on antioxidant activity in young wrestlers. *Biol Trace Elem Res*. 2010;134(1):55-56

32. Volpe SL. Minerals as ergogenic aids. *Curr Sports Med Rep*. 2008;7(4):224-229

33. Roberts LA, Beattie K, Close GL, Morton JP. Vitamin C consumption does not impair training-induced improvements in exercise performance. *Int J Sports Physiol Perform*. 2011;6(1):58-69

34. Yfanti C, Akerström T, Nielsen S, et al. Antioxidant supplementation does not alter endurance training adaptation. *Med Sci Sports Exerc*. 2010;42(7):1388-1395

35. McGinley C, Shafat A, Donnelly AE. Does antioxidant vitamin supplementation protect against muscle damage? *Sports Med*. 2009;239(12):1011-1032

36. Walsh NP, Gleeson M, Pyne DB, et al. Position statement. Part two: maintaining immune health. *Exerc Immunol Rev*. 2011;17:64-103

37. Hemilä H, Chalker E, Douglas B. Vitamin C for preventing and treating the common cold. *Cochrane Database Syst Rev*. 2007;(3):CD000980

38. Constantini NW, Dubnov-Raz G, Eyal BB, et al. The effect of vitamin C on upper respiratory infections in adolescent swimmers: a randomized trial. *Eur J Pediatr*. 2011;170(1):59-63

39. Constantini NW, Dubnov-Raz G, Chodick G, et al. Physical activity and bone mineral density in adolescents with vitamin D deficiency. *Med Sci Sports Exerc*. 2010;42(4):646-650

40. Chatzipapas C, Boikos S, Drosos GI, et al. Polymorphisms of the vitamin D receptor gene and stress fractures. *Hormone Metab Res*. 2009;41(8):635-640

41. Burgi AA, Gorham ED, Garland CF, et al. High serum 25-hydroxyvitamin D is associated with low incidence of stress fractures. *J Bone Miner Res*. 2011;26(10):2371-2377

42. Lappe J, Cullen D, Haynatzki G, et al. Calcium and vitamin D supplementation decreases incidence of stress fractures in female navy recruits. *J Bone Mineral Res*. 2009;23(5):741-749

43. Nieves JW, Melsop K, Curtis M, et al. Nutritional factors that influence change in bone density and stress fracture risk among young female cross-country runners. *PM R*. 2010;2(8):740-50

44. Larson-Meyer DE, Willis KS. Vitamin D and athletes. *Curr Sports Med Rep*. 2010;9(4):220-226

45. Pfeifer M, Begerow B, Minne HW. Vitamin D and muscle function. *Osteoporos Int.* 2002;13(3):187-189

46. Ward KA, Das G, Berry JL. Vitamin D status and muscle function in post-menarchal adolescent girls. *J Clin Endocrinol Metab.* 2009;94(2):559-563

47. Bartoszewska M, Kamboj M, Patel DR. Vitamin D, muscle function, and exercise performance. *Pediatr Clin N Am.* 2010;57(3):849-861

48. Constantini NW, Arieli R, Chodick G, Dubnov-Raz G. High prevalence of vitamin D insufficiency in athletes and dancers. *Clin J Sport Med.* 2010;20(5):368-371

49. Lovell G. Vitamin D status of females in an elite gymnastics program. *Clin J Sport Med.* 2008;18(2):159-161

50. National Collegiate Athletic Association. *NCAA 2010-2011 Sports Medicine Handbook.* Indianapolis, IN: National Collegiate Athletic Association; 2010. Available at: http://www.ncaapublications.com/productdownloads/MD11.pdf. Accessed October 9, 2012

51. Portal S, Rabinowitz J, Adler-Portal D, et al. Body fat measurements in elite adolescent volleyball players: correlation between skinfold thickness, bioelectrical impedance analysis, air-displacement plethysmography, and body mass index percentiles. *J Pediatr Endocrinol Metab.* 2010;23(4):395-400

52. Malina RM, Morano PJ, Barron M, et al. Growth status and estimated growth rate of youth football players: a community-based study. *Clin J Sport Med.* 2005;15(3):125-132

53. Malina RM, Morano PJ, Barron M, et al. Overweight and obesity among youth participants in American football. *J Pediatr.* 2007;151(4):378-382

54. Ghigiarelli JJ. Combine performance descriptors and predictors of recruit ranking for the top high school football recruits from 2001 to 2009: differences between position groups. *J Strength Cond Res.* 2011;25(5):1193-1203

55. Buell JL, Calland D, Hanks F, et al. Presence of metabolic syndrome in football linemen. *J Athl Train.* 2008;43(6):608-616

56. American Academy of Pediatrics, Committee on Sports Medicine and Fitness. Promotion of health weight-control practices in young athletes. *Pediatrics.* 2005;166(6):1557-1564

57. Mettler S, Mitchell N, Tipton KD. Increased protein intake reduces lean body mass loss during weight loss in athletes. *Med Sci Sports Exerc.* 2010;42(2):326-337

58. American Dietetic Association. Position of the American Dietetic Association: vegetarian diets. *J Am Diet Assoc.* 2009;109(7):1266-1282

59. Hoffman JR, Faigenbaum AD, Ratamess NA, et al. Nutritional supplementation and anabolic steroid use in adolescents. *Med Sci Sports Exerc.* 2008;40(1):15-24

60. American Academy of Pediatrics, Committee on Sports Medicine and Fitness. Use of performance-enhancing substances. *Pediatrics.* 2005;115(4):1103-1106

61. Babu KM, Church RJ, Lewander W. Energy drinks: the new eye-opener for adolescents. *Clin Pediatr Emerg Med.* 2008;9:35-42

62. Davis JK, Green JM. Caffeine and anaerobic performance: ergogenic value and mechanisms of action. *Sports Med.* 2009;39(10):813-832

63. Tarnopolsky MA. Caffeine and creatine use in sport. *Ann Nutr Metab.* 2010;57(Suppl 2):1-8

64. Del Coso J, Estevez E, Mora-Rodriguez R. Caffeine during exercise in the heat: thermoregulation and fluid-electrolyte balance. *Med Sci Sports Exerc*. 2009;41(1): 164-173

65. Rafferty K, Heaney RP. Nutrient effects on the calcium economy: emphasizing the potassium controversy. *J Nutr*. 2008;138(1):166S-171S

66. Ganio MS, Casa DJ, Armstrong LE, Maresh CM. Evidence-based approach to lingering hydration questions. *Clin Sports Med*. 2007;26(1):1-16

67. Myers MG. Caffeine and cardiac arrhythmias. *Ann Intern Med*. 1991;114(2):147-150

68. Reissig CJ, Strain EC, Griffiths RR. Caffeinated energy drinks – a growing problem. *Drug Alcohol Depend*. 2009;99(1-3):1-10

69. Dodge TL, Jaccard JJ. The effect of high school sports participation on the use of performance-enhancing substances in young adulthood. *J Adolesc Health*. 2006;39(3):367-373

70. Tang JE, Moore DR, Kujbida GW, et al. Ingestion of whey hydrolysate, casein, or soy protein isolate: effects on mixed muscle protein synthesis at rest and following resistance exercise in young men. *J Appl Physiol*. 2009;107(3):987-992

71. Tipton KD, Elliott TA, Cree MG, Wolf SE, Sanford AP, Wolfe RR. Ingestion of casein and whey proteins result in muscle anabolism after resistance exercise. *Med Sci Sports Exerc*. 2004;36(12):2073-2081

72. Lopez RM, Casa DJ, McDermott BP, et al. Does creatine supplementation hinder heat tolerance or hydration status? A systematic review with meta-analyses. *J Athl Train*. 2009;44(2):215-23

Chapter 13

Fast Foods, Organic Foods, Fad Diets, and Herbs, Herbals, and Botanicals

Fast Food

Fast Food Overview

Most people have a mental image of what fast food is; however, there is no standard definition. If you ask a child in Vietnam, he is likely to point to a street vendor selling Pho; if you ask a child in Peru, she is likely to tell you it is anticuchos, a spicy bit of grilled beef heart sold on a skewer on the street. In the United States, however, fast food and fast food restaurants are associated with hamburgers, French fries, and sweetened beverages; hot dogs or other sandwiches; pizza; and fried chicken. Orders can be placed and picked up within a few minutes and be taken away or consumed on the premises. Generally, fast food is eaten without cutlery, and fast food restaurants have no wait staff. Failure to have a standardized definition makes it difficult to compare studies or to set standards.

The origin of the fast food restaurant is unclear, but some food historians believe the first fast food restaurants were the Harvey Houses along the Santa Fe Railroad beginning in 1879, where food was served and consumed quickly by travelers. The growth of the "fast food" industry in this country has been phenomenal. Now, there are an estimated 160 000 fast food restaurants in the United States, serving more than 50 million Americans daily.[1] Fast food outlets are ubiquitous and found in local communities, public schools, military bases, and even hospitals.

In 2010, 47.9% of food dollars spent in the United States were spent away from home; there were approximately $594 billion in total expenditures outside the home, and 37.5% of these monies were spent in "limited-service eating places."[2] These figures are well up from the 25% spent on food away from home in 1970.[3] Using data from the Continuing Survey of Food Intake by Individuals (1994-1996, 1998), the proportion of children 4 to 8 years of age, 9 to 13 years of age, and 14 to 19 years of age consuming fast food on a typical day was 24.6%, 26.4%, and 39.0%, respectively.[4] Another study reported that 48% of California adolescents surveyed had consumed fast food one day prior to the survey. These data suggest that adolescents are the principal consumers of fast food.

Characteristics of Fast Food

Food consumed away from home is generally lower in dietary fiber, calcium, and iron and higher in energy, total and saturated fatty acids, cholesterol, sugars, and sodium than is food consumed at home,[4-9] and fast food restaurant meals have different quantities of fat and calories than do meals at full-service restaurants.[10] Fast food restaurants tend to promote meals low in fruits, vegetables, and dairy products,[11] although this is changing as the available menu items have changed to include more fruit, salad, and dairy options.

Fast food restaurants also tend to provide large portions of foods. Portion sizes are a critical issue for controlling energy intake. A single restaurant portion may offer close to the recommended daily number of food group servings in a single entree only. In infants, toddlers, and children up to 3 years of age, food intake is self-regulated.[12] By 4 years of age, larger portion sizes lead to increased consumption.[13] Fisher et al demonstrated that children consumed 25% more of an entree when a large portion was presented on their plates.[14] In general, the amount of food on a plate influenced consumption and lessened self-regulation of intake; in a restaurant setting, large portion sizes contributed to increased energy intake.[15] Portion size and energy density of food acted independently to increase intake.[16]

The Effect That Fast Food Has on Energy and Nutrient Intakes in the Diets of Children

Children consumed approximately 30% to 42% of energy from food away from home.[4,5,7,17] Food consumed away from home was associated with higher energy intakes and compromised diet quality, as measured by the Healthy Eating Index (HEI), especially in adolescents 13 to 18 years old. Sweetened beverages contributed to approximately 35% of this energy and approximately 20% of the decline in HEI scores. However, even after controlling for sweetened beverages, away-from-home meals contributed an extra 65 kcal to the diets of all children and 107 kcal to the diets of older children and lowered diet quality by 4%.[7] Table 13.1A shows the daily intake of food at home and away from home by children 2 to 19 years of age at different locations. Table 13.1A clearly demonstrates that fast foods contribute few servings of fruits, vegetables, whole grains, and dairy foods to the diets of children who consume them. Fast food is also high in added sugars and discretionary fats. It is also clear that children in this age group do not consume the recommended number of servings of dark green and orange vegetables—at home or away from home. Table 13.1B shows the density of foods at home and away from home. The density of foods consumed away from home was lower for fruits, dark green vegetables, and orange vegetables but higher for tomatoes and potatoes. The food density of whole grains and discretionary fats was also much lower for food consumed at fast food outlets when compared with foods consumed at home. Surprisingly, the food density from added sugars was higher at home than at fast food restaurants. The daily intake of nutrients, by food source (Table 13.1C) showed that food consumed at fast food restaurants was high in fat, saturated fatty acids, cholesterol, and sodium and low in calcium and iron.

Table 13.1A.
Daily Intake of Food at Home and Away From Home: 2003-2004

	Total	At Home	Away From Home				
			Total	Restaurant	Fast food	School	Other
Children age 2–19 y							
Calories (kcal)	2065	1421	644	106	324	159	101
Fruits (cups)	1.09	0.93	0.16	0.02	0.02	0.09	0.04
Vegetables total (cups)	1.17	0.74	0.44	0.09	0.24	0.10	0.04
Dark green (cups)	0.04	0.03	0.01	0.00	0.00	0.00	0.00
Orange color (cups)	0.04	0.03	0.01	0.00	0.00	0.00	0.00
Tomatoes (cups)	0.33	0.19	0.14	0.03	0.09	0.03	0.01
Potatoes (cups)	0.35	0.22	0.14	0.02	0.09	0.03	0.01
Dairy (cups)	2.26	1.62	0.64	0.08	0.27	0.29	0.05
Grains total (oz)	6.83	4.61	2.21	0.35	1.27	0.50	0.30
Whole grains (oz)	0.49	0.44	0.05	0.00	0.01	0.02	0.03
Meats (oz)	4.30	2.85	1.45	0.29	0.77	0.30	0.18
Added sugars (tsp)	21.40	15.45	5.95	0.96	2.45	1.16	1.69
Discretionary fats and oils (g)	62.87	40.39	22.48	3.68	12.32	5.30	2.96

Source: 2003-04 NHANES, 2-day averages for individuals 2 y and older who are not pregnant or lactating. Diet Quality and Food Consumption: Food and Nutrient Intake Tables. Available at: http://www.ers.usda.gov/briefing/dietquality/Data. Accessed October 15, 2012.

When the nutrient quality of "kids' meals" available at fast food restaurants was compared with the standards of meals from the National School Lunch Program (NSLP), it was demonstrated that only 3% of the fast food meals met the NSLP standards. Those that did provided 2 to 3 times the amounts of iron, vitamin A, and calcium but only one sixth the amount of added sugars of other fast food meals. Meals that met the NSLP standards offered fruit and milk and generally consisted of deli sandwich-based meals, whereas those that did not meet the standards included French fries and sweetened beverages.[18] Thus, kids' meals that are acceptable from a nutrient standpoint are available at fast food restaurants and could be selected by children or their parents.

In adolescents, fast food consumption was negatively associated with intakes of fruit and milk as well as the percentage of adolescents meeting the recommended servings of milk (boys), fruit (girls), and vegetables and discretionary calories (boys and girls). In girls only, fast food consumption was positively associated with discretionary energy and solid fat intake.[19] This is consistent with findings from an earlier study.[4]

Table 13.1B.
Density of Food at Home and Away From Home: 2003-2004

	Total	At Home	Away From Home				
			Total	Restaurant	Fast Food	School	Other
Children age 2–19 y							
Fruits (cups)	0.57	0.69	0.33	0.12	0.05	0.70	0.62
Vegetables total (cups)	0.57	0.51	0.66	1.01	0.80	0.78	0.30
Dark green (cups)	0.02	0.02	0.02	0.05	0.00	0.09	0.00
Orange color (cups)	0.02	0.02	0.01	0.04	0.00	0.05	0.01
Tomatoes (cups)	0.16	0.12	0.21	0.26	0.28	0.19	0.07
Potatoes (cups)	0.17	0.15	0.21	0.22	0.29	0.18	0.10
Dairy (cups)	1.11	1.14	1.03	0.74	0.86	1.88	0.39
Grains total (oz)	3.29	3.22	3.36	3.31	3.74	2.97	2.63
Whole grains (oz)	0.25	0.31	0.09	0.04	0.02	0.10	0.26
Meats (oz)	2.10	1.95	2.18	2.95	2.43	1.73	1.28
Added sugars (tsp)	10.26	11.39	9.45	8.17	7.48	7.33	20.06
Discretionary fats and oils (g)	30.06	27.80	34.31	34.36	37.83	32.08	26.72

Source: 2003-04 NHANES, 2-day averages for individuals 2 y and older who are not pregnant or lactating. Diet Quality and Food Consumption: Food and Nutrient Intake Tables. Available at: http://www.ers.usda.gov/briefing/dietquality/Data. Accessed October 15, 2012.

Accessibility of Nutrient Information on Food Consumed Away From Home

On March 23, 2010, the president signed into law the Patient Protection and Affordable Care Act (Pub L No. 111-148). Section 4205 of the Affordable Care Act amended section 403(q) of the Federal Food, Drug, and Cosmetic Act (FFDCA [21 USC 301]) to provide requirements for nutrition labeling for foods offered for sale at retail chains with 20 or more locations, regardless of ownership. On April 6, 2011, The Food and Drug Administration (FDA) published the Food Labeling; Nutrition Labeling of Standard Menu Items in Restaurants and Similar Retail Food Establishments; Proposed Rule in the *Federal Register*.[20] The rule states that the energy of menu items must be displayed on all menus and menu boards, including those at drive-through locations. The energy of variable menu items, such as combination meals, must be displayed in ranges. The energy content of self-serve meals must be posted on a sign next to the food. Additional written nutrition information, including total calories, calories from fat, total fat, saturated fatty acids, cholesterol, trans fat, sodium, total carbohydrates, sugars, dietary fiber, and

Table 13.1c.

Daily Intake of Nutrients by Food Source: 2005-08 National Health and Nutrition Examination Survey: Children 2-19 Years of Age

	Total	At Home	Away From Home				
			Total	Restaurant	Fast Food	School	Other
Energy (kcal)	1951.85	1310.16	641.69	100.32	266.39	140.26	134.71
Fiber (g)	12.84	8.99	3.86	0.62	1.46	1.01	0.77
Fiber (g/1000 kcal)	6.58	6.86	6.01	6.12	5.53	7.14	5.68
Total fat (g)	72.60	45.93	26.67	4.24	11.97	5.49	4.98
Total fat (% of energy)	33.48	31.55	37.41	37.87	40.47	35.37	33.21
SFA (g)	25.62	16.47	9.15	1.39	4.02	2.02	1.72
SFA (% of energy)	11.81	11.32	12.83	12.47	13.58	12.95	11.47
Cholesterol (mg)	223.39	148.74	74.65	15.94	31.10	14.70	12.91
Cholesterol (mg/1000 kcal)	114.45	113.53	116.34	159.74	116.00	103.78	97.55
Calcium (mg)	997.01	709.93	287.08	37.09	101.50	92.54	55.95
Calcium (mg/1000 kcal)	510.80	541.86	447.38	364.43	380.61	649.64	407.59
Iron (mg)	14.66	10.73	3.93	0.62	1.62	0.91	0.78
Iron (mg/1000 kcal)	7.51	8.19	6.12	6.22	6.12	6.44	5.83
Sodium (mg)	3062.48	1954.67	1107.81	192.71	467.30	237.40	210.40
Sodium (mg/1000 kcal)	1569.01	1491.93	1726.40	1899.93	1753.82	1681.09	1555.49

SFA indicates saturated fatty acids.

Note: Density measures intakes for each 1000 calorie intake.

Source: 2005-08 NHANES, 2-day averages for individuals 2 y and older who are not pregnant or lactating. Available at: http://www.ers.usda.gov/briefing/dietquality/Data. Accessed October 15, 2012.

protein of standard menu items must be available on request. The rule also states that state and local governments could not impose different or additional nutrition labeling requirements than those covered by the federal requirements but that they could establish nutrition labeling requirements for establishments not covered by this law. California, Maine, Massachusetts, New Jersey, Oregon, New York City,

Philadelphia, and other localities have laws pertaining to nutrition labeling already in effect or laws that are pending.

The benefits of nutrition labeling at fast food restaurants are unclear. Americans are less likely to be aware of ingredients and nutrient content of foods prepared away from home compared with foods prepared in their own homes.[21] Preliminary studies have, however, suggested that, at least for adults, menu labeling increased awareness of the energy content of fast foods[22-24] but did not always affect ordering habits.[22,25] Most studies have been conducted with adults; however, a study in adolescents demonstrated that when 106 adolescents (11-18 years of age) were asked to order from 3 different restaurant menus with and without energy and fat content posted beside each menu item, the majority of the adolescents did not modify their ordering behavior. Of the 27 who rated themselves as too fat or slightly overweight, only 9 (33%) changed their orders[26] in response to menu labeling. In another study of adolescents, it was reported that adolescents noticed calorie information at the same rate as adults but that it did not affect their ordering behavior.[27] For any nutrition labeling initiative to be successful, the public will need age-appropriate nutrition education.[28] A recent intervention study with a convenience sample showed that when provided with nutrition education and fast food menus with nutrition information, parents chose lower-energy meals for their children but not for themselves.[29]

Relationship of Weight to Fast Food

The parallel rise of the fast food industry with the obesity epidemic has suggested that fast food consumption is a causative agent. This has been difficult to demonstrate conclusively because of a lack of consistent findings; a recent review showed that only 1 in 5 studies in children demonstrated an association between body mass index (BMI) and the fast food environment.[30] A study of 7745 girls and 6610 boys (9-14 years of age) suggested that adolescents who consumed greater quantities of fried foods away from home were heavier, had higher total energy intakes, and had overall poorer diet quality than those who did not.[31] Project EAT (Eating Among Teens) showed that parents who purchased fast food for family meals at least 3 times per week had a higher mean BMI and were more likely to be overweight than parents who reported less frequent fast food purchases; however, these relationships were not found in their children.[32] Another study showed that children and adolescents 4 to 19 years of age who consumed fast food consumed an average of 187 kcals/day more than children who did not, and on days when fast food was eaten, the children consumed an average of 126 kcals more than on days they did not consume fast food. Children consuming fast food also had higher intakes of total fat, added sugars, and sugar-sweetened beverages and consumed less milk and fewer fruits and vegetables than did children not consuming fast food. The authors concluded that fast food affected diet quality in a way that was conducive to weight gain, but weight was not included as a variable in the study.[4] There are few longitudinal studies looking at the relationship between fast food intake and weight. One such study of 101 girls 8 and 12 years of age demonstrated that the frequency of eating quick-service food at baseline was positively associated with change in BMI z-score at the 11- and 19-year follow-up.[33]

The question, therefore, arises: If consuming fast food meals is causally related to the obesity epidemic, why aren't all children who eat fast food overweight? In part, this may relate to how often children eat fast food and how much energy they consume when they do. Recently, it was suggested that overweight adolescents consumed more energy at fast food restaurants than did their leaner counterparts and that their total energy intake was higher over a 24-hour period. Overweight adolescents were less likely to compensate for their higher energy intake. Study design should also be considered, because many of these studies were cross-sectional and, thus, cannot be used to show a cause-and-effect relationship.

Although some speculate that fast food consumption may be related to higher BMI, more longitudinal studies and randomized control trials are needed, particularly with larger samples of children from various ethnic groups and geographic locations, before any definitive conclusions can be made. Reducing the frequency of fast food consumption may be a strategy for individuals to decrease total energy intake, provided there is no compensation for consuming more energy at other times of the day. Despite the lack of a clear cause-and-effect relationship between consumption of fast food and overweight/obese status in children and adolescents, the American Academy of Pediatrics (AAP) recommends that eating at restaurants, particularly fast food restaurants, should be limited to help prevent pediatric obesity.[34]

Demographic and Other Factors Contributing to Fast Food Consumption
A number of studies have attempted to characterize who eats at fast food restaurants. Generally those who are younger, employed, and living in large households are more likely to report eating fast food. Attempts to link gender, BMI, educational level, income, and race/ethnicity to fast food consumption have been inconclusive.[35]

A recent study of a convenience sample of adolescents and adults[35] showed that overall, more than 50% of individuals (n=594) agreed or strongly agreed that they consumed fast food because it was quick (92.3%), it was easy to get to (80.1%), they like the taste of fast food (69.2%), they were too busy to cook (53.2%), or it was a "treat" (50.1%). Less than 50% of individuals agreed or strongly agreed that they consumed fast food because they do not like to prepare foods themselves (44.3%), their friends/family like fast food (41.8%), it is a way of socializing with friends and family (33.1%), they have many nutritious foods to offer (20.6%), and they are fun and entertaining (11.7%).

The family is a major influence on what children and adolescents eat. The traditional pattern of the family eating at the kitchen table has changed over the years, with fewer families eating meals at home together. There has been an increase in the number of single-parent households and substantial growth in maternal employment in the past few decades. Households in which both parents work or in which there is a single parent have less time to prepare meals. Reliance on fast food is a convenient and relatively cheap alternative for these parents to feed their families.

Media Influences and Product Branding and Fast Food Consumption

Public health experts have called for changes in the food environment to address the pediatric obesity epidemic and the overall poor diet in children and adolescents.[36] The volume of marketing for energy-dense, nutrient-poor foods targeted to children has been called one of the most "pernicious environmental influences on food consumption by youth,"[37] in part, because many children do not understand that the purpose of advertising is to sell them a product.[38,39] Studies on children's choices have shown consistently that children exposed to advertising choose advertised food products at significantly higher rates than those not exposed.[40]

US adolescents spend $155 billion a year; children younger than 12 years spend another $25 billion, but children and adolescents influence adults to spend an additional $200 billion per year.[41] It is projected that adolescents spend nearly $13 billion at fast food outlets.[42] Thus, there has been aggressive food marketing to children and adolescents. It is estimated that commercial enterprises spend more $11 billion dollars on food and beverage advertising. Fast food and snack foods dominate television advertising targeted to children, and the industry has been criticized for its strategies to create brand loyalty in children.[43] Some advertising campaigns targeted to children are remarkably successful; Ronald McDonald was introduced as the spokesman for McDonald's in 1963 and is recognized today by nearly 96% of American children. Fast food branding has been shown to influence children's taste, and greater effects were found in children with more televisions in their homes.[44] Older children and overweight children were most likely to recognize fast food logos.[43]

Children and adolescents live in a media-saturated environment. Television remains the principal vehicle for advertising.[45] Despite passage of the Children's Television Act of 1990 (Pub L No. 101-437), which places limits on advertising during children's TV programming hours, children are exposed to more than 40 000 television commercials/year,[41] of which approximately 5500 are food advertisements.[46] Television is often a constant presence; in households with youth 8 to 18 years of age, almost half (47%) reported that the television was on "most of the time," regardless of whether anyone was watching. Approximately two thirds of adolescents reported that the television was on during meals.[47] Increased television viewing has been associated with increased energy intake,[48,49] and adolescents who watched more television consumed more high-fat foods and fast food.[48] Half of children 6 to 17 years of age have a television in their bedroom; black youth (71.3%) are more likely to have a television in their room than are either Hispanic youth (56.2%) or white youth (44.4%).[50] In one study, children viewed an average of 21.3 commercials per hour, amounting to a viewing time of more than 10 minutes every hour. Food advertisements accounted for 47.8% of these commercials, and 91% of advertised foods were high in fat, sugar, or salt.[51]

Advertising targeted to children and adolescents is not limited to television, and fast food companies are using newer forms of interactive media—for example, Facebook's social ad system and online videos.[52] A recent Institute of Medicine Report[45] provided a comprehensive overview of the effect that media exposure can have on food preference, consumption, and obesity. Fig 13.1 shows how media exposure, coupled with product placement, promotion, and positioning, is related to health outcomes, such as overweight and obesity. Fig 13.1 also links media exposure with family and peers, as discussed previously, and with environmental influences, as discussed later, with health outcomes, including overweight and obesity.

Fig 13.1.
Influences on the diets and related health outcomes of children and youth.

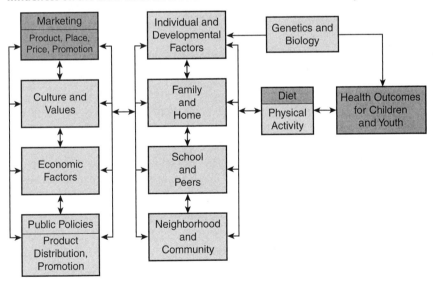

Used with permission from: Institute of Medicine, Committee on Food Marketing and the Diets of Children and Youth. *Food Marketing to Children and Youth: Threat or Opportunity?* McGinnis JM, Gootman JA, Kraak VI, eds. Washington, DC: National Academies Press: 2006:536.

On July 14, 2011, The Children's Food and Beverage Advertising Initiative (CFBAI) announced an agreement that will change the landscape of what is advertised to children by the nation's largest food and beverage companies. By December 31, 2013, these food and beverage companies, which do the vast majority of advertising to children, must follow uniform nutrition criteria for foods advertised to children. This agreement includes nutrition-specific criteria for 10 product categories typically marketed to children: juices; dairy products; grains, fruits, and vegetable products; soups and meal sauces; seeds, nuts, nut butters, and spreads; meat, fish, and poultry products; mixed dishes; main dishes and entrees; small meals; and meals. The 17 corporate participants of this initiative are Burger King Corporation, Cadbury Adams USA LLC, Campbell Soup Company, The Coca-Cola Company, ConAgra Foods Incorporated, The Dannon Company, General Mills Incorporated, The Hershey Company, Kellogg Company, Kraft Foods Global Incorporated, Mars Incorporated, McDonald's USA LLC, Nestlé USA, PepsiCo Incorporated, Post Foods LLC, Sara Lee Corporation, and Unilever United States.[a]

Environmental Influences on Fast Food Consumption

An obesigenic environment has been implicated in the dramatic increases in the prevalence of overweight in children of all racial and ethnic groups. Children and adolescents have wide access to fast food restaurants. Fast food restaurants are not the only source of "fast food" available to children and adolescents; neighborhood stores, convenience stores, gas stations, and even vending machines can provide similar fare.[53]

Studies have suggested that fast food restaurants were more likely to be found in low-socioeconomic status (SES) areas than in middle or upper SES areas and in areas with higher concentrations of ethnic minority groups than in those with a higher population of whites.[30] Locations of fast food restaurants have been implicated in the childhood obesity epidemic. In Chicago, IL, the median distance from any school to the nearest fast food restaurant was 0.52 km, and 78% of schools had at least 1 fast food restaurant within 800 m. It was estimated that there were 3 to 4 times as many fast food restaurants within 1.5 km from schools than would be expected if the restaurants were randomly distributed throughout the city.[54] Nearly all school children in New York City had high levels of access to fast food, and nearly 34% had a fast food restaurant within 400 m of the school. Low-income and Hispanic children had the highest level of access.[55] The effect that the proximity of fast food restaurants to schools may have on pediatric obesity is not clear. It has

---

[a] http://www.bbb.org/us/article/Council-of-Better-Business-Bureaus-Announces-Groundbreaking-Agreement-on-Ch-28325. Accessed August 11, 2011.

been assumed either that intake of these foods would be increased (and consumption has not been conclusively demonstrated to obesity in children) and that obesity would be more common[56] or that there would be higher levels of chronic disease, such as cardiac disease,[57] in children consuming fast foods. However, studies have failed to show these links.[58-60] Burdette and Whitaker,[59] for example, showed that there was no relationship to the prevalence of overweight and the location of fast food restaurants. However, their study was limited to preschool children, and further studies are needed to assess more fully the link between obesity in children and adolescents and the location of fast food outlets.

Virtually all schools participate in the NSLP, and approximately 50% of schools participate in the National School Breakfast Program. Schools participating in these programs are required to provide meals that meet strict dietary standards. Students participating in the NSLP have a higher nutrient intake than students who do not. Participation in the NSLP declines with age, with 66% of elementary school students but only 40% of high school students participating; overall, over the past decade, participation has declined. Middle and high schools often sell alternative options, including soft drinks and candy, to increase their profits; 17% of these schools have fast food outlets as a lunch alternative.[61] Less than 15% of parents and teachers believe that fast food options should be available for school lunch.[62] It is important to provide children with healthy food options at school and with the education to make informed choices.

Many high school students hold part-time jobs. At any given time, approximately one third of all high school students are employed. Restaurant work, particularly at fast food outlets, and retail sales jobs account for approximately 60% of all student jobs.[42] These work sites may provide employee food discounts or free beverages during the work day; thus, many adolescents may eat meals on site during their shift, which may compromise their nutritional intake.

Corporate Responsibility

In the popular press, McDonald's has been called "the most dominant fast food chain on the planet," and the company has taken steps to inform the public of the nutrient content of the food and to improve the menu items that they offer. In October, 2005 McDonald's announced it would begin printing nutrition facts information on food packages, and at the 2006 Winter Olympics, McDonald's unveiled the new packages. The new packaging was implemented in North America, Europe, Asia, and Latin America in the first half of 2006. Fast food restaurants, including McDonald's, Burger King, Wendy's, Subway, KFC, and Domino's Pizza have nutrition information available on their Web sites and available in their restaurants, but it is hoped that other fast food restaurants will follow McDonald's lead in product labeling.

On July 26, 2011, McDonald's issued a press release to inform the public of the company's "Commitments to Offer Improved Nutrition Choices." This comprehensive plan is structured to help customers, especially those with children, make healthier choices at their restaurants and others. As part of this initiative, McDonald's will automatically include produce or a low-fat dairy option in all Happy Meals, and by the end of 2012, McDonald's will provide apples in all Happy Meals and will promote the nutrition standards of the Council of Better Business Bureaus Food Pledge. By 2020, McDonald's will reduce added sugars, saturated fat, and energy through varied portion sizes, reformulations, and innovations. By 2015, it will reduce sodium an average of 15% overall across its national menu of food choices.

In response to the 2004 movie "Super Size Me," McDonald's announced that "supersized" beverages (42 oz, 410 kcal) and French fries (7 oz, 610 kcal) would no longer be available by the end of 2004, except in promotions. It should be noted that serving sizes available at McDonald's are still much larger than those available in 1955. The largest available meat portion at McDonalds is 8 oz, which exceeds the US Department of Agriculture (USDA) recommendations for 1 day (assuming a 2000-kcal diet) and is 500% larger than what was available in 1955.[63] Other fast food restaurants have very large portion sizes, which may be appealing to adolescents, especially boys. For example, in 2003, Hardee's introduced the Monster Thickburger with 11 oz of beef, 4 strips of bacon, and 3 slices of American cheese, providing 1320 kcals, 95 g of total fat, and 36 g of saturated fatty acids.[64] Although fast food restaurants continue to offer large portion sizes, an intervention in low-income New York City adolescents was effective in reducing the portion sizes ordered at fast food restaurants.[65]

Most fast food restaurant chains employ a registered dietitian or a fitness specialist at the corporate level. Providing healthful options in fast food restaurants is not new. Table 13.2 provides a list of options at fast food restaurants that are relatively healthy. It is clear that options are limited at these restaurants, and children or their parents need appropriate education to recognize healthy choices. It is also clear that fast food options are high in sodium. The lingering question is: When healthy food options are available at fast food restaurants, do people purchase them? Wendy's introduced its salad bar in 1979, Burger King test-marketed vegetarian burgers in the 1980s, and McDonald's introduced McLean Burgers in 1992; these products are no longer available because of lack of consumer demand.

Other ventures into healthful options by fast food chains have been more successful. Most chains have changed some of their preparation methods and added some new, healthier choices. In 2004, McDonald's improved their child-targeted

Happy Meals by allowing options of 1% milk or 100% apple juice instead of soft drinks and apple dippers instead of French fries.[66] In television advertising and on their Web site, these meals are shown with the milk and apple dippers; however, soft drinks and French fries remain as options for these meals. Wendy's,[67] Burger King,[68] and Subway[69] also provide a variety of kids' meals, which are shown on their Web sites with apple slices and either low-fat milk or 100% fruit juice. Hardee's meals for children, on the other hand, are offered with sweetened beverages and French fries and no healthier alternatives.[64]

McDonald's has introduced oatmeal, yogurt/fruit parfaits, and fruit smoothies and has 5 specialty salads.[66] Wendy's offers 4 main dish salad options and also allows patrons to substitute small salads for French fries in meal combinations.[67] Burger King has 3 salad options,[68] and Subway has 20 salad combinations.[69] Salad options may be perceived as being a healthy option, and those served at several fast food salads may be good choices (Table 13.2); however, as with all salads, dressings or add-ons, including avocado or guacamole, can add significant amounts of energy and fat. Some chains offer half portions of salads, and although this reduces the energy in the portion served, the percentage of energy from total fat remains high. Despite the finding that there appears to be greater consumer acceptance for salad options,[70] hamburgers and French fries continue to be the leaders in sales volume.[5]

The Subway brand was named the 2011 recipient of the MenuMasters Award by *Nation's Restaurant News* in the "Healthful Innovations" category for the introduction of "Build Your Better Breakfast."[69] The menu presents variations on 4 sandwich types with nutrition content of 185 to 427 kcal, 5 to 16 g of fat, 2 to 6 g of saturated fatty acids, 1 g of trans fat, 30 to 248 mg of cholesterol, 1 to 7 g of sugar, and 4 to 6 g of fiber. All however, are high in sodium, ranging from 641 to 1263 mg. Also provided on the Web site of fast food restaurants is information for children and adults about making healthy choices.

All major hamburger chains have switched from beef fat to vegetable oil for all frying; although this does not reduce energy intake, it does reduce the saturated fatty acids in the product. Virtually all chains now offer grilled and broiled foods alongside their fried dishes; for example, Burger King removed half the fat from its BK Broiler Chicken Sandwich; and Wendy's added a Grilled Chicken Sandwich. Subway advertises that many of its sandwiches have 6 g of fat or less (167 kcal for the Veggie Delight; 279 kcal for the Teriyaki Chicken); they also use a celebrity spokesperson to promote their products and the potential for weight loss. Restaurant chains are also working to reduce the sodium content of their product; however, virtually all foods available from fast food chains are high in sodium, and these efforts need to continue.

Table 13.2.

Selected Choices at Fast Food Restaurants That Are Relatively Low in Fat, Saturated Fatty Acids, and Cholesterol[a]

Food	Energy (kcal)	Total Fat (g)	Saturated Fat (g)	Chol (mg)	Fiber (g)	Total Sugar (g)	Sodium (mg)	Examples of Fast Food Menus for Children
Burger King[b]								
Apple Fries	70	0.5	0	0	NA	10	40	Small Hamburger
Small, Plain Hamburger	260	10	4	35	NA	6	490	Apple Fries
Tender Grill Garden Salad	230	7	3	85	NA	4	920	Low-fat Milk
Tender Crisp Garden Salad	410	22	5	65	NA	5	1060	Tender Grill Garden Salad
								Apple Fries
								Low-fat Milk
Jack in the Box[c]								
Chicken Fajita Pita made with whole grain	320	11	5	65	4	3	870	Chicken Fajita Pita
Chicken Teriyaki Bowl[d]	690	6	1	40	5	36	1700	Fruit Cup
Fruit Cup	50	0	0	0	1	11	10	Low-fat Milk
Grilled Chicken Salad	240	8	3.5	70	5	7	650	
Grilled Chicken Strips & Teriyaki Sauce	300	6	1	115	0	13	1510	Grilled Chicken Salad
Mango Smoothie	290	0	0	0	0	57	75	Mango Smoothie
Steak Teriyaki Bowl[d]	750	11	3	45	5	35	1750	
Strawberry Banana Smoothie	290	0	0	0	1	57	70	
KFC[e]								
Grilled Chicken Breast	210	8	2.5	105	0	0	460	Grilled Chicken Leg
Grilled Chicken Leg	80	4	4	55	0	0	230	Green Beans
Grilled Chicken Thigh	160	11	11	85	0	0	420	Corn
KFC Grilled Filet	140	1	1	70	0	1	560	Low-fat Milk
Doublicious with Grilled Fillet	340	8	3.5	80	2	6	880	Grilled Chicken Breast
Grilled Chicken Caesar Salad	220	7	3.5	85	3	4	740	Green Beans
Grilled Chicken BLT Salad	320	8	2.5	90	4	5	920	Mashed Potatoes
Green Beans	20	0	0	0	1	1	290	Corn (x2)
Mashed Potatoes without Gravy	90	3	0.5	0	1	0	320	Low-fat Milk
Corn on the Cob (3")	70	5	0	0	2	3	0	
BBQ Baked Beans	210	1.5	0	0	8	18	780	
Sargento Light String Cheese	50	2.5	1.5	10	0	0	160	

Item								Healthier Choices
McDonald's[f]								
Small Hamburger	250	9	3.5	25	2	6	520	Small Hamburger
Premium Grilled Chicken Classic	350	9	2	65	3	8	820	Apple Dippers
Premium Grilled Chicken Ranch BLT	380	10	3	25	3	9	1000	Low-fat Milk
Chipotle BBQ Snack Wrap Grilled	260	9	3.5	45	1	5	830	
Honey Mustard Snack Wrap	330	9	3.5	45	1	4	800	
Premium Southwest Salad/Grilled Chicken	320	9	3	70	6	11	960	Premium Grilled Chicken
Premium Southwest Salad—no Chicken	140	4.5	2	10	6	6	150	Classic
Snack Size Fruit and Walnut Salad	210	8	1.5	5	2	25	60	Snack Size Fruit and
Fruit & Maple Oatmeal without Br Sugar	260	4.5	2	10	5	18	115	Walnut Salad
Fruit & Yogurt Parfait	160	2	1	5	1	21	85	Low-fat Milk
Apple Dippers & Low-fat Caramel Sauce	100	0.5	0	5	0	11	35	
Pizza Hut[g] (1 slice servings)								
12" Fit and Delicious								1 slice thin and crispy pizza from the side list
Chicken, Red Onion, Gr Pepper	180	4.5	1.5	0	1	5	510	2 slices of any pizza on the side list
Chicken, Mushroom, Jalapeno	170	4.5	1.5	0	1	4	720	Sugar free beverage or low-fat milk if available
Ham, Red Onion, Mushroom,	160	4.5	1.5	0	1	4	550	
Ham, Pineapple, Diced Red Tomato	160	4.5	1.5	0	1	6	550	
Gr Pepper, Red Onion, Diced Tomato	150	4	1.5	0	2	5	400	Sugar free beverage
Diced Red Tomato, Mushroom, Jalapeno	150	4	1.5	0	2	4	610	or low-fat milk if it is available
Medium Thin Crispy Pizza								
Veggie Lovers	180	3	3	15	1	4	530	
Ham & Pineapple	180	3	3	20	1	5	540	
Medium Pan Pizza								
Veggie Lovers	230	3.5	3.5	15	2	3	500	

Table 13.2.
Selected Choices at Fast Food Restaurants That Are Relatively Low in Fat, Saturated Fatty Acids, and Cholesterol[a] *(continued)*

Food	Energy (kcal)	Total Fat (g)	Saturated Fat (g)	Chol (mg)	Fiber (g)	Total Sugar (g)	Sodium (mg)	Examples of Fast Food Menus for Children
Pizza Hut[g] (1 slice servings) *(continued)*								
Hand Tossed	200	3	3	20	1	5	550	
Ham & Pineapple	200	3	3	20	2	4	550	
Veggie Lover	240	4	4	25	1	5	640	
Subway[h]								
4" Deli Sandwiches for Kids' Meals								4" Deli Sandwich
Black Forest Ham	180	2.5	0.5	10	3	5	470	Apple Slices
Roast Beef	200	3	1	25	4	5	410	Yogurt or Low-fat Milk
Turkey Breast	180	2	1.5	10	3	5	460	
Veggie Delight	150	1.5	0	0	3	4	210	
Apple Slices	35	0	0	0	2	7	0	6" Deli Sandwich with
Light and Fit Yogurt	80	0	0	0	0	11	80	< 6 g fat
Baked Potato Chips	130	2	0	0	2	2	200	Apple Slices or Baked
Subway also serves 6" sandwiches with <6 g of fat, which would be suitable for an older child or adolescent								Potato Chips Low Fat Milk or Sugar Free Beverage
Taco Bell[i]								
Fresco Chicken Soft Taco	150	3.5	1	25	2	2	480	Chicken Soft Taco
Fresco Grilled Steak Soft Taco	150	4	1.5	15	2	2	520	Mexican Rice
Fresco Burrito Steak Supreme	340	8	2.5	15	7	4	1100	Lime Ade Sparkler
Fresco Burrito Chicken	340	8	2.5	25	7	4	1060	Fresco Burrito Chicken
Chicken Soft Taco	180	6	2.5	30	1	1	460	Mexican Rice
Bean Burrito	370	10	3.5	5	10	3	980	Lime Ade Sparkler
Mexican Rice	120	3.5	0	0	1	8	200	
Classic Lime Ade Sparkler	150	0	0	0	0	38	80	

Wendy's[j]							
Junior Hamburger	230	8	3.5	30	1	6	470
Junior Cheeseburger	270	11	5	40	1	6	670
Grilled Chicken Go Wrap	260	10	3.5	50	1	3	730
Ultimate Chicken Grill	360	7	1.5	80	2	9	1110
Sour Cream and Chives Potato	320	4	2	10	7	4	50
Small Chili	210	6	2.5	40	6	6	880
Apple Slices	40	0	0	0	2	7	0
100% Apple Juice	90	0	0	0	0	20	5

Meal suggestions:
- Junior Hamburger / Apple Slices / Low-fat Milk
- Two Chicken Go Wraps / Apple Slices / Low-fat Milk

NA indicates not available.

[a] Nutrient information is per serving and from company Web sites (accessed June 30, 2011). Salads are without dressing (low fat is available), sandwiches are without mayonnaise, and chicken products are without sauces. Most fast food restaurants also have 1% milk and 100% fruit juice, which are appropriate beverages for children. Note: Most entrees and sides have high sodium content. Menus in the top panel are suitable for young children and those in the bottom panel are suitable for older children or adolescents. These are presented as examples and are not intended to replace regular nutrient-dense meals prepared and consumed at home. These menu items are presented as examples and do not reflect all foods available; seasonal and regional options are also available. Overall, small, plain hamburgers, grilled chicken, plain side salads, fruit, low-fat milk, and 100% fruit juice are healthy options for young children a fast food restaurants. For breakfast, English muffins, plain pancakes, an egg, small servings of French toast, fruit, oatmeal, yogurt, 100% fruit juice, and 100% fruit juice are healthy options for young children. It is important to choose age-appropriate meals and snacks for children and adolescents.

[b] http://www.bk.com/en/us/menu-nutrition/index.html.

[c] http://www.jackinthebox.com. Menu items from Jack in the Box were from its "Healthy Choices" nutrition information. These purportedly meet the guidelines of Healthy Dining Finder (http://healthydiningfinder.com/learnmore/nutrition_criteria.asp), which identifies healthy entrees as having: at least 2 servings of fruit or vegetables, lean protein, or whole grain and ≤750 kcals, ≤25 g total fat or less, and ≤8 g saturated fatty acids. It should be noted that the Deluxe Hamburger, although conforming to these criteria, has 47% of energy from fat. Further, entree options are not low in sodium. Kics' meals are available.

[d] Menu items with this amount of energy are not suitable for young children but may be suitable as an entrée for adolescents.

[e] http://www.kfc.com/nutrition/pdf/kfc_nutrition.pdf.

[f] http://www.mcdonalds.com/us/en/food/food_quality/nutrition_choices.html

[g] http://www.pizzahut.com/nutrition.html. Low-fat milk or 100% fruit juice were not listed as a menu option; if customers dine in, the best available beverage would be a sugar-free soft drink; for meals delivered to the home for consumption, the best beverage options would be low-fat milk or 100% fruit juice.

[h] http://www.subway.com/applications/NutritionInfo/Files/NutritionValues.pdf.

[i] http://www.tacobell.com/nutrition/calculator. Kids' meals are available.

[j] http://www.wendys.com/food/Nutrition.jsp. Kids' meals with apple slices and low-fat milk are available

Fast food chains have instituted a variety of public health efforts. McDonald's and Subway have major initiatives to increase physical activity in children. Subway has teamed with My Weekly Reader, the largest and oldest educational magazine for students, to produce "*One Body! One Life! Eat Fresh! Get Fit!*"—an in-school curriculum designed to stress the importance of healthy eating and exercise.

Recommendations About Fast Food

Fast food restaurants are an integral and pervasive part of our society. Three of 10 consumers state that meals away from home, including fast food meals, are essential to the way they live. Restrictive feeding practices in children have been associated with an increased preference for the forbidden foods[71] and have resulted in an increased intake when these foods were available.[72] Thus, it is important not to totally restrict fast food from the diets of children and adolescents if they wish to consume it occasionally. Parents, with the help of nutrition professionals, must teach children and adolescents to make the best choices at fast food restaurants by instruction and by modeling. Healthful choices for children at fast food restaurants include oatmeal or egg sandwich wraps and low-fat milk or 100% fruit juice for breakfast. For lunch and dinner, kids' meals with deli sandwiches, plain hamburgers, or grilled chicken with apple slices and 100% fruit juice or low-fat milk are healthful choices for young children (Table 13.2). For older children and adolescents, healthful choices include plain hamburgers, grilled chicken, salads, chili, low-fat deli-style sandwiches, apple slices, 100% fruit juice, and low-fat milk. These foods should be associated with lower energy intake and improved diet quality. Overall, moderation is important, and fast food meals should not replace regular family meals at home.

Fast food restaurants and other outlets where these foods are sold must be sure that healthful foods and accurate nutrition information are available at the restaurant and on their Web sites. Responsible advertising to children must also be part of the corporate plan to improve the nation's health. This can be accomplished by advertising healthier menu options to children, emphasizing the importance of milk and other nutrient-dense foods in the diet. Sweden and Norway have an explicit ban on advertising targeted to children younger than 12 years; other countries have limits on advertising to children. Although accessibility to global media through cable and the Internet dilute the effect of this TV advertising ban somewhat, it is still an important step. If marketing of fast foods to children cannot be stopped, then innovative advertising of healthful foods to children needs to occur.[73] Advertisement of healthful foods, like fruit and vegetables, may serve to increase awareness of these foods and increase consumption.

Organic Foods

What Are Organic Foods?

The Organic Foods Production Act of 1990 (OFPA) (Title XXI of the 1990 Farm Bill [Pub L No. 101-624]) mandated that the USDA: (1) establish national standards governing the marketing of certain agricultural products as organically produced products; (2) assure consumers that organically produced products meet a consistent standard; and (3) facilitate interstate commerce in fresh and processed food that is organically produced. Foods covered by this act are fruits, vegetables, mushrooms, grains, dairy products, eggs, livestock feed, meats, poultry, fish and other seafood, and honey.

Regulations were proposed in 1997 and modified in 1998, with the first national standards being adopted in 2001. By October 21, 2002, 12 years after the OFPA was enacted, consumers buying foods bearing the USDA Organic Seal were assured that the food was produced and handled according to set standards. Regulations continue to be amended and producers must comply to be able to use the Organic Seal. The Organic Seal (Fig 13.2) can only appear on foods that are at least 95% organic; this means that a raw or processed agricultural product must contain (by weight or fluid volume, excluding water and salt) at least 95% of organically produced or processed agricultural products. The accompanying wording of "100% organic" reflects a product that is 100% organic. Products with at least 70% organic ingredients may say "made with organic ingredients," and products with less than 70% of organic ingredients may list specific organically produced ingredients on the side panel of the product packaging but may not make any organic claims on the front panel. The name and address of the government-approved certifier must be on all products that contain at least 70% organic ingredients. Use of the USDA Organic Seal is voluntary, and there is a fine of up to $11 000 per violation for misuse. When residue testing detects prohibited substances at levels that are greater than 5% of the Environmental Protection Agency's (EPA) tolerance for the specific residue detected or unavoidable residual environmental contamination, the agricultural product cannot be sold, labeled, or represented as organically produced. Despite these clear labeling laws, the public is unsure about the terms "organic," "natural," and other positively associated food terms (eg, "cage-free"),[74] and further education is needed.

III

Fig 13.2.
The USDA Organic Seal. http://www.ams.usda.gov/nop/Consumers/Seal.html.

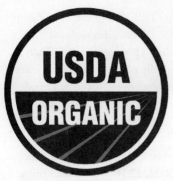

"Organic" is a production term and does not refer to characteristics of the foods themselves. Organic crop standards include that the land has had no prohibited substances applied to it for at least 3 years before the harvest of an organic crop. Use of genetic engineering, ionizing radiation, and sewage sludge is prohibited. Soil fertility and crop nutrients are managed through tillage and cultivation practices, crop rotations, and cover crops; soils can be supplemented with animal and crop waste materials and allowed synthetic materials. Crop pests, weeds, and diseases are controlled primarily through management practices including physical, mechanical, and biological controls. When these practices are not sufficient, a biological, botanical, or synthetic substance approved for use on the national list may be used.[75] Animals on organic farms eat organic feed, are not confined 100% of the time, and are raised without antibiotics or added hormones. Advantages to organic production are that it "promotes and enhances biodiversity, biological cycles, and soil biological activity."[76]

Purchasing Trends for Organic Foods

Once sold only in premium markets or health food stores, organic foods are now widely available year-round in conventional supermarkets, and half of all organic foods are purchased in supermarkets, club stores, or big-box stores.[77] Consumer demand for variety, convenience, and quality in fresh produce has boosted sales of organic foods and pressured farmers to expand acreage devoted to organic foods. In the past decade, the US organic food industry has grown substantially. In 2003, organic foods accounted for nearly $10.4 billion or approximately 1.8% of total food sales in the United States.[78] However, by 2010, organic food sales had increased to $26.7 billion or approximately 4% of all foods,[79] with fruits and vegetables making up the majority of all organic food sold. Periodic shortages have occurred as supply has struggled to keep up with demand.[77]

Organic produce is purchased at a premium price, with the cost ranging from 10% to 100% more than the cost of conventional produce.[77,80,81] The top selling organic fruits and vegetables are tomatoes, potatoes, carrots, onions, lettuce, apples, oranges, bananas, grapes, and strawberries in terms of their shares of fresh produce expenditures for home consumption. Dairy foods have been one of the fastest-growing segments of the organic market, with annual growth rates of retail sales ranging from 16% to 34% between 1997 and 2007. Organic milk is 60% to109% more expensive than conventional milk.[77] Sales of organic meat and eggs are low, but this is a rapidly expanding segment of the market, whereas grains and oilseeds face slow growth.[81]

Consumer Purchasing Behavior

Sixty-nine percent of adults bought organic food at least occasionally in 2008, and 28% bought organic food weekly.[81] The typical profile of a consumer varies; however, in general, consumer preference for organic foods has been associated with perceived benefits for environmental protection, supporting the local economy, animal welfare, food safety, perceived better taste, personal health or following an alternative lifestyle, and feelings of responsibility for one's family.[81-84] Consumers are also willing to pay more money for organic foods because of their perceived health benefits.[85] Those most likely to purchase organic foods were "mature" women with children younger than 18 years and those with higher levels of education.[86-88] Buyers and consumers were clearly willing to pay more for perceived benefits of organic foods. It is noteworthy that for organic baby food, the organic label was more important to consumers than the nutrient content.[89]

Barriers to purchasing organic foods included limited availability, high price, lack of knowledge, and lack of trust in organic labels.[74] In 2008, in response to weakening economic conditions, evidence suggested that consumers began buying conventional products or private-label organic products rather than branded organic products.[81]

Nutrients and Health Benefits of in Organic Versus Conventional Foods

It is widely believed that organic foods are healthier and safer than conventional foods.[82,83] However, the effects of organic growing systems on nutrient bioavailability and nonnutrient components have received little attention, so this belief is not evidence based. Many published studies comparing the nutrient content of organic to conventional produce have methodologic concerns. Natural products, including fruits and vegetables, vary in their nutrient content and nonnutrient substances. Moreover, it is difficult to compare studies performed over time, because regulations, recommendations, and analytical techniques vary.

The first systematic review of the literature that compared nutrient content between conventional and organic crops found that conventional crops had higher levels of nitrogen and organic crops had higher levels of phosphorus and higher titratable acidity. No other differences were found in the other 8 nutrient categories examined (vitamin C, magnesium, potassium, calcium, zinc, copper, phenolic compounds, and total soluble solids). Differences observed were likely attributable to differences in fertilizers and ripeness at harvest rather than to any specific organic techniques used in production.[90] This finding was in contrast to some previous studies that suggested higher levels of vitamin C were present in organically grown leafy green vegetables, peaches, tomatoes, and potatoes.[91] Overall, there is no convincing evidence that organic foods differ significantly in nutrient content when compared with conventional foods.[92] The Institute of Food Technologists Expert Panel on Food Safety and Nutrition[76] and the USDA do not promulgate organically grown food as more nutritious than conventional foods.

Health benefits of consuming recommended amounts of whole grains, produce, and low-fat dairy products cannot be underestimated, but there is no indication that organic foods offer an advantage over conventional foods. A recent systematic review of the literature did not find nutrition-based health benefits linked to consumption of organic produce.[93] However, that review did not compare the potential health effects of contaminants, such as pesticide or herbicide residues. Moreover, the number of articles available for review was small and further studies are clearly warranted.

Nitrate Content of Organic Versus Conventional Foods

An article appearing in *US News and World Report*[94] suggested that consumers believed that organic foods were free of the hazardous materials found in conventional foods. Nitrate is the main form of nitrogen fertilizer applied to crops. Nitrogenous fertilizers can, in turn, leech into the groundwater and contaminate well water and increase the nitrate content of food. Nitrate has low toxicity; however, conversion of nitrates to nitrites or nitrosamines can cause adverse health effects. Nitrate-contaminated well water and vegetables high in nitrates have been shown to cause methemoglobinemia in infants and has been addressed by the AAP[95] (see Chapter 54: Food Safety). The maximum contaminant level for nitrates is based on levels that reduce the risk of methemoglobinemia. The effects of the exposure to nitrates in drinking water on the incidence of birth defects, especially neural tube defects and cardiac anomalies, have also been reported[96,97]; however, the effect nitrate had in these studies was equivocal.

Lower nitrate concentrations have been found in some organically grown crops when compared with conventional ones, especially in leafy green vegetables.[85,91] Lower levels of nitrates have been shown for organically grown lettuce and rocket but not for arugula. Cereals, fruits, and bulb vegetables did not show any consistent difference in nitrate concentration.[91] In general, levels of nitrates in plant foods are inconsistent and depend on the producer, crop, season in which the plants are grown, storage conditions, geographic location, and postharvest processing. Thus, it seems that the use of organic farming to reduce dietary nitrate intake with the goal of reducing carcinogenesis is premature.

Pesticides

A detailed look at the effects of pesticides on health is beyond the scope of this chapter (see Chapter 54 for more information). However, some discussion is warranted as it relates specifically to organic foods. The 1993 National Research Council report "Pesticides in the Diets of Infants and Children" recognized that children have higher exposures and increased susceptibility to environmental toxicants, including pesticides[98] (Table 13.3). Exposure to organophosphorus pesticides have been reported to have neurologic and neurodevelopmental effects in infants and children.[99,100] Recently, data from the National Health and Nutrition Examination Survey (NHANES) have suggested that children exposed to low levels of organophosphate pesticides, presumably through diet, were at higher risk of developing attention-deficit/hyperactivity disorder; those data also suggested that children received a continuous exposure to these pesticides.[101] Children tended to have diets high in foods that were potentially high in pesticide residues, including juices, fruits, and vegetables.[98]

Table 13.3.
Children's Increased to Environmental Agents

Children have disproportionally higher exposures to many environmental agents.	Per unit weight, children drink more water, eat more food, and breathe more air than adults. Putting objects in their mouths and crawling or playing on the floor or ground also potentially contribute to higher exposures to pesticides.
A child's ability to metabolize, detoxify, or excrete environmental agents differs from adults.	Ironically, in some instances, children are protected against some agents, because they cannot make active metabolites required for toxicity.
Developmental processes are easily disrupted during rapid growth and development before and after birth.	
Children have more years of future life and this more time to develop diseases initiated by early exposures.	

Adapted with permission from Landrigan PJ, Kimmel CA, Correa A, Eskenazi B. Children's health and the environment: public health issues and challenges for risk assessment. *Environ Health Perspect.* 2004;112(2):257-265.

The Food Quality Protection Act (FQPA) of 1996 (Pub L No. 104-170, formerly known as HR 1627) amended the Federal Insecticide, Fungicide, and Rodenticide Act (FIFRA [Pub L No. 80-104]), and the FFDCA set high standards to protect infants and children from pesticide risks. Under the FIFRA, the EPA registers pesticides for use in the United States and prescribes labeling and other regulatory requirements to prevent unreasonable adverse effects on health or the environment. Under the FFDCA, the EPA establishes tolerances (maximum legally permissible levels) for pesticide residues in food. The Department of Health and Human Services/Food and Drug Administration enforces tolerances for most foods; the USDA Food Safety and Inspection Service enforce tolerances for meat, poultry, and some egg products. Conventional agricultural practices have changed over the past decade, and consumer exposure to organophosphate pesticides and paradichlorobenzene are within EPA regulations and are consistent with safe food standards.

The FQPA explicitly requires the EPA to address risks to infants and children and to publish a specific safety finding before a tolerance can be established. It also provides for an additional safety factor (tenfold, unless reliable data show that a different factor will be safe) to ensure that tolerances are safe for infants and children and requires collection of better data on food consumption patterns, pesticide residue levels, and pesticide use.

The Organic Seal does not guarantee that the food products are free of pesticides. In the United States, for foods to be certified as organic, no synthetic pesticides can have been applied to the land for at least 3 years, and a "sufficient buffer zone" must also be in place to reduce the risk of contamination from conventional farming operations. However, unless products were grown under cover, they could still become contaminated with pesticides. The persistence of pesticides in the environment was recently shown when organochlorine insecticides were shown to contaminate root crops[102] and tomatoes[103] despite the fact that these pesticides had been off the market for 20 years. Pesticide contamination of organic foods can occur from cultivation of previously contaminated soil, percolation of chemicals through soils, wind-drift, groundwater or irrigation water, or during transport, processing, or storage.

Organic foods have been shown to be contaminated by pesticide residues; however, they are less likely to be contaminated than foods grown using conventional methods.[104,105] One report that compared results from 3 studies showed that organic crops were 10 times less likely to be contaminated with multiple pesticide residues.[104] Levels of permitted pesticides are low—often undetectable—in both organic and conventional foods.

Consumption of organic foods is often assumed to reduce health risks by reducing exposure to pesticide residues.[106] Children can be exposed to pesticides via the diet.[107] Intuitively, it would seem that eating organic produce would reduce levels of pesticide residues in children; however, few data support this supposition. Several recent studies have used biological monitoring to examine dietary exposures to pesticides in children.[107-109] In a study of children 2 to 5 years of age (n=39), it was shown that those consuming primarily organic produce had levels of total dimethyl metabolites in their urine that were significantly lower than those who consumed conventional produce.[108] In a cross-over study of 23 children 3 to 11 years of age, Lu et al[109] demonstrated that children consuming a conventional diet during phases 1 (days 1-3) and 3 (days 9-15) of the study had significantly higher organophosphorus pesticide levels than when they ate an organic diet (phase 2, days 4-8). They also showed in a yearlong study that when children were switched to an organic diet, urinary organophosphorus residues were reduced.[110] Although small, these studies provide tantalizing information about the potential effects that consuming organic foods has on pesticide levels of children. What these studies did not demonstrate was a long-term health benefit to consuming organic foods.

Are There Adverse Health Concerns With Organic Foods?

Ironically, the use of composted manure and the reduced use of fungicides and antibiotics in organic food production could lead to a higher level of contamination by microorganisms or microbial products. Whether organic foods are more susceptible to microbial contamination or whether they take up microbial contamination from organic manure is controversial. It is clear, however, that organic foods, in common with conventionally produced foods, are not free from microbial contamination. Organically grown chickens have not been shown to have less *Salmonella*[111,112] or *Camplyobacter*[112] organisms than either conventional or free-range chickens. *Listeria monocytogenes* and *Escherichia coli* have been found on organically grown lettuce.[113] These studies suggest that foods bearing the Organic Seal must be treated, handled, and prepared in a manner consistent with reducing the risk of foodborne illness.

The FDA has consumer information available explaining how to wash fresh produce to reduce the risk of foodborne illnesses at: http://www.fda.gov/downloads/Food/ResourcesForYou/Consumers/UCM174142.pdf.

Recommendations About Organic Foods

Whether organic foods are safer or more nutritious or confer more health benefits than conventional foods is unclear, because studies are conflicting, but the preponderance of evidence suggests that organic foods are comparable in nutrient content and can be contaminated, albeit in lower levels than conventional foods, with pesticides. Organic foods are also subject to microbial contamination and must be treated, handled, and prepared in a manner consistent with practices that reduce the risk of foodborne illness. Because organic produce is not waxed, it may spoil more quickly—quick spoilage has been identified as a barrier to consumption of organic fruits and vegetables. However, the principal barrier to consuming organic foods is their higher cost.

It is important to consume a variety of foods to achieve nutrient adequacy and limit repeated exposure to a single contaminant, buy produce in season when possible, and use safe food–handling practices. Prepared products that use organic foods can also be high in fats and added sugars; thus, consumers need to read product labels to be able to make healthy selections.

At this time, there is no evidence-based information suggesting that organic foods have a nutrition or health advantage.[114]

AAP

"…organic diets have been convincingly demonstrated to expose consumers to fewer pesticides associated with human disease. Organic farming has been demonstrated to have less environmental impact than conventional approaches. However, current evidence does not support any meaningful nutritional benefits or deficits from eating organic compared with conventionally grown foods, and there are no well-powered human studies that directly demonstrate health benefits or disease protection as a result of consuming an organic diet. Studies also have not demonstrated any detrimental or disease-promoting effects from an organic diet. Although organic foods regularly command a significant price premium, well-designed farming studies demonstrate that costs can be competitive and yields comparable to those of conventional farming techniques. Pediatricians should incorporate this evidence when discussing the health and environmental impact of organic foods and organic farming while continuing to encourage all patients and their families to attain optimal nutrition and dietary variety consistent with the US Department of Agriculture's MyPlate recommendations."

Forman J; Silverstein J; American Academy of Pediatrics, Committee on Nutrition, Council on Environmental Health. Clinical report: organic foods: health and environmental advantages and disadvantages. *Pediatrics*. 2012; 130(5):e1406-e1415.

Fad Diets

Prevalence of Obesity in Adolescents and Dieting Behavior in Children and Adolescents

Using data from the 2009-2010 NHANES, 26.7% of children 2 to 5 years of age, 32.6% of children 6 to 11 years of age, and 33.6% of adolescents 12 to 19 years of age were overweight or obese. The prevalence was higher in boys than girls and highest in Mexican-American (2-5 years and 12-19 years of age) and Hispanic (6-11 years of age) children when compared with other ethnic/racial groups.[115] For adolescents, data from the 2011 Youth Risk Behavior Surveillance System (YRBSS) showed a slightly lower percentage (29.2%) of high school-aged students that self-described themselves as slightly or very overweight; the prevalence of obesity in these self-assessments was highest among girls, particularly Hispanic girls. However, a high percentage (46%) of students reported that they were trying to lose weight. The prevalence of those trying to lose weight was higher among girls (61.2%) than boys (31.6%) and higher among white girls (61.4%), black girls (55.2%), and Hispanic girls (66.4%) than among white boys (29.2%), black boys (26.6%), and Hispanic boys (49.6%). Overall, many students practiced dietary manipulation, including fasting, exercising, and purging to lose weight. The survey did not ask about the prevalence of fad diets or any specific type of diet. From 1991 to 2011, there was a significant linear increase in the percentage of students who reported trying to lose weight (41.8%-46.0%).[116]

There is clear disparity between the number of high school students who are overweight, those who perceive themselves as overweight, and those attempting to lose weight, suggesting that dieting practices to lose weight did not depend on overweight or perception of body shape. These perceptions may lead to unhealthy weight loss practices. Further, weight reduction practices among the nonoverweight are associated with "considerable risk to physical health and emotional well-being."[117]

The prevalence of dieting for weight loss cited previously from the YRBSS is similar to that shown in the Minnesota Adolescent Health survey, in which 62% of girls and 20% of boys in grades 7 through 12 reported dieting behavior.[118] In another study of 105 overweight children 6 to 13 years of age, 60% reported attempting at least 1 weight loss diet.[119] It is significant that many adolescents who reported dieting have BMIs within the normal range for height.[120] Also similar to the YRBSS, very few studies have asked adolescents who diet whether they have ever followed a "fad diet." One report of 146 high school students demonstrated that 36.5% of boys and 73.6% of girls reported trying to lose weight; however, of these, none of the boys and only 4.5% of the girls reported following a fad diet.[121] Only in the study of Calderon et al was the term "fad diet" described for the participants; thus, it was possible that adolescents did not understand what constituted a diet or fad diet or that low-carbohydrate diets are usually classified as fad diets.

It is concerning that girls as young as 5 years of age have reported body dissatisfaction, which was associated with the likelihood of dieting at 9 years of age.[122] Between 34% and 65% of girls 5 years of age had ideas about dieting[123] and expressed concerns about gaining weight.[124] Many factors, including parent's attitudes and practices about diet and weight,[123] peer pressure, and teasing or bullying by other children, influence a child's perception of body image or their decision to diet. Mothers, in particular, had an influence on girls' perceptions of dieting; thus, it is especially important that parents model healthy eating and maintain a healthy weight and perception of weight; however, all caregivers responsible for feeding children should also serve as good role models for healthy eating behaviors. The mass media has had a significant effect on girls' perception of weight and shape.[125] In one study of students in 5th through 12th grade (n=548), 69% of students reported that magazines influenced their idea of a perfect body shape, and 47% reported wanting to lose weight because of the pictures in these magazines.[125] Use of unhealthful weight loss practices in high school students was associated with reading women's beauty and fashion magazines.[126] Adolescents who diet are more likely to become overweight as adults,[127] suggesting a need to teach healthy eating habits at home and in the schools, rather than having students resort to the use of short-term weight loss diets, fad or otherwise.

An unresolved question is whether dieting behavior, especially in adolescent girls, leads to disordered eating.[128,129] Studies tend to be small; longitudinal studies are uncommon, and findings have been inconsistent.[128-130] Patton et al[129] found that adolescent girls who dieted at a severe level were 18 times more likely to develop an eating disorder than those who did not diet, and girls who dieted at a more moderate level were 5 times more likely to develop an eating disorder. Killen et al[130] also showed that girls with the highest level of dieting were more likely to develop disordered eating. A 5-year longitudinal study of adolescents (2516; 45% boys)[129] showed that both adolescent boys and girls who used unhealthy weight-control behaviors were at increased risk of binge eating with loss of control. Clearly, a large percentage of adolescents have tried to lose weight, either through diet or by more extreme weight loss measures, including self-induced vomiting or use of laxatives. Estimates for eating disorders in girls (who are at higher risk than boys) are between 1% and 4%. Parents and peers have been shown to influence body image perception, body dissatisfaction, and eating or dieting habits of children[131-134] and adolescents.[135-137]

Nutrient Intake in Restricted Eating

It is a challenge to follow a nutrient-dense, low energy diet. A recent study of adolescent girls showed that, on average, those who "often" used weight control measures had a BMI in the normal range but had serum markers suggesting chronic malnutrition when compared with those who "never" or "occasionally" dieted.[138] It is also difficult to obtain nutrient adequacy on diets that provide a limited variety of foods, as may occur on nutrient-restricted or specific food-restricted diets. Low-carbohydrate diets limit the variety of foods that can be eaten and, therefore, may be difficult to follow long-term. In general, low-carbohydrate diets require supplementation, because these diets are low in vitamins E, A, and B_6; thiamin, folate; calcium; magnesium; iron; potassium; and dietary fiber.[139] Few studies have looked at the effect that low-carbohydrate diets have on the intake of children or adolescents. Dietary intake data from children 10 years (n=568) in the Bogalusa Heart Study were stratified into 4 levels of carbohydrate intake: <45%, 45% to 50%, 50% to 55%, and >55% of energy. Investigators found that children in the low-carbohydrate group ate more meat, whereas children in the high-carbohydrate group ate more desserts and candy but also more fruits, grains, and milk.[140] The 1990 Ontario Health Survey collected dietary information, via a food frequency questionnaire, on 5194 adolescents 12 to 18 years of age. Low-carbohydrate diets were consumed by 27.6% of boys and 24.1% of girls. Fruit and vegetable intake was low and cholesterol and total fat intake was high in adolescents consuming these diets. Overweight status, smoking, and alcohol use were also associated with consuming a low-carbohydrate diet.[141]

Fad Diet Overview

"Fads" refer to something that enjoys temporary popularity. Fad diets have been described variously as diets that make unrealistic claims, promise a "quick fix" and rapid weight loss, or eliminate foods or food groups, often stating these are toxic. One problem with these diets is that they are usually undertaken without medical advice or under medical supervision. This is of special concern for children and adolescents, because they may not disclose to parents or medical professionals that they are on a "diet." Because the prevalence of pediatric obesity is so high, it is not surprising that children and adolescents may be driven to extreme weight loss regimens, including those that are untested or unsuitable for children or adolescents. It has been shown not only that fad diets are ineffective in children but also that they could ultimately lead to additional weight gain.

The goals and expectations of most dieters are unrealistic, and many look for a "quick fix." This has led many dieters to turn to self-prescribed weight loss regimens. In 2001, a search on Amazon.com with the key words "weight loss" brought up 1214 books.[139] In 2011, a similar search yielded 19 710 books, with 99 of these books specifically geared to children or adolescents.[138] The overwhelming majority of these books describe what can be termed a "fad diet." Table 13.4 describes how to determine whether a popular diet is actually a fad diet.

Table 13.4.

How to Determine Whether a Diet Is a Fad Diet

	Comment	Example = *Sugar Busters*
Step 1	Keep an open but informed mind. Many of the diets available on the market today are fad diets, but many are not. Do not automatically dismiss a popular diet as a fad diet.	*Sugar Busters* by H. Leighton Steward, Morrison C. Bethea, MD, Sam S. Andrews, MD, and Luis A. Balart, MD
Step 2	Look at the author(s) and their qualifications—are they trained in medicine or nutritional sciences or are they celebrity spokespeople?	3 medical doctors lend credence to this diet.
Step 3	Evaluate the overall tone of the writing—is it professional or is it biased?	The writing is casual, even for a popular press book—"How do I avoid getting arteriosclerosis? The answer is easy. Don't live long enough." And, "When the liver goes, 'Adios, Amigo'" are examples of this casual tone.
Step 4	Understand the premise of the diet—is the diet low carbohydrate, low energy, low fat, or something else?	Is the effect of the diet biologically plausible? Yes and no. The diet is based on the glycemic index but makes comments like "insulin is toxic."
Step 5	Does the peer-reviewed literature support the effectiveness of the diet? Or do the authors rely on testimonials?	The authors of this book rely principally on testimonials; however, it should be noted that articles linking weight loss to eating low-glycemic index foods are beginning to appear in the peer reviewed literature. Long-term studies on the safety and effectiveness of these diets are lacking. There are other comments in the book that are of concern. For example, "Yet the standard diet recommended for patients with or at risk for coronary disease is to consume 80 to 85% of calories from carbohydrates with very low amounts of fat and protein!" This is clearly not consistent with recommendations from the National Cholesterol Education Program.
Step 6	Look at the claims the authors make. If it seems too good to be true...it probably is not.	There are no fantastic claims for this diet.
Step 7	Are any foods or supplements required for the diet? Are the authors of the diet selling their own foods or supplements? Are any health risks associated with the supplements?	There is a line of *Sugar Buster* products.

Table 13.4. *(continued)*
How to Determine Whether a Diet Is a Fad Diet

	Comment	Example = *Sugar Busters*
Step 8	Are foods or food groups omitted?	Foods with high glycemic indices are omitted from this diet. Eliminating foods with simple sugars is an effective weight loss strategy; however, many wholesome foods like bananas, beets, and carrots are also eliminated.
Step 9	Is this diet potentially dangerous?	The diet is low in dairy and potentially low in fruits, vegetables, and fiber. The cumbersome schedule outlined for eating what fruits are allowed may limit intake.
Step 10	Are there any health warnings associated with the diet?	Yes, the authors do suggest that more carbohydrate foods may be needed for individuals with strenuous exercise schedules. There is no mention that insulin-dependent diabetics may need to adjust their insulin schedule. This diet should not be used by people with renal failure.
Step 11	Does the diet imply that weight loss and be maintained without physical activity and permanent lifestyle changes?	The diet encourages permanent lifestyle changes.
Step 12	Are there any good points associated with the diet?	Yes, there are many elements of this diet that can lead to weight loss. By omitting high-energy, simple carbohydrates, like cake and candy, as well as alcohol can eliminate many calories and lead to weight loss. *Sugar Busters* works principally because it is low energy.
Is this a fad diet? Yes, although elimination of foods high in simple sugars is likely to result in weight loss.		

Fad diets can be generally categorized as very low carbohydrate and, hence, high in fat and protein; moderate carbohydrate, which may incorporate principles of the glycemic index in carbohydrate selection; and high-carbohydrate and, hence, low fat. Low-carbohydrate diets have emerged as perhaps the "most popular" of the fad diets, but it is not clear how many children and adolescents actually self-prescribe these diets. As discussed later, low-carbohydrate diets are used for severely obese adolescents or those with obesity-related comorbid conditions under medical supervision.

Low-Carbohydrate Diets

Dr. Atkins' New Diet Revolution, a very low-carbohydrate diet, is perhaps the most recognizable of the low-carbohydrate diets. Atkins diet books have sold more than 45 million copies over a 45-year period. The proposed mechanism by which low-carbohydrate diets induce weight loss is that reduced carbohydrate intake lowers insulin levels, allows unrestrained lipolysis, increases lipid oxidation, and initiates ketone production, which in turn suppresses appetite. The Atkins diet is divided into 4 main phrases: induction, leading to rapid weight loss; ongoing weight loss when weight loss slows; premaintenance, with slow weight loss; and life-time maintenance. The carbohydrate content and the percent of energy from carbohydrates range from 15 g (3%) in the induction phase to 116 g (22%) of energy in the maintenance phase. Energy levels are lowest during the induction phase and highest during maintenance[139]; all phases of the diet are low energy.

The rapid weight loss that is usually found at the outset of starting most low-carbohydrate diets results from diuresis as a result of mobilization of glycogen stores. It is not clear what actually causes the longer-term weight loss found in subjects on a low-carbohydrate diet. Authors of the diet books have suggested weight loss results because ketosis suppresses appetite or because the high protein levels suppress hunger and increase satiety. None of these factors has been confirmed, although other studies suggest that protein preloads significantly increased subjective ratings of satiety.[142] It has also been suggested that low-carbohydrate diets have less variety and are, therefore, less palatable, leading people to eat less. It is generally assumed, in the scientific community, that these diets are effective because they are low in energy and that diet duration is longer than other weight loss diets. Freedman et al[139] reported energy levels of 3 popular low-carbohydrate diets—the Atkins' induction diet (1152 kcals), the Carbohydrate Addict's Diet (1476 kcals), and Sugar Busters (1462 kcals). The overwhelming majority of people will lose weight at these lower energy levels.

None of the low-carbohydrate diets have been studied adequately or studied long-term in children and adolescents. Studies have, however, looked at medically supervised low-carbohydrate diets in severely overweight adolescents. In one such study of adolescents (n=24), those on a low-carbohydrate diet lost more weight than those on a traditional low-fat weight loss diet (n=22), although both diets induced significant weight loss; however, by the 24-week follow-up, only the low-carbohydrate diet group's weight loss was significantly lower than baseline. There were no serious metabolic or cardiac adverse effects reported in this study. Further, both groups had significant improvement in total and low-density lipoprotein (LDL) levels, but only the low-carbohydrate group had a significant reduction in triglycerides. Sparing of lean tissue was not observed in the low-carbohydrate group, and nutrient adequacy was not assessed.[143] Another study of severely overweight adolescents also showed that the low-carbohydrate group lost more weight than the low-fat group. That study also showed no adverse effects on the lipid profiles of participants in either group; however, the low-carbohydrate group did not show an improvement in LDL levels.[144]

Are There Health Advantages Conferred by Low-Carbohydrate Diets?

If the end justifies the means, low-carbohydrate diets can be said to have health advantages, the principal one being that they result in weight loss. Weight loss is usually rapid at the outset, which may "jump start" some dieters and make them more likely to comply with a weight loss regimen. Because low-carbohydrate diets are generally associated with higher intakes of total fat, saturated fatty acids, and cholesterol, because the protein is provided mainly by animal sources, there were initial concerns that they would adversely affect lipid profiles; at least in the short-term, this fear has been shown to be unfounded. Some short-term studies have suggested that low-carbohydrate and low glycemic load diets have improved lipid profiles in children[145,146] and adolescents. The most notable improvements are in high-density lipoprotein and triglyceride levels; the diets do not appear as effective in lowering LDL levels, although studies are contradictory.[143,144]

Health Concerns of Low-Carbohydrate Diets

Short-term effects of low-carbohydrate diets have been summarized by Freedman et al[139] and include bad taste, constipation, diarrhea, dizziness, headache, nausea, thirst, tiredness, weakness, and fatigue. It is unclear whether these are related to the low energy content of the diets or the composition of the diet. Ketoacidosis has also been reported.[147] There is also some evidence that in children, dietary restraint may be associated with decreased cognitive function.[148] Over a longer term, low-carbohydrate diets or other fad diets may not provide adequate energy for growth. This is a concern in the ketogenic diets used to treat some children with epilepsy (discussed later in thus chapter and also in Chapter 49: Ketogenic Diets) or, under medical supervision, some severely overweight children and adolescents. It is unclear whether lean body mass is spared in ketogenic diets.[149]

Low-carbohydrate diets or other fad diets do not meet the dietary recommendations for children and adolescents[150,151] and are, therefore, not recommended for unsupervised use. Fruit and vegetable consumption in children is already low,[152] with some studies showing that when French fries are excluded, less than 20% of children ate the recommended number of fruits and vegetables a day.[153] If children or adolescents were to follow a low-carbohydrate diet, lack of fruits and vegetables could be exacerbated. Fruit and vegetable consumption has been associated with many health benefits; for example, fruit and salad consumption have been associated with lower diastolic blood pressure in adolescents.[154] It is important for children and adolescents to consume fruit and vegetables, because their dietary habits and health behaviors track into adulthood.[155] In adults, consumption of fruits or vegetables has been inversely related to the risk chronic disease including some cancers,[156] coronary heart disease,[157] hypertension,[158] and type 2 diabetes mellitus.[159] Primary prevention through diet in childhood and adolescence may reduce the risk of these diseases in adulthood.[155] Dairy foods, the major source of calcium in the diet, are also omitted from low-carbohydrate diets. In the 2010 Dietary Guidelines for Americans,[160] calcium was identified as a nutrient of public health concern, because intake is low in many groups. Because low-carbohydrate diets are low in many wholesome foods, they also provide lower than recommended levels of vitamins A, E, and B_6; folate; thiamin; calcium; magnesium; iron; potassium; and dietary fiber.[139] For children older than 2 years, a diet containing fruits and vegetables, whole grains, low-fat and nonfat dairy products, beans, fish, and lean meats is needed to maintain health and support growth.[151]

The high-protein aspects of these diets, coupled with the lack of fruits and vegetables in the diet, pose concerns about bone health. Observational studies suggest that the alkaline-forming properties of fruit and vegetables mediate the body's acid-base balance to improve bone health.[161] This may be especially important with the high renal acid loads that may occur with low-carbohydrate diets. There is also controversy whether high protein diets in patients without renal disease damages the kidneys, although there is no substance to this claim. Studies have not been performed in children or adolescents. It is clear that children with existing renal disease or diabetes with microalbuminuria or clinical albuminuria should not attempt a high-protein diet unless under medical supervision.

Medically Supervised Low-Carbohydrate Diets in Children: Lessons for Those on Fad Diets?

High-fat (90% of energy), low-carbohydrate (3% of energy) ketogenic diets are used to control seizures in children with epilepsy that are refractory to more traditional treatment. Ketogenic diets have been reviewed recently (see Chapter 49: The Ketogenic Diet).[162] In addition to the traditional ketogenic diet, a modified Atkins diet has been used successfully to treat these children.[163] Children with higher levels of urinary ketones seem to have better seizure control than subjects reporting variable ketosis. Children on these diets may be deficient in calcium, magnesium, and iron. A major concern about these diets is that they adversely affect growth. Recently, it was shown[164] that the higher the levels of urinary ketones, the more severely growth was affected.

Early-onset adverse effects of ketogenic diets include hypertriglyceridemia, transient hyperuricemia, hypercholesterolemia, various infectious diseases, symptomatic hypoglycemia, hypoproteinemia, hypomagnesemia, repetitive hyponatremia, low concentrations of high-density lipoprotein, aspiration pneumonia, hepatitis, acute pancreatitis, and persistent metabolic acidosis. Late-onset adverse effects include growth abnormalities, osteopenia, renal stones, cardiomyopathy, secondary hypocarnitinemia, and iron-deficiency anemia.[165] This suggests that diets, including low-carbohydrate (fad) diets that induce ketosis, have the potential to cause potentially severe adverse reactions in children and should not be undertaken lightly or without medical supervision.

Very low-energy ketogenic diets, introduced in the 1980s, for weight loss in moderate to severely overweight children and adolescents make no pretense of being nutritionally adequate. These diets usually provided 650 to 750 kcal/day, along with 80 to 100 g of protein and 25 g of carbohydrate and fat and had to be supplemented with potassium, calcium, and a multivitamin.[166] These diets were shown to be effective in inducing weight loss and, with short-term use (1-5 months), were not associated with grown abnormalities; however, with longer-term use, there may be some growth slowing. These low-energy diets are also associated with decreased bone mineral density.[166] These diets should not be undertaken unless under the guidance of a medical team. Children and adolescents, who self-select similar diets, should be counseled against this choice.

Other Types of Fad Diets

Very low-fat diets, such as the Pritikin diet or the Ornish diet, may not strictly constitute "fad diets" but are, nevertheless, worthy of mention. These diets contain <10% of energy from fat and are contraindicated in children. These diets are primarily fruits, vegetables, and grains with nonfat dairy or soy and egg whites and small amounts of sugar and white flour. The Pritikin diet allows no more than 3.5 oz of lean beef, poultry, or fish a day. Like their low-carbohydrate counterparts, these diets too are low in energy for most adolescents. The Ornish diet has been estimated at less than 1300 kcal/day,[139] and the New Pritikin program recommends 1000 to 1200 kcal/day. Weight loss is the result of a reduction in fat and lean body mass. As with other low-energy diets, there are concerns that children may not have adequate energy to grow. Very low-fat diets are also deficient in vitamins E, D, and B_{12} and zinc.[139]

There are other types of fad diets, and information is widely available on the Internet and through the popular press. These range from the "cabbage soup diet" to single-food diets, including the "chocolate ice cream diet." There is no information in the scientific literature about the number of children or adolescents attempting these diets or specific health concerns. Because of the wide availability of the diets to children and adolescents, studies are needed.

Recommendations for Fad Diets

The AAP[34] and the American Academy of Nutrition and Dietetics' Evidence Analysis Library[167] recommend that, if, in a medical or nutrition professional's judgment, an energy-restricted diet is needed as a component of the treatment plan for overweight or obese children and adolescents, the diet should be balanced in macronutrients. A balanced diet should also provide the recommended amounts of micronutrients.

No unsupervised weight loss program should be undertaken by children or adolescents. Overweight or obese children would be better served with medically supervised programs that rely on behavior modification techniques to improve diet and lifestyle. Because of the potential link to dieting, notably severe dieting and eating disorders, education programs in the schools should be established to alert children, adolescents, and their parents to potential dangers. It is also important that physicians discuss healthy weight and healthful dietary patterns with children, adolescents, and their parents.

Use of Botanicals by Children and Adolescents

Background

Complementary and alternative medicine (CAM) and health care practices are defined simply as those that are not presently part of conventional medicine. Included in CAM is phytotherapy, or using plant-derived substances to treat or prevent disease. Technically, plant parts, including leaves, stems, flowers, berries, rhizomes, or roots, are called botanicals. They are valued for their therapeutic qualities, flavor, or scent. The terms "herb" and "herbals" are often used interchangeably with botanicals; however, by definition, herbs are nonwoody seed-producing plants that die to the ground at the end of the growing season. For the purposes of this review, the terms "herbals" and "botanicals" are used interchangeably.

The Dietary Supplement Health and Education Act of 1994 (Pub L No. 103-417) created a new framework for supplements by defining a dietary supplement as "a product taken by mouth that contains a 'dietary ingredient' intended to supplement the diet. The 'dietary ingredients' in these products may include: vitamins, minerals, herbs or other botanicals, amino acids, and substances such as enzymes, organ tissues, glandulars, and metabolites. Dietary supplements can also be extracts or concentrates, and may be found in many forms such as tablets, capsules, softgels, gelcaps, liquids, or powders. They can also be in other forms, such as a bar, but if they are, information on their label must not represent the product as a conventional food or a sole item of a meal or diet. Whatever their form may be, DSHEA places dietary supplements in a special category under the general umbrella of 'foods,' not drugs, and requires that every supplement be labeled a dietary supplement. A 'new dietary ingredient' is one that meets the above definition for a 'dietary ingredient' and was not sold in the U.S. in a dietary supplement before October 15, 1994."[168]

Manufacturers are responsible for determining that the dietary supplements they produce or distribute are safe and that any representations or claims made about them are substantiated by adequate evidence to show that they are not false or misleading. Dietary supplements do not need approval from the FDA before they are marketed. Except in the case of a new dietary ingredient, for which premarket review for safety data and other information is required by law, a manufacturer does not have to provide the FDA with the evidence it relies on to substantiate safety or effectiveness before or after it markets its products. Manufacturers also need to register pursuant to the Bioterrorism Act with the FDA before producing or selling supplements. In June, 2007, the FDA published comprehensive regulations for Current Good Manufacturing Practices for those who manufacture, package, or hold dietary supplement products.[169] These regulations focus on practices that ensure the identity, purity, quality, strength, and composition of dietary supplements, including vitamins, minerals, and herbal preparations.

Information that must be on a dietary supplement label includes: a descriptive name of the product stating that it is a "supplement"; the name and place of business of the manufacturer, packer, or distributor; a complete list of ingredients; and the net contents of the product. In addition, each dietary supplement must have nutrition labeling in the form of a "Supplement Facts" panel, which must identify each dietary ingredient contained in the product. Because only drugs can make such claims, dietary supplements must bear on the label that "This statement has not been evaluated by the Food and Drug Administration. This product is not intended to diagnose, treat, cure, or prevent disease."[169]

Much of the information available about an herb or herbal supplement is available online, and it is important that parents and older children and adolescents can evaluate this information. The Office of Dietary Supplements of the National Institutes of Health provides information on how to assess information on the Internet and has a downloadable app to make the material more available. The site also explains how to spot a health fraud.

Herbal Medicines

Herbal medicines are widely available in drugstores, in supermarkets, and over the Internet, and their sales are increasing. In 2010, the total sales of dietary supplements were $5200 million, compared with $4230 million in 2000.[170] It is not clear what percentage of these sales were made to children and adolescents; however, it has been demonstrated that children are more likely to use CAM, including herbals, if their parents use them.[171]

Herbal medicines are available in several forms. Children may take teas or tisanes, which are made by pouring boiling water over herbal parts, such as the leaves or flowers, and allowing them to steep. Decoctions are similar; they are made by boiling parts of the herb, usually woody parts like roots or bark, in water and then straining and drinking the extract. Tinctures are hydroalcoholic or glycerol solutions that usually contain 1 to 2 g of active ingredient(s)/mL of solution. Fluid extracts contain a ratio of 1 part solvent to 1 part herb; these are more concentrated than tinctures. Powdered herbs can be pressed into tablets or made into capsules. Salves, ointments, shampoos, and poultices can also be used for external use. Aromatherapy uses inhalation of volatile oils from herbs to treat illnesses or reduce stress.

Aside from their classification as dietary supplements, herbal medicines differ from conventional medicines in other ways. In common with other plant extracts, herbals are not limited to a single agent, and the actual therapeutic component(s) and its mechanism of action may not be known. Herbs can be grown, harvested, processed, and sold by anyone. The concentration of active ingredients is influenced by growing conditions, time of harvest, and storage and processing. The species used may be in question if herbs are harvested locally using common names. Finally, herbal medicines have not been subjected to the rigorous clinical trials that traditional medicines have. Previously, "caveat emptor" (buyer beware) was advice that consumers needed to heed when purchasing herbals as studies showed that the assayed species content was inconsistent with the content on the label.[172,173] As regulatory controls, such as the FDA's comprehensive regulations for Current Good Manufacturing Practices, which have been implemented,[169] and improved analytical techniques to assess bioactive constituents of herbal preparations have been applied, the standardization of herbal preparations appears to have improved.

Use of Botanicals by Children and Adolescents

Seventy percent of the world's sick or injured children are treated, often by physicians, using CAM; these treatments include use of traditional herbal medicines. In the United States, use of botanicals is self–selected, and most dietary supplements marketed to children and adolescents are vitamin and mineral preparations, not herbals. However, there are some mixtures of herbal preparations marketed specifically to children. One such example includes: honeysuckle flower, European elder berry, lemon balm leaf, chamomile flower, catnip aerial parts, *Echinacea purpurea* root and leaf, cassia twig, and licorice root. Another, which is marketed as an "immune protect," contains astragalus root, baizhu atractylodes rhizome, and siler root. Another product, with extracts of ginger root, fennel seed, and chamomile flowers, is marketed for teething infants, including those as young as 0 to 1 month old.[174]

Botanicals are used by children and adolescents because of dissatisfaction with conventional medicine, fear of adverse effects of conventional medicine, perceived benefits, and the belief that herbals are "more natural" and, therefore, safer than conventional medications. Data from the 2007 National Health Interview Survey demonstrated that approximately 1 in 9 children (11.8%) had used CAM therapy in the past 12 months; the most commonly used therapy was taking nonvitamin, nonmineral, natural products (3.9%). Children with a parent who had used CAM were almost 5 times as likely (23.9%) to use CAM as children whose parents did not use CAM (5.1%). CAM use among children could be higher than reported, especially among adolescents, because some children and adolescents may neglect to tell their parents they are using CAM.[171]

In 2007, the most commonly used nonvitamin, nonmineral, natural products used by children for health reasons in the past 30 days were *Echinacea* (37.2%), fish oil or omega-3 or docosahexaenoic acid (30.5%), combination herb pill (17.9%), and flaxseed oil or pills (16.7%). Natural products were used for back or neck pain (6.7%), head or chest colds (6.6%), anxiety or stress (4.8%), other musculoskeletal problems (4.2%), and attention-deficit/hyperactivity disorder (2.5%).[171]

Another study showed that CAM use, including botanicals, by children and adolescents was common, with more than 70% of some populations using it.[175] CAM use was more common among children with chronic or recurrent conditions than healthy children or those with acute illnesses.[175] The percentage of children or adolescents using herbals that were surgical patients varies greatly; ranging from as few as 3.5% or 4%[176] to as many as 12.8%.[177] *Echinacea* was the most commonly reported herbal used by children presenting for elective surgery. Up to 42% of these children were also taking conventional medications. The recommended preoperative discontinuation times of botanical vary, but in general, it is recommended that herbals be discontinued 2 weeks in advance of elective surgery.

In children, use of nontraditional and potentially toxic products, such as turpentine, pine needles, and cow chip tea, has also been reported.[178] Other studies have reported aloe vera, chamomile, garlic, peppermint, lavender, cranberry, ginger, *Echinacea*, lemon balm/grass, licorice, goldenseal, St John wort, gingko, sweet oil, and milk thistle as common botanicals taken by children (and their caregivers).[178-180] Table 13.5 reviews herbals commonly used in pediatric populations.

Table 13.5.

Herbs and Herbal Products That Are Commonly Used by Pediatric Populations

Herb	Use	Comments
Aloe (*Aloe ferox*)	Internal: purgative External: burns and other skin conditions	Internal use is contraindicated in children younger than 12 y because of potential for diarrhea, dehydration, and electrolyte loss.
Chamomile (*Anthemis nobilis*)	Internal uses: gastrointestinal distress—indigestion, colic, heartburn, anorexia, diarrhea External: swelling, inflammation	Allergic reactions. Inhibits cytochromes, potentially leading to drug interactions or toxicities. May be effective in treatment of infantile colic.
Cranberry (*Vaccinium macrocarpon*)	Primarily used for urinary tract infections, also used for *Helicobacter* infections	Appears safe, but excess amounts can lead to stomach upset and diarrhea.
Echinacea (*Echinacea angustifolio; Echinacea purpurea*)	Colds, flu, coughs, bronchitis, fever, immune stimulant	Not recommended for individuals with autoimmune disorders. Allergic reactions may occur in some individuals. No benefit for upper respiratory infection has been shown for children from 2 to 11 y.
Garlic (*Allium sativum*)	Internal: colds, bronchitis, fever, hypertension, dyslipidemia External: antibacterial, antifungal	Not well studied in children. Possible adverse effects include: allergic reaction, stomach disorders, odor of skin or breath, diarrhea, and rash. Dysrhythmias have also been reported.
Ginger (*Zingiber officinale*)	Anti-nausea, motion sickness, indigestion, anti-inflammatory, headache	Has been used in children undergoing cancer chemotherapy. Allergic reactions are seen, as is heartburn, if taken in excess. Ginger may interfere with blood clotting, although there are no reports of interactions with blood-thinning medications; there is a report of a ginger and drug bezoar small bowel obstruction.
Ginkgo (*Ginkgo biloba*)	Asthma, bronchitis, tinnitus, multiple sclerosis, memory improvement	Adverse effects include headache, nausea, gastrointestinal upset, diarrhea, dizziness, and allergic skin reactions. There is an increased risk of bleeding, and ginkgo is contraindicated in patients taking anticoagulants.

Fewer than 50% of children, adolescents, or their parents informed their primary health care professional about herbal use, because they did not believe botanicals would have adverse effects or that they could interact with conventional medications. Many of those that did try to discuss use of botanicals with health care professionals were not given information to help them make an informed decision about use and instead got information from friends or relatives.[178] Although most pediatricians surveyed believe their patients use CAM, few ask about use.[181] Physicians with a higher comfort level discussing CAM therapies with patients were more likely to discuss it with patients; however, fewer than 5% of physicians surveyed felt very knowledgeable about CAM and its use, and most believe that they need more education.[182] Because use of botanicals can pose health risks, especially in children, it is important that physicians are knowledgeable about botanicals and ask parents and children about their use.

Botanical Use and Potential Risks and Benefits in Children With Chronic Health Problems

CAM use, including the use of botanicals, is up to 3 times more common in children with chronic disease, including asthma, inflammatory bowel disease, and cancer[176-182] or recurrent diseases. It is especially important to assess potential benefits and risks of botanical use in these children.

AAP

> Pediatricians should ask parents and adolescent patients whether any herbal medicines are being used. Parents and adolescents should also be encouraged to share this information with their pharmacists. Although especially important in children with chronic diseases, this should apply to all children.

Up to 29% of children with asthma use botanicals. Although they were perceived as being safe, use of botanicals has been associated with persistent asthma, use of high-dose inhaled or oral steroids, poor or very poor control of symptoms, more frequent doctor visits, and increased risk of hospitalization.[183,184] A recent meta-analysis suggested that there were insufficient data supporting the safety and efficacy of herbal preparations and what data were available were suggestive of only subjective improvement and were usually not supported by objective findings.[184] It should also be noted that although some treatments, like quail eggs, are benign, others, like lobelia, possibly pennyroyal mint, and tree tea oil, are potentially toxic.[185]

Botanicals have been used to treat allergic diseases in children, including atopic dermatitis.[186] Clinical trials are underway using an herbal preparation called Food Allergy Herbal Formula-2 (FAHF-2) to determine whether it is a safe and effective treatment for food-allergic reactions in children.[187,188]

A study in Australia suggested that as many as 72% of children with inflammatory bowel disease used CAM; each child used an average of 2.4 therapies. Probiotics (78%) and fish oil (56%) were the most commonly used products; however, (unidentified) herbal therapies were used by 8% of children. Only a minority of patients believed the treatments were efficacious.[188] Although other studies have shown a lower prevalence of children with inflammatory bowel disease using CAM treatments,[189] the prevalence is below that of generally healthy children.[170]

A wide variety of CAM therapies are used by children with cancer. One study showed that 35% of pediatric cancer patients used herbals.[190] In most surveys, these therapies are used as adjunct therapies rather than primary ones. Ginger, an antiemetic, may benefit children undergoing highly emetogenic cancer chemotherapy treatments.[191] However, herbals have the potential to interact with anticancer drugs. Herbs with the highest likelihood of this include those that modulate the activity of drug-metabolizing enzymes, especially cytochrome p450 isoenzymes and the drug transporter P-glycoprotein; these herbals include garlic, ginkgo, *Echinacea*, ginseng, St Johns wort, and kava.[192-194] Thus, it is critical for parents to discuss with health care professionals any herbal medications their children are taking.

Herbal medicines also have more novel uses in children. Recently, a sugar-free lollipop containing glycyrrhizol A from licorice roots was developed to reduce the risk of cariogenic bacteria[195] and, with twice-a-day use, was shown to work in children at high risk of dental caries.[196] Ginkgolide B complex has been shown to be a migraine prophylactic in children.[197]

Safety of Botanicals in Children

A wide variety of drug-herbal or food-herbal adverse effects and toxicities have been reported; however, very little is known about this in children and adolescents. Randomized controlled trials are lacking; the few that have been performed are difficult to interpret, because the herbals were not always characterized, making it difficult to understand fully any therapeutic effects or any adverse effects.[198]

Of major concern is that in the United States, herbals are self-prescribed, usually without an understanding of their potential toxicity or adverse effects. Moreover, dosages for children are unknown and may differ from those appropriate for adults. Infants and children differ from adults in the absorption, distribution, metabolism, and excretion of drugs, including herbals. The developing central nervous system and immune system of young children may make them more susceptible to adverse effects of herbals. Paradoxically, children have larger livers than adults and may be more efficient in detoxifying substances,[199] but the growing number of reports of hepatotoxicity of herbals is also of concern.[200] Laxatives, such as aloe and senna, and diuretics, including fennel and licorice, have the potential to cause dehydration and electrolyte imbalances in infants and young children.[199] Children are also at high risk of developing allergic reactions to commonly used herbs, such as *Echinacea* and chamomile, both members of the family Compositae.

The effect of long-term exposures of herbals on the fetus and breastfeeding infants is unknown. Woolf[199] reviewed a case of a newborn infant whose mother drank senecionine-containing herbal tea daily during her pregnancy. The infant was born with hepatic vaso-occlusive disease; senecionine is one of the pyrrolizidine alkaloids associated with hepatic venous injury. Comfrey is an example of an herb containing pyrrolizidine; although oral comfrey preparations have been banned from the United States and European markets, topical preparations are still available.

German Commission E[201] listed aloe, buckthorn, camphor, Cajeput oil, cascara sagrada bark, eucalyptus leaf and oil, fennel oil, horseradish, mint oils (external), nasturtium, rhubarb root, senna, and watercress as contraindicated in children. However, more research is clearly needed to establish the safety and efficacy of botanicals in children.

III

Recommendations for Herbals and Botanicals

Herbals have been used for centuries and are still used by the majority of the world's children. As use in the United States continues to grow, it is critical that reliable information be available to parents, adolescents, and physicians. Rigorous scientific studies should be conducted to determine the safety and efficacy of phytotherapy in children and adolescents.

Practitioners should be familiar with the Natural Medicines Comprehensive Database, which provides information on product specific efficacy and safety data.[202] Through links on the National Center for Complementary and Alternative Medicine Web site, the Dietary Supplements Labels Database can be accessed.[203] This site provides information on herbals, randomized controlled trials, adverse effects, and manufacturers. Courses on CAM, including phytotherapy, should be offered as part of the education of pediatricians and pharmacists, and health care professionals should be prepared to discuss CAM therapies with their patients.

Parents or caregivers may not tell pediatricians or other health care professionals that their child is receiving CAM. It is important, however, that parents or caregivers speak with their child's health care professional about any CAM therapy being used or considered. Full disclosure will help manage their child's health and will help ensure coordinated and safe care. The National Center for Complementary and Alternative Medicine provides online and printed information describing how patients can talk to their health care professional about CAM.[204] Points to consider for parent/health care professional discussions on CAM, taken from the National Center for Complementary and Alternative Medicine Web site, are shown in Table 13.6. Where to get reliable information about herbals is presented in Table 13.7. All health care professionals should ask pediatric surgical and medical patients about use of CAM, especially herbals.

Table 13.6.

Points to Consider When Considering Complementary and Alternative Medicine Use for Children

When seeking care from a CAM practitioner, it is important to ask about the practitioner's:
- Education and training
- Experience in delivering care to children
- Experience working with other providers, including physicians, to ensure coordinated care
- Licensing (some states have licensing requirements for certain CAM practitioners, such as chiropractors, naturopathic doctors, massage therapists, and acupuncturists).

Additional points to consider:
- Ensure that your child has received an accurate diagnosis from a licensed health care provider and that CAM use does not replace or delay conventional medical care.
- If you decide to use CAM for your child, do not increase the dose or length of treatment beyond what is recommended (more is not necessarily better).
- If your child experiences an effect from a CAM therapy that concerns you, contact your child's health care provider.
- Store herbal and other dietary supplements out of the sight and reach of children.
- If you are a woman who is pregnant or breastfeeding, remember that some CAM therapies may affect your fetus or nursing infant.

From: National Institutes of Health. National Center for Complementary and Alternative Medicine. Complementary and Alternative Medicine Use in Children. Available at: http://nccam.nih.gov/health/children. Accessed October 15, 2012.

Table 13.7.
Where To Get Reliable Information About Herbs

Books
Foster S, Tyler VE. *Tyler's Honest Herbal: a Sensible Guide to the Use of Herbs and Related Remedies.* 4th ed. London, England: The Hawthorn Press, Inc; 1999. ISBN: 0-789008750 Herr SM. *Herb-Drug Interaction Handbook.* 3rd ed. New York, NY: Church Street Books; 2005. ISBN: 0-9678773-2-6 *PDR for Herbal Medicine.* 3rd ed. Montvale, NJ: PDR Network; 2004. ISBN: 1563635127 Robbers JE, Tyler VE. *Tyler's Herbs of Choice: The Therapeutic Use of Phytochemicals.* 2nd ed. London, England: The Hawthorn Press, Inc; 1999. ISBN: 0-789001608
Online Databases
Agricola: http://agricola.nal.usda.gov Amazon Plants Tropical Plant Database: http://www.rain-tree.com/plants.htm American Indian Ethnobotany Database: http://herb.umd.umich.edu Botanical Dermatology Database: http://bodd.cf.ac.uk Community of Science: http://www.cos.com Cyberbotanica· Plant Compounds and Ethnobotanical Databases: http://biotech.icmb.utexas.edu/botany Dr. Duke's Phytochemical and Ethnobotanical Databases: http://www.ars-grin.gov/duke Garden Gate: Roots of Botanical Names: http://garden-gate.prairienet.org/botrts.htm Medical Herbalism: Poisonous Plant Database: http://medherb.com/POISON.HTM Medicinal Plant Databases: http://www.floridaplants.com/mdata.htm Medicinal and Poisonous Plant Database: http://www.biologie.uni-hamburg.de/b-online/ibc99/poison NAPRALERT: http://www.cas.org/ONLINE/DBSS/napralertss.html Natural Standard: http://www.naturalstandard.com Plants Database: http://plants.usda.gov Plants for a Future Database Search: http://www.ibiblio.org/pfaf/D_search.html Poisonous Plant Database (PLANTOX): http://www.cfsan.fda.gov/~djw/plantox.html PubMed: http://www.ncbi.nlm.nih.gov
Reliable Information About Botanicals on the Internet
The American Herbalist Guild: http://www.americanherbalistsguild.com American Herbal Products Association: http://www.ahpa.org American Botanical Council: http://www.herbalgram.org Herb Research Foundation: http://www.herbs.org Food and Drug Administration: http://www.fda.gov MedLine Plus Health Information Drugs and Supplements: http://www.nlm.nih.gov/medlineplus/druginformation.html National Center for Complementary and Alternative Medicine: http://nccam.nih.gov Office of Dietary Supplements, National Institutes of Health: http://dietary-supplements.info.nih.gov World Health Organization: http://www.who.int/en

III

References

1. NumberOf.net. Number of Fast Food Restaurants in America. Available at: http://www.numberof.net/number-of-fast-food restaurants-in-america. Accessed October 9, 2012

2. United States Department of Agriculture, Economic Research Service. Food Expenditures Overview. Available at: http://www.ers.usda.gov/data-products/food-expenditures.aspx. Accessed October 9, 2012

3. United States Department of Agriculture, Economic Research Service. Table 12—Food Expenditures at Constant Prices. Available at: http://www.ers.usda.gov/datafiles/Food_Expenditures/Food_Expenditures/table12.xls. Accessed October 9, 2012

4. Bowman SA, Gortmaker SL, Ebbeling CB, Pereira MA, Ludwig DS. Effects of fast-food consumption on energy intake and diet quality among children in a national household survey. *Pediatrics*. 2004;113(1 Pt 1):112-118

5. Paeratakul S, Ferdinand DP, Champagne CM, Ryan DH, Bray GA. Fast-food consumption among US adults and children: dietary and nutrient intake profile. *J Am Diet Assoc*. 2003;103(10):1332-1338

6. Pereira MA, Kartashov AI, Ebbeling CB, Van Horn L, Slattery ML, Jacobs DR Jr, Ludwig DS. Fast-food habits, weight gain, and insulin resistance (the CARDIA study): 15-year prospective analysis. *Lancet*. 2005;365(9453):36-42

7. Mancino L, Todd JE, Guthrie J, Lin B-H. How food away from home affects children's diet quality. Washington, DC: US Department of Agriculture, Economic Research Service; 2010. ERS Report Number 104. Available at: http://www.ers.usda.gov/Publications/err104/err104.pdf. Accessed October 9, 2012

8. Bowman SA, Vinyard BT. Fast food consumption of U.S. adults: impact on energy and nutrient intakes and overweight status. *J Am Coll Nutr*. 2004;23(2):163-168

9. Schmidt M, Affenito SG, Striegel-Moore R, et al. Fast-food intake and diet quality in black and white girls: the National Heart, Lung, and Blood Institute Growth and Health Study. *Arch Pediatr Adolesc Med*. 2005;159(7):626-631

10. Lin B, Frazao E. Nutritional quality of foods at and away from home. *Food Rev*. 1997;20(3):33-40

11. French SA, Story M, Neumark-Sztainer D, Fulkerson JA, Hannan P. Fast food restaurant use among adolescents: associations with nutrient intake, food choices and behavioral and psychosocial variables. *Int J Obes*. 2001;25(12):1823-1833

12. Fox MK, Devaney B, Reidy K, Razafindrakoto C, Ziegler P. Relationship between portion size and energy intake among infants and toddlers: evidence of self-regulation. *J Am Diet Assoc*. 2006;106(1 Suppl 1):S77-S83

13. Rolls BJ, Engell D, Birch LL. Serving portion size influences 5-year-old but not 3-year-old child's food intakes. *J Am Diet Assoc*. 2000;100(2):232-234

14. Fisher JO, Rolls BJ, Birch LL. Children's bite size and intake of an entrée are greater with large portions than with age-appropriate or self-selected portions. *Am J Clin Nutr*. 2003;77(5):1164-1170

15. Diliberti N, Bordi PL, Conklin MT, Roe LS, Rolls BJ. Increased portion size leads to increased energy intake in a restaurant meal. *Obes Res*. 2004;12(3):562-568

16. Fisher JO, Liu Y, Birch LL, Rolls BJ. Effects of portion size and energy density on young children's intake at a meal. *Am J Clin Nutr*. 2007;86(1):174-179

17. Guthrie JF, Lin BH, Frazao E. Role of food prepared away from home in the American diet, 1977-78 versus 1994-96: changes and consequences. *J Nutr Educ Behav*. 2002;34(3):140-150

18. O'Donnell SI, Hoerr SL, Mendoza JA, Tsuei Goh E. Nutrient quality of fast food kids meals. *Am J Clin Nutr*. 2008;88(5):1388-1395

19. Sebastian RS, Wilkinson Enns C, Goldman JD. US adolescents and MyPyramid: associations between fast-food consumption and lower likelihood of meeting recommendations. *J Am Diet Assoc*. 2009;109(2):226-235

20. Food Labeling; Nutrition Labeling of Standard Menu Items in Restaurants and Similar Retail Food Establishments; Proposed Rule. *Fed Regist*. 2011;76(66):19191-19236. Available at: http://edocket.access.gpo.gov/2011/2011-7940.htm. Accessed October 9, 2012

21. Variyam JN. *Nutrition Labeling in the Food-Away-From-Home Sector: An Economic Assessment*. Washington, DC: US Department of Agriculture, Economic Research Service; 2005. ERS Report No. 4

22. Elbel B, Kersh R, Brescoll VL, Dixon LB. Calorie labeling and food choices: a first look at the effects on low-income people in New York City. *Health Aff (Millwood)*. 2009;28(6):w1110-w1121

23. Dumanovsky T, Huang CY, Bassett MT, Silver LD. Consumer awareness of fast-food calorie information in New York City after implementation of a menu labeling regulation. *Am J Public Health*. 2010;100(12):2520-2525

24. Bassett MT, Dumanovsky T, Huang C, et al. Purchasing behavior and calorie information at fast-food chains in New York City, 2007. *Am J Public Health*. 2008;98(8):1457-1459

25. Harnack LJ, French SA. Effect of point-of-purchase calorie labeling on restaurant and cafeteria food choices: a review of the literature. *Int J Behav Nutr Phys Act*. 2008,5:51

26. Yamamoto JA, Yamamoto JB, Yamamoto BE, Yamamoto LG. Adolescent fast food and restaurant ordering behavior with and without calorie and fat content menu information. *J Adolesc Health*. 2005;37(5):397-402

27. Elbel B, Gyamfi J, Kersh R. Child and adolescent fast-food choice and the influence of calorie labeling: a natural experiment. *Int J Obes (Lond)*. 2011;35(4):493-500

28. Krukowski RA, Harvey-Berino J, Kolodinsky J, Narsana RT, Desisto TP. Consumers may not use or understand calorie labeling in restaurants. *J Am Diet Assoc*. 2006;106(6):917-920

29. Tandon PS, Wright, J, Zhou C, Rogers CB, Christakis DA. Nutrition menu labeling may lead to lower-calorie restaurant meal choices for children. *Pediatrics*. 2010;125(2):244-248

30. Fleischhacker SE, Evenson KR, Rodriguez DA, Ammerman AS. A systematic review of fast food access studies. *Obes Rev*. 2011;12(5):e460-e471

31. Taveras EM, Berkey CS, Rifas-Shiman SL, Ludwig DS, Rockett HR, Field AE, Colditz GA, Gillman MW. Association of consumption of fried food away from home with body mass index and diet quality in older children and adolescents. *Pediatrics*. 2005;116(4):e518-e524

III

32. Boutelle KN, Fulkerson JA, Neumark-Sztainer D, Story M, French SA. Fast food for family meals: relationships with parent and adolescent food intake, home food availability and weight status. *Public Health Nutr.* 2007;10(1):16-23

33. Thompson OM, Ballew C, Resnicow K, et al. Food purchased away from home as a predictor of change in BMI z-score among girls. *Int J Obes Relat Metab Disord.* 2004;28(2):282-289

34. Barlow SE; Expert Committee. Expert committee recommendations regarding the prevention, assessment, and treatment of child and adolescent overweight and obesity: summary report. *Pediatrics.* 2007;120(Suppl 4):S164-S192

35. Rydell SA, Harnack LJ, Oakes JM, Story M, Jeffery RW, French SA. Why eat at fast-food restaurants: reported reasons among frequent consumers. *J Am Diet Assoc.* 2008;108(12):2066-2070

36. Frieden TR, Dietz W, Collins J. Reducing childhood obesity through policy change: acting now to prevent obesity. *Health Aff (Millwood).* 2010;29(3):357-363

37. Andreyeva T, Kelly IR, Harris JL. Exposure to food advertising on television: Associations with children's fast food and soft drink consumption and obesity. *Econ Hum Biol.* 2011;9(3):221-233

38. Oates C, Blades M, Gunter B, Don J. Children's understanding of television advertising: a qualitative approach. *J Marketing Commun.* 2003;9:59-71

39. Carter OB, Patterson LJ, Donovan RJ, Ewing MT, Roberts CM. Children's understanding of the selling versus persuasive intent of junk food advertising: implications for regulation. *Soc Sci Med.* 2011;72(6):962-968

40. Coon KA, Tucker KL. Television and children's consumption patterns. A review of the literature. *Minerva Pediatr.* 2002;54(5):423-436

41. American Academy of Pediatrics, Committee on Communications. Policy statement: children, adolescents, and advertising. *Pediatrics.* 2006;118(6):2563-2569

42. Story M, Neumark-Sztainer D, French S. Individual and environmental influences on adolescent eating behaviors. *J Am Diet Assoc.* 2002;102(3 Suppl):S40-S51

43. Arredondo E, Castaneda D, Elder JP, Slymen D, Dozier D. Brand name logo recognition of fast food and healthy food among children. *J Community Health.* 2009;34(1):73-78

44. Robinson TN, Borzekowski DL, Matheson DM, Kraemer HC. Effects of fast food branding on young children's taste preferences. *Arch Pediatr Adolesc Med.* 2007;161(8):792-797

45. Institute of Medicine. *Food Marketing to Children and Youth: Threat or Opportunity? Committee on Food Marketing and the Diets of Children and Youth.* McGinnis JM, Gootman JA, Vivica I. Kraak VI, eds. Washington, DC: National Academies Press; 2006

46. Holt DJ, Ippolito PM, Desrochers DM, Kelley CR. *Children's Exposure to TV Advertising in 1977 and 2004: Information for the Obesity Debate.* Washington, DC: Federal Trade Commission; 2007

47. Ozer EM, Brindis CD, Millstein SG, Knopf DK, Irwin CEJ. *America's Adolescents: Are They Healthy?* San Francisco, CA: University of California, San Francisco, National Adolescent Health Information Center; 1998

48. French SA, Harnack L, Jeffery RW. Fast food restaurant use among women in the Pound of Prevention study: dietary, behavioral and demographic correlates. *Int J Obes Relat Metab Disord*. 2000;24(10):1353-1359

49. Crespo C, Smit E, Troiano R, Bartlett S, Macera C, Anderson R. Television watching, energy intake and obesity in US children. *Arch Pediatr Adolesc Med*. 2001;155(3):360-365

50. Sisson SB, Broyles ST, Newton RL Jr, Baker BL, Chernausek SD. TVs in the bedrooms of children: does it impact health and behavior? *Prev Med*. 2011;52(2):104-108

51. Taras HL, Gage M. Advertised foods on children's television. *Arch Pediatr Adolesc Med*. 1995;149(6):649-652

52. Montgomery KC, Chester J. Interactive food and beverage marketing: targeting adolescents in the digital age. *J Adolesc Health*. 2009;45(3 Suppl):S18-S29

53. Sharkey JR, Johnson CM, Dean WR, Horel SA. Focusing on fast food restaurants alone underestimates the relationship between neighborhood deprivation and exposure to fast food in a large rural area. *Nutr J*. 2011;10:10

54. Austin SB, Melly SJ, Sanchez BN, Patel A, Buka S, Gortmaker SL. Clustering of fast-food restaurants around schools: a novel application of spatial statistics to the study of food environments. *Am J Public Health*. 2005;95:1575-1581

55. Neckerman KM, Bader MD, Richards CA, et al. Disparities in the food environments of New York City public schools. *Am J Prev Med*. 2010;39(3):195-202

56. Block JP, Scribner RA, DeSalvo KB. Fast food, race/ethnicity, and income: a geographic analysis. *Am J Prev Med*. 2004;27(3):211-217

57. Alter DA, Eny K. The relationship between the supply of fast-food chains and cardiovascular outcomes. *Can J Public Health*. 2005;96(3):173-177

58. Sturm R, Datar A. Body mass index in elementary school children, metropolitan area food prices and food outlet density. *Public Health*. 2005;119(12):1059-1068

59. Burdette HL, Whitaker RC. Neighborhood playgrounds, fast food restaurants, and crime: relationships to overweight in low-income preschool children. *Prev Med*. 2004;38(1):57-63

60. Jeffery RW, Baxter J, McGuire M, Linde J. Are fast food restaurants an environmental risk factor for obesity? *Int J Behav Nutr Phys Act*. 2006;3:2

61. Pateman BC, McKinney P, Kann L, Small ML, Warren CW, Collins JL. School food service. *J Sch Health*. 1995;65(8):327-332

62. Kubik MY, Lytle LA, Story M. Soft drinks, candy, and fast food: what parents and teachers think about the middle school food environment. *J Am Diet Assoc*. 2005;105(2):233-239

63. Young LR, Nestle M. Portion sizes and obesity: responses of fast-food companies. *J Public Health Policy*. 2007;28(2):238-248

64. Hardee's. Available at: http://www.hardees.com/menu. Accessed October 9, 2012

65. Contento IR, Koch PA, Lee H, Calabrese-Barton A. Adolescents demonstrate improvement in obesity risk behaviors after completion of choice, control & change, a curriculum addressing personal agency and autonomous motivation. *J Am Diet Assoc*. 2010;110(12):1830-1839

III

66. McDonalds. Available at: http://www.mcdonalds.com/us/en/home.html. Accessed October 9, 2012

67. Wendy's. Available at: http://www.wendys.com. Accessed October 9, 2012

68. Burger King. Available at: http://www.bk.com/en/us/menu-nutrition/index.html. Accessed October 9, 2012

69. Subway. Available at: http://subwaykids.com/grownups/freshfit. Accessed October 9, 2012

70. Horovitz B. Fast-food giants hunt for new products to tempt consumers. *USA Today*. July 3–4, 2002

71. Birch LL, Zimmerman S, Hind H. The influence of social-affective context on preschool children's food preferences. *Child Dev*. 1980;51:856-861

72. Fisher JO, Birch LL. Restricting access to palatable foods affects children's behavioral response, food selection, and intake. *Am J Clin Nutr*. 1999;69(6):1264-1272

73. Nicklas TA, Goh ET, Goodell LS, et al. Impact of commercials on food preferences of low-income, minority preschoolers. *J Nutr Educ Behav*. 2011;43(1):35-41

74. Hughner RS, McDonagh P, Prothero A, Schultz C J II, Stanton J. Who are organic food consumers? A compilation and review of why people purchase organic food. *J Consum Behav*. 2007;6:94-110

75. United States Department of Agriculture. The National List of Allowed and Prohibited Substances. Available at: http://www.ams.usda.gov/AMSv1.0/getfile?dDocName=STELPRDC5068682. Accessed October 9, 2012

76. Winter CK, Davis SF. Organic foods. *J Food Sci*. 2006;71(9):R117-R124

77. Dimitri C, Oberholtzer L. *Marketing U.S. Organic Foods: Recent Trends From Farms to Consumers*. Washington, DC: US Department of Agriculture, Economic Research Service; 2009. Economic Information Bulletin No. 58

78. Nutrition Business Journal. NBJ's Organic Foods Report 2004. San Diego, CA: Nutrition Business Journal/Penton Media Inc; 2004. Available at: http://www.ccof.org/pdf/NBJ_Organic_Report_2004.pdf. Accessed October 9, 2012

79. Organic Trade Association. Industry Statistics and Projected Growth. Available at: http://www.ota.com/organic/mt/business.html. Accessed October 9, 2012

80. Oberholtzer L, Dimitri C, Greene C. Price Premiums Hold on as U.S. Organic Produce Market Expands. Washington, DC: US Department of Agriculture, Economic Research Service; 2005

81. Greene C, Dimitri C, Lin B-H, McBride W, Oberholtzer L, Smith T. Emerging issues in the U.S. Organic Industry. Washington, DC: US Department of Agriculture, Economic Research Service; 2009. Economic Information Bulletin No. 55

82. Magnusson MK, Arvola A, Hursti UK, Aberg L, Sjoden PO. Choice of organic foods is related to perceived consequences for human health and to environmentally friendly behaviour. *Appetite*. 2003;40(2):109-117

83. Shepherd R, Magnusson M, Sjoden PO. Determinants of consumer behavior related to organic foods. *Ambio*. 2005;34(4-5):352-359

84. Arvola A, Vassallo M, Dean M, et al. Predicting intentions to purchase organic food: the role of affective and moral attitudes in the Theory of Planned Behaviour. *Appetite.* 2008;50(2-3):443-454

85. Williams CM. Nutritional quality of organic food: shades of grey or shades of green? *Proc Nutr Soc.* 2002;61(1):19-24

86. Thompson G, Kidwell J. Explaining the choice of organic produce: cosmetic defects, prices, and consumer preferences. *Am J Agric Econ.* 1998;80:277-278

87. Dettmann RL, Dimitri C. Who's buying organic vegetables? Demographic characteristics of U.S. consumers. *J Food Prod Marketing.* 2010;16(1):79-91

88. Zepeda L, Li J. Characteristics of organic food shoppers. *J Agric Appl Econ.* 2007;39(1):17-28

89. Harris JM. Consumers pay a premium for organic baby foods. *Food Rev.* 1997;20(2):13-16

90. Dangour AD, Dodhia SK, Hayter A, Allen E, Lock K, Uauy R. Nutritional quality of organic foods: a systematic review. *Am J Clin Nutr.* 2009;90(3):680-685

91. Magkos F, Arvaniti F, Zampelas A. Organic food: buying more safety or just piece of mind? A critical review of the literature. *Crit Rev Food Sci Nutr.* 2006;46(1):23-56

92. Bourn D, Prescott J. A comparison of the nutritional value, sensory qualities, and food safety of organically and conventionally produced foods. *Crit Rev Food Sci Nutr.* 2002;42(1):1-34

93. Dangour AD, Lock K, Hayter A, Aikenhead A, Allen E, Uauy R. Nutrition-related health effects of organic foods: a systematic review. *Am J Clin Nutr.* 2010;92(1):203-210

94. Marcus MB. Organic foods offer peace of mind—at a price. *US News and World Report.* 2001;130:48-50

95. Greer FR; Shannon M; American Academy of Pediatrics, Committee on Nutrition, Committee on Environmental Health. Infant methemoglobinemia: the role of dietary nitrate in food and water. *Pediatrics.* 2005;116(3):784-786

96. Roberts JR; Karr CJ; American Academy of Pediatrics, Council on Environmental Health. Technical report: pesticide exposure in children. *Pediatrics.* 2012;130(6):e1765-e1788

97. American Academy of Pediatrics, Council on Environmental Health. Policy statement: pesticide exposure in children. *Pediatrics.* 2012;130(6):e1757-1763

98. National Research Council. *Pesticides in the Diets of Infants and Children.* Washington, DC: National Academies Press; 1993

99. Eskenazi B, Bradman A, Castorina R. Exposures of children to organophosphate pesticides and their potential adverse health effects. *Environ Health Perspect.* 1999;107(Suppl 3):409-419

100. Eskenazi B, Marks AR, Bradman A, et al. Organophosphate pesticide exposure and neurodevelopment in young Mexican-American children. *Environ Health Perspect.* 2007;115(5):792-798

101. Bouchard MF, Bellinger DC, Wright RO, Weisskopf MG. Attention-deficit/hyperactivity disorder and urinary metabolites of organophosphate pesticides. *Pediatrics.* 2010;125(6):e1270-e1277

102. Benbrook CM. Organochlorine residues pose surprisingly high dietary risks. *J Epidemiol Community Health*. 2002;56(11):822-823

103. Gonzales M, Miglioranza KS, Aizpun de Moreno JE, Moreno VJ. Occurrence and distribution of organochlorine pesticides (OCPs) in tomato (*Lycopersicon esculentum*) crops from organic production. *J Agric Food Chem*. 2003;51(5):1353-1359

104. Baker BP, Benbrook CM, Groth E, Benbrook L. Pesticide residues in conventional, integrated pest management (IPM)-grown and organic foods: insights from three US data sets. *Food Addit Contam*. 2002;19(5):427-446

105. Crinnion WJ. Organic foods contain higher levels of certain nutrients, lower levels of pesticides, and may provide health benefits for the consumer. *Altern Med Rev*. 2010;15(1):4-12

106. Williams PR, Hammitt JK. A comparison of organic and conventional fresh produce buyers in the Boston area. *Risk Anal*. 2000;20(5):735-746

107. MacIntosh DL, Kabiru C, Echols SL, Ryan PB. Dietary exposure to chlorpyrifos and levels of 3,5,6 trichloro-2-pyridinol in urine. *J Expo Anal Environ Epidemiol*. 2001;11(4):279-285

108. Curl CL, Fenske RA, Elgethun K. Organophosphorus pesticide exposure of urban and suburban preschool children with organic and conventional diets. *Environ Health Perspect*. 2003;111(3):377-382

109. Lu C, Toepel K, Irish R, Fenske RA, Barr DB, Bravo R. Organic diets significantly lower children's dietary exposure to organophosphorus pesticides. *Environ Health Perspect*. 2006;114(2):260-263

110. Lu C, Barr DB, Pearson MA, Waller LA. Dietary intake and its contribution to longitudinal organophosphorus pesticide exposure in urban/suburban children. *Environ Health Perspect*. 2008;116(4):537-542

111. Bailey JS, Cosby DE. *Salmonella* prevalence in free-range and certified organic chickens. *J Food Prot*. 2005;68(11):2451-2453

112. Cui S, Ge B, Zheng J, Meng J. Prevalence and antimicrobial resistance of *Campylobacter* spp. and *Salmonella* serovars in organic chickens from Maryland retail stores. *Appl Environ Microbiol*. 2005;71(7):4108-4111

113. Loncarevic S, Johannessen GS, Rorvik LM. Bacteriological quality of organically grown leaf lettuce in Norway. *Lett Appl Microbiol*. 2005;41(2):186-189

114. Forman J, Silverstein J; American Academy of Pediatrics, Committee on Nutrition and Council on Environmental Health. Organic foods: health and environmental advantages and disadvantages. *Pediatrics*. 2012;130(5):e1406-e1415

115. Ogden CL, Carroll MD, Kit BK, Flegal KM. Prevalence of obesity and trends in body mass index among US children and adolescents, 1999-2010. *JAMA*. 2012;307(5):483-490

116. Centers for Disease Control and Prevention. Youth Risk Behavior Surveillance, 2011. *MMWR Surveill Summ*. 2012;61(4):1-162

117. Kelly C, Molcho M, Nic Gabhainn S. Patterns in weight reduction behaviour by weight status in schoolchildren. *Public Health Nutr*. 2010;13(8):1229-1236

118. Serdula MK, Collins E, Williamson DF, Anda RF, Pamuk E, Byers TE. Weight control practices of US adolescents and adults. *Ann Intern Med*. 1993;119(7 Pt 2):667-671

119. Tanofsky-Kraff M, Faden D, Yanovski SZ, Wilfley DE, Yanovski JA. The perceived onset of dieting and loss of control eating behaviors in overweight children. *Int J Eat Disord.* 2005;38(2):112-122

120. Field AE, Austin SB, Taylor CB, et al. Relation between dieting and weight change among preadolescents and adolescents. *Pediatrics.* 2003;112(4):900-906

121. Calderon LL, Yu CK, Jambazian P. Dieting practices in high school students. *J Am Diet Assoc.* 2004;104(9):1369-1374

122. Davison KK, Markey CN, Birch LL. A longitudinal examination of patterns in girls' weight concerns and body satisfaction from ages 5 to 9 years. *Int J Eat Disord.* 2003;33(3): 320-332

123. Abramovitz BA, Birch LL. Five-year-old girl's ideas about dieting are predicted by their mother's dieting. *J Am Diet Assoc.* 2000;100(10):1157-1163

124. Feldman W, Feldman E, Goodman JT. Culture versus biology: children's attitudes toward fatness and thinness. *Pediatrics.* 1988;81(2):190-194

125. Field AE, Cheung L, Wolf AM, Herzog DB, Gortmaker SL, Colditz GA. Exposure to the mass media and weight concerns among girls. *Pediatrics.* 1999;103(3):e36

126. Thomsen SR, Weber MM, Brown LB. The relationship between reading beauty and fashion magazines and the use of pathogenic dieting methods among adolescent females. *Adolescence.* 2002;37(145):1-18

127. Irving LM, Neumark-Sztainer D. Integrating the prevention of eating disorders and obesity: feasible or futile? *Prev Med.* 2002;34(3):299-309

128. Neumark-Sztainer D, Wall M, Guo J, Story M, Haines J, Eisenberg M. Obesity, disordered eating, and eating disorders in a longitudinal study of adolescents: How do dieters fare 5 years later? *J Am Diet Assoc.* 2006;106(4):559-568

129. Patton GC, Selzer R, Coffee C, Carlin JB, Wolfe R. Onset of adolescent eating disorders: Population based cohort study over 3 years. *BMJ.* 1999:318:765-768

130. Killen JD, Taylor CB, Hayward C, et al. Weight concerns influence the development of eating disorders: a four year prospective study. *J Consult Clin Psychol.* 1996;64(5): 936-940

131. Killion L, Hughes SO, Wendt JC, Pease D, Nicklas TA. Minority mothers' perceptions of children's body size. *Int J Pediatr Obes.* 2006;1(2):96-102

132. Phares V, Steinberg AR, Thompson JK. Gender differences in peer and parental influences: body image disturbance, self-worth and psychological functioning in preadolescent children. *J Youth Adolesc.* 2004;33(5):421-429

133. Dohnt HK, Tiggemann M. Peer influences on body dissatisfaction and dieting awareness in young girls. *Br J Dev Psychol.* 2005;23(1):103-116

134. Lowes J, Tiggemann M. Body dissatisfaction, dieting awareness and the impact of parental influence in young children. *Br J Health Psychol.* 2003;8(Pt 2):135-147

135. Hutchinson DM, Rapee RM. Do friends share similar body image and eating problems? The role of social networks and peer influences in early adolescence. *Behav Res Ther.* 2007;45(7):1557-1577

III

136. Thompson JK, Shroff H, Herbozo S, Cafri G, Rodriguez J, Rodriguez M. Relations among multiple peer influences, body dissatisfaction, eating disturbance, and self-esteem: a comparison of average weight, at risk of overweight, and overweight adolescent girls. *J Pediatr Psychol*. 2007;32(1):24-29

137. Neumark-Sztainer D, Bauer KW, Friend S, Hannan PJ, Story M, Berge JM. Family weight talk and dieting: how much do they matter for body dissatisfaction and disordered eating behaviors in adolescent girls? *J Adolesc Health*. 2010;47(3):270-276

138. Guest J, Bilgin A, Pearce R, Baines S, Zeuschner C, Rossignol-Grant CL, Morris MJ, Grant R. Evidence for under-nutrition in adolescent females using routine dieting practices. *Asia Pac J Clin Nutr*. 2010;19(4):526-533

139. Freedman MR, King J, Kennedy E. Popular diets: a scientific review. *Obes Res*. 2001;9(Suppl 1):1S-40S

140. Nicklas TA, Myers L, Farris RP, Srinivasan SR, Berenson GS. Nutritional quality of a high carbohydrate diet as consumed by children: The Bogalusa Heart Study. *J Nutr*. 1996;126(5):1382-1388

141. Greene-Finestone LS, Campbell MK, Evers SE, Gutmanis IA. Adolescents' low-carbohydrate-density diets are related to poorer dietary intakes. *J Am Diet Assoc*. 2005;105(1):1783-1788

142. Halton TL, Hu FB. The effects of high protein diets on thermogenesis, satiety, and weight loss: a critical review. *J Am College Nutr*. 2004;23(5):373-385

143. Krebs NF, Gao D, Gralla J, Collins JS, Johnson SL. Efficacy and safety of a high protein, low carbohydrate diet for weight loss in severely obese adolescents. *J Pediatr*. 2010;157(2):252-258

144. Sondike SB, Copperman N, Jacobson MS. Effects of a low-carbohydrate diet on weight loss and cardiovascular risk factor in overweight adolescents. *J Pediatr*. 2003;142(3):253-258

145. Slyper A, Jurva J, Pleuss J, Hoffmann R, Gutterman D. Influence of glycemic load on HDL cholesterol in youth. *Am J Clin Nutr*. 2005;81(2):376-379

146. Starc TJ, Shea S, Cohn LC, Mosca L, Gersony WM, Deckelbaum RJ. Greater dietary intake of simple carbohydrate is associated with lower concentrations of high-density-lipoprotein cholesterol in hypercholesterolemic children. *Am J Clin Nutr*. 1998;67(6):1147-1154

147. Shah P, Isley WL. Ketoacidosis during a low-carbohydrate diet. *N Engl J Med*. 2006;354(1):97-98

148. Brunstrom JM, Davison CJ, Mitchell GL. Dietary restraint and cognitive performance in children. *Appetite*. 2005;45(3):235-241

149. Brehm BJ, Spang SE, Lattin BL, Seeley RJ, Daniels SR, D'Alessio DA. The role of energy expenditure in the differential weight loss in obese women on low-fat and low-carbohydrate diets. *J Clin Endocrinol Metab*. 2005;90(3):1475-1482

150. American Heart Association; Giddling SS, Dennison BA, Birch LL, Daniels SR, Gilman MW, Lichtenstein AH, Rattay KT, Steinberger J, Stettler N, Van Horn L. Dietary recommendations for children and adolescents: a guide for practitioners. *Pediatrics*. 2006;117(2):544-559

151. Nicklas TA, Hayes D. Position of the American Dietetic Association: nutrition guidance for healthy children aged 2 to 11 years. *J Am Diet Assoc.* 2008;108(6):1038-1047

152. Kimmons J, Gillespie C, Seymour J, Serdula M, Blanck HM. Fruit and vegetable intake among adolescents and adults in the United States: percentage meeting individualized recommendations. *Medscape J Med.* 2009;11(1):26

153. Dennison BA, Rockwell HL, Baker SL. Fruit and vegetable intake in young children. *J Am Coll Nutr.* 1998;17(4):371-378

154. McNaughton SA, Ball K, Mishra GD, Crawford DA. Dietary patterns of adolescents and risk of obesity and hypertension. *J Nutr.* 2008;138(2):364-370

155. Tercyak KP, Tyc VL. Opportunities and challenges in the prevention and control of cancer and other chronic diseases: children's diet and nutrition and weight and physical activity. *J Pediatr Psychol.* 2006;31(8):750-763

156. World Cancer Research Fund/American Institute for Cancer Research. *Food, Nutrition, Physical Activity, and the Prevention of Cancer: A Global Perspective.* Washington, DC: American Institute for Cancer Research; 2007

157. Mente A, de Koning L, Shannon HS, Anand SS. A systematic review of the evidence supporting a causal link between dietary factors and coronary heart disease. *Arch Intern Med.* 2009;169(7):659-669

158. Dauchet L, Amouyel P, Dallongeville J. Fruits, vegetables and coronary heart disease. *Nat Rev Cardiol.* 2009;6(9):599-608

159. Esposito K, Kastorini CM, Panagiotakos DB, Giugliano D. Prevention of type 2 diabetes by dietary patterns: a systematic review of prospective studies and meta-analysis. *Metab Syndr Relat Disord.* 2010;8(6):471-476

160. United States Department of Agriculture. *Dietary Guidelines for Americans 2010.* Available at: http://www.cnpp.usda.gov/DGAs2010-PolicyDocument.htm. Accessed October 9, 2012

161. McGartland CP, Robson PJ, Murray LJ, et al. Fruit and vegetable consumption and bone mineral density: the Northern Ireland Young Hearts Project. *Am J Clin Nutr.* 2004;80(4):1019-1023

162. Neal EG, Cross JH. Efficacy of dietary treatments for epilepsy. *J Hum Nutr Diet.* 2010;23(2):113-119

163. Kossoff EH, Dorward JL. The modified Atkins diet. *Epilepsia.* 2008;49(Suppl 8):37-41

164. Peterson SJ, Tangney CC, Pimentel-Zablah EM, Hjelmgren B, Booth G, Berry-Kravis E. Changes in growth and seizure reduction in children on the ketogenic diet as a treatment for intractable epilepsy. *J Am Diet Assoc.* 2005;105(5):718-724

165. Kang HC, Chung DE, Kim DW, Kim HD. Early- and late-onset complications of the ketogenic diet for intractable epilepsy. *Epilepsia.* 2004;45(9):1116-1123

166. Willi SM, Oexmann MJ, Wright NM, Collop NA, Key LL Jr. The effects of a high-protein, low-fat, ketogenic diet on adolescents with morbid obesity: Body composition, blood chemistries, and sleep abnormalities. *Pediatrics.* 1998;101(1 Pt 1):61-67

167. Academy of Nutrition and Dietetics, Evidence Analysis Library. *Pediatric Weight Management Evidence-Based Nutrition Practice Guideline.* Available at: http://www.adaevidencelibrary.com/topic.cfm?cat=2724. Accessed October 9, 2012

III

168. US Food and Drug Administration. Overview of Dietary Supplements. Available at: http://www.fda.gov/food/dietarysupplements/default.htm. Accessed October 9, 2012

169. US Food and Drug Administration. Current Good Manufacturing Practices (CGMPs). Dietary Supplements. Available at: http://www.fda.gov/Food/DietarySupplements/GuidanceComplianceRegulatoryInformation/RegulationsLaws/ucm079496.htm. Accessed October 9, 2012

170. Blumenthal M, Lindstrom A, Lynch ME, Rea P. Herb Sales Continue Growth – Up 3.3% in 2010. *HerbalGram*. 2011;90:64-67

171. Barnes PM, Bloom B, Nahin RL. Complementary and alternative medicine use among adults and children: United States, 2007. *Natl Health Stat Rep*. 2008;10(12):1-23

172. Gilroy CM, Steiner JF, Byers T, Shapiro H, Georgian W. Echinacea and truth in labeling. *Arch Intern Med*. 2003;163(6):699-704

173. Garrard J, Harms S, Eberly LE, Matiak A. Variations in product choices of frequently purchased herbs: caveat emptor. *Arch Intern Med*. 2003;163(19):2290-2295

174. National Institutes of Health. National Center for Complementary and Alternative Medicine. Complementary and Alternative Medicine Use in Children. Available at: http://nccam.nih.gov/health/children. Accessed October 9, 2012

175. Sanders H, Davis MF, Duncan B, Meaney FJ, Haynes J, Barton LL. Use of complementary and alternative medical therapies among children with special health care needs in southern Arizona. *Pediatrics*. 2004;111(3):584–587

176. Noonan K, Arensman RM, Hoover JD. Herbal medication use in the pediatric surgical patient. *J Pediatr Surg*. 2004;39(3):500-503

177. Lin YC, Bioteau AB, Ferrair LR, Berde CB. The use of herbs and complementary and alternative medicine in pediatric preoperative patients. *J Clin Anesth*. 2004;16(1):4-6

178. Lanski SL, Greenwald M, Perkins A, Simon HK. Herbal therapy use in a pediatric emergency department population: expect the unexpected. *Pediatrics*. 2003;111(5 Pt 1):981-985

179. Lohse B, Stotts JL, Priebe JR. Survey of herbal use by Kansas and Wisconsin WIC participants reveals moderate, appropriate use and identifies herbal education needs. *J Am Diet Assoc*. 2006;106(2):227-237

180. Wilson KM, Klein JD, Sesselberg TS, et al. Use of complementary medicine and dietary supplements among U.S. adolescents. *J Adolesc Health*. 2006;38(4):385-394

181. Kemper KJ, O'Connor KG. Pediatricians' recommendations for complementary and alternative medical (CAM) therapies. *Ambul Pediatr*. 2004;4(6):482-487

182. Ottolini MC, Hamburger EK, Loprieato JO, et al. Complementary and alternative medicine use among children in the Washington DC area. *Ambul Pediatr*. 2001;1(2):122-125

183. Shenfield G, Lim E, Allen H. Survey of the use of complementary medicines and therapies in children with asthma. *J Paediatr Child Health*. 2002;38(3):252-257

184. Clark CE, Arnold E, Lasserson TJ, Wu T. Herbal interventions for chronic asthma in adults and children: a systematic review and meta-analysis. *Prim Care Respir J*. 2010;19(4):307-314

185. Mazur LJ, De Ybarrondo L, Miller J, Colasurdo G. Use of alternative and complementary therapies for pediatric asthma. *Tex Med*. 2001;97(6):64-68

186. Hon KL, Lo W, Cheng WK, et al. Prospective self-controlled trial of the efficacy and tolerability of a herbal syrup for young children with eczema. *J Dermatolog Treat*. 2012;23(2):116-121

187. Nowak-Węgrzyn A, Sampson HA. Future therapies for food allergies. *J Allergy Clin Immunol*. 2011;127(3):558-573

188. Day AS, Whitten KE, Bohane TD. Use of complementary and alternative medicines by children and adolescents with inflammatory bowel disease. *J Paediatr Child Health*. 2004;40(12):681-684

189. Heuschkel R, Afzal N, Wuerth A, et al. Complementary medicine use in children and young adults with inflammatory bowel disease. *Am J Gastroenterol*. 2002;97(2):382-388

190. Neuhouser ML, Patterson RE, Schwartz SM, Hedderson MM, Bowen DJ, Standish LJ. Use of alternative medicine by children with cancer in Washington state. *Prev Med*. 2001;33(5):347-354

191. Pillai AK, Sharma KK, Gupta YK, Bakhshi S. Anti-emetic effect of ginger powder versus placebo as an add on therapy in children and young adults receiving high emetogenic chemotherapy. *Pediatr Blood Cancer*. 2011;56(2):234-238

192. Haidar C, Jeha S. Drug interactions in childhood cancer. *Lancet Oncol*. 2011;12(1):92-99

193. Sparreboom A, Cox MC, Acharya MR, Figg WD. Herbal remedies in the United States: potential adverse interactions with anticancer agents. *J Clin Oncol*. 2004;22(12): 2489-503

194. Kumar NB, Allen K, Bell H. Perioperative herbal supplement use in cancer patients: potential implications and recommendations for presurgical screening. *Cancer Control*. 2005;12(3):149-157

195. Hu CH, He J, Eckert R, et al. Development and evaluation of a safe and effective sugar-free herbal lollipop that kills cavity-causing bacteria. *Int J Oral Sci*. 2011;3(1):13-20

196. Peters MC, Tallman JA, Braun TM, Jacobson JJ. Clinical reduction of *S mutans* in pre-school children using a novel liquorice root extract lollipop: a pilot study. *Eur Arch Paediatr Dent*. 2010;11(6):274-278

197. Esposito M, Carotenuto M. Ginkgolide B complex efficacy for brief prophylaxis of migraine in school-aged children: an open-label study. *Neurol Sci*. 2011;32(1):79-81

198. Wolsko PM, Solondz DK, Phillips RS, Schachter SC, Eisenberg DM. Lack of herbal supplement characterization in published randomized controlled trials. *Am J Med*. 2005;118(10):1087-1093

199. Woolf AD. Herbal remedies and children: do they work? Are they harmful? *Pediatrics*. 2003;112(1 Pt 2):240-246

200. Pak E, Esrason KT, Wu VH. Hepatotoxicity of herbal remedies: an emerging dilemma. *Prog Transplant*. 2004;14(2):91-96

201. American Botanical Council. The Complete German Commission E Monographs Therapeutic Guide to Herbal Medicines. 1999. Available at: http://cms.herbalgram.org/commissione/intro/comm_e_int.html. Accessed October 9, 2012

III

202. Natural Medicines Comprehensive Database. Available at: http://naturaldatabase .therapeuticresearch.com/home.aspx. Accessed October 9, 2012

203. National Institutes of Health. National Center for Complementary and Alternative Medicine. Available at: http://dietarysupplements.nlm.nih.gov/dietary/herbIngred.jsp. Accessed October 9, 2012≠

204. National Institutes of Health. National Center for Complementary and Alternative Medicine. Time to Talk. Available at: http://nccam.nih.gov/timetotalk. Accessed October 9, 2012

Micronutrients and Macronutrients

Chapter 14

Energy

Introduction

Energy flow through living systems encompasses cellular respiration and metabolic processes that lead to production and utilization of energy in forms, such as adenosine triphosphate (ATP). Chemical energy in food is transformed and made available for biosynthesis, anabolic process, and mechanical work. Energy is required for all the biochemical and physiologic functions that sustain life—respiration, circulation, maintenance of electrochemical gradients across cell membranes, and maintenance of body temperature—as well as for growth and physical activity.[1,2] Energy provided in the diet by protein, carbohydrate, and fat is expressed as a unit of heat, the calorie. A calorie is defined as the amount of heat required to raise the temperature of 1 g of water by 1°C from 15°C to 16°C. The scientific international unit of energy is the joule (J), defined as the energy expended when 1 kg is moved 1 m by a force of 1 newton. In the field of nutrition, a kilocalorie (kcal), which is 1000 times the energy of a calorie (cal), is commonly used. Hence, 1 kcal = 4.184 kJ, and 1 kJ = 0.0239 kcal.

Energy Balance

Energy balance is the accounting for energy consumption; excretion in feces, urine, and combustible gases; expenditure; and retention of organic compounds (ie, protein and fat accretion).[3] Implicit in the definition of energy balance is that energy is conserved. Energy balance may be expressed as:

Energy Intake − Energy Excretion − Energy Expenditure = Energy Retention

Digestible energy is the dietary energy absorbed by the gastrointestinal tract after accounting for loss in feces.[4] Metabolizable energy is energy available after accounting for losses in feces, urine, and combustible gases. The Atwater factors of 4, 9, and 4 kcal of metabolizable energy per gram of protein, fat, and carbohydrate, respectively, are widely used to express the energy content of foods in food composition tables.[5] Atwater factors are applied to the protein estimated from its nitrogen content, fat determined by extraction, and carbohydrates determined by difference after taking into account the protein, fat, water, and ash in the food.

Although food intake is the result of complex interactions among central nervous system regulating regions (mainly hypothalamic) and peripheral neural (eg, vagal) and humoral (eg, gut peptides and insulin) signals and environmental factors, energy balance at all ages is regulated with a fair degree of precision. This is reflected in the observation that most infants and children grow in regular fashion, and many adults maintain stable body weight for long periods. Infants appear to eat to satisfy energy needs and will compensate for low food energy density and poor digestibility by increasing food intake.[6] Observations of young children fed ad libitum while recovering from malnutrition showed that their voracious appetites abated as they approached normal weight for height.[7] Despite the innate balancing of energy intake against energy expenditure and energy needs for growth, obesity (see Chapter 34), a consequence of long-term energy intake in excess of energy requirements, has become alarmingly prevalent among children in the United States.[8]

Most clinical problems involving energy balance can be approached by systematic evaluation of the terms in the energy balance equation, although specific macronutrient effects on metabolism may need to be considered in certain clinical settings.[6,9] Inadequate energy intake may be a consequence of insufficient provision of appropriate food by the child's caregivers or may be attributable to problems inherent to the child (eg, neurologic, behavioral, or certain gastrointestinal tract disorders). Fecal excretion of fat usually accounts for most of the energy excretion, although in some instances, carbohydrate and nitrogenous losses also may be clinically important. Clinically significant increased energy excretion most commonly is secondary to intestinal, pancreatic, or hepatobiliary disorders that result in macronutrient maldigestion and/or malabsorption. In some situations (eg, diabetes mellitus, ketosis), energy losses in urine may be significant.

Components of Energy Expenditure

Energy expenditure includes energy expended for basal metabolic processes, the thermic effect of food ingestion, energy expended for thermoregulation, and energy expended for physical activity.[1-3]

Basal Metabolism

Basal metabolic rate (BMR) is energy expenditure under standard conditions—for example, after a 12- to 18-hour fast, awake, but quietly lying down (in early morning after awakening), in a thermoneutral environment (eg, an environmental temperature at which the metabolic rate and, therefore, oxygen consumption are at a minimum), bodily and mentally at rest. BMR reflects energy required for vital body processes during physical, emotional, and digestive rest.[1] Important factors that affect energy expenditure at rest include age, body size and composition, and presence of disease (eg, infection, fever, or trauma). If the experimental conditions required for the measurement of BMR are not practical, resting metabolic rate is often measured instead. Resting metabolic rate, the energy expended by a person at rest in a thermoneutral environment, is 10% to 20% higher than the BMR because of recent food intake or physical activity. In the case of infants, sleeping metabolic rate is often measured to avoid uncontrollable body movement.

Because of the dominant contribution of the brain (60%-70%), BMR is highest during the first years of life.[10] BMR of term infants ranges from 43 to 60 kcal·kg^{-1}·day^{-1} or 2 to 3 times greater than that in adults.[11] BMR is influenced by age (greater in older than in younger children), gender (greater in males than in females), and feeding mode (less in breastfed than in formula-fed infants).[12] BMR of healthy children younger than 3 years may be predicted by the following equations derived by Schofield et al[11]:

Boys: BMR (kcal/day) = 0.1673 weight (kg) + 1517 length (m) − 618
Girls: BMR (kcal/day) = 16.25 weight (kg) + 1023 length (m) − 413

Similarly, the BMR for older children and adolescents may be estimated from the Schofield equations. These equations may not apply to sick children in whom metabolism and/or body composition may be altered. For children 3 to 10 years of age:

Boys: BMR (kcal/day) = 19.60 weight (kg) + 130.26 length (m) + 414.90
Girls: BMR (kcal/day) = 16.97 weight (kg) + 161.80 length (m) + 371.17

For children 10 to 18 years of age:

Boys: BMR (kcal/day) = 16.25 weight (kg) + 137.19 length (m) + 515.52
Girls: BMR (kcal/day) = 8.365 weight (kg) + 465.57 length (m) + 200.04

Thermic Effect of Food

The thermic effect of feeding (TEF) or specific dynamic action is the increase in energy expenditure resulting from ingestion of food.[3] The TEF is mainly attributable to the obligatory metabolic costs of processing a meal, which include nutrient digestion, absorption, transport, and storage. The remaining facultative TEF reflects heat production that does not result in net synthesis or mechanical work and likely involves uncoupling of oxidative phosphorylation (ie, substrates are oxidized but heat is produced instead of ATP). The TEF is computed as the increment in energy expenditure above BMR, divided by the energy content of the food consumed; TEF varies from 5% to 10% for carbohydrate, 0% to 5% for fat, and 20% to 30% for protein. A mixed meal elicits an increase in energy expenditure equivalent to approximately 10% of the calories consumed.

Thermoregulation

Humans, like all homeotherms, maintain an almost constant body temperature over a wide range of environmental temperatures.[3] Energy required to maintain body temperature depends on environmental temperature. When ambient temperatures are below or above the zone of thermoneutrality, energy expenditure will increase. The thermoneutral temperature range is higher for neonates, particularly for those born prematurely. However, beyond infancy, little additional energy is needed between environmental temperatures of 20°C and 30°C. Outside these limits, an additional 5% to 10% of total energy may be necessary to maintain body temperature.

IV

Physical Activity

Marked variability exists in the energy requirements of children and adolescents because of variable physical activity levels.[1,2] The amount of time children spend in recreational activities and domestic and productive work varies across societies. The energy costs of discrete physical activities have been measured using indirect calorimetry and are usually expressed in terms of metabolic equivalents (METs) or physical activity ratios.[13] The energetic efficiency for physical work is remarkably constant for nonweight-bearing activities.[14] Under optimal conditions, the net efficiency (external work/internal energy conversion rate necessary to accomplish the work) of the body is approximately 25%. However, this does not imply that the energy cost of activities is constant among individuals. Energy cost of activities among individuals varies because of differences in age, weight and skill. For weight-bearing physical activities, the cost is roughly proportional to body weight.

Ainsworth and colleagues provided comprehensive tables to estimate the energy expended in discrete physical activities for adults.[15] Energy expenditure per kilogram of body mass at rest or during exercise is greater in children than adults and varies with pubertal status; therefore, using the definition of an MET in the compendium of physical activities without adjustment is inappropriate for estimation of the energy cost of activity in children. Adjustment of the compendium MET increments for age and Tanner stage provides a better estimate of the actual energy cost of activities.[16] Examples of energy expenditure while performing various activities are given in Chapter 12: Sports Nutrition.

Measurement of Energy Expenditure

Energy expenditure can be measured by direct calorimetry, indirect calorimetry, and noncalorimetric methods.[17] For practical reasons, the most commonly used method is indirect calorimetry, in which energy expenditure is computed from oxygen consumption (VO_2), carbon dioxide production (VCO_2), and the respiratory quotient (RQ), which is equal to the ratio of VCO_2 to VO_2. Substrate utilization can be determined from rates of VO_2, VCO_2, and urinary nitrogen excretion.[18] The complete oxidation of glucose results in an RQ equal to 1.0. The complete oxidation of fat and protein results in an RQ averaging about 0.7 and 0.85, respectively, depending on the chemical structure of the foodstuff. The RQ for lipogenesis (conversion of carbohydrate to stored fat) is greater than 1. The ingestion or administration of a high percentage of calories as carbohydrate may cause difficulties for children with respiratory insufficiency, because excess carbon dioxide is produced. This is especially true if the energy intake from carbohydrate exceeds the energy expenditure.

The Weir equation[19] is the most widely used equation for the calculation of energy expenditure (EE):

$$EE \text{ (kcal)} = 3.941 \times VO_2 \text{ (L)} + 1.106 \, VCO_2 \text{ (L)} - (2.17 \times UrN \text{ (g))} \text{ or}$$
$$EE \text{ (kcal)} = 3.941 \times VO_2 \text{ (L)} + 1 \, VCO_2 \text{ (L)}/(1 + 0.082 \, p)$$

where UrN is urinary nitrogen and p is the fraction of calories resulting from protein. Weir demonstrated that the error in neglecting the effect of protein metabolism on the caloric equivalent of oxygen is 1% for each 12.3% of the total calories that arise from protein. Under usual conditions, approximately 12.5% of total calories will arise from protein; therefore, the foregoing equation can be reduced to the following:

$$EE \text{ (kcal)} = 3.9 \times VO_2 \text{ (L)} + 1.1 \, VCO_2 \text{ (L)}.$$

The doubly labeled water method, which provides an indirect measure of VCO_2, has been used to estimate total EE in a number of different research settings.[20,21] Doubly labeled water is a stable (nonradioactive) isotope method that provides an estimate of total EE in free-living individuals. Two stable isotopic forms of water ($H_2{}^{18}O$ and ^2H_2O) are administered to the individual, and their ^{18}O and ^2H disappearance rates from the body are monitored for 7 to 21 days. The disappearance rate of ^2H_2O reflects water flux, whereas that of $H_2{}^{18}O$ reflects water flux plus VCO_2, and the difference between the two disappearance rates is used to calculate VCO_2. Applying a value for RQ based on food intake, VO_2 is calculated ($VO_2 = VCO_2/ RQ$); hence, total EE is calculated using the Weir equation. The doubly labeled water method may be used to assess energy requirements in weight-stable individuals.

Energy Cost of Growth

The energy cost of growth also is a component of total energy requirements.[1] The energy needed for growth represents approximately 35% of total energy requirements at 1 month of age, decreases to approximately 3% at 12 months of age because of slower growth, and remains almost negligible until the onset of puberty. The energy cost of growth is estimated from the individual costs of protein and fat deposition and ranges from 2.4 to 6.0 kcal/g, depending on the composition of the tissues deposited.[22,23] For the US Dietary Reference Intakes, the energy cost of growth was estimated to be 175 kcal/day for the age interval 0 to 3 months, 60 kcal/day for 4 to 6 months, and 20 kcal/day for 7 to 35 months.[1] Although the composition of newly synthesized tissues varies in childhood and adolescence, these variations have a minor effect on total energy requirements, because approximately 20 to 25 kcal/day only are required for growth.

Energy Requirements of Infants, Children, and Adolescents

Energy requirements of infants, children, and adolescents are defined as the amount of food energy needed to balance total energy expenditure at a desirable level of physical activity and to support optimal growth and development consistent with long-term health.[1,2] In 2002, the Institute of Medicine published estimated energy requirements (EERs) for infants and children based on total energy expenditure measured by the doubly labeled water method.[1] EER equations for estimation of energy requirements are given for sedentary, low active, active, and very active categories of physical activity in Table 14.1. The sedentary level reflects BMR, TEF, and the minimal activity required for daily living. Incorporating approximately 120,

Table 14.1.
Estimated Energy Requirements

Estimated Energy Requirements (EERs)[a]	
0–3 mo	(89 × weight [kg] − 100) + 175 kcal
4–6 mo	(89 × weight [kg] − 100) + 56 kcal
7–12 mo	(89 × weight [kg] − 100) + 22 kcal
13–36 mo	(89 × weight [kg] − 100) + 20 kcal
3–8 y (boys)	88.5 − (61.9 × age [y]) + PA × (26.7 × weight [kg] + 903 × height [m]) + 20 kcal
3–8 y (girls)	135.3 − (30.8 × age [y]) + PA × (10.0 × weight [kg] + 934 × height [m]) + 20 kcal
9–18 y (boys)	88.5 − (61.9 × age [y]) + PA × (26.7 × weight [kg] + 903 × height [m]) + 25 kcal
9–18 y (girls)	135.3 − (30.8 × age [y]) + PA × (10.0 × weight [kg] + 934 × height [m]) + 25 kcal

Adapted with permission from Institute of Medicine. *Dietary Reference Intakes for Energy, Carbohydrate, Fiber, Fat, Fatty Acids, Cholesterol, Protein, and Amino Acids.* 5th ed. Washington, DC: National Academies Press; 2002.[1]

[a] EER = total energy expenditure + energy deposition.

Where PA is the physical activity coefficient:

For Boys 3 through 18 years:
PA = 1.00 (sedentary, estimated PAL ≥1.0<1.4)
PA = 1.13 (low active, estimated PAL ≥1.4<1.6)
PA = 1.26 (active, estimated PAL ≥1.6<1.9)
PA = 1.42 (very active, estimated PAL ≥1.9<2.5)
For Girls 3 through 18 years:
PA = 1.00 (sedentary, estimated PAL ≥1.0<1.4)
PA = 1.16 (low active, estimated PAL ≥1.4<1.6)
PA = 1.31 (active, estimated PAL ≥1.6<1.9)
PA = 1.56 (very active, estimated PAL ≥1.9<2.5)

230, and 400 minutes/day walking at 2.5 miles per hour or equivalent activity corresponds to the low active, active, and very active categories, respectively. Clearly, children in the active and very active categories are participating in moderate and vigorous activities, in addition to walking. Even though energy requirements also are presented for varying levels of physical activity, moderately active lifestyles are strongly encouraged to maintain fitness and health and to reduce the risk of developing obesity and its comorbidities.

Macronutrient Distribution Ranges

Acceptable macronutrient distribution ranges, as a percent of total energy intake, for fat are slightly higher in children than adults (30% to 40% for children 1 through 3 years of age, and 25% to 35% for children 4 to 18 years of age vs 20% to 35% in adults) and for protein are lower (5% to 20% for children 1 through 3 years of age and 10% to 30% for children 4 to 18 years of age vs 10% to 35% in adults).[1] The acceptable macronutrient distribution ranges for carbohydrates are the same for all ages—45% to 65% of energy intake from carbohydrates, with added sugars constituting no more than 25% of total energy intake. The average diet of individuals in the United States supplies 12% to 15% of calories from protein and the remainder from carbohydrates and fat. An appropriate balance of total calories and protein is required for adequate growth, especially in response to malnutrition. The more rapid the weight gain, the higher the dietary protein-to-energy (P:E) ratio required. Growth rates of 10, 30, and 50 g/day required P:E ratios of 5.6%, 6.9%, and 8.1%, respectively, in infants recovering from malnutrition.[7] Standard infant formulas and human milk have P:E ratios of approximately 12% and 8%, respectively.

Altered Energy Requirements

Many common pathologic conditions may alter energy requirements, interfere with nutrient availability, affect substrate utilization, or impair physical activity. Provision of adequate energy may be especially important in certain clinical situations, particularly if a patient's ability to regulate intake is impaired. Energy deficit in children leads to growth retardation; loss of fat and muscle; delayed motor, cognitive, and behavioral development; diminished immunocompetence; and increased morbidity and mortality.[2] Excess energy intake can lead to obesity and its comorbidities, including type 2 diabetes mellitus, hyperlipidemia, hypertension, hyperandrogenism in girls, sleep disorders, respiratory difficulties, nonalcoholic fatty liver disease, gall bladder disease, orthopedic problems, and idiopathic intracranial

IV

hypertension.[24] During infancy, childhood, and adolescence, growth rate may serve as a good "bioassay" for dietary adequacy in terms of meeting energy requirements. Careful consideration of the factors affecting energy balance (eg, energy intake, energy excretion, energy expenditure, and energy retention) can often clarify seemingly complex clinical problems.

Infection and Trauma

A characteristic response to infection and trauma is an increase in core body temperature and resting energy expenditure. Oxygen consumption was measured in adult patients with several febrile illnesses (eg, tuberculosis, typhoid fever, malaria, bacterial pneumonia, and rheumatic fever).[25] These studies indicated that for each degree centigrade increase in body temperature, the metabolic rate increased up to 13%.

During infection, fatty acids continue to be the major fuel source, but utilization of ketone bodies is decreased.[25] Uptake and utilization of branched-chain amino acids are accelerated in skeletal muscles to fuel gluconeogenesis in the liver and kidney.

When the energy cost of measles was estimated in Kenyan children 28 months of age, a 75% decrease was seen in energy intake and a slight decrease in absorption during acute illness.[26] BMR was similar during measles and after recovery. The energy density of the diet tolerated during illness decreased from 0.9 kcal/g to 0.6 kcal/g. Inadequate intake, not elevated expenditure, was responsible for the energy deficit with this infectious disease.

The degree of hypermetabolism with trauma varies with the extent of the injury, the most extensive being in burn patients.[27] A 50% total body surface burn may double the metabolic rate. If the burn patient's body temperature is regulated at a high set point, the patient must be kept warm and heat losses must be minimized during the febrile state. If heat production exceeds thermoregulatory needs, physical and pharmacologic measures should be used to lower body temperature. In either case, energy requirements should be determined and met with vigorous nutritional support.

Other Diseases

Bronchopulmonary dysplasia typically is associated with slow growth. The impaired growth rate has been attributed to decreased intake during acute illness and increased work of respiration. Oxygen consumption was 25% higher in infants with bronchopulmonary dysplasia than that in controls.[28] The increased energy requirements should be supported with aggressive nutritional therapy.

The metabolic rates of infants with congestive heart failure are elevated in proportion to their degree of growth retardation and heart failure. The oxygen consumption of infants with congestive heart failure was 9.4 mL/kg/min, compared with 6.5 mL/kg/min in infants with congenital heart disease but not in failure.[29] Infants with severe congenital heart disease who were markedly undergrown had abnormally high rates of oxygen consumption, whereas those with congenital heart disease whose growth was normal consumed oxygen at normal rates.[30]

References

1. Institute of Medicine. *Dietary Reference Intakes for Energy, Carbohydrate, Fiber, Fat, Fatty Acids, Cholesterol, Protein, and Amino Acids.* 5th ed. Washington, DC: National Academies Press; 2002

2. World Health Organization/Food and Agriculture Organization of the United Nations. *Expert Consultation: Human Energy Requirements.* Rome, Italy: World Health Organization; 2004

3. Blaxter K. *Energy Metabolism in Animals and Man.* Cambridge, United Kingdom: Cambridge University Press; 1989

4. Consolazio CF, Johnson RE, Pecora LJ. The computation of metabolic balances. In: Consolazio CF, Johnson RE, Pecora LJ, eds. *Physiological Measurements of Metabolic Functions in Man.* New York, NY: McGraw-Hill Book Company Inc; 1963:313-325

5. Watt BK, Merrill AL. *Composition of Foods.* ARS Handbook No. 8. Washington, DC: US Government Printing Office; 1963

6. Krieger JW, Sitren HS, Daniels MJ, Langkamp-Henken B. Effects of variation in protein and carbohydrate intake on body mass and composition during energy restriction: a meta-regression 1. *Am J Clin Nutr.* 2006;83(2):260-274

7. Ashworth A, Millward DJ. Catch-up growth in children. *Nutr Rev.* 1986;44(5):157-163

8. Ogden CL, Carroll MD, Curtin LR, Lamb MM, Flegal KM. Prevalence of high body mass index in US children and adolescents, 2007-2008. *JAMA.* 2010;303(3):242-249

9. Feinman RD, Fine EJ. "A calorie is a calorie" violates the second law of thermodynamics. *Nutr J.* 2004;3:9

10. Holliday M, Potter D, Jarrah A, Bearg S. Relation of metabolic rate to body weight and organ size. *Pediatr Res.* 1967;1(3):185-195

11. Schofield WN, Schofield C, James WPT. Basal metabolic rate-review and prediction, together with annotated bibliography of source material. *Hum Nutr Clin Nutr.* 1985;39C(Suppl 1):1-96

12. Butte NF, Wong WW, Hopkinson JM, Heinz CJ, Mehta NR, Smith EO. Energy requirements derived from total energy expenditure and energy deposition during the first 2 years of life. *Am J Clin Nutr.* 2000;72(6):1558-1569

13. Brooks GA, Fahey TD, Baldwin KM. *Exercise Physiology: Human Bioenergetics and its Applications.* 4th ed. New York: McGraw-Hill; 2004

14. McArdle WD, Katch FI, Katch VL. *Exercise Physiology, Energy Nutrition, and Human Performance.* 5th ed. Philadelphia, PA: Lippincott Williams & Wilkins; 2001

15. Ainsworth BE, Haskell WL, Whitt MC, et al. Compendium of physical activities: an update of activity codes and MET intensities. *Med Sci Sports Exerc.* 2000;32(9 Suppl):S498-S504

IV

16. Harrell JS, McMurray RG, Baggett CD, Pennell ML, Pearce PF, Bangdiwala SI. Energy costs of physical activities in children and adolescents. *Med Sci Sports Exerc*. 2005;37(2): 329-336

17. Jequier E, Acheson K, Schutz Y. Assessment of energy expenditure and fuel utilization in man. *Ann Rev Nutr*. 1987;7:187-208

18. Livesey G, Elia M. Estimation of energy expenditure, net carbohydrate utilization, and net fat oxidation and synthesis by indirect calorimetry: evaluation of errors with special reference to the detailed composition of fuels. *Am J Clin Nutr*. 1988;47(4):608-628

19. Weir JB. New methods for calculating metabolic rate with special reference to protein metabolism. *J Physiol*. 1949;109(1-2):1-9

20. Schoeller DA, Van Santen E. Measurement of energy expenditure in humans by doubly labeled water method. *J Appl Physiol*. 1982;53(4):955-959

21. Schoeller DA. Measurement of energy expenditure in free-living humans by using doubly labeled water. *J Nutr*. 1988;118(11):1278-1289

22. Butte NF, Wong WW, Garza C. Energy cost of growth during infancy. *Proc Nutr Soc*. 1989;48(2):303-312

23. Roberts SB, Young VR. Energy costs of fat and protein deposition in the human infant. *Am J Clin Nutr*. 1988;48(4):951-955

24. Barlow SE. Expert committee recommendations regarding the prevention, assessment, and treatment of child and adolescent overweight and obesity: summary report. *Pediatrics*. 2007;120(Suppl 4):S164-S192

25. Beisel WR, Wannemacher RW, Neufeld HA. Relation of fever to energy expenditure. In: *Assessment of Energy Metabolism in Health and Disease*. Columbus, OH: Ross Laboratories; 1980:144-150

26. Duggan MB, Milner RD. Energy cost of measles infection. *Arch Dis Child*. 1986;61(5): 436-469

27. Aulick LH. Studies in heat transport and heat loss in thermally injured patients. In: *Assessment of Energy Metabolism in Health and Disease*. Columbus, OH: Ross Laboratories; 1980:141-144

28. Weinstein MR, Oh W. Oxygen consumption in infants with bronchopulmonary dysplasia. *J Pediatr*. 1981;99(6):958-993

29. Krauss AN, Auld PAM. Metabolic rate of neonates with congenital heart disease. *Arch Dis Child*. 1975;50(7):539-541

30. Lees MH, Bristow JD, Griswold HE, Olmsted RW. Relative hypermetabolism in infants with congenital heart disease and undernutrition. *Pediatrics*. 1965;36:183-191

Chapter 15

Protein

Introduction

Proteins are the major structural and functional components of all cells in the body. They are macromolecules comprised of one or more chains of amino acids that vary in their sequence and length and are folded into specific 3-dimensional structures. The sizes and conformations of proteins, therefore, are infinitely diverse and complex, and this enables them to serve an extensive variety of functions in the cell. Dietary protein provides the amino acids required for both the synthesis of body proteins and the production of other nitrogenous compounds with important functional roles, such as glutathione, creatine, heme, nucleotides, hormones, nitric oxide, bile acids, and some neurotransmitters. Amino acids can exist as various stereoisomers in nature. Only the L-amino acids are biologically active and can be incorporated into proteins. Body proteins also can be catabolized and serve as an energy source when energy intake, in particular carbohydrate intake, is inadequate.

From the dietary perspective, it is the amino acid composition of a protein that is its most relevant property, although for some, the structure can dictate digestibility (eg, keratin, an insoluble protein that makes up hair, skin, and nails). Protein digestion begins in the stomach through the activity of pepsin in the presence of hydrochloric acid. In the young infant, pepsin and acid production are low, but this does not appear to limit the digestibility of protein. Protein digestion continues in the presence of pancreatic enzymes in the duodenum and the enzymes in the brush border of the jejunum and proximal ileum. Some of these enzymes, such as enterokinase, also have low activity during the newborn period, but the low activity does not appear to limit protein digestion. Digestion results in the hydrolysis of proteins to oligopeptides and amino acids that are absorbed. Oligopeptides are hydrolyzed to amino acids by enzymes in the cells of the intestinal epithelium. Protein that escapes digestion in the small intestine, including secreted proteins and sloughed off intestinal cells, can be broken down by bacteria in the colon, and the resulting ammonia can be absorbed and incorporated into amino acids.

Absorbed amino acids are first transported from the intestine to the liver and then enter the general amino acid pool of the body in the plasma and exchange with tissue pools. Some amino acids are used directly by the intestine itself, as an energy source, to synthesize gut proteins, or in the production of other nitrogen-containing biologic molecules. Indeed, the gut derives most of its energy from the metabolism of glutamate, glutamine, and aspartate. The gut's high capacity to metabolize glutamate serves to prevent excessive increases in plasma glutamate and the potential development of neurotoxicity from a high dietary intake of glutamate, such as when foods supplemented with monosodium glutamate are consumed.[1] In the growing organism, an influx of amino acids to the tissues from the diet rapidly stimulates protein synthesis.[2-4] This response is dampened as the organism matures, and in adults, protein consumption primarily reduces protein breakdown with only a moderate response in protein synthesis.[5,6] Dietary amino acids consumed in excess of the body's needs cannot be stored. The nitrogen component of amino acids is converted to urea, and the remaining keto acids are used directly for energy production or converted to glucose and fat when energy intake is adequate. Therefore, blood urea nitrogen is a good indicator of recent protein intake when hydration and renal function are normal. The stimulation of protein synthesis by the influx of amino acids from the diet, together with the body's inability to store excess dietary amino acids, are primary reasons for the recommendation that, in infants and children, the daily protein requirement should be consumed over several meals at regular intervals throughout the day.

Body proteins and the other nitrogenous compounds are continuously degraded and resynthesized. Several times more endogenous protein is turned over every day than is usually consumed. The rate of turnover can be rapid, as in bone marrow and in gastrointestinal mucosa, or it can be slow, as in muscle and collagen. Protein turnover also changes with age; it is highest during early life when tissues are maturing and their growth rates are at their highest.[6] The amino acids released from the breakdown of endogenous proteins are recycled, but this process is not completely efficient. Amino acids that are not reused are catabolized or lost in urine, feces, sweat, desquamated skin, hair, and nails. These losses create an obligatory requirement for dietary amino acids, in addition to any requirement for the net accretion of body protein. This obligatory fraction constitutes the maintenance or basal needs of the organism and, once growth has ceased, this fraction represents an individual's entire protein requirement. The magnitude of these basal losses is dictated by the individual's total lean mass and their basal metabolic rate.

Amino acids are usually categorized into 3 groups: indispensable, dispensable, and conditionally indispensable. Amino acids with carbon skeletons that cannot be synthesized de novo in adults are regarded as indispensable (essential) amino acids and must be provided by the diet; they include leucine, isoleucine, valine, threonine, methionine, phenylalanine, tryptophan, lysine, and histidine. To sustain normal growth and the maintenance of the body's protein mass after the requirements for indispensable amino acids have been met, the additional dietary nitrogen required must be provided as dispensable (nonessential) amino acids. Dispensable amino acids are those that can be synthesized in the body from other amino acids or nitrogen-containing molecules. These are usually divided into 2 categories—the truly dispensable amino acids and the conditionally indispensable ones. Conditionally indispensable amino acids and other nutrients are those that ordinarily can be synthesized, but an exogenous source is required under certain circumstances. The designation varies according to the age of the individual and the presence of genetic or acquired disease conditions. For all humans, alanine, aspartic acid, asparagine, serine, and glutamic acid can be classified as dispensable. Arginine, glutamine, proline, glycine, cysteine, and tyrosine are in the conditionally indispensable category. Cysteine, tyrosine, and arginine must be provided to the preterm infant because of the immaturity of the enzyme activities necessary for their synthesis from precursors. Recent studies suggest that by term, the necessary enzyme activities to generate these amino acids from their precursors is present, and they are no longer indispensable.[7] Glycine is required for the synthesis of creatine, porphyrins, glutathione, nucleotides, and bile salts; therefore, the requirement for this amino acid during times of rapid growth is relatively high.[8] Glycine is present in relatively small amounts in milk and may be a conditionally essential amino acid for the preterm infant and neonate.

Various disease conditions can also interfere with the synthesis of amino acids that can normally be synthesized from other amino acids. Arginine is essential in patients with defects of the urea cycle. Cysteine may be essential in patients with hepatic disease or homocystinuria. Tyrosine is essential for people with phenylketonuria and may be required for patients with hepatic disease. Glutamine is the preferred fuel for rapidly dividing cells, such as enterocytes and lymphocytes. Thus, during times of critical stress, such as after surgical procedures, nonsurgical trauma, or sepsis, or in patients with gastrointestinal mucosal injury, large amounts of glutamine are synthesized by the skeletal muscle from the amino acids of skeletal muscle proteins. Opinions are divided on the benefits of supplementary glutamine in these instances.[9] Taurine and carnitine are amino acids that serve important and specific functions in the cell but are not incorporated into proteins. They can be synthesized by the body from cysteine and lysine, respectively, and are present in a mixed diet containing proteins of animal origin. The rates of synthesis in infants fed by total parenteral nutrition or receiving synthetic formulas devoid of taurine and carnitine may be insufficient to meet all of their needs and may necessitate dietary supplementa-tion.[10,11] Nearly all infant formulas today contain added taurine and carnitine.

Recommended Dietary Intake for Protein and Amino Acids

The appropriate amount of protein that should be eaten is expressed in a number of different ways according to the information it is meant to convey, how the values are derived, and the purpose for which the information will be used. The Recommended Dietary Allowance (RDA) for protein is the average daily intake of protein that meets the nutrient needs of most healthy individuals in a particular life stage and gender group (Appendix E).[12-14] The RDA is derived from:

1. *The Estimated Average Requirement (EAR) for protein.* The EAR is the daily protein intake that meets the protein needs of 50% of all healthy individuals of a specific age and gender. The physiologic requirement is defined as the lowest level of protein intake needed to replace losses from the body when energy intake is in balance (maintenance requirement). In growing individuals and pregnant and lactating women, the protein requirement also includes the protein required for tissue accretion and milk production at a level associated with good health. The need for growth decreases from approximately 55% of total intake over the first 3 months of life to 10% or less by 8 years of age and accounts largely for the reduction with age in protein requirements (Table 15.1). These intakes assume that the protein source is of high quality on the basis of its amino acid composition.

Table 15.1.
Contribution of Maintenance and Growth to Protein Needs of Infants and Children[13,17,18]

Age	Protein Gain[a] (g/(kg.d⁻¹))	Intake	
		Growth	Maintenance
		(% of Total)	
0.5–3 months	0.49	55	45
3–6 months	0.30	43	57
6–12 months	0.18	31	69
1–3 years	0.10	20	80
4–8 years	0.046	10	90

[a] Average for boys and girls.

2. *The variability in protein needs for specific population groups.* The RDA defines the protein need of 97.5% of a particular age group. Thus, the EAR must be increased to account for the variability in the requirements among groups of similar individuals. This includes the variation in maintenance needs, the variation in protein accretion rate (if relevant), and the variation in the efficiency with which dietary protein is accumulated. It is important to note that because of this adjustment, the RDA exceeds the protein needs of most individuals within a specified group.

For some nutrients and/or certain populations, the scientific data (either average intakes or their variability) for estimating an EAR are not sufficiently robust to make a definitive recommendation. In these cases, a level defined as an Adequate

Intake (AI) is used. This value is based on the average protein intake of a group of individuals who appear to be healthy and in a good nutritional state. The recommendation for daily protein and amino acid intake of infants from birth to 6 months falls in this category and is based on the average daily protein intake of infants fed principally with human milk.

The Dietary Reference Intake guidelines[13] define 2 additional parameters that should be taken into consideration in the evaluation of diets and in making dietary recommendations. These are: the Tolerable Upper Intake Level (UL) and the Acceptable Macronutrient Distribution Ranges (AMDRs). No ULs have been set for protein or amino acid intakes because of the absence of sufficient data on which to base recommendations. This does not imply that high levels are not harmful; some of the current concerns regarding less beneficial effects of high protein intakes will be discussed later. The AMDRs were developed because of the increasing evidence that the dietary source from which individuals obtain their energy may play a role in the development of chronic diseases. Protein, fats, and carbohydrates can substitute for each other as sources of dietary energy; thus, for a given energy intake, if the proportion of one varies, so must the others. The AMDR for protein is the proportion of the total energy intake that is protein and that is associated with a reduced risk for chronic disease. The AMDR for protein is 5% to 20% of total energy intake in 1- to 3-year-old children and 10% to 30% of total energy intake for 4- to 18-year-old children.

For the 9 indispensable amino acids, EARs and RDAs have been developed for individuals from 7 months to 18 years of age, and AIs have been developed for infants from birth through 6 months of age. The requirement for methionine is frequently given as a composite value for total sulphur amino acids (ie, methionine and cysteine, the latter being a metabolic product of methionine catabolism). Thus, the requirement for cysteine is dependent on there being sufficient methionine in the diet to meet the needs of both amino acids, although it is clear that in some circumstances, such as in preterm infants, the metabolism of methionine to cysteine may not be sufficient to meet the entire cysteine requirement. Similarly, the requirements for phenylalanine and tyrosine, the aromatic amino acids, are pooled, because tyrosine can be formed from the metabolism of phenylalanine.

Methods for Determining Protein and Amino Acid Requirements

Protein
Protein requirements and balance data are frequently measured and expressed on the basis of nitrogen content. On average, nitrogen constitutes 16% of the weight of a protein, although the exact value varies from protein to protein. The

recommendations for protein intakes have used a factor of 6.25 to convert grams of nitrogen to grams of protein.

Protein needs have been estimated using various approaches.[12-16] During the first 6 months of life, human milk is the optimal source of protein for infants and, when freely fed, is sufficient to sustain good health and optimal growth. Thus, the average intake of breastfed infants has been used to define an AI for this age group. The intake of the infants was determined by test weighing and the average protein content of human milk.

Recommendations for dietary protein intakes of infants older than 6 months have been estimated using the factorial method. The factorial method provides an estimate of protein needs for maintenance and growth, and adjusts for the efficiency with which dietary protein is used according to age, size, and gender.

Maintenance protein requirements are derived from nitrogen balance studies (examples are described by Viteri[16]). This method involves determination of the difference between the intake and excretion of nitrogen in urine, feces, sweat, and minor losses via other routes for 1 to 3 weeks or longer. Several different levels of a quality protein source, such as milk or egg, legume and cereal mixes, or mixed vegetable and animal sources, are tested at a constant and adequate energy intake. From the relationship between intake and balance (intake minus excretion), the amount of nitrogen required for maintenance (zero balance) is extrapolated.

To the maintenance requirements, additional amounts of protein that would be sufficient to support appropriate body protein gains have been added. The mean rate of protein gain during growth has been estimated from the body composition data of children from 9 months to 3 years of age[17] and from 4 to 18 years of age.[18] In both studies, body composition was measured using a combination of water dilution, whole-body potassium, and dual-energy x-ray absorptiometry. The conversion of dietary protein to body proteins, however, is not 100% efficient. In growing individuals, the slope of the relationship between balance and intake provides a measure of the efficiency with which dietary protein is used for growth (58% from 0.5 to 13 years of age; 43% from 14 to 18 years of age[13]). Thus, the amount of dietary protein needed for growth must be adjusted to account for this inefficiency.

Amino Acids

Estimation of the requirements of amino acids can be determined by a number of approaches, including nitrogen balance, plasma amino acid concentrations, direct kinetic measurements of amino acid oxidation using stable isotope-labeled amino acids as tracers and balance, and indicator amino acid oxidation with balance. The values obtained, however, vary depending on the method used. Because of this uncertainty, together with the paucity of direct measurements of amino acid metabolism in the pediatric population, a factorial approach was used to estimate individual amino acid EARs from 0.5 to 18 years of age. For infants from birth through to 6 months of age, AIs have been defined based on data from human milk-fed infants.[12-15] These were calculated from the average volume of milk consumed and the amino acid composition of human milk proteins of normally growing, healthy infants.

To define the growth component of the requirement for individual amino acids, the factorial approach uses data for tissue protein accretion, and the amino acid composition of body tissues, corrected for the inefficiency of dietary utilization. Because the maintenance protein requirement does not vary with age in children and the values are very similar to adult values (expressed per unit of body weight), the values for the maintenance component of the amino acid requirements are based on adult maintenance values. The adult values are derived from direct measurements of amino acid kinetics and yield a different amino acid pattern from that of body proteins. Hence, as the total amount of amino acid deposited decreases with age, the composition of amino acids required changes (reflected in Table 15.2); the indispensable amino acids constitute approximately 42% of the tissue amino acid pattern but only 23% of the maintenance pattern.[15]

Table 15.2.
Amino Acid Scoring Patterns Based on the Estimated Average Requirements for Protein and Indispensable Amino Acids[13]

| Amino Acid | Protein (mg/g) | | |
	Infants	Children (1-3 y)	Adults (18 y)
Histidine	23	18	17
Isoleucine	57	25	23
Leucine	101	55	52
Lysine	69	51	47
Methionine + cysteine	38	25	23
Phenylalanine + tyrosine	87	47	41
Threonine	47	27	24
Tryptophan	18	7	6
Valine	56	32	29
Total indispensable amino acids	495	287	262

[a] Indispensable amino acid EAR/EAR for protein for an individual age group.

The RDA for amino acids adjusts the EAR to include an allowance for variability in the population in growth and maintenance requirements.

Protein Quality

In many respects, the ultimate test of the protein quality from a particular food is its ability to support appropriate growth of the individual consuming that food protein. When human milk is no longer the only source of protein, the quality and digestibility of food protein becomes important. Because of the wide variation in the amino acid composition and digestibility, proteins differ in their ability to provide the nitrogen and amino acids required for growth and maintenance. The amino acid composition of the food consumed is important, because if the content of a single indispensable amino acid is insufficient to meet an individual's need for that amino acid, it will limit the ability of the body to utilize the remaining amino acids in the diet even if the total amount of protein consumed would appear to be adequate. The recommendations for protein intake assume that the sources of protein are highly digestible (greater than 95%) and that the indispensable amino acid composition closely meets human needs. These properties apply to animal proteins, such as egg protein, milk protein, meat, and fish, whereas vegetable proteins often have a lower digestibility (70%–80%), and they often provide inadequate amounts of lysine (cereals) or the sulphur amino acids (legumes) (for examples, see Table 15.3).[12,13,19] Although plant proteins are generally of a lower quality than proteins of animal origin, equivalent amino acid patterns can be achieved by mixing plant proteins from different sources, such as legumes and cereals.[16] Processing of foods can also increase or decrease the digestibility of dietary proteins. An important example is the chemical modification to lysine with cooking, which renders it unavailable. Thus, to apply the recommendations for protein intake to mixed diets containing protein sources other than animal-based foods, it is necessary to adjust for the protein digestibility and correct for the adequacy of the amino acid composition of the food.

For the purpose of evaluating the adequacy of the amino acid content of food proteins, an amino acid scoring pattern that ideally must be provided by dietary protein can be derived by dividing the indispensable amino acid EAR by the EAR for protein for an individual age group (Table 15.2).[13] Thus, an ideal protein is one containing all the indispensable amino acids in amounts sufficient to meet requirements without any excess. For infants from birth to 1 year of age, the amino acid pattern of human milk proteins is considered the ideal and, provided the protein requirement is met with milk, the amino acid intake will be appropriate. The scoring pattern for children older than 1 year of age is significantly different from that for infants because of the smaller and different requirement pattern for growth. Thus, as maintenance requirements come to dominate, the requirement for indispensable amino acids diminishes. Because the scoring pattern is similar for young children and adults, the most recent recommendations propose that the scoring pattern for children from 1 to 3 years of age also be used for in the assessment of the diets of adolescents and adults.[13]

Table 15.3.
Mean Values for Digestibility and Amino Acid Scores of Various Protein Sources

Protein Source	True Digestibility[a]	Amino Acid Score[b]	
	(%)	6 mo to 1 y	School-Aged Child
Whole egg (hen)	97	0.74 (trp)	1.36 (his)
Cow milk	95	0.52 (thr)	0.90 (thr)
Beef (cooked)	94	0.54 (trp)	1.39 (trp)
Corn, whole	85	0.41 (lys)	0.55 (lys)
Rice, white, cooked	88	0.59 (lys)	0.80 (lys)
Wheat, flour, whole	86	0.40 (lys)	0.54 (lys)
Wheat, flour, refined	96	0.37 (lys)	0.50 (lys)
Peanut butter	95	0.40 (lys)	0.55 (lys)
Beans, navy cooked	78	0.60 (S)	0.91 (S)
Soy protein isolate	95	0.75 (S)	1.14 (S)
Rice and beans	78	0.70 (trp)	1.02 (lys)

[a] True digestibility in man (%) = $\dfrac{\text{Nitrogen intake} - (\text{Fecal N on test protein} - \text{Fecal N on nonprotein diet})}{\text{Nitrogen intake}} \times 100$

A factor of 6.25 is used to convert nitrogen to protein. Data taken from references 10 and 15.

[b] The amino acid score for various protein sources was derived using the amino acid requirement pattern shown in Table 15.2.

The amino acid of the protein sources was obtained from the USDA Nutrient Database for Standard Reference, Release 19, 2006. The abbreviation shown in parenthesis is for the most limiting amino acid; trp, tryptophan; lys, lysine; S, cysteine + methionine; thr, threonine; his, histidine. Values more than 1 indicate that the protein source contains relatively more of that amino acid than the ideal reference protein.

The effectiveness with which an absorbed dietary protein can meet the indispensable amino acid requirement is determined by the protein's amino acid score (Table 15.3). This is determined by the amino acid that least meets the individual's amino acid requirements. To determine the amino acid score, the amount of an amino acid in 1 g of the protein of interest is divided by the amount in 1 g of the reference protein for the relevant population (Table 15.2). The amino acid that has the lowest score is the limiting amino acid, and its value represents the amino acid score of that specific protein.

$$\text{amino acid score} = \frac{\text{mg of limiting amino acid in 1 g of food protein}}{\text{mg of amino acid in 1 g of reference pattern}}$$

The amino acid score corrected for the digestibility of the protein is termed the protein digestibility corrected amino acid score (PDCAAS)[12,13,19]:

$$\text{PDCAAS (\%)} = \text{true digestibility} \times \text{amino acid score} \times 100$$

Of the indispensable amino acids, only 4 are likely to affect the quality of a food protein: lysine, the sulfur amino acids (methionine + cysteine), threonine, and tryptophan. Examples of the amino acid score for various protein sources if they were the only protein source in the diet of a young child are shown in Table 15.3. In the formulation of special purpose diets in clinical practice, the scoring patterns for all essential amino acids should be considered.

Protein Requirements

Because of the differences in the quality of proteins available in the diet and other factors such as age, gender, activity levels, and methodologic limitations, confidence in the recommendations for protein and amino acid intakes for individuals or populations is somewhat tenuous. Nonetheless, recommendations are needed to guide the design of diets and the content of educational programs in nutrition and for planning specific intervention programs. The recommendations for protein are categorized by life stage and gender, because among healthy individuals, these are the 2 primary parameters that are responsible for variations in the body's need for protein. The pediatric stage of life has been subdivided into 6 groupings: infancy, 0 to 6 months of age; infancy, 7 to 12 months of age; toddlers, 1 to 3 years of age; early childhood, 4 to 8 years of age; puberty, 9 to 13 years of age; and adolescence, 14 to 18 years of age. Differences between boys and girls are only defined for the adolescent group.[13]

Infants

The optimal food for full-term infants is human milk, and it is recommended that this be the sole source of nutrition for infants during the first 6 months of life. Current recommendations are based on the average value determined from a number of different studies of exclusively breastfed infants. These results indicate that, on average, infants to 6 months of age consume 0.78 L of milk per day (reviewed by Institute of Medicine[13]). The protein content of human milk is the lowest of any species, with reported values varying from 9 to 14 g/L of true protein after the first few weeks postpartum, and an average value of 11.7 g/L was used to calculate the AI for protein. Milk also contains significant amounts of nonprotein nitrogen compounds, such as free amino acids, urea, and creatine, which constitute 20% to 27% of the nitrogen content of human milk, or 2 to 3 g/L. The proportion of the nonprotein nitrogen that is bioavailable and spares the utilization of milk protein amino acids is uncertain; estimates from 46% to 61% have been proposed.[14] The protein composition of human milk, in which the whey proteins rather than the caseins are the dominant protein constituents, is exceptional because of its high cysteine content and high cysteine-to-methionine ratio (Appendix R: Constituents of Human Milk). The nonprotein nitrogen component of human milk also contains substantial quantities of taurine, which is virtually absent from cow milk but is added to commercially prepared infant formulas.

Although the protein content of human milk is less than that of commercial infant formulas, the human milk proteins have a high nutritional quality and are digested and absorbed more efficiently than the cow milk proteins. Thus, a 6-kg infant ingesting 780 mL/day of human milk receives approximately 9.1 g of protein. This is approximately 1.52 g/kg/day of high-quality protein, the AI for infants up to 6 months of age. Because of the uncertainty of its availability, the contribution of nonprotein nitrogen is not included. On the other hand, data from infants freely fed commercial formulas consume more on the order of 2 g/kg/day.[14,15] The consensus from a number of studies seems to be that although the total weight and lean mass gain of formula-fed infants is higher than for exclusively human milk-fed infants after 3 months of age, this difference is not attributable specifically to the higher protein content of formulas but their higher food intake in general. Thus, after adjusting for differences in energy intake, differences in growth rate attributable to milk source are no longer evident.[13,14] There is no indication that the lower protein intake of breastfed infants has adverse effects.[15] Their protein intake appears to satisfy the infant requirements for maintenance and growth without an amino acid or solute excess.

Commercial infant formulas for term infants in the United States contain a protein equivalent of 14 to 16 g/L or 2.1 to 2.5 g/100 kcal (see Chapter 4: Formula Feeding of Term Infants). This concentration is higher than for human milk and provides a margin of safety for the lower digestibility of cow milk proteins. Additionally, most cow milk-based commercial infant formulas are supplemented with bovine milk whey to create a whey protein-to-casein ratio similar to that of human milk. Although the specific proteins of cow milk whey differ considerably from those of human milk whey, the amino acid composition (especially for cysteine and methionine) of these "humanized" formulas is closer to that of human milk proteins than are formulas with the whey protein-to-casein ratio of cow milk.

IV

Soy-based formulas, for which the digestibility of proteins is lower still,[20] contain even higher levels of protein to compensate (16.5–19 g/L).

For 7- to 12-month-old infants, nitrogen balance and body composition data are available, from which average requirements can be derived. Maintenance requirements for children from 9 months to 14 years of age were determined to be similar, and thus, a constant value equivalent to 0.688 g/kg/day is suggested for all ages. The growth requirement over this 6-month age range (corrected for the efficiency of utilization of dietary protein for growth—ie, 58%) yielded a value 0.312 g/kg/day, so that the EAR for the older infant was estimated at 1 g/kg/day, and the RDA is 1.2 g/kg/day. This is slightly lower than the measured AI of healthy older infants (1.6 g/kg/day) fed human milk supplemented with complementary foods.

Children

During the preschool and school years, there is a continuing decline in protein needs relative to body weight. This reflects the decreasing contribution of the growth requirement relative to the constant maintenance requirement. Current protein allowances have been derived from estimates of the average requirements by the factorial method and by assuming that the variability of protein needs among individual children is the same as that of other age groups.

Few data exist on the amino acid requirement of children and adolescents, and again these have been derived using the factorial approach. The requirement for growth (calculated from body composition measurements) contributes only a small proportion of total needs after the first few years of life (Table 15.1). As maintenance protein requirements have been demonstrated to change little with age, the amino acid requirement for maintenance has been based on the EAR for adults determined by direct amino acid oxidation measurements, which are generally believed to be more accurate than those derived from measuring obligatory losses or based on maintenance protein requirements at nitrogen equilibrium.

The amino acid requirement values for the 1- to 3-year-old child are only slightly higher than for adults. Thus, the scoring pattern for dietary proteins will also be very similar. Thus, the recommendation has been made that the reference amino acid pattern for preschool children should be used for assessing the protein components of foods for all individuals older than 1 year.[13] Food consumption surveys in the United States have established that the amino acid patterns and digestibility of proteins in foods commonly consumed is uniform from 1 year of age on and that no adjustment to the RDA is required for individuals consuming a typical US diet.[13] However, appropriate corrections must be made if a diet of lower quality than any acceptable reference protein is customarily consumed.[12]

Adolescents

Few data are available on the protein requirements of adolescents, specifically. Values have been estimated using the factorial approach, using the adult value for maintenance needs (0.656 g/kg/day), estimated from nitrogen balance studies. The growth component is derived from body composition studies corrected for the efficiency of utilization derived from the nitrogen balance studies (47%). Although the growth spurt is small relative to body size, the values are slightly higher for boys than girls; thus, the calculated EAR for 14- to 18-year-old boys is 0.73 g/kg/day compared with 0.71 g/kg/day for girls of the same age range. However, the RDA for adolescent boys and girls have both been set at 0.85 g/kg/day. There have been no further developments in identifying any specific amino acid needs for adolescents, and the same recommendations as for children have been adopted.

Factors Affecting Dietary Protein Requirements

Dietary requirements for protein are affected by a variety of factors, including gender, age, growth, pregnancy, lactation, illness, the adequacy of other nutrients in the diet, and possibly, genetic variation. These factors influence in various ways the maintenance needs of the organism and the efficiency with which amino acids can be used for growth. The primary factor that influences protein requirements is energy intake. All balance measurements and recommendations are based on the assumption that energy needs are adequately met. When energy intake is inadequate, proteins are catabolized for the provision of energy, effectively increasing protein requirements.

Protein requirements for pregnancy are increased to meet the need for maternal and fetal tissue deposition.[12,13] During the first trimester, the amount of tissue growth is insignificant, and requirements are the same as for nonpregnant females. During the second and third trimesters of pregnancy, higher protein intakes are required for both tissue deposition and the maintenance needs of the deposited, metabolically active tissue, and the fetus. The EAR to meet these needs is 0.88 g/kg/day, or 33% higher than for adult women, and the RDA for pregnancy is 1.1 g/kg/day. Whether adolescent mothers have different needs from adult mothers has not been definitively established, and no separate recommendation has been made. Protein supplementation studies demonstrating improved birth outcomes support the benefit of higher, but not excessive, protein intakes during pregnancy.[21]

Additional dietary protein also is required for lactation to supply amino acids for the production of milk proteins and nonprotein nitrogen. These values are adjusted for the efficiency of dietary protein utilization. The published recommendations specify the increase in the protein intake over the nonlactating value for adolescent girls and women that are necessary at different stages of lactation. Again, similar values (EAR, 1.05 kg/day; RDA, 1.3 kg/day) have been proposed for adolescent and adult females, even though the requirements for the nonpregnant adolescent are slightly higher than for the adult.

There are no data on the amino acid requirements of pregnancy and lactation specifically, so it is generally assumed that the indispensable amino acid needs are increased in the same proportions as the increased protein needs.

Infections and stressful stimuli, such as severe thermal or physical injury, are among factors that increase individual protein and amino acid needs.[12] In these conditions, maintenance needs are increased because of increased rates of protein and amino acid catabolism and increased losses, such as those that occur with burns. These responses are frequently compounded by a loss of appetite and reduced food intake. Despite the clear-cut evidence for a greater protein need during periods of infection and stress, exact recommendations are not available. On the basis of some studies, a reasonable estimate is a 20% to 30% increase in total protein after an infection (30% to 50% in the case of diarrhea) and during the recovery period, which is 2 to 3 times longer than the duration of the illness.[22]

Although athletic activity and heavy physical work increase energy needs, whether the need for protein is also increased once the energy needs are met is not clear (see also Chapter 12: Sports Nutrition). In theory, both endurance and resistance exercise increase protein and amino acid needs. With endurance exercise training, an acute increase in branched-chain amino acid oxidation has been measured, but in the resting state, a decrease has been observed and overall nitrogen balance is maintained when the RDA for protein is consumed, provided that energy intake is sufficient.[23] This is commensurate with the observation that endurance/aerobic exercise does not build muscle and improves protein utilization. Resistance exercise, in contrast, promotes muscle hypertrophy. Athletes undertaking intense exercise appear to require 1 to 1.5 g/kg/day to remain in nitrogen balance.[24] Nonetheless, chronic studies in which higher levels of protein have been provided have not been able to demonstrate significantly greater increases in muscle mass.[25] Recent studies have demonstrated that the timing of the feed in relation to the exercise, the amino acid composition of the protein, and the digestibility of the protein may interact to determine the degree of muscle anabolism.[26,27] Chronic, well-controlled studies in which the effects of these dietary variables on muscle accretion have been followed chronically have not been performed. It is fair to say, however, that provided individuals consume a well-balanced diet (in which approximately 15%–20% of the total energy content is from proteins), the increased food consumption that usually accompanies the increased energy needs of physical activity ensures that protein intake also is increased. Thus, any increased needs will be met without the need for specific supplements or a change in the composition of the diet. Increased protein intake in itself will not increase skeletal muscle protein deposition.

Protein requirements are increased in infants and children undergoing catch-up growth.[12,14] The additional amount of protein that must be supplied depends on the desired rate and composition of weight gain. With intensive supplementation, rates of weight gain up to 20 g/kg/day can be achieved in infants with severe wasting. The protein needs for depositing 1 g tissue/kg/day depend on the composition of the tissue gain. Assuming a composition of 14% protein and that the efficiency of conversion of dietary protein to body protein is 70% during catch-up growth, 0.2 g/kg/day of protein above the maintenance protein requirement will be needed. Along with the additional protein, energy must also be supplemented to support catch-up growth. The level of energy supplementation that is needed varies depending on whether the child has wasting or not. Weight gain in a child with wasting will have a larger proportion of fat, which carries a greater energy cost than an equivalent weight of lean body mass. However, when refeeding malnourished children, careful consideration also must be given to the overall protein-to-energy ratio of the diet, because it will influence the composition of the tissues deposited. Because children with severe wasting are often stunted, feedings with high protein-to-energy ratios to minimize the likelihood of excessive fat deposition are preferable. Catch-up growth also increases the requirements for micronutrients, such as zinc, magnesium, iron, and copper. Thus, the intake of these nutrients must be increased to maximize the efficiency of dietary protein utilization.

Effects of Insufficient and Excessive Protein Intake

Protein-energy malnutrition encompasses a wide spectrum of conditions, with kwashiorkor, the result of a greater deficiency of protein than energy intake, at one end of the spectrum and marasmus, resulting primarily from an inadequate energy intake, at the other. Especially in kwashiorkor, the condition is often precipitated by the development of conditions that increase the child's protein needs, such as an infection or diarrhea. A marginally adequate diet, as weaning diets often can be in less resource-rich countries, does not meet these increased needs. Although protein-energy malnutrition is observed even in industrialized countries, such as the United States, the cause is usually associated with the presence of clinical conditions that decrease food intake or impair the digestion or absorption of food.

The effects of too much dietary protein have not been studied extensively, and the findings are equivocal (summarized by Institute of Medicine[28]). Recently, the suggestion has been made that a high protein intake during the first 2 years life promotes more rapid growth and increases the risk of the development of obesity in later life.[29] The proposal is based on the comparison between the long-term growth of infants fed human milk or infant formula in early postnatal life as well as studies in older infants that relate protein intake and protein source to weight gain in later life. Although the findings are suggestive, they are by no means conclusive, and before changes in infant feeding practices are considered, a number of issues need to be delineated. These include a clearer understanding of the relationships between appetite control, food composition and energy intake,[30] accurate measurements of body composition to demonstrate increased adiposity rather than just greater body mass index values, and assessment of the contribution of differences in socioeconomic factors that frequently confound the comparison between formula-fed and breastfed infants. It has also been speculated that the protein source may be an important variable, with a high protein intake from animal but not vegetable or cereal protein sources being associated with the development of greater adiposity.[31] Thus, it is not possible to discern whether it is the protein intake per se or the composite nature of the protein-containing food that might be responsible for the observed associations between early protein intake and the risk of developing obesity in later life.

Urinary calcium excretion increases linearly at protein intakes above the RDA, with a doubling of protein intake leading to a 50% increase in urinary calcium in adults, in the absence of any change in other nutrients. This was thought to promote bone demineralization and to increase the risk of kidney stone formation. The increased bone demineralization was attributed to the increased acid load produced from the metabolism of the sulfur-containing amino acids, methionine and cysteine, when high-protein diets were consumed. Subsequently, it has been demonstrated that the increased excretion of urinary calcium with high-protein diets is attributable, in part, to increased intestinal calcium absorption. Thus, the net effect of dietary protein intake on bone appears to be a balance between the catabolic effects of a high acid load and an otherwise general anabolic effect of protein on bone formation.[32] Several studies have demonstrated that the beneficial effects of protein on bone are evident only in the presence of an adequate calcium intake. The presence of adequate fruit and vegetables which serve to "alkalinize" the diet, can further modulate the effects of dietary protein and calcium intake on bone mineralization.

There is little evidence for other adverse effects of high protein intakes in healthy individuals. As protein intake increases, plasma amino acids and urea concentrations increase. This might present difficulties to individuals in whom the mechanisms to eliminate nitrogen products are compromised, but not otherwise. High intakes of protein, especially casein, by small infants can result in acidosis, aminoacidemia, and cylindruria. For many years, a concern for the development of metabolic derangements limited the amount of amino acids that were administered to preterm infants. However, this practice is being abandoned rapidly, because it is clear that the provision of protein intakes as high as 4 g/kg/day can be tolerated and promote better short- and long-term outcomes.[33] Although in adults, some studies have shown a correlation between protein intake and the prevalence of atherosclerosis or risk of cancer, these findings have not been consistent. The positive associations seem to be more prevalent when meat is the source of dietary protein, and thus, a causative role for protein itself is uncertain. Given the paucity of data and the inconsistent nature of the conclusions derived from them, the only safe recommendation that can be made regarding high protein intakes is that the maximal levels of protein intake should be dictated by the overall macronutrient composition of the diet and should fall within the AMDR.[28]

References

1. Burrin DG, Stoll B. Metabolic fate and function of dietary glutamate in the gut. *Am J Clin Nutr.* 2009;90(3):850S-856S

2. Davis TA, Fiorotto ML. Regulation of muscle growth in neonates. *Curr Opin Clin Nutr Metab Care.* 2009;12(1):78-85

3. Denne SC, Kalhan SC. Leucine metabolism in human newborns. *Am J Physiol.* 1987;253(6 Pt 1):e608-e615

4. Denne SC, Rossi EM, Kalhan SC. Leucine kinetics during feeding in normal newborns. *Pediatr Res.* 1991;30(1):23-27

5. Matthews DE. Observations of branched-chain amino acid administration in humans. *J Nutr.* 2005;135(6 Suppl):1580S-1584S

6. Waterlow JC, Jackson AA. Nutrition and protein turnover in man. *Br Med Bull.* 1981;37(1):5-10

7. Kalhan SC, Bier DM. Protein and amino acid metabolism in the human newborn. *Annu Rev Nutr.* 2008;28:389-410

8. Jackson AA. The glycine story. *Eur J Clin Nutr.* 1991;45(2):59-65

9. Alpers DH. Glutamine: do the data support the cause for glutamine supplementation in humans? *Gastroenterology.* 2006;130(2 Suppl):S106-S116

10. Lourenco R, Camilo ME. Taurine: a conditionally essential amino acid in humans? An overview in health and disease. *Nutr Hosp.* 2002;17(6):262-270

11. Borum PR. Carnitine in neonatal nutrition. *J Child Neurol.* 1995;10(Suppl 2):S25-S31

12. World Health Organization/Food and Agriculture Organization of the United Nations. *Protein and Amino Acid Requirements in Human Nutrition: Report of a Joint WHO/FAO/UNU Expert Consultation.* Geneva, Switzerland: World Health Organization; 2007

13. Institute of Medicine, Food and Nutrition Board. Protein and Amino Acids. In: *Dietary Reference Intakes for Energy, Carbohydrates, Fiber, Fat, Fatty Acids, Cholesterol, Protein, and Amino Acids.* Washington, DC: The National Academies Press; 2005:589-768

14. Dewey KG, Beaton G, Fjeld C, Lonnerdal B, Reeds P. Protein requirements of infants and children. *Eur J Clin Nutr.* 1996;50(Suppl 1):S119-S147

IV

15. Nestle Nutrition Workshop Series Pediatric Program. *Protein and Energy Requirements in Infancy and Childhood.* Basel, Switzerland: Karger; 2006

16. Viteri FE. INCAP studies of energy, amino acids, and protein. *Food Nutr Bull.* 2010;31(1):42-53

17. Butte NF, Hopkinson JM, Wong WW, Smith EO, Ellis KJ. Body composition during the first 2 years of life: an updated reference. *Pediatr Res.* 2000;47(5):578-585

18. Ellis KJ, Shypailo RJ, Abrams SA, Wong WW. The reference child and adolescent models of body composition. A contemporary comparison. *Ann N Y Acad Sci.* 2000;904:374-382

19. Food and Agriculture Organization of the United Nations/World Health Organization. Protein Quality Evaluation. Rome, Italy: Food and Agriculture Organization of the United Nations; 1991

20. Lonnerdal B. Nutritional aspects of soy formula. *Acta Paediatr Suppl.* 1994;402:105-108

21. Dubois S, Coulombe C, Pencharz P, Pinsonneault O, Duquette MP. Ability of the Higgins Nutrition Intervention Program to improve adolescent pregnancy outcome. *J Am Diet Assoc.* 1997;97(8):871-878

22. Scrimshaw NS. Effect of infection on nutritional status. *Proc Natl Sci Counc Repub China B.* 1992;16(1):46-64

23. Gaine PC, Viesselman CT, Pikosky MA, et al. Aerobic exercise training decreases leucine oxidation at rest in healthy adults. *J Nutr.* 2005;135:1088-1092

24. Lemon PW. Effects of exercise on dietary protein requirements. *Int J Sport Nutr.* 1998;8(4):426-447

25. Lemon PW, Proctor DN. Protein intake and athletic performance. *Sports Med.* 1991;12(5):313-325

26. Lemon PW, Berardi JM, Noreen EE. The role of protein and amino acid supplements in the athlete's diet: does type or timing of ingestion matter? *Curr Sports Med Rep.* 2002;1(4):214-221

27. Tipton KD, Wolfe RR. Protein and amino acids for athletes. *J Sports Sci.* 2004;22(1):65-79

28. Institute of Medicine, Food and Nutrition Board. Macronutrients and Healthful Diets. In: *Dietary Reference Intakes for Energy, Carbohydrates, Fiber, Fat, Fatty Acids, Cholesterol, Protein, and Amino Acids.* Washington, DC: National Academies Press; 2005:769-879

29. Grote V, von Kries R, Closa-Monasterolo R, et al. Protein intake and growth in the first 24 months of life. *J Pediatr Gastroenterol Nutr.* 2010;51(Suppl 3):S117-S118

30. Kalhan SC. Optimal protein intake in healthy infants. *Am J Clin Nutr.* 2009;89(6):1719-1720

31. Gunther AL, Remer T, Kroke A, Buyken AE. Early protein intake and later obesity risk: which protein sources at which time points throughout infancy and childhood are important for body mass index and body fat percentage at 7 y of age? *Am J Clin Nutr.* 2007;86(6):1765-1772

32. Jesudason D, Clifton P. The interaction between dietary protein and bone health. *J Bone Miner Metab.* 2011;29(1):1-14

33. Ziegler EE. Meeting the nutritional needs of the low-birth-weight infant. *Ann Nutr Metab.* 2011;58(Suppl 1):8-18

Chapter 16

Carbohydrate and Dietary Fiber

Overview

Carbohydrate provides 50% to 60% of the calories consumed by the average American. Although relatively little carbohydrate is needed in the diet, carbohydrate spares protein and fat being metabolized for calories. The principal dietary carbohydrates are sugars and starches. In addition to providing energy, carbohydrates have numerous other potential effects, such as lowering cholesterol, increasing calcium absorption, acting as a source of short-chain fatty acids in the colon, and increasing fecal bulk (Table 16.1).

By convention, dietary carbohydrates can be classified by their chemical nature (Table 16.2).[1] Sugars are defined as monosaccharides or disaccharides. The monosaccharides include glucose, galactose, and fructose, and disaccharides include lactose, sucrose, maltose, and trehalose. Lactose is derived from milk, whereas fructose, glucose, and sucrose are contained in the cells of fruits and vegetables. Sucrose also is purified from cane or beet sources. Processed foods also may contain a significant amount of fructose and corn syrup, the latter also containing oligosaccharides and polysaccharides (see next paragraph), because it is derived from cornstarch. Fructose is the sweetest of the dietary carbohydrates. Besides being used as sweeteners, sugars also confer functional characteristics to foods (eg, viscosity, texture, control of moisture to prevent drying out).[1] The polyols (eg, sorbitol) are alcohols of sugars and found in some fruits but also made commercially as a replacement for sucrose in the diet of people with diabetes mellitus.[1]

Oligosaccharides contain between 3 and 9 sugars (3–9 degrees of polymerization or DP3-9; Table 16.1). Food oligosaccharides fall into 2 groups, maltodextrins (glucose-based) and oligosaccharides not composed solely of glucose molecules. Maltodextrins are mostly derived from starch and include maltotriose and a-limit dextrins, which contain both a-1-4 and a-1-6 bonds with an average DP8. They are used by the food industry as sweeteners, fat substitutes, and texture modifiers.[1] Oligosaccharides not made up of glucose molecules include raffinose, stachyose, and verbascose, which are sucrose molecules (glucose and fructose) joined to varying numbers of galactose molecules and are found in a variety of plant seeds.[1] Included in this group are inulin and fructo-oligosaccharides, which are used as prebiotics. Oligosaccharides in human milk, which are predominantly galactose based, also are prebiotics.

Polysaccharides are ≥10 sugars in length and consist of starches and nonstarch polysaccharides (Table 16.1). Starches are the storage carbohydrates of plants and consist of sugars (eg, glucose) linked together. Starches exist as either amylose

IV

Table 16.1.

Principal Physiological Properties of Dietary Carbohydrates

	Provide Energy	Increase Satiety	Glycemic	Cholesterol Lowering	Increase Calcium Absorption	Source of Short-Chain Fatty Acids	Prebiotic	Increase Stool Output	Immuno-modulatory
Monosaccharides	✓		✓						
Disaccharides	✓		✓		✓				
Polyols	✓					✓[a]		✓	
Maltodextrins	✓		✓						
Oligosaccharides (non-α-glucan)	✓				✓	✓	✓		✓
Starch	✓		✓			✓[b]		✓[b]	
Nonstarch polysaccharides	✓	✓		✓[c]		✓		✓	

Adapted with permission from Cummings and Stephen.[1]

[a] Except erythritol.

[b] Resistant starch.

[c] Some forms of nonstarch polysaccharides only.

Table 16.2.
Major Dietary Carbohydrates

Class (DP)	Subgroup	Principal Components
Sugars (1-2)	Monosaccharides Disaccharides Polyols (sugar alcohols)	Glucose, fructose, galactose Sucrose, lactose, maltose, trehalose Xylitol, erythritol, isomalt, maltitol
Oligosaccharides (3-9)	Malto-oligosaccharides (α-glucans) Non-α-glucan oligosaccharides	Maltodextrins Raffinose, stachyose, fructo- and galacto- oligosaccharides, polydextrose, inulin
Polysaccharides (≥10)	Starch (α-glucans) Nonstarch polysaccharides	Amylose, amylopectin, modified starches Cellulose, hemicellulose, pectin, arabinoxylans, b-glucan, glucomannans, plant gums and mucilages, hydrocolloids

Adapted with permission from Cummings and Stephen.[1]

(nonbranched with α-1-4 bonds) or amylopectin (branched with α-1-4 and α-1-6 bonds) (see section on Starches).

More recently, the National Academy of Sciences proposed a new definition of dietary fiber based on the concept that that the definition should determine the analytical methods needed to measure it rather than have the method determine what qualified as fiber or not.[2] The definition proposes that total fiber = dietary fiber + functional fiber. Dietary fiber consists of nondigestible carbohydrates and lignins, which are intrinsic and intact in plants (eg, gums, cellulose, oat, and wheat bran). Functional fiber consists of isolated, nondigestible carbohydrates that have beneficial physiological effects in humans and may be derived from plants (eg, resistant starches from bananas or potatoes) or animals (eg, chitin and chitosan from crab and lobster shells).

Digestion of Disaccharides and Starches

Lactose and sucrose are hydrolyzed to monosaccharides via lactase and sucrase, respectively (Fig 16.1). Lactase activity increases substantially during the third trimester in the fetus, whereas sucrase activity by the onset of the last trimester is already at levels found at birth.[3,4] Starch digestion is more complex. The production of amylase by the pancreas increases to mature levels during the first year of life.[5] Salivary, and more likely, mucosal enzymes (glucoamylase, sucrase, and isomaltase) are responsible for starch digestion in young infants.[5,6] Pancreatic and salivary amylase hydrolyze the interior α-1-4 bonds (Fig 16.1). Glucoamylase sequentially cleaves α-1-4 bonds from the nonreducing end of the molecule (Fig 16.1).[7] It is most active against starches between 5 and 9 glucose residues in length.[7] Isomaltase (α-dextrinase) and sucrase also have some activity in this regard. Isomaltase is primarily responsible for cleaving the α-1-6 bonds.

IV

Fig 16.1

Pancreatic and salivary amylase hydrolyze interior α-1-4 bonds 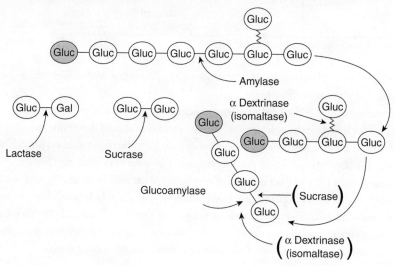. **Glucoamylase sequentially cleaves α-1-4 bonds from the nonreducing end of the molecule. The reducing end is designated** (Gluc). **Isomaltase and sucrase also have some activity in this regard. Isomaltase is primarily responsible for cleaving the α-1-6 bonds** (Gluc). **Lactose and sucrose are hydrolyzed by their respective hydrolases. Reproduced with permission from Shulman RJ. Intraluminal digestion and absorption in the small intestine. In: Gluckman P, Heymann MA, eds. *Pediatrics and Perinatology*. London, United Kingdom: Edward Arnold Ltd; 1996;630-637.**

Absorption of Monosaccharides

The end products of disaccharide and starch digestion are monosaccharides. These are absorbed in the small intestine (Fig 16.2).[8-10] Access into enterocytes occurs via carrier molecules. Glucose and galactose are actively transported via the sodium-glucose–linked transporter (SGLT1) located at the brush border.[11] Glucose and galactose entry is coupled to the entry of sodium along its electrochemical gradient.[11] This electrochemical gradient is maintained via sodium-potassium-adenosine triphosphatase (Na$^+$-K$^+$ ATPase) located at the basolateral surface.[11] SGLT1 has binding sites for both glucose and sodium.[11] Two sodium molecules are absorbed for every glucose molecule. Once both sites are occupied, the transporter translocates across the brush-border membrane and releases the glucose and sodium into the enterocyte.[11] The sodium-linked transport of glucose provides the basis for adding glucose or starches to oral rehydration solutions.[11]

Fig 16.2
Glucose and galactose are actively transported along with sodium across the brush border via SGLT1. Fructose is transported across the brush border via facilitated diffusion through the action of GLUT5. Fructose and glucose also appear to be transported via facilitated diffusion through the action of GLUT2. The transient upregulation of GLUT2 at the apical membrane in response to luminal sugar has been shown in murine models but not yet demonstrated in humans (designated by dotted lines). Glucose, galactose, and fructose exit the enterocyte via the action of GLUT2. Adapted with permission from Jones HF, Butler RN, Brooks DA. Intestinal fructose transport and malabsorption in humans. *Am J Physiol Gastrointest Liver Physiol.* 2011;300(2):G202-G206.[10]

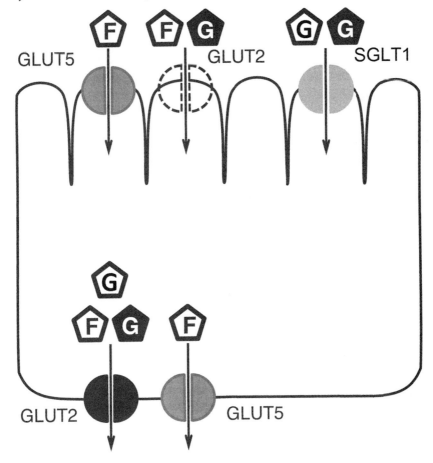

IV

Fructose transport across the brush-border membrane occurs passively down its concentration gradient via facilitated diffusion via GLUT5, a mechanism that is not sodium dependent.[8,10] Transport of glucose, galactose, and fructose across the basolateral membrane occurs by facilitated transport via the sodium-independent transporter, GLUT2.[8,10]

Recently, GLUT2 has been recognized in the brush-border membrane, and glucose transported by SGLT1 promotes the activation of GLUT2 already in the apical membrane and rapid insertion of GLUT2 from vesicles.[12] As a result, absorption of combinations of carbohydrates (eg, glucose and fructose, maltodextrin, and fructose) is more efficient than that of the single carbohydrate.[12,13] Exercise tolerance is increased as a consequence of the increased oxidative rate when the sugars are ingested at high rates (eg, 1 g/min) (Fig 16.3).[13] An additional metabolic effect to improve exercise tolerance may relate to the oxidation of fructose to lactate, which is used as an energy source in muscle.[13]

Fig 16.3
When multiple carbohydrates are ingested (squares), the total carbohydrate oxidation rate is increased compared with the ingestion of a single carbohydrate (circles). This is related, in part, to faster and more efficient intestinal absorption. Ingestion of multiple (eg, glucose and fructose) as opposed to single carbohydrates (eg, glucose) improves exercise performance. Reproduced with permission from Jeukendrup AE. Carbohydrate and exercise performance: the role of multiple transportable carbohydrates. *Curr Opin Clin Nutr Metab Care.* **2010;13(4):452-457.**

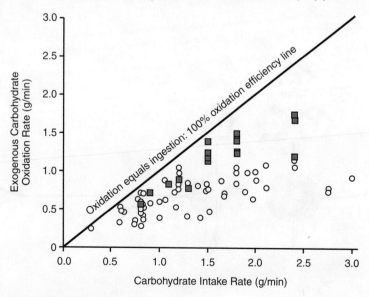

GLUT7 recently has been identified in the small intestine and colon.[14] Glucose and fructose, but not galactose, appear to be substrates.[14] Expression in the small intestine (but not colon) appears responsive to the amount of these hexoses in the diet, but its full role in absorption has yet to be elucidated.[14]

Carbohydrates not absorbed in the small intestine are fermented by colonic bacteria and converted to short-chain fatty acids, which are in turn absorbed by the colon.[15,16] Exceeding the ability of the fermentative rate results in the remaining mono-, di-, and oligosaccharides, creating an osmotic gradient that drives water into the lumen and results in an osmotic diarrhea.[17]

Metabolism of Glucose

Dietary carbohydrates are converted to glucose in the liver. It is the most abundant carbohydrate. The majority of glucose is metabolized for energy.[18] Quantitatively, the brain is the largest utilizer of glucose as an energy source. There are few data that allow the limits of carbohydrate intake to be defined.[18] Amino acids and glycerol from lipids can be converted to glucose. However, in the case of amino acids, this potentially shunts substrate away from protein synthesis. Glucose synthesis from both amino acids and glycerol is not very metabolically efficient. Estimates of minimum glucose requirements based on cerebral glucose utilization are shown in Table 16.3.

IV

Table 16.3.
Estimates of Glucose Consumption by the Brain

	Body Weight (kg)	Brain Weight (g)	Glucose Consumption		
			$(mg \cdot kg^{-1} \cdot min^{-1})$	$(g \cdot kg^{-1} \cdot d^{-1})$	(g/d)
Newborn	3.2	399	6.0	11.5	37
1 y	10.0	997	7.0	10.1	101
5 y	19.0	1266	4.7	6.8	129
Adolescent	50.0	1360	1.9	2.7	135
Adult	70.0	1400	1.0	1.4	98

Adapted with permission from Kalhan and Kilic.[18]

The upper limits of glucose requirements should be defined by the amount that defines a minimal need for fat and protein and maximum glucose oxidation rates (Table 16.4).[18] These are theoretical limits, because they presume the minimal intake of protein and fat with glucose providing essentially all energy needs. However, doing so can be associated with adverse effects, such as hyperglycemia.

Table 16.4.
Upper Limit of Carbohydrate Intake for Infants and Children[a]

Age	Total Energy Expenditure[b] (kcal·kg^{-1}·d^{-1})	Carbohydrate Equivalent[c] (g·kg^{-1}·d^{-1})
Newborn	73	19
1–3 y	85	22
4–6 y	68	18
12–13 y	55	14
18–19 y	44	12
Adult	35	9

Adapted with permission from Kalhan and Kilic.[18]

[a] Upper limit should be determined by the minimal need for protein and fat obtained. Therefore, the described upper limits here are theoretical maximal to meet all the energy needs.

[b] Average of data for boys and girls. Estimate based on double-labeled water method.

[c] Carbohydrate equivalent = total energy expenditure/3.8, assuming each g of carbohydrate yields 3.8 kcal.

Glucose that is not immediately oxidized can be polymerized to form glycogen. Current data suggest that in the human newborn infant, gluconeogenesis appears soon after birth and contributes 30% to 70% to glucose produced.[19] As noted previously, the majority of glucose is used by the central nervous system. Endogenous glucose can only provide 30% of glucose needed in very low birth weight infants because of the higher brain-to-body ratio.[20] Storage and mobilization of glycogen are under the hormonal control of insulin and glucagon (see Chapter 32: Hypoglycemia, and Chapter 31: Diabetes). During periods of fasting, the liver and kidney can mobilize glucose from glycogen. If fasting is prolonged, hepatic glycogen stores will be drained in a few hours and gluconeogenesis from lactate, alanine, glycerol, and glutamine must be stimulated to maintain euglycemia.[21] The newborn infant has approximately 34 g of glycogen, only 6 g of which is in the liver and is accumulated during the last weeks of fetal life. Hepatic glycogen is totally depleted during the first few days postnatally and then reaccumulates. Carbohydrate-free diets lead to ketosis, as does fasting. Ketosis occurs when carbohydrate intake drops below about 10% of total calories. It occurs more readily in children than in adults during fasting or when extremely low-carbohydrate diets are consumed. Low-carbohydrate diets and low-carbohydrate, high-fat diets (the ketogenic diet; see Chapter 49) have been used in the treatment of epilepsy and as a diagnostic test for ketotic hypoglycemia.

In addition to glycogen stores in the liver and skeletal muscle, the body contains carbohydrate in many different forms. These include mucopolysaccharides (structural carbohydrates that are important constituents of connective and collagenous tissues) and components of nucleic acids, glycoproteins, glycolipids, and various hormones and enzymes.

Recently, abnormalities in these structural carbohydrates have been associated with specific symptoms or disorders. Genetic defects in glycoprotein metabolism usually result in neurologic symptoms. However, defects in glycoprotein biosynthesis known as congenital disorders of glycosylation (formerly known as the carbohydrate-deficient glycoprotein syndromes) also present with hypoglycemia, protein-losing enteropathy, and hepatic pathology.[22] In these conditions, the N-glycosylation pathway is affected, resulting in alterations in the number or structure of sugar chains on the proteins. The diagnosis often can be made via isoelectric focusing of transferrin.[22]

Lactose

Lactose is present in almost all mammalian milks and is the major carbohydrate consumed by young infants.[23] However, at an early age, infants in the United States are fed a variety of other carbohydrates, including sucrose, natural and modified starches, starch hydrolysates, and small amounts of monosaccharides and indigestible carbohydrate (ie, fiber). Lactase, an enzyme on the brush border of the enterocyte in the small intestine, hydrolyzes the disaccharide lactose into the monosaccharides, glucose, and galactose (Fig 16.1).

Although a congenital form of lactase deficiency exists (also termed primary lactase deficiency), it is extremely rare. It manifests at birth in the presence of a lactose-containing diet. Lactase activity increases most rapidly during the last trimester of gestation.[4] Thus, developmental lactase deficiency is a temporary form of lactase deficiency that occurs in preterm infants (<34 weeks' gestation) and may be clinically significant.[24] Preterm infants do not digest lactose as well as glucose polymers.[25] Recent studies suggest that the feeding of formula containing lactose as the sole carbohydrate to very preterm infants may be associated with an increased risk of feeding intolerance and that the risk of feeding intolerance is inversely related to lactase activity.[26,27] However, one study in preterm infants reported increased lactase activity in breastfed infants when compared with formula-fed infants.[24] Thus, lactose from human milk may be less problematic than that from formula. Developmental lactase deficiency improves as the intestinal mucosa matures.[28]

Most commonly, lactase activity begins to decline in a genetically programmed (autosomal recessive) fashion so that by adulthood in many ethnic groups, it is low.[29] The highest prevalence of low lactase activity is found in the Far East. The prevalence in the United States varies according to race. In white US residents, the prevalence of low lactase activity is approximately 15% to 25%, in black US

IV

residents, it is approximately 80%, and in Asian US residents, it is approximately 90%.[23,29] The prevalence of low lactase activity also is related to ethnicity, with Hispanic people having a prevalence of approximately 53%. In the United States, the decline in lactase activity usually begins to occur around 3 to 7 years of age; ethnic groups with a higher prevalence of lactase deficiency typically have an earlier decline. People with low lactase activity often do not manifest symptoms of lactose intolerance, such as flatulence, bloating, abdominal pain, and nausea and diarrhea (also see Chapter 1).[23] In fact, most people with low lactase activity can tolerate some lactose intake, particularly when it is part of a meal.

Symptoms of lactase intolerance are caused by lactose that escapes digestion in the small intestine, passing into the colon, where it is fermented by enteric bacteria, forming organic acids, hydrogen, methane, and other gases.[15,16,23] The gases may cause bloating and pain, and the unabsorbed sugar and acids may cause an increase in osmotic pressure, which may result in osmotic diarrhea. As noted previously, however, the likelihood of developing symptoms depends on the amount of residual lactase activity, the amount of lactose ingested, and the composition of the meal. Lactose malabsorption may be detected by an increase in expired breath hydrogen after lactose ingestion, although clinical lactose intolerance does not always correlate with an abnormal breath hydrogen test.[23] Specific evaluation for lactose intolerance can be achieved relatively easily by dietary elimination and challenge.[23]

Lactase activity also can be diminished secondary to mucosal injury in the small intestine (also termed secondary lactase deficiency). This occurs most commonly in infants with viral gastroenteritis. It is a consequence of damage to the intestinal villi and resolves with resolution of the illness. In the otherwise healthy infant, the lactase deficiency may not be clinically significant. For example, most infants with rotavirus are not lactose intolerant.[23]

However, infants who have had inadequate weight gain or prolonged diarrhea may have clinical lactose intolerance until the illness resolves. Using a lactose-free formula until the infant recovers from diarrhea may be beneficial.[23] The intolerance usually lasts 1 to 2 weeks, except in severe cases. Carbohydrate malabsorption (including that from lactose) is detected by testing the pH of the stool by using nitrazine paper (pH <5.5 indicates carbohydrate fermentation attributable to malabsorption) and testing for glucose (based on copper reduction) using the same products used to test for glucose in the urine.[23] The glucose derives from the breakdown of lactose by the colonic microbiota. It is important to test the watery part of the stool, because the formed part of the stool is likely to give a false-negative result. This test can be used to detect the presence of other sugars, such as sucrose and starches, because the bacteria will degrade some proportion of these sugars to glucose. Detectable carbohydrate malabsorption should be treated to reduce fluid losses attributable to osmotic diarrhea with the consequent risks of dehydration and acidosis.

Starches

As noted previously, starches are the storage carbohydrate of plants consisting of amylose (a linear α-1-4 polysaccharide of glucose molecules) and amylopectin (an α-1-4 polysaccharide of glucose molecules with α-1-6 branch points). Chains between DP3 and DP9 and those $\geq$DP10 are termed oligosaccharides and polysaccharides, respectively (Table 16.1). The larger the starch, the less osmotically active it is.

Corn syrup is a generic term for products derived from cornstarch by hydrolysis with acid or enzymes. These products are classified according to their chemical-reducing power relative to glucose, which has a dextrose equivalent (DE) of 100%. The DE of corn syrups ranges from less than 20% to more than 95%. A low-DE corn syrup is somewhat hydrolyzed and is, therefore, more like starch than a high-DE corn syrup. Glucose polymer (or maltodextrin) is another term for corn syrup that has been hydrolyzed to (usually) a high DE carbohydrate. They often are added to formulas to provide additional calories without greatly increasing the osmolality of the feeding. Approximately 20% to 25% of infants in the United States are fed lactose-free soy isolate formulas containing sucrose or corn syrup solids or a combination of both as the carbohydrate source(s).

Modified food starches possess certain technical properties, such as altered viscosity and "mouth feel," freeze-thaw stability, gel clarity, and stability in acid products. In animal models, caloric availability of modified food starches is similar to unmodified starches. Modified food starches appear to be safe and reasonably well digested by human infants, although concern has been raised about the long-term implications of their feeding.[30,31] Many powdered special formulas and strained foods contain modified corn or tapioca starches. Special formulas may provide approximately 15% of the total calories in the form of modified starch, which is used to facilitate suspension of insoluble nutrients during feeding. The amount of modified starch in a few commercial infant desserts may amount to as much as 45% of the total content of the solids.

Fiber

The term fiber has multiple definitions in the nutrition world but generally refers to intrinsic plant cell polysaccharides, which are derived from the cellular walls and are poorly digestible.[1] Fiber is also called bulk or roughage. Fiber is composed predominantly of nonstarch polysaccharides and nonpolysaccharides (mainly lignins).

Nonstarch polysaccharides are the most diverse of all the carbohydrate groups and include cellulose (β1-4 linkages) and noncellulosic polysaccharides (eg, hemicelluloses, pectins, gums, and mucilages), which contain a mixture of hexose and pentose sugars. Pectin often is used to improve the gel consistency of jams. Gums also are used as thickeners. Mucilages are used as thickeners in mayonnaise, soups, and toothpaste. Carrageenan, derived from algae, is used in dairy products and chocolate. The definition of nonstarch polysaccharides excludes other substances in the plant materials, such as phytates, cutins, saponins, lectins, proteins, waxes, silicon, and other organic constituents. Fibers are present in the cell walls of all plants.

Fiber also is classified as soluble (some hemicelluloses, pectins, gums, and mucilages) or insoluble (most hemicelluloses, celluloses, and lignins). Soluble fiber, found in beans, fruits, psyllium, and oat products, dissolves in water. Soluble fiber is metabolized in the colon and, to a lesser extent, in the small intestine by the enzymatic action of anaerobic bacteria. Soluble fibers have been shown to increase stool size moderately and to decrease intestinal transit time, gastric emptying, glucose absorption, and serum cholesterol concentration (see Potential Benefits of Fiber Intake).[32] Insoluble fiber, found in whole-grain products and vegetables, does not dissolve. It consists of nondigestible polysaccharide and lignins. The intestinal microbiota does not significantly metabolize insoluble fibers. Insoluble fibers significantly increase fecal bulk, decrease intestinal transit time, delay glucose absorption, and slow down the process of starch hydrolysis.[32]

Crude fiber refers to the residue left after strong acid and base hydrolysis of plant material. This process dissolves pectin, gums, mucilages, and most of the hemicellulose. Thus, crude fiber is mainly a measure of cellulose and lignin and tends to underestimate the total amount of fiber in the food. Most food composition tables give only crude fiber values. Appendix I lists the fiber content of common foods. It has been estimated in adults that 5% to 10% of dietary starch (20–40 g in a Western diet) is "resistant starch," which is not digested in the small intestine and, therefore, reaches the colon in its intact form.[16,33] Young infants have a limited ability to digest starches such as those in cereal.[6,34,35]

Glycemic Index

The Glycemic Index (GI) is a numerical scale first introduced by Jenkins et al in 1981 to determine how rapidly affected and elevated blood glucose will be after consuming a particular food.[36] The index is calculated by first measuring the area under the 2-hour blood glucose response curve after ingestion of a fixed portion of carbohydrate (usually 50 g).[36] This area is then divided by the area under the curve of a standard, based on ingestion of an equal amount of carbohydrate (commonly glucose). This value is then multiplied by 100 to determine the index value.[36] Per equal gram of carbohydrate, a high-GI food will elevate blood glucose concentration higher than a low-GI food. Disaccharides have a high GI, whereas fiber generally has a low GI.[37] Evidence suggests that long-term consumption of a diet with a high GI may predict the risk of developing type 2 diabetes mellitus and cardiovascular disease.[37] Thus, many groups recommend a diet rich in foods with a low GI.[37] However, there are limitations to the GI. For example, GI can be significantly altered depending on the variety of a specific food, storage conditions, cooking methods, and ripeness as well as differences in testing techniques.[37]

Potential Benefits of Fiber Intake

The current interest in fiber was stimulated in part by the suggestion that fiber could help prevent certain diseases common in the United States, such as cancer of the colon, irritable bowel syndrome, constipation, obesity, and coronary heart disease. Epidemiologic studies noted that Africans in rural areas where the fiber intake was high rarely had these diseases. However, as urban migration has increased, the adoption of Western habits and dietary patterns has coincided with the increased incidence of Western diseases. A high-fiber diet increases fecal bulk, produces softer and more frequent stools, and speeds transit through the intestine.

A number of hypotheses have been put forth with regard to how increased dietary fiber could reduce the risk of colorectal carcinoma. These include dilution of potential carcinogens, reduced contact time with carcinogens because of fiber-induced faster transit, and inhibition of tumor cell lines. Although still controversial, current data suggest that consistent adherence to a low-fat, high-fiber, high-fruit, and high-vegetable diet may be effective in preventing recurrence of colorectal adenomas and possibly in preventing colorectal cancer.[38-40]

Increasing fiber intake has been used as a treatment in children with recurrent abdominal pain.[41] In a double-blind study, supplementation with corn fiber was associated with a 50% decrease in the frequency of abdominal pain.[41] To relieve constipation, a recent study suggested an intake of approximately 10 g/day and 14.5 g/day in children 3 through 7 years of age and 8 through 14 years of age, respectively.[42]

Adherence to a high-fiber diet leads to a better heart health as well. Fiber plays an important role in inflammation, weight control, blood pressure, and glycemic control and can affect cardiovascular disease biomarkers. Because fiber can be a dietary addition, rather than a restriction, adherence to this goal may be enhanced if routinely recommended.[40] The fiber content of various foods is provided in Appendix I.

Obesity is less prevalent in populations that consume most carbohydrate as complex carbohydrates and have a high fiber intake. The lower energy density of

IV

this type of diet may increase satiety. However, in many cultures in which this type of diet is common, the total energy intake is low by Western standards. Given the increasing prevalence of childhood obesity in the United States, there is interest in the role of fiber in reducing the risk of obesity. There are several explanations for the role of fiber in preventing obesity, but none have been proven unequivocally. These include effects on: (1) reducing food intake because of earlier satiety achieved with a larger volume in the stomach and intestine but reduced caloric density compared with a high-fat diet as well as slower gastric emptying; (2) reducing absorption of carbohydrate and protein (but not fat) related to faster small intestinal transit; and (3) flattening the insulin response curve to carbohydrate, thereby reducing the appetite-stimulating effects of insulin.[43]

Interpretation of the potential relationship between fiber intake and the development of obesity in children is problematic because of a lack of data and limitations on the interpretation of the available data. A recent study evaluating a possible relationship between fiber intake and adiposity in overweight Latino youths concluded that a decrease in fiber intake over a 1- to 2-year period can inversely lead to increase in adipose tissue.[44]

Atherosclerosis has its origins in childhood. Fatty streaks begin in the coronary arteries before 10 years of age and are almost universal after 20 years of age and are present in the aorta of almost all children by 10 years of age, according to some studies.[45] Given that research suggests a direct correlation between the percent of calories from saturated fat and cholesterol in children's diets and their blood cholesterol concentrations, the potential effects of fiber on reducing blood lipids and, thereby, the risk of heart disease are of great interest.[46]

The lipid-lowering effect is seen with soluble fiber but not with the insoluble form (Table 16.1). A review of the current data strongly suggests that the addition of soluble fiber to a step 1 lipid-lowering diet can reduce further certain fractions of blood lipids and/or increase serum high-density lipoprotein concentration (HDL).[46] The degree of reduction, the fraction of lipid that is reduced, and the effect on serum HDL may be dependent on the type of soluble fiber used. Supplementation with psyllium appeared to decrease serum low-density lipoprotein concentration (LDL) and increase HDL in 48 children 2 to 11 years of age with moderate hypercholesterolemia.[47,48]

Potential Adverse Effects of Fiber Intake

Objections have been made to an increased fiber intake for children. One of the concerns has been that fiber may compromise intake of other nutrients. It has been shown in young infants that addition of cereal in the amounts used to treat gastroesophageal reflux decreases total daily formula intake.[34] On the other hand, the addition of a soy fiber to infant formula to treat diarrhea does not appear to affect the intake of infants with diarrhea.[49]

Another concern is that fiber supplementation will affect the absorption of nutrients, particularly micronutrients.[2] Some plant foods contain phytate (inositol hexaphosphate), which serves as the storage form of phosphorus for plants and may form insoluble compounds with minerals, such as calcium, iron, copper, magnesium, and zinc, rendering them unavailable for normal absorption and metabolism.[50] Although phytate is destroyed in the process of leavening in the making of bread, it remains intact in many foods, such as legumes and grains. Consumption of primarily plant-based diets is considered to be a major etiologic factor for mineral deficiencies on a global basis.

Although it is possible that children on high-fiber diets may have a deficiency of these minerals, especially in situations in which mineral intake is low, children in the United States on a varied complete dietary regimen are unlikely to have mineral deficiencies irrespective of fiber intake.[2,50] Some foods also contain oxalic acid (spinach, rhubarb, chards, etc), which interferes with absorption of iron and calcium especially in individuals on high-fiber diets.[50] A review of the data suggests that addition of fiber to an otherwise normal omnivorous diet for a child in the United States does not adversely affect micronutrient status including that of iron.[50] This has recently been confirmed by a study in adolescents using dietary recall to evaluate fiber intake.[51]

Current Dietary Recommendations

Over the years, the amount of recommended dietary fiber has been increasing. Previous recommendations suggested that between 6 to 12 months of age, whole cereals, green vegetables, and legumes be introduced gradually, increasing to 5 g/day by the first year.[52] The American Health Foundation had set forth a suggested guideline for the recommended amount of fiber in a child's diet.[53] The recommendation suggested that children older than 2 years consume an amount of fiber approximately equivalent to the child's age plus 5 g/day. A safe range was believed to be age plus 10 g/day.[53] This "age plus 5" guideline results in a gradual increase of fiber intake over time, with 17-year-olds eating 22 g/day. The amount that was recommended for an older adolescent was also within the range recommended by the National Cancer Institute.[50] These older recommendations were endorsed by a conference that was held on dietary fiber in childhood in 1995.[54]

The Institute of Medicine report on Dietary Reference Intakes in 2002 established the Allowable Intake for fiber for children.[55] Table 16.5 provides the daily recommended fiber intake by age and gender.

Table 16.5.
Daily Recommended Intake of Fiber*

Gender/Age (y)	Fiber (g)
0-1	ND
≥1-3	19
4-8	25
9-13	
Female	26
Male	31
14-18	
Female	26
Male	38

Sources: United States Department of Agriculture and Trumbo et al.[55]

ND indicates not determinable.

More recently, the Dietary Guideline Advisory Committee of the US Department of Agriculture published *Dietary Guidelines for Americans in 2010*. It recommended a total fiber intake of greater than or equal to 14 g/1000 kcal consumed, or 25 g/day for women and 38 g/day for men. As the report points out, most Americans do not eat an adequate amount of dietary fiber. Average dietary fiber intake can be as low as 15 g/day. A recent survey of toddlers and preschoolers suggested that their intake is in the range of 9 g/day, which is below the current allowable intake of 19 g/day, although the use of this recommendation (14 g/1000 kcal) has been questioned.[56] Similarly, low intake of dietary fiber has been reported in Canadian adolescents.[57]

Refined flour commonly found in breads, rolls, buns, and pizza crust contribute substantially to dietary fiber consumption, even though they are not the best sources of dietary fiber. The report recommends, as do others, that one should increase the consumption of beans and peas, other vegetables, fruits, whole grains, and other foods with naturally occurring fiber as opposed to fiber supplementation.[58] Whole grains vary in fiber content.

With all this in mind, the European Society for Pediatric Gastroenterology, Hepatology, and Nutrition has pointed out that our lack of knowledge regarding the physiologic impact of fiber makes it difficult to define precisely quantitative and qualitative recommendations for infants and young children.[58]

The fiber content of common foods as well as over-the-counter fiber preparations is presented in Appendix I.

References

1. Cummings JH, Stephen AM. Carbohydrate terminology and classification. *Eur J Clin Nutr.* 2007;61(Suppl 1):S5-S18

2. Williams CL. Dietary fiber in childhood. *J Pediatr.* 2006;149(5):S121-S130

3. Weaver LT, Laker MF, Nelson R. Neonatal intestinal lactase activity. *Arch Dis Child.* 1986;61(9):896-899

4. Antonowicz I, Chang SK, Grand RJ. Development and distribution of lysosomal enzymes and disaccharidases in human fetal intestine. *Gastroenterology.* 1974;67(1):51-58

5. Raul F, Lacroix B, Aprahamian M. Longitudinal distribution of brush border hydrolases and morphological maturation in the intestine of the preterm infant. *Early Hum Dev.* 1986;13(2):225-234

6. Shulman RJ, Kerzner B, Sloan HR, Boutton TW, Wong WW, Klein PD. Absorption and oxidation of glucose polymers of different lengths in young infants. *Pediatr Res.* 1986;20(8):740-743

7. Eggermont E. The hydrolysis of the naturally occurring alpha-glucosides by the human intestinal mucosa. *Eur J Biochem.* 1969;9(4):483-487

8. Augustin R. The protein family of glucose transport facilitators: it's not only about glucose after all. *IUBMB Life.* 2010;62(5):315-333

9. Bialostosky K, Wright JD, Kennedy-Stephenson J, McDowell M, Johnson CL. *Dietary Intake of Macronutrients, Micronutrients, and Other Dietary Constituents: United States 1988-94.* Hyattsville, MD: National Center for Health Statistics; 2002. DHHS Publication No. PHS 2002-1695

10. Jones HF, Butler RN, Brooks DA. Intestinal fructose transport and malabsorption in humans. *Am J Physiol Gastrointest Liver Physiol.* 2011;300(2):G202-G206

11. Wright EM, Hirayama BA, Loo DF. Active sugar transport in health and disease. *J Intern Med.* 2007;261(1):32-43

12. Kellett GL, Brot-Laroche E. Apical GLUT2: a major pathway of intestinal sugar absorption. *Diabetes.* 2005;54(10):3056-2062

13. Jeukendrup AE. Carbohydrate and exercise performance: the role of multiple transportable carbohydrates. *Curr Opin Clin Nutr Metab Care.* 2010;13(4):452-457

14. Cheeseman C. GLUT7: a new intestinal facilitated hexose transporter. *Am J Physiol Endocrinol Metab.* 2008;295(2):e238-e241

15. Cummings JH, Macfarlane GT. Role of intestinal bacteria in nutrient metabolism. *JPEN J Parenter Enteral Nutr.* 1997;21(6):357-365

16. Elia M, Cummings JH. Physiological aspects of energy metabolism and gastrointestinal effects of carbohydrates. *Eur J Clin Nutr.* 2007;61(Suppl 1):S40-S74

17. Grabitske HA, Slavin JL. Gastrointestinal effects of low-digestible carbohydrates. *Crit Rev Food Sci Nutr.* 2009;49(4):327-360

18. Kalhan SC, Kilic I. Carbohydrate as nutrient in the infant and child: range of acceptable intake. *Eur J Clin Nutr.* 1999;53(Suppl 1):S94-S100

19. Kalhan S, Parimi P. Gluconeogenesis in the fetus and neonate. *Semin Perinatol.* 2000;24(2):94-106

IV

20. Bodamer OA, Halliday D. Uses of stable isotopes in clinical diagnosis and research in the paediatric population. *Arch Dis Child*. 2001;84(5):444-448

21. Halliday D, Bodamer OA. Measurement of glucose turnover--implications for the study of inborn errors of metabolism. *Eur J Pediatr*. 1997;156(Suppl 1):S35-S38

22. Jaeken J. Congenital disorders of glycosylation. *Ann N Y Acad Sci*. 2010;1214:190-198

23. Heyman MB. Lactose intolerance in infants, children, and adolescents. *Pediatrics*. 2006;118(3):1279-1286

24. Shulman RJ, Schanler RJ, Lau C, Heitkemper M, Ou CN, Smith EO. Early feeding, feeding tolerance, and lactase activity in preterm infants. *J Pediatr*. 1998;133(5):645-649

25. Stathos TH, Shulman RJ, Schanler RJ, Abrams SA. Effect of carbohydrates on calcium absorption in premature infants. *Pediatr Res*. 1996;39(4 Pt 1):666-670

26. Griffin MP, Hansen JW. Can the elimination of lactose from formula improve feeding tolerance in premature infants? *J Pediatr*. 1999;135(5):587-592

27. Shulman RJ, Ou CN, Smith EO. Evaluation of potential factors predicting attainment of full gavage feedings in preterm infants. *Neonatology*. 2011;99(1):38-44

28. Shulman RJ, Wong WW, Smith EO. Influence of changes in lactase activity and small-intestinal mucosal growth on lactose digestion and absorption in preterm infants. *Am J Clin Nutr*. 2005;81(2):472-479

29. Sahi T. Genetics and epidemiology of adult-type hypolactasia. *Scand J Gastroenterol Suppl*. 1994;202:7-20

30. Filer LJ, Jr. Modified food starch—an update. *J Am Diet Assoc*. 1988;88(3):342-344

31. Lanciers S, Mehta DI, Blecker U, Lebenthal E. Modified food starches in baby foods. *Indian J Pediatr*. 1998;65(4):541-546

32. Hillemeier C. An overview of the effects of dietary fiber on gastrointestinal transit. *Pediatrics*. 1995;96(5 Pt 2):997-999

33. Stephen AM, Haddad AC, Phillips SF. Passage of carbohydrate into the colon. Direct measurements in humans. *Gastroenterology*. 1983;85(3):589-595

34. Shulman RJ, Wong WW, Irving CS, Nichols BL, Klein PD. Utilization of dietary cereal by young infants. *J Pediatr*. 1983;103(1):23-28

35. Shulman RJ, Gannon N, Reeds PJ. Cereal feeding and its impact on the nitrogen economy of the infant. *Am J Clin Nutr*. 1995;62(5):969-972

36. Jenkins DJ, Wolever TM, Taylor RH, et al. Glycemic index of foods: a physiological basis for carbohydrate exchange. *Am J Clin Nutr*. 1981;34(3):362-366

37. Foster-Powell K, Holt SH, Brand-Miller JC. International table of glycemic index and glycemic load values: 2002. *Am J Clin Nutr*. 2002;76(1):5-56

38. Sansbury LB, Wanke K, Albert PS, Kahle L, Schatzkin A, Lanza E. The effect of strict adherence to a high-fiber, high-fruit and -vegetable, and low-fat eating pattern on adenoma recurrence. *Am J Epidemiol*. 2009;170(5):576-584

39. Dahm CC, Keogh RH, Spencer EA, et al. Dietary fiber and colorectal cancer risk: a nested case-control study using food diaries. *J Natl Cancer Inst*. 2010;102(9):614-626

40. Mann J, Cummings JH, Englyst HN, et al. FAO/WHO scientific update on carbohydrates in human nutrition: conclusions. *Eur J Clin Nutr*. 2007;61(Suppl 1):S132-S137

41. Feldman W, McGrath P, Hodgson C, Ritter H, Shipman RT. The use of dietary fiber in the management of simple, childhood, idiopathic, recurrent abdominal pain. Results in a prospective, double-blind, randomized, controlled trial. *Am J Dis Child*. 1985;139(12):1216-1218

42. Chao HC, Lai MW, Kong MS, Chen SY, Chen CC, Chiu CH. Cutoff volume of dietary fiber to ameliorate constipation in children. *J Pediatr*. 2008;153(1):45-49

43. Papathanasopoulos A, Camilleri M. Dietary fiber supplements: effects in obesity and metabolic syndrome and relationship to gastrointestinal functions. *Gastroenterology*. 2010;138(1):65-72

44. Davis JN, Alexander KE, Ventura EE, Toledo-Corral CM, Goran MI. Inverse relation between dietary fiber intake and visceral adiposity in overweight Latino youth. *Am J Clin Nutr*. 2009;90(5):1160-1166

45. Strong JP. The natural history of atherosclerosis in childhood. *Ann N Y Acad Sci*. 1991;623:9-15

46. Kwiterovich PO Jr. Recognition and management of dyslipidemia in children and adolescents. *J Clin Endocrinol Metab*. 2008;93(11):4200-4209

47. Kwiterovich PO Jr. The role of fiber in the treatment of hypercholesterolemia in children and adolescents. *Pediatrics*. 1995;96(5 Pt 2):1005-1009

48. Williams CL, Bollella M, Spark A, Puder D. Soluble fiber enhances the hypocholesterolemic effect of the step I diet in childhood. *J Am Coll Nutr*. 1995;14(3):251-257

49. Vanderhoof JA, Murray ND, Paule CL, Ostrom KM. Use of soy fiber in acute diarrhea in infants and toddlers. *Clin Pediatr (Phila)*. 1997;36(3):135-139

50. Williams CL, Bollella M. Is a high-fiber diet safe for children? *Pediatrics*. 1995;96(5 Pt 2):1014-1019

51. Nicklas TA, Myers L, O'Neil C, Gustafson N. Impact of dietary fat and fiber intake on nutrient intake of adolescents. *Pediatrics*. 2000;105(2):e21

52. Agostoni C, Riva E, Giovannini M. Dietary fiber in weaning foods of young children. *Pediatrics*. 1995;96(5 Pt 2):1002-1005

53. Williams CL, Bollella M, Wynder EL. A new recommendation for dietary fiber in childhood. *Pediatrics*. 1995;96(5 Pt 2):985-988

54. A summary of conference recommendations on dietary fiber in childhood. Conference on Dietary Fiber in Childhood, New York, May 24, 1994. *Pediatrics*. 1995;96(5 Pt 2):1023-1028

55. Trumbo P, Schlicker S, Yates AA, Poos M. Dietary reference intakes for energy, carbohydrate, fiber, fat, fatty acids, cholesterol, protein and amino acids. *J Am Diet Assoc*. 2002;102(11):1621-1630

56. Butte NF, Fox MK, Briefel RR, et al. Nutrient intakes of US infants, toddlers, and preschoolers meet or exceed dietary reference intakes. *J Am Diet Assoc*. 2010;110(12 Suppl):S27-S37

IV

57. Schenkel TC, Stockman NK, Brown JN, Duncan AM. Evaluation of energy, nutrient and dietary fiber intakes of adolescent males. *J Am Coll Nutr*. 2007;26(3):264-271

58. Aggett PJ, Agostoni C, Axelsson I, et al. Nondigestible carbohydrates in the diets of infants and young children: a commentary by the ESPGHAN Committee on Nutrition. *J Pediatr Gastroenterol Nutr*. 2003;36(3):329-337

Chapter 17

Fats and Fatty Acids

General Considerations

The absolute fat requirement of the human species is the amount of essential fatty acids needed to maintain optimal fatty acid composition of all tissues and normal eicosanoid synthesis. At most, this requirement is no more than approximately 5% of an adequate energy intake. However, fat accounts for approximately 50% of the nonprotein energy content of both human milk and currently available infant formulas. This is thought to be necessary to ensure that total energy intake is adequate to support growth and optimal utilization of dietary protein. In theory, the energy supplied by fat could be supplied by carbohydrate, from which all fatty acids except the essential ones can be synthesized. In practice, however, it is difficult to ensure an adequate energy intake without a fat intake considerably in excess of the requirement for essential fatty acids. In part, this is because the osmolality of such a diet containing simple carbohydrates (eg, monosaccharides and disaccharides) will be sufficiently high to result in diarrhea and because such a diet containing more complex carbohydrates may not be fully digestible, particularly during early infancy. Moreover, because approximately 25% of the energy content of carbohydrate that is converted to fatty acids is consumed in the process of lipogenesis, metabolic efficiency is greater if nonprotein energy is provided as a mixture of fat and carbohydrate rather than predominately carbohydrate. Fat also facilitates the absorption, transport and delivery of fat-soluble vitamins and is an important satiety factor. Considering these issues, the lower limit of fat intake that has been recommended for infants and young children is 15% of total energy intake, but that a more practical recommendation is in the range of 30% to 35% of energy intake.[1] These issues are important in consideration of the age at which a prudent (ie, lower-fat) diet to reduce the risks of cardiovascular disease is recommended (see Chapter 46: Cardiac Disease).

Dietary Fats

Triglycerides account for the largest proportion of dietary fat. Structurally, these have 3 fatty acid molecules esterified to a single molecule of glycerol. They usually contain at least 2, often 3, different fatty acids. Other dietary fats include phospholipids, free fatty acids, monoglycerides and diglycerides, and small amounts of sterols and other nonsaponifiable compounds.

Naturally occurring fatty acids contain from 4 to 26 carbon atoms. Some of these are saturated (ie, no double bonds in the carbon chain), some are monounsaturated (ie, 1 double bond), and some are polyunsaturated (ie, 2 or more double bonds). All have common names but, by convention, are identified by their number of carbon atoms, their number of double bonds, and the site of the first double bond from the terminal methyl group of the molecule. For example, palmitic acid, a saturated, 16-carbon fatty acid, is designated 16:0, and oleic acid, an 18-carbon, monounsaturated fatty acid with the single double bond located between the ninth and tenth carbon from the methyl terminal, is designated 18:1ω-9. Linoleic acid, 18:2ω-6, is an 18-carbon fatty acid with 2 double bonds, the first between the sixth and seventh carbon from the methyl terminal. The common names as well as the shorthand numerical designations of a number of common fatty acids are shown in Table 17.1.

Table 17.1.
Common Names and Numerical Nomenclature of Selected Fatty Acids

Common Name	Numerical Nomenclature
Caprylic acid	8:0
Capric acid	10:0
Lauric acid	12:0
Myristic acid	14:0
Palmitic acid	16:0
Stearic acid	18:0
Oleic acid	18:1ω-9[a]
Linoleic acid	18:2ω-6[a]
Arachidonic acid	20:4ω-6[a]
Linolenic acid[b]	18:3ω-3[a]
Eicosapentaenoic acid	20:5ω-3[a]
Docosahexaenoic acid	22:6ω-3[a]

[a] ω-9, ω-6, and ω-3 are used interchangeably with n-9, n-6, and n-3.
[b] Usually designated α-linolenic acid to distinguish it from 18:3ω-6 or γ-linolenic acid.

Unsaturated fatty acids are folded at the site of each double bond; in this configuration, they are said to be in the cis form. During processing, the molecules may become unfolded, transforming them to trans fatty acids, which have been implicated in development of atherosclerosis. In general, the amount of trans fatty acids in infant formulas and foods is low; however, some processed fats (eg, margarines) may have a higher content. The trans fatty acid content of human milk also is reasonably low unless the mother's diet is high in trans fatty acids.

Fat Digestion, Absorption, Transport, and Metabolism

At birth, the infant must adjust from using carbohydrate as the major energy source to using a mixture of carbohydrate and fat. Hence, some aspects of fat digestion and metabolism are not fully developed, even at term. However, most term infants have sufficient fat digestive capacity to adjust satisfactorily. The limitations of fat digestion are somewhat more serious in the preterm infant but there is little evidence that these infants have significant limitations beyond the first few weeks of life.

Fat digestion begins in the stomach, where lingual lipase hydrolyzes short- and medium-chain fatty acids from triglycerides and gastric lipase hydrolyzes long- as well as medium- and short-chain fatty acids.[2] The intragastric release of fatty acids with formation of monoglycerides delays gastric emptying and facilitates emulsification of fat in the intestine. Further, some of the released short- and medium-chain fatty acids can be absorbed directly from the stomach.[3] On entry into the duodenum, the monoglycerides and free fatty acids stimulate release of a number of enteric hormones; among these is cholecystokinin, which stimulates contraction of the gall bladder and secretion of pancreatic enzymes.[4] Lingual and gastric lipases are largely inactivated in the duodenum, and fat digestion continues through the action of pancreatic lipase and colipase, which may be somewhat limited during the first few weeks of life. Like lingual and gastric lipase, pancreatic lipase hydrolyzes triglycerides into free fatty acids and a monoglyceride.

Human milk contains 2 additional lipases, lipoprotein lipase and bile salt-stimulated lipase. The former is essential for formation of milk lipid in the mammary gland but plays little role in intestinal fat digestion.[5] The latter is present in much larger amounts. It is stable at a pH as low as 3.5 if bile salts are present and it is not affected by intestinal proteolytic enzymes.[6] However, it is heat labile and, hence, is inactivated by pasteurization. This is thought to be a major factor in the poor fat absorption of infants fed pasteurized human milk.

Bile salt-stimulated lipase hydrolyzes triglyceride molecules into free fatty acids and glycerol rather than into free fatty acids and a monoglyceride. In theory, the bile salt-stimulated lipase of human milk can substitute for limited pancreatic lipase[7]; however, this does not appear to be of great importance for fat digestion of most infants. On the other hand, because bile salt-stimulated lipase is much more effective than pancreatic lipase in hydrolyzing esters of vitamin A, the primary form of this vitamin in human milk and many other foods, it may be important for optimal vitamin A absorption.[6]

IV

The bile acids released by contraction of the gall bladder help emulsify the intestinal contents, thereby facilitating triglyceride hydrolysis and fat absorption. They are released primarily as salts of taurine or glycine and, hence, have both a water-soluble and a lipid soluble portion. Alone, bile salts are poor emulsifiers, but in combination with monoglycerides, fatty acids, and phospholipids, they are quite effective. Thus, the fat hydrolysis that occurs in the stomach is an important adjunct to intestinal fat digestion.

The rate of synthesis of bile salts by newborn infants is less than that of adults, and the bile salt pool of newborn infants is only about one quarter that of adults.[8] However, an intraduodenal concentration of bile salts below 2 to 5 mM, the critical concentration required for the formation of micelles, is unusual.[9] Bile salts are actively reabsorbed in the distal ilium, transported back to the liver, and eventually reappear in bile.[10] This enterohepatic circulation occurs approximately 6 times daily, with loss of only approximately 5% of the bile salts with each circulation.[11]

The monoglycerides and diglycerides and long-chain fatty acids resulting from lipolysis as well as phospholipids, cholesterol, and fat-soluble vitamins are insoluble in water but are solubilized by physicochemical combination with bile salts to form micelles.[11] Because of their amphiphilic nature, bile salts aggregate with their hydrophobic region to the interior, or core, of the micelle and their hydrophilic region to the exterior. The components of the micelle are transferred into the enteric mucosal cell, where long-chain fatty acids and monoglycerides are re-esterified into triglycerides and subsequently combined with protein, phospholipid and cholesterol to form chylomicrons or very low density lipoproteins. In this form, they enter the intestinal lymphatics, then the thoracic duct and, finally, the peripheral circulation.

Medium-chain triglycerides can be absorbed into the enteric cells without being hydrolyzed.[11] However, they also are rapidly hydrolyzed in the duodenum, and because the released medium-chain fatty acids are relatively soluble in the aqueous phase of the intestinal lumen, they can be absorbed without being incorporated into micelles. This makes them particularly useful in treatment of infants and children with a variety of pancreatic, hepatic, biliary, and/or intestinal disorders.

In general, long-chain unsaturated fatty acids are absorbed more readily than long-chain saturated fatty acids. The ease of absorption of palmitic acid (16:0), the most common dietary saturated fatty acid, is further related to its position on the triglyceride molecule.[12] The 2-monoglyceride of palmitic acid is well absorbed, but free palmitic acid released from the terminal positions of the triglyceride molecule is not. The palmitic acid content of human milk is esterified primarily to the 2-position of glycerol, and this is thought to account for the better absorption of palmitic acid from human milk than from formulas containing butterfat. Synthetic fats that contain palmitic acid, primarily in the 2 position, are available[13-16] but, as yet, have not been used extensively in infant formula.

In the circulation, chylomicrons acquire a specialized apoprotein from high-density lipoproteins.[11] This enables the triglycerides of the chylomicron to be hydrolyzed by lipoprotein lipase, the major enzyme responsible for intravascular hydrolysis of chylomicrons and very low-density lipoproteins.[17] Lipoprotein lipase is synthesized in most tissues, and the flow of fatty acids to tissues reflects its activity on the tissue's capillary bed. Levels of lipoprotein lipase are somewhat low in preterm and small-for-gestational-age infants, but this does not appear to impose major difficulties except, perhaps, in tolerance of intravenously administered lipid emulsions.[18]

The phospholipid and most of the apoproteins remaining after hydrolysis of chylomicron triglyceride are transferred to high-density lipoprotein, and the remainder of the apoproteins is transferred to other lipoprotein particles. This reduces the chylomicron to a fraction of its original mass, resulting in a chylomicron remnant that is removed from the circulation by specialized hepatic receptors.

Essential Fatty Acids

Fatty acids with double bonds in the ω-6 and ω-3 positions cannot be synthesized endogenously by the human species.[19] Therefore, specific ω-6 and ω-3 fatty acids or their precursors with double bonds at these positions—that is, linoleic acid (LA [18:2ω-6]) and α-linolenic acid (ALA [18:3ω-3])—must be provided in the diet. The precursor fatty acids are metabolized by the same series of desaturases and elongases to longer-chain, more unsaturated fatty acids,[20] referred to collectively as long-chain polyunsaturated fatty acids (LC-PUFAs). This pathway is outlined in Fig 17/1. Important metabolites of 18:2ω-6 and 18:3ω-3 include 18:3ω-6 (gamma linolenic acid [GLA]), 20:3ω-6 (dihomogamma linolenic acid [DHLA]), 20:4ω-6 (arachidonic acid [ARA]), 20:5ω-3 (eicosapentaenoic acid [EPA]), and 22:6ω-3 (docosahexaenoic acid [DHA]).

LA (18:2ω-6) and ALA (18:3ω-3) are present in many vegetable oils (see Table 17.2). In vivo, they are found in storage lipids, cell membrane phospholipids, intracellular cholesterol esters, and plasma lipids. The longer-chain, more unsaturated fatty acids synthesized from these precursors, in contrast, are found primarily in specific cell membrane phospholipids. DHLA, ARA, and EPA are immediate precursors of eicosanoids,[19,21] and DHA is the precursor of the docosanoids,[22] each being converted to a different series with different biological activities and/or functions.

IV

Table 17.2.
Fatty Acid Composition of Common Vegetable Oils[a]

Fatty Acid	Canola	Corn	Coconut	Palm Olein	Safflower[b]	Soy	High-Oleic Sunflower
6:0–12:0	-	0.1	62.1	0.2	-	-	-
14.0	-	0.1	18.1	1.0	0.1	0.1	-
16:0	4.0	12.1	8.9	39.8	6.8	11.2	3.7
18:0	2.0	2.4	2.7	4.4	2.4	0.4	5.4
18:1ω-9	55.0	32.1	6.4	42.5	76.8	22.0	81.3
18:2ω-6	26.0	50.9	1.6	11.2	12.5	53.8	9.0
18:3ω-3	10.0	0.9	-	0.2	0.1	7.5	-
Other	2.0	1.0	-	<1.6	<1.0	<1.0	<1.0

[a] Percent of total fatty acids (g/100 g).

[b] High-oleic safflower oil: approximately 77% 18:1ω-9 and 12.5% 18:2ω-6.

The same series of desaturases and elongases that catalyze desaturation and elongation of ω-6 and ω-3 fatty acids also catalyze desaturation and elongation of ω-9 fatty acids. The substrate preference of these enzymes is ω-3, ω-6, and finally, ω-9.[20] Thus, competition between the ω-9 fatty acids and either the ω-6 or ω-3 fatty acids is not an issue unless LA and/or ALA concentrations are very low, as occurs in deficiency states. In this case, oleic acid (18:1ω-9) is readily desaturated and elongated to eicosatrienoic acid (20:3ω-9). The ratio of this fatty acid to 20:4ω-6, ie, the triene-to-tetraene ratio, is a useful diagnostic index of ω-6 fatty acid deficiency. This ratio usually is <0.1. A ratio of >0.4 is usually cited as indicative of deficiency,[23] but most believe that an even lower value (eg, >0.2) might be more reasonable. In the few documented cases of isolated 18:3ω-3 deficiency in which the triene-to-tetraene ratio was measured (see later discussion), it was not elevated.

LA (18:2ω-6) has been recognized as an essential nutrient for the human species for more than 75 years.[24,25] The most common symptoms of deficiency are poor growth and scaly skin lesions. These symptoms are usually preceded by an increase in the triene/tetraene ratio of plasma lipids. It is now clear that ALA (18:3ω-3) also is an essential nutrient. In animals, deficiency of this fatty acid results in visual and neurologic abnormalities.[26-29] Neurologic abnormalities also were observed in a human infant who had been maintained for several weeks on a parenteral nutrition regimen lacking ALA[30] and in elderly nursing home residents who were receiving intragastric feedings of an elemental formula with no ALA.[31]

Although symptoms related to deficiency of the 2 series of fatty acids seem to differ, many studies on which the description of ω-6 fatty acid deficiency are based used a fat-free or very low-fat diet rather than a diet deficient in only 18:2ω-6.

Thus, there may be some overlap in the symptoms of LA and ALA deficiency. The clinical symptoms of ω-6 fatty acid deficiency can be corrected by LA or ARA; those related to ALA deficiency can be corrected by ALA, EPA, or DHA. Thus, it is not clear whether LA and ALA serve specific functions other than as precursors of LC-PUFAs.

LA usually represents between 8% and 20% of the total fatty acid content of human milk, and ALA usually represents between 0.5% and 1%.[32] Human milk also contains small amounts of a number of longer-chain, more unsaturated metabolites of both fatty acids, primarily ARA (20:4ω-6) and DHA (22:6ω-3). Maternal diet has a marked effect on the concentration of all fatty acids in human milk. The concentration of DHA in the milk of women consuming a typical North American diet is generally in the range of 0.1% to 0.3% of total fatty acids, and the level of ARA ranges from 0.4% to 0.6%.[32] The milk of vegetarian women contains less DHA,[33] and that of women whose dietary fish consumption is high or who take DHA supplements is higher.[34-36] The ARA content of human milk is less variable and appears to be less dependent on maternal ARA intake, perhaps reflecting the relatively high LA intake of most populations.

Corn, coconut, safflower, and soy oils as well as high-oleic safflower and sunflower oils and palm olein oil are commonly used in the manufacture of infant formulas (see Table 17.2). All except coconut oil contain adequate amounts of LA, but only soybean oil contains an appreciable amount of ALA (6% to 9% of total fatty acids). Canola oil, a component of many formulas available outside the United States, contains somewhat less LA and more ALA. Until the 1990s, little emphasis was placed on the ALA content of infant formulas, and many with virtually no ALA were available. Current recommendations specify minimal intakes of LA ranging from 2.7% to 8% of total fat and maximum intakes ranging from 21% to 35% of total fatty acids.[37,38] The most recent recommendations for the minimum and maximum contents of ALA in term infant formulas are 1.75% and 4% of total fatty acids, respectively.[38] To maintain a reasonable balance between the 2 fatty acids, it is recommended that the LA-to-ALA ratio be between 5 to 6 and 15 to 16.[37,38] Term and preterm infant formulas currently available in the United States contain approximately 20% of total fatty acids as LA and approximately 2% as ALA; hence, their LA-to-ALA ratios are approximately 10.

Long-Chain Polyunsaturated Fatty Acids

LC-PUFAs are fatty acids with a chain length of more than 18 carbons and 2 or more double bonds. Those of primary interest for infant nutrition are ARA (20:4ω-6) and DHA (22:6ω-3), the plasma and erythrocyte lipid contents of which are higher in breastfed than formula-fed infants.[39,40] Because human milk contains these fatty acids but, until 2002, formulas did not, the lower content of these fatty acids in plasma lipids of formula-fed infants were interpreted as indicating that the infant cannot synthesize enough of these fatty acids to meet ongoing needs. Prior and concurrent observations of better cognitive function of breastfed versus formula-fed infants[41-44] focused attention on the possibility that the lower cognitive function of formula-fed infants might be related, in part, to inadequate LC-PUFA intake.

The possibility that cognitive function is related to LC-PUFA intake is supported by the facts that ARA and DHA are the major ω-6 and ω-3 fatty acids of neural tissues[45-47] and that DHA is a major component of retinal photoreceptor membranes.[47] Further, the major supply of these fatty acids to the fetus during development is from maternal plasma.[48] Thus, the need for these fatty acids by the infant born before or during the third trimester of pregnancy and, hence, receiving a limited supply of LC-PUFA prior to birth is thought to be greater than that of the term infant. However, the daily rates of accumulation of these fatty acids in the developing central nervous system change minimally between mid-gestation and 1 year of age.[47]

On the basis of postmortem studies,[49,50] the cerebral content of DHA, but not ARA, is minimally but significantly lower in formula-fed term infants. However, the DHA content of the retina does not differ between breastfed and formula-fed infants,[50] perhaps because the content of this fatty acid in retina reaches adult levels at approximately term, whereas adult levels in cerebrum are not reached until much later. In piglets, the cerebral DHA content of formula-fed infants reflected the ALA content of the formula received before death.[51] In this study, ALA intakes less than 0.7% of total energy resulted in low brain levels of DHA.[51] Further, studies in infants have shown a positive relationship between ALA intake and rates of DHA synthesis.[52]

Both term and preterm infants can convert LA to ARA and ALA to DHA.[53-57] This has been established by studies in which the precursor fatty acids labeled with stable isotopes of either carbon (^{13}C) or hydrogen (^{2}H) were administered to the infant and blood concentrations of the labeled fatty acids as well as labeled metabolites of each were measured by gas chromatography/mass spectroscopy (see Fig 17.1). The studies of Sauerwald et al[52,56] and Uauy et al[57] suggested that the overall ability of preterm infants to convert LA and ALA to LC-PUFAs is at least as good as that of term infants. On the other hand, there is considerable variability in conversion among both preterm and term infants fed the same formula. Moreover, because measurements of enrichment have been limited to plasma, which represents only a small fraction of the body pool of precursor as well as product fatty acids and may not be representative of fatty acid pools of other tissues, including the central nervous system, the amount of LC-PUFAs that either preterm or term infants can synthesize is not known.

Fig 17.1
Metabolism of ω-6 and ω-3 Fatty Acids

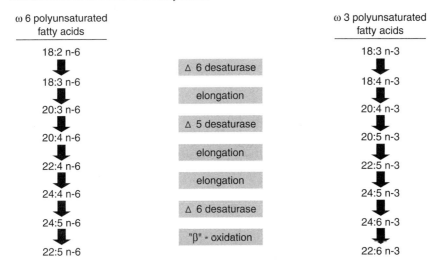

The higher DHA content of plasma and erythrocyte lipids of breastfed infants and infants fed formulas supplemented with LC-PUFAs versus infants fed unsupplemented formulas, including those with a relatively high ALA content,[58-60] suggests that the amounts of LC-PUFAs formed endogenously are less than the amounts provided by human milk or supplemented formulas. However, the extent to which the concentration of individual LC-PUFAs in plasma reflects the content of these fatty acids in tissues, particularly the brain, is not known.

In this regard, animal studies have demonstrated that the content of LC-PUFAs in plasma is much less highly correlated with the content of these fatty acids in brain than with the content in erythrocytes and liver.[61] In contrast, postmortem studies in human infants have demonstrated a weak but statistically significant, correlation between erythrocyte and brain contents of DHA.[50] Correlation between the content of this fatty acid in erythrocyte membranes and the contents of other tissues was not reported. Studies in isolated cell systems suggest that precursors of DHA are transferred from plasma to astrocytes where they are converted to DHA, which is subsequently transferred to neurons.[62,63] This pathway for direct synthesis of DHA within the central nervous system appears to occur in vivo in some animal species,[64] but the extent to which it occurs in the human is not known.

Importance of LC-PUFAs in Development

The findings discussed previously, although far from definitive, are compatible with the possibility that failure to provide preformed LC-PUFAs during early infancy, perhaps longer, may compromise development of tissues/organs with a high content of these fatty acids, particularly 22:6ω-3. However, the specific roles of LC-PUFAs in normal development are not clear.[65-68] These fatty acids affect gene transcription and may produce post-translational modifications. Moreover, many are precursors of eicosanoids and docosanoids that, in turn, modify a number of processes. These fatty acids also have effects on signal transduction, and the amount of these fatty acids in cell membranes can modify membrane fluidity, membrane thickness, and the microenvironment of the membrane as well as interactions between the fatty acid and membrane proteins. Such changes, in turn, can affect receptor function, and the fatty acids also may exert direct effects on receptor function. Although the degree of unsaturation of membrane fatty acids affects fluidity, this effect is most marked by substituting a monounsaturated or polyunsaturated fatty acid for a saturated fatty acid. In 22:6ω-3 deficiency, 22:5ω-6 replaces 22:6ω-3 with little effect on fluidity. Possible mechanisms for the effects of LC-PUFAs have been reviewed by Uauy et al,[68] Lauritzen et al,[66] Heird and Lapillonne,[65] and McCann and Ames.[67]

Despite the lack of a clear mechanism of the role of LC-PUFAs in development, a number of studies over the past several years have focused on differences in visual acuity and neurodevelopmental indices between breastfed and formula-fed infants. Because human milk contains a number of factors other than LC-PUFAs that might affect visual acuity and/or neurodevelopmental indices, studies comparing breastfed versus formula-fed infants cannot help resolve the specific role of LC-PUFAs in infant development. Rather, intervention studies comparing infants fed LC-PUFA-supplemented and unsupplemented formulas and studies comparing different LC-PUFA intakes of breastfed infants secondary to maternal supplementation can provide important insights into cause-and-effect relationships between LC-PUFA intake and early childhood outcomes.

LC-PUFA Intake and Visual Function

Early studies in rodents established the importance of ω-3 fatty acids for normal retinal function,[26,29] and subsequent studies established this in primates.[27,28] More recently, studies have focused on the effect of ω-3 fatty acids on retinal function and/or overall visual function of human infants. However, whereas the abnormal retinal/visual function of ω-3 fatty acid-deficient animals clearly resulted from an inadequate intake of 18:3ω-3 and were partially reversed by adding this fatty acid or DHA, the more recent studies in human infants have focused primarily on the effects of 22:6ω-3 intake on retinal and/or visual function. Studies have been conducted in both term and preterm infants and have used both behaviorally based and electrophysiologically based methods for assessing visual function.

The most commonly used behaviorally based method for assessing visual acuity, the Teller Acuity Card procedure, is based on the innate tendency to look toward a discernible pattern rather than a blank field.[69,70] This rapid measure of resolution acuity combines forced-choice and operant preferential looking procedures. The infant is shown a series of cards with stripes (gratings) of different widths on one side and a blank field on the other, and his or her looking behavior is observed through a peephole in the center of the card.[71] Cards with wider stripes are shown initially followed by cards with progressively decreasing stripe widths. The subject's visual acuity is the finest grating toward which he or she clearly looks preferentially (ie, the finest grating that he or she is able to resolve).

The electrophysiologically based tests use visual evoked potentials (VEPs) that measure the activation of the visual cortex in response to visual information that is processed by the retina and transmitted to the visual cortex.[72,73] The presence of a reliable evoked response indicates that the stimulus information was resolved up to the visual cortex, where the response is processed. Use of VEPs to assess visual acuity requires measuring the electrical potentials of the visual cortex in response to patterns of contrast reversal with vertical square wave gratings or checkerboards. The frequency of the gratings or checkerboards is decreased from low (large) to high (small), and the visual acuity threshold is estimated by linear regression of the VEP amplitudes versus the frequency, or size, of the grating or checkerboard stimulus.[72,73] Data are recorded as the $\log_{10}$ of the minimum angle of resolution (logMAR), which is the smallest grating that results in a measurable amplitude. Thus, smaller logMAR values indicate better visual acuity. A rapid VEP method (sweep VEP) has been developed for use in infant populations.[74]

The transient VEP also allows assessment of latency, or the time between presentation of a stimulus and the peak of the electrical potential. This reflects the rate of transmission of the stimulus and, hence, should be useful for assessing the effects of LC-PUFAs (or other intervention). However, it has been used for this purpose by only a few investigators,[75-78] perhaps because it does not provide an assessment of acuity.

Electroretinography, unlike the above procedures that measure the response of the entire visual system, measures only the activity of the retina.[79-81] However, this methodology is somewhat more invasive and time consuming than the other methods and has been used to assess effects of LC-PUFAs in only a few studies. The primary components of the electroretinogram generated in response to a flash of light are the a-wave, which is produced by hyperpolarization of the photoreceptor, and the b-wave, which reflects the subsequent activation of retinal neurons.

IV

Performance is quantified by parameters[70,73] such as the threshold (the minimal intensity of light necessary to elicit a small amplitude), the implicit time or peak latency (the time from the presentation of a brief flash of light to the response peak), the maximal amplitude, and the sensitivity (the intensity of light that elicits a response of half the maximal amplitude).

To date, there have been 9 trials assessing the effect of LC-PUFA supplementation of infant formulas for term infants that have included a measure of visual acuity. VEP acuity was assessed in 6 trials, the behavioral method of Teller Acuity Cards was used in 2 studies, and another trial used both electrophysiological and behavioral methods. These have recently been summarized in a Cochrane systematic review.[82] Four of the 9 included studies reported a beneficial effect of supplementation on visual acuity, and the 5 remaining studies reported no effect of supplementation. All of the included studies have compared a low to modest dose of DHA supplementation (up to approximately 0.3% of total fatty acids) with no supplementation. The results of the meta-analyses were inconsistent, although all meta-analyses assessing visual acuity using Teller Acuity Cards at different ages consistently showed no effect of supplementation. Because the electrophysiological protocols for assessing visual acuity were different between trials, it is not possible to ascertain whether the inconsistent results are attributable to methodologic differences, random error, or some other factor.

Some have suggested that dietary DHA dose may be an important factor and that at least 0.3% of total fatty acids as DHA is required in the infant diet to document a beneficial effect of supplementation on visual acuity.[59,60] This view has recently been supported in a dose-response trial involving 4 different doses of DHA. This was a 2-site trial in which formula-fed infants were randomly allocated to equivalent formulas containing either 0%, 0.32%, 0.64%, or 0.96% DHA as total fatty acids.[83] All formulas also contained 0.64% total fatty acids as ARA. Infants fed the control formula (0% DHA) had poorer visual evoked potential acuity compared with DHA-supplemented infants. There were no differences in the visual acuity between the groups fed the 3 different doses of DHA at any time point.[83] Although the overall data from this trial are suggestive that a dose of at least 0.3% DHA may be needed to maximize visual acuity development, a significant study site by formula group interaction suggested that the visual acuity response to the formulas varied by enrolling site, with differences between control and DHA-supplementation being most marked in only one of the study sites. Interestingly, a dose-response trial conducted in breastfed infants some 13 years earlier reported that supplementation of lactating women to increase the average DHA concentration of their human milk from a mean of approximately 0.2% total fatty acids as DHA to 0.35%, 0.46%,

0.86%, or 1.13% DHA as total fatty acids resulted in no differences in infant visual evoked potential acuity or latency between groups.[84] Unfortunately, the visual acuity estimates from the 2 trials do not appear to be directly comparable because of methodologic differences.[83,84]

Maternal supplementation with DHA during pregnancy has been investigated in 4 randomized controlled trials, including 467 infants, with visual outcomes in term infants.[85-88] Three of the 4 studies reported no differences in VEP latency[87,88] and no difference in visual acuity measured either using VEPs[88] or the card procedure.[85] Only 1 study with a small sample size suggested improvement with Teller acuity card acuity at 4 but not 6 months of age.[86]

Infants born preterm are considered to be at greatest risk of dietary LC-PUFA insufficiency, because they miss the large and active accumulation of LC-PUFAs that occurs during the last trimester of pregnancy, they are born with few fat reserves, and their feeding regimens often contain minimal LC-PUFA. Therefore, it follows that any beneficial effects of LC-PUFAs will be more obvious in preterm infants rather than their counterparts who are born at term. However, this has not been the case with regard to studies investigating the effects on LC-PUFA supplementation of infant formulas and visual outcomes. The relevant trials have been summarized in a recent Cochrane systematic review.[89] Eight randomized trials were included; 3 tested the addition of only ω-3 LC-PUFAs to infant formulas, 4 tested the addition of ω-3 LC-PUFAs and ARA, and another had 2 intervention groups – 1 with ω-3 LC-PUFAs only and 1 with ω-3 LC-PUFAs and ARA. Seven trials have visual acuity outcomes, and 4 of these studies reported beneficial effects of supplementation during early infancy,[79,90-92] although in 2 cases this was confined to specific subgroups.[91,92] It is important to note that the methodologies of assessing acuity differed, the sample sizes were generally small, and some of the randomization processes were not adequately reported. Similar issues were apparent in the 2 trials that assessed electroretinographic responses, with 1 study reporting a positive effect of supplementation and the other reporting no effect.[60,76]

Most recently, the dose of DHA in milks fed to preterm infants has been assessed in a randomized trial based on realistic feeding practices in which infants are fed a combination of expressed human milk and infant formula.[93] This trial tested a high dose of DHA (1% total fatty acid) against a standard dose of DHA (0.3% total fatty acids), with the ARA concentration being held constant in both groups at about 0.4% of total fatty acids and found that infants fed the high-DHA diet had better visual acuity at 4 months' corrected age compared with control infants. No differences were noted at 2 months' corrected age, and there were no differences in VEP latency.[93]

LC-PUFAs and Cognitive/Behavioral Development

Most studies addressing the cognitive/behavioral development of infants fed LC-PUFA-supplemented versus unsupplemented formulas have used the Bayley Scales of Infant and Toddler Development, which are considered the "gold standard" for assessing global abilities of infants from birth to about 42 months of age. They provide standardized indices of both mental/cognitive and psychomotor development. However, they are intended to distinguish between "normal" and "abnormal," not degrees of either. Thus, unless cognitive and/or psychomotor function as assessed by the Bayley Scales early in life is abnormal, the relationship between these early scores and later function is relatively poor.[94]

The Fagan Test of Infant Intelligence also has been used, either alone or in combination with the Bayley Scales. This test, which assesses novelty preference,[95] involves showing the infant a single image (usually a face) for a standardized, age-based period and, then, showing this image paired with a "novel" one. If the infant has "learned" the original image prior to the novelty test, the typical response is to look selectively toward the "novel" versus the "familiar" image. Scores on this test during infancy are somewhat more predictive of later cognitive function than scores on the Bayley Scales of Infant Development; however, its internal consistency (reproducibility), unlike that of the Bayley Scales, is relatively poor.[96] Look duration during the familiarization and the paired comparison phases of the test also is a modest predictor of both concurrent performance on other tests during infancy and later tests of intelligence[96]; shorter look durations during the familiarization phase predict better concurrent as well as subsequent cognitive performance.

One or both of these tests has been used to evaluate the effect of LC-PUFA supplementation on cognitive/behavioral development. Some of the studies utilizing these tests have shown advantages of LC-PUFA supplementation with both tests, some with one but not the other, and still others with neither. Available studies in term infants were reviewed in 1998 by an expert panel appointed by the Life Sciences Research Organization to assess the nutrient requirements for term infant formulas.[38] These studies were criticized by consultants to the panel for including too few infants, failing to control adequately for confounding factors, failing to assess function at more than one age, failing to examine individual differences in development, and failing to follow the infants for a sufficiently long period (eg, none of the studies available at that time included data beyond 1 year of age). Partially on the basis of these criticisms, the panel did not recommend addition of LC-PUFA to term infant formulas but suggested that the issue be reevaluated in approximately 5 years.

The randomized trials involving term infants published since 1998[38,97-101] have not resolved many of these criticisms. The trials have differed with respect to the source of LC-PUFA supplementation, the duration of supplementation, the amounts of 22:6ω-3 and 20:4ω-6 supplementation, and the ratio of 22:6ω-3 to 20:4ω-6. There also were differences in the 18:2ω-6 and 18:3ω-3 contents of the control and experimental formulas. The variance in Bayley mental and psychomotor scores also varied among studies, being smallest in the one study that showed an advantage of 22:6ω-3 and 20:4ω-6 supplementation for the first 4 months of life on the Bayley mental development score at 18 months of age.[98]

Relevant data from LC-PUFA intervention trials involving term formula-fed infants have been summarized in 2 meta-analyses, one including data from 6 trials[102] and the other more recent meta-analysis including data from 9 trials.[82] Both reported no effect of LC-PUFA supplementation of infant formula for term infants on Bayley mental or psychomotor scores.

Two recent systematic reviews and meta-analyses are also available summarizing the randomized controlled trials assessing LC-PUFA–supplemented versus unsupplemented formulas for preterm infants.[89,103] Both reviews included the same 7 trials with Bayley outcomes, and both reported no overall effect of LC PUFA supplementation on Bayley mental or psychomotor scores, although these trials are subject to many of the same criticisms levied against the studies in term infants.[89,103] Indeed, some sensitivity analyses have suggested that the heterogeneity between trials may be related to the administration of different versions of the Bayley Scales, the sample population studied, the way the intervention was applied, or trial methodology.[103] Interestingly, the subgroup of 5 of the 7 studies using the second version of the Bayley Scales and including the majority of infants tested (n=879) demonstrated that supplementation of preterm formula with LC-PUFAs resulted in an increase in mental development scores by 3.4 points (95% CI, 0.6–6.3) compared with control.[103] Further high-quality trials are clearly needed to substantiate these findings but are probably unlikely to occur, because most infant formulas for preterm infants are now supplemented with LC-PUFAs.

Of more current clinical relevance are 2 recent trials in which DHA doses reflective of the estimated in utero accretion rate were used.[104-106] These trials also included infants fed human milk. Both trials reported no differences in mental development scores at 18 to 20 months of age.[105,106] However, the larger and more robust of the 2 trials demonstrated that girls had a 4.5 point (approximately 0.3 standard deviations) improvement in mental development scores (95% confidence interval [CI], 0.5–8.5) and significant mental delay (mental development scores <70) was reduced from 10.5% in the control group to 5% in the higher DHA group (relative risk, 0.50; 95% CI, 0.26–0.93).[105] Although there was some suggestion of benefit with LC-PUFA supplementation at 18 months of age, the long-term benefits of LC-PUFA supplementation in preterm children remains unclear.

The effects of maternal supplementation with ω-3 LC-PUFAs, either in pregnancy or during lactation, on childhood developmental outcomes has also been investigated in randomized controlled trials, and the available systematic reviews indicate no consistent benefit of supplementation.[107-109]

LC-PUFAs and Other Aspects of Central Nervous System Development

The effects of LC-PUFA supplementation on other aspects of brain function and/or development also have been examined using auditory evoked potentials, problem-solving ability, measures of attention, measures of general movements, and most recently, assessment of brain structure using magnetic resonance imaging. Few consistent effects are apparent, although beneficial effects of LC-PUFA supplementation on problem-solving tasks have been noted in 10-month-old term infants[110] and 6-month-old preterm infants.[104]

Effects of LC-PUFAs on Allergy Outcomes

Outside the sphere of neurologic development, interest has focused on the anti-inflammatory and immune-modulating effects of ω-3 LC-PUFAs and the possibility that increased ω-3 LC-PUFA status may be associated with a lower risk of developing childhood allergies. The rationale is that ω-3 LC-PUFAs, particularly EPA, antagonize the actions of ARA, leading to a range of biochemical and immunologic changes that limit inflammatory responses. Some postnatal dietary intervention studies designed to increase ω-3 LC-PUFA status through a combination of DHA-rich tuna oil supplementation and a reduction in dietary LA intake have suggested that dietary intervention lowers the prevalence of early asthma symptoms, such as cough and wheeze, but follow-up studies have generally failed to detect an effect.[111,112]

Randomized trials that have commenced ω-3 LC-PUFA intervention during pregnancy, mainly as fish oil, are producing interesting results. One of the earliest prenatal supplementation studies involved high-risk infants and showed changes in neonatal immune responses that were consistent with a less-allergic phenotype in the fish oil group compared with the control group.[113] More recently, 2 studies have demonstrated that ω-3 LC-PUFA supplementation with at least 1 g during the last half of pregnancy reduced the risk of atopic eczema during the first year of life and reduced the frequency of egg sensitization in infants who are at high hereditary risk of allergies.[114,115] Of interest are the findings by Olsen et al,[116] who demonstrated that ω-3 LC-PUFA supplementation during pregnancy reduced asthma in adolescence in a study including families at normal risk of allergies. However, the allergy outcomes from the trial of Olsen et al[116] were obtained through linkage to a national registry of doctor visits. The expected event rates in the study by Olsen et al[116] were low, and it was not known whether diagnoses were made according to standard definitions.

Effects of LC-PUFAs on Growth

The observation in the early 1990s that preterm infants assigned to a formula supplemented with fish oil (0.3% of total fatty acids as 20:5ω-3 and 0.2% as 22:6ω-3) versus an unsupplemented formula had lower normalized weight and lower normalized length at various times during the first year of life[117] generated considerable concern. In this study, weight at 12 months' corrected age was correlated with plasma phospholipid 20:4ω-6 content at various times during the first year of life.[118] This led to the assumption that the lower rate of weight gain was related in some way to the 20:5ω-3 content of the fish oil. Two additional studies in preterm infants[91,119] demonstrated an adverse effect of ω-3 LC-PUFAs on growth, whereas another trial suggested a positive effect,[120] and yet others demonstrated no effects.[59] These confusing data may be the result of random error and/or the small sample sizes in most trials. It is difficult to think of a biologic mechanism by which ω-3 fatty acids may inhibit growth. Possibilities that have been suggested include inhibition of desaturation and elongation of 18:2ω-6 to 20:4ω-6 by the ω-3 fatty acids, inhibition of eicosanoid synthesis from 20:4ω-6 by the intake of preformed 20:5ω-3 or endogenous synthesis of 20:5ω-3 from a moderately high intake of 18:3ω-3, and effects of ω-3 and ω-6 fatty acids on transcription of genes controlling lipolysis and lipogenesis.[121]

Trials of infant formula feeding for preterm infants including a combination of ω-3 LC-PUFAs with ARA have generally been of higher quality than the earlier trials of formula feeding that have included only ω-3 LC-PUFAs, and these trials most consistently have demonstrated no effect of LC-PUFA supplementation on the growth of preterm infants, as summarized in the most recent Cochrane systematic review.[89] Interestingly, the only growth effects noted are higher weights and higher lengths in infants at 2 months post-term, and the meta-analysis included a combination of trials that supplemented infants with ω-3 LC-PUFAs alone or in combination with ARA.[89]

The single largest trial of LC-PUFA supplementation to assess growth, involving more than 650 infants born at <33 weeks' gestation, compared supplementation with DHA of approximately 1% total fatty acids with and supplementation with DHA of approximately 0.3% total fatty acids, supplied either through human milk, infant formula, or a combination of both to mimic typical feeding practices in neonatal intensive care units.[122] All milks contained approximately 0.5% total fatty acids. There was no effect of higher dietary DHA on weight or head circumference

IV

at any age, but infants given more DHA were 0.7 cm (95% CI, 0.1–1.4 cm; *P* =.02) longer at 18 months' corrected age. There was an interaction effect between treatment and birth weight strata for weight and length. Higher DHA supplementation resulted in increased length in infants born weighing ≥1250 g at 4 months' corrected age and in both weight and length at 12 and 18 months' corrected age.[122] Although complex, these data indicate that DHA up to 1% total dietary fatty acids does not adversely affect growth.

The situation regarding LC-PUFA supplementation and growth of term infants is more straightforward. A recent meta-analysis of growth data from 14 (from a total of 21 known trials) generally high-quality trials that involved LC-PUFA supplementation of infant formula fed to term infants found no evidence that such supplementation influences the growth of term infants in either a negative or a positive way.[123] Subgroup analyses showed that neither supplementation with only ω-3 LC-PUFAs nor source of LC-PUFA supplementation affected infant growth. This analysis of data from 1846 infants should put to rest the question of growth inhibition by ω-3 LC-PUFAs.

Other Adverse Effects of LC-PUFAs

In addition to concerns about adverse effects of ω-3 fatty acids on growth, a number of theoretical concerns related to the known biologic effects of ω-6 and ω-3 LC-PUFAs must be considered.[124] Among these is the possibility that supplementation with highly unsaturated oils will increase the likelihood of oxidant damage. This is because peroxidation occurs at the site of double bonds, making membranes with unsaturated fatty acids more vulnerable to oxidant damage. Thus, it is possible that LC-PUFA supplementation will increase the incidence of conditions thought to be related to oxidant damage (eg, necrotizing enterocolitis, bronchopulmonary dysplasia, retrolental fibroplasia). There also is concern that unbalanced supplementation with ω-3 and/or ω-6 LC-PUFAs will result in altered eicosanoid metabolism with potential effects on a variety of physiological mechanisms (eg, blood clotting, infection). Further, more polyunsaturated fatty acids in muscle cell membranes has been related to enhanced insulin sensitivity,[125] and specific LC-PUFAs have been shown to inhibit as well as to enhance transcription of a variety of genes.[126] There are few data to either support these theoretical concerns with respect to the small amounts of LC-PUFAs that are added to infant formulas.

Many of the randomized controlled trials comparing the outcomes of preterm infants receiving supplemented formulas with either DHA or both DHA and ARA from a variety of sources (single-cell oils, fish oil, egg yolk triglyceride, egg yolk phospholipids) with infants receiving unsupplemented formula have reported a range of clinical outcomes, including necrotizing enterocolitis, sepsis, retinopathy of prematurity, intraventricular hemorrhage, and bronchopulmonary dysplasia. The relevant trials have been summarized in a systematic review and meta-analysis specifically designed to consider the effects of LC-PUFA supplementation of infant formula on the typical diseases of prematurity.[103] The clinical signs and symptoms used to diagnose a disease may differ between neonatal units and may change with improvements in clinical practice over time. Thus, the reported meta-analyses included all outcomes according to any definition as well as sensitivity analyses including trials only using internationally accepted definitions or trials with a low risk of bias on the basis of reporting adequate concealment of randomization and analysis according to the intention-to-treat principle. In meta-analyses of data from approximately 1500 preterm infants, the risk of necrotizing enterocolitis and sepsis did not differ between infants fed LC-PUFA–supplemented or control formula when all available data were included, when necrotizing enterocolitis or sepsis were confirmed, or in sensitivity analysis.[103] There were also no clear differences in rates of retinopathy of prematurity, intraventricular hemorrhage, or bronchopulmonary dysplasia between preterm infants fed LC-PUFA–supplemented or control formula in overall analyses or when trials reported diseases according to the prespecified definitions or in sensitivity analysis.[103] However, in many cases, the small numbers of infants and low disease rates limited these analyses. Collectively, these data together with those from LC-PUFA supplementation of infant formulas have not resulted in a greater incidence of adverse conditions and suggest that the amounts and the sources of LC-PUFAs used in these studies are safe. Furthermore, supplementation with DHA at higher doses (up to 1% of total fatty acids) has also had no effect on the incidence of sepsis, necrotizing enterocolitis, or intraventricular hemorrhage and, in fact, may result in lower rates of bronchopulmonary dysplasia, particularly in infants born weighing <1250 g and male infants.[105,127]

IV

Sources for LC-PUFA Supplementation

Available sources for LC-PUFA supplementation include egg yolk lipid, phospholipid, and triglyceride, all of which contain ω-6 as well as ω-3 LC-PUFAs; fish oils; and oils produced by single-cell organisms (ie, microalgal and fungal oils). Aside from the early reports of an adverse effect of fish oil on growth of infants (as discussed earlier), few untoward effects of the available supplements have been noted. In vitro and animal studies of toxicity also have revealed little toxicity of any of these sources. In fact, the US Food and Drug Administration has recently accepted the conclusion of a manufacturer of a combination of algal and fungal oils as well as that of a manufacturer of a combination of low-EPA tuna and a fungal oil that their products are generally regarded as safe sources of DHA and ARA for addition to formulas intended for normal infants.

Supplementation of Infant Formulas With LC-PUFAs

The American Academy of Pediatrics has no official position on supplementation of term or preterm infant formulas with LC-PUFAs. The Life Sciences Research Organization Expert Panel on Nutrient Composition of Term Infant Formulas recommended neither a minimum nor maximum content of either ARA or DHA.[38] The Life Sciences Research Organization Expert Panel on Nutrient Composition of Preterm Formulas specified a maximum amount of ARA and DHA for preterm infant formulas but did not specify a minimum amount of either fatty acid.[128] In contrast, regulatory and advisory groups from other countries recommend that infant formulas, particularly those intended for preterm infants, be supplemented with these 2 fatty acids,[37] and such formulas are now available in most countries, including the United States. It has been estimated that approximately 75% of the term formulas and 100% of the preterm formulas sold in the United States are supplemented with DHA and ARA.

The evidence for efficacy of supplementing term infant formulas with these fatty acids is only modestly different from that available to the Life Sciences Research Organization term formula panel in 1998, but the evidence for efficacy of supplementation of preterm formulas is more convincing, with a few studies suggesting that there are advantages with respect to level of general development. Moreover, most of the theoretical safety concerns expressed earlier have been resolved. Most notably, no recent study has documented an adverse effect of formulas supplemented with both ARA and DHA on growth and supplementation with DHA alone or DHA plus ARA does not appear to result in a higher incidence of conditions such as necrotizing enterocolitis, sepsis, and bronchopulmonary dysplasia, which, theoretically, might be higher with addition of these bioactive compounds to formulas.

Finally, considering the marked variability among infants of apparent conversion of ALA to DHA and LA to ARA, it is conceivable that some infants will benefit from supplementation, whereas others will not. Such a scenario certainly would help explain the marked variability in outcomes documented by virtually every study. It also is likely that any beneficial effects of LC-PUFA supplementation will be subtle and possibly not detectable with all methodologies.

References

1. Bier DM, Brosnan JT, Flatt JP, et al. Report of the IDECG Working Group on lower and upper limits of carbohydrate and fat intake. International Dietary Energy Consultative Group. *Eur J Clin Nutr*. 1999;53(Suppl 1):S177-S178

2. Hamosh M. A review. Fat digestion in the newborn: role of lingual lipase and preduodenal digestion. *Pediatr Res*. 1979;13(5 Pt 1):615-622

3. Faber J, Goldstein R, Blondheim O, et al. Absorption of medium chain triglycerides in the stomach of the human infant. *J Pediatr Gastroenterol Nutr.* 1988;7(2):189-195

4. Linscheer WG, Vergroesen AJ. Lipids. In: Shils ME, Shike M, Ross AC, Caballero B, Cousins RJ, eds. *Modern Nutrition in Health and Disease.* Philadelphia, PA: Lea & Febiger; 1988:72-1007

5. Hernell O, Olivecrona T. Human milk lipases. I. Serum-stimulated lipase. *J Lipid Res.* 1974;15:367-374

6. Fredrikzon B, Hernell O, Blackberg L, Olivecrona T. Bile salt stimulated lipase in human milk and lipid digestion during the neonatal period. In: Lebenthal E, ed. *Textbook of Gastroenterology and Nutrition in Infancy.* New York, NY: Raven Press, 1987:465-471

7. Hernell O. Human milk lipases. III. Physiological implications of the bile salt-stimulated lipase. *Eur J Clin Invest.* 1975;5(3):267-272

8. Watkins JB, Ingall D, Szczepanik P, et al. Bile salt metabolism in the newborn: Measurement of pool size and synthesis by stable isotape technique. *N Engl J Med.* 1972;288(9):431-434

9. Watkins JB. Lipid digestion and absorption. *Pediatrics.* 1985;75(1 Pt 2):151-156

10. Hofmann AF, Roda A. Physicochemical properties of bile acids and their relationship to biological properties: an overview of the problem. *J Lipid Res.* 1984;25(13):1477-1489

11. Gray GM. Mechanisms of digestion and absorption of food. In: Sleisenger MH, Fordtran JS, eds. *Gastrointestinal Disease: Pathophysiology, Diagnosis, Management.* Philadelphia, PA: WB Saunders; 1983:844-858

12. Filer LJ Jr, Mattson FH, Fomon SJ. Triglyceride configuration and fat absorption by the human infant. *J Nutr.* 1969;99(3):293-298

13. Carnielli VP, Luijendijk IH, van Beek RH, Boerma GJ, Degenhart HJ, Sauer PJ. Effect of dietary triacylglycerol fatty acid positional distribution on plasma lipid classes and their fatty acid composition in preterm infants. *Am J Clin Nutr.* 1995;62:776-781

14. Carnielli VP, Luijendijk IH, van Goudoever JB, et al. Structural position and amount of palmitic acid in infant formulas: effects on fat, fatty acid, and mineral balance. *J Pediatr Gastroenterol Nutr.* 1996;23(5):553-560

15. Carnielli VP, Luijendijk IHT, van Goudoever JB, et al. Feeding premature newborn infants palmitic acid in amounts and stereoisomeric position similar to that of human milk: Effects on fat and mineral balance. *Am J Clin Nutr.* 1995;61(5):1037-1042

16. Lucas A, Quinlan P, Abrams S, Ryan S, Meah S, Lucas PJ. Randomised controlled trial of a synthetic triglyceride milk formula for preterm infants. *Arch Dis Child Fetal Neonatal Ed.* 1997;77(3):F178-F84

17. Bensadoun A. Lipoprotein lipase. *Annu Rev Nutr.* 1991;11:217-237

18. Griffin EA, Bryan MH, Angel A. Variations in intralipid tolerance in newborn infants. *Pediatr Res.* 1983;17(6):478-481

19. Innis SM. Essential fatty acids in growth and development. *Prog Lipid Res.* 1991;30(1):39-103

20. Holman RT. Nutritional and biochemical evidences of acyl interaction with respect to essential polyunsaturated fatty acids. *Prog Lipid Res* 1986;25(1-4):29-39

IV

21. Oliw E, Gramstrom E, Anggard E. The prostaglandins and related substances. In: Pace-Asciak C, Gramstron E, eds. *Prostaglandins and Related Substances*. Amsterdam, The Netherlands: Elsevier; 1983:1-19

22. Calder PC. Immunomodulation by omega-3 fatty acids. *Prostaglandins Leukot Essent Fatty Acids*. 2007;77(5-6):327-335

23. Holman RT. The ratio of trienoic: tetraenoic acids in tissue lipids as a measure of essential fatty acid requirement. *J Nutr* 1960;70:405-410

24. Burr GO, Burr MM. A new deficiency disease produced by the rigid exclusion of fat from the diet. *J Biol Chem*. 1929;82(8):345-367

25. Hansen AE, Stewart RA, Hughes G, Soderhjelm L. The relation of linoleic acid to infant feeding. *Acta Paediatr Suppl*. 1962;137:1-41

26. Benolken RM, Anderson RE, Wheeler TG. Membrane fatty acids associated with the electrical response in visual excitation. *Science*. 1973;182(4118):1253-1254

27. Neuringer M, Connor WE, Lin DS, Barstad L, Luck S. Biochemical and functional effects of prenatal and postnatal omega-3 fatty acid deficiency on retina and brain in rhesus monkeys. *Proc Natl Acad Sci U S A*. 1986;83(11):4021-4025

28. Neuringer M, Connor WE, Van Petten C, Barstad L. Dietary omega-3 fatty acid deficiency and visual loss in infant rhesus monkeys. *J Clin Invest*. 1984;73(1):272-276

29. Wheeler TG, Benolken RM, Anderson RE. Visual membranes: specificity of fatty acid precursors for the electrical response to illumination. *Science*. 1975;188(4195):1312-1314

30. Holman RT, Johnson SB, Hatch TF. A case of human linolenic acid deficiency involving neurological abnormalities. *Am J Clin Nutr*. 1982;35(3):617-623

31. Bjerve KS, Fischer S, Alme K. Alpha-linolenic acid deficiency in man: effect of ethyl linolenate on plasma and erythrocyte fatty acid composition and biosynthesis of prostanoids. *Am J Clin Nutr*. 1987;46(4):570-576

32. Jensen RG. Lipids in human milk. *Lipids*. 1999;34(12):1243-1271

33. Sanders TAB, Reddy S. The influence of a vegetarian diet on the fatty acid composition of human milk and the essential fatty acid status of the infant. *J Pediatr*. 1992;120(4 Pt 2):S71-S7

34. Henderson RA, Jensen RG, Lammi-Keefe CJ, Ferris AM, Dardick KR. Effect of fish oil on the fatty acid composition of human milk and maternal and infant erythrocytes. *Lipids*. 1992;27(11):863-869

35. Jensen CL, Maude M, Anderson RE, Heird WC. Effect of docosahexaenoic acid supplementation of lactating women on the fatty acid composition of breast milk lipids and maternal and infant plasma phospholipids. *Am J Clin Nutr*. 2000;71(1 Suppl):292S-299S

36. Makrides M, Neumann MA, Gibson RA. Effect of maternal docosahexaenoic acid (DHA) supplementation on breast milk composition. *Eur J Clin Nutr*. 1996;50(6):352-357

37. Aggett PJ, Haschke F, Heine W, et al. Comment on the content and composition of lipids in infant formulas. ESPGAN Committee on Nutrition. *Acta Paediatr Scand*. 1991;80(8-9):887-896

38. Raiten DJ, Talbot JM, Waters JH. Assessment of nutrient requirements for infant formulas. *J Nutr.* 1998;128(Suppl):S2110-S2130

39. Carlson SE, Rhodes PG, Ferguson MG. Docosahexaenoic acid status of preterm infants at birth and following feeding with human milk or formula. *Am J Clin Nutr.* 1986;44(6):798-804

40. Innis SM, Akrabawi SS, Diersen-Schade DA, Dobson MV, Guy DG. Visual acuity and blood lipids in term infants fed human milk or formulae. *Lipids.* 1997;32(1):63-72

41. Lucas A, Morley R, Cole TJ. Randomised trial of early diet in preterm babies and later intelligence quotient. *BMJ.* 1998;317(7171):1481-1487

42. Lucas A, Morley R, Cole TJ, et al. Early diet in preterm babies and developmental status at 18 months. *Lancet.* 1990;335(8704):1477-1481

43. Morrow Tlucak M, Haude RH, Ernhart CB. Breastfeeding and cognitive development in the first 2 years of life. *Social Sci Med.* 1988;26(6):635-639

44. Rogan WJ, Gladen BC. Breast-feeding and cognitive development. *Early Hum Dev.* 1993;31(3):181-193

45. Clandinin MT, Chappell JE, Leong S, Heim T, Swyer PR, Chance GW. Intrauterine fatty acid accretion rates in human brain. implications for fatty acid requirements. *Early Hum Dev.* 1980;4(2):121-129

46. Clandinin MT, Chappell JE, Leong S, Heim T, Swyer PR, Chance GW. Extrauterine fatty acid accretion in infant brain: implications for fatty acid requirements. *Early Hum Dev.* 1980;4(2):131-138

47. Martinez M. Tissue levels of polyunsaturated fatty acids during early human development. *J Pediatr.* 1992;120(4 Pt 2):S129-S138

48. Dutta-Roy AK. Transport mechanisms for long-chain polyunsaturated fatty acids in the human placenta. 2000;71(1 Suppl):315S-322S

49. Farquharson J, Cockburn F, Patrick WA, Jamieson EC, Logan RW. Infant cerebral cortex phospholipid fatty-acid composition and diet. *Lancet.* 1992;340(8823):810-813

50. Makrides M, Neumann MA, Byard RW, Simmer K, Gibson RA. Fatty acid composition of brain, retina, and erythrocytes in breast- and formula-fed infants. *Am J Clin Nutr.* 1994;60(2):189-194

51. Arbuckle LD, MacKinnon MJ, Innis SM. Formula 18:2(n-6) and 18:3(n-3) content and ratio influence long-chain polyunsaturated fatty acids in the developing piglet liver and central nervous system. *J Nutr.* 1994;124(2):289-298

52. Sauerwald TU, Hachey DL, Jensen CL, Chen H, Anderson RE, Heird WC. Effect of dietary alpha-linolenic acid intake on incorporation of docosahexaenoic and arachidonic acids into plasma phospholipids of term infants. *Lipids.* 1996;31(Suppl):S131-S135

53. Carnielli VP, Wattimena DJL, Luijendijk IHT, Boerlage A, Degenhart HJ, Sauer PJJ. The very low birth weight premature infant is capable of synthesizing arachidonic and docosahexaenoic acids from linoleic and linolenic acids. *Pediatr Res.* 1996;40(1):169-174

54. Demmelmair H, von Schenck U, Behrendt E, Sauerwald T, Koletzko B. Estimation of arachidonic acid synthesis in fullterm neonates using natural variation of 13C-abundance. *J Pediatr Gastroenterol Nutr.* 1995;21(1):31-36

IV

55. Salem N Jr, Wegher B, Mena P, Uauy R. Arachidonic and docosahexaenoic acids are biosynthesized from their 18-carbon precursors in human infants. *Proc Natl Acad Sci U S A.* 1996;93(1):49-54

56. Sauerwald TU, Hachey DL, Jensen CL, Chen HM, Anderson RE, Heird WC. Intermediates in endogenous synthesis of C22:6 omega 3 and C20: 4 omega 6 by term and preterm infants. *Pediatr Res.* 1997;41(2):183-187

57. Uauy R, Mena P, Wegher B, Nieto S, Salem N Jr. Long chain polyunsaturated fatty acid formation in neonates: effect of gestational age and intrauterine growth. *Pediatr Res.* 2000;47(1):127-135

58. Carlson SE, Cooke RJ, Rhodes PG, Peeples JM, Werkman SH, Tolley EA. Long-term feeding of formulas high in linolenic acid and marine oil to very low birth weight infants: phospholipid fatty acids. *Pediatr Res.* 1991;30(5):404-412

59. Uauy R, Hoffman DR, Birch EE, Birch DG, Jameson DM, Tyson J. Safety and efficacy of omega-3 fatty acids in the nutrition of very low birth weight infants: Soy oil and marine oil supplementation of formula. *J Pediatr.* 1994;124(4):612-620

60. Uauy RD, Birch DG, Birch EE, Tyson JE, Hoffman DR. Effect of dietary omega-3 fatty acids on retinal function of very-low-birth-weight neonates. *Pediatr Res.* 1990;28(5):485-492

61. Rioux FM, Innis SM, Dyer R, MacKinnon M. Diet-induced changes in liver and bile but not brain fatty acids can be predicted from differences in plasma phospholipid fatty acids in formula- and milk-fed piglets. *J Nutr.* 1997;127(2):370-377

62. Moore SA. Cerebral endothelium and astrocytes cooperate in supplying docosahexaenoic acid to neurons. *Adv Exp Med Biol.* 1993;331:229-233

63. Moore SA, Yoder E, Murphy S, Dutton GR, Spector AA. Astrocytes, not neurons, produce docosahexaenoic acid (22:6-omega-3) and arachidonic acid (20:4-omega-6). *J Neurochem.* 1991;56(2):518-524

64. Pawlosky RJ, Denkins Y, Ward G, Salem N Jr. Retinal and brain accretion of long-chain polyunsaturated fatty acids in developing felines: the effects of corn oil-based maternal diets. 1997;65(2):465-472

65. Heird WC, Lapillonne A. The role of essential fatty acids in development. *Annu Rev Nutr.* 2005;25:549-571

66. Lauritzen L, Hansen HS, Jorgensen MH, Michaelsen KF. The essentiality of long chain n-3 fatty acids in relation to development and function of the brain and retina. *Prog Lipid Res.* 2001;40(1-2):1-94

67. McCann JC, Ames BN. Is docosahexaenoic acid, an n-3 long-chain polyunsaturated fatty acid, required for development of normal brain function? An overview of evidence from cognitive and behavioral tests in humans and animals. *Am J Clin Nutr.* 2005;82(2):281-295

68. Uauy R, Hoffman DR, Peirano P, Birch DG, Birch EE. Essential fatty acids in visual and brain development. *Lipids.* 2001;36(9):885-895

69. Dobson V. Clinical applications of preferential looking measures of visual acuity. *Behav Brain Res.* 1983;10(1):25-38

70. Dobson V, Teller DY. Visual acuity in human infants: a review and comparison of behavioral and electrophysiological studies. *Vision Res.* 1978;18(11):1469-1483

71. McDonald MA, Dobson V, Sebris SL, Baitch L, Varner D, Teller DY. The acuity card procedure: a rapid test of infant acuity. *Invest Ophthalmol Vis Sci.* 1985;26(8):1158-1162

72. Sokol S, Hansen VC, Moskowitz A, Greenfield P, Towle VL. Evoked potential and preferential looking estimates of visual acuity in pediatric patients. *Ophthalmology.* 1983;90(5):552-562

73. Uauy R, Birch E, Birch D, Peirano P. Visual and brain function measurements in studies of n-3 fatty acid requirements of infants [published erratum appears in *J Pediatr.* 1992;121(2):329]. *J Pediatr.* 1992;120(4 Pt 2):S168-S180

74. Norcia AM, Tyler CW. Spatial frequency sweep VEP: visual acuity during the first year of life. *Vision Res.* 1985;25(10):1399-1408

75. Bougle D, Denise P, Vimard F, Nouvelot A, Penneillo MJ, Guillois B. Early neurological and neuropsychological development of the preterm infant and polyunsaturated fatty acids supply. *Clin Neurophysiol.* 1999;110(8):1363-1370

76. Faldella G, Govoni M, Alessandroni R, et al. Visual evoked potentials and dietary long chain polyunsaturated fatty acids in preterm infants. *Arch Dis Child Fetal Neonatal Ed.* 1996;75(2):F108-F12

77. Jensen CL, Prager TC, Fraley JK, Chen HM, Anderson RE, Heird WC. Effect of dietary linoleic/alpha-linolenic acid ratio on growth and visual function of term infants. *J Pediatr.* 1997;131(2):200-209

78. van Wezel-Meijler G, van der Knaap MS, Huisman J, Jonkman EJ, Valk J, Lafeber HN. Dietary supplementation of long-chain polyunsaturated fatty acids in preterm infants: effects on cerebral maturation. *Acta Paediatr.* 2002;91(9):942-950

79. Birch DG, Birch EE, Hoffman DR, Uauy RD. Retinal development in very-low-birth-weight infants fed diets differing in omega-3 fatty acids. *Invest Ophthalmol Vis Sci.* 1992;33(8):2365-2376

80. Hood DC, Birch DG. The A-wave of the human electroretinogram and rod receptor function. *Invest Ophthalmol Vis Sci.* 1990;31(10):2070-2081

81. Naka KI, Rushton WA. S-potentials from colour units in the retina of fish (Cyprinidae). 1966;185(3):536-555

82. Simmer K, Patole SK, Rao SC. Long-chain polyunsaturated fatty acid supplementation in infants born at term. *Cochrane Database Syst Rev.* 2011;(12):CD000376

83. Birch EE, Carlson SE, Hoffman DR, et al. The DIAMOND (DHA Intake And Measurement Of Neural Development) Study: a double-masked, randomized controlled clinical trial of the maturation of infant visual acuity as a function of the dietary level of docosahexaenoic acid. *Am J Clin Nutr.* 2010;91(4):848-859

84. Gibson RA, Neumann MA, Makrides M. Effect of increasing breast milk docosahexanoic acid on plasma and erythrocyte phospholipid fatty acids and neural indices of exclusively breast fed infants. *Eur J Clin Nutr.* 1997;51(9):578-584

85. Innis SM, Friesen RW. Essential n-3 fatty acids in pregnant women and early visual acuity maturation in term infants. *Am J Clin Nutr.* 2008;87(3):548-557

86. Judge MP, Harel O, Lammi-Keefe CJ. A docosahexaenoic acid-functional food during pregnancy benefits infant visual acuity at four but not six months of age. *Lipids.* 2007;42(2):117-122

IV

87. Malcolm CA, McCulloch DL, Montgomery C, Shepherd A, Weaver LT. Maternal docosahexaenoic acid supplementation during pregnancy and visual evoked potential development in term infants: a double blind, prospective, randomised trial. *Arch Dis Child Fetal Neonatal Ed.* 2003;88(5):F383-F390

88. Smithers LG, Gibson RA, Makrides M. Maternal supplementation with docosahexaenoic acid during pregnancy does not affect early visual development in the infant: a randomized controlled trial. *Am J Clin Nutr.* 2011;93(6):1293-1299

89. Schulzke SM, Patole SK, Simmer K. Long-chain polyunsaturated fatty acid supplementation in preterm infants. *Cochrane Database Syst Rev.* 2011;(2):CD000375

90. Carlson SE, Werkman SH, Rhodes PG, Tolley EA. Visual-acuity development in healthy preterm infants: effect of marine-oil supplementation. *Am J Clin Nutr.* 1993;58(1):35-42

91. Carlson SE, Werkman SH, Tolley EA. Effect of long-chain n-3 fatty acid supplementation on visual acuity and growth of preterm infants with and without bronchopulmonary dysplasia. *Am J Clin Nutr.* 1996;63(5):687-697

92. O'Connor DL, Hall R, Adamkin D, et al. Growth and development in preterm infants fed long-chain polyunsaturated fatty acids: a prospective, randomized controlled trial. *Pediatrics.* 2001;108(2):359-371

93. Smithers LG, Gibson RA, McPhee A, Makrides M. Higher dose of docosahexaenoic acid in the neonatal period improves visual acuity of preterm infants: results of a randomized controlled trial. *Am J Clin Nutr.* 2008;88(4):1049-1056

94. McCall RB, Mash CW, Dobbing J. Long-chain polyunsaturated fatty acids and the measurement and prediction of intelligence (IQ). In: Dobbing J, ed. *Developing Brain and Behaviour: the Role of Lipids in Infant Formula.* London, England: Academic Press; 1997:295-338

95. Fagan JF, Singer LT. Infant recognition memory as a measure of intelligence. *Adv Infant Res.* 1983;2:31-78

96. Colombo J, Dobbing J. Individual differences in infant cognition: methods, measures, and models. In: Dobbing J, ed. *Developing Brain and Behaviour: The Role of Lipids in Infant Formula.* London, England: Academic Press; 1997:339-385

97. Auestad N, Halter R, Hall RT, et al. Growth and development in term infants fed long-chain polyunsaturated fatty acids: a double-masked, randomized, parallel, prospective, multivariate study. *Pediatrics.* 2001;108(2):372-381

98. Birch EE, Garfield S, Hoffman DR, Uauy R, Birch DG. A randomized controlled trial of early dietary supply of long-chain polyunsaturated fatty acids and mental development in term infants. *Dev Med Child Neurol.* 2000;42(3):174-181

99. Bouwstra H, Dijck-Brouwer DA, Wildeman JA, et al. Long-chain polyunsaturated fatty acids have a positive effect on the quality of general movements of healthy term infants. *Am J Clin Nutr.* 2003;78(2):313-318

100. Lucas A, Stafford M, Morley R, et al. Efficacy and safety of long-chain polyunsaturated fatty acid supplementation of infant-formula milk: a randomised trial. *Lancet.* 1999;354(9194):1948-1954

101. Makrides M, Neumann MA, Simmer K, Gibson RA. A critical appraisal of the role of dietary long-chain polyunsaturated fatty acids on neural indices of term infants: A randomized, controlled trial. *Pediatrics.* 2000;105(1 Pt 1):32-38

102. Makrides M, Smithers LG, Gibson RA. Role of long-chain polyunsaturated fatty acids in neurodevelopment and growth. *Nestle Nutr Workshop Ser Pediatr Program*. 2010;65:123-133

103. Smithers LG, Gibson RA, McPhee A, Makrides M. Effect of long-chain polyunsaturated fatty acid supplementation of preterm infants on disease risk and neurodevelopment: a systematic review of randomised controlled trials. *Am J Clin Nutr*. 2008;87(4):912-920

104. Henriksen C, Haugholt K, Lindgren M, et al. Improved cognitive development among preterm infants attributable to early supplementation of human milk with docosahexaenoic acid and arachidonic acid. *Pediatrics*. 2008;121(6):1137-1145

105. Makrides M, Gibson RA, McPhee AJ, et al. Neurodevelopmental outcomes of preterm infants fed high-dose docosahexaenoic acid: a randomized controlled trial. *JAMA*. 2009;301(2):175-182

106. Westerberg AC, Schei R, Henriksen C, et al. Attention among very low birth weight infants following early supplementation with docosahexaenoic and arachidonic acid. *Acta Paediatr*. 2011;100(1):47-52

107. Delgado-Noguera MF, Calvache JA, Bonfill Cosp X. Supplementation with long chain polyunsaturated fatty acids (LCPUFA) to breastfeeding mothers for improving child growth and development. *Cochrane Database Syst Rev* 2010;(12):CD007901

108. Gould J, Smithers LG, Makrides M. The effect of omega-3 LCPUFA supplementation during pregnancy, or pregnancy and lactation, on infant cognitive and visual development: a systematic review and meta analysis of randomised controlled trials. Presented at: 10th Congress of the International Society for the Study of Fatty Acids and Lipids; Vancouver, British Columbia, Canada; May 26-30, 2012

109. Dziechciarz P, Horvath A, Szajewska H. Effects of n-3 long-chain polyunsaturated fatty acid supplementation during pregnancy and/or lactation on neurodevelopment and visual function in children: a systematic review of randomized controlled trials. *J Am Coll Nutr* 2010;29(5):443-454

110. Willatts P, Forsyth JS, DiModugno MK, Varma S, Colvin M. Effect of long-chain polyunsaturated fatty acids in infant formula on problem solving at 10 months of age. *Lancet* 1998;352(9129):688-691

111. Marks GB, Mihrshahi S, Kemp AS, et al. Prevention of asthma during the first 5 years of life: a randomized controlled trial. *J Allergy Clin Immunol*. 2006;118(1):53-61

112. Peat JK, Mihrshahi S, Kemp AS, et al. Three-year outcomes of dietary fatty acid modification and house dust mite reduction in the Childhood Asthma Prevention Study. *J Allergy Clin Immunol*. 2004;114(4):807-813

113. Dunstan JA, Mori TA, Barden A, et al. Fish oil supplementation in pregnancy modifies neonatal allergen-specific immune responses and clinical outcomes in infants at high risk of atopy: a randomized, controlled trial. *J Allergy Clin Immunol*. 2003;112(3):1178-1184

114. Furuhjelm C, Warstedt K, Larsson J, et al. Fish oil supplementation in pregnancy and lactation may decrease the risk of infant allergy. *Acta Paediatr*. 2009;98(9):1461-1467

115. Palmer DJ, Sullivan T, Gold MS, et al. Effect of n-3 long chain polyunsaturated fatty acid supplementation in pregnancy on infants' allergies in first year of life: randomised controlled trial. *BMJ*. 2012;344:e184

IV

116. Olsen SF, Osterdal ML, Salvig JD, et al. Fish oil intake compared with olive oil intake in late pregnancy and asthma in the offspring: 16 y of registry-based follow-up from a randomized controlled trial. *Am J Clin Nutr.* 2008;88(1):167-175

117. Carlson SE, Cooke RJ, Werkman SH, Tolley EA. First year growth of preterm infants fed standard compared to marine oil n-3 supplemented formula. *Lipids.* 1992;27(11):901-907

118. Carlson SE, Werkman SH, Peeples JM, Cooke RJ, Tolley EA. Arachidonic acid status correlates with first year growth in preterm infants. *Proc Natl Acad Sci U S A.* 1993;90(3):1073-1077

119. Ryan AS, Montalto MB, Groh-Wargo S, et al. Effect of DHA-containing formula on growth of preterm infants to 59 weeks postmenstrual age. *Am J Human Biol.* 1999;11(4):457-467

120. Fewtrell MS, Abbott RA, Kennedy K, et al. Randomized, double-blind trial of long-chain polyunsaturated fatty acid supplementation with fish oil and borage oil in preterm infants. *J Pediatr.* 2004;144(4):471-479

121. Lapillonne A, Clarke SD, Heird WC. Plausible mechanisms for effects of long-chain polyunsaturated fatty acids on growth. *J Pediatr.* 2003;143(4 Suppl):S9-S16

122. Collins CT, Makrides M, Gibson RA, et al. Pre- and post-term growth in pre-term infants supplemented with higher-dose DHA: a randomised controlled trial. *Br J Nutr.* 2011(11):1635-1643

123. Makrides M, Gibson RA, Udell T, Ried K, International LCPUFA Investigators. Supplementation of infant formula with long-chain polyunsaturated fatty acids does not influence the growth of term infants. *Am J Clin Nutr.* 2005;81(5):1094-1101

124. Heird WC. Biological effects and safety issues related to long-chain polyunsaturated fatty acids in infants. *Lipids.* 1999;34(2):207-214

125. Borkman M, Storlien LH, Pan DA, Jenkins AB, Chisholm DJ, Campbell LV. The relationship between insulin sensitivity and the fatty-acid composition of skeletal-muscle phospholipids. *N Engl J Med.* 1993;328(4):238-244

126. Clarke SD, Jump DB. Polyunsaturated fatty acid regulation of hepatic gene transcription. *J Nutr.* 1996;126(4 Suppl):1105S-1109S

127. Manley BJ, Makrides M, Collins CT, et al. High-dose docosahexaenoic acid supplementation of preterm infants: respiratory and allergy outcomes. *Pediatrics* 2011;128(1):e71-e77

128. Klein CJ. Nutrient requirements for preterm infant formulas. *J Nutr.* 2002;132(6 Suppl 1):1395S-1577S

Chapter 18

Calcium, Phosphorus, and Magnesium

Basic Physiology/Homeostasis

The minerals calcium, magnesium, and phosphorus participate in many of the body's most important functions. These elements play prominent roles in energy processes and transport of metabolites in a host of molecular biochemical reactions. In addition, calcium and phosphorus constitute the principal components of the skeleton in the form of hydroxyapatite $Ca_{10}(PO_4)_6(OH)_2$. Magnesium, which is mainly an intracellular cation, is a cofactor in a wide variety of enzymatic reactions. Thus, these minerals are essential nutrients for life processes and for forming the mineral skeleton.[1-3]

Naturally occurring calcium sources include milk and other dairy products, animal bones, and in lesser amounts, a number of vegetables (Appendix J). In addition, calcium is widely found in fortified food products, such as breakfast cereals and fruit juices, especially orange juice. Phosphorus is abundantly available from virtually all animal and vegetable sources. Magnesium, like phosphorus, is abundant in animal and plant cells. Together, these 3 elements constitute 98% of body minerals by weight. Bone accounts for 99% of the calcium, 80% of the phosphorus, and 60% of the magnesium in the body.

Both calcium and phosphorus appear in the serum and extracellular fluid in low concentrations. Total serum calcium concentration is closely maintained in a narrow range of 2.13 to 2.63 mmol/L (8.5–10.5 mg/dL). Approximately half of the calcium in the serum is bound to albumin at normal levels of the latter; most of the remainder is ionized. The ionized fraction is the physiologically active portion, and, in health, the concentration is constant. If hypoalbuminemia should occur, the total calcium concentration decreases, but the ionized portion remains undisturbed. The phosphorus concentration varies and is age and diet dependent. The normal range is 1.6 to 2.4 mmol/L (5.0–7.5 mg/dL) in infants, 1.3 to 1.78 mmol/L (4–5.5 mg/dL) in older children, and 0.8 to 1.6 mmol/L (2.5–4.5 mg/dL) in adolescents and adults.[4]

Calcium is regulated by various hormones (parathyroid hormone, calcitonin, vitamin D) and a number of organs (skin, small intestine, kidney, and bone). The gastrointestinal tract regulates calcium absorption; a portion of the calcium is absorbed by passive diffusion, and a portion of it is actively transported. Parathyroid hormone enhances serum calcium primarily by releasing calcium from bone. The concentration of ionized calcium in the fluid perfusing the parathyroid gland is a major determinant of the rate of synthesis and release of this hormone. Calcitonin, a hormone elaborated by the parafollicular cells of the thyroid, inhibits bone

IV

reabsorption.[4-6] The kidney is an important site of action of parathyroid hormone and is also the site of synthesis of the active form of vitamin D, 1,25-dihydroxyvitamin D ($1,25\text{-OH}_2\text{-D}$).

Vitamin D facilitates transcellular calcium intestinal absorption. To achieve this effect, it must undergo sequential hydroxylation in the liver to calcidiol and in the kidney to the final product, calcitriol ($1,25\text{-OH}_2\text{-D}$).[7,8] Calcidiol (25-hydroxyvitamin D [25-OH-D]) represents the primary circulatory and storage form of vitamin D. Anticonvulsant drugs, such as phenobarbital and phenytoin, can interfere with vitamin D hydroxylation and metabolism, increasing the daily requirement. The large reservoir of calcium in bone is important in maintaining calcium homeostasis, because a portion of bone calcium exchanges readily with the calcium of extracellular fluid.

Factors other than calcium and vitamin D that are important in maintaining bone health are physical activity and genetic factors. In children, evidence suggests that a combination of adequate mineral intake and weight-bearing physical activity are optimal for bone formation and mineralization.[9] Disuse osteoporosis, as may occur in children with chronic illnesses, also leads to marked bone loss. Although only partially understood, bone formation and calcium metabolism are also regulated via genetic factors. Recent data implicate specific vitamin D receptor genes as affecting calcium absorption in children.[10] Other data indicate that race and gender also affect calcium absorption.[11,12]

Less is known about the regulation of phosphorus. Phosphorus is absorbed efficiently in the small intestine, and its absorption is inhibited by aluminum-containing antacids. It is filtered and reabsorbed in the kidney, and parathyroid hormone inhibits its renal reabsorption. A significant aspect of phosphorus regulation is by renal excretion, such that renal insufficiency leads to decreased renal phosphate excretion and hyperphosphatemia.[8]

Only a small fraction of total body magnesium is present in serum. The normal serum total magnesium concentration is 1.6 to 2.5 mg/dL. Approximately half of this magnesium is protein bound, principally to albumin. Magnesium homeostasis is maintained partly by control of intestinal absorption, but also by control of renal excretion. Magnesium appears to be absorbed principally in the ileum by 3 mechanisms: passive diffusion, "solvent drag," and probably, active transport.[8] Absorption of magnesium is inversely related to intake and is minimally affected by vitamin D.

Parathyroid hormone decreases renal reabsorption of filtered magnesium. Release of parathyroid hormone is modestly suppressed by increased concentrations of magnesium in extracellular fluid, an action that may be mediated by an increase in calcium in the cytosol of parathyroid cells. Conversely, acute (but not chronic) hypomagnesemia stimulates the release of parathyroid hormone.[8,13-16]

Transient neonatal hypomagnesemia has been observed in association with both hypocalcemia and hyperphosphatemia. Transient neonatal hypomagnesemia is more common in infants with intrauterine growth retardation and infants of mothers with diabetes, hypophosphatemia, or hyperparathyroidism. Magnesium supplementation or even intravenous magnesium may be required for these infants. Rarely, severe hypomagnesemia associated with convulsions occurs in early infancy as a result of a genetically determined disorder of magnesium metabolism. This disorder probably results from a defective intestinal absorption of magnesium. Long-term magnesium supplementation is necessary.[14]

Calcium Requirements

The specific requirements for calcium intake by full-term infants, children, and adolescents have been extensively reviewed in recent years.[17,18] The current Recommended Dietary Allowances (RDAs)[18] for children 1 year of age and older, as well as the new Tolerable Upper Intake Level (ULs), are shown in Appendix E.

Multiple approaches are used to assess the requirements for calcium in older children. They include the following: (1) measurement of calcium balance in people with various levels of calcium intake; (2) measurement of bone mineral content, by dual-energy x-ray absorptiometry or other techniques, in groups of children before and after calcium supplementation; and (3) epidemiologic studies relating bone mass or fracture risk in adults with childhood calcium intake.[15] The interactions of these factors make identification of a single optimal daily calcium "requirement" for all children impossible.[19]

The calcium balance technique consists of measuring the effects of any given calcium intake on the net retention of calcium by the body. This approach is commonly used to estimate the minimal requirement. Its usefulness is based on the principle that all retained calcium is used, and that which is not is excreted and, thus, unnecessary. In children, optimizing calcium retention from the diet should lead to the highest degree of skeletal mineralization and, thus, decrease the relative risk of osteoporosis in adults.[19-22]

The substantial limitations involved in obtaining and interpreting data about calcium balance are well known. These include substantial technical problems with measuring calcium excretion and the difficulty obtaining dietary intake control in children. These problems have been partly overcome by the development of stable isotopic methods to assess calcium absorption and excretion.[21] Because the majority of these data are from studies in infants and adolescent girls, more data are needed to establish the "optimal" level of calcium retention at different ages. Recent data have clarified that very low calcium intakes, such as those <600 mg/day, lead to much lower levels of total calcium absorption and retention than recommended intake levels.[23]

A major advance in the field during the last 25 years has been improved methods of measuring total body and regional bone mineral content by various radiologic techniques. Currently, the technique used in the majority of studies is dual-energy x-ray absorptiometry (DXA). This technique can rapidly measure the bone mineral content and bone mineral density of the entire skeleton or of regional sites with a minimal level of radiation exposure. Furthermore, enhancements in the precision of the technique have made it suitable for assessing the short- and long-term effects of calcium supplementation on bone mass in children of all ages.[24,25] Nonetheless, substantial limitations in current DXA technology has led to increased interest in the use of newer techniques, including quantitative computed tomography and bone ultrasonography.[26]

Preterm Infants

Calcium and phosphorus accretion rates increase exponentially during the third trimester in utero. Decreased calcium intake is common in preterm infants and may be less than the postconceptional requirement. This places preterm infants at risk of osteopenia of prematurity. It is a common problem in infants with birth weight less than 1000 g who have relatively low intakes of calcium and phosphorus. The frequency of osteopenia is also increased in preterm infants who require long-term parenteral nutrition or who require medications, such as diuretics, which may adversely affect mineral metabolism.[27] In small preterm infants fed parenterally, the danger of calcium-phosphorus precipitation in the solution limits the amount of these minerals that can be administered intravenously. As a result, prenatal retention rates of calcium and phosphorus are not achieved in preterm infants.[28]

The presence of osteopenia can be assessed by direct radiologic evaluation. Increased lucency of the cortical bone with or without epiphyseal changes is characteristic of significant osteopenia. Although the presence of a fracture can be the presenting sign of osteopenia of prematurity, most infants with decreased bone mineralization, including some with severe rickets, do not have fractures. The American Academy of Pediatrics has published a clinical report that addresses the importance of calcium and vitamin D intake in the preterm infant to prevent osteopenia.[29]

Human milk is relatively low in calcium and phosphorus relative to the in utero accretion rates of these minerals. Although minerals are well absorbed from human milk (60%-70%), the net retention of calcium and phosphorus are far below the rates in utero, which leads to the development of undermineralized bones. Supplementary calcium and phosphorus are needed to sustain optimal calcium balance. Currently, human milk fortifiers (for human milk-fed infants) and special formulas with added minerals are marketed in the United States for feeding preterm infants (see Appendix D). Use of these products has led to net calcium retention comparable to that achieved in utero.[29] After preterm infants with birth weight <1500 g are discharged from the hospital, there may be benefits to providing a higher mineral intake than is available from human milk or from routine cow milk-based formulas.[30-32] This is particularly true for infants who require oxygen or fluid restriction after hospital discharge. Multiple strategies are in clinical use for this situation without clear identification of an optimal approach. One recent randomized control study has shown the benefit of continuing human milk fortifier in preterm infants after hospital discharge.[33]

Full-Term Infants and Children

The optimal primary nutritional source during the first year of life for healthy full-term infants is human milk. No available evidence shows that exceeding the amount of calcium retained by the exclusively breastfed full-term infant during the first 6 months of life or the amount retained by the human milk-fed infant given complementary foods during the second 6 months of life is beneficial to achieving long-term increases in bone mineralization. Cow milk-based formulas contain more calcium than does human milk. Relatively greater calcium concentrations are found in specialized formulas, such as soy formulas and casein hydrolysates, to account for the potential lower bioavailability of the calcium from these formulas relative to cow milk-based formula.[14] Of note is the fact that the fractional absorption of calcium from some formulas is similar to that of human milk. Thus, the much higher calcium content in such formulas may lead to greater net calcium retention in the formula-fed infant than in the breastfed infant.[34,35]

Some variations exist in the amount of calcium absorbed by infants from different formulas and the bone mineral mass accumulated during infancy.[36,37] Studies comparing the bone mineral content of full-term infants during the first year of life have generally found a slightly greater value for those fed infant formulas than those fed human milk, likely because of the usual greater net calcium retention as noted previously.[34,35,38] However, there are no data suggesting that such a difference is maintained through adolescence, and there is no evidence at present that these differences lead to clinically significant differences in bone mass.[39] Longer-term studies are needed to evaluate these issues, but at the present time, the bone mass of the breastfed infant remains the reference standard for appropriate bone mineral mass accumulation in infancy.

One should be cautious about using the Adequate Intake (AI) guidelines of the Institute of Medicine to determine the appropriate intake of calcium for formula-fed infants. The AI guidelines are specific to breastfed infants, and the AI value for calcium does not hold for infants who are not breastfed. The concentration of

IV

calcium (and phosphorus and the calcium-to-phosphorous ratio) in infant formulas is set by the Infant Formula Act, and there is no specific science-based rationale for specific AIs of calcium for formula-fed infants.[40] The IOM did not make any specific recommendations in this regard in its 2011 guidelines.[18]

Few data are available about the calcium requirements of children before puberty.[17] Calcium retention is relatively low in toddlers and slowly increases as puberty approaches. The benefits of intakes above the AI in this age group are uncertain. High levels of calcium intake may negatively affect other minerals, especially iron, although adaptation to this effect may occur.[41] Because these minerals are important for growth and development and may be marginal in toddlers and preschool-aged children, more data regarding the risks and benefits of higher calcium intake are needed before it can be recommended before puberty.

Perhaps of most importance in young children is the development of eating patterns that will be associated with adequate calcium intake later in life. As such, it is important that families learn to identify the calcium content of foods (see Appendix J) based on the food label and incorporate this information into their food-buying habits. The most readily available source of calcium (70%–80% of calcium content in US diets) is from dairy products, and the current dietary guidelines recommend 3 to 4 servings a day.

Preadolescents and Adolescents

The majority of research in children about calcium requirements has been directed toward 9- to 18-year-old females. The efficiency of calcium absorption is increased during puberty, and the majority of bone formation occurs during this period. Data from balance studies suggest that for most healthy children in this age range, an intake of 1300 mg/day will support optimal bone growth.[18,42] Virtually all the data used to establish this intake level are from white children; minimal data are available for other ethnic groups.

Numerous controlled trials have found an increase in the bone mineral content in children in this age group who have received calcium supplementation.[8,43-47] However, the available data suggest that if calcium intake is augmented only for relatively short periods (ie, 1 to 2 years), there may be minimal or no long-term benefits to establishing and maintaining a maximum peak bone mass.[48,49] Even longer-term increased intake of calcium may only lead to relatively small benefits in bone mass.[46] Recent results indicate that calcium supplementation may be more beneficial in some subgroups of children, such as those with early puberty or those of greater height.[46,50,51] The implications of such findings for dietary guidance are unclear. In general, the available data emphasize the importance of a well-balanced diet in achieving adequate calcium intake and in establishing dietary patterns with a calcium intake at or near recommended levels throughout childhood and adolescence.[17]

In addition to calcium intake, exercise is an important aspect of achieving maximal peak bone mass. There is evidence that childhood and adolescence may represent an important period for achieving long-lasting skeletal benefits from regular exercise.[45] Recent data support the possibility that a low bone mass may be a contributing factor to some fractures in children.[52]

Although virtually all data regarding the importance of calcium intake has focused on the bone health benefits, emerging evidence, both in adults and in some studies performed in children, suggest that calcium intake may be important in both blood pressure and weight regulation. However, some but not all evidence supports the conclusion that children who have an adequate intake of calcium are more likely to have an optimal weight for age.[53-55]

It is recommended that pediatricians actively discuss issues of bone health with families during routine visits. Recommended ages for such discussions are 2 to 3 years of age, 8 to 9 years of age, and then later during adolescence. An emphasis should be placed on preventing inadequate calcium intake, encouraging weight-bearing exercise, and ensuring adequate vitamin D status.[17]

Adolescent Pregnancy and Lactation

At birth, the fetus contains approximately 30 g of calcium. This represents approximately 2.5% of typical maternal body calcium stores.[14] Evidence suggests that, in adult women, much of this 30 g comes from increases in dietary calcium absorption during pregnancy.[56] A recent study demonstrated a similar increase in calcium absorption during pregnancy in adolescents.[57]

During lactation, a period of 6 months of exclusive breastfeeding would lead to an additional 45 g of calcium secreted by the mother. Although some of this is accounted for by decreased urinary calcium excretion during lactation, there is extensive evidence demonstrating a loss of maternal bone calcium during lactation.[58-60] In adult women, however, bone remineralization occurs after weaning, and neither pregnancy nor lactation is associated with persistent bone loss. Because of data demonstrating that calcium supplementation is not effective in preventing lactation-associated bone loss or enhancing postweaning bone mass recovery,[58] dietary recommendations do not suggest increases in calcium for healthy adult women who are pregnant or lactating above the 1000 mg/day RDA for nonlactating adult women.[18]

The situation for pregnant and lactating adolescents is less clear. Current guidelines do not recommend an increased intake above the age-appropriate maximum for adolescents (1300 mg/day) who are either pregnant or lactating.[8] Shorter femur length in the fetuses of pregnant African American adolescents with low dairy intake compared with those with higher intakes has been shown.[61] This is

IV

consistent with earlier similar data demonstrating a lower neonatal bone mineral density associated with low calcium intake during pregnancy in adults.[62]

At the present time, the available evidence supports the recommendation that the benefits of breastfeeding greatly outweigh any demonstrated risks to adolescents in terms of achieving either optimal growth or peak bone mass.[57,63] No available data suggest that calcium intakes above the recommended amounts are beneficial to pregnant or lactating adolescents. However, it should be noted that these recommended intake levels are far above those typical of the diet of even most nonpregnant adolescents.

Phosphorous Requirements

As with calcium, the recommended AI for phosphorus for infants was based on usual dietary intakes of breastfed infants. These values are 100 mg/day from ages 0 through 6 months and 275 mg/day from ages 7 through 12 months. The higher value in older infants reflects the considerable contribution of solid foods to usual phosphorus intakes of these infants. There are few data on which to base estimates of phosphorus requirements for older children. Dietary guidelines[8] used a factorial approach based on limited estimates of phosphorus absorption, excretion, and accretion to determine average requirements. An allotment of an additional 20% was provided to calculate the RDA. Using this method, values for the RDA of 460 mg/day for children 1 through 3 years of age and 500 mg/day for children 4 through 8 years of age were derived. These values are well below typical intakes for children of these ages, suggesting that deficient phosphorus intake is an uncommon problem in small children. Dietary requirements for phosphorus were not considered by the recent RDA committee evaluating calcium and vitamin D requirements.[18] Thus, the recommendations from 1997 were not changed (see Appendix E).

For adolescents, both the factorial method and estimates of intake needed to maintain typical serum phosphorus were used to determine RDAs. An RDA of 1250 mg/day was calculated for boys and girls ages 9 through 18 years.[8] This value is much closer to typical intake values for adolescents and reflects the rapid bone and muscle growth during this time period. No increase was added for pregnant or lactating adolescents (see Appendix E).

Magnesium Requirements

Current dietary guidelines for infants are based on the intakes of human milk-fed infants. The recommended AI is 30 mg/day for infants in the first 6 months of life and 75 mg/day from 7 through 12 months of age (see Appendix E). Commercial cow-milk based infant formulas are generally higher in magnesium concentration (40-50 mg/L) than is human milk (34 mg/L). Soy-based formulas may have even higher levels of magnesium (50-80 mg/L).[8,10] In a large series of studies, Fomon and Nelson reported approximately 40% absorption of magnesium in infants fed soy- or cow milk-based formulas (based on total intake of 53-59 mg/day) with a net retention of 9 to 10 mg/day.[8,14]

Few metabolic balance studies have been performed for magnesium in children, especially those 1 through 8 years of age. On the basis of limited available data, it appears that a magnesium intake of 5 mg/kg/day should lead to positive magnesium balances in most children. Using average weight-for-age data, this leads to an RDA of 80 mg/day for ages 1 through 3 years, 130 mg/day for ages 4 through 8 years, and 240 mg/day for 9 through 13 years. For adolescents ages 14 through 18 years, slightly greater average intakes are needed (5.3 mg/kg/day) to account for increased pubertal magnesium needs. Differences in average weights of boys and girls were used to calculate RDAs of 410 mg/day for boys and 360 mg/day for girls[8] (see Appendix E).

Because of efficient homeostatic mechanisms, especially renal conservation of magnesium, low dietary magnesium alone does not usually cause clinically apparent magnesium deficiency. Magnesium deficiency is, however, quite common in young children with protein-energy malnutrition, especially when accompanied by gastroenteritis. Muscle magnesium is depressed, but serum magnesium may be normal. Hypomagnesemia sometimes occurs in malabsorption syndromes, and magnesium depletion may develop in subjects with severe diarrhea. Convulsions are the most clearly documented feature of hypomagnesemia with or without total body magnesium deficiency in infants and young children. Neuropsychiatric disorders are well documented in magnesium-depleted adults. Hypocalcemia associated with magnesium deficiency may be the result of defective synthesis or release of parathyroid hormone. Hypokalemia also occurs secondarily to magnesium deficiency.[64]

Numerous conditions may be related to subacute magnesium deficiency, however. For example, recent evidence has also linked magnesium deficiency with insulin resistance and worsening diabetic regulation. Increased blood pressure, migraines, and inadequate bone mineralization may also be linked to habitually low magnesium intake, although data for these relationships continues to be incomplete.[8]

Dietary Sources: Calcium and Phosphorus

Knowledge of dietary calcium sources is a first step toward increasing the intake of calcium-rich foods. The largest source of dietary calcium for most people is milk

IV

and other dairy products. Most vegetables contain calcium, although at low density. Therefore, relatively large servings are needed to equal the total intake achieved with typical servings of dairy products. The bioavailability of calcium from vegetables is generally high. An exception is spinach, which is high in oxalate, making the calcium virtually nonbioavailable. Several products have been introduced that are fortified with calcium. These products, most notably orange juice, are fortified to achieve a calcium concentration similar to that of milk. Breakfast foods also are frequently fortified with minerals, including calcium. The gap between the recommended calcium intakes and the typical intakes of children and adolescents is substantial. A list of foods relatively high in calcium is given in Appendix J. Most adolescents, especially females, have calcium intakes below the recommended levels (see Table 18.1). Preoccupation with being thin is common in this age group, especially among females, as is the misconception that all dairy foods are fattening. Many children and adolescents are unaware that low-fat milk contains at least as much calcium as whole milk.[17]

Table 18.1.
Calcium Intake From the Diet and All Sources Compared with AI Recommendations Among Children in the United States, 2003-2006

					Calcium	
	Age group, y	n	AI	UL	Total Intake,[a] mg/d	% Above AI[b]
Males	1-3	758	500	2500	1008 ± 28.3	96 ± 1.0
	4-8	807	800	2500	1087 ± 31.0	83 ± 2.5
	9-13	1009	1300	2500	1093 ± 32.9	23 ± 4.2
	14-18	1351	1300	2500	1296 ± 41.1	42 ± 3.2
Females	1-3	745	500	2500	977 ± 28.1	97 ± 0.9
	4-8	869	800	2500	974 ± 27.1	67 ± 4.9
	9-13	1039	1300	2500	988 ± 47.1	15 ± 4.4
	14-18	1249	1300	2500	918 ± 29.7	13 ± 2.8

[a] Data are mean ± SE for total intake: food, water, antacids, and dietary supplements.

[b] Data are percent ± SE.

Adapted from Bailey RL, Dodd KW, Goldman JA, et al. Estimation of total usual calcium and vitamin D intakes in the United States. *J Nutr*. 2010;140(4):817-822.

For children with lactose intolerance, several alternatives exist. Lactose intolerance is more common in African-American, Mexican-American, and Asian-Pacific Islander individuals than in white individuals. Many children with lactose intolerance can drink small amounts of milk without discomfort. Other alternatives include the use of other dairy products, such as solid cheeses and yogurt, which may be better tolerated than milk. Lactose-free and low-lactose milks are available.

In general, dietary sources of calcium, including fortified foods, are preferred to calcium supplementation via pill or similar nondietary supplements because of the range of nutrients and the establishment of good dietary habits that are enhanced by use of natural dietary calcium sources. Furthermore, nutrient interactions may be decreased and tolerance may be greater for minerals provided from food sources.

Dietary Sources: Magnesium

Quantities in infant formulas range from 40 to 70 mg/L (3.3–5.8 mEq/L). Whole grains, beans, and legumes are good sources of magnesium. Because magnesium is a component of chlorophyll, green leafy vegetables are high in magnesium. Other dietary sources include milk, eggs, and meat. Depending on its "hardness," water may also significantly contribute to dietary magnesium intake.

References

1. Cohn SH, Vaswani A, Zanzi I, Aloia JF, Roginsky MS, Ellis KJ. Changes in body chemical composition with age measured by total-body neutron activation. *Metabolism.* 1976;25(1):85-95

2. Widdowson EM, Spray CM. Chemical development in utero. *Arch Dis Child.* 1951;26(127):205-214

3. Widdowson EM, McCance RA, Spray CM. The chemical composition of the human body. *Clin Sci.* 1951;10:113-125

4. Broadus AE. Physiological functions of calcium, magnesium, and phosphorus and mineral ion balance. In: Favus MJ, ed. *Primer on the Metabolic Bone Diseases and Disorders of Mineral Metabolism.* 5th ed. New York, NY: Raven Press; 2003:105-111

5. Salle BL, Delvin EE, Lapillonne A, Bishop NJ, Glorieux FH. Perinatal metabolism of vitamin D. *Am J Clin Nutr.* 2000;71(5 Suppl):1317S-1324S

6. Bronner F, Pansu D. Nutritional aspects of calcium absorption. *J Nutr.* 1999;129(1):9-12

7. Kim Y, Linkswiler HM. Effect of level of protein intake on calcium metabolism and on parathyroid and renal function in the adult human male. *J Nutr.* 1979;109(8):1399-1404

8. Institute of Medicine, Food and Nutrition Board. *Dietary Reference Intakes for Calcium, Phosphorus, Magnesium, Vitamin D, and Fluoride.* Washington, DC: National Academies Press; 1997

9. Specker BL, Mulligan L, Ho M. Longitudinal study of calcium intake, physical activity, and bone mineral content in infants 6-18 months of age. *J Bone Miner Res.* 1999;14(4):569-576

10. Abrams SA, Griffin IJ, Hawthorne KM, et al. Vitamin D receptor Fok1 polymorphisms affect calcium absorption, kinetics and bone mineralization rates during puberty. *J Bone Miner Res.* 2005;20(6):945-953

11. Wigertz K, Palacios C, Jackman LA, et al. Racial differences in calcium retention in response to dietary salt in adolescent girls. *Am J Clin Nutr.* 2005;81(4):845-50

12. Abrams SA, O'Brien KO, Liang LK, Stuff JE. Differences in calcium absorption and kinetics between black and white girls age 5-16 years. *J Bone Miner Res.* 1995;10(5):829-833

13. Hardwick LL, Jones MR, Brautbar N, Lee DB. Magnesium absorption: mechanisms and the influence of vitamin D, calcium, and phosphate. *J Nutr.* 1991;121(1):13-23

14. Fomon SJ, Nelson SE. Calcium, phosphorus, magnesium, and sulfur. In: Fomon SJ, ed. *Nutrition of Normal Infants.* St Louis, MO: Mosby-Year Book Inc; 1993:192-218

15. Shils ME. Magnesium in health and disease. *Annu Rev Nutr.* 1988;8:429-460

16. Yamamoto T, Kabata H, Yagi R, Takashima M, Itokawa Y. Primary hypomagnesemia with secondary hypocalcemia: report of a case and review of the world literature. *Magnesium.* 1985;4(2-3):153-164

17. Greer FR; Krebs NF; American Academy of Pediatrics, Committee on Nutrition. Optimizing bone health and calcium intakes of infants, children, and adolescents. *Pediatrics.* 2006;117(2):578-585

18. Institute of Medicine, Food and Nutrition Board. *Dietary Reference Intakes for Calcium and Vitamin D.* Washington, DC: The National Academies Press; 2011

19. Miller GD, Weaver CM. Required versus optimal intakes; a look at calcium. *J Nutr.* 1994;124(8 Suppl):1404S-1405S

20. Jackman LA, Millane SS, Martin BR, Wood OB, McCabe GP, Peacock M, Weaver CM. Calcium retention in relation to calcium intake and postmenarcheal age in adolescent females. *Am J Clin Nutr.* 1997;66(2):327-333

21. Abrams SA, Stuff JE. Calcium metabolism in girls: current dietary intakes lead to low rates of calcium absorption and retention during puberty. *Am J Clin Nutr.* 1994;60(5):739-743

22. Abrams SA, Grusak MA, Stuff J, O'Brien KO. Calcium and magnesium balance in 9-14-y-old children. *Am J Clin Nutr.* 1997;66(5):1172-1177

23. Abrams SA, Griffin IJ, Hicks PD, Gunn SK. Pubertal girls only partially adapt to low dietary calcium intakes. *J Bone Min Res.* 2004;19(5):759-763

24. Ellis KJ, Abrams SA, Wong WW. Body composition of a young, multiethnic female population. *Am J Clin Nutr.* 1997;65(3):724-731

25. Christiansen C, Rodbro P, Nielsen CT. Bone mineral content and estimated total body calcium in normal children and adolescents. *Scand J Clin Lab Invest.* 1975;35(6):507-510

26. Wren TA, Liu X, Pitukcheewanont P, Gilsanz V. Bone densitometry in pediatric populations: discrepancies in the diagnosis of osteoporosis by DXA and CT. *J Pediatr.* 2005;146(6):776-779

27. Atkinson SA. Human milk feeding of the micropremie. *Clin Perinatol.* 2000;27(1):235-247

28. Prestridge LL, Schanler RJ, Shulman RJ, Burns PA, Laine LL. Effect of parenteral calcium and phosphorus therapy on mineral retention and bone mineral content in very low birth weight infants. *J Pediatr.* 1993;122(5 Pt 1):761-768

29. Abrams SA: American Academy of Pediatrics. Calcium and vitamin D requirements of enterally fed preterm infants. *Pediatrics.* 2013;131(5):e1676-e1683

30. Carver JD, Wu PY, Hall RT, et al. Growth of preterm infants fed nutrient-enriched or term formula after hospital discharge. *Pediatrics.* 2001;107(4):683-689

31. Hawthorne KM, Griffin IJ, Abrams SA. Nutritional approaches to the care of preterm infants. *Minerva Pediatr.* 2004;56(4):359-372

32. Lapillonne A, Salle BL, Glorieux FH, Claris O. Bone mineralization and growth are enhanced in preterm infants fed an isocaloric, nutrient-enriched preterm formula through term. *Am J Clin Nutr.* 2004;80(6):1595-1603

33. Almone A, Rovet J, Ward W, et al. Growth and body composition of human milk-fed premature infants provided with extra energy and nutrients early after hospital discharge:1-year follow-up. *J Pediatr Gastroenterol Nutr.* 2009;49(4):456-466

34. Abrams SA, Griffin IJ, Davila PM. Calcium and zinc absorption from lactose-containing and lactose-free infant formulas. *Am J Clin Nutr.* 2002;76(2):442-446

35. Abrams SA, Wen J, Stuff JE. Absorption of calcium, zinc and iron from breast milk by 5- to 7-month-old infants. *Pediatr Res.* 1997;41(3):384-390

36. Nelson SE, Frantz JA, Ziegler EE. Absorption of fat and calcium by infants fed a milk-based formula containing palm-olein. *J Am Coll Nutr.* 1998;17(4):327–333

37. Koo WW, Hammami M, Margeson DP, Nwaesei C, Montalto MB, Lasekan JB. Reduced bone mineralization in infants fed palm olein-containing formula: a randomized, double-blinded, prospective trial. *Pediatrics.* 2003;111(5 Pt 1):1017-1023

38. Specker BL, Beck A, Kalkwarf H, Ho M. Randomized trial of varying mineral intake on total body bone mineral accretion during the first year of life. *Pediatrics.* 1997;99(6):e12

39. Young RJ, Antonson DL, Ferguson PW, Murray ND, Merkel K, Moore TE. Neonatal and infant feeding: effect on bone density at 4 years. *J Pediatr Gastroenterol Nutr.* 2005;41(1):88-93

40. Abrams SA. What are the risks and benefits to increasing dietary bone minerals and vitamin D intake in infants and small children? *Annu Rev Nutr.* 2011;31:285-297

41. Ames SK, Gorham BM, Abrams SA. Effects of high vs low calcium intake on calcium absorption and red blood cell iron incorporation by small children. *Am J Clin Nutr.* 1999;70(1):44-48

42. Vatanparast H, Bailey DA, Baxter-Jones AD, Whiting SJ. Calcium requirements for bone growth in Canadian boys and girls during adolescence. *Br J Nutr.* 2010;103(4):575–580

43. Lloyd T, Andon MB, Rollings N, et al. Calcium supplementation and bone mineral density in adolescent girls. *JAMA.* 1993;270(7):841-844

44. Lee WTK, Leung SSF, Leung DMY, Cheng JCY. A follow-up study on the effects of calcium-supplement withdrawal and puberty on bone acquisition of children. *Am J Clin Nutr.* 1996;64(1):71-77

45. Lloyd T, Petit MA, Lin HM, Beck TJ. Lifestyle factors and the development of bone mass and bone strength in young women. *J Pediatr.* 2004;144(6):776-782

46. Matkovic V, Goel PK, Badenhop-Stevens NE, et al. Calcium supplementation and bone mineral density in females from childhood to young adulthood: a randomized controlled trial. *Am J Clin Nutr.* 2005;81(1):175-188

IV

47. Matkovic V, Landoll JD, Badenhop-Stevens NE, et al. Nutrition influences skeletal development from childhood to adulthood: a study of hip, spine, and forearm in adolescent females. *J Nutr.* 2004;134(3):701S-705S

48. Lanou AJ, Berkow SE, Barnard ND. Calcium, dairy products, and bone health in children and young adults: a reevaluation of the evidence. *Pediatrics.* 2005;115(3):736-743

49. Abrams SA. Calcium supplementation during childhood: long-term benefits on bone mineralization. *Nutr Rev.* 2005;63(7):251-255

50. Abrams SA, Griffin IJ, Hawthorne KM, Liang L. Height and height Z-score are related to calcium absorption in 5 to 15 yr-old girls. *J Clin Endocrinol Metab.* 2005;90(9):5077-5081

51. Ferrari SL, Chevalley T, Bonjour JP, Rizzoli R. Childhood fractures are associated with decreased bone mass gain during puberty: an early marker of persistent bone fragility? *J Bone Miner Res.* 2006;21(4):501-507

52. Goulding A, Cannan R, Williams SM, Gold EJ, Taylor RW, Lewis-Barned NJ. Bone mineral density in girls with forearm fractures. *J Bone Miner Res.* 1998;13(1):143-148

53. Dixon LB, Pellizzon MA, Jawad AF, Tershakovec AM. Calcium and dairy intake and measures of obesity in hyper- and normocholesterolemic children. *Obes Res.* 2005;13(10):1727-1738

54. Huang TT, McCrory MA. Dairy intake, obesity, and metabolic health in children and adolescents: knowledge and gaps. *Nutr Rev.* 2005;63(3):71-80

55. Lorenzen JK, Molgaard C, Michaelsen KF, Astrup A. Calcium supplementation for 1 y does not reduce body weight or fat mass in young girls. *Am J Clin Nutr.* 2006;83(1):18-23

56. Heaney RP, Skillman TG. Calcium metabolism in normal human pregnancy. *J Clin Endocrinol Metab.* 1971;33(4):661-670

57. O'Brien KO, Nathanson MS, Mancini J, Witter FR. Calcium absorption is significantly higher in adolescents during pregnancy than in the early postpartum period. *Am J Clin Nutr.* 2003;78(6):1188-1193

58. Kalkwarf HJ, Specker BL, Bianchi DC, Ranz J, Ho M. The effect of calcium supplements on bone density during lactation and after weaning. *N Engl J Med.* 1997;337(8):523-528

59. Kalkwarf HJ, Specker BL. Bone mineral loss during lactation and recovery after weaning. *Obstet Gynecol.* 1995;86(1):26-32

60. Hopkinson JM, Butte NF, Ellis K, Smith EO. Lactation delays postpartum bone mineral accretion and temporarily alters its regional distribution in women. *J Nutr.* 2000;130(4):777-783

61. Chang SC, O'Brien KO, Nathanson MS, Caulfield LE, Mancini J, Witter FR. Fetal femur length is influenced by maternal diary intake in pregnant African American adolescents. *Am J Clin Nutr.* 2003;77(5):1248-1254

62. Koo WW, Walters JC, Esterlitz J, Levine RJ, Bush AJ, Sibai B. Maternal calcium supplementation and fetal bone mineralization. *Obstet Gynecol.* 1999;94(4):577-584

63. Bezerra FF, Mendonca LM, Lobato EC, O'Brien KO, Donangelo CM. Bone mass is recovered from lactation to postweaning in adolescent mothers with low calcium intakes. *Am J Clin Nutr.* 2004;80(5):1322-1326

64. Rude RK. Magnesium deficiency: a cause of heterogeneous disease in humans. *J Bone Miner Res.* 1998;13(4):749-758

Chapter 19

Iron

Introduction

Iron deficiency (ID) and iron deficiency anemia (IDA) continue to be of worldwide concern. Among children in the developing world, iron is the most common single-nutrient deficiency.[1] Even in industrialized countries, despite a demonstrable decline in prevalence, IDA remains a common cause of anemia in young children.[2] Even more important is that even ID without anemia may adversely affect long-term neurodevelopment and behavior, and some of these effects may be irreversible.[3,4] In November 2010, the Committee on Nutrition of the American Academy of Pediatrics (AAP) issued its first-ever clinical report concerning the iron needs of infants and young children.[5] Previous statements dealt almost exclusively with the iron content of infant formula.[6,7] The new clinical report advocated for iron fortification of infant formulas and iron supplementation for breastfed infants and toddlers. It also recommended routine monitoring of iron status at 12 months of age. The report suggested that toddlers found to be iron deficient should be treated with iron supplements and that these toddlers should be followed until their deficiency resolves.[5] Although the report came at a time when ID and IDA are at a nadir among children in the United States, ID occurs in 6.6% to 15.2% of toddlers, and IDA occurs in 0.9% to 4.4% of toddlers, depending on race/ethnicity and socioeconomic status.[8] The reason for these precautions now, when ID as a cause of anemia among children appears to be waning, is the growing amount of information pointing to subtle behavioral and developmental consequences of ID, even without anemia. These deficits seem to persist for decades, if not for life.[3,4,9,10]

Iron Metabolism

Iron is a highly regulated metal. Absorption occurs in the apical surfaces of the enterocytes of the duodenum. Heme iron is transported into the enterocyte via the recently described heme carrier protein 1 (HCP1),[11] although it is less likely to be relevant in newborn infants exclusively fed human milk or infant formula without heme iron. The exact pathway is incompletely described, although the heme oxygenase enzyme known to free iron from the protoporphyrin ring is present in the microsomal fraction of the enterocyte.[12] More is known about the absorption of nonheme iron (iron 3+ or ferric iron), relevant to the exclusively breastfed or formula-fed infant. One pathway involves the reduction of iron 3+ to iron 2+ (ferrous iron) at the enterocyte brush border via the enzyme duodenal ferric reductase. Subsequently, the divalent metal transporter 1 (DMT-1) shuttles the iron 2+ across the apical membrane.[13,14] Once iron enters the enterocyte, it can be stored as ferritin for later use in the mitochondria or sloughed into the lumen with the senescent enterocyte. Alternatively, the intracellular nonheme iron can be exported across the basolateral membrane after oxidation via the nonheme iron transporter, ferroportin, into the villus capillary circulation. In addition to enterocytes, ferroportin is an important exporter of intracellular iron from hepatocytes and macrophages.[13,14] Once in circulation, iron is transported bound to transferrin to the site of use or storage. Erythrocyte precursors express high levels of transferrin receptor 1 (TfR1) and, thus, have preferred access to circulating iron. Another source of iron, the senescent erythrocytes, are taken up by macrophages, and iron is made available for use or storage. This is especially true right after birth. Macrophages export the recovered iron via ferroportin, the same transporter found on duodenal enterocytes. Iron is stored in the liver, which takes up the absorbed iron from the portal system via TfR1.[15]

Another important aspect of regulation of body iron is the communication that is needed between transport and storage iron and the cells that consume iron, such as erythrocyte precursors. This communication is mediated by hepcidin, an antimicrobial peptide synthesized in hepatocytes, and the major negative feedback regulator of iron homeostasis—for example, when erythrocyte precursors do not need iron, hepcidin induces internalization and degradation of enterocyte ferroportin, which then limits the entry of iron into the extracellular fluid and villus capillaries. On the other hand, low levels of hepcidin lead to increased activity of ferroportin and increased iron absorption by intestinal enterocytes. How exactly hepcidin expression is in turn regulated, especially in human development, is unknown at this time.[13]

It is clear that the human body is able to prioritize available iron both between and within organs. As iron is prioritized to erythrocytes, its role in oxygen transport is clearly its most critical function. When iron is deficient in the breastfed infant, hepatic stores are depleted first, followed by other lower-priority tissues, such as skeletal muscle and intestine. With a greater degree of iron deficiency, cardiac iron is compromised, followed by brain iron, and finally erythrocyte iron. Thus, IDA represents a severe form of ID, and the prioritization of iron for erythrocytes even over the brain accounts for the adverse neurodevelopmental effects seen in ID without anemia, as is seen in infants after 4 to 6 months of age who were not receiving supplemental iron. Intraorgan prioritization also occurs, and this has been demonstrated in the developing rat brain, with selective hippocampal and cortical vulnerability to perinatal iron deficiency, resulting in critical loss of recognition memory.[16]

Nutritional Requirements for Iron

Iron requirements of healthy children have been established by the Institute of Medicine (IOM) and published in the Dietary Reference Intakes (DRIs).[17] These values are given in Table 19.1. The strengths of the recommendations are listed in the first column. When the recommendation is based on sound and adequate scientific evidence, a Recommended Dietary Allowance (RDA) is given. If sufficient scientific evidence is lacking, the best estimate based on the available information is listed as the Adequate Intake (AI). Both the RDA and the AI should supply adequate amounts of the nutrient to cover the needs of almost all (97%-98%) healthy individuals. Levels of iron intake are given in mg of elemental iron per day.

Table 19.1.
Dietary Recommended Intake: Iron

Strength of Recommendation	Age	Gender	Level of Iron Intake[a]
AI	0-6 mo	Male and female	0.27 mg/day
RDA	7-12 mo	Male and female	11 mg/day
RDA	1-3 y	Male and female	7 mg/day
RDA	4 8 y	Male and female	10 mg/day
RDA	9-13 y	Male	8 mg/day
RDA	9-13 y	Female	8 mg/day
RDA	14-18 y	Male	11 mg/day
RDA	14-18 y	Female	15 mg/day

AI indicates Adequate Intake; RDA, Recommended Dietary Allowance.

[a] Iron is given in milligrams of elemental iron.

Source: Institute of Medicine, Food and Nutrition Board. *Dietary Reference Intakes for Vitamin A, Vitamin K, Arsenic, Boron, Chromium, Copper, Iodine, Iron, Manganese, Molybdenum, Nickel, Silicon, Vanadium, and Zinc.* Washington, DC: National Academies Press; 2003.

Full-Term Infants

Infants born at term have sufficient iron stores to last until 4 to 6 months of age, largely because of high hemoglobin (Hb) concentrations and high blood volume in proportion to body weight. They experience a physiological decline in both blood volume and Hb concentration during the first months of life, which diminishes the requirement for iron and likely accounts for the low iron content of human milk— on average, 0.35 mg/L. The iron concentration of human milk is also variable from day to day and it varies from mother to mother. The IOM used the average iron content of human milk and an average intake of human milk (0.78 L/day) to determine the AI of 0.27 mg/day for the full-term breastfed infant through 6 months of age[17] (Table 19.1). The IOM recommendations, however, do not take into account infants who are born with lower-than-usual iron stores (low birth weight infants, infants of diabetic mothers).[18] A number of studies have shown that exclusively breastfed infants supplemented with iron before 6 months of age have higher Hb concentrations at 6 months of age compared with peers who did not receive iron supplementation.[19,20] Supplementation also resulted in improved visual acuity and higher Bayley psychomotor developmental indices by 13 months of age.[19] These were some of the reasons the AAP recommended that all exclusively breastfed term infants receive an iron supplementation of 1 mg/kg/day starting at 4 months of age and continuing until appropriate iron-containing complementary foods are introduced[5] (Table 19.2 and Appendix K). For partially breastfed infants, the proportion of human milk versus formula is uncertain. Therefore, the AAP has recommended that, beginning at 4 months of age, infants receiving more than one half of their daily feedings as human milk and who are not receiving iron-containing complementary foods should also receive 1 mg/kg/day of supplemental iron. These AAP recommendations will ensure that breastfeeding infants will not be affected by iron deficiency.[5]

Table 19.2.
Foods That Help Prevent Iron Deficiency

Table Food	Iron (mg of Elemental Iron)
Selected Heme Iron Sources	
Clams, canned, drained solids, 3 oz	23.8
Chicken liver, cooked, simmered, 3 oz	9.9
Oysters, Eastern canned, 3 oz	5.7
Beef liver, cooked, braised, 3 oz	5.6
Shrimp, cooked moist heat, 3 oz	2.6
Beef, composite of trimmed cuts, lean only, all grades, cooked, 3 oz	2.5
Sardines, Atlantic, canned in oil, drained solids with bone, 3 oz	2.5
Turkey, all classes, dark meat, roasted, 3 oz	2.0
Lamb, domestic, composite of trimmed retail cuts, separable lean only, choice, cooked, 3 oz	1.7
Fish, tuna, light, canned in water, drained solids, 3 oz	1.3
Chicken, broiler or fryer, dark meat, roasted, 3 oz	1.1
Turkey, all classes, light meat, roasted, 3 oz	1.1
Veal, composite of trimmed cuts, lean only, cooked, 3 oz	1.0
Chicken, broiler or fryer, breast, roasted, 3 oz	0.9
Pork, composite of trimmed cuts (leg, loin, shoulder), lean only, cooked, 3 oz	0.9
Fish, salmon, pink, cooked, 3 oz	0.8

Table Food	Iron (mg of Elemental Iron)
Commercial Baby Food[a]	
Meat	
Baby food, lamb, junior, 1 jar (2.5 oz)	1.2
Baby food, chicken, strained, 1 jar (2.5 oz)	1.0
Baby food, lamb, strained, 1 jar (2.5 oz)	0.8
Baby food, beef, junior, 1 jar (2.5 oz)	0.7
Baby food, beef, strained, 1 jar (2.5 oz)	0.7
Baby food, chicken, junior, 1 jar (2.5 oz)	0.7
Baby food, pork, strained, 1 jar (2.5 oz)	0.7
Baby food, ham, strained, 1 jar (2.5 oz)	0.7
Baby food, ham, junior, 1 jar (2.5 oz)	0.7
Baby food, turkey, strained, 1 jar (2.5 oz)	0.5
Baby food, veal, strained, 1 jar (2.5 oz)	0.5
Selected Nonheme Iron Sources	
Oatmeal, instant, fortified, cooked, 1 cup	14.0
Blackstrap molasses,[b] 2 tbsp	7.4
Tofu, raw, regular, ½ cup	6.7
Wheat germ, toasted, ½ cup	5.1
Ready-to-eat cereal, fortified at different levels, 1 cup	approx 4.5 to 18
Soybeans, mature seeds, cooked, boiled, ½ cup	4.4
Apricots, dehydrated (low moisture), uncooked, ½ cup	3.8
Sunflower seeds, dried, ½ cup	3.7
Lentils, mature seeds, cooked, ½ cup	3.3
Spinach, cooked, boiled, drained, ½ cup	3.2
Chickpeas, mature seeds, cooked, ½ cup	2.4
Prunes, dehydrated (low moisture), uncooked, ½ cup	2.3
Lima beans, large, mature seeds, cooked, ½ cup	2.2
Navy beans, mature seeds, cooked, ½ cup	2.2
Kidney beans, all types, mature seeds, cooked, ½ cup	2.0
Molasses, 2 tbsp	1.9
Pinto beans, mature seeds, cooked, ½ cup	1.8

IV

Table 19.2. *(continued)*
Foods That Help Prevent Iron Deficiency

Table Food	Iron (mg of Elemental Iron)
Selected Nonheme Iron Sources *(continued)*	
Raisins, seedless, packed, ½ cup	1.6
Prunes, dehydrated (low moisture), stewed, ½ cup	1.6
Prune juice, canned, 4 fluid oz	1.5
Green peas, cooked, boiled, drained, ½ cup	1.2
Enriched white rice, long grain, regular, cooked, ½ cup	1.0
Whole egg, cooked (fried or poached), 1 large egg	0.9
Enriched spaghetti, cooked, ½ cup	0.9
White bread, commercially prepared, 1 slice	0.9
Whole wheat bread, commercially prepared, 1 slice	0.7
Spaghetti or macaroni, whole wheat, cooked, ½ cup	0.7
Peanut butter, smooth style, 2 tbsp	0.6
Brown rice, medium grain, cooked, ½ cup	0.5
Commercial Baby Food[a]	
Vegetables	
Baby food, green beans, junior, 1 jar (6 oz)	1.8
Baby food, peas, strained, 1 jar (3.4 oz)	0.9
Baby food, green beans, strained, 1 jar (4 oz)	0.8
Baby food, spinach, creamed, strained, 1 jar (4 oz)	0.7
Baby food, sweet potatoes, junior (6 oz)	0.7
Cereals	
Baby food, brown rice cereal, dry, instant, 1 tbsp	1.8
Baby food, oatmeal cereal, dry, 1 tbsp	1.6
Baby food, rice cereal, dry, 1 tbsp	1.2
Baby food, barley cereal, dry, 1 tbsp	1.1
Selected Good Vitamin C Sources	
Fruits	**Vegetables**
Citrus fruits (eg, orange, tangerine, grapefruit)	Green, red, and yellow peppers
Pineapples	Broccoli

Selected Good Vitamin C Sources	
Fruits	**Vegetables**
Fruit juices enriched with vitamin C	Tomatoes
Strawberries	Cabbages
Cantaloupe	Potatoes
Kiwifruit	Leafy green vegetables
Raspberries	Cauliflower

[a] Baby food values are generally based on generic jar, not branded jar; 3 oz table-food meat = 85 g; a 2.5-oz jar of baby food = 71 g (an infant would not be expected to eat 3 oz [approximately the size of a deck of cards] of pureed table meat at a meal).

[b] Source of iron value was obtained from a manufacturer of this type of molasses.

Note: Figures are rounded. Source of iron values in foods: US Department of Agriculture, Agricultural Research Service. *USDA National Nutrient Database for Standard Reference, Release 20*. Nutrient Data Laboratory Home Page. Available at: http://www.nal.usda.gov/fnic/foodcomp/search/. Accessed July 29, 2011.

For infants 7 to 12 months of age, the RDA for iron is 11 mg/day[17] (Table 19.1). This was determined by a factorial approach from the amount of iron lost (skin, intestinal track, urine) and amount of iron required for the increased blood volume, for increased tissue mass, and for storage iron in the second 6 months of life. The disjuncture that occurs when going from 0.27 mg/day to 11 mg/day by 6 months of age results from the very different methods of determining these values (see Table 19.1). Infants in the second 6 months of life would not need iron supplements if they were receiving adequate amounts of iron from formula or appropriate amounts of iron-rich complementary foods[5] (Table 19.2). Meats containing heme iron should be encouraged, not only for their increased amount of iron absorption (20%-35%),[21] but also because they contain other minerals, including zinc.

Full-term, formula-fed infants do not need additional iron. For the last 20 years, routinely fed infant formulas in the United States have contained 12 mg of iron/L. This amount was calculated to supply all of the exogenous iron requirements of a normal formula-fed full-term infant for the first year of life. Because a normal infant has iron sources other than formula (especially cereal and meats), the 12 mg/L iron formula appears to supply more iron than is necessary.[5] Concerns have been expressed that this amount of iron may have associated risks; however, it is the conclusion of the AAP that infant formula containing 12 mg of elemental iron/L is safe for its intended use.[5] Although there is some concern about linear growth in in iron-replete infants given medicinal iron, no published studies have convincingly documented decreased linear growth in iron-replete infants receiving formulas containing high amounts of iron.[22] Evidence is also insufficient to associate formulas containing 12 mg of iron/L with gastrointestinal tract symptoms. At least 4 studies have shown no adverse effects.[23-26] Reports have conflicted on whether iron fortification is associated with increased risk of infection. Decreased incidence, increased incidence, and no change in number of infections have all been reported.[27,28] A recent systematic review concluded that "iron supplementation has no apparent harmful effect on the overall incidence of infectious illnesses in children, though it slightly increases the risk of developing diarrhea."[29]

Preterm Infants

Accretion of iron occurs predominantly in the last 3 months of intrauterine life; therefore, preterm infants lack sufficient iron. This iron deficit increases with decreasing gestational age. Additional factors that negatively affect iron status at birth include intrauterine growth restriction, maternal anemia, hypertension, and maternal diabetes. To complicate the issue, postnatal events can drastically alter the infant's iron status. Sick preterm infants undergo frequent blood sampling. If not compensated for, this can further deplete body iron. The use of erythropoietin to avoid transfusions can dramatically increase the need for exogenous iron. On the other hand, sick preterm infants frequently receive multiple blood transfusions that can result in iron overload. How the iron should be supplied, how much iron should be supplied, and in what form it should be supplied are all relatively unknown and vary from infant to infant. This makes establishing recommendations difficult. The AAP has recommended that all preterm infants have an intake of iron of at least 2 mg/kg/day through 12 months of age, which is the amount of iron supplied by iron-fortified formulas.[5] Despite the use of iron-containing formulas, 14% of preterm infants develop ID between 4 and 8 months of age.[30] Preterm infants fed human milk should receive an iron supplement of 2 mg/kg/day by 1 month of age, and this should be continued until infants are weaned to iron-fortified formula or begin eating complementary foods that supply 2 mg/kg/day of iron. An exception to this practice would be infants who have received an iron load from multiple transfusions of packed red blood cells during their hospitalization.[5]

Toddlers 1 Through 3 Years of Age

Toddlers 1 through 3 years of age should have an intake of iron of 7 mg/day[17] (Table 19.1). Toddlers go through many dietary changes that affect their iron status. In their transition from "infant food" to more adult-like food, they leave behind iron-fortified formula and cereal, but they gain a variety of naturally iron-containing foods, such as meats and some vegetables, which should be encouraged (Table 19.2). Fruits containing vitamin C, which augments iron absorption, should also be encouraged. Many toddlers are labeled as "picky eaters," and their food choices may select against iron-rich foods. Therefore, the iron status of toddlers is variable and not predictable. "At-risk" characteristics include low socioeconomic status, Mexican-American heritage, history of prematurity, early introduction of cow milk, and poor growth.[5] Because of a these uncertainties, universal screening of toddlers for ID at approximately 12 months of age is recommended by the AAP.[5]

ID and lead poisoning are associated in this age group. IDA increases lead absorption and hinders lead chelation. Correction of ID restores response to chelation and returns lead absorption to normal. Thus, primary ID prevention could act to reduce the risk of lead intoxication as well. This prospect is all the more important as very low concentrations of lead have been shown to be neurotoxic.[31] For toddlers not receiving 7 mg/day of iron or who are at risk of ID, liquid supplements are suitable for children 12 to 36 months of age, and chewable vitamins can be used for children 3 years and older.[5]

AAP

Diagnosis and Prevention of Iron Deficiency and Iron-Deficiency Anemia in Infants and Young Children (0-3 Years of Age)

1. Full-term, healthy infants have sufficient iron for at least the first 4 months of life. Human milk contains very little iron. Exclusively breastfed infants are at increasing risk of ID after 4 completed months of age. Therefore, at 4 months of age, breastfed infants should be supplemented with 1 mg/kg/day of oral iron beginning at 4 months of age until appropriate iron-containing complementary foods (including iron-fortified cereals) are introduced in the diet (see Table 19.3). For partially breastfed infants, the proportion of human milk versus formula is uncertain; therefore, beginning at 4 months of age, partially breastfed infants (more than half of their daily feedings as human milk) who are not receiving iron-containing complementary foods should also receive 1 mg/kg/day of supplemental iron.

2. For formula-fed infants, the iron needs for the first 12 months of life can be met by a standard infant formula (iron content, 10-12 mg/dL) and the introduction of iron-containing complementary foods after 4 to 6 months of age, including iron-fortified cereals (Table 19.3). Whole milk should not be used before 12 completed months of age.

3. The iron intake between 6 and 12 months of age should be 11 mg/day. When infants are given complementary foods, red meat and vegetables with higher iron content should be introduced early (Table 19.3). To augment the iron supply, liquid iron supplements are appropriate if iron needs are not being met by the intake of formula and complementary foods.

4. Toddlers 1 through 3 years of age should have an intake of iron intake of 7 mg/day. This would be best delivered by eating red meats, cereals fortified with iron, vegetables that contain iron, and fruits with vitamin C, which augments the absorption of iron (Table 19.3). For toddlers not receiving this iron intake, liquid supplements are suitable for children 12 through 36 months of age, and chewable multivitamins can be used for children 3 years and older.

5. All preterm infants should have an intake of iron of at least 2 mg/kg/day through 12 months of age, which is the amount of iron supplied by iron-fortified formulas. Preterm infants fed human milk should receive an iron supplement of 2 mg/kg/day by 1 month of age, and this should be continued until the infant is weaned to iron-fortified formula or begins eating complementary foods that supply the 2 mg/kg of iron. An exception to this practice would include infants who have received an iron load from multiple transfusions of packed red blood cells during their hospitalization.

6. Universal screening for anemia should be performed at approximately 12 months of age with determination of Hb concentration and an assessment of risk factors associated with ID/IDA. These risk factors would include low socioeconomic status (especially children of Mexican-American descent [Table 19.1]), a history of prematurity or low birth weight, exposure to lead, exclusive breastfeeding beyond 4 months of age without supplemental iron, and weaning to whole milk or complementary foods that do not include iron-fortified cereals or foods naturally rich in iron (Table 19.3). Additional at-risk factors are feeding problems, poor growth, and inadequate nutrition, typically seen in infants with special health care needs. For infants and toddlers (1 through 3 years of age), additional screening can be performed at any time if there is a risk of ID/IDA, including inadequate dietary iron intake.

7. If Hb concentration is less than 11.0 mg/dL at 12 months of age, then further evaluation for IDA is required to rule this out as a cause of anemia. If there is a high risk of dietary iron deficiency as described in recommendation 6, then further testing for ID should be performed, given the potential adverse effects on neurodevelopmental outcomes. Additional screening tests for ID or IDA should include:
   - serum ferritin (SF) and C-reactive protein concentration (CRP); or
   - reticulocyte hemoglobin concentration (CHr)

8. If a child has mild anemia (Hb 10-11 mg/dL) and can be closely monitored, an alternative method of diagnosis would be to document a 1 g/dL increase in plasma Hb concentration after 1 month of appropriate iron replacement therapy, especially if the history indicates that the diet is likely to be iron deficient.

9. Use of the TfR1 assay as screening for ID is promising, and the AAP supports the development of TfR1 standards for use of this assay in infants and children.

10. If IDA (or any anemia) or ID has been confirmed by history and laboratory evidence, a means of carefully tracking and following infants and toddlers with a diagnosis of ID/IDA should be implemented. Electronic health records could be used not only to generate reminder messages to screen for IDA and ID at 12 months of age but also to document that IDA and ID have been adequately treated once diagnosed.

Baker RD, Greer FG; American Academy of Pediatrics, Committee on Nutrition. Diagnosis and prevention of iron deficiency and iron-deficiency anemia in infants and young children (0–3 years of age) *Pediatrics.* 2010;126(5):1040-1050

School-Aged Children Four Through Eight Years of Age

The recommended iron intake for this age group is 10 mg/day.[17] All of the risk factors for an iron-deficient diet during the toddler years persist, plus there is increasing independence in food choices and decreasing supervision of meals and snacks. Thus, risk of ID and IDA continues. Iron-containing foods need to be encouraged, and this may be best accomplished by limiting foods available in the household to those of high iron content and high in ascorbic acid to promote iron absorption (Table 19.2). If anemia or an iron-deficient diet is suspected, these children should be screened by measuring Hb concentration. Low Hb concentration should be investigated further for type and cause of anemia (see Screening for ID and IDA). ID should be treated with iron supplements and followed to resolution.

School-Aged Children 9 Through 13 Years of Age

The recommended iron intake for this age group is 8 mg/day (Table 19.1). School-aged children have a lot of discretion in food selection. Skipped meals are common. Some children eat almost all of their food outside the home. Breakfast, lunch, and snacks are available at school and at after-school activities. Eating on the go or at fast food restaurants can become the norm. These circumstances can result in poor nutrition and little parental supervision of the quality and content of meals (see Chapter 8: Adolescent Nutrition). Some children in this age group will be entering a phase of rapid growth. Iron needs in this group must take into account basal losses, increase in Hb mass, increase in tissue/muscle mass, and menstrual loss in adolescent girls. Thus, increased demands may exceed what is available in the diet and deplete iron stores. There is a wide range of actual iron needs in this group, reflecting their heterogeneity. Some, but not all, individuals will have entered their adolescent growth spurt. Some girls will have reached menarche. For those who are

IV

menstruating, the quantity of iron lost during menstruation varies widely. Foods of high iron content should be encouraged (Table 19.2). If ID is suspected, especially if the child follows an alternative diet, such as vegetarian or vegan, or if the diet is of poor overall quality, the adolescent should be screened for anemia (see Screening for ID and IDA). If the Hb concentration is low, further investigations to define the type of anemia and search for an underlying cause should be undertaken, including ID. ID should be treated and followed to resolution.

Adolescents 14 Through 18 Years of Age

Iron needs in this group must take into account basal losses, increase in hemoglobin mass, increase in muscle mass, and menstrual loss in adolescent girls. The risk of iron deficiency in girls of this age is significantly higher than the risk in boys, not only because of menstrual losses but also because of food preferences and lifestyle. Girls are more likely than boys to avoid meat and are more likely than boys to adhere to alternative diets that may be deficient in iron (see Chapter 8: Adolescent Nutrition). Thus, the RDA for iron in this age group is 11 mg for males and 15 mg for females (Table 19.1). There is a tendency for all teenagers, boys as well as girls, to skip breakfast, thereby missing out on iron-fortified cereal and orange juice that increases iron absorption. ID without anemia may be important as it has been demonstrated that iron fortification in this group improved verbal learning and memory.[32] A decrease in aerobic capacity has also been documented among iron deficient, nonanemic girls.[33] Many males and females in this group are involved in vigorous athletic activities. Adequate iron will improve their performance, however, especially early in training, "sports anemia" has been described and is unresponsive to iron supplementation.[34] Healthy diets, regular meals, including foods that are iron rich should be encouraged (Table 19.2). Adolescents with restricted diets and unhealthy eating patterns should be screened for anemia (see below). Anemia, when identified, should be characterized and treated. IDA should be followed until resolution.

Screening for ID and IDA

Iron status varies from a mild ID to a deficiency severe enough to result in life-threatening anemia. It also includes iron overload that, in the context of overdose, can also be life threatening. ID and IDA are attributable to an imbalance between iron needs and available iron. This may result in a deficiency of mobilizable iron stores and is accompanied by changes in laboratory measurements that include Hb concentration, mean corpuscular Hb concentration, mean corpuscular volume, reticulocyte Hb concentration (abbreviated in the literature as CHr), total iron-binding capacity, transferrin saturation, serum ferritin concentration, and serum TfR1 concentration. The characteristics of tests that are used to describe iron status are listed in Table 19.3.

Table 19.3.
Measurement of Iron Status

Parameter	Iron Overload	Depleted Iron Stores	ID Without Anemia	IDA
SF	↑	↓	↓	↓↓
Transferrin saturation	↑↑	Normal	↓	↓
TfR1	↓	↑	↑↑	↑↑↑
CHr	Normal	↓	↓	↓
Hemoglobin	Normal	Normal	Normal	↓
MCV	Normal	Normal	Normal	↓

SF indicates serum ferritin; CHr, reticulocyte hemoglobin concentration; MCV, mean corpuscular volume.

No single test value will completely characterize iron status. A set of tests is required to establish the iron status of an individual. Each set of tests requires interpretation. The tests most easily obtained are a Hb concentration to establish presence of anemia, serum ferritin concentration to suggest iron as the cause of the anemia, and a CRP to ensure that an elevated serum ferritin concentration is truly attributable to lack of iron and not secondary to an inflammatory state. These 3 tests are widely available and relatively easy to interpret. Two alternative sets of tests offer some advantages but are not as widely available: (1) Hb and serum TfR1; and (2) Hb and CHr. TfR1 is not influenced by inflammatory states and reflects iron status across the spectrum of iron nutriture. It is the test favored by the World Health Organization but it is not widely available, and normal values in children are lacking.[35] CHr is more widely available and has been standardized in children. It, like TfR1, is free from influence by inflammation.[36] If ID is suspected, especially if the child follows an alternative diet, such as vegetarian or vegan, or if the diet is of poor quality, the child should be screened for anemia. Screening for IDA initially requires a Hb concentration to establish the presences of anemia. In the presence of anemia, follow-up includes: (1) serum ferritin and CRP; (2) serum TfR1; or (3) CHr.

Iron Supplements

Oral iron supplementation has been blamed for a host of unwanted adverse effects. Some of these have not been verified when looked at scientifically. Gastrointestinal tract symptoms, such as nausea, vomiting, abdominal pain, and constipation, are the most frequently reported unwanted effects of iron supplementation. Approximately half of adults receiving high-dose iron supplementation (50 mg or more of elemental iron per day) report one or more of these gastrointestinal tract adverse effects. The incidence of adverse effects is decreased if the iron is taken with food and at lower doses. Adverse effects of supplemental iron are not well documented in children. The alleged constipation associated with iron fortification of infant formula could not be confirmed when evaluated systematically.[26] Similarly, an increase in infections in children receiving iron supplements appears to be clinically insignificant.[29]

Many forms of oral iron are available (Table 19.4). In children younger than 12 years, the prophylactic dose of iron is 1 to 2 mg of elemental iron/kg/day in 1 to 2 divided doses, with a maximum of 15 mg/day. For mild to moderate ID, an oral dose of elemental iron of 3 mg/kg/day in 1 to 2 divided doses is usually well tolerated. For more severe anemia, 4 to 6 mg/kg/day of elemental iron in 3 divided doses is recommended. For older children and adults, the prophylactic dose of elemental iron is 60 to 100 mg/day in 1 to 2 divided doses. To treat anemia in the older child and adults under medical supervision, the dose is 60 to 180 mg/day of elemental iron, not to exceed 60 mg per dose.[37]

Summary

ID and IDA continue to be of worldwide concern. Among children in the developing world, iron is the most common single-nutrient deficiency.[1] Even in industrialized countries, despite a demonstrable decline in prevalence, IDA remains a common cause of anemia in young children.[2] Even more important is that even ID without anemia may adversely affect long-term neurodevelopment. Because of evidence that lack of iron is associated with numerous and sometimes subtle detrimental effects, the AAP recommends iron supplementation or fortification for infants and screening all infants at 12 months of age for anemia by determining Hb concentration. Further testing for ID with additional tests is recommended if the infant is anemic or has risk factors for ID (see AAP sidebar, pp 457-458). Older children and teenagers should be screened for unhealthy dietary practices that put them at risk of ID and IDA and tested appropriately. The initial screening test is determination of Hb concentration. If anemia is present, further investigations are necessary to establish the type and cause of anemia (Table 19.3). When ID is detected, the reason for the deficiency (inadequate intake, poor absorption, or increased losses) needs to be determined. Once a diagnosis of iron deficiency is established, it should be corrected with exogenous iron and followed until resolution.

Table 19.4.
Oral Iron Preparations for Children

Compound	Trade Name	Formulation	Compound Quantity	Elemental Fe (mg)	Other Ingredients	Product Web Sites
Ferrous Sulfate	Fer-in-sol	Drops	75 mg/1 mL	15 mg/1 mL	0.2% alcohol Sugar, sorbitol	www.enfamil.com
	Tri-Vi-Sol w/ iron	Drops	50 mg/mL	10 mg/mL	glycerin	www.enfamil.com
	Poly-Vi-Sol with iron	Drops	50 mg/mL	10 mg/mL	glycerin	www.enfamil.com
	Ferrous sulfate (generic)	Elixer	220 mg/5 mL	44 mg/5 mL	5% alcohol	
	MyKidz Iron 10	Drops	75 mg/1.5 mL	15 mg/1.5 mL	No alcohol, dye, or sugar	www.mykidziron.com/ productMyKidzIron10.cfm
	Feosol	Tablets	324 mg	65 mg		feosol.com/
	Slow-Fe	Slow-release tablets	142 mg	45 mg		www.novartis.com
Ferrous Gluconate	Fergon	Tablets	240 mg	27 mg		www.bayercare.com/fergon.cfm
	Nature's Way Iron	Tablets	160 mg	18 mg		www.naturesway.com/Products/ Minerals/41041-Iron.aspx
Ferrous Fumarate	Ircon	Tablets	200 mg	66 mg		dailymed.nlm.nih.gov/ dailymed/fda/fdaDrugXsl. cfm?id=24946&type=display
	Ferretts	Tablets	325 mg	106 mg		
	Ferrocite	Tablets	324 mg	106 mg		dailymed.nlm.nih.gov/dailymed/ drugInfo.cfm?id=24857
Polysaccharide Iron Complex	Nu-Iron 150	Capsules	219 mg	150 mg		
	Ferrex Forte	Capsule	219 mg	150 mg	Folic Acid 1 mg Vitamin B_{12} 25 µg	dailymed.nlm.nih.gov/dailymed/ drugInfo.cfm?id=40323

IV

References

1. United Nations, Administrative Committee on Coordination, Sub-Committee on Nutrition, and International Food Policy Research Institute. *Fourth Report of the World Nutrition Situation*. Geneva, Switzerland: United Nations, Administrative Committee on Coordination, Sub-Committee on Nutrition; 2000

2. Sherry B, Mei Z, Yip R. Continuation of the decline in prevalence of anemia in low-income infants and children in five states. *Pediatrics*. 2001;107(4):677-682

3. Lozoff B, Jimenez E, Smith JB. Double burden of iron deficiency in infancy and low socioeconomic status: a longitudinal analysis of cognitive test scores to age 19 years. *Arch Pediatr Adolesc Med*. 2006;160(11):1108-1113

4. Bruner AB, Joffe A, Duggan AK, Casella JF, Brandt J. Randomized study of cognitive effects of iron supplementation in non-anemic iron-deficient adolescent girls. *Lancet*. 1996;348(9033):992-996

5. Baker RD; Greer FR; American Academy of Pediatrics, Committee on Nutrition. Clinical report: diagnosis and prevention of iron deficiency and iron deficiency anemia in infants and young children (0-3 years of age). *Pediatrics*. 2010;126(5):1040-1050

6. American Academy of Pediatrics, Committee on Nutrition. Iron fortification of infant formulas. *Pediatrics*. 1999;104(1 Pt 1):119-123

7. American Academy of Pediatrics, Committee on Nutrition. Iron-fortified infant formulas. *Pediatrics*. 1989;84:1114-1115

8. Centers for Disease Control and Prevention, National Center for Health Statistics. National Health and Nutrition Examination Survey. Available at: http://www.cdc.gov/nchs/nhanes.htm. Accessed October 22, 2012

9. Lozoff B, De Andraca I, Castillo M, Smith JB, Walter T, Pino P. Behavioral and developmental effects of preventing iron-deficiency anemia in healthy full-term infants. *Pediatrics*. 2003;112(4):846-854

10. McCann JC, Ames BN. An overview of evidence for a causal relation between iron deficiency during development and deficits in cognitive or behavioral function. *Am J Clin Nutr*. 2007;85(4):931-945

11. Shayeghi M, Latunde-Dada GO, Oakhill JS, et al. Identification of an intestinal heme transporter. *Cell*. 2005;122(5):789-780

12. Rouault TA. The intestinal heme transporter revealed. *Cell*. 2005;122(5):649-651

13. Collard KJ. Iron homeostasis in the neonate. *Pediatrics*. 2009;123:1208-1216

14. Andrews NC. Understanding heme transport. *N Engl J Med*. 2005;353(23):2508-2509

15. Andrews NC. Iron deficiency and related disorders. In: Greer JP, Foerster J, Rodgers GM, et al, eds. *Wintrobe's Clinical Hematology*. 11th ed. Philadelphia, PA: Lippincott Williams & Wilkins; 2004:979-1009

16. Siddappa AJ, Rao RB, Wobken JD, et al. Iron deficiency alters iron regulatory protein and iron transport protein expression in the perinatal rat brain. *Pediatr Res*. 2003;53(5):800-807

17. Institute of Medicine. *Dietary Reference Intakes for Vitamin A, Vitamin K, Arsenic, Boron, Chromium, Copper, Iodine, Iron, Manganese, Molybdenum, Nickel, Silicon, Vanadium, and Zinc*. Washington, DC: National Academies Press; 2003

18. Georgieff MK, Wewerke SW, Nelson CA, deRegnier RA. Iron status at 9 months of infants with low iron stores at birth. *J Pediatr*. 2002;141(3):405-409

19. Friel JK, Aziz K, Andrews WL, Harding SV, Courage ML, Adams RJ. A double-masked, randomized control trial of iron supplementation in early infancy in healthy term breast-fed infants. *J Pediatr*. 2003;143(5):582-586

20. Dewey KG, Domellof M, Cohen RJ, Landa Rivera R, Hornell O, Lönnerdal B. Iron supplementation effects growth and morbidity of breast-fed infants: results of a randomized trial in Sweden and Honduras. *J Nutr*. 2002;132(11):3249-3255

21. Bjom-Rasmussen E, Hallberg L, Isaksson B, Arvidsson B. Food iron absorption in man. Applications of the two-pool extrinsic tag method to measure heme and nonheme iron absorption from the whole diet. *J Clin Invest*. 1974;53:247-255

22. Iannotti LL, Tielsch JM, Black MM, Black RE. Iron supplementation in early childhood: health benefits and risks. *Am J Clin Nutr*. 2006;84(6):1261-1276

23. Iron-fortified formulas and gastrointestinal symptoms in infants: a controlled study, with the cooperation of The Syracuse Consortium for Pediatric Clinical Studies. *Pediatrics*. 1980;66(2):168-170

24. Nelson SE, Ziegler EE, Copeland AM, Edwards BB, Fomon SJ. Lack of adverse reactions to iron-fortified formula. *Pediatrics*. 1988;81(3):360-364

25. Bradley CK, Hillman L, Sherman AR, Leedy D, Cordano A. Evaluation of two iron-fortified, milk-based formulas during infancy. *Pediatrics*. 1993;91(5):908-914

26. Hyams JS, Treem WR, Etienne NL, et al. Effect of infant formula on stool characteristics of young infants. *Pediatrics*. 1995;95(1):50-54

27. Murray MJ, Murray AB, Murray MB, Murray CJ. The adverse effect of iron repletion on the course of certain infections. *Br Med J*. 1978;2(6145):1113-1115

28. Baqui AH, Zaman K, Persson LA, et al. Simultaneous weekly supplementation of iron and zinc is associated with lower morbidity due to diarrhea and acute lower respiratory infection in Bangladeshi infants. *Nutrition*. 2003;133(12):4150-4157

29. Gera T, Sachdev HP. Effect of iron supplementation on incidence of infectious illness in children: systematic review. *BMJ*. 2002;325(7373):1142

30. Griffin IJ, Cooke RJ, Reid MM, McCormick KP, Smith JS. Iron nutritional status in preterm infants feed formulas fortified with iron. *Arch Dis Child*. 1999;81(1):F45-F49

31. Canfield RL, Henderson CR Jr, Cory-Slechta DA, Cox C, Jusko TA, Lanphear PB. Intellectual impairment in children with blood lead concentration below 10 micrograms per deciliter. *New Engl J Med*. 2003;348(16):1517-1526

32. Bruner AB, Joffe A, Duggan AK, Casella JF, Brandt J. Randomised study of cognitive effects of iron supplementation in non-anemic iron-deficient adolescent girls. *Lancet*. 1996;348:993-996

33. Zhu YI, Haas JD. Iron depletion without anemia and physical performance in young women. *Am J Clin Nutr*. 1997;66(2):334-341

34. Schumacher YO, Schmid A, Konig D, Berg A. Effects of exercise on soluble transferrin receptor and other variables of the iron status. *Br J Sports Med*. 2002;36(3):195–199

IV

35. World Health Organization. *Assessing the Iron Status of Populations: Report of a Joint World Health Organization/Centers for Disease Control and Prevention Technical Consultation on the Assessment of Iron Status at the Population Level.* Geneva, Switzerland; World Health Organization; April 6-8; 2004. Available at: http://www.who.int/nutrition/publications/micronutrients/anaemia_iron_deficiency/9789241596107.pdf. Accessed October 22, 2012

36. Brugnara C, Schiller B, Moran J. Reticulocyte hemoglobin equivalent (Ret He) and assessment of iron-deficient states. *Clin Lab Haematol.* 2006;28(5):303-308

37. Institute of Medicine, Food and Nutrition Board. *Iron Deficiency Anemia: Recommended Guidelines for Prevention, Detection, and Management Among US Children and Women of Childbearing Age.* National Academies Press; 1993

Chapter 20

Trace Elements

Introduction

A trace element can be arbitrarily defined as a mineral that constitutes less than 0.01% of total body weight or one for which requirements in adults are in the 1- to 100-mg/day range. Some trace elements are clearly essential for human health, such as iron, zinc, copper, manganese, molybdenum, chromium, iodine, selenium, and vanadium. Others are not essential but are beneficial for human health (fluoride), of uncertain importance (arsenic, boron, cobalt, silicon, manganese, and nickel), or important mostly in terms of their potential toxicity (aluminum, manganese). Iron and fluoride are discussed in Chapters 19 and 50, respectively; the rest are discussed in this chapter.

The Food and Nutrition Board of the Institute of Medicine has established Dietary Reference Intakes (DRIs) for humans for iron, zinc, copper, manganese, chromium, iodine, molybdenum, and selenium, using a framework containing 4 sets of dietary intake levels: Estimated Average Requirements (EARs), Recommended Dietary Allowances (RDAs), Adequate Intakes (AIs), and Tolerable Upper Intake Levels (ULs).[1] The EAR is the intake expected to be adequate for 50% of a population, and the RDA is the nutrient intake that is sufficient to meet the needs for nearly all individuals (approx 97%) in an age and gender group. If insufficient data are available to determine the EAR and RDA, an AI is determined, the intake expected to meet the needs of the vast majority of people within a population. The RDAs or the AIs of the major trace minerals discussed in this chapter are shown in Table 20.1 (see also Appendix E). The table also summarizes normal serum values, biochemical actions, effects of deficiency, effects of excess, and food sources of the trace elements.

Zinc

Basic Science/Background

Zinc is an essential cofactor for several hundred enzymes with a multitude of functions.[2] These enzymes are involved in nucleic acid and protein metabolism, histone stability, apoptosis, cell division, and energy metabolism. Zinc is also important for the maintenance of protein stability (especially beta-pleated sheets) and is a component of several transcription factors (in so-called zinc fingers). In light of these varied effects, it is not surprising that in many species, including humans, zinc deficiency limits growth in utero as well as in infancy and childhood. Nor is it unexpected that cells and tissues that are turning over rapidly are affected

Table 20.1.
Trace Elements

Name/Normal Serum Values	Biochemical Action	Effects of Deficiency	Effects of Excess	RDA or AI[a]	Food Sources
Zinc (Zn)/0.75–1.20 mg/L or 11.5–18.5 μmol/L	Components of many enzymes and transcription factors	Anorexia, hypogeusia, retarded growth, delayed sexual maturation, impaired wound healing, skin lesions	Few toxic effects; may aggravate marginal copper deficiency	Infants, 0–6 mo: 2 mg/d[a]; 7–12 mo: 3 mg/d Children, 1–3 y: 3 mg/d; 4–8 y: 5 mg/d Males, 9–13 y: 8 mg/d; 14–18 y: 11 mg/d Females, 9–13 y: 8 mg/d; 14–18 y: 9 mg/d	Oysters, liver, meat, cheese, legumes, whole grains
Copper (Cu)/1.10–1.45 mg/L or 11–22 μmol/L	Constituent of ceruloplasmin; component of key metalloenzymes; role in connective tissue biosynthesis	Sideroblastic anemia, retarded growth, osteoporosis, neutropenia, decreased pigmentation	Few toxic effects; Wilson disease, liver dysfunction	Infants, 0–6 mo: 0.20 mg/d[a]; 7–12 mo: 0.22 mg/d[a] Children, 1–3 y: 0.34 mg/d; 4–8 y: 0.44 mg/d Adolescents, 9–13 y: 0.70 mg/d; 14–18 y: 0.89 mg/d	Shellfish, meat, legumes, nuts, cheese
Manganese (Mn)[b] 4–12 μg/L or 73–210 μmol/L	Activator of metal-enzyme complexes important for synthesis of polysaccharides and glycoproteins; constituent of pyruvate carboxylase and Mn-superoxide dismutase	Human, not documented; animals, growth retardation, ataxia of newborn, bone abnormalities, reduced fertility	Few toxic effects; neurologic manifestations from industrial contamination and in long-term total parenteral nutrition	Infants, 0–6 mo: 0.003 mg/d[a]; 7–12 mo: 0.6 mg/d[a] Children, 1–3 y: 1.2 mg/d; 4–8 y: 1.5 mg/d Males, 9–13 y: 1.9 mg/d; 14–18 y: 2.2 mg/d Females, 9–13 y: 1.6 mg/d; 14–18 y: 1.6 mg/d	Nuts, whole grains, tea

Element	Function	Deficiency	Toxicity	Recommended intake	Sources
Selenium (Se)/30-75 μg/L or 0.35-1.00 μmol/L	Component of enzymes: glutathione peroxidase and deiodinase	Humans, cardiomyopathy; animals, hepatic necrosis, muscular dystrophy, exudative diathesis, pancreatic fibrosis	Irritation of mucous membranes (nose, eyes, upper respiratory tract), pallor, irritability, indigestion	Infants, 0-6 mo: 15 μg/d[a]; 7-12 mo: 20 μg/d[a] Children, 1-3 y: 20 μg/d; 4-8 y: 30 μg/d Adolescents, 9-13 y: 40 μg/d; 14-18 y: 55 μg/d	Seafood, meat, whole grains
Chromium (Cr)	Required for maintenance of normal glucose metabolism; potentiates the action of insulin	Humans, impairment of glucose utilization; animals, impaired growth, disturbances of carbohydrate, protein, and lipid metabolism	Few toxic effects; humans, not well documented; animals, growth retardation, hepatic and kidney damage	Infants, 0-6 mo: 0.2 μg/d[a]; 7-12 mo: 5.5 μg/d[a] Children, 1-3 y: 11 μg/d; 4-8 y: 15 μg/d Males, 9-13 y: 25 μg/d; 14-18 y: 35 μg/d Females, 9-13 y: 21 μg/d; 14-18 y: 24 μg/d	Meat, cheese, whole grains, brewer's yeast
Cobalt (Co)	Component of vitamin B_{12}	Humans, unknown; animals, anemia, growth retardation	Few toxic effects; polycythemia, myocardial degeneration	Not established	Green leafy vegetables
Molybdenum (Mo)	Component of enzymes involved in production of uric acid (xanthine oxidase) and in oxidation of aldehydes and sulfides	Humans, unknown; animals: growth retardation, anorexia	Humans, gout-like syndrome, antagonist of copper	Infants, 0-6 mo: 2 μg/d[a]; 7-12 mo: 3 μg/d[a] Children, 1-3 y: 17 μg/d; 4-8 y: 22 μg/d Adolescents, 9-13 y: 34 μg/d; 14-18 y: 43 μg/d	Meats, grains, legumes
Iodine (I)	Essential element in production of thyroid hormones (T_3, T_4)	Goiter; impaired mental function, delayed development	"Toxic goiter"	Infants, 0-6 mo: 110 μg/d[a]; 7-12 mo: 130 μg/d[a] Children, 1-3 y: 90 μg/d; 4-8 y: 90 μg/d Adolescents, 9-13 y: 120 μg/d; 14-18 y: 150 μg/d	Iodized salt, dairy products, saltwater fish, seafood

[a] For healthy breastfed infants, the AI is the mean intake.

[b] Whole blood.

IV

relatively early in zinc deficiency, with the immune system, the intestinal mucosa, and the skin being particularly susceptible. Zinc is vitally important for proper immune function,[3] both in its roles in barrier function (because of its importance in skin and mucosal function) as well as in humoral and cellular immunity.

Zinc is known to reduce the mortality and morbidity from acute and chronic diarrhea in high-risk populations, both as a treatment of established diarrhea and as a preventive public health measure.[4-6] It may have beneficial effects on other diseases, such as lower respiratory tract infections.[7-9] Furthermore, zinc has also been shown to have a positive effect on physical activity of preschool children[10] and on cognition and neurodevelopment.[11-13]

Zinc is absorbed in the small intestine by active transport, is resecreted into the gastrointestinal tract, and is excreted in the urine. Biliary and pancreatic secretions contain large amounts of zinc, most of which is reabsorbed more distally in the gastrointestinal tract. There is homeostatic regulation of absorption, both by uptake and endogenous secretion.[14] Reductions in urinary zinc excretion appear to be an extremely late sign of deficiency. Small amounts of zinc are also lost in sweat and in desquamated skin cells.

Two large families of zinc transporters have been described. The ZIP family appears to be responsible for zinc influx into cells and intracellular compartments, and the ZnT family regulates zinc efflux across the plasma membrane and out of intracellular organelles.[15-17] The regulation of these transporters by hormonal and dietary modifiers is complex, and there appears to be a large degree of duplication and redundancy in the system. Zinc is transported in serum bound to serum albumin and α_2-macroglobulin, and further homeostasis of zinc metabolism occurs in the liver, where zinc may be stored as metallothionein.

Zinc Deficiency

For many years, it was believed that free-living humans consuming self-selected diets would not be zinc deficient, because zinc was so widely spread throughout the environment and in the food supply. Therefore, the first reports of zinc deficiency from Egypt and Iran were surprising.[18] Although uncommon in children, severe zinc deficiency is well characterized. Its clinical features include acro-orificial skin lesions, diarrhea, increased susceptibility to infection, diarrhea, immune dysfunction, delayed pubertal development, short stature, and slow growth.[19] These features are found in the autosomal-recessive genetic disorder of zinc metabolism, acrodermatitis enteropathica (AE), which causes severe zinc deficiency by decreased cellular retention of zinc. AE is caused by a mutation in ZIP4, a key zinc transporter in the brush-border membrane, regulating zinc uptake into the enterocyte.[20] People with AE require daily zinc supplements for alleviation of all symptoms. In children, the proper daily dose may be difficult to determine, particularly during periods of rapid growth, and there is a risk of excessive doses causing copper deficiency.[21] A dose of 20 to 30 mg/day of elemental zinc should usually be adequate to meet the zinc requirements of AE infants and children. Recovery from zinc deficiency is rapid after introduction of oral zinc, and the dermatitis often completely resolves within 4 to 5 days of adequate treatment. Severe zinc deficiency may also be observed in infants, particularly those with mothers with a defect in mammary gland zinc secretion[22] (see Zinc Requirements) and in preterm infants with excessive losses—for example, those with proximal ileostomies because of necrotizing enterocolitis or intestinal resections. In the latter case, the loss of bilious fluid from an ostomy should caution that zinc is probably also being lost, and zinc intake should be increased by between 2 and 3 times the maintenance requirements.

Since Prasad's first description of severe human zinc deficiency,[18] severe zinc deficiency is now well recognized. What remains problematic is diagnosing and understanding the true incidence and importance of milder forms of zinc deficiency, largely because of the lack of reliable measures of zinc status in individuals. Although the incidence of stunting and plasma zinc measurements are useful for assessing the zinc status of populations, they perform poorly as measures of the zinc status of an individual.[23,24]

Mild zinc deficiency in infants was first described by Walravens and Hambidge, who found slower-than-normal growth in male formula-fed infants[25] and lower plasma zinc concentrations[26] than in breastfed infants. Fortification of formula to a zinc content of 5.8 mg/L led to normal growth. Several recent studies have shown a positive effect of zinc supplements on the growth of infants and children,[27-29] but others have failed to show an effect.[30] Zinc status at baseline, the dose of zinc given, growth rate, infections, compliance, and other factors may affect the outcome.[31] Whether growth impairment in children with suboptimal zinc status is attributable to effects on hormonal mediators of growth, reduced appetite, and food intake or more frequent infections is not yet known. Preterm infants are born with lower stores of zinc, and 2 small studies on such infants demonstrated beneficial effects of zinc supplementation on their growth rate.[32,33]

During the last decade, the significance of zinc deficiency in childhood growth, morbidity, and mortality has been recognized by a number of large-scale, randomized, controlled supplementation trials in developing countries, and zinc deficiency has been identified as a leading cause of preventable deaths in children worldwide.[34] Systematic reviews have shown that in children with stunting, zinc supplementation was associated with significantly increased height and weight.[30] Similar reviews in young children evaluating the effect of daily or weekly zinc supplementation on infectious disease have reported a robust decrease (approximately 40%) in treatment failure and death secondary to diarrhea and pneumonia.[6,9,35] The consistent positive

IV

effects on diarrhea prompted the inclusion of zinc into oral rehydration solution (ORS),[36] which showed beneficial effects on stool output and diarrhea duration,[37] although successful implementation has proved difficult.[38] Zinc supplements may have benefits in other infectious diseases, but the data are insufficient to draw meaningful conclusions for either malaria or tuberculosis at the current time.[18]

Mild to moderate zinc deficiency can be difficult to diagnose because of the lack of specific features. Slow growth, frequent infections, minor rashes, lack of appetite, and compromised immune function may be suggestive of zinc deficiency. Zinc status is often evaluated by measurement of the plasma or serum zinc concentration. However, neither is a sensitive indicator, and infection, stress, growth rate, and other factors can affect these values.[39] Hair zinc concentration is sometimes used, but it is difficult to analyze and may be affected by factors other than zinc status.[40] When zinc deficiency is suspected, a zinc supplementation trial (usually 1 mg/kg per day) may provide a measurable response.[41] The supplement can be administered as an oral solution of zinc acetate (30 mg of zinc acetate in 5 mL of water). For term infants receiving total parenteral nutrition, intravenous requirements have been estimated to 100 µg/kg/day, and in preterm infants, up to 300 µg/kg/day has been recommended to prevent zinc deficiency.[42] Infants with cystic fibrosis have been shown to have low plasma zinc and abnormal zinc homeostasis[43] and may, therefore, have a higher requirement for zinc, as may those with Crohn disease or sickle cell disease.[44,45]

Zinc Requirements

Zinc intake from human milk averages 0.5 to 1.0 mg/day but decreases over time as the human milk zinc content decreases with increasing duration of lactation. Infant formulas are fortified with zinc to a level higher than that of human milk (to compensate for lower bioavailability). Thus, intake is usually around 3 to 5 mg/day (or 1 mg/kg per day). Lower zinc intakes may be adequate for healthy term infants, because human milk zinc concentrations as low as 1.1 mg/L do not result in zinc deficiency.[46] However, overt zinc deficiency can occur in some infants receiving human milk with a lower than normal level of zinc.[47] This is of particular concern in preterm infants, because their rapid growth increases their zinc requirement. In preterm infants, deficiency because of low human milk content of zinc can occur quickly. Maternal zinc supplementation does not increase the content of zinc in the milk. Some women with abnormally low milk zinc have a genetic defect in ZnT-2, one of the transporters regulating mammary zinc metabolism.[48] It is not yet known how common this specific mutation is among afflicted mothers, but these infants may present with features of AE that respond to relatively low levels of zinc supplementation or to the introduction of other sources of zinc into the diet (eg, complementary foods or infant formula). Unlike children with AE, zinc supplements are not required lifelong but for only as long as they rely on their human milk as a source of dietary zinc.

The RDA for zinc for older (7-12 months of age) infants and toddlers (1-3 years of age) is 3 mg/day. Exclusively breastfed infants ingest only 0.4 to 0.6 mg of zinc per day at 6 months of age without signs of overt zinc deficiency.[49] Little is known about the infant's capacity to homeostatically regulate zinc metabolism, but several of the zinc transporters described previously are affected by zinc intake and zinc status. Stable isotope studies in infants have suggested that zinc absorption is increased and fecal losses decreased when zinc intake is low.[14] For several age groups, the margin between the estimated average intake (EAR) and the tolerable upper limit (UL) is relatively narrow. Among preschool-aged children in the United States, zinc intakes are relatively high compared with recommended intakes and are more likely to exceed the UL than be below the EAR.[50] For example, data from the Feeding Infants and Toddlers Study reveal that intakes below the EAR are seen in 6% of 5- to 11-month-old US children but <1% of 12- to 47-month-old children.[51] Conversely, the number of children consuming diets containing more than the UL for zinc varies between 47% (12- to 23-month-olds) and 74% (24- to 47-month-olds).[51] Although the incidence of low zinc intakes is more common in adolescents,[52,53] the absence of obvious adverse effects in young children from this nominally "excessive" zinc intakes does raise questions about the UL for zinc for young children. The UL was set on the basis of concerns that zinc may impair copper absorption, and this interaction is exploited clinically in the early management of Wilson disease (see Zinc Toxicity).

Dietary Sources/Bioavailability

Zinc absorption from human milk has been shown to be high compared with that from cow milk-based formula or cow milk.[54] The higher bioavailability of zinc from human milk may be because zinc is loosely bound to citrate and serum albumin in human milk[55] rather than tightly bound to casein as in cow milk and cow milk-based formula. Citrate-bound zinc is readily absorbed, and the limited digestive capacity of neonates may be sufficient to release zinc from serum albumin but possibly inadequate for complete digestion of casein, resulting in unabsorbed zinc.[56] Zinc absorption from soy formula and infant cereals is even lower than from milk formula, most likely because of the high phytate content of these diets.[54,57] Phytic acid contains several negative charges and can bind divalent cations like zinc, iron, and calcium. Because humans cannot digest phytate to any significant degree, fecal zinc losses increase. Because removal of phytate increases zinc absorption considerably,[58] efforts are being made to reduce the phytate content of staple foods (corn, rice, barley) by fermentation, precipitation, phytase treatment, or genetic selection.[59] However, such products are not yet commercially available, and phytate

IV

reduction of food crops is problematic, because it may have adverse effects on crop yields. High intake of phytate-containing foods (cereals, legumes) and the low intake of zinc-rich foods such as meat (see Appendix L) are the most important reasons for the high prevalence of low zinc status in developing countries.

When oral supplements are given, iron may partially inhibit zinc absorption,[60] and combined supplements of iron and zinc have been shown to be less effective in preventing low zinc status in infants than zinc supplementation alone.[61]

During the second 6 months of life, zinc requirements remain relatively high, and the amount of zinc provided from human milk may be inadequate. The concentration of zinc in human milk is approximately 2 to 3 mg/L during early lactation but by 6 months postpartum usually is only approximately 0.5 mg/L.[62] The quantity of zinc provided from human milk may be too low to meet the requirement; however, another likely reason for the beneficial effect of zinc supplements on growth of these infants may be that phytate-containing weaning foods reduce the bioavailability of zinc from human milk. It is apparent that zinc intake is a limiting factor during recovery from malnutrition and during rapid catch-up growth after stunting.[63] This was considered when new recommendations for complementary foods were issued by the World Health Organization (WHO)/ United Nations Children's Fund.[64]

Zinc Toxicity

Acute zinc toxicity is rare but may occur from ingestion of pharmacologic preparations of zinc. Symptoms are usually diarrhea and vomiting. The Institute of Medicine used data on zinc intake and copper status to determine UL for zinc, and high amounts of oral zinc do reduce copper absorption. This may lead to desirable effects, such as when oral zinc is used as a treatment for Wilson disease (a disorder of inappropriate copper absorption and hyperaccumulation; see Copper), and undesirable effects, such as the case report of copper deficiency in an adolescent boy given excessive amounts of zinc for the treatment of AE.[21]

Copper

Basic Science/Background

Copper is essential in several physiologically important enzymes, such as lysyl oxidase, elastase, monoamine oxidases, cytochrome oxidase, ceruloplasmin, and copper-zinc-superoxide dismutase.[65] Lysyl oxidase and elastase are involved in connective tissue synthesis and collagen cross-linking, cytochrome oxidase is involved in the electron transport system as well as energy metabolism, ceruloplasmin (ferroxidase) is involved in iron metabolism, and superoxide dismutase is an antioxidant and scavenger of free radicals. The signs of copper deficiency can all be related to impaired activities of these enzymes.[65,66] Our knowledge regarding copper absorption and homeostasis is limited, but recently, several novel copper transporters (ATP7A, ATP7B, Ctr1) have been discovered,[65] in part because of their role in genetic disorders of copper metabolism.

Copper Deficiency

An x-linked recessive genetic disorder of copper metabolism, Menkes syndrome, usually manifests early in life and is characterized by depigmentation, anemia, steely hair, and a progressive degeneration of the brain.[67] Patients become copper deficient at a very young age, and aggressive treatment with copper should be used, but the long-term outcome for these patients is poor.[67,68] The gene involved has now been identified by work on mouse models of Menkes disease.[69] The defective protein is a P-type ATPase, ATP7A, which is involved in cellular copper metabolism, particularly the export of copper out of the cell.[70] Thus, copper enters the enterocyte, but insufficient copper is transported out of the enterocyte and into the systemic circulation, resulting in severe copper systemic deficiency.

Risk factors for copper deficiency include low hepatic stores and rapid growth, malabsorption syndromes, and increased copper losses, but deficiency is usually not precipitated unless the dietary intake of copper is also low.[65,71]

Preterm infants have substantially lower hepatic stores of copper (which mainly accumulate during the third trimester); these prenatal stores are normally used during neonatal life by copper being incorporated into ceruloplasmin and exported into the bloodstream, causing an early increase in serum copper and ceruloplasmin.[72] Thus, many of the first descriptions of copper deficiency were from preterm infants who had been fed low-copper diets for prolonged periods. Iatrogenic copper deficiency continues to be seen in preterm infants, particularly those with short gut syndrome and parenteral nutrition-associated liver disease or parenteral nutrition-associated cholestasis (PNALD/ PNAC, aka "TPN cholestasis"), in whom copper is often removed from or severely reduced in the parenteral nutrition. Copper deficiency has also been found in malnourished infants and children.[65] Signs of copper deficiency include neutropenia, hypochromic anemia (which does not respond to iron supplementation), bone abnormalities (osteoporosis, metaphyseal cupping), skin disorders, and depigmentation of skin and hair.[65,66] The immune system is also affected, reflected by decreased phagocytic capacity of neutrophils and impaired cellular immunity.[73] The anemia is caused by the low levels of ceruloplasmin, which is needed in several steps leading to the incorporation of iron into hemoglobin. Patients with aceruloplasminemia (a genetic defect in ceruloplasmin production) have normal copper status but pronounced iron deficiency anemia[74] resulting from decreased incorporation of iron into developing erythrocytes.

IV

Anemia attributable to copper deficiency may be mistaken for iron deficiency anemia, although it will not respond to iron supplementation.

Patients with copper deficiency usually respond rapidly to adequate treatment. Clinical parameters that are used to assess copper status include serum copper and ceruloplasmin, hair copper, and erythrocyte superoxide dismutase.[66] In infants older than 1 or 2 months, serum copper concentrations lower than 0.5 µg/mL or ceruloplasmin concentrations lower than 15 µg/100 mL should be considered abnormally low. However, serum copper and ceruloplasmin are not very responsive to marginal copper deficiency and are affected by other conditions, such as infection, which may raise concentrations. The level of hair copper also has limited value, because it may be affected by external factors.[40] The erythrocyte level of superoxide dismutase has been suggested as a good indicator of long-term copper status,[66] but the measurement has not reached routine clinical use.

Copper Requirement

The copper intake of infants is usually low, because human milk contains only 0.2 to 0.4 mg copper/L, and infant formulas are usually fortified to a similar level (0.4–0.6 mg/L).[71] This level of copper intake appears adequate in healthy term infants, because copper deficiency is rare.[19] In fact, even formula that had not been fortified with copper and only contained 0.08 mg/L resulted in adequate copper status in term infants.[75] The WHO has set the minimum recommended intake for infants at 60 µg/kg per day, and the current RDA for copper is 200 µg/day.[1]

After weaning, cereals and other foods provide more copper than does milk, and copper intake increases rapidly. Studies with older infants and children[76] indicate that copper intake at this age meets the requirements for growth and maintenance. Although there has been some concern that drinking water may be excessively high in copper in some areas, either because of the environment (eg, copper-mining areas) or copper pipes, infants fed formula at the current maximum copper content according to the WHO (2 mg/L) exhibited no signs of copper excess after 6 months of exposure.[77]

Dietary Sources/Bioavailability

Copper absorption in infants is high, approximately 80%, and does not appear to be dependent on age.[78] Increasing the copper intake of infants did not affect copper absorption, suggesting no or limited homeostatic regulation at a young age.[78] Stable isotope studies in preterm infants,[79] balance studies in term infants,[80] and radioisotope studies in experimental animals[81] demonstrated higher bioavailability of copper from human milk than from cow milk-based formula and cow milk. Copper bioavailability from soy formula and infant cereals appears to be even lower than that of cow milk, although phytate present in these products does not seem to have the same strong inhibitory effect on the absorption of copper as found for zinc absorption.[82] Dietary factors known to decrease copper absorption include high levels of ascorbic acid, zinc, iron, and cysteine. However, levels of these nutrients used in infant diets are moderate and usually exert no pronounced effects on copper absorption[83] Some types of heat processing of infant formula, however, may have a negative effect on copper absorption,[84] possibly by formation of unabsorbable complexes.

Copper Toxicity

Acute copper toxicity is rare and is usually attributable to the consumption of contaminated foods or beverages or accidental or deliberate ingestion of large quantities of copper salts.[85] Symptoms include nausea, vomiting, and diarrhea. Chronic toxicity is also rare but appears to appear in geographic clusters. Indian childhood cirrhosis has been reported in families consuming milk boiled or stored in brass or copper containers,[86] and the Institute of Medicine selected changes in liver enzymes as a measure of excessive copper intake.[1] In the Austrian Tyrol, infants and children were reported to have died from liver cirrhosis resulting from high chronic copper intake.[87,88] In these cases, inheritance followed the typical pattern of a Mendelian recessive trait, suggesting that these individuals were particularly sensitive to copper exposure. This was supported by the observation that many children who had similar copper exposure were determined to have no liver damage. Sporadic cases have been reported in other areas, and some of these cases have occurred in consanguineous marriages.[89] Cases were much more frequent in boys, and a genetic origin is possible.

IV

Wilson disease is an autosomal-recessive genetic disorder of copper metabolism that results in copper hyperaccumulation. Excessive amounts of copper are accumulated in the body, particularly in the liver and brain, and lead to liver cirrhosis, eye lesions (Kayser-Fleisher ring), renal impairment, and neurologic problems.[90] Despite very high levels of copper in the liver, serum copper and ceruloplasmin are low. Treatment includes a variety of chelating agents and large doses of oral zinc to reduce copper absorption.[91] In advanced cases, hepatic transplantation may be required. This disorder of copper metabolism has also been shown to be attributable to a defective transporter, in this case ATP7B,[92] which is responsible for copper trafficking and excretion of excess copper into the biliary canalicular system. Several different mutations of ATP7B have been described, and the severity of the disease varies with the type of mutation.[93] Genotyping of presymptomatic infants and children is, therefore, important for early and appropriate medical intervention. Copper absorption does not appear to be dysregulated in these patients; rather, tissue copper metabolism, particularly in the liver, is affected, causing excessive cellular accumulation of copper.[90] The outcome for these patients under treatment is usually good, but continuous monitoring of copper, zinc, and iron status is needed.

Manganese

Basic Science/Background

The essentiality of manganese in humans has not been fully established, although it has been determined for most other species. Manganese is a cofactor for enzymes including arginase, glutamate-ammonia ligase, manganese superoxide dismutase, and pyruvate carboxylase. In many cases, magnesium ions can replace manganese with continued enzyme activity.[94] Only one potential case of human manganese deficiency has been described.[95] It is possible that manganese deficiency does not occur in infants and children and that, instead, concern should be directed toward toxic effects of manganese excess.

Manganese Requirements

Requirements for manganese of infants and children are likely very small, and the current AI for 0- to 6-month-old infants is 3 µg/day.[1] However, for 9- to 13-year-old children, the AI is 1.6 to 1.9 mg/day, and this considerably higher level reflects the fact that manganese at this age is retained by the body to a very limited extent.

Assessment of Status

Manganese status is difficult to assess because of the very low concentrations of manganese in biological tissues and fluids; blood concentrations are only 10 µg/L, and serum concentrations are approximately 1 µg/L,[96] making analysis impossible for most laboratories. Because few of the manganese-dependent enzymes are found in blood, they are not helpful in the evaluation of manganese status.

Dietary Sources/Bioavailability

The concentration of manganese in human milk is very low, only 4 to 8 µg/L,[97] and most is bound to lactoferrin.[98] Cow milk and cow milk-based formula are about 10 times higher in manganese concentration (30 to 60 µg/L), and soy formula is about 50 to 75 times higher in manganese than is human milk.[99] Although in the past, some formulas were fortified with manganese,[96] the present levels of manganese in cow's milk formula and soy formula reflect the natural levels of manganese in the protein sources used. Of potential concern is the increasing use of soy and rice beverages ("milks") for feeding infants. These beverages contain 2 to 17 times the manganese content of soy formula and exceed the UL for 1- to 3-year-old children (there is no established UL for infants).[100]

Drinking water can contain significant concentrations of manganese.[101,102] In a recent US Geological Survey of glacial aquifers, manganese was the metal most commonly seen at levels above "benchmark," with 18.5% of samples containing >300 µg/L of manganese.[102] This source needs to be taken into account when estimating the manganese intake of children and also of infants fed powdered infant formula diluted in such water.

Manganese Toxicity

Although the bioavailability of manganese from human milk appears high relative to that from cow milk-based formula and soy formula,[103] there appears to be little regulation of manganese absorption at young ages, and it is strongly correlated with dietary intake.[104] Thus, the body burden of absorbed and retained manganese will be much larger in infants fed cow milk-based formula or, in particular, soy formula than in breastfed infants.[99] This is reflected in higher whole blood manganese concentrations in formula-fed infants.[105]

Toxic effects of manganese in human adults are manifested by central nervous system dysfunction, such as lack of coordination and balance, mental confusion, and muscle cramps.[106] The major site for the toxic effects of manganese is the extrapyramidal tracts. Although most reports on manganese toxicity in humans are on workers exposed to manganese by inhalation, there are cases of manganese toxicity in children who have ingested high doses of manganese.[107,108] In such cases, lack of attention, poor memory test results, and an epileptic syndrome were described. It has been shown in young animals that the brain may be particularly sensitive to manganese. Ingestion of modest amounts of manganese during early life caused a dose-dependent depletion of striatum dopamine and adverse effects on motor development and behavior in rats.[109] A negative correlation between blood manganese and cord blood monoamine metabolites was has been reported in healthy women.[110] It was also shown that cord blood manganese was negatively correlated to nonverbal psychomotor scores in 3-year-old children of these women. Behavioral studies in infant rhesus monkeys exposed to high levels of manganese in soy formula demonstrated that these infant monkeys engaged in less play behavior and more affiliative clinging and had shorter wake cycles and shorter daytime inactivity than controls,[111] suggesting signs of attention-deficit/hyperactivity disorder. Higher levels of manganese in drinking water have been shown to be associated with poor developmental scores in children.[101,112]

In North America, drinking water may be sufficient to meet the manganese requirements of formula-fed infants.[113] Indeed, in the United States, some household wells have water manganese levels exceeding 300 µg/L, the current lifetime health advisory level set by the US Environmental Protection Agency. It should be noted that soy formulas usually contain manganese at amounts exceeding this level.

Children receiving long-term parenteral nutrition may be at risk of excessive manganese exposure, parenteral nutrition solutions frequently are high in

IV

manganese.[114] In such patients, cholestatic disease and nervous system disorders have been associated with high blood concentrations of manganese. The normal homeostatic mechanisms of the liver and gut are bypassed in these patients, leading to hypermanganesemia, and a reduction in the manganese concentration of parenteral nutrition solutions has been advocated.[115] Manganese is excreted via bile, so elevated plasma manganese concentrations are seen in children with biliary obstruction.[116] Given the questionable need for parenteral manganese and the risk of manganese toxicity, there is a good case for arguing that manganese should not be added to parenteral nutrition.[117]

Balance studies in infants show that breastfed infants accumulate little manganese, but formula-fed infants are in positive balance.[80] Little is known about the threshold for development of toxic effects of manganese, but because manganese absorption is high at young ages,[104] the possibility should be considered. This high absorption of manganese may be accentuated, because manganese absorption increases substantially during iron deficiency,[99] which is not uncommon in children.

Selenium

Basic Science/Background

Selenium is required in a limited number of proteins, including selenium-dependent glutathione peroxidase, selenoprotein P in serum, and iodothyronine-5'-deiodinase. In these proteins, selenium is incorporated into the proteins as selenocysteine, via a unique transfer-RNA.[118] Thus, the number of selenocysteine residues in each protein is tightly regulated. Selenium can also be incorporated nonspecifically into methionine. A typical US diet consists of organic selenium (largely selenomethionine) and inorganic selenium in the form of selenite and selenate. Knowledge is limited about the metabolism of these different forms of selenium in humans, but they appear to be metabolized quite differently.[119,120] Glutathione peroxidase participates in the antioxidant defense and helps to scavenge free radicals that may cause tissue damage. Selenium is an integral part of cellular glutathione peroxidase, serum glutathione peroxidase, and a membrane-bound form of glutathione peroxidase, but there are also selenium-independent glutathione peroxidases.[118] Type I iodothyronine-5'-deiodinase catalyzes the conversion of thyroxine (T_4) to triiodothyronine (T_3) in liver and other tissues[121] and is, therefore, involved in thyroid function.

In children with goiter, selenium deficiency limited their response to iodine supplementation and, therefore, the improvement in thyroid size and function.[5]

Selenium Deficiency

The essentiality of selenium in human nutrition was discovered recently, although selenium deficiency in animals had been known for some time. In Keshan province of China, a cardiomyopathy of unknown etiology was known to lead to high mortality in children.[122] Because of similarities between the pathologic changes of Keshan disease and selenium deficiency in cattle and the fact that the local soil was found to be low in selenium, deficiency of selenium was suspected as a cause. A large study evaluating the effects of selenium fortification of salt was begun, and mortality decreased significantly; selenium fortification has since been used routinely. However, other factors may have contributed to the cause of Keshan disease, because Keshan disease is not evident in other areas with similarly low intakes of selenium, and there is evidence to support a viral etiology.[123] It has been suggested that the low-selenium environment puts evolutionary pressure on normally harmless viruses (such as Coxsackie virus), causing them to mutate, which makes them pathogenic.[124] Evidence for such mutations in Coxsackie virus that can cause cardiomyopathy has been obtained at the molecular level.[125] Selenium deficiency has also been found in children receiving long-term total parenteral nutrition solutions that were not supplemented with selenium.[126] Signs of deficiency include macrocytosis and loss of skin and hair pigmentation. In severe pediatric cases, cardiomyopathy is also observed.[127] Selenium supplementation of parenteral solutions is, therefore, recommended at 2 μg/kg/day.

Low levels of erythrocyte glutathione peroxidase activity and serum and hair selenium concentrations have been found in low birth weight infants,[128] but the clinical significance of these observations is questionable. Low selenium status in pediatric patients with HIV has been shown to be a predictor of more rapid disease progression and mortality,[129] and selenium supplementation of such patients may, therefore, be beneficial.

Selenium Requirements

Tissue selenium and plasma selenium concentrations are lower in preterm infants than in term infants.[130] A selenium intake of at least 1 μg/kg/day is recommended to achieve intrauterine tissue accretion. However, evaluation of the selenium status of preterm infants is difficult. When preterm infants were fed human milk (containing 24 μg/L selenium) or infant formula with or without selenium fortification (34.8 and 7.8 μg/L selenium, respectively), no differences were found in plasma selenium, erythrocyte selenium, or glutathione peroxidase concentrations.[130] However, all of these infants may have had suboptimal selenium status, and selenium may have been quickly removed from the circulation and incorporated into newly synthesized tissue. Selenium fortification of infant formula improves selenium status of preterm infants,[131] and selenium supplementation may reduce the risk of sepsis.[132]

There is also limited evidence that low maternal selenium concentrations in the first trimester may increase the risk of preterm birth and maternal pregnancy-induced hypertension[133] and that selenium supplementation may reduce the risk of pregnancy-induced hypertension.[134]

Dietary Sources/Bioavailability

Selenium in the diet is strongly affected by local conditions; soil and water selenium levels affect plant selenium levels and the levels in grazing animals and their milk.[119] Similarly, selenium in human milk is affected by maternal selenium intake.[135] Thus, the selenium intake of infants and children is affected by geographic location. Some areas of the United States have high levels of selenium, and other areas have considerably lower levels. The raw materials used for infant formulas, such as skim milk powder, whey protein, and soy protein isolate, strongly affect the selenium content of the formulas.

The selenium concentration of human milk has been shown to be as low as 3 µg/L in some areas of China, while levels in other low-selenium areas, such as Finland and New Zealand, are around 10 µg/L.[119] Selenium levels in human milk from women in the United States vary but are usually approximately 15 µg/L.[136] A lower level of selenium was shown in formula-fed infants than in breastfed infants in several studies.[136,137] Infant formulas that are not fortified with selenium often contain considerably lower selenium levels (2 to 6 µg/L) than the level in human milk. Furthermore, the bioavailability of selenium in human milk, which is mostly in protein-bound form,[138] seems higher than that of selenium-fortified formula. A study in which the selenium status of formula-fed infants was lower than the that in breastfed infants, even though the formula was fortified with selenium to a level higher than that of human milk, supports this.[137] At least part of the difference in selenium bioavailability may be related to the form of selenium in the diet; selenite or selenate (ie, inorganic selenium) is used in infant formula, whereas most selenium in human milk is protein bound (organic selenium). A difference in utilization of selenium given in different forms was shown in a study in which lactating women were given selenium supplements. Yeast selenium (ie, organic selenium) resulted in higher selenium levels in human milk than when selenite was given.[135] These differences were also manifested in the selenium status of the breastfed infants of mothers in the study.

Soy formula often provides even less selenium than does cow milk-based formula. Again, this depends on the soy protein source used, but several commercial soy formulas have been reported to contain only 2 to 6 µg selenium/L.[139,140] Selenium fortification of soy formula has, therefore, recently been implemented.

Both selenite[131] and selenate[141] have been studied; stable isotope studies in infants show that the latter form is better absorbed, but selenium retention is similar from both forms.[142] The level of fortification has been chosen to provide the infant with an amount equal to the RDA of 15 to 20 µg/kg per day for infants from birth to 6 months of age. Another factor to consider is the selenium status of infants at birth. Markedly different concentrations of plasma selenium in infants in Finland and the United States may explain why increases after birth were seen in one study[137] but not in another.[143]

Selenium Toxicity

Acute selenium toxicity is very rare in humans, and cases are usually caused by ingestion of selenium supplements. Signs include diarrhea and garlic-smelling breath. Chronic selenium toxicity also appears rare, with signs such as brittle nails, hair loss, and fatigue.

Iodine

Basic Science/Background

The primary biological role of iodine is in the synthesis of thyroid hormones, particularly T_4. Iodine deficiency is a particular concern in pregnant women and in children, because it may lead to irreversible growth impairment and developmental delays.[144] Iodine is readily absorbed and then is rapidly taken up by the thyroid gland, as well as other tissues. Excess iodine is excreted via the urine, and urinary iodine is often used as an indicator of iodine status.[145]

Iodine Deficiency

Although iodine deficiency is one of the most common nutrient deficiencies worldwide, it is very uncommon among infants and children in the United States. Common use of iodine in baked goods and in dairy cattle management, together with iodination of table salt, makes the dietary iodine intake of the US population more than sufficient to meet the requirements.[145,146] However, in other industrialized countries, there are concerns about the possible reemergence of childhood iodine deficiency.[147]

Goitrous children with iron-deficiency anemia do not respond to iodine supplementation,[148] suggesting that iron may be important for some vital step in iodine metabolism. Oral iron supplementation of such children led to a significantly improved response to iodine supplementation.[149]

Adequate selenium status is also vital for normal iodine metabolism, as the enzyme converting T_4 to T_3 (deiodinase) is selenium dependent (see Selenium). It may, therefore, be prudent to evaluate T_4 and T_3 status of infants and children with suspected selenium deficiency. Human milk, infant formulas, and parenteral nutrition solutions appear to contain insufficient iodine to meet the requirement of the preterm infant.[150] A Cochrane review found only one randomized controlled trial on iodine supplementation of preterm infants and morbidity and neurodevelopment and found insufficient data to make any conclusions.[151]

Iodine Requirement

The RDA of iodine for infants up to 6 months of age is 110 µg/day and for those 6 to 12 months of age, 130 µg/day. The concentration of iodine in human milk depends on maternal intake and, therefore, varies, but values of 50 to 60 µg/L were found in a multicenter international study.[152] The iodine concentration in human milk of women in the United States appears to be higher, with a mean value of 130 µg/L[153]; maternal dietary intake strongly influences the iodine concentration.[154] Cow milk is a rich source of iodine, and cow milk-based infant formula is, therefore, a good source of iodine. Soy formula usually contains approximately 70 to 100 µg/L. Thus, it is evident that formula-fed and breastfed infants will receive adequate quantities of iodine. Children in the United States will get an ample supply of iodine from salt, dairy products, and baked goods. For areas that are not reached by iodine fortification, low-dose oral iodized oil has been developed for children.[155,156]

Iodine Toxicity

Although goiter attributable to iodine deficiency is rare in the United States, there is an increasing risk of goiter attributable to excessive iodine intake. Several sources contribute to the iodine intake of children, and it is possible that iodination of salt is no longer needed.[155]

Other Trace Elements

Chromium functions as a cofactor for insulin. In experimental animals, chromium deficiency is characterized by impaired growth and longevity and by impaired glucose, lipid, and protein metabolism. However, chromium deficiency in infants is rare and has only been reported associated with protein-calorie malnutrition. The only reliable indicator of chromium deficiency is the demonstration of a beneficial effect of chromium supplementation.

Cobalt is considered essential for humans only because it is a component of the vitamin B$_{12}$ molecule. Cobalt deficiency has never been demonstrated in humans or laboratory animals, and the requirement for cobalt is considered minute.

Molybdenum's biochemical functions are in the synthesis and function of xanthine oxidase, aldehyde oxidase, and sulfite oxidase. Molybdenum deficiency has not been reported under any natural conditions in humans, but it has recently been suggested that low birth weight infants may not meet their molybdenum requirement, particularly when receiving parenteral nutrition.[157]

Arsenic, nickel, silicon, and vanadium are probably not nutritionally important. Human deficiency states have not been demonstrated, and dietary requirements have not been set because of insufficient evidence.

Aluminum, although poorly absorbed, can accumulate in patients with renal insufficiency, and this accumulation has been associated with osteomalacia and encephalopathy. Preterm infants accumulate aluminum[158] during their initial hospital care as contamination in parenteral nutrition exceeds losses in the urine. Of concern is that one study in preterm infants has shown that higher aluminum intakes are associated with both poorer neurodevelopmental outcome at 18 months[159] and lower bone mineral density at 15 years.[160] Care should be taken when administering aluminum-containing antacids to children with renal insufficiency (who may be less able to excrete aluminum). Although many commercial infant formulas contain relatively high levels of aluminum,[161] particularly soy formulas,[162] the functional effects (if any) of this are unclear, and has not been associated with negative consequences.[163]

References

1. Institute of Medicine, Food and Nutrition Board. *Dietary Reference Intakes for Vitamin A, Vitamin K, Arsenic, Boron, Chromium, Copper, Iodine, Iron, Manganese, Molybdenum, Nickel, Silicon, Vanadium, and Zinc.* Washington, DC: National Academies Press; 2001

2. Prasad AS. Clinical and biochemical spectrum of zinc deficiency in human subjects. In: Prasad AS, ed. *Clinical, Biochemical, and Nutritional Aspects of Trace Elements.* New York, NY: Alan R Liss Inc; 1982:3-62

3. Shankar AH, Prasad AS. Zinc and immune function: the biological basis of altered resistance to infection. *Am J Clin Nutr.* 1998;68(2 Suppl):447S-463S

4. Sazawal S, Black RE, Bhan MK, et al. Efficacy of zinc supplementation in reducing the incidence and prevalence of acute diarrhea—a community-based, double-blind, controlled trial. *Am J Clin Nutr.* 1997;66(2):413-418

5. Ruel MT, Rivera JA, Santizo, MC, Lonnerdal B, Brown KH. Impact of zinc supplementation on morbidity from diarrhea and respiratory infections among rural Guatemalan children. *Pediatrics.* 1997;99(6):808-813

6. Bhutta ZA, Bird SM, Black RE, et al. Zinc Investigators Collaborative Group. Therapeutic effects of oral zinc in acute and persistent diarrhea in children in developing countries: pooled analysis of randomized controlled trials. *Am J Clin Nutr.* 2000;72(6):1516-1522

7. Sazawal S, Black RE, Jalla S, et al. Zinc supplementation reduces the incidence of acute lower respiratory infections in infants and preschool children: a double-blind, controlled trial. *Pediatrics.* 1998;102(1 Pt 1):1-5

8. Black RE. Therapeutic and preventive effects of zinc on serious childhood infectious diseases in developing countries. *Am J Clin Nutr.* 1998;68(2 Suppl):476S-479S

IV

9. Bhutta ZA, Black RE, Brown KH, et al. Prevention of diarrhea and pneumonia by zinc supplementation in children in developing countries: pooled analysis of randomized controlled trials. Zinc Investigators Collaborative Group. *J Pediatr*. 1999;135(6):689-697

10. Sazawal S, Bentley M, Black RE, Dhingra P, George S, Bhan MK. Effect of zinc supplementation on observed activity in low socioeconomic Indian preschool children. *Pediatrics*. 1996;98:1132-1137

11. Sandstead HH, Penland JG, Alcock NW, et al. Effects of repletion with zinc and other micronutrients repletion on neuropsychological performance and growth of Chinese children. *Am J Clin Nutr*. 1997;16(2 Suppl):268-272

12. Castillo-Duran C, Perales CG, Hertrampf ED, et al. Effect of zinc supplementation on development and growth of Chilean infants. *J Pediatr*. 2001;138(2):229-235

13. Frederickson CJ, Suh SW, Frederickson CJ, et al. Importance of zinc in the central nervous system: the zinc-containing neuron. *J Nutr*. 2000;130(5 Suppl):S1471-S1483

14. Hambidge KM, Krebs NF, Westcott JE, Miller LV. Changes in zinc absorption during development. *J Pediatr*. 2006;149(5 Suppl):S64-S68

15. McMahon RJ, Cousins RJ. Mammalian zinc transporters. *J Nutr*. 1998;128(4):667-670

16. Gaither LA, Eide DJ. The human ZIP1 transporter mediates zinc uptake in human K562 erythroleukemia cells. *J Biol Chem*. 2001;276(25):22258-22264

17. Eide DJ. Zinc transporters and the cellular trafficking of zinc. *Biochim Biophys Acta*. 2006;1763(7):711-722

18. Prasad AS. Impact of the discovery of human zinc deficiency on health. *J Am Coll Nutr*. 2009 Jun;28(3):257-265

19. Walravens PA. Nutritional importance of copper and zinc in neonates and infants. *Clin Chem*. 1980;26(2):185-189

20. Wang K, Zhou B, Kuo YM, et al. A novel member of a zinc transporter family is defective in acrodermatitis enteropathica. *Am J Hum Genet*. 2002;71(1):66-73

21. Sandström B, Cederblad Å, Lindblad BS, Lönnerdal B. Acrodermatitis enteropathica, zinc metabolism, copper status and immune function. *Arch Pediatr Adolesc Med*. 1994;148(9):980-985

22. Zimmerman AW, Hambidge KM, Lepow MI, et al. Acrodermatitis in breast-fed premature infants: evidence for a defect of mammary zinc secretion. *Pediatrics*. 1982;69:176-183

23. Gibson RS, Hess SY, Hotz C, Brown KH. Indicators of zinc status at the population level: a review of the evidence. *Br J Nutr*. 2008;99(Suppl 3):S14-S23

24. de Benoist B, Darnton-Hill I, Davidsson L, et al. Conclusions of the Joint WHO/UNICEF/IAEA/IZiNCG Interagency Meeting on Zinc Status Indicators. *Food Nutr Bull*. 2007;(3 Suppl):S480-S484

25. Walravens PA, Hambidge KM. Growth of infants fed a zinc supplemented formula. *Am J Clin Nutr*. 1976;29(10):1114-1121

26. Hambidge KM, Walravens PA, Casey CE, et al. Plasma zinc concentrations of breast-fed infants. *J Pediatr*. 1979;94(4):607-608

27. Ruz M, Castillo-Duran C, Lara X, et al. A 14-mo zinc-supplementation trial in apparently healthy Chilean preschool children. *Pediatrics*. 1997;66(6):1406-1413

28. Rivera JA, Ruel MT, Santizo MC, et al. Zinc supplementation improves the growth of stunted rural Guatemalan infants. *J Nutr*. 1998;128(3):556-562

29. Umeta M, West CE, Haidar J, et al. Zinc supplementation and stunted infants in Ethiopia: a randomized controlled trial. *Lancet*. 2000;355(9220):2021-2026

30. Brown KH, Peerson JM, Rivera J, Allen LH. Effect of supplemental zinc on the growth and serum zinc concentrations of prepubertal children: a meta-analysis of randomized controlled trials. *Am J Clin Nutr*. 2002;75(6):1062-1071

31. Brown KH. Commentary: zinc and child growth. *Int J Epidemiol*. 2003;32(6):1103-1104

32. Diaz-Gomez NM, Domenech E, Barroso F, et al. The effect of zinc supplementation on linear growth, body composition, and growth factors in preterm infants. *Pediatrics*. 2003;115(5 Pt 1):1002-1009

33. Islam MN, Chowdhury MA, Siddika M, et al. Effect of oral zinc supplementation on the growth of preterm infants. *Indian Pediatr*. 2010;47(10):845-849

34. Jones G, Steketee RW, Black RE, et al. How many child deaths can we prevent this year? *Lancet*. 2003;362(9377):65-71

35. Brooks WA, Santosham M, Naheed A, et al. Effect of weekly zinc supplements on incidence of pneumonia and diarrhea in children younger than 2 years in an urban, low-income population in Bangladesh: randomised controlled trial. *Lancet*. 2005;366(9490):999-1004

36. Robberstad B, Strand T, Black RE, Sommerfelt H. Cost-effectiveness of zinc as adjunct therapy for acute childhood diarrhea in developing countries. *Bull World Health Organ*. 2004;82(7):523-531

37. Bhatnagar S, Bahl R, Sharma PK, et al. Zinc with oral rehydration therapy reduces stool output and duration of diarrhea in hospitalized children: a randomized controlled trial. *J Pediatr Gastroenterol Nutr*. 2004;38(1):34-40

38. Fischer Walker CL, Fontaine O, Young MW, Black RE. Zinc and low osmolarity oral rehydration salts for diarrhoea: a renewed call to action. *Bull World Health Organ*. 2009;87(10):780-786

39. Brown KH. Effect of infections on plasma zinc concentration and implications for zinc status in low-income populations. *Am J Clin Nutr*. 1998;68(2 Suppl):S425-S429

40. Hambidge KM. Hair analyses: worthless for vitamins, limited for minerals. *Am J Clin Nutr*. 1982;36(5):943-949

41. Hotz C, Brown KH. Identifying populations at risk of zinc deficiency: the use of supplementation trials. *Nutr Rev*. 2001;59(3 Pt 1):80-84

42. Greene HL, Hambidge KM, Schanler R, Tsang R. Guidelines for the use of vitamins, trace elements, calcium, magnesium, and phosphorus in infants and children receiving total parenteral nutrition. Report of Subcommittee. Committee on Clinical Practice Issues of the ASCN. *Am J Clin Nutr*. 1988;48(5):1324-1342

43. Krebs NF, Westcott JE, Arnold TD, et al. Abnormalities in zinc homeostasis in young infants with cystic fibrosis. *Pediatr Res*. 2000;48(2):256-261

44. Solomons NW, Rosenberg IH, Sandstead HH, Vo-Khactu KP. Zinc deficiency in Crohn's disease. *Digestion*. 1977;16(1-2):87-95

IV

45. Zemel BS, Kawchak DA, Fung EB, et al. Effect of zinc supplementation on growth and body composition in children with sickle cell disease. *Am J Clin Nutr.* 2002;75(2):300-307

46. Krebs NF, Reidinger CJ, Robertson AD, Hambidge KM. Growth and intakes of energy and zinc in infants fed human milk. *J Pediatr.* 1994;124(1):32-39

47. Atkinson SA, Whelan D, Whyte RK, Lönnerdal B. Abnormal zinc content in human milk. *Am J Dis Child.* 1989;143(5):608-611

48. Chowanadisai W, Lonnerdal B, Kelleher SL. Identification of a mutation in SLC30A2 (ZnT-2) in women with low milk zinc concentration that results in transient neonatal zinc deficiency. *J Biol Chem.* 2006;281(51):39699-36707

49. Krebs NF, Hambidge KM. Zinc requirements and zinc intakes of breast-fed infants. *Am J Clin Nutr.* 1986;43(2):288-292

50. Arsenault JE, Brown KH. Zinc intake of US preschool children exceeds new dietary reference intakes. *Am J Clin Nutr.* 2003;78(5):1011-1017

51. Butte NF, Foz MK, Briefel RR, et al. Preshoolers meet or exceed dietary reference intakes. *J Am Diet Assoc.* 2010;110(12 Suppl):S27-S37

52. Affenito SG, Thompson DR, Franko DL, et al. Longitudinal assessment of micronutrient intake among African American and White girls: The National Heart, Lung, and Blood Institute Growth and Health Study. *J Am Diet Assoc.* 2007;107(7):1113-1123

53. Schenkel TC, Stockman NKA, Brown JN, Duncan Am. Evaluation of energy, nutrient and dietary fiber intakes in adolescents males. *J Am Coll Nutr.* 2007;26(3):264-271

54. Sandstrom B, Cederblad A, Lonnerdal B. Zinc absorption from human milk, cow's milk, and infant formulas. *Am J Dis Child.* 1983;137(8):726-729

55. Lönnerdal B, Hoffman B, Hurley LS. Zinc and copper binding proteins in human milk. *Am J Clin Nutr.* 1982;36:1170-1176

56. Lönnerdal B. Dietary factors influencing zinc absorption. *J Nutr.* 2000;130(6):1378S-1383S

57. Lonnerdal B, Cederblad A, Davidsson L, Sandstrom B. The effect of individual components of soy formula and cow's milk formula on zinc bioavailability. *Am J Clin Nutr.* 1984;40(6):1064-1070

58. Lönnerdal B, Bell JG, Hendrickx AG, Burns RA, Keen CL. Effect of phytate removal on zinc absorption from soy formula. *Am J Clin Nutr.* 1988;48(5):1301-1306

59. Gibson RS, Yeudall F, Drost N, et al. Dietary interventions to prevent zinc deficiency. *Am J Clin Nutr.* 1998;68(2 Suppl):484S-487S

60. Sandström B, Davidsson L, Cederblad Å, Lönnerdal B. Oral iron, dietary ligands and zinc absorption. *J Nutr.* 1985;115(3):411-414

61. Lind T, Lönnerdal B, Stenlund H, et al. A community-based randomized controlled trial of iron and zinc supplementation in Indonesian infants: interactions between iron and zinc. *Am J Clin Nutr.* 2003;77(3):883-890

62. Krebs NF, Reidinger CJ, Hartley S, et al. Zinc supplementation during lactation: effects on maternal status and milk zinc concentrations. *Am J Clin Nutr.* 1995;61(5):1030-1036

63. Castillo-Duran C, Heresi G, Fisberg M, Uauy R. Controlled trial of zinc supplementation during recovery from malnutrition: effects on growth and immune function. *Am J Clin Nutr.* 1987;45(3):602-608

64. Brown KH. WHO/UNICEF review on complementary feeding and suggestions for future research: WHO/UNICEF guidelines on complementary feeding. *Pediatrics.* 2000;106(5):1290

65. Olivares M, Araya M, Uauy R. Copper homeostasis in infant nutrition: deficit and excess. *J Pediatr Gastroenterol Nutr.* 2000;31(2):102-111

66. Milne DB. Copper intake and assessment of copper status. *Am J Clin Nutr.* 1998;67(5 Suppl):1041S-1045S

67. Kaler SG. Diagnosis and therapy of Menkes syndrome, a genetic form of copper deficiency. *Am J Clin Nutr.* 1998;67(5 Suppl):1029S-1034S

68. Sheela SR, Latha M, Liu P, Lem K, Kaler SG. Copper-replacement treatment for symptomatic Menkes disease: ethical considerations. *Clin Genet.* 2005;68:278-283

69. Mercer JF, Livingston J, Hall B, et al. Isolation of a partial candidate gene for Menkes disease by positional cloning. *Nat Genet.* 1993;3:20-25

70. Camakaris J, Petris MJ, Bailey L, et al. Gene amplification of the Menkes (MNK; ATP7A) P-type ATPase gene of CHO cells is associated with copper resistance and enhanced copper efflux. *Hum Mol Genet.* 1995;4(11):2117-2123

71. Lönnerdal B. Copper nutrition during infancy and childhood. *Am J Clin Nutr.* 1998;67(5 Suppl):1046S-1053S

72. Salmenperä L, Perheentupa J, Pakarinen P, Siimes MA. Cu nutrition in infants during prolonged exclusive breast-feeding: low intake but rising serum concentrations of Cu and ceruloplasmin. *Am J Clin Nutr.* 1986;43(2):251-257

73. Percival SS. Copper and immunity. *Am J Clin Nutr.* 1998;67(5 Suppl):1064S-1068S

74. Harris ZL, Takahashi Y, Miyajima H, et al. Aceruloplasminemia: molecular characterization of this disorder of iron metabolism. *Proc Natl Acad Sci U S A.* 1995;92(7):2539-2543

75. Salmenperä L, Siimes MA, Näntö V, Perheentupa J. Copper supplementation: failure to increase plasma copper and ceruloplasmin concentrations in healthy infants. *Am J Clin Nutr.* 1989;50(4):843-847

76. Sorenson AW, Butrum RR. Zinc and copper in infant diets. *J Am Diet Assoc.* 1983;83(3):291-297

77. Olivares M, Pizarro F, Speisky H, Lönnerdal B, Uauy R. Copper in infant nutrition: safety of World Health Organization provisional guideline value for copper content of drinking water. *J Pediatr Gastroenterol Nutr.* 1998;26(3):251-257

78. Olivares M, Lönnerdal B, Abrams SA, Pizarro F, Uauy R. Age and copper intake do not affect copper absorption, measured with the use of stable isotopes. *Am J Clin Nutr.* 2002;76(3):641-645

79. Ehrenkranz RA, Gettner PA, Nelli CM, et al. Zinc and copper nutritional studies in very low birth weight infants: comparison of stable isotopic extrinsic tag and chemical balance methods. *Pediatr Res.* 1989;26(4):298-307

80. Dörner K, Dziadzka S, Hohn A, et al. Longitudinal manganese and copper balances in young infants and preterm infants fed on breast-milk and adapted cow's milk formulas. *Br J Nutr.* 1989;61:559-572

IV

81. Lönnerdal B, Bell JG, Keen CL. Copper absorption from human milk, cow's milk and infant formulas using a suckling rat model. *Am J Clin Nutr*. 1985;42(5):836-844

82. Lönnerdal B, Jayawickrama L, Lien EL. Effect of reducing the phytate content and of partially hydrolyzing the protein in soy formula on zinc and copper absorption and status in infant rhesus monkeys and rat pups. *Am J Clin Nutr*. 1999;69(3):490-496

83. Stack T, Aggett PJ, Aitken E, Lloyd DJ. Routine L-ascorbic acid supplementation does not alter iron, copper, and zinc balance in low birthweight infants fed a cow's milk formula. *J Pediatr Gastroenterol Nutr*. 1990;10(3):351-356

84. Lönnerdal B, Kelleher SL, Lien EL. Extent of thermal processing of infant formula affects copper status in infant rhesus monkeys. *Am J Clin Nutr*. 2001;73(5):914-919

85. Pizarro F, Olivares M, Uauy R, et al. Acute gastrointestinal effects of graded levels of copper in drinking water. *Environ Health Perspect*. 1999;107(2):117-121

86. Tanner MS, Kantarjian AH, Bhave SA, Pandit AN. Early introduction of copper-contaminated animal milk feeds as a possible cause of Indian childhood cirrhosis. *Lancet*. 1983;2(8357):992-995

87. Müller T, Feichtinger H, Berger H, Müller W. Endemic Tyrolean infantile cirrhosis: an ecogenetic disorder. *Lancet*. 1996;347(9005):877-880

88. Müller T, Müller W, Feichtinger H. Idiopathic copper toxicosis. *Am J Clin Nutr*. 1998;67(5 Suppl):1082S-1086S

89. Müller-Höcker J, Meyer U, Wiebecke B, et al. Copper storage disease of the liver and chronic dietary copper intoxication in two further German infants mimicking Indian childhood cirrhosis. *Pathol Res Pract*. 1988;183(1):39-45

90. Danks DM. Disorders of copper transport. In: Scriver CL, Beaudet AL, Sly WS, Valle D, eds. *The Metabolic and Molecular Bases of Inherited Disease*. New York, NY: McGraw-Hill; 1995:2211-2235

91. Brewer GJ, Hill GM, Prasad AS, et al. Oral zinc therapy for Wilson's disease. *Ann Intern Med*. 1983;99(3):314-319

92. Petrukhin K, Lutsenko S, Chernov I, et al. Characterization of the Wilson disease gene encoding a P-type copper transporting ATPase: genomic organization, alternative splicing, and structure/function predictions. *Hum Mol Genet*. 1994;3(9):1647-1656

93. Panagiotataki E, Tzetis M, Manolaki N, et al. Genotype-phenotype correlations for a wide spectrum of mutations in the Wilson disease gene (ATP7B). *Am J Med Genet*. 2004;131(1):168-173

94. Tian G, Kane LS, Holmes WD, Davis ST. Modulation of cyclin-dependent kinase 4 by binding of magnesium (II) and manganese (II). *Biophys Chem*. 2002;95(1):79-90

95. Doisy EA. Effects of deficiency in manganese upon plasma levels of clotting proteins and cholesterol in man and chick. In: Hoekstra WG, Suttie JW, Ganther HE, Mertz W, eds. *Trace Elements in Man and Animals: 2*. Baltimore, MD: University Park Press; 1974:668-670

96. Stastny D, Vogel RS, Picciano MF. Manganese intake and serum manganese concentration of human milk-fed and formula-fed infants. *Am J Clin Nutr*. 1984;39(6):872-878

97. Vuori E. A longitudinal study of manganese in human milk. *Acta Paediatr Scand.* 1979;68:571-573

98. Lönnerdal B, Keen CL, Hurley LS. Manganese binding proteins in human and cow's milk. *Am J Clin Nutr.* 1985;41:550-559

99. Lönnerdal B. Manganese nutrition of infants. In: Klimis-Tavantzis DJ, ed. *Manganese in Health and Disease.* Boca Raton, FL: CRC Press Inc; 1994:175-191

100. Cockell KA, Bonacci G, Belonje B. Manganese content of soy or rice beverages is high in comparison to infant formulas. *J Am Coll Nutr.* 2004;23(2):124-130

101. Wasserman GA, Liu X, Parvez F, et al. Water manganese exposure and children's intellectual function in Araihazar, Bangladesh. *Environ Health Perspect.* 2006;114(1):124-129

102. Groschen GE, Arnold TL, Morrow WS, Warner KL. Occurrence and distribution of iron, manganese, and selected trace elements in ground water in the glacial aquifer system of the Northern United States. US Geological Survey Scientific Investigations Report 2009–5006. Washington, DC: US Department of the Interior; 2008. Available at: http://pubs.usgs.gov/sir/2009/5006/. Accessed October 22, 2012

103. Davidsson L, Cederblad Å, Lönnerdal B, Sandström B. Manganese absorption from human milk, cow's milk and infant formulas in humans. *Am J Dis Child.* 1989;143(7):823-827

104. Keen CL, Bell JG, Lönnerdal B. The effect of age on manganese uptake and retention from milk and infant formulas in rats. *J Nutr.* 1986;116(3):395-402

105. Hatano S, Aihara K, Nishi Y, Usui T. Trace elements (copper, zinc, manganese, and selenium) in plasma and erythrocytes in relation to dietary intake during infancy. *J Pediatr Gastroenterol Nutr.* 1985;4(1):87-92

106. Mena I. Manganese. In: Bronner F, Coburn JW, eds. *Disorders of Mineral Metabolism.* Orlando, FL: Academic Press Inc; 1981:233-270

107. Woolf A, Wright R, Amarasiriwardena C, Bellinger D. A child with chronic manganese exposure from drinking water. *Environ Health Perspect.* 2002;110(6):613-616

108. Herrero Hernandez E, Discalzi G, Dassi P, et al. Manganese intoxication: the cause of an inexplicable epileptic syndrome in a 3 year old child. *NeuroToxicology.* 2003;24(4-5):633-639

109. Tran TT, Chowanadisai W, Crinella FM, et al. Effect of high dietary manganese intake of neonatal rats on tissue mineral accumulation, striatal dopamine levels, and neurodevelopmental status. *NeuroToxicology.* 2002;23(4-5):635-643

110. Takser L, Mergler D, Hellier G, Sahuquillo J, Huel G. Manganese, monoamine metabolite levels at birth, and child psychomotor development. *NeuroToxicology.* 2003;24(4-5):667-674

111. Golub MS, Hogrefe CE, Germann SL, et al. Neurobehavioral evaluation of rhesus monkeys fed cow's milk formula, soy formula, or soy formula with added manganese. *Neurotoxicol Teratol.* 2005;27(4):615-627

112. Bouchard MF, Sauvé S, Barbeau B, et al. Intellectual impairment in school-age children exposed to manganese from drinking water. *Environ Health Perspect.* 2011;119(1):138-143

IV

113. Deveau M. Contribution of drinking water to dietary requirements of essential metals. *J Toxicol Environ Health A*. 2010;73(2):235-241

114. Dickerson RN. Manganese intoxication and parenteral nutrition. *Nutrition*. 2001;17*7-8):689-693

115. Fell JM, Reynolds AP, Meadows N, et al. Manganese toxicity in children receiving long-term parenteral nutrition. *Lancet*. 1996;347(9010):1218-1221

116. Bayliss EA, Hambidge KM, Sokol RJ, et al. Hepatic concentrations of zinc, copper and manganese in infants with extrahepatic biliary atresia. *J Trace Elem Med Biol*. 1995;9(1):40-43

117. Hardy IJ, Gillanders L, Hardy G. Is manganese an essential supplement for parenteral nutrition? *Curr Opin Clin Nutr Metab Care*. 2008;11(3):289-296

118. Sunde RA. Molecular biology of selenoproteins. *Annu Rev Nutr*. 1990;10:451-474

119. Litov RE, Combs GF Jr. Selenium in pediatric nutrition. *Pediatrics*. 1991;87(3):339-351

120. Thomson CD, Robinson MF. Urinary and fecal excretion and absorption of a large supplement of selenium: superiority of selenate over selenite. *Am J Clin Nutr*. 1986;44(5):659-663

121. Berry MJ, Banu L, Larsen PR. Type I iodothyronine deiodinase is a selenocysteine-containing enzyme. *Nature*. 1991;349(6308):438-440

122. Observations on effect of sodium selenite in prevention of Keshan disease. *China Med J (Engl)*. 1979;92(7):471-476

123. Peng T, Li Y, Yang Y, Niu C, Morgan-Capner P, Archard LC, Zhang H. Characterization of enterovirus isolates from patients with heart muscle disease in a selenium-deficient area of China. *J Clin Microbiol*. 2000;38(10):3538-3543

124. Nelson HK, Shi Q, Van Dael P, et al. Host nutritional status as a driving force for influenza virus. *FASEB J*. 2001;15(10):U488-U499

125. Peng T, Li Y, Yang Y, et al. Characterization of enterovirus isolates from patients with heart muscle disease in a selenium deficient area of China. *J Clin Microbiol*. 2000;38(10):3538-3543

126. Vinton NE, Dahlström KA, Strobel CT, Ament ME. Macrocytosis and pseudoalbinism: manifestations of selenium deficiency. *J Pediatr*. 1987;111(5):711-717

127. Lockitch G, Taylor GP, Wong LT, et al. Cardiomyopathy associated with nonendemic selenium deficiency in a Caucasian adolescent. *Am J Clin Nutr*. 1990;52(3):572-577

128. Lockitch G, Jacobson B, Quigley G, Dison P, Pendray M. Selenium deficiency in low birth weight neonates: an unrecognized problem. *J Pediatr*. 1989;114(5):865-870

129. Campa A, Shor-Posner G, Indacochea F, et al. Mortality risk in selenium-deficient HIV-positive children. *J Acquire Immune Defic Syndr Hum Retrovirol*. 1999;20(5):508-513

130. Smith AM, Chan GM, Moyer-Mileur LJ, Johnson CE, Gardner BR. Selenium status of preterm infants fed human milk, preterm formula, or selenium-supplemented preterm formula. *J Pediatr*. 1991;119(3):429-433

131. Tyrala EE, Borschel MW, Jacobs JR. Selenate fortification of infant formulas improves the selenium status of preterm infants. *Am J Clin Nutr*. 1996;64(6):860-865

132. Darlow BA, Austin NC. Selenium supplementation to prevent short-term morbidity in preterm neonates. *Cochrane Database Syst Rev*. 2003;(4):CD003312

133. Rayman MP, Wijnen H, Vader H, Kooistra L, Pop V. Maternal selenium status during early gestation and risk for preterm birth. *CMAJ*. 2011;183(5):549-555

134. Tara F, Maamouri G, Rayman MP, et al. Selenium supplementation and the incidence of preeclampsia in pregnant Iranian women: a randomized, double-blind, placebo-controlled pilot trial. *Taiwan J Obstet Gynecol*. 2010;49(2):181-187

135. Kumpulainen J, Salmenperä L, Siimes MA, Koivistoinen P, Perheentupa J. Selenium status of exclusively breast-fed infants as influenced by maternal organic or inorganic selenium supplementation. *Am J Clin Nutr*. 1985;42:829-835

136. Smith AM, Picciano MF, Milner JA. Selenium intakes and status of human milk and formula fed infants. *Am J Clin Nutr*. 1982;35:521-526

137. Kumpulainen J, Salmenperä L, Siimes MA, et al. Formula feeding results in lower selenium status than breast-feeding or selenium-supplemented formula feeding: a longitudinal study. *Am J Clin Nutr*. 1987;45:49-53

138. Milner JA, Sherman L, Picciano MF. Distribution of selenium in human milk. *Am J Clin Nutr*. 1987;45(3):617-624

139. Johnson CE, Smith AM, Chan GM, Moyer-Mileur LJ. Selenium status of term infants fed human milk or selenite-supplemented soy formula. *J Pediatr*. 1993;122(5 Pt 1):739-741

140. Smith AM, Chen LW, Thomas MR. Selenate fortification improves selenium status of term infants fed soy formula. *Am J Clin Nutr*. 1995;61(1):44-47

141. Ehrenkranz RA, Gettner PA, Nelli CM, et al. Selenium absorption and retention by very-low-birth-weight infants: studies with the extrinsic stable isotope tag [74]Se. *J Pediatr Gastroenterol Nutr*. 1991;13(2):125-133

142. Van Dael P, Davidsson L, Ziegler EE, Fay LB, Barclay D. Comparison of selenite and selenate apparent absorption and retention in infants using stable isotope methodology. *Pediatr Res*. 2002;51(1):71-75

143. Litov RE, Sickles VS, Chan GM, Hargett IR, Cordano A. Selenium status in term infants fed human milk or infant formula with or without added selenium. *Nutr Res*. 1989;9(6):585-596

144. Zimmermann MB. The adverse effects of mild-to-moderate iodine deficiency during pregnancy and childhood: a review. *Thyroid*. 2007;17(9):829-835

145. Caldwell KL, Miller GA, Wang RY, Jain RB, Jones RL. Iodine status of the US population, National health and Nutrition Examination Survey 2003-2004. *Thyroid*. 2008;18(11):1207-1214

146. Zimmermann MB. The impact of iodised salt or iodine supplements on iodine status during pregnancy, lactation and infancy. *Public Health Nutr*. 2007;10(12A):1584-1595

147. Vanderpump MP, Lazarus JH, Smyth PP, Laurberg P, Holder RL, Boelaert K, Franklyn JA; British Thyroid Association UK Iodine Survey Group. Iodine status of UK schoolgirls: a cross-sectional survey. *Lancet*. 2011;377(9782):2007-2012

148. Zimmermann M, Adou P, Torresani T, Zeder C, Hurrell R. Low dose oral iodized oil for control of iodine deficiency in children. *Br J Nutr*. 2000;84(2):139-141

149. Zimmermann M, Adou P, Torresani T, Zeder C, Hurrell R. Persistence of goiter despite oral iodine supplementation in goitrous children with iron deficiency anemia in Cote d'Ivoire. *Am J Clin Nutr*. 2000;71(1):88-93

150. Ares S, Quero J, Morreale de Escobar G. Neonatal iodine deficiency: clinical aspects. *J Pediatr Endocrinol Metab*. 2005;18(Suppl 1):1257-1264

151. Ibrahim M, Sinn J, McGuire W. Iodine supplementation for the prevention of mortality and adverse neurodevelopmental outcomes in preterm infants. *Cochrane Database Syst Rev*. 2006;(2):CD005253

152. Parr RM, DeMaeyer EM, Lyengar VG, et al. Minor and trace elements in human milk from Guatemala, Hungary, Nigeria, Philippines, Sweden and Zaire. *Biol Trace Elem Res*. 1991;29(1):51-75

153. Bruhn JC, Franke AA. Iodine in human milk. J Dairy Sci. 1983;66:1396-1398

154. Gushurst CA, Mueller JA, Green JA, Sedor F. Breast milk iodide: reassessment in the1980s. *Pediatrics*. 1984;73(3):354-357

155. Zimmermann MB, Adou P, Torresani T, Zeder C, Hurrell RF. Effect of oral iodized oil on thyroid size and thyroid hormone metabolism in children with concurrent selenium and iodine deficiency. *Eur J Clin Nutr*. 2000;54(3):209-213

156. Fomon SJ. *Nutrition of Normal Infants*. St. Louis, MO: Mosby-Year Book, 1993:294-298

157. Friel JK, MacDonald AC, Mercer CN, et al. Molybdenum requirements in low-birth-weight infants receiving parenteral and enteral nutrition. *J Parenteral Enteral Nutr*. 1999;23(3):155-159

158. Bohrer D, Oliveira SM, Garcia SC, Nascimento PC, Carvalho LM. Aluminum loading in preterm neonates revisited. *J Pediatr Gastroenterol Nutr*. 2010;51(2):237-241

159. Bishop NJ, Morley R, Day JP, Lucas A. Aluminum neurotoxicity in preterm infants receiving intravenous-feeding solutions. *N Engl J Med*. 1997;336(22):1557-1561

160. Fewtrell MS, Bishop NJ, Edmonds CJ, Isaacs EB, Lucas A. Aluminum exposure from parenteral nutrition in preterm infants: bone health at 15-year follow-up. *Pediatrics*. 2009;124(5):1372-1379

161. Burrell SA, Exley C. There is (still) too much aluminium in infant formulas. *BMC Pediatr*. 2010;10:63

162. Agostoni C, Axelsson I, Goulet O, et al. Soy protein infant formulae and follow-on formulae: a commentary by the ESPGHAN Committee on Nutrition. *J Pediatr Gastroenterol Nutr*. 2006;42(4):352-361

163. Litov RE, Sickles VS, Chan GM, Springer MA, Cordano A. Plasma aluminum measurements in term infants fed human milk or a soy-based infant formula. *Pediatrics*. 1989;84(6):1105-1107

Chapter 21.I

Fat-Soluble Vitamins

Introduction

Intestinal absorption of the fat-soluble vitamins (A, D, E, and K) is strongly dependent on adequate secretion of pancreatic enzymes and of bile acids from the liver into the intestinal lumen. In addition, vitamin A and vitamin E esters require hydrolysis before intestinal absorption by an intestinal esterase that is bile acid dependent. Therefore, each of these vitamins may be poorly absorbed if any phase of fat digestion, absorption, or transport is interrupted. Therefore, deficiency, during conditions associated with fat malabsorption, such as cystic fibrosis, celiac disease, and cholestatic liver diseases is common.[1] Deficiency in these vitamins is also associated with inadequate intake in specific clinical situations. A detailed description of each fat-soluble vitamin is given in this chapter.

Vitamin A

The term vitamin A refers to retinol and derivatives that have the same β-ionone ring and qualitatively similar biologic activities. The principal vitamin A compounds—retinol, retinal (retinaldehyde), retinoic acid, and retinyl esters—differ in the terminal C-15 group at the end of the side chain. The functions of vitamin A are maintenance of proper vision, epithelial cell integrity, and regulation of glycoprotein synthesis and cell differentiation.

Vitamin A is present in the diet as retinyl esters derived almost exclusively from animal sources (liver and fish liver oils, dairy products, kidney, and eggs) and as provitamin A carotenoids (mainly beta-carotene) that are distributed widely in green and yellow vegetables. A report by the Institute of Medicine suggested that carotene-rich fruits and vegetables (carrots, sweet potatoes, broccoli) provide the body with half as much vitamin A as previously thought.[2] Vitamin A activity is expressed as retinol activity equivalents (RAEs; 1 RAE = 3.3 IU of vitamin A activity). The recommended intakes for vitamin A (Adequate Intake [AI] for infants 0–12 months of age and Recommended Dietary Allowance [RDA] for children 1–18 years) vary with age and are given in Table 21.1 in international units. (To convert to RAEs, divide IU by 3.3.) Human milk, cow milk, and commercial infant formulas are excellent sources of vitamin A.

Deficiency

Vitamin A deficiency may occur in children receiving less than the AI and in those with fat malabsorption. Deficiency may lead to xerophthalmia, keratomalacia, and irreversible damage to the cornea as well as night blindness and pigmentary retinopathy. Deficiency may also increase morbidity and mortality from various infections, such as measles. Administration of the vitamin may be lifesaving in children with chronic deficiency and malnutrition.[3] Additionally, routine supplementation with vitamin A during early childhood has decreased visual complications of malnutrition and measles, as well as childhood mortality from measles in developing countries.[4]

The role of supplementation in infectious diseases other than measles is less clear. In several studies and a Cochrane review, vitamin A supplementation made no difference in clinical symptoms in non-measles infections (pneumonia, respiratory syncytial virus infection, infectious diarrhea)[5-8] and, in several instances, worsened clinical symptoms.[9-11]

Assessment

Vitamin A status is monitored by serum retinol and retinol-binding protein (RBP) concentrations. In children with chronic liver disease, a modified relative dose response test may be a more specific means of assessing deficiency,[12] although this approach should be validated in prospective studies. In developing countries, screening has been performed using conjunctival impression cytology.[13,14]

Prevention and Treatment

The AI for infants is approximately 1320 to 1650 IU/day. The RDA for older children varies with age and peaks at 3000 IU/day (21.1).[2] Children with conditions associated with fat malabsorption (cystic fibrosis, cholestatic liver disease) may require supplemental oral doses (2000–5000 IU/day) of a water miscible preparation to prevent deficiency. Treatment of frank vitamin A deficiency depends on the clinical manifestations. Significant eye findings, such as the presence of Bitot spots, xerophthalmia, and/or keratomalacia, should be treated with 50 000 to 100 000 IU of vitamin A administered parenterally. In patients without deficiency, supplementation with 1500 to 3000 μg (4950–9900 IU) of vitamin A during acute measles infection has been shown to be associated with lower morbidity and mortality.[15] Additionally, the World Health Organization (WHO) recommends administration of an oral dose of vitamin A (100 000 IU in infants and 200 000 IU in children older than 1 year) each day for 2 consecutive days to children with measles when they live in areas where vitamin A deficiency may be present. A Cochrane review revealed that this approach was associated with a decrease in mortality in children younger than 2 years with measles.[16]

Toxicity

Claims that extremely high doses of vitamin A (24 750–49 500 IU/day) improve visual acuity in those who work in bright or dim light are unsubstantiated. As little

Table 21.1.

Vitamin Deficiency States, Recommended Intake, Deficiency Symptoms, Deficiency Risk Factors, Diagnostic Tests, and Therapeutic Dosages

Nutrient	Recommended Intake	Deficiency Name	Deficiency Symptoms	Deficiency Risk Factors	Diagnostic Tests	Food Sources	Recommended Therapeutic Dosage
Vitamin A AI infants RDA 1-18 y	0-6 mo 1320 IU/d 7-12 mo 1650 IU/d 1-3 y 1000 IU/d 4-8 y 1430 IU/d 9-13 y 2000 IU/d 14-18 y 2310-3000 IU/d		Night blindness, Infection (measles), keratomalacia	Fat malabsorption	Serum retinol Serum retinol-binding protein	Liver, eggs, dairy, vegetables	100 000 to 200 000 IU, orally
Vitamin D AI infants RDA 1-18y	400 IU infants 600 IU >1 y	Rickets	Rickets, hypocalcemia, tetany, osteomalacia, hypophosphatemia	Fat malabsorption, lack of sunshine	X-ray, serum 25-OH-D	Fatty fish egg yolk	2000-5000 IU day (see text)
Vitamin E RDA all ages	0-6 mo 4 mg/d 7-12 mo 5 mg/d 1-3 y 6 mg /d 4-8 y 7 mg/d 9-13 y 11 mg/d 14-18 y 15 mg/d		Neuropathy, ataxia	Fat malabsorption	Serum alpha-tocopherol	Grain and vegetable oils	25 IU/kg/day for fat malabsorption

IV

Table 21.1. *(continued)*

Vitamin Deficiency States, Recommended Intake, Deficiency Symptoms, Deficiency Risk Factors, Diagnostic Tests, and Therapeutic Dosages

Nutrient	Recommended Intake	Deficiency Name	Deficiency Symptoms	Deficiency Risk Factors	Diagnostic Tests	Food Sources	Recommended Therapeutic Dosage
Vitamin K All ages	0-6 mo 2 μg/d 7-12 mo 2.5 μg/d 1-3 y 30 μg/d 4-8 y 55 μg/d 9-18 y 60-75 μg/d	Newborn deficiency bleeding	Bleeding	Fat malabsorption, breast feeding	PT, PIVKA, clotting factors	Green vegetables, soy oil, seeds, fruits	1 mg, intramuscularly, in newborn infants
Thiamine (B₁) AI infants RDA 1-18y	0-6 mo 0.2 mg/d 7-12 mo 0.3 mg/d 1-3 y 0.5 mg/d 4-8 y 0.6 mg/d 9-13 y 0.9 mg/d 14-18 y 1-1.2 mg/d	Beriberi or Wernicke encephalopathy	Beriberi: symmetrical, peripheral neuropathy, edema; Wernicke: ophthalmoplegia, nystagmus, ataxia	HIV, alcohol abuse, dialysis, gastrointestinal tract disease, total parenteral nutrition, anorexia, furosemide, food faddism; inflammation in pediatric intensive care unit	Whole blood/RBC transketolase activation test, baseline and after thiamine pyrophosphate (TPP); or TPP level, urinary total thiamine	Unrefined grain, liver, pork, vegetables, dairy, peanuts, legumes, fruits, eggs	Severe: 50-100 mg, parenterally, X 1, followed by 10-25 mg/day, parenterally, X 2 wk, followed by 5-10 mg/day, orally, X 1 mo. Mild: 10 mg/day, orally, until resolution.
Riboflavin (B₂) AI infants RDA 1-18y	0-6 mo 0.3 mg/d 7-12 mo 0.4 mg/d 1-3 y 0.5 mg/d 4-8 y 0.6 mg/d 9-13 y 0.9 mg/d 14-18 y 1-1.3 mg/d		Pharyngitis, cheilosis, angular stomatitis, glossitis, seborrheic dermatitis	Weaning from breast-feeding, breastfed from deficient mother, alcoholism, phototherapy, cystic fibrosis, malnutrition, thyroid insufficiency, adrenal insufficiency	RBC or 24-h urine riboflavin level or RBC glutathione reductase (but of limited value in glutathione reductase deficiency, G6PD deficiency, or beta-thalassemia)	Milk, cheese, eggs, liver, lean meats, green vegetables	Infants: 0.5 mg, orally, twice/wk. Children: 1-3 mg, orally, dose 3 X/day until resolution.

Vitamin / Dose	Deficiency	Symptoms	Causes	Laboratory	Food Sources	Treatment
Niacin (B₃) AI infants; RDA 1–18y: 0-6 mo 2 mg/d; 7-12 mo 4 mg/d; 1-3 y 6 mg/d; 4-8 y 8 mg/d; 9-13 y 12 mg/d; 14-18 y 14-16 mg/d	Pellagra	Diarrhea, dermatitis, dementia, glossitis, angular stomatitis, sun-exposed	Crohn disease; anorexia nervosa; Hartnup disease; Carcinoid syndrome; immigrant from area with nonfortified grains; medications isoniazid, anticonvulsants, antidepressants, 5-fluorouracil, 6-mercaptopurine, chloramphenicol, sulfas	24-h niacin and N-methylnicotinamide; or RBC NAD/NADP niacin number	Beef, liver, fish, pork, wheat flour, eggs	10-50 mg/dose, orally, 4 X/day for several wk.
Pantothenic acid (B₅) AI all ages: 0-6 mo 1.7 mg/d; 7-12 mo 1.8 mg/d; 1-3 y 2 mg/d; 4-8 y 3 mg/d; 9-13 y 4 mg/d; 14-18 y 5 mg/d		Not characterized		24-h pantothenic acid	Chicken, beef, potatoes, oats, tomatoes, liver, kidney, yeast, egg yolk, broccoli	
Pyridoxine (B₆) AI infants; RDA 1-18y: 0-6 mo 0.1 mg/d; 7-12 mo 0.3 mg/d; 1-3 y 0.5 mg/d; 4-8 y 0.6 mg/d; 9-13 y 1 mg/d; 14-18 y 1.2-1.3 mg/d		Glossitis, cheilosis, angular stomatitis, depression, confusion	Chronic renal failure; leukemia; pyridoxine-dependent seizure; alcoholism; medications isoniazid, hydralazine, penicillamine, theophylline	Plasma pyridoxal 5'-phosphate; 24-h urine 4-pyridoxic acid	Meat, liver, kidneys	Without neuropathy: 5-25 mg orally/day X 3 wk, with neuropathy: 10-50 mg/day, orally X 3 wk; then followed by 1.5-2.5 mg/day, orally. Seizures: 50-100 mg, intravenously or intramuscularly.

IV

Table 21.1. (continued)

Vitamin Deficiency States, Recommended Intake, Deficiency Symptoms, Deficiency Risk Factors, Diagnostic Tests, and Therapeutic Dosages

Nutrient	Recommended Intake	Deficiency Name	Deficiency Symptoms	Deficiency Risk Factors	Diagnostic Tests	Food Sources	Recommended Therapeutic Dosage
Biotin (B_7) AI all ages	0-6 mo 5 µg/d 7-12 mo 6 µg/d 1-3 y 8 µg/d 4-8 y 12 µg/d 9-13 y 20 µg/d 14-18 y 25 µg/d		Hypotonia, exfoliative dermatitis	Infants on total parenteral nutrition without biotin, eating large amounts of undercooked eggs, holocarboxylase synthase deficiency, biotinidase deficiency, biotin transport defect, anticonvulsants	Urinary biotin or urinary 3-hy-roxyisovaleric acid; lymphocyte propionyl-CoA carboxylase con-centration, or leu-kocyte LSC19A3 transporter	Chard, toma-toes, romaine lettuce, carrots	Acquired deficiency: 150 µg/d.
Folate (B_9) AI infants RDA 1-18y	0-6 mo 65 µg/d 7-12 mo 80 µg/d 1-3 y 150 µg/d 4-8 y 200 µg/d 9-13 y 300 µg/d 14-18 y 400 µg/d		Megaloblastic anemia, neural tube defect, cleft lip/palate	Poor intakes relatively common at 12 mo; consuming carbonated beverages, fruit, and carb; Crohn disease; diarrhea; HIV; medica-tions methotrexate, trimethoprim, oral contraceptives, pyri-methamine, phenobar-bital, phenytoin	Plasma or serum folate (acute); RBC folate (chronic deficiency); 5-me-thyltetrahydro-folate; or urinary total folate	Cauliflower, green veg-etables, yeast, liver, kidney	Infants: 15 µg/kg/day, orally or intramuscularly. Children: 1 mg/day, orally or intramuscularly, followed by 0.1 mg/d until recovery.

Cobalamin (B$_{12}$) AI infants RDA 1-18y 0-6 mo 0.4 µg/d 7-12 mo 0.5 µg/d 1-3 y 0.9 µg/d 4-8 y 1.2 µg/d 9-13 y 1.8 µg/d 14-18 y 2.4 µg/d		Megaloblastic anemia, ataxia, muscle weakness, spasticity, incontinence, hypotension, vision problems, dementia, psychosis, mood disturbance, neural tube defect	Breastfed children of strict vegans; post bariatric surgery or stomach or ileal resection; pernicious anemia; bacterial overgrowth of gut; phenylketonuria; Whipple disease; Zollinger-Ellison syndrome; celiac disease; medications H$_2$ blockers	Serum cobalamin concentration, plasma homocysteine or serum methylmalonic acid in patient with phenylketonuria	Fish, eggs, cheese	Children: 30-100 µg/day, intramuscularly, X 2 wk, followed by 100 µg, intramuscularly, every mo, or 1 mg orally/day.
Vitamin C AI infants RDA 1-18y 0-6 mo 40 mg/d 7-12 mo 50 mg/d 1-3 y 15 mg/d 4-8 y 25 mg/d 9-13 y 45 mg/d 14-18 y 65-75 mg/d	Scurvy	Osmotic diarrhea, bleeding gums, arthropathy, perifollicular hemorrhage	Overcooked foods, with minimal fruits and vegetables, anorexia nervosa, autism, ulcerative colitis, Whipple disease, dialysis, alcoholism, tobacco use, total parenteral nutrition without vitamin C	White blood cell ascorbate concentration, urinary ascorbate, capillary fragility, widening of zone of provisional calcification bone ends on x-rays	Citrus fruits	Children: 25-100 mg, orally, intramuscularly or intravenously, 3X/day × 1 wk, followed by 100 mg orally/day.

IV

References for the table

Institute of Medicine, Food and Nutrition Board. *Dietary Reference Intakes for Thiamin, Riboflavin, Niacin, Vitamin B6 Folate, Vitamin B$_{12}$, Pantothenic Acid, Biotin, And Choline.* Washington, DC: National Academies Press; 1998

Institute of Medicine, Food and Nutrition Board. *Dietary Reference Intakes for Vitamin C, Vitamin E, Selenium, and Carotenoids.* Washington, DC: National Academies Press; 2000

Institute of Medicine, Food and Nutrition Board. *Dietary Reference Intakes for Calcium and Vitamin D.* Washington, DC: National Academies Press; 2011

Institute of Medicine, Food and Nutrition Board. *Dietary Reference Intakes for Vitamin A, Vitamin K, Arsenic, Boron, Chromium, Copper, Iodine, Manganese, Molybdenum, Nickel, Silicon, Vanadium, and Zinc.* Washington, DC: National Academies Press. 2001

Setharaman U. Vitamins. *Pediatr Rev.* 2006;27(2):44-55

TABLE 21.2.

Vitamin Tolerable Upper Limits, Adverse Effects/Overdose Symptoms, Overdose Risk Factors, and Drug Interactions

Nutrient	Tolerable Upper Limits	Adverse Effects/Overdose Symptoms	Drug Interactions (Rogovick et al)
Vitamin A	2000 to 10 000 IU dependent on age in children	Anorexia, increased intracranial pressure, painful bone lesions, hepatotoxicity	Iron, retinoids, hepatotoxic drugs, tetracycline, warfarin
Vitamin D	1000 to 4000 IU dependent on age in children	Hypercalcemia	Aluminum, calcipotriene, digoxin, magnesium, thiazides, verapamil
Vitamin E	0-12 mo not established 1-3 y 200 mg/d 4-8 y 300 mg/d 9-13 y 600 mg/d 14-18 y 800 mg/d	Toxicity is rare—see text	Aspirin, chemotherapy, ibuprofen, iron, naproxen, warfarin
Vitamin K	Not established	Toxicity is rare—see text	Warfarin
Thiamine (B_1)	Not established, but symptoms can occur with parenteral dosing	Parenteral may cause dermatitis, hypersensitivity, tenderness, tingling, pruritus, pain, weakness, sweating, nausea, gastrointestinal tract distress, restlessness, respiratory distress, pulmonary edema, vascular collapse, death; high dose, with pantothenic A, eosinophilic pleuropericardial effusion	High dose >10 mg/d × 2 mo with pantothenic acid; chemotherapy agents
Riboflavin (B_2)	Not established but >400 mg/d suggested	Diarrhea, polyuria, orange urine	Sulfamethoxazole
Niacin (B_3)	0-12 mo unknown 1-3 y unknown 4-8 y 15 mg/d 9-13 y 20 mg/d 14-18 y 30 mg/d	Flushing (niacin flush), pruritus, nausea, headache, vomiting, bloating, diarrhea, anorexia, peptic ulcer, impaired glucose control, impaired uric acid excretion, rare hepatotoxicity	Ibuprofen, insulin, oral diabetes drugs, nonsteroidal anti-inflammatory drugs, aspirin, carbamazepine, primidone, valproic acid, clobazam, clonidine, statins, warfarin
Pantothenic Acid (B_5)	Not established	Diarrhea, peripheral sensory neuropathy with paresthesia, high dose with riboflavin, eosinophilic pleuropericardial effusion	High dose >10 mg/d × 2 mo with riboflavin, statins, nicotinic acid

Pyridoxine (B$_6$)	0-12 mo unknown 1-3 y 30 mg/d 4-8 y 40 mg/d 9-13 y 60 mg/d 14-18 y 80 mg/d	Peripheral sensory neuropathy, nausea, vomiting, somnolence, allergic reactions, breast soreness and enlargement, increased ulcerative colitis; high dose combined with B$_{12}$, rosacea fulminans	High dose combined with B$_{12}$, corticosteroids, phenobarbital, phenytoin, levodopa
Biotin (B$_7$)	Not established	High dose combined with pantothenic A, eosinophilic pleuropericardial effusion	High dose combined with pantothenic A
Folate (B$_9$)	1-3 y 300 mg/d 4-8 y 400 mg/d 9-13 y 600 mg/d 14-18 y 800 mg/d	Abdominal cramps, diarrhea, rash, high doses altered sleep patterns, irritability, confusion, exacerbation of seizures, nausea, flatulence, worsening B12 deficiency, increased risk of adverse coronary events	Corticosteroids, nonsteroidal anti-inflammatory drugs, aspirin, methotrexate, phenobarbital, phenytoin, primidone, pyrimethamine, alcohol, oral contraceptives, trimethoprim
Cobalamin (B$_{12}$)	Not established	Diarrhea, peripheral vascular thrombosis, itching, urticaria, anaphylaxis; 20 μg/d, combined with 80 mg/d pyridoxine, may cause rosacea fulminans with nodules, papules, pustules; skin cream with avocado oil may cause itching	Combined with high-dose pyridoxine; corticosteroids; ibuprofen; antiretroviral drugs; H2 blockers; proton pump inhibitors
Vitamin C	Children not established Adults 2 g/d	Nausea, vomiting, esophagitis, heartburn, abdominal cramps, gastrointestinal tract obstruction, fatigue, flushing, headache, insomnia, sleepiness, diarrhea, urinary tract stones, increased coronary events	Acetaminophen, aspirin, warfarin, aluminum hydroxide, beta blockers, chemotherapy, estrogens, fluphenazine, protease inhibitors, antiviral drugs, iron

IV

References for the table

Institute of Medicine, Food and Nutrition Board. *Dietary Reference Intakes for Thiamin, Riboflavin, Nicacin, Vitamin B6, Folate, Vitamin B12, Pantothenic Acid, Biotin, And Choline.* Washington, DC: National Academies Press; 1998

Institute of Medicine, Food and Nutrition Board. *Dietary Reference Intakes for Vitamin C, Vitamin E, Selenium, and Carotenoids.* Washington, DC: National Academies Press; 2000

Institute of Medicine, Food and Nutrition Board. *Dietary Reference Intakes for Calcium and Vitamin D.* Washington, DC: National Academies Press; 2011

Institute of Medicine, Food and Nutrition Board. *Dietary Reference Intakes for Vitamin A, Vitamin K, Arsenic, Boron, Chromium, Copper, Iodine, Manganese, Molybdenum, Nickel, Silicon, Vanadium, and Zinc.* Washington, DC: National Academies Press. 2001

Rogovik AL, Vohra S, Goldman RD. Safety considerations and potential interactions of vitamins: should vitamins be considered drugs? *Ann Pharmacother.* 2010;44(2):311-324

Setharaman U. Vitamins. *Pediatr Rev.* 2006;27(2):44-55

Table 21.3.

Multivitamin Preparations for Children

Formulation	Content Given Per	A (IU)	C (IU)	D (IU)	E (mg)	B$_1$ (mg)	B$_2$ (mg)	B$_3$ (mg)	B$_6$ (mg)	Folate (μg)	B$_{12}$ (μg)	Elemental Fe (mg)	Sweetener	Other	Product Web sites
Drops															
Poly-Vi-Sol[a]	1 mL	1500	35	400	5	0.5	0.6	8	0.4		2		Glycerin		www.enfamil.com
Poly-Vi-Sol w/ Iron[a]	1 mL	1500	35	400	5	0.5	0.6	8	0.4		10		Glycerin		www.enfamil.com
Tri-Vi-Sol	1 mL	1500	35	400									Glycerin		
Tri-Vi-Sol w/ Iron	1 mL	1500	35	400								10	Glycerin		
AquADEK Pediatric Liquid	1mL	5751	45	400	50	0.6	0.6	6	0.6				Corn starch, mannitol	Biotin 15 μg, pantothenic acid, Zn, Se, vit K 400 μg, coenzyme Q10	www.yasoo.com/products/aquadeks/
TwinLab Infant Care w/ DHA	1 mL	1500	35	400	5	0.5	0.6	8	0.4		2		Glycerin	DHA 20.0 mg, pantothenic acid 3.0 mg	www.twinlab.com/product/

[a]Various generic formulations are available with same composition of vitamins.

	Serving													Others	Website
Tablets															
Flintstones Complete	1 tab	3000	60	400	30	1.5	1.7	15	2	400	6	18	Sorbitol, sucrose, xylitol, aspartame	Biotin 40 µg, pantothenic acid, Ca, P, I, Zn, Mg, Cu, Na, choline	www.flintstones-vitamins.com/en/products.php
Centrum Kids	1 tab	3500	60	400	30	1.5	1.7	20	2	400	6	18	Sucrose, dextrose, lactose, mannitol, aspartame	Vit K 10 µg, Biotin 45 µg, pantothenic acid, Zn, Ca, Mg, Mn, P, I, Cu, Cr, Mo	www.centrum.com/centrum-kids#chewables
Windmill Bite-A-Mins	1 tab	2500	60	400	15	1.05	1.2	13.5	1.05	300	4.5		Sucrose, mannitol		www.windmillvitamins.com
AquADEK Chewable Tablets	2 tabs	18167	70	800	100	1.5	1.7	10	1.9		12		Sorbitol, fructose, corn starch, sucrose 15 calories	Vit K 700 µg, biotin 100 µg, pantothenic acid, Zn, Se, co-enzyme Q10	www.yasoo.com/products/aquadeks/
Gummies															
Flintstones Complete	2 gummies	2000	30	400	18				1	200	3		Glucose syrup, sucrose 15 calories	Biotin 75 µg, pantothenic acid, I, Zn, choline	www.flintstones-vitamins.com/en/products.php
L'il Critters Gummy Vites	2 gummies	2100	20	400	16.5				2	260	6		Glucose syrup, sucrose 10 calories	Biotin 60 µg, pantothenic acid, I, Zn, choline, inositol	www.nnpvitamins.com/lilcritters/
Disney Gummies	2 gummies	1500	15	400	15				0.5	200	3		Sugar, corn syrup 15 calories	Biotin 45 µg, pantothenic acid, I, Mg, Zn, inositol, DHA 100 µg	Unknown

IV

as 19 800 IU (6000 μg RAE) daily can produce serious toxic effects in children, and the UL in children is 2000 to 10 000 IU depending on age (Table 21.2). Vitamin A toxicity is manifested by anorexia, increased intracranial pressure (vomiting and headaches), painful bone lesions, precocious bone growth, desquamative dermatitis, and hepatotoxicity.[17-19] Caffey warned that the hazards of vitamin A poisoning from the routine prophylactic use of concentrates of vitamins A in well-fed healthy infants and children in the United States are considerably greater than the hazards of vitamin A deficiency in healthy infants and children not fed vitamin concentrates.[20] Toxic effects of vitamin A were found in young children who were fed large amounts of chicken liver, which contains 300 IU (90 μg RAE) of vitamin A per gram, for 1 month or longer.[21] Vitamin A excess, including vitamin A derivatives, such as retinoic acid, are teratogenic; teenagers who may become pregnant should be informed of the dangers of vitamin A or derivatives used in the treatment of acne.[22]

Assessment

To monitor for vitamin A toxicity during high-dose vitamin A therapy, serum retinyl esters, normally not present, should be monitored. Plasma concentrations of retinol and RBP are not always reliable means of detecting vitamin A toxicity.[19,23]

Vitamin D

Vitamin D (calciferol) refers to 2 secosteroids, vitamin D_2 (ergocalciferol) and vitamin D_3 (cholecalciferol). Vitamin D_2 is derived from plants and fungi, and its use as a food or dietary supplement has largely been replaced by vitamin D_3. Vitamin D_3 is synthesized in the skin from 7-dehydrocholesterol on exposure to sunlight and is present in nature primarily in the fat of ocean-dwelling fish. Vitamin D_2 and D_3 are considered prohormones and subsequently undergo 25-hydroxylation in the liver to form 25-hydroxyvitamin D (25-OH-D, calcidiol), which is the major circulating form of vitamin D. From the liver, 25-OH-D is transported to the kidney for hydroxylation to form the biologically active hormone 1,25-dihydroxyvitamin D (1,25-OH$_2$-D, calcitriol).[24] Calcitriol is the biologically active form of vitamin D, which stimulates intestinal absorption of calcium and phosphorous, renal reabsorption of filtered calcium, and the mobilization of calcium and phosphorous from bone. Vitamin D is, therefore, essential for bone formation and mineral homeostasis. Although some recent evidence suggests that vitamin D may have other nonskeletal actions and health benefits, such as modulating the risk of heart disease, cancer, multiple sclerosis, and diabetes, a recent report from the Institute of Medicine (IOM) stated that the evidence was inconclusive and that no true cause-and-effect relationship could be proven.[24]

Vitamin D is synthesized in the skin by the action of ultraviolet light on a cholesterol precursor (the most effective wavelengths are in the range of 290–315 nm); therefore, the requirement for dietary vitamin D depends exposure to sunlight, taking into account the effects of the environment. The actual requirement for vitamin D in the absence of sunlight is unknown. The heightened awareness of the hazards of ultraviolet radiation exposure, highlighted in the policy statement from the American Academy of Pediatrics (AAP) on the subject, have resulted in revised recommendations for sunlight exposure as a means of maintaining adequate vitamin D stores.[25] Therefore, exposure to sunlight should not be used as a method to ensure adequate vitamin D status. Accordingly, ensuring adequate vitamin D status while promoting sun-protection strategies requires attention to the use of dietary supplementation of vitamin D.[26]

Deficiency

The primary manifestations of vitamin D deficiency are related to the effects on calcium metabolism. Hypocalcemia, hypophosphatemia, tetany, osteomalacia, and rickets are the most common clinical features. Children at higher risk of deficiency include exclusively breastfed infants, children with dark skin pigmentation, and children with dietary fat malabsorption. More recently, obese children have been identified as being at risk of vitamin D deficiency.[24]

Assessment

The best indicator of vitamin D status is serum 25-OH-D concentration, which reflects absorption from the diet and synthesis by the skin. Other potentially useful tests include serum calcium, phosphorous, and alkaline phosphatase concentrations. The AAP, the IOM, and the Pediatric Endocrine Society recommend a target for serum 25-OH-D concentration of ≥50 nmol/L (20 ng/mL).[24,27,28] The diagnosis of rickets is made on the basis of a history of inadequate intake and clinical findings (craniotabes, enlargement of the costochondral junctions, beading of the ribs) and is confirmed by biochemical indices and radiographic findings. Parathyroid hormone is generally elevated in rickets associated with vitamin D deficiency.

Prevention and Treatment

In 2011, the IOM increased the recommended intake of vitamin D, establishing an AI of 400 IU/day for infants up to 1 year of age and an RDA of 600 IU/day for children 1 to 18 years of age.[24] This new RDA for children older than 1 year of 600 IU/day is higher than the amount provided by food fortification and above typical dietary intakes for most children. Although the vitamin D content of human milk is low (22 IU/L), most infant formulas contain 1.5 mg (62 IU) of vitamin D/100 kcal or 10 mg/L (400 IU/L), as do cow milk and evaporated milks.

IV

Consequently, the use of vitamin D supplementation will be needed for many children, in addition to exclusively breastfed infants.[24,26]

Patients with diseases associated with fat malabsorption (cystic fibrosis, cholestatic liver disease) may become vitamin D deficient despite an intake of 400 IU/day. Higher doses of vitamin D supplementation may be necessary to achieve normal vitamin D status in these children. Vitamin D deficiency can be treated with oral vitamin D supplementation (ergocalciferol [Drisdol], 50 000 IU/capsule [800 U/mL]), at a dose range of 600 to 2000 IU/day. If a vitamin supplement is prescribed, 25-OH-D concentrations should be measured at 3-month intervals until normal concentrations have been achieved.[28]

Several approaches have been utilized for the treatment of nutritional or vitamin D deficient rickets, including daily oral administration of 2000 to 5000 IU of ergocalciferol in children with normal gastrointestinal tract function or oral administration of 10 000 to 25 000 IU/day in children with malabsorption for 2 to 4 weeks. Vitamin D supplementation guidance for children with renal failure is given in Chapter 42.

Toxicity

The principal manifestations of vitamin D intoxication are hypercalcemia, leading to depression of the central nervous system and ectopic calcification, and hypercalciuria, leading to nephrocalcinosis and nephrolithiasis. The UL, or the highest daily intake that is likely to pose no risk, was recently revised by the IOM to 1000 IU/day for infants 0 to 6 months of age, 1500 IU/day for infants 6 to 12 months of age, 2500 IU/day for children 1 through 3 years of age, 3000 IU for children 4 through 8 years of age, and 4000 IU/day for children 9 years and older[24] (Table 21.2). It should be noted that the UL is not intended as a target intake; rather, the risk of harm begins to increase once intake surpasses this level.

Vitamin E

There are 4 major forms (alpha, beta, delta, and gamma) of tocopherol and tocotrienols, the 2 main forms of vitamin E. Alpha tocopherol has the highest biological activity and is the predominant form in foodstuffs, with the exception of soybean oil, which contains high levels of gamma tocopherol. The major function of vitamin E is its role as an antioxidant, protecting cell membrane polyunsaturated fatty acids, thiol-rich proteins, and nucleic acids from oxidant damage initiated by free radical reactions. Vitamin E is essential for the maintenance of structure and function of the human nervous system, retina, and skeletal muscle. The common dietary sources of vitamin E are the oil-containing grains, plants, and vegetables. Vitamin E supplementation prevents severe neuropathy in infants with biliary atresia and other forms of chronic cholestatic liver disease, and it prevents muscle weakness in children with cystic fibrosis. [29] Little or no basis exists for the claims that high dietary intakes of vitamin E prolong life, increase sexual potency, or prevent cancer. Although it was suggested that vitamin E supplementation may play a role in prevention of cardiovascular disease,[30] recent large-scale prospective studies have not shown any beneficial effect.[31,32]

Deficiency

The wide distribution of vitamin E in vegetable oils and cereal grains makes deficiency in humans from developed countries unlikely. Vitamin E supplements are necessary for those with malabsorption (eg, pancreatic insufficiency or cystic fibrosis), biliary atresia and other biliary tract disorders, cirrhosis, and lipid transport disorders. Uncorrected vitamin E deficiency during childhood leads to a progressive neurologic disorder, including truncal and limb ataxia, hyporeflexia, depressed vibratory and position sensation, impairment in balance and coordination, peripheral neuropathy, proximal muscle weakness, ophthalmoplegia, and retinal dysfunction.[29] Significant cognitive and behavioral abnormalities have been described in association with prolonged vitamin E deficiency. The neurologic lesions may be irreversible to a substantial degree if vitamin E deficiency remains untreated. Congenital deficiency of the hepatic tocopherol transport protein also results in vitamin E deficiency and ataxia, despite normal absorption of vitamin E.[33]

IV

Assessment

Vitamin E status is monitored by serum a-tocopherol concentrations and serum α-tocopherol-to-total lipid ratios.

Prevention and Treatment

The AI for α-tocopherol is 4 mg/day for infants 0 through 6 months of age and 5 mg/day for infants 7 to 12 months of age. The RDA for α-tocopherol is 6 mg/day for children 1 through 3 years of age, 7 mg/day for children 4 through 8 years of age, and 11 to 15 mg/day for children 9 through 18 years of age[34] (see Table 21.1).

During conditions associated with fat malabsorption (cystic fibrosis, cholestatic liver disease), supplemental doses (25 IU/kg/day) of vitamin E are required to prevent deficiency. The water miscible form of vitamin E, a-tocopherol polyethylene glycol succinate (TPGS) is the preferable form for oral supplementation during cholestasis and may even improve the absorption of other fat-soluble vitamins or drugs when given concurrently.[35,36]

Toxicity

Vitamin E toxicity is rare, and there have been no reports in children. Normal adults appear to tolerate oral doses of 100 to 800 mg/day without clinical signs or biochemical evidence of toxicity.[34] The IOM has set the UL in children at 200 to 800 mg/day depending on age, although no limit has been established for the first 12 months of life (Table 21.2).[34]

Vitamin K

Vitamin K belongs to the family of 2 methyl-1,4 naphthoquinones and exists naturally in 2 forms.[37] Phylloquinone (vitamin K_1) is obtained from leafy vegetables, soybean oil, fruits, seeds, and cow milk. Menaquinone (vitamin K_2), which has 60% of the activity of vitamin K_1, is synthesized by intestinal bacteria. Vitamin K is necessary for the post-translational carboxylation of glutamic acid residues of the vitamin K-dependent coagulation proteins (Factors II, VII, IX, and X, protein C, and protein S). Carboxylation allows these proteins to bind calcium, thus, leading to activation of the clotting factors.[37,38] Other proteins undergoing this carboxylation of glutamic acid residues include osteocalcin, which is involved in bone mineralization.

Deficiency

Vitamin K deficiency leads to hypoprothrombinemia and hemorrhagic disorders. Newborn infants are especially at risk of newborn deficiency bleeding secondary to the inherently poor placental transport of vitamin K and the low concentration of vitamin K in human milk (20 IU/L compared with 60 IU/L in cow milk).[38] Common sites of bleeding include the gastrointestinal tract, the umbilicus, or at the site of circumcision. In older children and adults, hypoprothrombinemia associated with vitamin K deficiency is usually secondary to disorders of fat malabsorption or chronic liver disease.[39] Vitamin K deficiency may also be seen in children on highly restricted diets or following bariatric surgery. Several studies have suggested an association between low vitamin K concentrations and abnormal bone mineral density, bone turnover, and even osteoarthritis, although a causal relationship has not been definitively established.[40,41]

Assessment

Vitamin K status is monitored by prothrombin time, the measurement of vitamin K-dependent factors (factors II, VII, IX, X), plasma phylloquinone (vitamin K_1), or the analysis of proteins-induced-in-vitamin K absence (PIVKA).[2]

Prevention and Treatment

The newborn infant is usually given vitamin K soon after birth for prophylaxis against hemorrhagic disease of the newborn. Vitamin K should be given as a single intramuscular dose of 1 mg (0.3–0.5 mg/kg for preterm infants with birth weights <1000 g). If this is not possible, then an oral dose of 2 mg should be administered at birth, 1 to 2 weeks of age, and 4 weeks of age.[38,42] Following the prophylactic dose of vitamin K at birth, most infants receive adequate vitamin K from cow milk-based formulas, and the formula-fed infant ordinarily does not need additional vitamin K. The AI for infants is 2 μg/day of phylloquinone or menaquinone for the first 6 months and 2.5 μg/day for the second 6 months of life. The AI for older children is 30 μg/day for children 1 through 3 years of age, 55 μg/day for children 4 through 8 years of age, and 60 to 75 μg/day for older children and adolescents[2] (Table 21.1).

In conditions associated with fat malabsorption (cystic fibrosis, cholestatic liver disease), supplemental doses of 2.5 to 5 mg, 2 to 7 times/week, may be required to prevent deficiency. Hypoprothrombinemia associated with chronic liver disease may be corrected by the administration of 5 to 10 mg of vitamin K given intramuscularly. Failure of the prothrombin time to improve following adequate administration of vitamin K suggests severe liver synthetic dysfunction. There have not been any prospective studies of vitamin K treatment for gastrointestinal bleeding in patients with liver disease, as highlighted by a Cochrane database review.[43] Vitamin K does not appear to be an effective treatment for the reversal of excessive anticoagulation secondary to oral anticoagulants.[44]

Toxicity

Vitamin K toxicity is rare. In newborn infants, large parenteral administration of water soluble synthetic vitamin K (Vitamin K_3) has been associated with hemolytic anemia, hyperbilirubinemia, and kernicterus.[38] No toxicity states have been associated with administration of the natural forms of vitamin K (K_1 and K_2).[2]

A Note on Vitamin K and Cancer Risk

In 1990, Golding et al reported on a study of a 1970 birth cohort in Great Britain in which they noted an unexpected association between childhood cancer and pethidine administered during labor and the neonatal administration of vitamin K.[45] Subsequently, they reported in a retrospective, case-controlled study a significant association between intramuscular vitamin K and cancer when compared with no vitamin K or oral vitamin K.[46] Draper and Stiller have questioned this study on the basis of other data from Great Britain and have called for large cohort studies.[47] The AAP formed a Vitamin K Ad Hoc Task Force to study this area in greater detail. The task force in 1993 found no convincing links between vitamin K administration and childhood cancer.[42] On the basis of these observations, the AAP continues to recommend the routine administration of vitamin K to newborn infants.[48]

AAP

Recommendations Concerning the Administration of Vitamin K to Newborn Infants

Because parenteral vitamin K prevents a life-threatening disease of the newborn infant, and the risks of cancer are unproven, the AAP recommends:

1. Vitamin K should be given to all newborn infants as a single, intramuscular dose of 0.5 to 1 mg.
2. Additional research should be conducted on the efficacy, safety, and bioavailability of oral formulations and optimal dosing regimens of vitamin K to prevent late vitamin K deficiency bleeding.
3. Health care professionals should promote awareness among families of the risks of late vitamin K deficiency bleeding associated with inadequate vitamin K prophylaxis from current oral dosage regimens, particularly for newborns who are breastfed exclusively.

American Academy of Pediatrics, Committee on Fetus and Newborn. Controversies concerning vitamin K and the newborn. *Pediatrics*. 2003;112(1):191-192. Reaffirmed May 2006

Reference List

1. Sokol RJ. Fat-soluble vitamins and their importance in patients with cholestatic liver diseases. *Gastroenterol Clin North Am*. 1994;23(4):673-705

2. Institute of Medicine, Food and Nutrition Board. *Dietary Reference Intakes for Vitamin A,Vitamin K, Arsenic, Boron, Chromium, Copper, Iodine, Manganese, Molybdenum, Nickel, Silicon, Vanadium, and Zinc*. Washington, DC: National Academies Press; 2001

3. Rahmathullah L, Underwood BA, Thulasiraj RD, et al. Reduced mortality among children in southern India receiving a small weekly dose of vitamin A. *N Engl J Med*. 1990;323(14):929-935

4. Underwood BA, Arthur P. The contribution of vitamin A to public health. *FASEB J*. 1996;10(9):1040-1048

5. Kjolhede CL, Chew FJ, Gadomski AM, Marroquin DP. Clinical trial of vitamin A as adjuvant treatment for lower respiratory tract infections. *J Pediatr*. 1995;126(5 Pt 1):807-812

6. Bresee JS, Fischer M, Dowell SF, et al. Vitamin A therapy for children with respiratory syncytial virus infection: a multicenter trial in the United States. *Pediatr Infect Dis J*. 1996;15(9):777-782

7. Henning B, Stewart K, Zaman K, Alam AN, Brown KH, Black RE. Lack of therapeutic efficacy of vitamin A for non-cholera, watery diarrhoea in Bangladeshi children. *Eur J Clin Nutr*. 1992;46(6):437-443

8. Ni J, Wei J, Wu T. Vitamin A for non-measles pneumonia in children. *Cochrane Database Syst Rev*. 2005;(3):CD003700

9. Stephensen CB, Franchi LM, Hernandez H, Campos M, Gilman RH, Alvarez JO. Adverse effects of high-dose vitamin A supplements in children hospitalized with pneumonia. *Pediatrics*. 1998;101(5):e3

10. Fawzi WW, Mbise RL, Fataki MR, et al. Vitamin A supplementation and severity of pneumonia in children admitted to the hospital in Dar es Salaam, Tanzania. *Am J Clin Nutr*. 1998;68(1):187-192

11. Long KZ, Montoya Y, Hertzmark E, Santos JI, Rosado JL. A double-blind, randomized, clinical trial of the effect of vitamin A and zinc supplementation on diarrheal disease and respiratory tract infections in children in Mexico City, Mexico. *Am J Clin Nutr*. 2006;83(3):693-700

12. Feranchak AP, Gralla J, King R, et al. Comparison of indices of vitamin A status in children with chronic liver disease. *Hepatology*. 2005;42(4):782-792

13. Tseng SC. Staging of conjunctival squamous metaplasia by impression cytology. *Ophthalmology*. 1985;92(6):728-733

14. medee-Manesme O, Luzeau R, Wittepen JR, Hanck A, Sommer A. Impression cytology detects subclinical vitamin A deficiency. *Am J Clin Nutr*. 1988;47(5):875-878

15. Hussey GD, Klein M. A randomized, controlled trial of vitamin A in children with severe measles. *N Engl J Med*. 1990;323(3):160-164

16. Huiming Y, Chaomin W, Meng M. Vitamin A for treating measles in children. *Cochrane Database Syst Rev*. 2005;(4):CD001479

17. Rubin E, Florman AL, Degnan T, Diaz J. Hepatic injury in chronic hypervitaminosis A. *Am J Dis Child*. 1970;119(2):132-138

18. Lippe B, Hensen L, Mendoza G, Finerman M, Welch M. Chronic vitamin A intoxication. A multisystem disease that could reach epidemic proportions. *Am J Dis Child*. 1981;135(7):634-636

19. Mobarhan S, Russell RM, Underwood BA, Wallingford J, Mathieson RD, Al-Midani H. Evaluation of the relative dose response test for vitamin A nutriture in cirrhotics. *Am J Clin Nutr*. 1981;34(10):2264-2270

20. Caffey J. Chronic poisoning due to excess of vitamin A; description of the clinical and roentgen manifestations in seven infants and young children. *Pediatrics*. 1950;5(4):672-688

21. Mahoney CP, Margolis MT, Knauss TA, Labbe RF. Chronic vitamin A intoxication in infants fed chicken liver. *Pediatrics*. 1980;65(5):893-897

22. Lammer EJ, Chen DT, Hoar RM, Agnish ND, Benke PJ, Braun JT, et al. Retinoic acid embryopathy. *N Engl J Med*. 1985;313(14):837-841

23. Smith FR, Goodman DS. Vitamin A transport in human vitamin A toxicity. *N Engl J Med*. 1976;294(15):805-808

IV

24. Institute of Medicine, Food and Nutrition Board. *Dietary Reference Intakes for Calcium and Vitamin D*. Washington, DC: National Academies Press; 2011

25. Balk SJ. Ultraviolet radiation: a hazard to children and adolescents. *Pediatrics*. 2011;127(3):e791-e817

26. Abrams SA. Dietary guidelines for calcium and vitamin D: a new era. *Pediatrics*. 2011;127(3):566-568

27. Misra M, Pacaud D, Petryk A, Collett-Solberg PF, Kappy M. Vitamin D deficiency in children and its management: review of current knowledge and recommendations. *Pediatrics*. 2008;122(2):398-417

28. Wagner CL, Greer FR. Prevention of rickets and vitamin D deficiency in infants, children, and adolescents. *Pediatrics*. 2008;122(5):1142-1152

29. Sokol RJ. Vitamin E and neurologic deficits. *Adv Pediatr*. 1990;37:119-148

30. Pryor WA. Vitamin E and heart disease: basic science to clinical intervention trials. *Free Radic Biol Med*. 2000;28(1):141-164

31. Tornwall ME, Virtamo J, Korhonen PA, et al. Effect of alpha-tocopherol and beta-carotene supplementation on coronary heart disease during the 6-year post-trial follow-up in the ATBC study. *Eur Heart J*. 2004;25(13):1171-1178

32. Hercberg S, Galan P, Preziosi P, et al. The SU.VI.MAX Study: a randomized, placebo-controlled trial of the health effects of antioxidant vitamins and minerals. *Arch Intern Med*. 2004;164(21):2335-2342

33. Traber MG, Sokol RJ, Burton GW, et al. Impaired ability of patients with familial isolated vitamin E deficiency to incorporate alpha-tocopherol into lipoproteins secreted by the liver. *J Clin Invest*. 1990;85(2):397-407

34. Institute of Medicine, Food and Nutrition Board. *Dietary Reference Intakes for Vitamin C, Vitamin E, Selenium, and Carotenoids*. Washington, DC: National Academies Press; 2000

35. Sokol RJ, Butler-Simon N, Conner C, et al. Multicenter trial of d-alpha-tocopheryl polyethylene glycol 1000 succinate for treatment of vitamin E deficiency in children with chronic cholestasis. *Gastroenterology*. 1993;104(6):1727-1735

36. Sokol RJ, Johnson KE, Karrer FM, Narkewicz MR, Smith D, Kam I. Improvement of cyclosporin absorption in children after liver transplantation by means of water-soluble vitamin E. *Lancet*. 1991;338(8761):212-214

37. Shearer MJ, Newman P. Metabolism and cell biology of vitamin K. *Thromb Haemost*. 2008;100(4):530-547

38. Greer FR. Vitamin K the basics—what's new? *Early Hum Dev*. 2010;86(Suppl 1):S43-S47

39. Mager DR, McGee PL, Furuya KN, Roberts EA. Prevalence of vitamin K deficiency in children with mild to moderate chronic liver disease. *J Pediatr Gastroenterol Nutr*. 2006;42(1):71-76

40. Conway SP, Wolfe SP, Brownlee KG, White H, Oldroyd B, Truscott JG, et al. Vitamin K status among children with cystic fibrosis and its relationship to bone mineral density and bone turnover. *Pediatrics*. 2005;115(5):1325-1331

41. Neogi T, Booth SL, Zhang YQ, et al. Low vitamin K status is associated with osteoarthritis in the hand and knee. *Arthritis Rheum*. 2006;54(4):1255-1261

42. American Academy of Pediatrics, Vitamin K Ad Hoc Task Force. Controversies concerning vitamin K and the newborn. *Pediatrics*. 1993;91(5):1001-1003

43. Marti-Carvajal AJ, Marti-Pena AJ. Vitamin K for upper gastrointestinal bleeding in patients with liver diseases. *Cochrane Database Syst Rev*. 2005;(3):CD004792

44. DeZee KJ, Shimeall WT, Douglas KM, Shumway NM, O'Malley PG. Treatment of excessive anticoagulation with phytonadione (vitamin K): a meta-analysis. *Arch Intern Med*. 2006;166(4):391-397

45. Golding J, Paterson M, Kinlen LJ. Factors associated with childhood cancer in a national cohort study. *Br J Cancer*. 1990;62(2):304-308

46. Golding J, Greenwood R, Birmingham K, Mott M. Childhood cancer, intramuscular vitamin K, and pethidine given during labour. *BMJ*. 1992;305(6849):341-346

47. Draper GJ, Stiller CA. Intramuscular vitamin K and childhood cancer. *BMJ*. 1992;305(6855):709

48. American Academy of Pediatrics, Committee on Fetus and Newborn. Controversies concerning vitamin K and the newborn. *Pediatrics*. 2003;112(1):191-192. Reaffirmed May 2006

IV

Water-Soluble Vitamins

Introduction

Deficiencies of the water-soluble vitamins (WSVs) are rare. Most children and adolescents who eat a diet consisting of fruits, vegetables, animal protein (meat, dairy, and egg), cereals, and breads consume sufficient WSVs to meet daily allowances. This includes formula-fed infants and breastfed infants of mothers consuming a diverse and healthy diet. Appreciating who might be at risk of deficiency of WSVs, however, is important because of limited total body stores and lack of endogenous synthesis of most WSVs. Not all WSV deficiency states in infancy and childhood are caused by dietary deficiency, because diseases caused by WSV deficiency can result from inborn errors of metabolism and nucleotide polymorphisms. Additionally, medical conditions that may predispose someone to deficiency of WSVs include malabsorption secondary to celiac disease, Crohn disease, cystic fibrosis, anorexia nervosa, HIV/AIDS, and having undergone bariatric surgery. Adolescent athletes, especially females with disorded eating habits or vegetarians, may suffer from poorer WSV status as a result of the twofold increased need for B-complex vitamins.[1] Table 21.1 shows a list of WSVs and their recommended intakes, deficiency symptoms, deficiency risk factors, diagnostic tests, and therapeutic dosages.

Health and dietary fads may influence WSV status even in the pediatric population. The increasing utilization of complementary and alternative medicine (CAM) in the United States and abroad highlights this notion.[2,3] Children and adolescents have been reported to account for one third of visits to homeopathic and naturopathic providers,[4] and 68% of adolescents use CAM.[3] Nearly one third of children with autism are treated with multivitamin therapy,[5] the most common form of CAM prescribed for children and adults by a naturopathic provider.[3,4] Single fat-soluble or water-soluble vitamin preparations are also commnly prescribed.[3,6,7] Energy drinks, vitamin water products, and energy drinks (shot-sized) contain variable amounts of WSVs and may contain extremely high amounts. For example, the label of a 2-ounce energy shot product (5-Hour Energy) reports an excess of the daily requirement of 2000% for vitamin B_6 and more than 8000% for vitamin B_{12}. A widely held belief is that WSVs are safe if given in excess; however, they have the potential for serious toxicity if given in excessive quantities, especially in combinations with other medications and over a prolonged period of time.[3] Table 21.2 shows tolerable upper limits, adverse effects/overdose symptoms, and risk factors for symptoms and drug interactions for WSVs.

IV

The increasing population of overweight children and adolescents in the United States is also changing WSV intakes.[8,9] Analysis of data from the National Health and Nutrition Examination Survey III reveals that low-nutrient density foods contribute more than 30% of the daily energy to the diets of children and adolescents. Studies show that the mean intake of vitamins A, C, and B$_6$; folate; and riboflavin decreased as low-nutrient density or high-fat foods increased.[10,11] Conversely, research in Scandinavian children showed that diets low in fat positively correlated with increased intake of several WSVs.[12] In US adolescents, a low-fat and high-fiber diet was associated with a greater likelihood of adequate vitamin B$_6$, B$_{12}$, and C; niacin; thiamin; riboflavin; and folicin intakes.[13] Not surprisingly, children and adolescents who regularly eat meals with their family ingested higher amounts of vitamins B$_6$, B$_{12}$, and C and folate. Taken together, these studies demonstrate that diets high in fat or with a preponderance of low-nutrient density foods will place children and adolescents at risk of WSV deficiency.

Thiamine (Vitamin B$_1$)

Thiamine is an essential coenzyme involved in carbohydrate metabolism. Thiamine pyrophosphate (TPP) is the primary active form, as TPP and nicotinamide adenine dinucleotide (NAD) are coenzymes to pyruvate dehydrogenase in the oxidative decarboxylation of pyruvate to acetyl coenzyme A (CoA). Thiamine also plays an integral role with transketolase in the pentose phosphate pathway, which provides substrates for nucleic acid and fatty acid synthesis. In addition to being a coenzyme, thiamine also plays a key a role in nerve impulse conduction and voluntary muscle action.[14]

Foods rich in thiamine include yeast, legumes, pork, rice, and whole-grain cereals. Dairy products, milled white flour, milled white rice, and most fruits contain little thiamine. Deficiency of thiamine can result in the clinical syndromes of beriberi and Wernicke encephalopathy. Beriberi is traditionally classified as 2 forms: dry beriberi, which is characterized by a symmetrical peripheral neuropathy, and wet beriberi, in which cardiac involvement predominates. The neuropathy seen in dry beriberi is progressive, with increasing weakness, muscle wasting, loss of ambulation, ataxia, painful parasthesias, and loss of deep tendon reflexes. Edema is the hallmark symptom of wet beriberi because of cardiomyopathy, which progresses to congestive heart failure and death if untreated. Infantile beriberi generally occurs in breastfed children whose mothers have subclinical thiamine deficiency and is characterized by the sudden onset of shock in a 2- to 3-month-old previously well infant. These symptoms may be preceded by a hoarse, weak cry; poor feeding; and vomiting.[15] Wernicke encephalopathy is characterized by the triad of ophthalmoplegia, nystagmus, and ataxia in addition to altered consciousness and has been reported with thiamine deficiency in infants and children as well during a parenteral multivitamin preparation shortage.[15,16]

Thiamine deficiency may result from inadequate dietary intake of the vitamin, malabsorption, excessive loss, or defective transport of the vitamin. Mothers at risk of thiamine deficiency include those with a poor thiamine intake, alcohol abuse, gastrointestinal disease, hyperemesis gravidarum, and HIV/AIDS. Other children and adolescents at particularly high risk of the development of thiamine deficiency include those who follow fad diets, have anorexia nervosa, have undergone gastric bypass surgery, have kidney disease for which they are undergoing chronic dialysis, are hospitalized in the pediatric intensive care unit, or have congenital heart disease and potentially those receiving long-term parenteral nutrition.[16-21]

Several tests are used to detect thiamine deficiency. These include the measurement of thiamine dependent enzymes with the blood transketolase activation test at baseline and after added TPP[22] or erythrocyte TPP concentration.[23] Infantile beriberi is treated with 50 to 100 mg of parenteral thiamine as a 1-time dose and withholding breastfeeding until maternal diet is supplemented with thiamine.[24] Beriberi in children is treated with 10 to 25 mg of parenteral thiamine, once daily, for 2 weeks followed by 5 to 10 mg of oral thiamine, daily, for 1 month. When mild, beriberi can be treated with 10 mg of oral thiamine daily. Tolerable upper limits for thiamine have not been established, but in high doses, interactions with chemotherapy agents or other high-dose vitamins have been reported.[3] Although rare, injections of thiamine may cause hypersensitivity dermatitis, tenderness, tingling, pruritus, pain, weakness, sweating, nausea, gastrointestinal tract distress, restlessness, respiratory distress, pulmonary edema, vascular collapse, or even death.[3]

IV

Riboflavin (Vitamin B$_2$)

Riboflavin is a precursor of the enzyme cofactors flavin mononucleotide (FMN) and flavin adenine dinucleotide (FAD), involved in oxidation-reduction reactions integral to carbohydrate, protein, and fat metabolism. FAD is an essential component of the antioxidant enzymes glutathione reductase and xanthine oxidase. Riboflavin is found in abundance in animal protein (meat, dairy, and eggs), as well as green vegetables and fortified cereals. Riboflavin deficiency is generally accompanied by deficiencies of one or more B complex vitamins, in part because of riboflavin's role in the metabolism of folate, pyridoxine, and niacin.[25,26] Signs and symptoms are nonspecific in the mildly deficient state but progress to more characteristic symptoms with increasing severity, including pharyngitis, cheilosis, angular stomatitis, glossitis (magenta tongue), and seborrheic dermatitis involving the nasolabilal folds, the flexural area of extremities, and the genital area.

Children at risk of deficiency include the economically disadvantaged with limited dietary meat or dairy intake but also include breastfed infants who have not yet weaned to cow milk. Studies also document decreased serum riboflavin in neonates undergoing phototherapy.[27] Ariboflavinosis has been described in protein-energy malnutrition states, such as kwashiorkor and anorexia nervosa, and prolonged malabsorptive disease, such as celiac disease and short-bowel syndrome. Riboflavin deficiency has been reported in patients with cystic fibrosis.[28] Additionally, children who have undergone bariatric surgery are at risk of thiamine deficiency.[29] Thyroid and adrenal insufficiency can impair the synthesis of riboflavin cofactors and may precipitate the deficiency state.

Deficiency can be directly assessed with a 24-hour urine collection for riboflavin or measurement of riboflavin in red blood cells (RBCs).[30,31] Deficiency can also be assessed indirectly by RBC glutathione reductase activity coefficient,[32,33] but the test is of limited value in patients with glutathione reductase deficiency, gluclose-6-phosphate dehydrogenase (G6PD) deficiency and β-thalassemia. Deficiency in children is treated with oral riboflavin, 1 mg, 3 times daily until signs of deficiency resolve. Infants may respond to 0.5 mg twice weekly.

Although tolerable upper limits of dosing have not been established, doses greater than 400 mg daily may cause diarrhea, polyuria, and/or orange urine and exacerbate or precipitate acneiform eruptions.[34] High doses of riboflavin decrease the effectiveness of sulfonamide antibiotics.[3] Although more studies are necessary, riboflavin as complementary and alternative medicine for migraine prophylaxis (25, 200, or 400 mg daily) has been prescribed alone or with magnesium and feverfew. Additionally, 25 mg alone has been reported to achieved a 50% reduction in migraines in 44% of people studied.[35,36]

Niacin (Vitamin B$_3$)

Nicotinic acid and nicotinamide are the 2 vitamins commonly referred to as niacin. These 2 forms of niacin are chemically modified in the mitochondria to form the coenzymes NAD and NAD phosphate (NADP). Enzymes involved in oxidation-reduction reactions require the coenzymes NAD and NADP to accept or donate electrons. Unlike most WSVs, half of the body's niacin can be synthesized in the liver and kidney from tryptophan in a series of reactions dependent on riboflavin and pyridoxine. Animal protein (dairy, eggs, and meat), beans, and fortified cereals are excellent sources of niacin, and many of these foods are also good sources of tryptophan. However, sugars and high leucine present in some nonfortified grains may bind to niacin, reducing bioavailablity.[9]

Deficiency of niacin results in the clinical syndrome known as pellagra, or "rough skin" in Italian. Pellagra is characterized by the triad of diarrhea, dermatitis, and dementia or, in the case of advanced stages, a tetrad including death. The gastrointestinal tract symptoms associated with niacin deficiency include glossitis, angular stomatitis, cheilitis, and diarrhea in one third to one half of patients.[37] The skin lesions in pellagra are quite characteristic, with painful erythema in areas of sun-exposed skin (dorsal surface of the hands, face, and neck), which can progress to an exudatitve phase. Repeated sun exposure may result in vesicles coalescing into bullae, eventually becoming rough, hard, and scaly, giving pellagra its name.[38] Hair and nails are spared. This rash differs from the generalized dermatitis found in kwashiorkor, which is found in both sun-exposed and nonsun-exposed skin. The early neuropsychiatric symptoms of pellagra may include insomnia, fatigue, nervousness, irritability, depression, mental dullness, apathy, and memory impairment. Untreated, these symptoms may progress to dementia and, ultimately, death.

With few exceptions, pellagra is a disease limited to malnourished children from developing countries. In the industrialized regions of the world, those at risk include the homeless, individuals with malabsorptive conditions, such as Crohn disease, and people with nutritional self-deprivation states, such as anorexia nervosa.[39,40] Pellagra has been reported in Hartnup disease, a disorder of neutral amino acid transport resulting in tryptophan malabsorption; in the carcinoid syndrome from depleted tryptophan stores; in patients with treated with isoniazid, 5-fluorouracil, or 6-mercaptopurine from inadequate conversion of tryptophan to niacin; and in patients receiving long-term anticonvulsants.[9,41,42]

Niacin status can be evaluated by 24-hour urinary excretion of niacin and its metabolite N_1-methylnicotinamide[43] and RBC NAD and NADP levels to determine whether the "niacin number" (NAD/NADP x 100) is deficient (ie, less than 130).[44-46] The treatment for pellagra in children is an oral dose of 50 to 100 mg nicotinamide, 3 times daily. Use of nicotinamide avoids the uncomfortable flushing associated with nicotinic acid. Therapy should be continued until resolution of acute symptoms. High-dose niacin, as seen in energy drinks and energy shots, also causes flushing. Niacin is used to treat dyslipidemia in adults and children, with daily dosage of 20 to 40 mg/kg/day, up to 3 g. However, pharmacologic doses of niacin for the treatment of dyslipidemia in children has been inadequately studied. Adverse effects of pharmacologic doses of niacin include flushing, pruritus, nausea, vomiting, headache, bloating, diarrhea, anorexia, peptic ulcer, and rarely, hepatotoxicity. Chronic administration can also impair glucose control and impair uric acid excretion.[3] Niacin can interfere with commonly administered drugs, such as insulin, oral diabetes drugs, nonsteroidal anti-inflammatory drugs, warfarin, and seizure medications by increasing blood concentrations and increasing risk of toxicity (see Table 21.2).

IV

Pyridoxine (Vitamin B₆)

There are 3 naturally occurring forms of vitamin B_6: pyridoxine, pyridoxal, and pyridoxamine. These pyridines are activated to the coenzyme form by phophorylation. Pyridoxal 5'-phosphate is the most ubiquitous form of the vitamin and is integral to a multitude of enzymes necessary for human amino acid and carbohydrate metabolism. It is required for the conversion of tryptophan to both niacin and serotonin. Similarly, vitamin B_6 is also required for the conversion of dopa to dopamine as well as the synthesis of the inhibitory neurotransmitter gamma-aminobutyric acid (GABA). Hematologically, pyridoxine is a necessary cofactor in the rate-limiting step of heme biosynthesis. Foods rich in pyridoxine include bananas, fish, milk, yeast, eggs, and fortified cereals.

Isolated deficiency of pyridoxine is rare because of its interaction with other WSVs. Pyridoxine metabolism requires adequate levels of riboflavin, niacin, and zinc, and biosynthesis and metabolism of niacin and folate requires pyridoxine. As with other WSVs, children in developing countries with marginal nutrition are at risk of deficiency.[47] In the 1950s, a manufacturing error in infant formula resulted in severe vitamin B_6 deficiency and seizures in a cohort of infants. Deficiency has been described in childhood leukemia and chronic renal failure.[48,49] Mild deficiency of vitamin B_6 can result from the covalent binding of certain drugs (isoniazid, hydralazine, oral contraceptives, penicillamine, cycloserine, theophylline) to pyridoxal 5'-phosphate. The manifestations of pyridoxine deficiency are nonspecific and include seborrheic eruption on face and scalp, neck, and shoulders as well as glossitis, angular stomatitis, cheilosis, irritability, depression, and confusion.

There are several rare vitamin B_6 dependency syndromes, including vitamin B_6-responsive anemia, xanthurenic aciduria, cystathionuria, and homocystinuria. Pyridoxine-dependent seizure disorder is a deficiency of alpha aminoadipic semialdolase dehyrodgenase (antiquitin) encoded by ALDH7A1, an autosomal-recessive disorder presenting with intractable seizures, because byproducts degrade pyridoxine, making it unavailable to function as a cofactor in the conversion of glutamic acid to the inhibitory neurotransmitter GABA.[50] Despite a normal serum vitamin B_6 concentration, the seizures in these infants respond to 10 to 500 mg of parenteral vitamin B_6. Oral folinic acid (3–5 mg/kg/day) may be added to treat pyridoxine-dependent seizures because of improved response in some patients. Maintenance pyridoxine therapy is required indefinitely with this seizure disorder with doses as high as 15 to 18 mg/kg/day, orally (maximum of 500 mg), well above the RDA.[51] Recently, a second pyridoxine-resposive seizure disorder has also been found to respond to pyridoxine, but discontinuation of the vitamin can occur later.[50] Additionally, a third and rare disorder, pyridoxal phosphate-dependent seizure disorder caused by deficiency of pyridox(am)ine 5' phosphate oxidase

(PNPO), also presents as retractable seizures, hypoglycemia, and lactic acidosis. It is treated with 30 to 50 mg/kg/day of pyridoxal 5'-phosphate divided in 4 to 6 doses. A fourth seizure disorder, infantile spasms (West syndrome), can also be treated with pyridoxal 5'-phosphate and adrenocorticotropic hormone. Because pyridoxal 5'-phosphate treats all conditions, experts recommend that pyridoxine, pyridoxal 5'-phosphate, and folate be given for intractable seizures in newborn infants until biochemical and genetic testing allow final diagnosis and optimal treatment.[50]

Vitamin B$_6$ has been utilized at pharmacologic doses with little proof of efficacy to remedy the symptoms of carpal tunnel syndrome, depression, hyperoxaluria, and dysmenorrhea, among others.[52-57] High-dose vitamin B$_6$ is also used to treat children with autism spectrum disorders, as plasma pyridoxine concentrations are high and pyridoxal 5'-phosphate concentrations are low in these children because of deficient activity of the enzyme pyrodoxal kinase. A Cochrane review found data insufficient to recommend treatment of autism with vitamin B$_6$ because of heterogeneous and poor-quality studies.[58] Despite the lack of evidence, vitamin B$_6$ continues to be used for many of the aforementioned conditions, including autism, with a potential for toxicity when given in excess. When taken in excess on a chronic basis, vitamin B$_6$ can exacerbate or precipitate acneiform eruptions and cause a peripheral sensory neuropathy characterized by bilateral parasthesias, hyperaesthesia, limb pain, ataxia, somnolence, and poor coordination.[5] Nausea, vomiting, allergic reactions, breast soreness and enlargement, and increased risk of ulcerative colitis can also be seen. The combination of high doses of both vitamin B$_6$ with vitamin B$_{12}$ may result in a severe rosacea fulminans.[3]

Various methods have been used to assess vitamin B$_6$ status, including 24-hour urine assay for the pyridoxine metabolic product 4-pyridoxic acid or plasma pyridoxal 5'-phosphate, the predominant B$_6$ vitamer present in the plasma.[59] Children deficient in vitamin B$_6$ without neuritis should receive 5 to 25 mg/day of oral pyridoxine for 3 weeks, followed by 1.5 to 2.5 mg/day, orally, contained in a multivitamin product (Table 21.3). With peripheral neuropathy, the dosing is increased to 10 to 50 mg/day of oral pyridoxine for 3 weeks, then decreased to 1 to 2 mg/day. Vitamin B$_6$ therapy has been shown to slow the development of nephropathy and vascular disease in type 2 diabetes mellitus, and higher plasma concentrations of vitamin B$_6$ protected against coronary artery disease in the Nurses Health Study and other studies.[60]

Folate

Folic acid carries hydroxymethyl and formyl groups necessary for the synthesis of purines and thymine required for DNA formation. The vitamin is necessary for RBC maturation and promotion of cellular growth in general. Total serum homocysteine is increased in the presence of folate deficiency in neonates.[61] Supplemental folate, taken alone or added to food, is better absorbed than folate normally present in food, and many cereals, grains, and breads are now fortified with folate. Natural sources include fresh green vegetables, liver, yeast, and some fruits. Megaloblastic anemia is the primary sign of deficiency.

Low serum and RBC folic acid concentrations in women of childbearing potential increase the risk of fetal birth defects, particularly neural tube defects. Some evidence also supports maternal deficiency of either folic acid or vitamin B_{12} as independent risk factors for this phenomena.[62] Since the identification of a single nucloetide polymorphism (SNP) C677T of the 5,10–methylenetetrahydrofolate reductase gene as a risk factor for neural tube defects,[63] work has proceeded to investigate the relationship between SNPs in folate metabolic pathways and the occurrence of neural tube defects. C677T homozygosity in either mother or fetus increases fetal risk of neural tube defects. Many other SNPs in the folate pathway have been investigated, and a small number have also been linked to neural tube defects.[64] Additionally, the risk of stroke in children with the C677T allele may be double that of age-matched controls,[65] so studies to determine whether folate supplementation also prevents recurrent stroke in this group are needed. Some additional data also support that low periconceptual folate intake by pregnant women is also associated with fetal orofacial clefts and congenital heart disease.[66,67]

In contrast to the other WSVs, inadequate intake of folate in children and adolescents is common. In one study of white preschool children of middle and upper socioeconomic status 2 to 5 years of age, mean folate intake was consistently below recommended amounts.[68] Foods most commonly eaten were fruit drinks, carbonated beverages, 2% milk, and french fries, with folate intakes only 79% of recommended amounts.[68,69] Over the last 30 years, the diets of US adolescents include greater consumption of soft drinks and noncitrus fruit juices and consumption of fruits and vegetables well below the recommended 7 to 9 servings per day, especially in girls, resulting in inadequate folate intake.[70]

Other patients at risk of folate deficiency are those with malabsorption syndromes, including Crohn disease, and patients with HIV infection.[71,72] In pediatric and adolescent patients on chronic dialysis, folate deficiency promotes erythropoietin resistance.[73] There are also several inherited diseases of folate metabolism. Methylenetetrahydrofolate reductase deficiency, described in 4 siblings, presented as retarded psychomotor development, poor social contact, and seizures with low serum and RBC folate concentrations.[74] Cerebral folate deficiency is a disorder in which serum and RBC folate concentrations are normal but folate transport from plasma to the central nervous system (CNS) is prevented either by an inherited defect in CNS transporter or by autoantibodies[75]; however, the disease is responsive to folinic acid treatment. In children with autism spectrum disorders, vitamin B_{12} and folinic acid therapy has been studied because of a previously identified dysfunctional folate-methionine metabolic pathway crucial for DNA synthesis, DNA methylation, and cellular redox balance.[5] Although a subset showed improvement in glutathione-mediated redox status,[5] systematic reviews of the studies of children with autism spectrum disorders are underpowered with clinical heterogeneity that make findings inconclusive.[76]

Adverse effects of folate deficiency include abdominal cramps, nausea, diarrhea, rash, altered sleep patterns, irritability, worsening of seizures, and worsening of B_{12} deficiency. Low serum folate indicates short-term deficiency, and low RBC folate indicates chronic folate deficiency. Measurement of 5-methyltetrahydrofolate, the principal circulating form of plasma folate, may be clinically useful,[75] as is the meaurement of the serum concentration of homocysteine, which is elevated in folic acid deficiency. Folic acid deficiency is treated with daily administration of oral supplements of 0.1 mg in infants and 1.0 mg in children, followed by maintenance of 0.1 to 0.5 mg daily. Folic acid can also be given parenterally. Adverse interactions with other medications have been reported, including methotrexate, seizure medications, oral contraceptives, and trimethoprim.[3] Nonsteroidal anti-inflammatory drugs inhibit folate enzymes.

Cobalamin (Vitamin B_{12})

Cobalamin functions as a coenzyme for a number of enzymes involved in RBC maturation and central nervous system development. Cobalamin and folate are necessary for the remethylation of homocysteine to methionine by methionine synthase. Higher concentrations of cobalamin are found in colostrum compared with those in the third month of lactation. Levels of cobalamin and its binding protein in human milk are similar over the course of a day and in fore versus hind milk.[77] Cobalamin is found in foods of animal origin only. Good sources are meat, fish, poultry, cheese, milk, eggs, and vitamin B_{12}-fortified soy milk. Signs and symptoms of deficiency include macrocytic megaloblastic anemia and neurologic problems (ataxia, muscle weakness, spasticity, incontinence, hypotension, vision problems, dementia, psychoses, and mood disturbances). Vitamin B_{12} deficiency is accompanied by hyperhomocysteinemia, which is a reported risk factor for cardiovascular disease.[78] Vitamin B_{12} and folate have been studied as a treatment for autism spectrum disorders[74] (See Folate).

Breastfed infants of strict vegan mothers are at risk of vitamin B_{12} deficiency. Elevated plasma methylmalonic acid and total homocysteine are useful indicators of functional cobalamin deficiency in infants, and administration of either oral or intramuscular vitamin B_{12} can normalize urinary values of methylmalonic acid in vitamin B_{12}-deficient infants.[79] Megaloblastic anemia secondary to vitamin B_{12} deficiency in children consuming alternative diets has also been reported.[80] Other subjects at risk of vitamin B_{12} deficiency include those with resection of stomach and/or ileum, because gastric intrinsic factor is necessary for ileal absorption of vitamin B_{12}. Pernicious anemia is an autoimmune disease characterized by megaloblastic anemia secondary to intrinsic factor deficiency. Patients with phenylketonuria on an unrestricted or relaxed diet are at risk of vitamin B_{12} deficiency.[81] Vitamin B_{12}-responsive inborn errors of metabolism exist, including transcobalamin II deficiency, homocysteinuria, and hereditary juvenile cobalamin deficiency caused by mutations in gastric intrinsic factor.[82,83] Imerslund-Grasbeck syndrome, a familial selective vitamin B_{12} malabsorption disorder, can be successfully treated by intramuscular administration of vitamin B_{12}. Maternal vitamin B_{12} deficiency has also been associated with neural tube defects in offspring.[84]

The diagnosis of cobalamin deficiency is made by determination of the serum cobalamin concentration. If serum concentration is borderline low, finding elevated plasma homocysteine and urinary methylmalonic acid would be confirmatory.[85,86] Treatment is large doses of cobalamin given orally or, in the case of malabsorption syndromes, periodic administration via the intramuscular or intranasal route. The dose for treatment of vitamin B_{12} deficiency in children is 30 to 50 µg, intramuscularly or deep subcutaneously, daily for 2 weeks, followed by maintenance injection of 100 µg monthly. Energy drinks and shots contain vitamin B_{12} with variable amounts but can contain more than 8000% of the daily value. Toxic reactions include urticaria, anaphylaxis, and exacerbation of and precipitation of acneiform eruptions. High-dose vitamin B_{12} in combination with pyridoxine may cause the severe skin lesion rosacea fulminans.[87] Antiretroviral drugs may lower vitamin B_{12} concentrations.[3]

Vitamin C

Vitamin C is essential for many biological functions, including folate metabolism, collagen biosynthesis, bone formation, neurotransmitter synthesis, and iron absorption. Dietary sources include papaya, citrus fruits, tomatoes, cabbage, potatoes, cantaloupe, and strawberries. In the recent Dietary Reference Intakes (DRIs) recommended by the Institute of Medicine, the Recommended Dietary Allowance (RDA) for vitamin C for adults was established on the basis of maintenance of near-maximal concentration of vitamin C in neutrophils with minimal urinary excretion of ascorbate. Because similar data in infants were not available, Adequate Intakes for vitamin C in infants was based on mean vitamin C intake of breastfed infants. RDAs for children and adolescents were estimated on the basis of relative body weight. Signs and symptoms of deficiency include fatigue, malaise, and lethargy, followed by abnormal hyperkeratotic hair follicles and brittle, coiled hair. As the deficiency state progresses, perifollicular hemorrhage, osmotic diarrhea, bleeding gums, ocular hemorrhages, and anemia occur, followed by the development of frank scurvy with painful bones, joint hemorrhage, and arthropathy.[9,88]

Intakes of vitamin C by school-aged children has been studied. After defining marginal vitamin C intake as less than 30 mg/day, 12% of boys and 13% of girls between 7 and 12 years of age as well as 14% of boys and 20% of girls between 14 and 18 years of age reported intakes of vitamin C as submarginal.[89] Children with low vitamin C intake tended to have greater energy-adjusted intakes of fat and saturated fat, and children with desirable vitamin C intakes consumed more high-vitamin C fruit juices and whole milk, more high-vitamin C containing vegetables, and more citrus fruits than did children with low vitamin C intake.[89] In a group of children receiving long-term dialysis, dietary intake of vitamin C was less than 100% of the RDA in most children not receiving supplementation.[90] Vitamin C is removed by dialyzation, so ongoing adequate intake is necessary in dialysis patients. Low intake can also result from unsupplemented parenteral nutrition, anorexia nervosa, autism, ulcerative colitis, and Crohn disease. Although scurvy is increasingly rare in children, it is still reported in children who ingest only well-cooked foods and few fruits or vegetables. Use of alcohol and tobacco can decrease vitamin C absorption and increase its metabolism. Low periconceptual intake of vitamin C has been associated with low birth weight.[91] Vitamin C deficiency may play a role in oxidant stress in children with chronic renal disease and in children with sickle cell anemia.[92,93] In addition to dietary deficiencies, a hereditary methemoglobinemia in infants that is responsive to vitamin C has been described.

Vitamin C status is best assessed by measuring the concentration of ascorbate in blood leukocytes, considered a better measure of tissue reserves than plasma ascorbate.[94] In children, scurvy is treated with 100 mg of ascorbic acid given 3 times daily for 1 week, then 100 mg daily for several weeks until tissue saturation is normal. The regimen may be administered intramuscularly, intravenously, or orally. High-dose vitamin C as a CAM has been touted to prevent the common cold, but data are unsupportive unless under extreme physcial stress. However, vitamin C may have a modest effect in reducing the duration but not the severity of the common cold in adults and children.[95] Excessive vitamin C intake may cause nausea, vomiting, esophagitis, abdominal cramps, constipation, headache, insomnia, and kidney stones. High doses can increase the blood concentrations of acetaminophen, aspirin, warfarin, and estrogens while decreasing blood concentrations of some antiviral medicines and decreasing enteral absorption of beta blockers.[3]

IV

Other Water-Soluble Vitamins

Information on human needs for pantothenic acid is limited. Pantothenic acid is a component of CoA and is involved in many enzymatic reactions. It is found in liver, yeast, egg yolk, fresh vegetables, whole grains, and legumes. Deficiency symptoms have not been characterized. In one survey, 49% of female adolescents and 25% of male adolescents consumed less than 4 mg/day, the amount recommended by the Institute of Medicine.[96] However, average blood concentrations for both groups were in the normal range.

Biotin is the CoA for 5 mammalian carboxylases. Dietary sources include liver, egg yolk, soybeans, milk, and meat. Clinical biotin deficiency is characterized by hypotonia and severe exfoliative dermatitis. To date, symptomatic nutritional deficiency has been described only in infants receiving total parenteral nutrition that was free of biotin and in children consuming undercooked eggs containing large amounts of avidin, a biotin-binding protein. However, children receiving long-term anticonvulsant therapy exhibit impaired biotin concentrations but not overt deficiency.[97] The growing list of inborn errors of metabolism that exhibit biotin dependency and various degrees of neurologic and dermatologic abnormalities include holocarboxylase synthetase deficiency, biotinidase deficiency, and a defect in biotin transport.[98] Diagnosis of deficiency is made by measuring urinary biotin, urinary 3-hydroxyisovaleric acid, and lymphocyte proprionyl-CoA carboxylase. Expression of the potential biotin transporter SLC19A3 in leukocytes may prove to be a useful indicator of marginal biotin deficiency.[99]

Conclusion

WSV deficiency states occur as a result of decreased intake but can also be secondary to inborn errors of metabolism in which pharmacologic doses of WSVs may ameliorate signs of disease. The genetic polymorphisms responsible for some diseases relating to WSVs have been delineated, with more genetic polymorphisms with disease potential to be identified in the future. Other future research priorities include investigation of the global prevalence of WSV deficiencies, the role of WSVs in autism and cognitive development, the importance of nutrient-nutrient interactions, effects of excessive WSV ingestion, and the effects of age, gender, and genetics on WSV status in the pediatric age group.[100,101]

- Supplemental WSVs are probably unnecessary for the healthy child older than 1 year who consumes a varied diet.
- Children at-risk of WSV deficiencies may benefit from supplemental multivitamin preparations (Table 21.3) providing 50% to 100% of the RDA with minimal risks when given as recommended. At-risk children include

those following a fad diet or a diet high in fat; those with anorexia, gastrointestinal tract malabsorptive diseases, chronic illness, history of bariatric surgery, HIV/AIDS, and obesity; and those receiving chemotherapeutic, antituberculosis, or anticonvulsant medications.

- Several gene polymorphism and inherited metabolic defects can also lead to deficiency states and have been described for thiamine, pyridoxine, folic acid, vitamin B_{12}, biotin, niacin, riboflavin, and vitamin C.

- Because of the interrelationships of WSV metabolic pathways, deficiencies of multiple WSVs can be seen.

- Symptoms of WSV deficiencies overlap and commonly include skin disorders, anemia, diarrhea, and impaired neurologic function.

REFERENCES

1. Position of the American Dietetic Association and the Canadian Dietetic Association: nutrition for physical fitness and athletic performance for adults. *J Am Diet Assoc.* 1993;93(6):691-696

2. Eisenberg DM, Davis RB, Ettner SL, et al. Trends in alternative medicine use in the United States, 1990-1997: results of a follow-up national survey. *JAMA.* 1998;280(18):1569-1575

3. Rogovik AL, Vohra S, Goldman RD. Safety considerations and potential interactions of vitamins: should vitamins be considered drugs? *Ann Pharmacother.* 2010;44(2):311-324

4. Lee AC, Kemper KJ. Homeopathy and naturopathy: practice characteristics and pediatric care. *Arch Pediatr Adolesc Med.* 2000;154(1):75-80

5. James SJ, Melnyk S, Fuchs G, et al. Efficacy of methylcobalamin and folinic acid treatment on glutathione redox status in children with autism. *Am J Clin Nutr.* 2009;89(1):425-430

6. Wilson K, Busse JW, Gilchrist A, Vohra S, Boon H, Mills E. Characteristics of pediatric and adolescent patients attending a naturopathic college clinic in Canada. *Pediatrics.* 2005;115(3):e338-e343

7. Boon HS, Cherkin DC, Erro J, et al. Practice patterns of naturopathic physicians: results from a random survey of licensed practitioners in two US States. *BMC Complement Altern Med.* 2004;4:14

8. Ogden CL, Flegal KM, Carroll MD, Johnson CL. Prevalence and trends in overweight among US children and adolescents, 1999-2000. *JAMA.* 2002;288(14):1728-1732

9. Jen M, Yan AC. Syndromes associated with nutritional deficiency and excess. *Clin Dermatol.* 2010;28(6):669-685

10. Kant AK. Reported consumption of low-nutrient-density foods by American children and adolescents: nutritional and health correlates, NHANES III, 1988 to 1994. *Arch Pediatr Adolesc Med.* 2003;157(8):789-796

11. Lee Y, Mitchell DC, Smiciklas-Wright H, Birch LL. Diet quality, nutrient intake, weight status, and feeding environments of girls meeting or exceeding recommendations for total dietary fat of the American Academy of Pediatrics. *Pediatrics.* 2001;107(6):e95

IV

12. Tonstad S, Sivertsen M. Relation between dietary fat and energy and micronutrient intakes. *Arch Dis Child*. 1997;76(5):416-420

13. Nicklas TA, Myers L, O'Neil C, Gustafson N. Impact of dietary fat and fiber intake on nutrient intake of adolescents. *Pediatrics*. 2000;105(2):e21

14. Ishibashi S, Yokota T, Shiojiri T, et al. Reversible acute axonal polyneuropathy associated with Wernicke-Korsakoff syndrome: impaired physiological nerve conduction due to thiamine deficiency? *J Neurol Neurosurg Psychiatry*. 2003;74(5):674-676

15. Luxemburger C, White NJ, ter Kuile F, et al. Beri-beri: the major cause of infant mortality in Karen refugees. *Trans R Soc Trop Med Hyg*. 2003;97(2):251-255

16. Hahn JS, Berquist W, Alcorn DM, Chamberlain L, Bass D. Wernicke encephalopathy and beriberi during total parenteral nutrition attributable to multivitamin infusion shortage. *Pediatrics*. 1998;101(1):e10

17. Towbin A, Inge TH, Garcia VF, et al. Beriberi after gastric bypass surgery in adolescence. *J Pediatr*. 2004;145(2):263-267

18. Hung SC, Hung SH, Tarng DC, Yang WC, Chen TW, Huang TP. Thiamine deficiency and unexplained encephalopathy in hemodialysis and peritoneal dialysis patients. *Am J Kidney Dis*. 2001;38(5):941-947

19. Shamir R, Dagan O, Abramovitch D, Abramovitch T, Vidne BA, Dinari G. Thiamine deficiency in children with congenital heart disease before and after corrective surgery. *JPEN J Parenter Enteral Nutr*. 2000;24(3):154-158

20. Winston AP, Jamieson CP, Madira W, Gatward NM, Palmer RL. Prevalence of thiamin deficiency in anorexia nervosa. *Int J Eat Disord*. 2000;28(4):451-454

21. Lima LF, Leite HP, Taddei JA. Low blood thiamine concentrations in children upon admission to the intensive care unit: risk factors and prognostic significance. *Am J Clin Nutr*. 2011;93(1):57-61

22. Bayoumi RA, Rosalki SB. Evaluation of methods of coenzyme activation of erythrocyte enzymes for detection of deficiency of vitamins B1, B2, and B6. *Clin Chem*. 1976;22(3):327-335

23. Talwar D, Davidson H, Cooney J, St JO'Reilly D. Vitamin B(1) status assessed by direct measurement of thiamin pyrophosphate in erythrocytes or whole blood by HPLC: comparison with erythrocyte transketolase activation assay. *Clin Chem*. 2000;46(5):704-710

24. Reid DH. Acute infantile beriberi. *J Pediatr*. 1961;58:858-863

25. Powers HJ. Riboflavin (vitamin B-2) and health. *Am J Clin Nutr*. 2003;77(6):1352-1360

26. McCormick DB. Two interconnected B vitamins: riboflavin and pyridoxine. *Physiol Rev*. 1989;69(4):1170-1198

27. Amin HJ, Shukla AK, Snyder F, Fung E, Anderson NM, Parsons HG. Significance of phototherapy-induced riboflavin deficiency in the full-term neonate. *Biol Neonate*. 1992;61(2):76-81

28. McCabe H. Riboflavin deficiency in cystic fibrosis: three case reports. *J Hum Nutr Diet*. 2001;14(5):365-370

29. Pratt JS, Lenders CM, Dionne EA, et al. Best practice updates for pediatric/adolescent weight loss surgery. *Obesity (Silver Spring)*. 2009;17(5):901-910

30. Floridi A, Palmerini CA, Fini C, Pupita M, Fidanza F. High performance liquid chromatographic analysis of flavin adenine dinucleotide in whole blood. *Int J Vitam Nutr Res*. 1985;55(2):187-191

31. Graham JM, Peerson JM, Haskell MJ, Shrestha RK, Brown KH, Allen LH. Erythrocyte riboflavin for the detection of riboflavin deficiency in pregnant Nepali women. *Clin Chem*. 2005;51(11):2162-2165

32. Tillotson JA, Baker EM. An enzymatic measurement of the riboflavin status in man. *Am J Clin Nutr*. 1972;25(4):425-431

33. Sauberlich HE, Judd JH Jr, Nichoalds GE, Broquist HP, Darby WJ. Application of the erythrocyte glutathione reductase assay in evaluating riboflavin nutritional status in a high school student population. *Am J Clin Nutr*. 1972;25(8):756-762

34. Schoenen J, Jacquy J, Lenaerts M. Effectiveness of high-dose riboflavin in migraine prophylaxis. A randomized controlled trial. *Neurology*. 1998;50(2):466-470

35. Maizels M, Blumenfeld A, Burchette R. A combination of riboflavin, magnesium, and feverfew for migraine prophylaxis: a randomized trial. *Headache*. 2004;44(9):885-890

36. Schiapparelli P, Allais G, Castagnoli Gabellari I, Rolando S, Terzi MG, Benedetto C. Non-pharmacological approach to migraine prophylaxis: part II. *Neurol Sci*. 2010;31(Suppl 1):S137-S139

37. Spivak JL, Jackson DL. Pellagra: an analysis of 18 patients and a review of the literature. *Johns Hopkins Med J*. 1977;140(6):295-309

38. Hegyi J, Schwartz RA, Hegyi V. Pellagra: dermatitis, dementia, and diarrhea. *Int J Dermatol*. 2004;43(1):1-5

39. Kertesz SG. Pellagra in 2 homeless men. *Mayo Clin Proc*. 2001;76(3):315-318

40. Pollack S, Enat R, Haim S, Zinder O, Barzilai D. Pellagra as the presenting manifestation of Crohn's disease. *Gastroenterology*. 1982;82(5 Pt 1):948-952

41. Darvay A, Basarab T, McGregor JM, Russell-Jones R. Isoniazid induced pellagra despite pyridoxine supplementation. *Clin Exp Dermatol*. 1999;24(3):167-169

42. Kaur S, Goraya JS, Thami GP, Kanwar AJ. Pellagrous dermatitis induced by phenytoin. *Pediatr Dermatol*. 2002;19(1):93

43. Carpenter KJ, Kodicek E. The fluorimetric estimation of N1-methylnicotinamide and its differentiation from coenzyme. *Biochem J*. 1950;46(4):421-426

44. Jacobson EL, Jacobson MK. Tissue NAD as a biochemical measure of niacin status in humans. *Methods Enzymol*. 1997;280:221-230

45. Shah GM, Shah RG, Veillette H, Kirkland JB, Pasieka JL, Warner RR. Biochemical assessment of niacin deficiency among carcinoid cancer patients. *Am J Gastroenterol*. 2005;100(10):2307-2314

46. Fu CS, Swendseid ME, Jacob RA, McKee RW. Biochemical markers for assessment of niacin status in young men: levels of erythrocyte niacin coenzymes and plasma tryptophan. *J Nutr*. 1989;119(12):1949-1955

47. Setiawan B, Giraud DW, Driskell JA. Vitamin B-6 inadequacy is prevalent in rural and urban Indonesian children. *J Nutr*. 2000;130(3):553-558

48. Pais RC, Vanous E, Hollins B, et al. Abnormal vitamin B6 status in childhood leukemia. *Cancer*. 1990;66(11):2421-2428

IV

49. Mydlik M, Derzsiova K, Guman M, Hrehorovsky M. Vitamin B6 requirements in chronic renal failure. *Int Urol Nephrol*. 1992;24(4):453-457

50. Gospe SM, Jr. Neonatal vitamin-responsive epileptic encephalopathies. *Chang Gung Med J*. 2010;33(1):1-12

51. Baxter P. Pyridoxine-dependent seizures: a clinical and biochemical conundrum. *Biochim Biophys Acta*. 2003;1647(1-2):36-41

52. Findling RL, Maxwell K, Scotese-Wojtila L, Huang J, Yamashita T, Wiznitzer M. High-dose pyridoxine and magnesium administration in children with autistic disorder: an absence of salutary effects in a double-blind, placebo-controlled study. *J Autism Dev Disord*. 1997;27(4):467-478

53. Aufiero E, Stitik TP, Foye PM, Chen B. Pyridoxine hydrochloride treatment of carpal tunnel syndrome: a review. *Nutr Rev*. 2004;62(3):96-104

54. Williams AL, Cotter A, Sabina A, Girard C, Goodman J, Katz DL. The role for vitamin B-6 as treatment for depression: a systematic review. *Fam Pract*. 2005;22(5):532-537

55. Malouf R, Grimley Evans J. The effect of vitamin B6 on cognition. *Cochrane Database Syst Rev*. 2003;(4):CD004393

56. Kaelin A, Casez JP, Jaeger P. Vitamin B6 metabolites in idiopathic calcium stone formers: no evidence for a link to hyperoxaluria. *Urol Res*. 2004;32(1):616-618

57. Proctor ML, Murphy PA. Herbal and dietary therapies for primary and secondary dysmenorrhoea. *Cochrane Database Syst Rev*. 2001;(3):CD002124

58. Adams JB, George F, Audhya T. Abnormally high plasma levels of vitamin B6 in children with autism not taking supplements compared to controls not taking supplements. *J Altern Complement Med*. 2006;12(1):59-63

59. Bor MV, Refsum H, Bisp MR, et al. Plasma vitamin B6 vitamers before and after oral vitamin B6 treatment: a randomized placebo-controlled study. *Clin Chem*. 2003;49(1):155-161

60. Jain SK. Vitamin B6 (pyridoxamine) supplementation and complications of diabetes. *Metabolism*. 2007;56(2):168-171

61. Minet JC, Bisse E, Aebischer CP, Beil A, Wieland H, Lutschg J. Assessment of vitamin B-12, folate, and vitamin B-6 status and relation to sulfur amino acid metabolism in neonates. *Am J Clin Nutr*. 2000;72(3):751-757

62. Kirke PN, Molloy AM, Daly LE, Burke H, Weir DG, Scott JM. Maternal plasma folate and vitamin B12 are independent risk factors for neural tube defects. *Q J Med*. 1993;86(11):703-708

63. Botto LD, Yang Q. 5,10-Methylenetetrahydrofolate reductase gene variants and congenital anomalies: a HuGE review. *Am J Epidemiol*. 2000;151(9):862-877

64. van der Linden IJ, Afman LA, Heil SG, Blom HJ. Genetic variation in genes of folate metabolism and neural-tube defect risk. *Proc Nutr Soc*. 2006;65(2):204-215

65. Cardo E, Monros E, Colome C, et al. Children with stroke: polymorphism of the MTHFR gene, mild hyperhomocysteinemia, and vitamin status. *J Child Neurol*. 2000;15(5):295-298

66. Pei LJ, Zhu HP, Li ZW, et al. Interaction between maternal periconceptional supplementation of folic acid and reduced folate carrier gene polymorphism of neural tube defects. *Zhonghua Yi Xue Yi Chuan Xue Za Zhi*. 2005;22(3):284-287

67. Pei L, Zhu H, Zhu J, Ren A, Finnell RH, Li Z. Genetic variation of infant reduced folate carrier (A80G) and risk of orofacial defects and congenital heart defects in China. *Ann Epidemiol*. 2006;16(5):352-356

68. Skinner JD, Carruth BR, Houck KS, et al. Longitudinal study of nutrient and food intakes of white preschool children aged 24 to 60 months. *J Am Diet Assoc*. 1999;99(12):1514-1521

69. Picciano MF, Smiciklas-Wright H, Birch LL, Mitchell DC, Murray-Kolb L, McConahy KL. Nutritional guidance is needed during dietary transition in early childhood. *Pediatrics*. 2000;106(1 Pt 1):109-114

70. Cavadini C, Siega-Riz AM, Popkin BM. US adolescent food intake trends from 1965 to 1996. *Arch Dis Child*. 2000;83(1):18-24

71. Jeejeebhoy KN. Clinical nutrition: 6. Management of nutritional problems of patients with Crohn's disease. *CMAJ*. 2002;166(6):913-918

72. Meira DG, Lorand-Metze I, Toro AD, Silva MT, Vilela MM. Bone marrow features in children with HIV infection and peripheral blood cytopenias. *J Trop Pediatr*. 2005;51(2):114-119

73. Bamgbola OF. Pattern of resistance to erythropoietin-stimulating agents in chronic kidney disese. *Kidney Int*. 2011;80(5):464-474

74. Tonetti C, Burtscher A, Bories D, Tulliez M, Zittoun J. Methylenetetrahydrofolate reductase deficiency in four siblings: a clinical, biochemical, and molecular study of the family. *Am J Med Genet*. 2000;91(5):363-367

75. Ramaekers VT, Rothenberg SP, Sequeira JM, et al. Autoantibodies to folate receptors in the cerebral folate deficiency syndrome. *N Engl J Med*. 2005;352(19):1985-1991

76. Main PA, Angley MT, Thomas P, O'Doherty CE, Fenech M. Folate and methionine metabolism in autism: a systematic review. *Am J Clin Nutr*. 2010;91(6):1598-1620

77. Donangelo CM, Trugo NM, Koury JC, et al. Iron, zinc, folate and vitamin B12 nutritional status and milk composition of low-income Brazilian mothers. *Eur J Clin Nutr*. 1989;43(4):253-266

78. Chambers JC, Seddon MD, Shah S, Kooner JS. Homocysteine--a novel risk factor for vascular disease. *J R Soc Med*. 2001;94(1):10-13

79. Specker BL, Miller D, Norman EJ, Greene H, Hayes KC. Increased urinary methylmalonic acid excretion in breast-fed infants of vegetarian mothers and identification of an acceptable dietary source of vitamin B-12. *Am J Clin Nutr*. 1988;47(1):89-92

80. Dagnelie PC, van Staveren WA, Hautvast JG. Stunting and nutrient deficiencies in children on alternative diets. *Acta Paediatr Scand Suppl*. 1991;374:111-118

81. Vugteveen I, Hoeksma M, Monsen AL, et al. Serum vitamin B12 concentrations within reference values do not exclude functional vitamin B12 deficiency in PKU patients of various ages. *Mol Genet Metab*. 2011;102(1):13-17

82. Bibi H, Gelman-Kohan Z, Baumgartner ER, Rosenblatt DS. Transcobalamin II deficiency with methylmalonic aciduria in three sisters. *J Inherit Metab Dis*. 1999;22(7):765-772

83. Tanner SM, Li Z, Perko JD, et al. Hereditary juvenile cobalamin deficiency caused by mutations in the intrinsic factor gene. *Proc Natl Acad Sci U S A*. 2005;102(11):4130-4133

IV

84. Steen MT, Boddie AM, Fisher AJ, et al. Neural-tube defects are associated with low concentrations of cobalamin (vitamin B12) in amniotic fluid. *Prenat Diagn.* 1998;18(6):5455-55

85. Yetley EA, Coates PM, Johnson CL. Overview of a roundtable on NHANES monitoring of biomarkers of folate and vitamin B-12 status: measurement procedure issues1,5. *Am J Clin Nutr.* 2011;94(1):297S-302S

86. Yetley EA, Pfeiffer CM, Phinney KW, et al. Biomarkers of vitamin B-12 status in NHANES: a roundtable summary. *Am J Clin Nutr.* 2011;94(1):313S-321S

87. Jansen T, Romiti R, Kreuter A, Altmeyer P. Rosacea fulminans triggered by high-dose vitamins B6 and B12. *J Eur Acad Dermatol Venereol.* 2001;15(5):484-485

88. Fain O. Musculoskeletal manifestations of scurvy. *Joint Bone Spine.* 2005;72(2):124-128

89. Hampl JS, Taylor CA, Johnston CS. Intakes of vitamin C, vegetables and fruits: which schoolchildren are at risk? *J Am Coll Nutr.* 1999;18(6):582-590

90. Pereira AM, Hamani N, Nogueira PC, Carvalhaes JT. Oral vitamin intake in children receiving long-term dialysis. *J Ren Nutr.* 2000;10(1):24-29

91. Lee BE, Hong YC, Lee KH, et al. Influence of maternal serum levesl of vitamins C and E during eh second trimester on birth weight and length. *Eur J Clin Nutr.* 2004;58(10):1365-1371

92. Amer J, Ghoti H, Rachmilewitz E, Koren A, Levin C, Fibach E. Red blood cells, platelets and polymorphonuclear neutrophils of patients with sickle cell disease exhibit oxidative stress that can be ameliorated by antioxidants. *Br J Haematol.* 2006;132(1):108-113

93. Zwolinska D, Grzeszczak W, Szczepanska M, Kilis-Pstrusinska K, Szprynger K. Vitamins A, E and C as non-enzymatic antioxidants and their relation to lipid peroxidation in children with chronic renal failure. *Nephron Clin Pract.* 2006;103(1):c12-c18

94. Thurnham DI. Micronutrients and immune function: some recent developments. *J Clin Pathol.* 1997;50(11):887-891

95. Douglas RM, Hemila H, Chalker E, Treacy B. Vitamin C for preventing and treating the common cold. *Cochrane Database Syst Rev.* 2007;(3):CD000980

96. Eissenstat BR, Wyse BW, Hansen RG. Pantothenic acid status of adolescents. *Am J Clin Nutr.* 1986;44(6):931-937

97. Krause KH, Bonjour JP, Berlit P, Kynast G, Schmidt-Gayk H, Schellenberg B. Effect of long-term treatment with antiepileptic drugs on the vitamin status. *Drug Nutr Interact.* 1988;5(4):317-343

98. Mardach R, Zempleni J, Wolf B, et al. Biotin dependency due to a defect in biotin transport. *J Clin Invest.* 2002;109(12):1617-1623

99. Vlasova TI, Stratton SL, Wells AM, Mock NI, Mock DM. Biotin deficiency reduces expression of SLC19A3, a potential biotin transporter, in leukocytes from human blood. *J Nutr.* 2005;135(1):42-47

100. Bryan J, Osendarp S, Hughes D, Calvaresi E, Baghurst K, van Klinken JW. Nutrients for cognitive development in school-aged children. *Nutr Rev.* 2004;62(8):295-306

101. Viteri FE, Gonzalez H. Adverse outcomes of poor micronutrient status in childhood and adolescence. *Nutr Rev.* 2002;60(5 Pt 2):S77-S83

Chapter 22

Federal Regulation of Foods and Infant Formulas, Including Addition of New Ingredients: Food Additives and Substances Generally Recognized as Safe (GRAS)

Introduction

It is imperative that infants and children consume foods that are safe and nutritionally adequate for optimal health. In consuming a healthful diet, infants and children are exposed to food additives and "generally recognized as safe" (GRAS) substances. Such ingredients may be found in infant formulas, toddler foods, or foods that are marketed for the general population.

The American Academy of Pediatrics (AAP) supports exclusive breastfeeding (in which all fluid, energy, and nutrients come from human milk, with the possible exception of small amounts of medicinal/nutrient supplements) for approximately 6 months.[1] The US Department of Health and Human Services also recommends that infants be exclusively breastfed for the first 4 to 6 months of an infant's life, preferably 6 months.[2] Similarly, the World Health Organization recommends exclusive breastfeeding for the first 6 months of life,[3] but for many reasons, including medical conditions, human milk may not be available to all infants. In the absence of human milk, iron-fortified infant formulas are the most appropriate substitutes for feeding healthy, full-term infants during the first year of life. By 3 months of age, despite the improving rates of breastfeeding initiation, nearly 40% of US infants are exclusively formula fed, and 65% are receiving some infant formula at 6 months of age.[4]

Although infant formulas do not duplicate the composition of human milk, formulas are reformulated as new nutritional information, ingredients, and technology become available. Infant formula manufacturers often consider the composition of human milk in trying to improve their products. When used as the sole source of nourishment during the first 6 months of life, infant formulas meet all the energy and nutrient requirements of healthy, term infants. After 6 months of age, formulas complement the increasing variety of solid foods being introduced into the diet and continue to supply a significant part of the infant's nutritional requirements.[5,6]

Preterm infants consume infant formulas specially designed to meet their needs. These infants, typically defined as those born before 37 weeks of gestation, are at risk of medical complications attributable to their premature births. Ordinarily, preterm infants are hospitalized in neonatal intensive care units, where their care often includes nutrition via parenteral administration and specialized formulas.[7]

Preterm infant formulas are higher in calories and provide additional vitamins and minerals relative to term infant formulas. Preterm follow-up formulas may be used at home after discharge; such formulas are nutrient-dense, being higher in protein and some vitamins and minerals. Multiple factors must be considered in determining the appropriate formula for an infant, including the infant's body weight and overall health status.

Complementary feeding is defined as providing nutrient-containing foods or liquids along with human milk[8] and includes both solid foods and infant formula.[9] Complementary foods are generally introduced between 4 and 6 months of age. The age at which first foods are introduced to an infant and the type of food offered varies considerably and is largely determined by cultural practices and perceptions.

Beyond infancy, children may consume toddler foods for 1 or 2 years while learning to transition to foods that are marketed for the general population. Under its regulations, the US Food and Drug Administration (FDA) considers toddlers to be children 1 to 3 years of age.

Federal Regulation of Ingredients Added To Food

The Center for Food Safety and Applied Nutrition of the FDA is responsible for promoting and protecting public health by making sure that the food supply is safe and wholesome. Its food safety mission is broad in scope and includes regulatory and research programs to address health risks associated with foodborne chemical and biological contamination, proper labeling of foods, including health claims, dietary supplements, food industry compliance, and international harmonization efforts. An important part of the Center for Food Safety and Applied Nutrition's mission is to review the safety of ingredients added to food, including infant formula and other foods developed for children. It also reviews substances contacting food, including materials used to package infant formula and baby food. These reviews are within the mission of the Office of Food Additive Safety.

Food from plant or animal sources contains carbohydrates, proteins, lipids, vitamins, minerals, and other nutrients. As such, food is a complex mixture of hundreds or thousands of chemical substances. Under the Federal Food, Drug, and Cosmetic Act (FD&C Act),[a] whole foods are presumed to be safe on the basis of their history of common use. This presumption is not extended to ingredients added to food, which must undergo a safety assessment and meet the safety standard of "reasonable certainty of no harm."

---

[a] http://www.fda.gov/RegulatoryInformation/Legislation/FederalFoodDrugandCosmeticActFDCAct/default.htm.

The term "food ingredients," as used in this chapter, includes food additives, color additives, and other substances that are GRAS under specified conditions of use. These ingredients are intentionally added to food for technical reasons, including: (1) to maintain or improve safety and freshness; (2) to improve or maintain nutritional value; or (3) to improve taste, texture, and appearance. In addition, some ingredients are added to conventional foods for their effects on the human body. It is important to understand that the regulatory framework for foods defines a standard of safety and not the efficacy of the food additive. Thus, the evaluation of ingredients by the FDA is limited to consideration of risks rather than benefits.

Materials used to package or transport food are called food contact substances. Although not intentionally added to food, food contact substances are subject to the same safety standard as food ingredients. Some food contact substances (eg, plastic packaging materials, can coatings, and sealants for lids and caps) are also relevant to the packaging of infant formula. Further consideration of food contact substances is beyond the scope of this chapter.

The FDA has several programs to ensure the safety of food ingredients, including a mandatory review processes for food and color additives and a voluntary notification program for GRAS substances. When a petition for GRAS status is filed for new food ingredients (eg, docosahexaenoic acid [DHA]), the notice of filing and the agency's final action on a petition are published in the *Federal Register*. An inventory of GRAS notices and the agency's response to those notices is posted on the FDA Web site: http://www.fda.gov/Food/FoodIngredientsPackaging/ucm112642.htm.

Food Ingredients: Food Additive or GRAS Substance?

In 1958, Congress enacted the Food Additives Amendment to the FD&C Act. A food additive is broadly defined as a substance that, when added to food, becomes a component or otherwise affects the characteristics of food. Food additives must undergo premarket review and approval by the FDA to be added to foods. This includes a substance that imparts color to a food. In addition, a source of radiation is explicitly defined by the law as a food additive, thus, giving the FDA regulatory power over the use of irradiation of food. Of note, infant formulas are not irradiated and do not contain color additives.

On the other hand, the FD&C Act states that substances that are GRAS for their intended use by experts qualified by scientific training and experience to evaluate their safety are excluded from the food additive definition. Put simply, GRAS substances are not "food additives" and do not require premarket review and approval by the FDA. As noted previously, irrespective of whether a substance is deemed to be GRAS or is a food additive, the safety determination is always limited to the substance's intended conditions of use, not its efficacy. In other words, the GRAS substance does not have to be shown to be beneficial to use in food but has to be shown not to be harmful.

For approval of a food additive, data and information, which may be proprietary, must be sent to the FDA to evaluate the safety of the additive. Thus, for a food additive, the FDA determines the safety of the ingredient, whereas a determination that an ingredient is GRAS can be made by any qualified experts, including those outside government.

A food substance may be GRAS either through scientific procedures or, for a substance used in food before passage of the FD&C Act, through experience based on common use in food prior to 1958. General recognition of safety for a GRAS substance through scientific procedures requires the same quantity and quality of scientific evidence required to obtain approval of the substance as a food additive and ordinarily is based on published studies, which may be corroborated by unpublished studies and other data and information. General recognition of safety through experience based on common use in foods prior to 1958 requires a substantial history of widespread consumption for food by a significant number of consumers.

Voluntary Submissions for GRAS Substances

A substance that will be added to food is subject to mandatory premarket review and approval by the FDA unless its use is determined by qualified experts to be GRAS. On April 17, 1997, the FDA issued a proposed rule[10] to establish a voluntary notification procedure whereby any person may notify the FDA of a determination by that person that a particular use of a substance is GRAS. Although the proposed rule for GRAS notification was never finalized, the FDA accepts voluntary GRAS notices for use in human food. Thus, submission of a GRAS notice is voluntary, and in the case of an ingredient intended for use in infant formula, establishing the safety prior to infant formula notification (see Regulation of Infant Formula and Table 22.1) is advantageous to the industry and the FDA.

As described in the GRAS proposed rule, the agency evaluates whether each submitted notice provides a sufficient basis for a GRAS determination and whether information in the notice or otherwise available to the FDA raises issues that lead the agency to "question" whether use of the substance is GRAS. Following this evaluation, the FDA responds to the notifier by letter.

More information about the universe of food additives and GRAS substances can be found on the FDA Web site (http://www.fda.gov/Food/GuidanceComplianceRegulatoryInformation/GuidanceDocuments/FoodIngredientsandPackaging/ucm061846.htm).

Ingredient Review Focuses on Safety

The term "safe," as it refers to food additives and ingredients (including food contact substances), is defined by legislation as a "reasonable certainty in the minds of competent scientists that a substance is not harmful under the intended conditions of use." The concept of safety involves the question of whether a substance is hazardous to the health of man or animal and takes into consideration that in reality it is impossible to establish with complete certainty the absolute harmlessness of the use of any substance.[11]

The safety data considered in reviewing a food ingredient include, at a minimum, chemical information and toxicologic data. Microbiologic information is also needed when a microorganism is used in the production of an ingredient. Clinical studies designed for purposes other than safety may still provide information pertaining to the safe use of an ingredient in infant formula.

Chemical Information

Information provided for the ingredient includes composition as well as information on the method of manufacture that allows identification and characterization of both the intended component(s) and any likely impurities (eg, residual starting materials, products of side reactions, and decomposition products of reactants or of the additive) in the food ingredient (Table 22.2). For food ingredients of natural origin that might contain known toxicants, consideration of the ability of the manufacturing process to control, reduce, or concentrate toxicant levels is important. In addition, food grade specifications include identification and quantification of components of the ingredient as well as limitations for impurities or contaminants if needed (eg, lead, residual solvents, microorganisms, etc).

IV

Table 22.1.

Ingredients New to Infant Formula That Have Been the Subject of a GRAS Notice (GRN) Submitted to the FDA GRAS Notification Program as of 2011

GRN Number	Ingredient	Intended Use
Fatty Acids and Lipids		
GRN 41	DHASCO from *Crypthecodinium cohnii* (docosahexaenoic acid-rich single-cell oil) and ARASCO from *Mortierella alpina* (arachidonic acid-rich single-cell oil)	Term infant formula
GRN 94	Docosahexaenoic acid-rich oil from tuna (DHA-rich tuna oil) and arachidonic acid-rich oil from *M alpina* (AA-rich fungal oil)	Preterm infant formula used by hospitalized preterm infants and term infant formula
GRN 80	ARASCO (arachidonic acid-rich single-cell oil) from *M alpina*	Term infant formula
GRN 326	Arachidonic acid rich oil from *M alpina* strain I49-N18	Preterm and term infant formula containing docosahexaenoic acid
GRN 379	Tuna oil	Preterm and term infant formula containing an appropriate source of arachidonic acid
GRN 131	High 2-palmitic vegetable oil	Term and preterm infant formula
GRN 192	High 2-palmitic vegetable oil	Term infant and preterm infant formulas; also for use in baby and toddler foods, including meat and poultry products
GRN 216	Lipase enzyme preparation from *Rhizopus oryzae*	As an enzyme to produce tailored triglycerides for use in infant formula

Probiotics and Prebiotics		
GRN 49	Bifidobacterium lactis strain Bb12 and Streptococcus thermophilus strain Th4	Milk-based infant formula that is intended for consumption by infants 4 months a nd older
GRN 231	Lactobacillus casei subspecies rhamnosus strain GG	Term infant formul'a
GRN 268	Bifidobacterium longum strain BB536	Milk-based powdered infant formula for term infants 9 months and older; also for use in weaning foods
GRN 281	Lactobacillus rhamnosus strain HN001 produced in a milk-based medium	Milk-based powdered term infant formula that is intended for consumption from the time of birth, as well as in milk-based powdered follow-up formula
GRN 233	Combination of galacto-oligosaccharides and polydextrose	Milk-based term infant formula
GRN 236	Galacto-oligosaccharides	Term infant formula; also for use in baby foods
GRN 286	Galacto-oligosaccharides	Term infant formula and follow-up formula
GRN 334	Galacto-oligosaccharides	Term infant formula
Carotenoids		
GRN 221	Suspended lutein	Term infant formula
GRN 390	Suspended lutein	Preterm infant formula

IV

Table 22.2.

Types of Chemistry Data and Information Typically Evaluated for New Ingredients or New Uses of Ingredients

Identity	• Chemical name and CAS number • Structure and molecular weigh • Physical characteristics
Manufacturing process	• Full description of process • List of chemicals/reagents used
Specifications	• Typically proposed or references published specifications • Includes description of the ingredients, identification tests, purity assay, and limits for impurities/contaminants
Stability	• Data demonstrating the stability • Discussion of the fate of the ingredient
Technical effect and intended use	• Type of food and use level • Data to show that the use level accomplishes the technical effect
Analytical methodology	• If a use limitation of the additive is required for safe use, the petition must include a method able to quantify the substance for the purpose of enforcing the limit

As part of the chemist's evaluation of the intended use of an ingredient, the dietary exposure is estimated by considering the amount of a substance added to various foods and the amount of such foods generally consumed by the population at large on a daily basis over a lifetime.

Toxicologic Information

For a safety assessment, the types and number of safety studies needed depends primarily on the chemical nature of the substance being evaluated and the dietary exposure estimated from the conditions of intended use. The fate of the substance in the gut and other metabolic considerations (ie, absorption, distribution, metabolism, and elimination) are important as well. Toxicologic studies play a prominent role. Other specialized studies may be needed as determined on a case-by-case basis. Types of toxicologic studies typically evaluated for new ingredients or new uses of ingredients are listed in Table 22.3. The FDA has provided guidance documents to assist individuals who wish to submit data for the safety assessment of a food ingredient (http://www.fda.gov/FoodRedbook).

Table 22.3.

Type of Toxicological Studies Typically Evaluated for New Ingredients or New Uses of Ingredients

- Short-term tests for genetic toxicity (in vivo and in vitro testing).
- Metabolism and pharmacokinetic studies.
- Subchronic feeding studies (at least 90 days) in a rodent (eg, rat) and nonrodent (eg, dog) species.
- Two-generation reproduction study with a teratology phase (developmental toxicity study) in a rodent (eg, rat).
- Chronic feeding studies (at least 1 year) in a rodent (eg, rat) and nonrodent (eg, dog) species (may be conducted as a component of a lifetime carcinogenicity study in rodents).
- Two-year carcinogenicity studies in two rodent species (eg, rats and mice). The rat carcinogenicity study should also include an in utero phase.
- Other studies as needed (eg, neurotoxicity and immunotoxicity) on the basis of available data and information about the substance.

Microbiological Information

Microorganisms used in the production of ingredients should be taxonomically identified and shown to be nonpathogenic and nontoxigenic. However, certain strains of microorganisms normally considered to be nontoxigenic may be capable of producing toxins when cultured under certain conditions. When such microorganisms are used as sources of ingredients, the fermentation conditions should be adjusted to prevent toxin synthesis, and appropriate tests should be conducted to ensure that the final ingredients do not contain toxins at unsafe levels. Alternatively, such microorganisms may be genetically modified to inactivate biochemical pathways involved in toxin synthesis. All the information relevant to the identity and safety of the microorganisms used as sources of ingredients should be described, including current and previous uses in food or in the production of food ingredients, if applicable. Microbiological considerations relevant to an ingredient safety assessment are discussed further by Mattia and Merker.[12]

Other Information, Including Human Studies

Scientific reviewers at the Center for Food Safety and Applied Nutrition do not use a checklist of required studies for a given food ingredient safety review. Although general guidelines exist, all safety reviews are approached on a case-by-case basis. In evaluating the safety of any ingredient, all scientific issues relevant to the intended use of the ingredient must be resolved. Therefore, a wide variety of study types could be included in an ingredient data package. Some additional examples of the types of studies that may bear on the safe use of an ingredient in foods include epidemiologic and clinical studies as well as specialized studies in well-defined scientific disciplines. Human studies that are not conducted for safety assessment per se may be relevant sources of information for safety evaluations. For example, efficacy studies of food ingredients conducted primarily for substantiating claims may contain relevant safety information.

For infant formula, human studies are often conducted to determine whether the formula supports normal physical growth when the formula is fed as the sole source of nutrition. Such testing is discussed by a 1998 report of the Life Sciences Research Organization.[13] Although growth studies are not safety studies, they are evaluated as part of the safety assessment of an ingredient added to infant formula.

"Functional Foods" and Provisions for Claims

In recent years, the food industry has been developing and marketing foods that it refers to as "functional foods." Although there is no formal definition of what the industry means by functional food, one report[14] defines functional foods as "foods and food components that provide a health benefit beyond basic nutrition (for the intended population). …These substances provide essential nutrients often beyond quantities necessary for normal maintenance, growth, and development, and/or other biologically active components that impart health benefits or desirable physiological effects."

Currently, the FDA has neither a definition nor a specialized regulatory rubric for foods being marketed as functional foods. Rather, the FDA regulates foods that are marketed as functional foods under the same regulatory framework as other conventional foods. Thus, any ingredient in a functional food needs to be safe and lawful, in accordance with the existing provisions of the FD&C Act.[14] As with a safety assessment for any food ingredient, the purported benefits of a "functional" ingredient are not relevant, except to the extent that such effects might negatively affect health.

In the FD&C Act, a food is misbranded if its labeling is false or misleading in any way. The FD&C Act also lays out the statutory framework for the use of labeling claims that characterize the level of a nutrient in a food or that characterize the relationship of a nutrient to a disease or health-related condition. If products bear any claims on the label or in labeling, those claims are the purview of the Office of Nutrition, Labeling, and Dietary Supplements (see the FDA Web site for more information on claims at http://www.fda.gov/Food/LabelingNutrition/LabelClaims/default.htm).

Another type of claim is a structure/function claim, which historically has appeared on products including conventional foods. The FDA defines structure/function claims as claims that describe the role of a food or food component (such as a nutrient) that is intended to affect the structure or function of the human body (eg, "builds stronger bones"). There is a regulatory process for structure/function claims for dietary supplements; however, there is no process for structure/function claims made for food ingredients or conventional foods, including infant formula. Examples of structure/function claims on infant formulas include "easy-to-digest comfort proteins," "calcium for stronger bones," and "proven to build a stronger immune system."

Regulation of Infant Formula

In the United States, infant formula is regulated as food by the FDA. Therefore, the laws and regulations governing all foods also apply to infant formula. The FD&C Act defines infant formula as "a food which purports to be or is represented for special dietary use solely as food for infants by reason of its simulation of human milk or its suitability as a complete or partial substitute for human milk." Infant formulas are formulated to meet the differing nutritional needs of term infants, preterm infants, and infants with inborn errors of metabolism or other medical or dietary problems.

Infant formula is subject to specific additional statutory and regulatory requirements, because it often provides the sole source of nutrition during a critical period of growth and development. For this reason, infant formula is manufactured using specific standards and critical measures to ensure the safety and nutritive value of the product. Prior to marketing, infant formula manufacturers must notify the FDA of a change in formulation or processing (eg, addition of new ingredients, changes in packaging, a new manufacturing plant, etc).

The Center for Food Safety and Applied Nutrition is responsible for regulation of infant formula. Within the Center for Food Safety and Applied Nutrition, 2 offices share the responsibility for evaluating information regarding infant formula. The Office of Nutrition, Labeling, and Dietary Supplements has program responsibility for infant formula, and the Office of Food Additive Safety has program responsibility for the safety of food ingredients added directly to formula as well as substances used in the packaging of infant formula. The Office of Nutrition, Labeling, and Dietary Supplements evaluates whether the infant formula manufacturer has met the requirements of the FD&C Act. The Office of Nutrition, Labeling, and Dietary Supplements consults with the Office of Food Additive Safety regarding the safety of ingredients in infant formula and packaging materials for infant formula. Together, the regulatory programs of the 2 offices ensure that infant formulas available in the United States have adequate nutritional quality and are safe. For additional information on the FDA's regulation of infant formula, consult http://www.fda.gov/Food/GuidanceComplianceRegulatoryInformation/GuidanceDocuments/InfantFormula/ucm056524.htm.

IV

Infant Formula Ingredients, Including New Ingredients

It is estimated that 40% of infants in the United States are exclusively formula fed by 3 months of age.[4] As the sole source of nutrition, infant formula, by itself, must provide adequate nutrition. Serious adverse effects can result in infants who do not receive adequate nutrition. On the basis of these considerations, infant formula is more highly regulated than other types of foods.

The need for greater regulatory oversight of infant formula became apparent after a reformulation error caused hypochloremic metabolic alkalosis in infants fed chloride-deficient soy formulas.[15] Following this incident, Congress passed the Infant Formula Act (IFA) of 1980 (Pub L No. 96-359), which amended the FD&C Act. The FDA's implementing regulations set out recall procedures, quality control procedures, and labeling and nutrient requirements. In 1986, Congress again amended the FD&C Act, among other things, to specify that an infant formula is adulterated unless it provides certain required nutrients and unless it meets quality factor requirements. In 1996, the FDA proposed a regulation[16] that included provisions for good manufacturing practices, quality-control procedures, quality factors, notification requirements, and reports and records for the production of infant formula. The proposed rule is still under review by the FDA.

The regulations implementing the IFA are consistent with the general food provisions of the FD&C Act. Any ingredient added to infant formula must be GRAS or covered by a food additive regulation for this intended use. The entire formulation must be suitable for its intended use as a sole source of nutrition to support the healthy growth of infants. If this is not the case, the FDA has the authority to remove the product from the marketplace.

Since enactment of the IFA, manufacturers' changes to infant formula formulations first focused on changes in macronutrients. Over the last decade, the changes have focused more on the addition of substances with the intention of more closely mimicking the advantages associated with consumption of human milk. Other changes focus on new sources of ingredients. Table 22.1 contains examples of new ingredients and new sources. As previously noted in the section on Voluntary Submissions for GRAS Substances, in the case of an ingredient intended for use in infant formula, establishing the safety prior to infant formula notification is advantageous to the industry and the FDA. A way to establish the safety of an ingredient intended for use in infant formula prior to the submission to Office of Nutrition, Labeling, and Dietary Supplements is to submit a GRAS notice to the Office of Food Additive Safety. Examples of substances intended for use in infant formula that have been evaluated in the GRAS notification program and received a "no questions" letter regarding the GRAS status from FDA are discussed later (see Table 22.1).

Required Nutrients

According to the FD&C Act, infant formula must provide infants with 29 essential substances, which include macronutrients, vitamins, and minerals (Table 22.4). This includes minimum levels of required nutrients and maximum levels that cannot be exceeded in all infant formula products. If these nutrient requirements are not met, the infant formula would be considered adulterated, unless the infant formula is classified as "exempt." An exempt infant formula is "any infant formula which is represented and labeled for use by an infant who has an inborn error of metabolism or low birth weight, or who otherwise has an unusual medical or dietary problem."

Table 22.4.

Recommended Nutrient Levels of Infant Formulas (per 100 kcal)[a]

Nutrient	Range	
	Minimum	Maximum
Protein, g	1.8[b]	4.5[b]
Fat, g	3.3 (30% of kcal)	
Linoleic acid (18:2 ω6), mg	300 (2.7% of kcal)	6.0 (54% of kcal)
Vitamins		
A, IU	250 (75μg)[c]	750 (225 μg)[c]
D, IU	40 (1 μg)[d]	100 (2.5 μg)[d]
K, μg[e]	4	...
E, IU	0.7 (0.5 mg)[f] at least 0.7 IU (0.5 mg)/g linoleic acid	
C (ascorbic acid), mg	8	...
B$_1$ (thiamine), μg	40	...
B$_2$ (riboflavin), μg	60	...
B$_6$ (pyridoxine), μg	35[g]	...
B$_{12}$, μg	0.15	...
Niacin, μg	250 (or 0.8 mg niacin equivalents)	
Folic acid, μg	4	...
Pantothenic acid, μg	300	...
Biotin, μg	1.5[h]	...
Choline, mg	7[h]	...
Inositol, mg	4[h]	...

Table 22.4. (continued)
Recommended Nutrient Levels of Infant Formulas (per 100 kcal)[a]

Nutrient	Range	
	Minimum	Maximum
Minerals		
Calcium, mg	60[i]	...
Phosphorus, mg	30[i]	...
Magnesium, mg	6	...
Iron, mg[j]	0.15	3.0
Iodine, μg	5	75
Zinc, mg	0.5	...
Copper, μg	60	...
Manganese, μg	5	...
Sodium, mg	20 (0.9 mEq)	60 (2.6 mEq)
Potassium, mg	80 (2.1 mEq)	200 (5.1 mEq)
Chloride, mg	55 (1.6 mEq)	150 (4.2 mEq)

[a] From the US Infant Formula Act of 1980 (Pub L No. 96-359), amended 1986 (Pub L No. 99-570).

[b] Biologically equivalent to or better than casein. If protein of lower quality used, minimum is increased in proportion. In no case, protein with biological value <70%.

[c] Retinol equivalents.

[d] Cholecalciferol.

[e] Any vitamin K added shall be in the form of phylloquinone.

[f] All rac-α-tocopherol equivalents.

[g] At least 15 μg for each g protein in excess of 18 g/100 kcal.

[h] Naturally present in cow milk-based formulas; addition required only in non-cow milk-based formulas.

[i] Calcium-to-phosphorus ratio should be no less than 1.1 and more than 2.

[j] If contains ≥1 mg/100 kcal, must be labeled as formula "with iron."

Other Added Ingredients

Compositional analyses have shown that human milk contains nutrients already required in infant formula manufacturing, such as carbohydrates, fats, proteins, vitamins, and minerals,[17] and other components not required by the IFA. Human milk contains bioactive components, such as enzymes, antibodies, white blood cells, prebiotics, and microorganisms. These substances are thought to be important in the early stages of development of the gastrointestinal and immune systems.[18] Manufacturers now add the following categories of ingredients to infant formula:

lipids (docosahexaenoic acid [DHA] and arachidonic acid [ARA]), probiotics and prebiotics, and carotenoids. The FDA has received GRAS notices for such ingredients (see New Fatty Acids and Lipids and Table 22.1). Among new ingredients in infant formula are new sources of traditional ingredients.[19]

New Fatty Acids and Lipids

Fatty acids are important components of the structural part of cell membranes; they also provide energy and play a role in cell signaling. Alpha-linolenic acid (an omega-3 fatty acid) and linoleic acid (an omega-6 fatty acid) are "essential fatty acids," because humans cannot synthesize them.[20] These 2 essential polyunsaturated fatty acids must be obtained from the diet from foods rich in these fatty acids, such as eggs, seeds, nuts, fish, and green leafy vegetables.[21] Alpha-linolenic acid and linoleic acid are present in human milk and in infant formula. The consumption of omega-6 fatty acids has overtaken the consumption of omega-3 fatty acids in the diet. It is considered important for the intake of these fatty acids to be balanced in the diet.[22]

Polyunsaturated fatty acids with a carbon chain of 18 or longer are called long-chain polyunsaturated fatty acids (LC-PUFAs). LC-PUFAs are naturally present in human milk, and like other components in human milk, their levels can be modulated through the mother's dietary intake. DHA and ARA are 2 LC-PUFAs that are abundant in tissues, such as the brain, retina, and heart. The infant body can synthesize DHA and ARA by elongation of alpha-linoleic acid and linolenic acid, respectively, which are present in infant formulas. However, it is unclear whether infants can synthesize sufficient levels of DHA and ARA from their precursor fatty acids for optimal development. Furthermore, some studies suggest that some infants, particularly preterm infants, may benefit from direct consumption of DHA and ARA. For that reason, infant formula manufacturers have added lipids containing DHA and ARA to infant formulas at concentrations comparable to those found in human milk.[23] In evaluating the safety of these lipids, manufacturers specify maximum amounts as percentages of the total dietary fat and specify the ratio of DHA to ARA.

Since the introduction of lipids containing DHA and ARA as new ingredients to infant formula in the United States in 2002, the market penetration of formulas with DHA and ARA has increased to approximately 98%.[24] Manufacturers are also adding lipids containing DHA and ARA to follow-up formulas and lipids containing DHA to foods likely to be consumed by toddlers and young children, such as cereals, yogurts, and snack foods.

The first sources of DHA and ARA added to infant formula were oils extracted from the microalga *Crypthecodinium cohnii* and the fungus *Mortierella alpina*, respectively. The industry has been keen to identify additional commercial sources

IV

of omega-3 fatty acids. To date, only tuna oil has been evaluated for use as an alternative source of DHA in infant formula.

The FDA has also reviewed GRAS notices for "tailored" lipids (Table 22.1). Tailored lipids are chemically or enzymatically modified using lipases; their fatty acid composition is modified to increase the levels of a specific fatty acid. Tailored lipids may also be modified to enhance absorption by the body and increase the delivery of essential fatty acids. Some lipids have been modified to resemble the fatty acid composition of fats in human milk.

An example of a tailored lipid for use in infant formula is high 2-palmitic vegetable oil for use in term and preterm infant formula. Triglycerides are a type of lipid with a glycerol backbone to which 3 fatty acids are attached. High 2-palmitic vegetable oil is enzyme-modified to largely replace palmitic acid with oleic acid at the 1 and 3 positions and increase the content of palmitic acid at the 2 position of the triglyceride. Palmitic acid in 1 and 3 positions is hydrolyzed in the gut, forming insoluble calcium soaps, which can cause constipation; palmitic acid in the 2 position is not hydrolyzed extensively in the gut. The lower availability of free palmitic acid in the gut is thought to reduce soap formation in the gut of the infant.

New Ingredients: Probiotics and Prebiotics

Probiotics are viable, nonpathogenic microorganisms, usually bacteria, added to food for their effects on the human intestinal tract; prebiotics are carbohydrates known to encourage the grown of certain commensal microorganisms. The gastrointestinal tract of the human body represents a complex ecosystem; current evidence suggests a dynamic environment of perhaps a thousand distinct bacterial species along with many specialized human cells.[25] Studies on germ-free animals have established that the normal structure and function of the gastrointestinal tract, and indeed the whole body, rests on the presence of an adequate intestinal microbiome, a term that is used to convey this ecosystem and the complex relationships among the microflora. Addition of representative species can reconstitute these functions in germ-free animals.[26] Similarly, current evidence suggests that the microflora may be altered by diet and certain diseases and also by obesity.[27]

The intestine is relatively sterile prior to birth; after birth, inoculation occurs quite rapidly with microorganisms from both the mother and the environment. The relative proportions of microorganisms in infants vary depending on the type of birth (vaginal vs Cesarean delivery) and source of nutrition (human milk vs different types of infant formula).[28] In newborn infants, the immune system develops tolerance as a result of its interactions with the commensal microorganisms in the infant's gut.[29]

The consumption of microorganisms in food dates back thousands of years; fermented foods and beverages have been consumed throughout history. In comparison, the science of microbiology is relatively new, and the microorganisms involved in these food fermentations were not identified until the early 20th century. In 1906, Dr. Elie Metchnikoff published a book titled *The Prolongation of Life,* proposing that acid-producing organisms in foods could prevent the proliferation of other, harmful organisms in the intestine.[30] Some of his observations were based on the long-lived peoples of Northern Europe who consumed yogurts and other fermented dairy products. Later, the organisms used to ferment yogurt were identified as streptococci and lactobacilli. Nowadays, many believe that by altering the microbial content of the gut, either through consuming foods containing certain microorganisms (ie, probiotics) or foods containing ingredients (ie, prebiotics) intended to encourage growth in the gut of certain microorganism, a variety of health parameters can be improved.

The FDA has not defined probiotic as a regulatory term. The term probiotics has been proposed to denote "live microorganisms, which, when administered in adequate amounts, confer a health benefit on the host."[31] Most organisms commonly considered to be probiotics are lactic acid bacteria of the genera *Bifidobacterium* and *Lactobacillus,* although particular strains of *Bacillus coagulans, Escherichia coli,* and a single yeast, *Saccharomyces boulardii,* have been described in the literature as probiotics.[32]

In recent years, interest in the use of "friendly" nonpathogenic microorganisms has increased, and research and case reports on microorganisms purported to be probiotics have proliferated. Research on probiotics varies widely, from studies on the ability of probiotics to interact with or potentially eliminate intestinal pathogens to studies bearing on the ability of some microorganisms to improve certain disease states. More is known about the effects of probiotics on individuals with disease states, although some studies have investigated their effects on healthy individuals. Fewer studies are available in infants and young children than in adults. Bibliographies in the GRAS notices on various probiotics in FDA's Inventory of GRAS Notices (http://www.fda.gov/grasnoticeinventory) provide a wealth of references on these topics.

Aureli et al reviewed various mechanisms by which purported probiotics may promote human health.[25] One proposed mechanism is that the absorption of organic acids, produced as end-products of anaerobic fermentation of carbohydrates by probiotic bacteria, influence human mood, energy level, and even cognitive abilities. Other possible mechanisms are competition by probiotic bacteria with pathogens, directly or by providing incompatible conditions for their growth, and stimulating host immune responses by producing specific polysaccharides. In general, although the consumption of probiotic bacteria is thought to stimulate the immune system, any specific effects are thought to be strain-based, with differences

IV

even among related organisms, and dependent on the levels of microorganisms added.

The composition of the fecal microflora has been compared in infants fed regular formula and infants fed formula containing bifidobacteria. The levels of bifidobacteria were higher in the feces of infants fed the formula containing bifidobacteria.[33] In some other studies, consumption of formula with bifidobacteria or lactobacilli resulted in fewer and shorter episodes of rotavirus-associated diarrhea in children.[34]

Currently, labels on food products marketed as probiotic rarely specify the minimum levels of the organism that should be present. However, experience in GRAS notices is that use levels are based on the numbers of viable bacteria, typically expressed as colony-forming units (CFUs); the use levels in most notices is for a maximum level of 10^8 CFUs/g of powdered infant formula. The FDA has evaluated several GRAS notices for the safe use of probiotics in infant formula (Table 22.1) and other foods.

The FDA does not distinguish between microorganisms used as "probiotics" and those used for fermentation purposes in safety reviews.[12] As noted previously, the FDA's authority is limited to consideration of safety. For microorganisms, the major safety considerations focus on the lack of pathogenicity and absence of toxin production in the microorganisms. Clear identification of the species and strain using molecular techniques is also extremely important. Many of the genomes of these microorganisms have been sequenced, and comparisons with known pathogens can be made. Animal feeding studies, tolerance studies in humans, and efficacy studies also provide relevant safety data. In infants, growth studies may be used to confirm the absence of adverse effects predicted using preclinical data. Many uses of microorganisms in the production of various foods are considered GRAS on the basis of history of use prior to 1958.

Prebiotics are typically carbohydrate compounds that are have been shown to enhance the growth of beneficial bacteria, such as *Bifidobacterium* species and lactobacilli, in the gastrointestinal tract. Prebiotics were first described by Gibson and Roberfroid in 1995.[35] In a publication in 2007, Roberfroid revisited prebiotics and offered the following definition: "A prebiotic is a selectively fermented ingredient that allows specific changes, both in the composition and/or activity in the gastrointestinal microflora that confers benefits upon host well-being and health."[36] Similar to probiotics, the FDA does not have a regulatory definition for prebiotics.

Complex carbohydrates (oligosaccharides) that encourage growth of bifidobacteria and other resident microorganism are present in human milk. To emulate the function of these carbohydrates in human milk, infant formula manufacturers have begun adding prebiotics to infant formula. Prebiotics with GRAS status added to infant formula include fructo-oligosaccharides and galacto-oligosaccharides (see

Table 22.1). Some prebiotics, such as fructo-oligosaccharides, are short-chain molecules with fewer linked saccharides compared with long-chain molecules, such as inulin. It is thought that molecules of differing chain length nourish bacteria in different locations of the colon.[37,38] As a result, prebiotics are being added to infant formula in combination with each other.

Carotenoids

Carotenoids are light-gathering pigments that participate in photosynthesis in plants. They also function as antioxidants in plants and other organisms. Carotenoids naturally occur in plant-derived foods, so they have been consumed for ages. Humans cannot synthesize carotenoids and must rely on fruits and vegetables or other dietary sources for intake.

Some carotenoids are added to processed foods as color additives. Carotenoids that are approved for coloring foods, in amounts consistent with good manufacturing practice, include beta carotene and tomato lycopene extract and concentrate. All color additives require FDA approval, because there is no GRAS exemption for the use of a color additive, as discussed previously. Carotenoids, however, are present in human milk and have GRAS status when added to infant formula for intended effects other than coloring food.

Carotenoids are divided into 2 classes on the basis of whether or not they contain oxygen; xanthophylls (yellow in color) contain oxygen, and carotenes (orange to red in color) do not. Lutein and zeaxanthin are xanthophylls and are the only carotenoids present in the macular region of the human retina.[39,40] In the retina, xanthophylls may serve a protective function by absorbing damaging frequencies of light (ie, blue light filtration). Lutein and zeaxanthin are reported to reduce the risk of age-related macular degeneration.[40] Carotenes include the vitamin A precursors, alpha-carotene and beta-carotene, and lycopene. Lycopene, primarily found in tomatoes, accounts for approximately 50% of the carotenoids in human serum, and it may be the most potent antioxidant in the group.[41,42]

The carotenoids that have been used as ingredients in infant formula are lutein (with a minor zeaxanthin component), beta-carotene, and lycopene. Lutein, the most abundant xanthophyll in human serum, is present in human milk, as are beta-carotene and lycopene.[43] As with some other human milk constituents, the levels of carotenoids in human milk vary depending on maternal diet. The specific carotenoids are added to infant formula at levels that simulate the levels found in human milk.[44] Some studies have shown that the addition of these ingredients to foods, including infant and toddler foods, is beneficial to visual function.[40,45,46]

The FDA has recently evaluated GRAS notices for the use of suspended lutein derived from the marigold flower (*Tagetes erecta*) for use in formulas for term and

IV

preterm infants (Table 22.1). Beta-carotene is regulated for use as a source of vitamin A in infant formula.

Newer Food Ingredients for the General Population

Once infants and toddlers transition away from infant formula and toddler foods, they consume food intended for the general population and are, therefore, exposed to the same food additives and GRAS substances that older children and adults consume. In this section, newer ingredients now being added to foods are highlighted.

New Ingredients in Infant Formula That Cross Over to Foods for the General Population

Sources of LC-PUFAs, probiotics and prebiotics, and carotenoids, ingredients that are added to infant formula, are also added to foods for consumption by the general population. Industry has been eager to add omega-3 fatty acids, generally DHA and eicosapentaenoic acid (EPA), to foods for consumption by the general population. Marine sources of DHA and EPA include tuna oil, small planktivorous pelagic fish oil, salmon oil, and krill oil. Because market demand may exceed availability from marine sources, nonmarine sources (ie, algae and fungi) could be potentially more sustainable. For example, algal oils from *Schizochytrium* species and *Ulkenia* species are more recent sources of DHA food ingredients. The FDA considers that the uses and amounts of oils containing omega-3 fatty acids in foods must be consistent with the GRAS regulation for menhaden oil. The industry has submitted a number of GRAS notices for omega-3 fatty acid-containing oils for which the FDA has issued response letters. Of note, however, infant formula is not among the foods in which the use of menhaden oil is affirmed as GRAS.

Industry has also been eager to add probiotics and prebiotics to food. The inclusion of certain species of bacteria in yogurt is a common example of probiotics in food. FDA regulations for various types of yogurt state that yogurt must be fermented by *Lactobacillus delbrueckii* subspecies *bulgaricus* (formerly *Lactobacillus bulgaricus*) and *Streptococcus thermophilus*. Most yogurt manufacturers also add *Lactobacillus acidophilus,* and some manufacturers add *Bifidobacterium* species, *Lactobacillus casei,* and *Lactobacillus rhamnosus* as well. These additional cultures are also added for purported probiotic effects. Such yogurt products are formulated for consumers of all ages, although some are specifically targeted for consumption by young children. Prebiotic ingredients for use in foods generally include fructo-oligosaccharides, galacto-oligosaccharides, fibers from various plant sources (ie, oats, potato, carrot, wheat, and barley), a wheat bran extract composed largely of xylo- and arabino-galactans, and yeast beta glucan. The combined use of prebiotics and probiotics, such as in some yogurt products containing additional fiber, is becoming commonplace. The industry has submitted a number of GRAS notices for probiotic ingredients or prebiotic ingredients for which the FDA has issued response letters.

Likewise, the FDA has evaluated several GRAS notices for use of lutein and lycopene in foods in general. Lutein, lycopene, and other carotenoids are readily available from tomatoes and other fruits and vegetables. For ingredient use, sources vary. For example, a source of lutein is the marigold flower, and sources of lycopene include concentrated tomato extract and *Blakeslea trispora*.

Sterols, Stanols, and Their Esters

Plant sterols, stanols, and their fatty acid esters are added to a variety of foods, such as vegetable oil spreads, dressings for salad, drinks, bars, yogurt, and other dairy products. The sterols include beta-sitosterol, campesterol, and stigmasterol. Sources of fatty acids and the sterols or stanols to which they are esterified include vegetable oils and oils from pine trees. The FDA has evaluated GRAS notices for uses of these ingredients. These ingredients have been associated with health claims for lowering the risk of coronary heart disease.[47]

Nonnutritive Sweeteners

Artificial Sweeteners

Artificial sweeteners are many times sweeter than sugar. Therefore, it takes a smaller amount of them to create the same sweetness as sugar, resulting in negligible calories to achieve the same sweetening effect. To date, 5 sugar substitutes have been approved by the FDA for use in a variety of foods—saccharin, sucralose, aspartame, acesulfame K, and neotame.[48]

Saccharin was discovered in 1879 and was used to help compensate for sugar rationing during both world wars. Saccharin is the chemical 1,2-benzisothiazolin-3-one 1,1–dioxide ($C_7H_5NO_3S$) and specified salts.[49] It is 300 times sweeter than sugar but is only used in 3% of food products containing a nonnutritive sweetener.[50] Because of animal studies suggesting saccharin caused bladder cancer in rats, the FDA proposed in 1977 to ban the use of saccharin as a food additive. Congress responded by passing the Saccharin Study and Labeling Act (Pub L No. 95-203 [1983]), which placed a moratorium on any ban of the sweetener while additional safety studies were conducted. The law also originally required that any foods containing saccharin must carry a label that stated, "Use of this product may be hazardous to your health. This product contains saccharin which has been determined to cause cancer in laboratory animals." However, in 2001, Congress repealed the requirement for the warning label. The Environmental Protection Agency has officially removed saccharin and its salts from their list of hazardous constituents and commercial chemical products. In a December 2010 release, the Environmental

Protection Agency stated that saccharin is no longer considered a potential hazard to human health.[51]

Sucralose is the chemical 1,6-dichloro-1,6-beta-D-fructofuranosyl-4-chloro-4-deoxy-alpha-D-galactopyranoside. Sucralose is 600 times sweeter than sugar.[49] It is also known by its trade name, Splenda (McNeil Nutritionals, Washington, PA). Sucralose tastes and looks like sugar because it is made from table sugar. Because it cannot be digested, it adds no calories. It is now used in approximately 40% of food products that contain nonnutritive sweeteners.[50]

Aspartame is the chemical 1-methyl N-L-alpha-aspartyl-L-phenylalanine ($C_{14}H_{18}N_2O_5$). Aspartame is sold under trade names such as NutraSweet (The NutraSweet Company, Chicago, IL) and Equal (Merisant Company, Chicago, IL). Aspartame is 180 times sweeter than sugar. Because aspartame contains phenylalanine, its use is potentially harmful to people with phenylketonuria.[49] Therefore, all products containing aspartame are required to bear a warning that the product contains phenylalanine. It is an ingredient in 23% of the food products containing an artificial sweetener.[50]

Acesulfame potassium, also called acesulfame K, is also known by its trade name Sunett (Nutrinova, Celanese, Dallas, TX). It is about 200 times sweeter than sucrose.[49] Acesulfame K is the potassium salt of 6-methyl-1,2,3-oxathiazine-4(3H)-one-2,2-dioxide. It is currently used in 35% of the food products containing nonnutritive sweeteners.[50]

Neotame is chemically similar to aspartame and is 7000 to 13 000 times sweeter than sucrose and not widely used in food products to date.[50]

Sugar Alcohols

Sugar alcohols are used as anti- or reduced-cariogenic substitutes for sugars, as reduced-calorie substitutes for starch or sugar, and as bulking agents when starch or sugar is removed from foods.[49] Sugar alcohols are naturally present in fruits and vegetables. For commercial food ingredient purposes, they are generally prepared by the catalytic hydrogenation of the parent sugars. The digestion, absorption, and metabolism of the sugar alcohols differ among the alcohols and are generally less complete than the parent sugars. Bioavailability in the upper gastrointestinal tract varies significantly among the alcohols. The portion of the ingested sugar alcohols that reaches the colon undergoes anaerobic fermentation by the colonic micro flora to product methane, hydrogen, and short-chain fatty acids. Fermentation in the colon generates some usable energy but generally less than would be obtained from the parent sugar. The production of short-chain fatty acids and lactic acid also lowers the pH of colonic material and may change the species distribution of colonic microorganisms. The reduced- and anticariogenic properties of sugar alcohols, as compared with the caloric sweeteners, is related to their resistance to fermentation by the oral microflora and production of reduced quantities of plaque. The most widely used sugar alcohols in foods are sorbitol, maltitol, mannitol, xylitol, and erythritol.[50]

SORBITOL

Approximately 50% of ingested sorbitol is absorbed through passive diffusion in the small intestine, and up to 85% of this is metabolized.[49] Sorbitol is absorbed more slowly than glucose. When consumed in large quantities, a laxative effect may be observed. Approximately 50% of ingested sorbitol reaches the colon, where it is rapidly fermented to short-chain fatty acids, hydrogen, and methane. Estimates of the caloric value of sorbitol range from 2.0 to 3.9 kcal/g. It is the most widely used of the sugar alcohols in food products—31% of foods containing nonnutritive sweeteners.[50]

MALTITOL

In the stomach, maltitol is hydrolyzed to glucose and sorbitol, both of which are readily absorbed.[49] A substantial portion of maltitol reaches the large intestine and is fermented to short-chain fatty acids. The net energy value for maltitol is approximately 3 kcal/g. It is used in 12% of the food products containing non-nutritive sweeteners.[50]

MANNITOL

Approximately 25% of ingested D-mannitol is absorbed via passive diffusion.[49] Once absorbed, it is oxidized by mannitol dehydrogenase or L-iditol 2-dehydrogenase to fructose and undergoes normal fructose metabolism. The net energy value of mannitol may be as low as 1.5 kcal/g, and it is used in 6% of foods containing nonnutritive sweeteners.[50]

XYLITOL

The absorption of xylitol occurs by simple diffusion and ranges from 13% to 95%.[49] The unabsorbed xylitol is completely fermented in the colon. Most of the absorbed xylitol is metabolized in the liver. The metabolizable energy from xylitol is approximately 2.5 to 2.9 kcal/g, and it is used in less than 5% of foods containing nonnutritive sweeteners.[50]

ERYTHRITOL

Erythritol has a unique metabolic fate in animals, presumably because of its low molecular weight. The sugar alcohol is almost completely absorbed in the small intestine and quantitatively excreted unchanged in the urine.[49] The result is a bulking agent with no caloric value. It has the least gastrointestinal adverse effects of any of the sugar containing alcohols and is only used in 2.6% of the food products with nonnutritive sweeteners.[50]

IV

New High-Intensity Sweeteners From the Stevia Plant

The leaves of the stevia plant (*Stevia rebaudiana*) contain a class of compounds, steviol glycosides, that are known for their intense sweet taste. In fact, steviol glycosides are about 200-fold sweeter than sugar. In 2008, the FDA responded to 2 GRAS notices on rebaudioside A from the stevia plant. These notices provided data and information supporting the conclusion of the notifiers that rebaudioside A is GRAS for use as a sweetener in various foods. Among the information provided by the notifiers were published scientific studies and the conclusions of various panels that, although the data were incomplete regarding the safety of whole leaf stevia, the data were adequate to establish the safety of preparations of highly purified steviol glycosides.[52]

Since 2008, the FDA has responded to a series of GRAS notices on other highly purified preparations of steviol glycosides and has had no questions about the conclusions of the notifiers that the substances are GRAS for their intended uses. Typically, rebaudioside A and stevioside are major components in these preparations. However, it is important to note that an import alert originally issued by the FDA in 1991 and revised in 2010 prohibits the entry of stevia leaves and crude stevia extracts that do not meet the specifications for highly purified steviol glycosides into the United States for use as a food additive or GRAS substance.[53] The import alert does not prohibit the importation of stevia leaves for use solely as a dietary ingredient in the manufacture of a dietary supplement product. At the present time, steviol glycosides are in chocolate milk and multivitamins targeting the pediatric population, and their use is increasing at the present time.

Other New Sweeteners

The FDA has also responded to GRAS notices on other substances, including trehalose, ribose, tagatose, and isomaltulose, and an isomalto-oligosaccharide mixture. The sweetness and caloric value of these compounds are generally lower than those of sucrose (table sugar). These other sweet substances have a variety of purposes, including use as lower-calorie nutritive sweeteners, bulking agents, or prebiotics. Most of these products are derived from fermentation processes carried out by well characterized and safe production organisms, usually bacteria, although some are produced synthetically. However, none of these sweeteners has garnered the level of commercial interest generated by the steviol glycosides, likely because of the perception that steviol glycosides are "natural" sweeteners, because they are derived from the stevia plant.

Fat Replacers

Three types of substitutes have been developed to replace fat.[49] Fat mimetics are proteins or carbohydrates that imitate the organoleptic or physical properties of fat.

Therefore, they provide 4 kcal/g rather than the 9 kcal/g provided by food fats. Fat substitutes are synthetic or enzymatically modified lipids that chemically resemble conventional fats. They can replace food fat on a gram-for-gram basis while providing no, or significantly fewer, calories than food fat. Structured triglycerides are similar to conventional fats in that they contain fatty acids attached to a glycerol backbone. However, they are designed to provide fewer calories than normal (<9 kcal/g) by substituting poorly absorbed fatty acids and short-chain fatty acids with lower caloric value than the usual fatty acids found in foods.[49]

Fat Mimetics

The typical constituents of fat mimetics are carbohydrates (eg, starch, cellulose, pectin, protein, hydrophilic colloids, dextrins, and polydextrose) and proteins (eg, egg, milk, whey, soy, gelatin, and wheat gluten).[49] These materials are frequently microparticulated to emulate the particle size and mouth feel of emulsified fats. Most of the fat mimetic materials are fully digestible, providing 4 kcal/g as compared with the 9 kcal/g for the food fats they replace. However, some mimetics are not digested (eg, cellulose, seaweed, some gums) and contribute no calories. Many fat mimetics are highly hydrated; thus, part of the caloric advantage comes from the replacement of fat with water. One of the mimetics, Simplesse (CP Kelco, Chicago, IL), is manufactured from whey protein concentrate by a patented microparticulation process. It retains any antigenic/allergenic properties of the parent protein.

Fat Substitutes

Fat substitutes are macromolecules that can replace food fat on a one-to-one basis.[49] Olestra is one example of a fat substitute. Olestra contains a mixture of octa-, hepta-, and hexa-esters of sucrose with fatty acids derived from edible fats and oils. It is formed by chemical transesterification or interesterification of sucrose with 6 to 8 conventional food fatty acids. Because humans lack enzymes to break the sucrose/fatty acid bonds, olestra is not absorbed or metabolized. Therefore, olestra provides no calories. However, because this is a nonabsorbed lipid, products containing olestra are required to add vitamins A, D, E, and K to compensate for any interference with the absorption of these fat-soluble vitamins. These added nutrients, because they are unlikely to be physiologically available, will not be considered in nutrient declarations in the food label nutrition facts box but will be listed in the ingredient list. Products are also required to carry a warning label for potential adverse gastrointestinal tract effects.

Structured Lipids

Structured lipids are triglycerides that are designed to provide fewer than 9 kcal/g.[49] Examples of structured lipids include salatrim and medium-chain triglycerides

IV

(MCTs). Salatrim represents a family of low-calorie fats constituting a mixture containing at least 1 short-chain fatty acid (eg, C2:0, C3:0, C4:0) and at least 1 long-chain fatty acid (predominately C18:0) attached to the glycerol backbone.[49] Because short-chain fatty acids have a lower caloric value than do long-chain fatty acids and because stearic acid is incompletely absorbed, the caloric value of salatrim is about five ninths the value of conventional fats. It is used as a substitute for cocoa butter in chocolate production.

MCTs predominately contain saturated fatty acids of chain length C8:0 (caprylic acid) and C11:0 (capric acid), with traces of C6:0 and C12:0 fatty acids.[49] MCTs are absorbed intact into the intestine as free fatty acids without the need for enzymes or bile salts. They bind to serum albumin and are transported to the liver via the portal system. They are oxidized to ketone bodies in the liver. They are less likely to be stored in adipose tissue. They have been used clinically in enteral and parenteral diets for individuals with lipid absorption, digestion, or transport disorders. They provide approximately 8.3 kcal/g. Most MCTs used in food products, including infant formula, are derived from coconut oil.

Biotechnology in the Development of New Food Ingredients

Biotechnology is a field of applied biology that uses a variety of scientific techniques, such as cross-breeding, molecular cloning, and bioengineering, to modify living organisms. Since the 1990s, recombinant DNA (rDNA) techniques have been used to introduce new genes or to modify the expression of genes in plants used as food and in microorganisms used in food, in fermentations, and as sources of food ingredients or processing aids.

Bioengineered plant varieties intended for food use include corn, soybean, cotton (used for cottonseed oil and animal feed), and canola (used largely for oil and grown largely in Canada), as well as other commodity and specialty crops. According to a 2011 US Department of Agriculture (USDA) survey, 94% of soybean, 90% of cotton, and 88% of corn grown in the United States were bioengineered varieties.[54] As of 2011, the most common traits in these bioengineered varieties were for agronomic enhancement (ie, herbicide tolerance and pest resistance). These crops are generally handled as bulk commodities, and consequently, conventional varieties and bioengineered varieties are not segregated, except when intended for use in products certified by the USDA organic program (see Chapter 13). Consequently, corn-, cotton-, and soy-derived ingredients added to processed foods are largely derived from bioengineered varieties. The composition of ingredients from bioengineered, agronomically enhanced crops is comparable to those produced from conventional varieties.

FDA Regulation of Foods Derived From New Plant Varieties

In 1992, the FDA published its "Statement of Policy: Foods Derived from New Plant Varieties."[55] The FDA explained its use of existing provisions of the FD&C Act to evaluate the safety of and other regulatory issues regarding human foods and animal feed derived from new plant varieties, including bioengineered plants. Before genetically modified food products are commercialized, the FDA, the Environmental Protection Agency, and the USDA conduct scientific reviews to help ensure the safety of these products. Although the FDA is responsible for food and feed safety of bioengineered plants, the USDA is responsible for their planting and environmental issues. In addition, the Environmental Protection Agency is responsible for bioengineered crops that contain pesticides. Thus, the oversight of bioengineered plants is a shared federal endeavor under a coordinated framework.[56]

In the 1992 policy document, the FDA stated that new methods of genetic modification, such as rDNA techniques, extend the capabilities of conventional breeding by allowing the transfer of DNA across organisms and the expression of nonnative proteins by recipient plants. The FDA considers DNA as GRAS on the basis of its consumption as a component of most whole foods and that the vast majority of proteins are neither toxins nor food allergens. Ordinarily, on the basis of this broad understanding of protein safety, the introduction of a new protein into a food crop would not need to be evaluated in a food additive petition. A food additive petition might be needed, for example, if safety could not be supported by publicly available information. The FDA considers that the characteristics of the food should be the focus of the FDA's safety evaluation, rather than the method used to impart those characteristics. In the 1992 policy document, the FDA offered developers guidance on food safety and nutritional concerns for new plant varieties, including decision trees that indicate when developers should consult the FDA.

In 1996, the FDA developed a voluntary consultation program and released guidance for industry regarding consultations under its 1992 policy. Through 2011, the FDA had completed more than 85 consultations under this policy. The traits addressed in these consultations are summarized in Table 22.5. Developers have indicated that the next generation of traits will favor varieties that appeal to consumers. Consumer appeal may be enhanced as a result of nutritional or visual improvements to food; agronomic traits in most currently marketed varieties benefit growers.

Table 22.5.

Food Crops With New Traits Introduced by Recombinant DNA Technology That Have Been the Subject of 85 Biotechnology Consultations With the FDA Through 2011

Crops	Trait
Alfalfa, canola, corn, cotton, soybean, sugar beet, creeping bent grass, flax, rice	Herbicide tolerance
Squash, plum, papaya	Virus resistance[a]
Corn, cotton, potato, soybean, tomato	Insect resistance[a]
Soybean, canola	Altered composition oils, 3 consultations to date
Corn, canola, radicchio	Male sterility
Tomato, cantaloupe	Delayed ripening
Corn (increased lysine), canola (reduced phytate)	Altered composition, 2 consultations to date
Corn	Drought tolerance

[a] Regulated as a pesticide by the United States Environmental Protection Agency.

Products of Bioengineered Microorganisms Reviewed by the FDA

The FDA has evaluated the safety of enzymes and other products produced by microorganisms modified through rDNA techniques in a number of GRAS notices and, prior to the GRAS notification program, in GRAS affirmation petitions that resulted in regulations.

Enzymes are proteins used by food processors to confer chemical changes to foods or ingredients, including ingredients used in infant formula and other foods consumed by infants and children. Examples of enzymes used in food processing include amylases, glycosidases, and lipases. Today, food enzyme manufacturers commonly introduce genes encoding well-known enzymes from microorganisms into host organisms considered safe for enzyme production. The food safety assessments of enzyme preparations focus on the safety of the host organism and the safety of the expressed protein. The host organism should not produce toxic substances related to pathogenic strains. Frequently used hosts for enzyme production include bacteria (eg, *Bacillus subtilis*) and fungi (eg, *Aspergillus niger* and *Aspergillus oryzae*). Because fungal strains are known to produce mycotoxins, most commercial fungal strains (*Aspergillus* species and *Trichoderma reesei*) have been modified to block mycotoxin production.[57] Pariza and Johnson[58] provided a strategy for toxicity testing of proteins produced by a bioengineered microorganism.

Bioengineered microorganisms can be used directly in food fermentations or used to produce nonprotein substances used in food. For example, several yeast varieties with modified traits primarily for use in winemaking have been developed. Also, a strain of the yeast *Yarrowia lipolytica* was genetically augmented with a number of genes derived from a variety of organisms to produce EPA-rich triglyceride oil for use in food.

Hormones Used in Animal Production

Hormones used in animal production are also regulated by the FDA. Most of these are sex steroids. Such hormones may be of endogenous or exogenous origin and have been used as growth stimulants to increase lean muscle mass. Animals treated with these sex steroids have included steers, heifers, veal calves, sheep, swine, and poultry.[59] Although there has been concern about the relative contribution of meat from hormone-treated animals to the total consumption of hormones in humans, it is clear that the contribution from meat of treated animals is insignificant when hormones have been properly used and must be considered biologically without effect.

One of the most controversial hormones has been bovine somatotrophin (bST) or bovine growth hormone. Since 1994, it has been possible to synthesize the hormone using rDNA technology with genetically engineered *Escherichia coli* to create recombinant bovine somatotrophin (rBST). This is injected into cows to increase milk yield. There is no evidence that the composition of milk is altered by treatment of cows with rBST.[60] Approximately 90% of the hormone is destroyed during pasteurization, and there is also no evidence that the milk of treated cows has a significantly increased amount of bovine growth hormone. Furthermore, growth hormone is destroyed in the gastrointestinal tract when given orally and must be injected to retain biologic activity. Bovine growth hormone is very specific and is biologically inactive in humans. Thus, any bovine growth hormone present in food products has no physiological effect on humans, and its safety in humans was recently reconfirmed by the FDA.[61]

Although not a hormone but a hormone antagonist, gonadotrophin-releasing factor analog-diphtheria toxoid conjugate is used as a chemical castrator in male pigs. When injected into pigs, the immune system is stimulated to produce antibodies that neutralize the pigs' own gonadotrophin-releasing factor. This improves the quality of the meat. Because there have been no demonstrated residues in the meat that affect human health, its use has been approved by the FDA.[62]

Conclusions

The definition of food is broad and includes infant formula. Any ingredient added to food in the United States must be approved by the FDA for such use, or the intended use of the ingredient must be GRAS. Over many years, the FDA has gained much experience in conducting safety assessments for a variety of ingredients to provide safe and wholesome foods. Although chemical, toxicologic, and microbiological studies are typically reviewed, a variety of types of studies, including studies conducted in humans and specialized studies, may be used to address all of the issues that arise in conducting a safety evaluation.

No area of ingredient testing or safety assessment is more critical to public health than assessing the safety of ingredients added to infant formula or, for that matter, for foods specifically marketed to young children. Infants may rely on infant formula as their sole source of nutrition, and young children who are transitioning to eating adult foods cannot choose from the full range of dietary products available. Both infants and young children have high energy demands to support their rapid growth and development. Poor nutrition or unsafe foods could have adverse health effects that persist throughout life. As science and technology change over time, it will be important to refine toxicity testing paradigms with infants and children in mind to ensure the safety of the products they consume; likewise, refined methods for estimating dietary exposure in infants and children will be needed. As manufacturers continue to research and to develop new ingredients for use in foods for consumers of all ages, regulatory agencies will need to keep pace with developments to continually improve their assessments to protect and promote public health.

To emulate the functionality of human milk, manufacturers of infant formulas are adding ingredients that are present in human milk, such as LC-PUFAs, prebiotics and probiotics, and carotenoids. What is contentious is whether the addition of these ingredients confers additional benefits, beyond ordinary nutrition, to infants who consume them. Similar ingredients are being added to foods targeted to the adult population, albeit with somewhat less concern. In evaluating the safety of ingredients added to foods, the FDA does not consider benefits. However, with the advent of "functional ingredients" and "functional foods," risk assessment strategies for the future may be designed to more directly address purported beneficial effects on the human body. In other words, assessments may need to consider the risk of adding a new ingredient relative to the risk of not adding it if a benefit has been convincingly demonstrated in infants, children, or adults.

Many of the ingredients that have been added to foods in recent years are common components of food with new uses. As a result, use of these ingredients fall under the GRAS provisions of the FD&C Act. Some of the more interesting ingredients to enter the market place include LC-PUFAs, probiotics and prebiotics, carotenoids, sterols and stanols, and steviol glycosides. These are components of foods that are present in the diet; however, their intended uses in foods have changed. For example, certain bacteria have been used in fermentation processes for millennia, but the addition of these microorganisms directly to food to transiently inhabit the gut is relatively new. Innovations in the sourcing of ingredients and the methods of manufacture of ingredients have also changed in the last decade. For example, oils previously obtained from marine sources are now produced by culturing single-cell organisms, such as algae or fungi. It is now commonplace to produce enzymes using bioengineered microorganisms and biotechnology is moving in the direction of modifying food crops to enhance their nutritive value. As food science continues to evolve, the FDA will continue to ensure the safety and wholesomeness of foods and food ingredients in the US marketplace.

References

1. American Academy of Pediatrics, Section on Breastfeeding. Policy statement: breastfeeding and the use of human milk. *Pediatrics*. 2012;129(3):e827-e841

2. Department of Health and Human Services. HHS Blueprints and Breastfeeding Policy Statements. Available at: http://www.womenshealth.gov/breastfeeding/government-in-action/hhs-blueprints-and-policy-statements. Accessed November 15, 2012

3. World Health Organization. The World Health Organization's infant feeding recommendation. Available at: http://www.who.int/nutrition/topics/infantfeeding_recommendation/en/index.html. Accessed November 15, 2012

4. Grummar-Strawn LM, Scanlon KS, Fein SB. Infant feeding and feeding transitions during the first year of life. *Pediatrics*. 2008;122(Suppl 2):S36-S42

5. Montalto MB, Benson JD, Martinez GA. Nutrient intakes of formula-fed infants and infants fed cow milk. *Pediatrics*. 1985;75(2):343-351

6. Martinez GA, Ryan AS, Malec DJ. Nutrient intakes of American infants and children fed cow's milk or infant formula. *Am J Dis Child*. 1985;139(10):1010-1018

7. Institute of Medicine, Committee on Understanding Premature Birth and Assuring Healthy Outcomes. *Preterm Birth: Causes, Consequences, and Prevention*. Behrman RE, Butler AS, ed. Washington, DC: National Academies Press; 2007

8. Brown K, Dewey K, Allen L. *Complementary Feeding of Young Children in Developing Countries: A Review of Current Scientific Knowledge*. Geneva, Switzerland: World Health Organization; 1998. Available at: http://www.who.int/nutrition/topics/complementary_feeding/en/. Accessed November 15, 2012

9. Foote KD, Marriott LD. Weaning of infants. *Arch Dis Child*. 2003;88(3):488-492

10. US Food and Drug Administration. Substances generally recognized as safe. *Federal Register*. 1997;62(74):18938-18964

11. *Scott v FDA*, 728 F 2d 322, 6th Cir 1984

12. Mattia A, Merker R. Regulation of probiotic substances as ingredients in foods: premarket approval or "generally recognized as safe" notification. *Clin Infect Dis*. 2008;46(Suppl 2):S115-S118

13. Raiten DJ, Talbot JM, Waters JH, ed. LSRO Report: Assessment of nutrient requirements for infant formulas. *J Nutr*. 1998;128(Suppl 11):2200S-2201S

IV

14. Institute of Food Technologists. *Functional Foods: Opportunities and Challenges.* Washington, DC: Institute of Food Technologists; 2005. Available at: http://www.ift.org/knowledge-center/read-ift-publications/science-reports/expert-reports/~/media/Knowledge%20Center/Science%20Reports/Expert%20Reports/Functional%20Foods/Functionalfoods_expertreport_full.pdf. Accessed November 15, 2012

15. Linshaw MA, Harrison HL, Gruskin AB, et al. Hypochloremic alkalosis in infants associated with soy protein formula. *J Pediatr.* 1980;96(4):635-640

16. US Food and Drug Administration. Current good manufacturing practice, quality control procedures, quality factors, notification requirements, and records and reports, for the production of infant formula. *Federal Register.* 1996;61(132):361543-36219

17. Institute of Medicine, Committee on the Evaluation of the Addition of Ingredients New to Infant Formula. *Infant Formula: Evaluating the Safety of New Ingredients.* Washington, DC: National Academies Press; 2004

18. Wagner CL. Human Milk and Lactation. Medscape, Drugs, Diseases & Procedures Web site. 2010. Available at: http://emedicine.medscape.com/article/1835675-overview. Accessed November 15, 2012

19. Food Advisory Committee Meeting on Infant Formula Briefing Materials Overview. April, 2002. Available at: http://www.fda.gov/OHRMS/DOCKETS/ac/02/briefing/3852b1_01.htm. Accessed November 15, 2012

20. Panickar KS, Bhathena SJ. Control of fatty acid intake and the role of essential fatty acids in cognitive function and neurological disorders. In: Montmayeur JP, le Coutre J, eds. *Fat Detection: Taste, Texture, and Post Ingestive Effects.* Boca Raton, FL: CRC Press Inc; 2010; chapter 18. Available at: http://www.ncbi.nlm.nih.gov/books/NBK53554/. Accessed November 15, 2012

21. Huffman SL, Harika RK, Eilander A, Osendarp SJ. Essential fats: how do they affect growth and development of infants and young children in developing countries? A literature review. *Matern Child Nutr.* 2011;7(Suppl 3):44-65

22. Simopoulos A. Evolutionary aspects of diet: the omega-6/omega-3 ratio and the brain. *Mol Neurobiol.* 2011;44(2):203–215

23. US Food and Drug Administration. Infant Formula Q&A. Consumer Questions. Available at: http://www.fda.gov/Food/FoodSafety/Product-SpecificInformation/InfantFormula/ConsumerInformationAboutInfantFormula/ucm108079.htm. Accessed November 15, 2012

24. Oliviera V, Davis D. Recent Trends and Economic Issues in the WIC Infant Formula Rebate Program. Washington, DC: US Department of Agriculture, Economic Research Service; 2006. Available at: http://www.ers.usda.gov/Publications/ERR22/. Accessed November 15, 2012

25. Aureli P, Capurso L, Castellazzi AM, et al. Probiotics and health: an evidence-based review. *Pharmacol Res.* 2011;63(5):366-376

26. O'Hara AM, Shanahan F. The gut flora as a forgotten organ. *EMBO Rep.* 2006;7(7):688-693

27. Ley RE, Hamady M, Lozupone C, et al. Evolution of mammals and their gut microbes. *Science.* 2008;320(5883):1647-1651

28. Guarner F, Malagelada JR. Gut flora in health and disease. *Lancet.* 2003;361(9356):512-519

29. Renz H, Brandtzaeg P, Hornef M. The impact of perinatal immune development on mucosal homeostasis and chronic inflammation. *Nature Rev Immunol.* 2012;12(1):9-23

30. Figueroa-Gonzalez I, Quijano G, Ramirez G, Cruz-Guerrero A. Probiotics and prebiotics—perspectives and challenges. *J Sci Food Agric*. 2011;91(8):1341-1348

31. Joint FAO/WHO Working Group Report on Drafting Guidelines for the Evaluation of Probiotics in Food. London, Ontario, Canada: Food and Agriculture Organization of the United Nations/World Health Organization; 2002

32. Saxelin M. Probiotic formulations and applications, the current probiotics market, and changes in the marketplace: a European perspective. *Clin Infect Dis*. 2008;46(Suppl 2):S76-S79

33. Mountzouris KC, McCartney AL, Gibson GR. Intestinal microflora of human infants and current trends for its nutritional modulation. *Br J Nutr*. 2002;87(5):405–420

34. Rowland I, Capurso L, Collins K, et al. Current level of consensus on probiotic science. *Gut Microbes*. 2010;1(6):436–439

35. Gibson GR, Roberfroid MB. Dietary modulation of the human colonic microbiota: introducing the concept of prebiotics. *J Nutr*. 1995;125(6):1401-1412

36. Roberfroid MB. Prebiotics: the concept revisited. *J Nutr*. 2007;137(3 Suppl 2):830S-837S

37. Kleessen B, Hartmann L, Blaut M. Oligofructose and long-chain inulin: influence on the gut microbial ecology of rats associated with a human faecal flora. *Br J Nutr*. 2001;86(2):291-300

38. Bouhnik Y, Vahedi K, Achour L, et al. Short-chain fructo-oligosaccharide administration dose-dependently increases fecal bifidobacteria in healthy humans. *J Nutr*. 1999;129(1):113-116

39. O'Connell E, Neelam K, Nolan J, Au Eong KG, Beatty S. Macular carotenoids and age-related maculopathy. *Ann Acad Med Singapore*. 2006;35(11):821-830

40. SanGiovanni JP, Chew EY, Clemons TE, et al. The relationship of dietary carotenoid and vitamin A, E, and C intake with age-related macular degeneration in a case-control study: AREDS Report No. 22. *Arch Ophthalmol*. 2007;125(9):1225–1232

41. Agarwal S, Rao AV. Tomato lycopene and its role in human health and chronic diseases. *CMAJ*. 2000;163(6):739-744

42. Gerster H. The potential role of lycopene for human health. *J Am Coll Nutr*. 1997;16(2):109-126

43. Jewell VC, Mayes CB, Tubman TR, et al. A comparison of lutein and zeaxanthin concentrations in formula and human milk samples from Northern Ireland mothers. *Eur J Clin Nutr*. 2004;58:90-97

44. Gossage CP, Deyhim M, Yamani S, Douglass L, Moser-Veillon PB. Carotenoid composition of human milk during the first month postpartum and the response to β-carotene supplementation1–3. *Am J Clin Nutr*. 2002;76(1):193-197

45. Dutta D, Chaudhuri UR, Chakraborty R. Structure, health benefits, antioxidant property and processing and storage of carotenoids. *Afr J Biotechnol*. 2005;4(13):1510-1520

46. Weigert G, Kaya S, Pemp B, et al. Effects of lutein supplementation on macular pigment optical density and visual acuity in patients with age-related macular degeneration. *Invest Ophthalmol Vis Sci*. 2011;52(11):8174-8178

47. US Food and Drug Administration. Food labeling: health claims; plant sterol/stanol esters and coronary heart disease; interim final rule. *Federal Register*. 2000;65(175):54685-54739

IV

48. Mattes RD, Popkin BM. Nonnutritive sweetener consumption in humans: effects on appetite and food intake and their putative mechanisms. *Am J Clin Nutr*. 2009;89(1):1-14

49. Finley JW, Leville GA. Macronutrient substitutes. In: Ziegler EE, Filer LJ Jr, eds. Present Knowledge in Nutrition. 7ᵗʰ Ed. Washington, DC: International Life Sciences Institute; 1996:581-595

50. US Department of Agriculture, National Agricultural Library. Nutritive and Nonnutritive Sweetener Resources. Available at: http://fnic.nal.usda.gov/food-composition/nutritive-and-nonnutritive-sweetener-resources. Accessed November 15, 2012

51. US Environmental Protection Agency. Removal of Saccharin from the Lists of Hazardous Constituents and Hazardous Wastes Under RCRA and from the List of Hazardous Substances Under CERCLA. Available at: http://www.epa.gov/waste/hazard/wastetypes/wasteid/saccharin/index.htm. Accessed November 15, 2012

52. World Health Organization. Safety evaluation of certain food additives. *WHO Food Additives Series 59*. Geneva, Switzerland: World Health Organization; 2008

53. US Food and Drug Administration. What Refined Stevia Preparations Have Been Evaluated by the FDA to Be Used as a Sweetener? Available at: http://www.fda.gov/AboutFDA/Transparency/Basics/ucm214865.htm. Accessed November 15, 2012

54. USDA, National Agricultural Statistics Service. Biotechnology Varieties. Available at: http://usda.mannlib.cornell.edu/usda/nass/Acre//2010s/2011/Acre-06-30-2011.pdf#page=25. Accessed November 15, 2012

55. US Food and Drug Administration. Statement of policy: foods derived from new plant varieties. *Federal Register*. 1992;57(104):22984-22992

56. US Executive Office of the President, Office of Science and Technology Policy. Coordinated framework for regulation of biotechnology. *Federal Register*. 1986;51(123):23302-23309

57. Olempska-Beer ZS, Merker RI, Ditto MD, DiNovi MJ. Food-processing enzymes from recombinant microorganisms—a review. *Regul Toxicol Pharmacol*. 2006;45(2):144-158

58. Pariza MW, Johnson EA. Evaluating the safety of microbial enzyme preparations used in food processing: update for a new century. *Regul Toxicol Pharmacol*. 2001;33(2):173-186

59. Velle W. The Use of Hormones in Animal Production. Geneva, Switzerland: Food and Agriculture Organization of the United Nations, Agriculture and Consumer Protection. Available at: http://www.fao.org/DOCREP/004/X6533E/X6533E01.htm. Accessed November 15, 2012

60. American Academy of Pediatrics, Committee on Environmental Health. Food safety. In: Etzel RA, Balk SJ, eds. *Pediatric Environmental Health*. 3rd ed. Elk Grove Village, IL: American Academy of Pediatrics; 2012:247-267

61. US Food Drug Administration. Report on the Food and Drug Administration's review of the safety of recombinant bovine somatotropin. Available at: http://www.fda.gov/AnimalVeterinary/SafetyHealth/ProductSafetyInformation/ucm130321.htm. Accessed November 15, 2012

62. US Food and Drug Administration. Freedom of Information Summary: Improvest. Gonadotropin Releasing Factor Analog - Diphtheria Toxoid Conjugate sterile solution for injection: Swine, intact males. Available at: http://www.fda.gov/downloads/AnimalVeterinary/Products/ApprovedAnimalDrugProducts/FOIADrugSummaries/UCM292021.pdf. Accessed November 15, 2012

Nutrient Delivery Systems V

Chapter 23

Parenteral Nutrition

Introduction

Appropriate nutrition is of paramount importance during infancy and childhood. Parenteral nutrition may be required as a supplement or as a complete substitute for enteral nutrition. This chapter will review parenteral nutrition as a nutritional strategy to ensure appropriate growth and development for the pediatric patient.

Indications for Parenteral Nutrition

Effective use of parenteral nutrition will meet metabolic demands and improve response to medical and surgical therapy.[1] Common indications for the use of parenteral nutrition are listed in Table 23.1.

Table 23.1.
Common Indications for the Use of Parenteral Nutrition

1. Intestinal insult: surgery, or trauma
2. Intestinal inflammation: necrotizing enterocolitis, inflammatory bowel disease
3. Intestinal obstruction: imperforate anus, ileus, atresias
4. Intestinal malabsorption: short-bowel syndrome, chronic diarrhea, chemotherapy, bone marrow transplant
5. Intestinal immaturity: preterm infant
6. Intestinal dysmotility: intractable emesis, intestinal pseudo-obstruction syndrome
7. Extraintestinal disorders resulting in malnutrition: cardiac or renal failure, severe burns, cancer

A nutrition support team is required for all patients receiving parenteral nutrition. The team should include medical, surgical, nursing, dietary, and pharmacy staff with expertise in parenteral nutrition. The team is invaluable in decreasing costs and morbidities associated with parenteral nutrition therapy. Guidelines available from the American Society of Parenteral and Enteral Nutrition (http://www.nutritioncare.org/library.aspx) include critical elements of screening, establishing nutrition care plans, and providing enteral and parenteral nutritional support, including home specialized nutritional support.

Routes of Administration

Parenteral nutrition can be administered through peripheral or central veins. For peripheral veins, using standard intravenous catheters, the solutions are limited to a dextrose concentration of ≤12.5%, and a larger volume of fluid is required for adequate caloric intake. Peripheral veins are used for short-term parenteral nutrition, which is usually associated with fewer complications. Central venous parenteral nutrition is usually reserved, by consensus, for patients who are or will be intolerant of enteral feedings for more than 2 weeks and for whom solutions with osmolarity >1250 mOsm/L are necessary. Large central veins will tolerate solutions of higher osmolarity and concentrations of up to 20% to 30% glucose. The tip of the central venous catheter is typically placed near the junction of the superior vena cava and the right atrium. Two techniques are commonly used for central catheter placement: (1) a percutaneously inserted central catheter (PICC), positioned in an upper or lower extremity vein or external jugular vein, is advanced into the superior or inferior vena cava to lie at the junction of the right atrium and the large vein; or (2) a catheter is placed surgically in the internal or external jugular or subclavian vein. The second approach is largely used when a longer duration of parenteral nutrition is required or percutaneous placement is not possible. The catheter also comes with a cuff to secure it and is tunneled subcutaneously to exit in the anterior chest remote from the site of insertion. Strict aseptic technique should be used for both percutaneous and surgical approaches. Chlorhexidine cleansing of the skin site is performed to reduce the likelihood of catheter-related bloodstream infections. Meticulous attention to catheter maintenance by a specialized nursing team is a recommended practice for patients receiving parenteral nutrition. Parenteral nutrition-related complications are summarized in Table 23.2.

Table 23.2.
Complications of Parenteral Nutrition[a]

Mechanical Malposition Pleural/pericardial effusion and cardiac tamponade Pneumothorax Brachial plexus injury, diaphragmatic palsy Air embolus Thrombotic events and thrombophlebitis Skin sloughing and subcutaneous injury
Infectious Sepsis: bacterial, fungal
Metabolic Hepatic dysfunction (cholestasis, steatosis, cirrhosis) Metabolic bone disease (osteopenia to frank rickets or fractures) Errors of commission or omission (electrolyte imbalance, hypo- or hyperglycemia, essential fatty acid deficiency, trace mineral deficiencies)

[a] Adapted with permission from Baisden B, Bunyapen C, Bhatia J. Feeding the preterm infant. In: Bernadier CD, Dwyer J, Feldman EB, eds. *Handbook of Nutrition and Food*. 2nd ed. Boca Raton, FL: CRC Press; 2008:259-270.

Catheter occlusions can be thrombotic or nonthrombotic, with most being the former.[2] Nonthrombotic occlusions can be attributable to calcium precipitates. Various treatment options have been attempted. Currently, alteplase (tissue plasminogen activator) is recommended for catheter-related thrombosis or occlusion that cannot otherwise be treated.[3]

Composition of Solutions for Infants and Children

In the current era of aggressive nutrition, numerous studies have been published establishing the efficacy and safety of parenteral nutrition early in life.[4-8] In these studies, amino acid intakes ranging from 2.4 to 3.5 g/kg/day between days 1 and 2 have been recommended for preterm infants to establish positive nitrogen balance and improve energy intakes. Preterm and term infants receiving 3 g/kg/day of amino acids demonstrate plasma amino acid concentrations similar to those observed in the fetus.[9]

Overall energy intakes for preterm infants on parenteral nutrition should be between 90 and 100 kcal/kg/day. Higher energy intakes, whether through the use of intravenous lipids or excess amounts of glucose, will lead to increased fat deposition. Tables 23.3 through 23.5 summarize parenteral nutrition requirements beyond the neonatal period.[10,11]

Table 23.3.

Components of Maintenance Parenteral Nutrition in Infants and Children[a,b]

	Weight		
Base Components	**<10 kg**	**10–20 kg**	**>20 kg**
Fluid	100–150 mL/kg	1000 mL + 50 mL/kg >10 kg	1500 mL + 20 mL/kg >20 kg
Calories, kcal/kg[c] Dextrose, g/kg (3.4 kcal/g)	90–100 10–30	75–90 8–28	30–75 5–20
Protein, g/kg[c] (1 g protein = 0.16 g nitrogen)	1.5-3.0	1.0–2.5	0.8–2.0
Fat, g/kg	0.5–3	1–3	1–3
Additive	**Infants and Toddlers**	**Children**	**Adolescents**
Sodium	2–4 mEq/kg	2–4 mEq/kg	60–150 mEq
Potassium	2–4 mEq/kg	2–4 mEq/kg	70–180 mEq
Chloride	2–4 mEq/kg	2–4 mEq/kg	60–150 mEq
Magnesium (125 mg/mEq)	0.25–1 mEq/kg	0.25–1 mEq/kg	8–32 mEq
Calcium[d] (20 mg/mEq)	0.45–4 mEq/kg	0.45–3.15 mEq/kg	10–40 mEq

Table 23.3. *(continued)*
Components of Maintenance Parenteral Nutrition in Infants and Children[a,b]

Additive	Infants and Toddlers	Children	Adolescents
Phosphorus (31 mg/mmol)	0.5–2 mmol/kg	0.5–2 mmol/kg	9–30 mmol/kg
Heparin (optional)	0.5–1 U/mL	0.5–1 U/mL	0.5–1 U/mL
Trace elements	0.2 mL/kg (pediatric trace elements)[e]	0.2 mL/kg (pediatric trace elements)[e]	5 mL (adult trace elements)[e,f]
Selenium (maximum 30 µg/d)	2 µg/kg	2 µg/kg	2 µg/kg
Molybdenum (maximum 5 µg/d)	0.25 µg/kg	0.25 µg/kg	0.25 µg/kg
Adult multivitamin (maximum 10 mL/d)[g]	NA	NA	10 mL[h]
Pediatric multivitamin (maximum 5 mL/d)[g]	<2.5 kg 2 mL/kg	2.5–40 kg 5 mL	>40 kg use adult multivitamin

IU indicates International Units; NA, not applicable.
[a] Adapted from Chan[10]; Kowalski and Nucci[11]; Persinger M. Pediatric nutrition support in critical care. In: Nevin-Folino NL, ed. *Pediatric Manual of Clinical Dietetics*. Chicago, IL: American Dietetic Association; 2003; and Wesley JR, Coran AG. Intravenous nutrition for the pediatric patient. *Semin Pediatr Surg*. 1992;1(3):212-230.
[b] See Chapter 5 for preterm infants.
[c] Ideal weight (50th percentile for length or height).
[d] If given as calcium gluconate: 1 mL of a 10% solution of calcium gluconate provides 9.3 mg of elemental calcium.
[e] See Table 23.4. If patient receives parenteral nutrition for more than 30 days with no significant enteral intake, the addition of trace elements is advisable.
[f] Omit copper and manganese in patients with obstructive jaundice; omit selenium, chromium, and molybdenum in patients with renal dysfunction. Maximum pediatric trace elements: 5 mL/day.
[g] See Table 23.5.
[h] Add 200 µg vitamin K (phytonadione).

Table 23.4.
Parenteral Trace Element Solutions

Ingredient	Adult Trace/mL[a]	Pediatric Trace/mL[b]
Zinc	5 mg	1.0 mg
Copper	1.0 mg	0.1 mg
Manganese	0.5 mg	25 µg
Chromium	10 µg	1 µg
Selenium	60 µg	NA

NA indicates not applicable.
[a] Multitrace-5 Concentrate, USP, American Regent Laboratories Inc, Shirley, NY.
[b] Multitrace-4 Pediatric Trace Elements Injection 4, USP, American Regent Laboratories Inc, Shirley, NY.

Table 23.5.
Parenteral Vitamin Solutions

Ingredient	Adult MVI/5 mL[a]	Pediatric MVI/4 mL[b]
Vitamin A	1 mg 3300 IU	0.7 mg 2300 IU
Vitamin D	5 µg 200 IU	10 µg 400 IU
Vitamin E	10 mg 10 IU	7 mg 7 IU
Vitamin B_1	6 mg	1.2 mg
Vitamin B_2	3.6 mg	1.4 mg
Vitamin B_6	6 mg	1 mg
Niacin	40 mg	17 mg
Dexpanthenol	15 mg	5 mg
Folic acid (per mL)	600 µg	140 µg
Vitamin B_{12} (per mL)	5 µg	1 µg
Biotin (per mL)	60 µg	20 µg
Ascorbic acid	200 mg	80 mg
Vitamin K_1	150 µg	200 µg

[a] Infuvite Adult, Sandoz Canada, Boucherville, Quebec, Canada.

[b] Pediatric MVI, AAI Pharma, Wilmington, NC.

Macronutrients

Protein

Crystalline amino acids provide the nitrogen in current solutions and can be diluted to meet the requirements of patients at different ages. Pediatric amino acid formulations (TrophAmine [B. Braun Medical Inc, Irvine, CA], Aminosyn PF [Hospira Inc, Lake Forest, IL], and Premasol [Baxter Healthcare Corp, Deerfield, IL]) have been specially formulated to meet the requirements of neonates. The latter is a sulfite-free amino acid preparation that includes N-acetyl-L-tyrosine. A listing of the currently available amino acid solutions and their amino acid contents can be found in Appendix M. These solutions contain taurine, tyrosine, histidine, aspartic acid, and glutamic acid, all of which are found in human milk. They contain lower concentrations of methionine, glycine, and phenylalanine than are found in amino acid solutions intended for older patients. The plasma amino acid profile of infants receiving these solutions for nutritional maintenance is similar to that of term breastfed infants. In addition, greater weight gain and positive nitrogen balance are achieved by infants receiving these formulations than by infants receiving standard adult amino acid solutions.

V

Commercial solutions do not contain cysteine, although separate preparations of cysteine can be added to the solutions. Cysteine must be added during compounding, because it converts to its dimeric form and precipitates over time in solution. Cysteine may be an essential amino acid in infants with low activity of hepatic cystathionine gamma-lyase, which converts methionine to cysteine.[12]

Taurine, which is formed from cysteine and is present in human milk, may also be important in preterm infants. Tyrosine is provided as N-acetyl-L-tyrosine (0.24%).[13]

No commercially available parenteral nutrition amino acid solution currently contains glutamine (primarily because of its short shelf-life when placed in solution), the most abundant amino acid in both plasma and human milk.[14] Glutamine is a primary fuel for enterocytes, lymphocytes, and macrophages and is a precursor for nucleotide synthesis and glutathione, an important antioxidant. Previous studies in animals and critically ill adults have suggested that parenteral nutrition supplemented with glutamine reduces the risk of sepsis and mortality.[15] However, in a large, multicentered, randomized, double-masked clinical trial, glutamine supplementation of infants between 401 and 1000 g did not decrease mortality or the incidence of late-onset sepsis. Although well tolerated, routine supplementation is, therefore, not recommended.[16] Although there is some evidence that glutamine supplementation may be of value to very-low-birth-weight infants and pediatric patients with short-bowel syndrome, more studies are needed before its routine use can be recommended.[17,18]

Most infants tolerate available solutions and grow well while receiving them. Complications are rarely encountered with the recommended intake of 2.5 to 3.5 g of protein equivalent per kg per day. The metabolic complications related to amino acids, such as azotemia and acidosis, have occurred when infants have received more than 4 g of protein equivalent per kg per day. In a recent study, preterm infants were either provided a maximum of 3 or 4 g/kg/day, parenterally, within the first few days of life.[19,20] (All infants were maintained on 3.5 g/kg/day after 7 days.) Six infants in the early and high amino acid group (4 g/kg/day) were withdrawn by 3 to 4 days because of elevated blood urea nitrogen and ammonia concentrations. Further, in a preliminary follow-up study, Blanco et al reported worse anthropometric measurements and cognitive scores in infants at 18 months who received early and high amino acid infusions.[20] In a 2-year follow-up study of 32 of 61 infants of the same cohort, infants provided the early and high amino acid intake of 4 g/kg/day had significantly lower group z-score means for weight, length, and head circumference, compared with the standard regimen. However, the lower mental development index scores observed at 18 months were no longer observed at 24 months. Amino acid concentrations negatively correlated with mental development index and poor postnatal growth.[21] Therefore, it appears that limiting extremely low birth weight infants to 2.5 to 3.5 g/kg/day of intravenous amino acids after birth is a reasonable approach until more information is available.

For older, critically ill children, provision of adequate protein may be the single most important nutritional intervention that can be made in their care. A lack of adequate protein has been associated with respiratory failure, muscle weakness, and sepsis.[22] Protein requirements will vary with the age or weight of the patient, as depicted in Table 23.3.

Carbohydrate

Glucose (dextrose), fructose, galactose, sorbitol, glycerol, and ethanol all have been used as sources of carbohydrate calories in infants. The small amount of glycerol present in lipid emulsions contributes to carbohydrate calories. Other carbohydrate sources have no advantage over glucose and can produce serious complications in preterm infants. The quantity of infused glucose that preterm infants tolerate varies. Infusing glucose at 5 mg/kg/min and advancing gradually to 15 mg/kg/min over several days may reduce intolerance. This is best accomplished by increasing the concentration of glucose in the solution while keeping the volume of infusate constant at between 80 and 150 mL/kg/day, depending on the infant's fluid requirements. Gradual increases of 2.5% to 5% dextrose per day are usually well tolerated. The consequences of acute intolerance to glucose are serum hyperosmolarity and osmotic diuresis, which can be avoided by careful monitoring. Hypoglycemia is usually related to the sudden cessation of the parenteral nutrition solution. In adult postsurgical patients, an increase in the glucose infusion rate from 4 to 7 mg/kg/min is associated with an increased rate of glucose oxidation; at higher infusion rates, fat is synthesized from the glucose without a further increase in oxidation.[23]

Higher glucose loads delivered by solutions containing more than 25% dextrose at 150 mL/kg/day (>26 mg/kg/min) may not be beneficial to infants and children and may contribute to fatty infiltration of the liver. Continuous insulin infusion (0.01-0.1 unit/kg/h) has been shown to be tolerated and effective in managing hyperglycemia in the neonate and in promoting greater weight gain.[24-27] However, little is known about its effects on quality of weight gain and counterregulatory hormone concentrations. One study demonstrated a significant elevation in plasma lactate as a result of insulin therapy.[28] Further study of the effects of insulin in infants is suggested before it is recommended for routine use.

Lipids

The composition, use, and complications of intravenous fat emulsions have been published previously.[29,30] Intravenous lipid preparations are a concentrated source of energy (2 kcal/mL in the 20% solution), provide essential fatty acids, and are iso-osmolar. When lipid and amino acid-glucose solutions are infused simultaneously into the same vein, the patient receives a higher-energy and lower-osmolar solution (which helps spare peripheral veins) than with a glucose and amino acid solution alone.

In adults and older children, a 3-in-1 solution (also called a total nutrient ad-mixture) in which the lipid emulsion is mixed with the amino acid-glucose solution and continuously administered through a single line. This method of delivery has certain advantages: (1) simplified administration, which may prove to be a cost savings; (2) less manipulation of the delivery system (reduced opportunity for contamination); and (3) lessened loss of vitamin A. One retrospective study of 3-in-1 solutions in infants younger than 1 year found them safe, efficacious, and cost-effective.[31]

If these infusates are administered without an in-line filter, the presence of lipid in the infusate will obscure any visual precipitation that may occur on removal from refrigeration (4°C) and warming before or during administration. However, a 1.2-Tm (maximal tubular transport rate) in-line filter is available that can be used with lipids. The use of 3-in-1 solutions in low birth weight infants may compromise efforts to maximize calcium and phosphate intakes to meet their high requirements. The addition of lipid emulsion to the amino acid-glucose solution increases the pH of the solution, which may result in a decrease in solubility of calcium and phosphorus, and therefore, a lower concentration of these nutrients is available to the infant. Although 3-in-1 solutions are widely and safely used in pediatrics, iron is not compatible with 3-in-1 solutions, and patients who receive long term 3-in-1 solutions will likely need iron supplementation.[32,33] This is particularly relevant for home total parenteral nutrition therapy, for which 3-in-1 formulations are commonly used.

The requirement for alpha-linoleic acid (an essential fatty acid) can be achieved by supplying as little as 0.5 to 1 g/kg of body weight per day of intravenous lipid. Alpha-linolenic acid is also an essential fatty acid that is found in the intravenous lipid, in amounts approximately one tenth that of linoleic acid. Preterm infants younger than 32 weeks' gestation may be unable to clear lipid doses in excess of 2 g/kg/day, especially in the early weeks of life and during exacerbations of clinical disease.[34] This requires monitoring of the serum triglyceride concentration as the intravenous lipid doses are advanced (Table 23.6). Continuous infusion of no more than 3 g/kg/day of intravenous lipid should minimize the chance of lipid intolerance. Neonates <32 weeks' postconceptional age appear to tolerate continuous infusion better than intermittent infusion on the basis of concentrations of triglycerides, free fatty acids, and free fatty acids-to-albumin ratios.[35] Moreover, infants >32 weeks' postconceptional at age tolerated the continuous infusion better when lipid doses greater than 2 g/kg/day were provided. Under certain circumstances (eg, sepsis), the lowest dose that meets essential fatty acid requirements should be used to avoid potential complications.

Table 23.6.
Suggested Clinical and Laboratory Monitoring Schedule During Total Parenteral Nutrition in the Hospitalized Patient[a,b]

Variable Monitored	Initial Period[c]	Later Period[d]
Serum electrolytes		
(and carbon dioxide)	3–4 times/wk	Weekly
Serum urea nitrogen	Weekly	Weekly
Serum calcium, magnesium, phosphorous	3 times/wk	Weekly
Serum glucose	e	e
Serum protein or albumin		Weekly or biweekly
Liver function studies		Biweekly
Hematocrit	Weekly	Weekly
Urine glucose	optional	optional
Clinical observations (eg, activity, temperature)	Daily	Daily
Blood cell count and differential count	As indicated	As indicated
Cultures	As indicated	As indicated
Serum triglyceride	After every increase	Weekly

[a] Adapted with permission from Baisden B, Bunyapen C, Bhatia J. Feeding the premature infant. In: Bernadier CD, Dwyer J, Feldman EB, eds. *Handbook of Nutrition and Food*. 2nd ed. Boca Raton, FL: CRC Press; 2008:259-270

[b] Schedule may vary with age and underlying medical condition of the patient.

[c] Initial period is the period before full glucose, protein, and lipid intake is achieved or any period of metabolic instability.

[d] Later period is the period during which patient is in a metabolic steady state.

[e] Blood glucose should be monitored closely during a period of glucosuria and for 2 to 3 days after cessation of parenteral nutrition to determine the degree of hypoglycemia. In the latter instance, frequent determination of blood glucose levels in fingertip venous blood constitutes adequate screening. After a month or more of receiving total parenteral nutrition, measurements can be made once a week or less frequently.

A practical way of monitoring parenteral nutrition may simply include the measurement of direct bilirubin (specific but least sensitive marker for cholestasis) and alkaline phosphatase (sensitive measure of metabolic bone disease in the absence of hepatic dysfunction) at 2 to 4 weeks. If they are increased, a full "liver panel," calcium, phosphorous measurements can be obtained, achieving the same endpoint.

Twenty percent intravenous fat is cleared more efficiently than 10% fat emulsions and is the preparation of choice. The phospholipid-to-triglyceride ratio is 0.12 in 10% intravenous emulsion and 0.06 in 20% intravenous emulsion. Phospholipid is believed to inhibit lipoprotein lipase, the main enzyme for intravenous fat clearance; therefore, using a fat emulsion with the lowest ratio of phospholipid to triglyceride (eg, 20% fat emulsions) is preferable.

There have been concerns about products of lipid metabolism and the development of chronic lung disease in preterm infants.[36,37] The toxic lipid peroxidation products in the fat emulsions may increase the risk of developing of chronic lung disease, and the exposure of total parenteral nutrition solutions to ambient light and phototherapy increases lipid oxidation.[38] Data to date are conflicting but disturbing. This may be additive to the previously known photo-oxidation of amino acids and has implications for the development of hepatic dysfunction as well.[39] However, a meta-analysis did not show any difference in rates of chronic lung disease between infants given intravenous lipid soon after birth compared with those cases in which lipids were delayed.[40] Older studies have demonstrated decreased pulmonary membrane diffusion in adults infused with 500 mL of 10% intralipid over a 4-hour period.[41] These alterations reverted to basal levels when serum lipids cleared. In preterm infants, a significant decrease in blood oxygen levels was observed when 1 g of lipids/kg was infused over a 4-hour period and correlated with increased levels of triglyceride.[42] Using more clinically relevant infusion times of 16 or 24 hours at doses ranging from 1 to 4 g/kg/day, no changes in pH or alveolar-arteriolar gradient of oxygen were demonstrated, and the authors concluded that an infusion rate of 24 hour be used to avoid overloading the clearance mechanism of fat in small infants.[43]

No available parenteral solutions contain carnitine, which is required for the optimal metabolism of fatty acids. Infants have a poorly developed capacity to synthesize and store carnitine. Some experts do recommend carnitine supplementation (2.4–10 mg/kg/day in preterm and term infants), but the lack of carnitine in parenteral nutrition formulations has not been associated with any clinical deficiency syndrome, and the results of clinical studies of its addition to parenteral nutrition formulations have been contradictory.[44,45]

Alternate lipid emulsions have become available in infants and children.[46-50] Olive oil preparations contain decreased concentrations of omega-6 polyunsaturated fatty acids, which have been noted to adversely affect leukocyte recruitment. On the other hand, olive oil contains alpha-tocopherol, with its antioxidant properties. In adults, the use of parenteral nutrition fish-oil emulsions containing omega-3 fatty acids has been studied, and these lipid solutions are under investigation in infants and children.[47] Omegaven (Fresnenius-Kabi, Bad Homburg,

Germany) is a 10% emulsion with 100 g of lipid/L, of which 27 to 59 g is eicosapentaenoic acid (EPA) plus docosahexaenoic acid (DHA) and has a low ratio of omega-6 to omega-3 polyunsaturated fatty acids. Other new DHA-containing lipid emulsions include Lipoplus (soybean oil, medium-chain triglycerides [MCTs], fish oil) and SMOFlipid (soybean oil, MCTs, olive oil, fish oil). Studies in animals show that an inclusion of omega-3 polyunsaturated fatty acids in mixed lipid emulsions increases blood clearance and extrahepatic tissue uptake of lipid, despite the fact that fish oil is a poor substrate for lipoprotein lipase.[48-50] Omega-3 fatty acids have important effects on the developing retina and brain.[51,52] Preterm infants may particularly benefit from supplemental omega-3 fatty acids, because they may not be capable of synthesizing these metabolites in amounts necessary to support the needs of the rapidly growing central nervous system, making preterm infants more vulnerable to long-chain polyunsaturated fatty acid deficiency (DHA and arachidonic acid [AHA]; see Chapter 17: Fats and Fatty Acids).

Vitamins, Minerals, and Trace Elements

Vitamins, minerals, and trace elements must be supplied in parenteral solutions. Metabolic complications have been described for deficiencies and excesses of some of these nutrients. Intravenous dose requirements are not fully known. Guidelines from an expert panel for multivitamin and trace element preparations for parenteral use are shown in Tables 23.4 and 23.5.[53] A higher, more physiologic calcium-to-phosphorus ratio of 1.7:1 by weight (1.3:1 by molar ratio, similar to the fetal mineral accretion ratio) allows for the highest absolute retention of both minerals. This ratio provides 76 mg/kg/day of elemental calcium and 45 mg/kg/day of phosphorus.[54] Dunham et al have generated calcium and phosphorus precipitation curves for parenteral nutrition using TrophAmine (its low pH allows for the maximum possible calcium and phosphorous in solution) to help pharmacists and clinicians avoid compounding total parenteral nutrition solutions that will precipitate.[55]

Other precipitation curves for parenteral nutrition will be needed if other amino acid preparations are used or cysteine is added to the base amino acid solution. Precipitation information can also be found in the package inserts of the amino acid solutions.

Vitamin A supplementation beyond generally recommended intakes for VLBW infants have been recommended to decrease the risk of bronchopulmonary dysplasia.[56,57] Supplemental vitamin A must be delivered intramuscularly, not in parenteral nutrition solutions.

A number of substances commonly administered intravenously, including calcium and phosphorus salts and albumin, contain relatively large amounts of aluminum. Preterm infants receiving intravenous fluid therapy may accumulate aluminum and show evidence of aluminum toxicity,[58] but on the basis of the current recommendations, parenteral nutrition manufacturers exceed the range of Food and Drug Administration protocols to limit aluminum in parenteral nutrition in both calculated and measured aluminum.[59] Calcium gluconate can contribute up to 80% of the total aluminum load from parenteral nutrition. Bishop et al demonstrated developmental delay in preterm infants receiving 45 μg/kg/day of aluminum in parenteral nutrition solutions.[60] Findings have been conflicting with regard to bone health. Naylor et al[61] did not find a decrease in bone formation in preterm infants, whereas Fewtrell et al[62] found that neonates exposed to aluminum via the parenteral route may have reduced lumbar spine and hip bone mass during adolescence, suggesting that these are potential risk factors for later osteoporotic disease. Aluminum intake should be determined in children at high risk of toxicity: preterm infants, infants or children with impaired renal function, and patients receiving prolonged parenteral nutrition. It is currently recommended that all parenteral nutrition solutions have aluminum content stated.

Ordering Parenteral Nutrition

Parenteral nutrition formulations must be prepared using current and established policies and procedures regarding sterility, compatibility, and labeling. There are specific standards for nutrition support, including the order of compounding additives, to prevent crystallization in the solutions.[63] Preprinted parenteral nutrition order sheets or those now available in electronic health records save time and errors of order entry. Electronic order entry has the advantage of providing algorithms for computing nutrient intakes and automatically screening for errors. There has been a trend in the medical profession to move toward having qualified pharmacists perform order entry in the electronic health record for parenteral nutrition as well.

Gastrointestinal and Hepatic Effects of Parenteral Nutrition

Hepatic disease is the major complication of parenteral nutrition, particularly in infants and young children. When the liver is examined histologically, cholestasis, hepatocellular necrosis, and in advanced cases, cirrhosis may be found.[64-66] Cholestasis, steatosis, and steatohepatitis may progress to cirrhosis and end-stage liver disease. In infants, the first clinical indication of parenteral nutrition-induced liver injury is hepatomegaly followed by biochemical evidence of cholestasis. The first biochemical abnormality is an increase in serum bile salts followed by an increase in direct serum bilirubin concentration, which may develop any time after

2 to 3 weeks of parenteral nutrition. Serum alkaline phosphatase and transaminases increase days to weeks later.

Enteral starvation is a critical factor in the pathogenesis of parenteral nutrition-related hepatic disease. The most severe hepatic pathologic changes are seen in patients with the poorest enteral intake. Significantly less significant and progressive hepatic disease is being documented in recent years, likely because of earlier initiation of enteral feeding (stimulating bile flow and secretion of gastrointestinal hormones). In all patients receiving parenteral nutrition, enteral feedings should be initiated as soon as possible, even if only in minimal amounts (trophic feedings), to minimize the risk of hepatic dysfunction. Once liver disease has developed, "lipid-reducing" strategies, providing lipid infusions only 2 to 3 times per week or limiting the quantity of infused lipid to 1 to 2 g/kg/day may be useful to reverse the disorder.[66] Another potential treatment for parenteral nutrition cholestasis has been the use of fish oil-based emulsions, which in limited, small studies have been demonstrated to reverse total parenteral nutrition-induced cholestasis when compared with historical controls.[47] In animal models, a reduction in fat deposits in the liver occurred when intravenous omega-3 fatty acid emulsion was given.[67,68] To date, however, no study has demonstrated prevention of hepatic dysfunction with the use of these fish oil-based emulsions in infants and children.

Less is known about the long-term effects of total parenteral nutrition on the stomach, pancreas, and small bowel. Studies in animals have documented decreased pancreatic secretion and intestinal mucosal atrophy, which are reversible on resumption of enteral feeding. A few studies in humans suggest that exocrine pancreatic secretion and gastric parietal cell mass are decreased and that the small intestine atrophies during total parenteral nutrition, although the observed changes are minor.[69,70] Intragastrically fed rats demonstrated a greater increase in immunoreactive insulin and a smaller increase in serum immunoreactive glucagon compared with intravenously fed rats.[70]

Preterm infants are at high risk of the development of metabolic bone disease, most commonly as a result of inadequate intakes of calcium and phosphorus during parenteral nutrition. In general, serum concentrations of calcium are maintained even as there is increasing hypophosphatemia and increasing alkaline phosphatase is observed, while bones appear more osteopenic on radiographs. Rising alkaline phosphatase in the absence of elevated liver enzymes is often used as an indicator of metabolic bone disease. The incidence of rickets/metabolic bone disease is inversely proportional to birth weight and gestational age and has been reported to be as high as 55% in very low birth weight infants.[71] The major predisposing factor is deficiency of both calcium and phosphorus. This cannot be diagnosed without radiography, which demonstrates a decreased lucency of the cortical bone with or without epiphyseal changes, and in rare cases, a fracture may also be seen.

Approaches to interrupting parenteral nutrition therapy during drug administration differs from institution to institution and should be carefully discussed with pharmacy staff and the institution's parenteral nutrition committee. Acyclovir, amphotericin B, metronidazole, and trimethoprim-sulfamethoxazole are just a few of the drugs that are incompatible with parenteral nutrition solutions. Drugs may be given in the central catheter with 10% dextrose with the parenteral nutrition turned off. Bicarbonate also should not be given with the parenteral nutrition solution. Although ranitidine is compatible with parenteral nutrition solutions, no studies in infants and children have demonstrated that this is of any benefit. On the contrary, the association of the use of ranitidine and the increased risk of sepsis and necrotizing enterocolitis in neonates should be considered before any decision to use ranitidine is made.[72] Information about the compatibility of individual drugs with parenteral nutrition is available through the pharmacies of all major hospitals.

Transition to Enteral Feedings

Initiation of enteral feedings should begin as soon as the gastrointestinal tract is functional. Small amounts of trophic feedings have been demonstrated to promote gastrointestinal tract function in the preterm infant. Enteral feedings can be used to supplement parenteral nutrition. Parenteral nutrition should not be discontinued until the patient tolerates enteral feedings well enough to meet nutritional requirements. Enteral feedings provide less risk of infection, are less expensive, are associated with fewer metabolic abnormalities, and facilitate recovery of intestinal morphology and enzymes. See Chapter 24 for further details.

Conclusion

The nutritional requirements of young infants, preterm and term, can be met better by recognizing their limitations in absorption and digestion. Poor in-hospital nutrition is one of the most frequently recognized morbidities in very low birth weight and sick infants.[73] Extrauterine growth restriction remains a serious problem in preterm neonates. Poor nutrition and poor growth are associated with adverse neurocognitive outcomes. When gastrointestinal tract disease is superimposed on an immature digestive system, special nutritional support is needed to maintain adequate growth. This support can be given with parenteral or specialized enteral feeding techniques and formulations. Because parenteral nutrition solutions can provide complete nutrition support, they may be used for extended periods.

Summary Recommendations for the Use of Parenteral Nutrition

1. If a central line is used, the catheter should be placed carefully, and its intravenous position should be confirmed by imaging; aseptic techniques and established guidelines of catheter care should be adhered to strictly.

2. Protein (nitrogen) in the form of crystalline amino acids should be provided as noted in Table 23.3 by body weight. The concentration of glucose should be advanced methodically to ensure tolerance. Essential fatty acid requirements can be met by infusing 0.5 to 1 g/kg/day of intravenous lipid. The continuous infusion (over 24 hours) of up to 3 g/kg/day of intravenous lipid should maximize tolerance. Vitamins, minerals, and trace elements are essential nutrients and should be provided in parenteral nutrition solutions.

3. Patients should be monitored clinically and with laboratory tests for intolerance to components of the parenteral nutrition solution (see Table 23.6).

4. The transition to enteral nutrition should begin as soon as possible, with continuation of parenteral nutrition until near full enteral nutritional support is achieved.

5. Nutritional status and anthropometric measurements should be monitored continuously to ensure the adequacy of nutritional support. A nutrition support team with expertise in parenteral nutrition provides optimal care, decreases costs and complications, and potentially shortens the length of hospitalization.

References

1. Shulman RJ, Phillips S. Parenteral nutrition: indications, administration, and monitoring. In: Baker SS, Baker RD, Davis AM, eds. *Pediatric Nutrition Support*. Sudbury, MA: Jones and Bartlett Publishers; 2007:273-286

2. Fuhrman MP. Complication management in parenteral nutrition. In: Matarese LE, Gottschlich MM, ed. *Contemporary Nutrition Support Practice*. St Louis, MO: WB Saunders; 2003:242-262

3. Haire WD, Herbst SL. Use of Alteplase [t-PA] for the management of thrombotic catheter dysfunction: guidelines from a consensus conference of the National Association of Vascular Access Networks [NAVAN]. *Nutr Clin Pract*. 2000;15(6):265-275

4. Ehrenkranz RA, Das A, Wrage LA, et al. Early nutrition mediates the influence of severity of illness on extremely LBW infants. *Pediatr Res*. 2011;69(6):522-529

5. Thureen PJ, Melara D, Fennessey PV, Hay WW Jr. Effect of low versus high intravenous amino acid intake on very low birth weight infants in the early neonatal period. *Pediatr Res*. 2003;53(1):24-32

6. te Braake FW, van den Akker CH, Wattimena DJ, et al. Amino acid administration to premature infants directly after birth. *J Pediatr*. 2005;147(4):457-461

7. Poindexter BB, Langer JC, Dusick AM, et al. Early provision of parenteral amino acids in extremely low birth weight infants: relation to growth and neurodevelopmental outcome. *J Pediatr*. 2006;148(3):300-305

8. Valentine CJ, Fernandez S, Rogers LK, et al. Early amino-acid administration improves preterm infant weight. *J Perinatol*. 2009;29(6):428-432

9. Zlotkin SH, Bryan MH, Anderson GH. Intravenous nitrogen and energy intakes required to duplicate in utero nitrogen accretion in prematurely born human infants. *J Pediatr*. 1981;99(1):115-120

10. Chan DS. Recommended daily allowance of maintenance parenteral nutrition in infants and children. *Am J Health Syst Pharm*. 1995;52(6):651-653

11. Kowalski L, Nucci A. Pediatrics. In: Cresci G, ed. *Nutrition Support for the Critically Ill Patient: A Guide to Practice*. Boca Raton, FL: CRC Press; 2005:389-405

12. Viña J, Vento M, García-Sala F, et al. L-cysteine and glutathione metabolism are impaired in premature infants due to cystathionase deficiency. *Am J Clin Nutr*. 1995;61(5):1067-1069

13. Van Goudoever JB, Sulkers EJ, Timmerman M, et al. Amino acid solutions for premature neonates during the first week of life: the role of N-acetyl-L-cysteine and N-acetyl-L-tyrosine. *JPEN J Parenter Enteral Nutr*. 1994;18(5):404-408

14. Griffiths RD, Jones C, Palmer TE. Six-month outcome of critically ill patients given glutamine-supplemented Parenteral nutrition. *Nutrition*. 1997;13(4):295-302

15. Ziegler TR, Young LS, Benfell K. Clinical and metabolic efficacy of glutamine-supplemented parenteral nutrition after bone marrow transplantation. *Ann Intern Med*. 1992;116(10):821-828

16. Poindexter BB, Erenkranz RA, Stoll BJ, et al. Parenteral glutamine supplementation does not reduce the risk of mortality or late-onset sepsis in extremely low birth weight infants. *Pediatrics*. 2004;113(5):1209-1215

17. LeLeiko NS, Walsh MJ. The role of glutamine, short chain fatty acids, and nucleotides in intestinal adaptation to gastrointestinal disease. *Pediatr Clin North Am*. 1996;43(2):451–469

18. Lacey JM, Crouch JB, Benfell K, et al. The effects of glutamine supplemented parenteral nutrition in premature infants. *JPEN J Parenter Enteral Nutr*. 1996;20(1):74–80

19. Blanco CL, Falck A, Green BK, Cornell JE, Gong AK. Metabolic responses to early and high protein supplementation in a randomized trial evaluating the prevention of hyperkalemia in extremely low birth weight infants. *J Pediatr*. 2008;153(4):535-540

20. Blanco CL, Gong AK, Leichty EA. Plasma amino acid concentrations (conPIAA) in ELBW infants during 1st week of life correlate inversely with 18-month Bailey MDI (MDI) and anthropometrics [abstr 2155.3]. Presented at Pediatric Academic Societies Annual Meeting; May 1-2, 2009; Baltimore, MD

21. Blanco CL, Gong AK, Schoolfield J, Green BK, Daniels W, Liechty EA, Ramamurthy R. The impact of early and high amino acid supplementation on ELBW infants at two years. *J Pediatr Gastroenterol Nutr*. 2012;54(5):601-607

22. Deitch EA, Ma WJ, Ma L, Berg RD, Specian RD. Protein malnutrition predisposes to inflammatory-induced gut-origin septic states. *Ann Surg*. 1990;211(5):560-567

23. Wolfe RR, Allsop JR, Burke JF. Glucose metabolism in man: responses to intravenous glucose infusion. *Metabolism.* 1979;28(3):210–220

24. Heron P, Bourchier D. Insulin infusions in infants of birthweight less than 1250 g and with glucose intolerance. *Aust Pediatr J.* 1988;24(6):362-365

25. Kanarek KS, Santeiro ML, Malone JI. Continuous infusion of insulin in hyperglycemic low-birth-weight infants receiving parenteral nutrition with and without lipids. *JPEN J Parenter Enteral Nutr.* 1991;15(4):417-420

26. Collins JW Jr, Hoppe M, Brown L, et al. A controlled trial of insulin infusion and parenteral nutrition in extremely low birth weight infants with glucose intolerance. *J Pediatr.* 1991;118(6):921-927

27. Ostertag SG, Javanovic L, Lewis B, et al. Insulin pump therapy in the very-low-birth-weight infant. *Pediatrics.* 1986;78(4):625-630

28. Poindexter BB, Karn CA, Denne SC. Exogenous insulin reduces proteolysis and protein synthesis in extremely-low-birth-weight infant. *J Pediatr.* 1998;132(6):948-953

29. Mascarenhas MR, Kerner JA Jr, Stallings VA. Parenteral and enteral nutrition. In: Walker WA, Durie PR, Hamilton JR, Walker-Smith JA, Watkins JB, eds. *Pediatric Gastrointestinal Disease.* 3rd ed. Toronto, Canada: BC Decker Inc. 2000,1705 1752

30. American Academy of Pediatrics, Committee on Nutrition. Use of intravenous fat emulsions in pediatric patients. *Pediatrics.* 1981;68(5):738–743

31. Rollins CJ, Elsberry VA, Pollack KA, Pollack PF, Udall JN Jr. Three-in-one parenteral nutrition: a safe and economical method of nutritional support for infants *JPEN J Parenter Enteral Nutr.* 1990;14(3):290–294

32. Leung FY. Trace elements in parenteral micronutrition. *Clin Biochem.* 1995;28(6):561-566

33. Driscoll DF, Bhargava HN, Li L, et al. Physiochemical stability of total nutrient admixtures. *Am J Hosp Pharm.* 1995;52(6):623-634

34. Schanler TJ. Parenteral nutrition in premature infants. *UpToDate.* October 7, 2011. Available at: http://www.uptodate.com/contents/parenteral-nutrition-in-premature-infants. Accessed November 16, 2012

35. Kao LC, Cheng MH, Warburton D. Triglycerides, free fatty acids, free fatty acids/albumin molar ratio, and cholesterol levels in serum of neonates receiving long-term lipid infusions: controlled trial of continuous and intermittent regimens. *J Pediatr.* 1984;104(3):429-435

36. Sosenko IR. Intravenous lipids and the management of chronic lung injury: helpful or harmful? *Semin Neonatal Nutr Metab.* 1995;3:3–5

37. O'Donovan DJ, Fernandes. Free Radicals and diseases in premature infants. Antioxidants and redox Signaling 2004;6(1):169-176

38. Neuzil J, Darlow BA, Inder TE, Sluis KB, Winterbourn CC, Stocker R. Oxidation of parenteral lipid emulsion by ambient and phototherapy lights: potential toxicity of routine parenteral feeding. *J Pediatr.* 1995;126(5 Pt 1):785–790

39. Bhatia J, Moslen MT, Haque AK, McCleery R, Rassin DK. Total parenteral nutrition-associated alterations in hepatobiliary function and histology in rats; is light exposure a clue? *Pediatr Res.* 1993;33(5):487-492

40. Simmer K, Rao SC. Early introduction of lipids in parenterally-fed preterm infants. *Cochrane Database Syst Rev.* 2005;(1):CD000376

41. Greene HL, Hazlett D, Demaree R. Relationship between intralipid-induced hyperlipemia and pulmonary function. *Am J Clin Nutr.* 1976;29(2):127

42. Periera GR, Fox WW, Stanley CA, Baker L, Schwartz JG. Decreased oxygenation and hyperlipemia during intravenous fat infusions in premature infants. *Pediatrics.* 1980;66(1):26-30

43. Brans YW, Dutton EB, Andrew DS, Menchaca EM, West DL. Fat emulsion tolerance in very low birth weight neonates: effect on diffusion of oxygen in the lungs and on blood pH. *Pediatrics.* 1986;78(1):79-84

44. Koo WK, Cepeda EE. Parenteral nutrition in neonates. In: Rombeau JL, Rolandelli RH, eds. *Clinical Nutrition: Parenteral Nutrition.* 3rd ed. Philadelphia, PA: WB Saunders Co; 2001;463–475

45. Falcone RA Jr, Warner BW. Pediatric parenteral nutrition. In: Rombeau JL, Rolandelli, RH, eds. *Clinical Nutrition: Parenteral Nutrition.* 3rd ed. Philadelphia, PA: W.B. Saunders Co; 2001;476–496

46. Sala-Vila A, Barbosa VM, Calder PC. Olive oil in parenteral nutrition. *Curr Opin Clin Nutr Metab Care.* 2007;10(2):165-174

47. Gura K M, Lee S, Valim C, Zhou J, et al. Safety and efficacy of a fish-oil-based fat emulsion in the treatment of parenteral nutrition -associated liver disease. *Pediatrics.* 2008;121(3):e678-e686

48. Le HD, de Meijer VE, Zurakowski D, Meisel JA, Gura KM, Pruder M. Parenteral fish oil as monotherapy improves lipid profiles in children in parenteral nutrition associated liver disease. J Parenter Enteral Nutr 2010a;34(5):477-484

49. Qi K, Al-Haideri M, Seo T, Carpentier YA, Deckelbaum RJ. Effects of particle size on blood clearance and tissue uptake of lipid emulsions with different triglyceride compositions. *JPEN J Parenter Enteral Nutr.* 2003;27(1):58-64

50. Ton M, Chang C, Carpentier Y, Deckelbaum RJ. In vivo and in vitro properties of an intravenous lipid emulsion containing only medium chain and fish oil triglycerides. *Clin Nutr.* 2005;24(4):492-501

51. SanGiovanni JP, Chew EY. The role of omega-3 long chain poly unsaturated fatty acids in health and disease of the retina. *Prog Retin Eye Res.* 2005;24(1):87-138

52. McNamara RK, Carlson SE. Role of omega-3 fatty acids in brain development and function: potential implications for the pathogenesis and prevention of psychopathology. *Prostaglandins Leukot Essent Fatty Acids.* 2006;75(4-5):329-349

53. Greene HL, Hambidge KM, Schanler R, Tsang RC. Guidelines for the use of vitamins, trace elements, calcium, magnesium and phosphorous in infants and children receiving total parenteral nutrition: report of the Subcommittee of Pediatric Parenteral Nutrient Requirements from the Committee on Clinical Practice Issues of the American Society for Clinical Nutrition. *Am J Clin Nutr.* 1988;48(5):1324–1342

54. Pelegano JF, Rowe JC, Carey DE, et al. Effect of calcium/phosphorous ratio on mineral retention in parenterally fed premature infants. *J Pediatr Gastroenterol Nutr.* 1991;12(3):351–355

55. Dunham B, Marcuard S, Khazanie PG, Meade G, Craft T, Nichols K. The solubility of calcium and phosphorus in neonatal total parenteral nutrition solutions. *JPEN J Parenter Enteral Nutr.* 1991;15(6):608–611

56. Hazinski TA. Vitamin A treatment for the infant at risk for bronchopulmonary dysplasia. *NeoReviews.* 2000;1(1):e11–e15

57. Tyson JE, Wright LL, Oh W, et al. Vitamin A supplementation for extremely-low-birth-weight infants. *N Engl J Med.* 1999;340(25):1962–1968

58. American Academy of Pediatrics, Committee on Nutrition. Aluminum toxicity in infants and children. *Pediatrics.* 1996;97(3):413–416

59. Poole RL, Hintz SR, MacKenzie NI, Kerner JA Jr. Aluminum exposure from pediatric parenteral nutrition: meeting the new FDA regulation. *J Parenter Enteral Nutr.* 2008;32(3):242-246

60. Bishop NJ, Morley R, Chir B, Day JP, Lucas A. Aluminum neurotoxicity in preterm infants receiving intravenous-feeding solutions. *N Engl J Med.* 1997;36(22):1557–1561

61. Naylor KE, Eastell R, Shattuck KE, Alfrey AC, Klein GL. Bone turnover in preterm infants. *Pediatr Res.* 1999;45(3):363-366

62. Fewtrell MS, Bishop NJ, Edmonds CJ, et al. Aluminum exposure from parenteral nutrition in preterm infants: bone health at 15-year follow-up. *Pediatrics.* 2009;124(5):1372-1379

63. Wessel J, Balint J, Crill C, Klotz K; American Society for Parenteral and Enteral Nutrition, Task Force on Standards for Specialized Nutrition Support for Hospitalized Pediatric patients. Standards for specialized nutrition support: hospitalized pediatric patients. *Nutr Clin Pract.* 2005;20(1):103-116

64. Whitington PF. Cholestasis associated with total parenteral nutrition in infants. *Hepatology.* 1985;5(4):693–696

65. Quigley EM, Marsh MN, Shaffer JL, Markin RS. Hepatobiliary complications of total parenteral nutrition. *Gastroenterology.* 1993;104(1):286–301

66. Colomb V, Jobert-Giraud A, Lacailee F, Goulet, Fournet JC, Ricour C. Role of lipid emulsions in cholestasis associated with long-term parenteral nutrition in children. *JPEN J Parenter Enteral Nutr.* 2000;24(6):345-350

67. Alwayn IP, Gura K, Nose V, et al. Omega-3 fatty acid supplementation prevents hepatic steatosis in a murine model of nonalcoholic fatty liver disease. *Pediatr Res.* 2005;57(5):445-452

68. Van Aerde JE, Duerksen DR, Gramlich L, et al. Intravenous fish oil emulsion attenuates total parenteral nutrition-induced cholestasis in newborn piglets. *Pediatr Res.* 1999;45(2):202-208

69. Lo CW, Walker WA. Changes in the gastrointestinal tract during enteral or parenteral feeding. *Nutr Rev.* 1989;47(7):193-198

70. Lickley HL, Track NS, Vranic M, Bury KD. Metabolic responses to enteral and parenteral nutrition. *Am J Surg.* 1978;135(2):172-176

71. Backstrom MC, Kuusela AL, Maki R. Metabolic bone disease of prematurity. *Ann Med.* 1996;28(4):275-282

V

72. Passariello TG, De Curtis M, Manguso F, Salvia G, Lega L, Messina F, Paludetto R, Canani RB. Ranitidine is associated with infection, necrotizing enterocolitis, and fatal outcome in newborns. *Pediatrics*. 2012;129(1):e40-50

73. Clark RH, Thomas P, Peabody J. Extrauterine growth restriction remains a serious problem in prematurely born neonates. *Pediatrics*. 2003;111(5 Pt 1):986-990

Chapter 24

Enteral Nutrition

Introduction

Pediatric patients who do not have adequate growth on oral intake may be supported by enteral nutrition for nutritional management. Commonly used enteral tube feeding routes include nasogastric, gastrostomy, nasojejunal, gastrojejunal, and jejunostomy. Although enteral and parenteral routes can be used to provide nutritional support to pediatric patients, enteral nutrition support is preferred, because it is more "physiologic," more affordable, easier, and safer than parenteral feedings. Enteral nutrition produces fewer metabolic and infectious complications and better supports the integrity of the barrier function of the gastrointestinal tract. Enteral nutrition also allows for better physiologic control of electrolyte levels and serves as effective prophylaxis against stress-induced gastropathy and gastrointestinal (GI) tract hemorrhage. Enteral nutrition also can provide a more complete range of nutrients, including glutamine, long-chain polyunsaturated fatty acids, short-chain fatty acids, and fiber. Finally, enteral nutrition provides a trophic effect on the gut by promoting pancreatic and biliary secretions as well as endocrine, paracrine, and neural factors that help promote the physiologic and immunologic integrity of the intestine. Timely initiation of enteral nutrition is also important, with the greatest metabolic benefits resulting from initiating early enteral nutrition within less than 72 hours of injury or admission. Within the setting of critical illness, however, enteral nutrition should not be initiated until the child achieves hemodynamic stability, thus minimizing the risk of bowel ischemia.[1]

Indications for Enteral Tube Feedings: Management of Nutrition-Related Disorders (Table 24.1)

Prematurity

A feeding method for preterm infants should be individualized to gestational age, birth weight, and medical status. Preterm infants present a unique nutritional challenge because of their GI tract immaturity, limited fluid tolerance, high nutrient requirements, limited renal function, and predisposition to specific metabolic and clinical complications, such as hypoglycemia and necrotizing enterocolitis. Because the coordination of sucking and swallowing appears at approximately 34 weeks of gestation, intragastric or jejunal feedings are often used before this time. These techniques may be useful beyond 34 weeks' gestation in selected infants who are unable to achieve and/or tolerate adequate oral feedings. Studies in preterm infants suggest that minimal enteral feedings (2–8 mL/kg per day) administered soon after birth promote a GI tract hormonal response and, thus, mediate intestinal adaptation.[2] In sick preterm infants requiring parenteral nutrition support, these small-volume, hypocaloric enteral feedings are used to prime the gut and are thought to promote maturation of GI tract motor patterns, increase general growth and feeding tolerance, and encourage earlier progression to full enteral feedings and hospital discharge. For further information about feeding the preterm infant, see Chapter 5.

Table 24.1.
Conditions Under Which Enteral Tube Feeding May Be Warranted[a]

Prematurity
Cardiorespiratory illness
Chronic lung disease
Cystic fibrosis
Congenital heart disease
Gastrointestinal tract disease and dysfunction
Inflammatory bowel disease
Short-bowel syndrome
Biliary atresia
Gastroesophageal reflux (GER) disease
Protracted diarrhea of infancy
Chronic nonspecific diarrhea
Renal disease
Hypermetabolic states
Burn injury
Severe trauma or closed head injury
Cancer
Neurologic disease or cerebral palsy
Oral motor dysfunction
Inadequate spontaneous oral intake

[a] Adapted with permission from: Abad-Sinden, A, Sutphen J. Enteral nutrition. In: Walker WA, Goulet O, Kleinman RE, et al, eds. *Pediatric Gastrointestinal Disease: Pathophysiology, Diagnosis, Management*. 4th ed. Burlington, Ontario: BC Decker Inc; 2004:1981-1994

Cardiorespiratory Illness

Infants and children with pulmonary disease often require enteral nutrition support during acute exacerbations of their primary disease, as well as for nutritional rehabilitation of chronic secondary malnutrition. Growth failure in patients with neonatal chronic lung disease can be caused by hypoxia, hypercapnia, elevated metabolic rates, inefficient suck and swallow mechanisms, poor appetite, decreased intake, and recurrent emesis with decreased gastric motility. Children with cystic fibrosis (CF) (see also Chapter 48: Cystic Fibrosis) have increased energy needs and poor intake resulting from their lung disease, malabsorption, and chronic infection. Nocturnal nasogastric feedings using elemental or polymeric nutrient formulas supplemented with pancreatic enzymes are used in children and adolescents with

CF in whom conservative nutritional supplement measures have failed. Short-term nasogastric feedings have resulted in increased caloric intake and significant weight gain for patients with CF, but long-term effectiveness may be limited by noncompliance. Gastrostomy feedings are more appropriate when long-term (beyond 3 months) infusions are required.

Infants with congenital heart disease (CHD) (see also Chapter 46: Cardiac Disease) are also at significant nutritional risk. Growth failure resulting from inadequate intake and elevated energy expenditure may be caused by respiratory distress, increased metabolic needs, tissue hypoxia, and impaired absorption, including protein-losing enteropathy. Because of their elevated nutritional needs and limited fluid tolerance, these infants often require high-caloric–density formulas (Appendix C). Increased caloric density of formula up to 30 kcal/oz has been used in these infants. Concentration above 24 kcal/oz with increased formula-to-water ratio increases the renal solute load but may not allow enough free water for excretion of the renal solute load by immature kidneys. If necessary, additional calories may also be provided through carbohydrate (eg, Polycose [Abbott Nutrition, North Chicago, IL) or fat supplementation (eg, Microlipid [Nestlé, Vevey, Switzerland). Consultation with a registered dietitian will guide customization of this recipe to safely meet an individual infant's needs. Infants with CHD often experience delayed gastric emptying that may result in early satiety and/or promote gastroesophageal reflux (GER).[3] Continuous nocturnal nasogastric feedings or 24-hour enteral feedings of infants, particularly those with acyanotic CHD, may result in significant catch-up growth.[4] Alternatively, providing intermittent oral feedings with nasogastric supplementation of the remainder of the required volume may also facilitate achievement of the nutritional goals.[5]

Gastrointestinal Tract Disease and Dysfunction

Pediatric patients with acute and chronic gastrointestinal tract disease and dysfunction often benefit from enteral feeding regimens (see Chapter 44: Inflammatory Bowel Disease). Growth failure in children with Crohn's disease is multifactorial in origin but is most often related to inadequate nutrient intake and the increased energy requirements associated with chronic inflammation and malabsorption. In addition to encouraging higher-calorie oral intake, the use of elemental and semi-elemental diets administered orally and/or nasogastrically have been demonstrated to produce a significant improvement in nutritional status. Clinical remission of Crohn's disease of the small bowel with the use of enteral nutrition has been reported and may be equally as effective as steroids, with the additional benefit of improved linear growth.[6,7]

The nutritional management of short-bowel syndrome is particularly challenging and usually involves the artful implementation of both enteral and parenteral nutrition. Total parenteral nutrition is often used initially. As soon as possible after recovery from surgery, enteral feedings should begin at a slow, continuous rate and be advanced as tolerated. The period of transition to complete enteral feedings may take weeks to years, depending on the length and function of the residual intestine. If the ileocecal valve is preserved, the outcome may be improved, but overall length and function of the remaining intestine are the most important determinants of intestinal adaptation. In the early stages of enteral nutrition support and particularly in cases in which the formula is delivered directly into the small bowel distal to the ligament of Treitz, elemental or semi-elemental formulas are preferred to polymeric formulas.[8] Long-term parenteral nutrition for infants with short-bowel syndrome can lead to parenteral nutrition-associated liver disease (PNALD), which is a significant cause of morbidity and mortality in infants and children with short-bowel syndrome. In fact, end-stage PNALD involving cirrhosis is one of the direct consequences of short-bowel syndrome and may be fatal unless a combined liver-intestine transplantation can be performed. Sepsis, bacterial overgrowth, and absence of enteral intake are some of the many factors that increase the probability of PNALD. Enteral nutrition helps prevent and/or ameliorate hepatic disease in this situation. Cyclic (10 to 12 hours) customized parenteral nutrition with lipid minimization[9] plus continuous and/or intermittent enteral feedings and oral intake as tolerated, as well as the early identification and treatment of catheter-related infections, are usually the most successful strategies to avoid PNALD.[10] Some patients with PNALD who remain dependent on parenteral nutrition may also benefit from the use of fish oil derived intravenous lipid emulsion instead of the standard soybean derived lipid emulsion.[11] However, this product can only be used through compassionate-use protocols, because it is not approved by the US Food and Drug Administration at the time of this publication. Eventual weaning off parenteral nutrition onto full enteral nutrition is the major goal and will often allow for recovery of PNALD if it has not reached end-stage liver disease.[10]

When children with short-bowel syndrome are fed enterally, they will inevitably have diarrhea, and in general, this should be tolerated as long as there is adequate weight gain, appropriate electrolyte and fluid balance, and no perineal complications from skin contact with fecal fluid. In particular, extra sodium should be provided if the serum sodium concentration is not well into the normal range. Prevention and careful management of perineal skin breakdown and infection is critical in this situation. In infants, it is useful to monitor the number of diapers that have urine alone without fecal material as a measure of the adequacy of fluid balance. As the concentration or volume of formula is advanced, ultimately, the maximum absorptive capability of the remaining intestine will be exceeded, and an abrupt increase in stool output will occur or the maximum rate of gastric emptying will be exceeded and emesis will occur. At this point, the feedings should be decreased and a variable amount of time should be allowed for the intestine to adapt to the increased intake. Judicious, often empirical, treatment of bacterial overgrowth with periodic antibiotics may facilitate the advancement of enteral feeding volumes.

Continuous feedings may provide the best nutrient absorption when the intestinal length is shortened, but it is important to allow a break of a few hours in both enteral and parenteral feedings each day. During this time, oral intake, especially in infants, should be encouraged to promote the development and maintenance of oral motor function (see Chapter 47: Short-Bowel Syndrome).

Several other illnesses affecting GI tract function and nutritional status can be managed successfully with enteral tube feedings. For selected infants and children who undergo surgery for whatever cause and who encounter difficulty feeding in the perioperative period, enteral nutrition can be a valuable adjunct to support nutritional needs and enhance recovery. Infants with biliary atresia frequently experience reduced intake associated with hepatic disease and infection. Nutritional support with nasogastric tube feedings using a semi- or elemental formula rich in medium-chain triglycerides can promote energy and nitrogen balance in preparation for and after hepatic transplantation. Once the clinical condition of the infant or child is stable after transplantation, transition to a polymeric formula or an oral diet should be made. Infants with GER disease and poor weight gain may benefit from continuous nasogastric tube feedings with improved weight gain, reduction or cessation of vomiting, and catch-up growth.[12] However, one should be cautious in attributing poor weight gain to GER disease alone, and other underlying diseases, such as CF, should be ruled out with appropriate tests before embarking on aggressive enteral feeding regimens. Children with chronic nonspecific or protracted diarrhea and malnutrition may also benefit from continuous enteral tube feedings.

Renal Disease

Chronic renal failure in infants and children commonly results in growth failure and developmental delay, particularly in patients with congenital renal disease early in life.[13] The cause of growth failure is thought to be related to protein-energy malnutrition, renal osteodystrophy, chronic metabolic acidosis, and endocrine dysfunction. Despite aggressive medical management and specialized high–caloric-density formulas, inadequate weight gain often persists. Early nutritional intervention can augment the effect of dialysis by improving anabolism and reducing nitrogen losses (see Chapter 42: Renal Disease).

Critical Illness and Hypermetabolic States

Patients with extensive trauma, head or spinal cord injury, or burn injury and hypermetabolic states, such as cancer, HIV infection, AIDS, or sickle cell anemia (see Chapter 40: HIV, and Chapter 41: Sickle Cell Disease and Thalassemia), often require specialized nutritional support. Children with advanced cancer (see Chapter 43: Cancer) who are at high nutritional risk and who have minimal GI tract symptoms may be enterally fed via nocturnal or 24-hour nasogastric or gastrostomy tube feedings, depending on the extent of oral intake.[14] Enteral nutrition support is the preferred method for the nutritional support of children with uncomplicated trauma, such as severe head and spinal cord injuries, who have a significant elevation in their basal metabolic rates in the initial days following injury.[15] Enteral nutrition can be used to support infants and children with critical illness to meet their initial energy and protein needs. Careful consideration of nutrient needs in these patients will avoid the consequences of overfeeding of calories, including hypercapnia, difficulty weaning from the ventilator, hepatotoxicity, hyperglycemia, and increased infection rates[15] (see Chapter 38: Nutrition of Children Who Are Critically Ill). Metabolic effects associated with burn wounds leading to malnutrition include accelerated rate of energy expenditure, increased urine and wound nitrogen losses, and abnormal protein and glucose metabolism. Pediatric patients with burns of >20% total body surface area are often provided nutritional support using continuous enteral feedings.[16]

Neurologic Disease or Impairment

The specific nutritional requirements and feeding approach for neurologically impaired children are highly variable and depend on the degree of impairment, oral motor function, mobility, and muscle control. Children and infants with chromosomal disorders, including Down syndrome, Prader-Willi syndrome, or myelomeningocele, may have decreased energy needs, growth rates, and motor activity compared with healthy children.[17] Children with cerebral palsy are generally underweight for height and may have increased energy needs, particularly if they have spasticity, severe contractures, or choreoathetoid movements. The nutritional goals for feeding the child with devastating neurologic disease may be less than those predicted by standard growth charts. Excessive intake may place the child at risk of aspiration. Obesity can compromise neuromuscular and respiratory function. The concerns of primary caregivers about lifting heavy children must also be considered. Often, a general children's multivitamin, preferably in liquid form, as well as calcium, phosphorous, and iron supplements, may be needed for children with special needs with restricted volume intake to ensure that their vitamin and mineral requirements are being met.

Finally, but perhaps most importantly, one must remember to provide adequate water for children with neuromuscular disease. These children may not be able to communicate thirst to the caregiver. Often in an attempt to decrease risk of aspiration, more concentrated formulas are utilized with a resultant decrease in water intake. Fluid balance is important in the pediatric patient who is fed by tube, because several metabolic complications can be related to inadequate intake. Fluid requirements can be calculated by estimating normal water requirements adjusted for specific disease-related factors. Special consideration must be given to monitoring the fluid balance of children receiving high-calorie, high-protein formulas and children with excess water loss resulting from emesis, diarrhea, fever, or polyuria[18] (see Chapter 37: Nutritional Support for Children With Developmental Disabilities).

Enteral Formula Selection for Children 1 to 13 Years of Age

When children are older, they are often more capable of expressing their own preferences for favorite foods. It is important to remember that few children will spontaneously decide that they prefer nutritional supplements to other favorite foods that they see other children eating and/or see advertised in the media. Before one embarks on a control struggle to force or tube feed a high-calorie supplement to a thin child who does not want to eat, it is useful to first try commonly available high-calorie foods that are appetizing. If these foods lead to adequate weight gain, they can be very helpful. After nutritional status improves, less calorie-dense, "healthier" dietary options may be provided.

If it is not possible for a child to gain weight on his or her favorite energy-dense foods and enteral feedings are necessary, they should be started in a timely manner, optimally within the first 48 to 72 hours after injury or hospitalization, depending on the child's clinical status.[13] They should be offered first by mouth, preferably by a trusted caregiver. If the child refuses them, enteral tube feedings can be used. Formula selections for children younger than 1 year are discussed in Chapter 4. A variety of pediatric formulas are available with energy distribution of protein, carbohydrate, and fat between that of infant and adult formulas and age-appropriate vitamin and mineral content. Most of these pediatric formulas can provide the Dietary Recommended Intakes (DRIs) for most children 1 to 13 years of age (see Appendix N-1). At a caloric density of approximately 1 kcal/mL, these formulas are useful for children with increased metabolic needs or for those with fluid restrictions. In addition, the vitamin and mineral concentrations in 1000 to 1200 mL of most pediatric formulas meet or exceed 100% of the Recommended Dietary Allowances (RDAs) for children in this age range. "Predigested" or elemental formulas are only necessary when there is a deficiency in the digestive and/or absorptive process. They have no advantage for the child with normal digestive function. It is important to note that in the past, adult formulas were used for the enteral nutrition support of children older than 1 year, because enteral formulas for young children were not available. The primary disadvantages of using adult formulas for young children are the elevated renal solute load and insufficient vitamin and mineral levels. Dilution of these adult formulas to reduce the renal solute load further decreased the vitamins and minerals provided, which was suboptimal. However, there may be situations when a higher-protein adult formula is appropriate to use in a child younger than 13 years because of higher protein needs, as may be encountered in heavier children or children with certain types of injuries.

Enteral Formulas for Use in Children Older Than 13 Years of Age: Standard Tube-Feeding Formulas

Standard adult tube-feeding formulas can generally be used in children older than 13 years and are presented in Appendix N. These formulas, most of which are lactose free and low residue, vary in osmolality from 300 to 650 mOsm/kg and in caloric density from 1.0 to 2.0 kcal/mL. Isotonic formulas, such as Osmolite (Abbott Nutrition), which contain medium-chain triglyceride oil, are often useful for people with a history of delayed gastric emptying, dumping syndrome, or osmotic diarrhea. Tube-feeding formulas with added fiber, such as Jevity (Abbott Nutrition) are often useful in the management of patients with chronic constipation and diarrhea. Because of their low osmolality, caloric density, and moderate protein content, isotonic tube feedings, including those with added fiber, are the formulas of choice for general use with pediatric patients older than 13 years. Although high-calorie, high-nitrogen, hypertonic formulations are often well tolerated by adults with elevated metabolic needs, they are usually not tolerated by children and may lead to diarrhea, emesis, abdominal distention, and delayed gastric emptying. Children and adolescents with markedly elevated calorie and protein requirements attributable to severe trauma or burn injury are best managed with high-calorie formulations such as Jevity 1.5 (17% protein, Abbott Nutrition) and Nutren 1.5 (16% protein, Nestlé Nutrition). Because of the elevated protein levels in these formulas, however, hydration status must be closely monitored.

Peptide-Based and Elemental Formulas

Peptide-based (hydrolysate) and elemental formulas with predigested nutrients can be used for the nutritional support of pediatric patients with short-bowel syndrome, inflammatory bowel disease, and/or food protein sensitivity (Appendices D and N). Peptide-based formulas may be used in the enteral nutrition support of patients with cystic fibrosis, although the use of intact protein formulas with appropriate pancreatic enzyme administration may be just as effective. Amino acid-based formulas may offer further protection from feeding intolerance over protein hydrolysate formulas in some children. However, there is a significant increase in cost to purchase amino acid-based formulas. Immunonutrition, the use of enteral formula supplemented with possible immune-modulating nutrients, such as glutamine, arginine, antioxidants, and omega-3 fatty acids, has been considered for use in critically ill pediatric patients. Data are limited on safety and efficacy, and there are no guidelines or standardized formulas for pediatric patients[19,20] (see Chapter 38: Nutrition of Children Who Are Critically Ill).

Oral Supplements

Various flavored polymeric formulas may be used as oral supplements for pediatric patients. As noted previously, high-calorie commercially available foods may be more palatable and affordable than specialized supplements for most children. The constant supervision required to enforce frequent intake of commercial supplements can be a source of considerable family conflict. Oral supplements mixed with milk, such as Carnation Breakfast Essentials (Nestlé Nutrition), are often better accepted by children than are the lactose-free commercial supplements. Tips for increasing the nutrient and caloric density of foods are given in Tables 24.2 and 24.3. Flavored polymeric formulas that contain intact proteins, long-chain fatty acids, and simple carbohydrates are usually marketed as oral supplements because of their palatability. These products, which have osmolalities ranging from 450 to 600 mOsm/kg, are often not sufficiently palatable for long-term voluntary supplementation for children. Some examples of polymeric oral supplements include Pediasure, Pediasure 1.5, Ensure Plus (Abbott Nutrition), Boost, Boost Kids Essentials, and Boost Kids Essentials 1.5 (Nestlé Nutrition). It is useful to remember that salt is an appetite stimulant and that the combination of salty foods with sugary fluids to slake the resultant thirst can stimulate oral intake and initiate insulin surges that may be useful in further increasing appetite.

Table 24.2.
Increasing the Nutrient Density of Foods

Use cream, whole milk, or evaporated whole milk instead of water for baking whenever possible.
Use liberal portions of butter, margarine, oil, and cheeses on vegetables, on breads, and in soups and hot cereals. Add sauces and gravies to foods.
Add sugar, jelly, or honey to toast and cereals. Use fruits canned in heavy syrup, or sweeten fresh fruits with added sugar.
Add skim milk powder or instant breakfast powder to regular whole milk for use as a beverage or for cooking. Add powdered milk to puddings, potatoes, soups, and cooked cereals.
Use peanut butter (after 3 years of age) or cheese on fruit or crackers. Make finger sandwiches for meals or snacks.
Provide a variety of high-calorie salad dressings for addition to vegetables or other foods to increase caloric density.
Emphasize variety with all high-calorie foods to decrease flavor fatigue and increase exploratory behavior with foods.

Table 24.3.
Energy and Protein Content of Selected Energy-Dense Foods[a]

	Energy, kcal	Protein, g
Instant breakfast powder (1 packet)	130	5
Mixed with 1 cup whole milk	276	13
Powdered milk (1 tbsp)	25	3
Evaporated milk (1 tbsp)	20	1
Cheese (1 oz)	100	7
Peanut butter (1 tbsp)	95	4
Butter or margarine (1 tsp)	45	0[b]

[a] See also Appendix O .

[b] Not "spreads," which have a lot of air and water added and, therefore, are lower in kcal.

Blenderized Formulas

Commercially available blenderized diets, such as Compleat Pediatric (Nestlé Nutrition), consist of meats, eggs, milk, cereal, fruits, vegetables, and vegetable oils. These formulas, which contain a moderate to high level of residue, have osmolalities usually ranging from 300 to 500 mOsm/kg. Blenderized feedings are beneficial for chronically ill patients who have normal digestive function and require long-term enteral nutrition; however, they may not be well tolerated by the malnourished pediatric patient with compromised gastrointestinal tract function. Often, these products are expensive. Their high viscosity may cause obstruction of pediatric enteral feeding tubes.

Blenderized feedings can be prepared at home from milk, juices, cereals, and baby food. Parents of neurologically impaired children who require long-term feeding through a gastrostomy tube are often interested in learning how to prepare blenderized feedings at home because of the economic and psychosocial advantages. The help of a registered dietitian is important to ensure that adequate free water, macronutrient, and micronutrient concentrations are provided with these mixtures.

Formula Concentration and Supplementation With Use of Modular Components

Because of the unique and often elevated nutritional requirements of the enterally fed pediatric patient, modification of enteral formulas through either formula concentration or supplementation with modular components is often necessary. Formula concentration with the use of liquid formula concentrates or liquid modular products is usually the preferred modality for increasing formula concentration. Infant formula powder may also be used as a convenient and economical way to increase the caloric density of human milk and infant formulas. However, within the hospital setting, use of liquid formula concentrates and liquid modular components are preferred to minimize the risk of formula contamination (see Appendix N-2). It is important to remember that formula concentration may lead to decreased intake in patients who are voluntarily drinking the formula and may lead to vomiting if they prolong gastric emptying in patients who are being tube fed. Therefore, fluid and electrolyte balance must be monitored.

Tube Feeding

When the requirement for enteral nutrition support has been established, the optimal route for delivering nutrients must be determined. Many practitioners recommend the placement of nasogastric or nasoduodenal feeding tubes when the estimated course of therapy will not exceed 3 months (a size 6F tube is usually adequate). These tubes should be changed from one nostril to the other every 1 to 3 weeks to decrease associated sinus and ear disease. During upper respiratory tract infections, extra care should be taken to avoid airway compromise. Tube placement should be verified after episodes of emesis before restarting feedings. If the risk of aspiration is not significant, gastric feedings are preferable, because they are more physiologic and easier to manage. Tubes made of polyurethane and silicone rubber are soft and pliable and may be left in place for longer time periods. Polyvinyl chloride tubes become stiff and nonpliable when left in place for more than a few days; however, they are useful for intestinal decompression or short-term feeding. They should be changed every 2 to 3 days to avoid skin necrosis or intestinal perforation.

Some feeding tubes made of polyurethane or silicone rubber have a tungsten or mercury weight at the tip that makes them useful for duodenal or jejunal feedings. Placement of transpyloric tubes can be greatly facilitated by the use of an intravenous prokinetic drug, such as metoclopramide. Children who require long-term tube feeding for longer than 3 months are potential candidates for placement of a gastrostomy tube. GER disease, which may occur in neurologically disabled children or healthy infants after gastrostomy tube placement, may necessitate an operative antireflux procedure (eg, Nissen fundoplication).[21] Although the procedure is effective in reducing GER disease, postoperative complications can be troublesome. Intractable retching episodes, dumping syndrome, continued problems with swallowing, impaired esophageal emptying, slow feeding, and gas bloating have all been reported. Controversy exists over the necessity of an antireflux procedure in neurologically impaired children who require a feeding gastrostomy tube. A trial of nasogastric feedings to determine whether they are well tolerated without significant GER before the placement of the gastrostomy tube can help the clinician determine the need for a simultaneous Nissen fundoplication. During the trial of nasogastric feeding, documented pulmonary disease associated with GER disease in the face of maximal medical therapy is an indication for a Nissen fundoplication when a subsequent gastrostomy tube placement is performed.

A common problem with all gastrostomy tubes is inward migration of the standard gastrostomy tube through the ostomy site. Ultimately, the tip of the catheter may contact the pylorus, where it can induce retching as it passes in and out of the gastric outlet. These problems may be minimized by firmly attaching the tube and placing a mark on the tube to detect inward migration. When a urinary catheter is used as a temporary gastrostomy tube, migration (caused by lack of an effective external bolster) remains a common problem. The low-profile gastrostomy button tube is a feeding device that can be used to form an effective 1-way valve at the gastrostomy site. The button fits flush with the skin and attaches to commercial feeding tubes that lock onto the button in a variety of ways. Gastrostomy buttons generally do not migrate through the pylorus or cause retching and are also less prone to accidental removal. Buttons may be placed in standard percutaneous gastrostomies after the site has matured by healing for at least 12 weeks. There are also newer devices that allow for percutaneous placement of a low-profile gastrostomy button at the time of the initial gastrostomy.

To overcome problems related to gastric emptying and frequent GER, transpyloric feedings offer potential benefit. Feeding jejunostomies can be placed through existing gastrostomies. If a modified (eg, urinary catheter) tube is used to convert a gastrostomy to a jejunostomy, extreme care must be exercised to be certain that retching or emesis has not moved the tip of the tube into the esophagus. Even commercial gastrojejunostomy feeding tubes can accidentally migrate retrograde into an esophageal position when persistent emesis occurs. Retrograde continuous delivery of formula into the esophagus presents an extreme risk of aspiration. Nasal transpyloric tubes can be used but are relatively easily displaced and are uncomfortable as a long-term approach to enteral nutrition support. Operative direct feeding jejunostomies overcome these difficulties and may be indicated for selected patients. Patients with direct-feeding jejunostomies generally do not tolerate large bolus feedings over short intervals without experiencing dumping syndrome. Also, button adapters by virtue of the large internal bolster are often precluded for direct feeding jejunostomies.

The transition from enteral feeding to full oral feeding can be prolonged. If infants and children are completely deprived of oral feeding during critical maturation phases, feeding refusal and oral aversion often occur when oral feedings are resumed.[22] Reinstituting oral feedings in children who have been fed exclusively by a gastrostomy tube for a long period of time can evoke a resistant response, such as gagging, choking, or vomiting. To preserve oral motor function during prolonged tube feedings, it is important to continue to offer oral intake whenever possible. This may require interrupting the infusion to allow a sufficient amount of hunger to develop to facilitate oral intake. Generally, this may require several hours. Speech pathologists and occupational therapists can help provide oral motor stimulation exercises for such children. Without frequent oral stimulation, infants can lose the suckle reflex within a few weeks, which severely limits their ability to control oral intake and also compromises language and oral motor development. They may also develop oral defensiveness as a result of prolonged absence of oral stimulation.

Continuous Versus Intermittent Enteral Feeding

Two methods are used for delivery of enteral feedings. Intermittent bolus feedings deliver the formula over a relatively short period of time similar to that for an oral feeding—10 to 20 minutes. This technique is simple, requires minimal supplies, and may facilitate the transition to home care. Generally, bolus feedings are used during the day and are not used at night because of the greater tendency for gastroesophageal reflux with the bolus feed. Gastric distension by bolus feeding can lead to a better gastrocolic reflex and aid the prevention of constipation, which is a frequent problem in tube-fed patients. When intermittent bolus feeding is not tolerated, a continuous infusion using an infusion pump may be effective. To improve patient mobility, a backpack pump may be of considerable benefit. Continuous feeding may be particularly beneficial when used for patients who have impaired absorption. In some situations, a combination of bolus feeding during the day and continuous feeding at night is beneficial.

One Final Note of Caution

Specialized formulas are very expensive, and their cost can easily exceed the food budget of an entire family. Many patients have discovered that it is possible to buy large quantities of expensive elemental and other specialized formulas on the Internet from people who have "left-over" quantities that were prescribed for them. Although this can represent an enormous savings, it is important to remember that the bidder is depending on the integrity of the seller for Internet purchases from private individuals. Counterfeit nutritional products sold online pose the same problems that are encountered with counterfeit medications.

V

References

1. Canete A, Duggan C. Nutritional support of the pediatric intensive care unit patient. *Curr Opin Pediatr*. 1996;8(3):248-255

2. Meetze W, Valentine C, McGuigan JE, Conlon M, Sacks N, Neu J. Gastrointestinal priming prior to full enteral nutrition in very low birth weight infants. *J Pediatr Gastroenterol Nutr*. 1992;15(2):163-170

3. Cavell B. Effect of feeding an infant formula with high energy density on gastric emptying in infants with congenital heart disease. *Acta Paediatr Scand*. 1981;70(4):513-516

4. Schwarz SM, Gewitz MH, et al. Enteral nutrition in infants with congenital heart disease and growth failure. *Pediatrics*. 1990;86(3):368-373

5. Abad-Sinden A, Sutphen A. Growth and nutrition. In: Emmanoullides GC, Riemenschneider, TA, Allen HD, Gutgessel HP, eds. *Moss and Adams Heart Diseases in Infants, Children and Adolescents, Including the Fetus and Young Adult*. Philadelphia, PA: Williams & Wilkins; 2001;325–332

6. Bernstein CN, Shanahan F. Braving the elementals in Crohn's disease. *Gastroenterology*. 1992;103(4):1363-1364

7. Wiskin AE, Wotton SA, Beattie RM. Nutrition issues in pediatric Crohn's disease. *Nutr Clin Pract*. 2007;22:214-222

8. Olieman JF, Penning C, Ijsselstijn H, et al. Enteral nutrition in children with short-bowel syndrome: current evidence and recommendations for the clinician. *J Am Diet Assoc*. 2010;110(3):420-426

9. Cober MP, Teitelbaum DH. Prevention of parenteral nutrition-associated liver disease: lipid minimization. *Curr Opin Organ Transplant*. 2010;15(3):330-333

10. Javid PJ, Collier S, Richardson D, et al. The role of enteral nutrition in the reversal of parenteral nutrition-associated liver dysfunction in infants. *J Pediatr Surg*. 2005;40(6):1015-1018

11. De Meijer VE, Gura KM, Meisel JA, Le HD, Puder M. Parenteral fish oil monotherapy in the management of patients with parenteral nutrition-associated liver disease. *Arch Surg*. 2010;145(6):547-551

12. Ferry GD, Selby M, Pietro TJ. Clinical response to short-term nasogastric feeding in infants with gastroesophageal reflux and growth failure. *J Pediatr Gastroenterol Nutr*. 1983;2(1):57-61

13. Spinozzi NS. Chronic renal disease. In: Queen Samour P, King Helm K, Lang CE, eds. *Handbook of Pediatric Nutrition*. Gaithersburg, MD: ASPEN Publishers Inc; 1999:385-394

14. Barale KV, Charuhas PM. Oncology and bone marrow transplant. In: Queen Samour P, King Helm K, Lang CE, eds. *Handbook of Pediatric Nutrition*. Gaithersburg, MD: ASPEN Publishers Inc; 1999:465-492

15. Chwals W. Overfeeding the critically ill child: fact or fantasy? *New Horizons*. 1994;2(2):147–155

16. Trocki O, Michelini JA, Robbins ST, Eichelberger MR. Evaluation of early enteral feeding in children less than 3 years old with smaller burns (8-25 percent TBSA). *Burns*. 1995;21(1):17–23

17. Cloud HH. Developmental disabilities. In: Queen Samour P, King Helm K, Lang CE, eds. *Handbook of Pediatric Nutrition*. Gaithersburg, MD: ASPEN Publishers Inc; 1999:293–314

18. Schwenk WF, Olson D. Pediatrics. In: Gottschlich MM, ed. *The Science and Practice of Nutrition Support: A Case-Based Core Curriculum*. Dubuque, IA: Kendall/Hunt Publishing Co; 2001:347–372

19. Heyland DK, Novak F, Drover JW, Jain M, Su X, Suchner U. Should immunonutrition become routine in critically ill patients? A systematic review of the evidence. *JAMA*. 2001;286(8):944-953

20. Briassoulis G, Filippou O, Hatzi E, Papassotiriou I, Hatzis T. Early enteral administration of immunonutrition in critically ill children: results of a blinded randomized controlled clinical trial. *Nutrition*. 2005;21(7-8):799-807

21. Albanese CT, Towbin RB, Ulman I, Lewis J, Smith SD. Percutaneous gastrojejunostomy versus Nissen fundoplication for enteral feeding of the neurologically impaired child with gastroesophageal reflux. *J Pediatr*. 1993;123(3):371-375

22. Ramasamy M, Perman JA. Pediatric feeding disorders. *J Clin Gastroenterol*. 2000;30(1): 34-46

V

Nutrition in Acute and Chronic Illness

Chapter 25

Assessment of Nutritional Status

Introduction

Assessment of nutritional status should be an integral part of the evaluation and management of all children with acute and chronic disease and is the primary step in the evaluation of all children whose growth differs from the norm.[1] A complete nutritional assessment includes the evaluation of dietary intake, physical characteristics, biochemical parameters, body size, and composition compared with age-appropriate norms, as available. During a prolonged hospital stay, nutritional disturbances can occur, particularly when oral intake is suspended or limited. This chapter discusses nutritional assessment methods and their practical application. For most patients, dietary history, physical examination, and longitudinal changes in height, weight, and relative weight, such as body mass index (BMI), are sufficient to assess nutritional status.

Assessment of Dietary Intake

An assumption cannot be made that all children eat normally, so a detailed diet history (including factors such as timing of meals, food choices, site [home or out of home], preparation, use of supplements) is important as an initial evaluation of intake. Children on a strict vegetarian diet may ingest inadequate amounts of protein, vitamin B_{12}, iron, or pyridoxine if their meals are not properly planned. Adolescents often skip meals, and athletic children may not ingest adequate calories, or they may become involved in fad diets associated with some sports. Older children and adolescents may attempt weight loss by starvation, and anorexia nervosa or bulimia may develop. On the other hand, children may snack frequently throughout the day and ingest large amounts of sugar-containing beverages and energy-dense snack foods; combined with sedentary behavior, this pattern may lead to obesity.

For a more quantitative evaluation of dietary intake, 3- to 5-day food records may be used. This method allows for an assessment of usual intake, which is important when trying to identify nutrient inadequacies and evaluate relationships between diet and biological parameters or chronic disease.[2] Ideally, the child and/or caregiver should be trained on how to estimate or measure food portions for the food records, and the dietary analysis is best performed by a registered dietitian. Some medications can cause nutritional disturbances (see Appendix G: Food-Drug Interactions).

VI

Clinical Assessment

Careful inspection of the patient remains a valid method of nutritional assessment.[3] The current epidemic of childhood obesity has begun to distort perceptions of what is the normal appearance of children. Distinguishing wasting from stunting in the young child is also difficult. Obesity and wasting are not necessarily obvious and need to be confirmed by weight-for-length or BMI reference charts. Visual assessment is a useful screening test for gross changes in body composition by which edema, dehydration, excess or inadequate subcutaneous fat, and increase or decrease of the muscle mass can be detected. Some of the findings of vitamin and mineral deficiencies are listed in Tables 25.1 and 25.2. Deficiency of any trace substance can result in growth failure. The clinical signs and symptoms of specific vitamin or mineral deficiencies or toxic effects are usually not pathognomonic.

Table 25.1.
Signs and Symptoms of Vitamin Deficiency or Excess

Vitamin	Deficiency	Excess
A	Night blindness, xerophthalmia, keratomalacia, follicular hyperkeratosis	Scaly skin, bone pain, pseudotumor cerebri, hepatomegaly
C	Scurvy: capillary hemorrhage of gingiva, skin, bone, poor wound healing	"Rebound" deficiency after high intake
D	Rickets, osteomalacia	Constipation, renal stones, myositis ossificans, hypercalcemia
E	Hemolysis (in preterm infant), peripheral neuropathy	Suppresses hematologic response to iron in anemia
K	Bruising, bleeding	Jaundice
Thiamine	Beriberi: cardiomyopathy, peripheral neuropathy, and encephalopathy	None known
Riboflavin	Cheilosis, glossitis, angular stomatitis	None known
Niacin	Pellagra: dementia, diarrhea, and dermatitis	Flushing
Pyridoxine	Seizures, anemia, irritability	Neuropathy
Biotin	Dermatitis, alopecia, muscle pain	None known
Folate	Macrocytic anemia, stomatitis paresthesia, glossitis, neural tube defects of fetus	None known
B_{12}	Megaloblastic anemia, neuropathy, paresthesia, glossitis	None known

Table 25.2.
Signs and Symptoms of Mineral Deficiency or Excess

Mineral	Deficiency	Excess
Aluminum	None known	Central nervous system disorder
Boron	Calcification abnormalities	None known
Calcium	Osteomalacia, tetany	Constipation, heart block, vomiting
Chloride	Alkalosis	Acidosis
Chromium	Diabetes (in animals)	None known
Cobalt	Vitamin B_{12} deficiency	Cardiomyopathy
Copper	Anemia, neutropenia, osteoporosis, neuropathy, depigmentation of hair and skin	Cirrhosis, central nervous system effects, Fanconi nephropathy, corneal pigmentation
Fluoride	Dental caries	Fluorosis
Iodine	Goiter, cretinism	Goiter
Iron	Anemia, behavioral abnormalities	Hemosiderosis
Lead	None known	Encephalopathy, neuropathy, stippled red blood cells
Magnesium	Hypocalcemia, hypokalemia, tremor, weakness, arrhythmia	Weakness, sedation, hypotension, nausea, vomiting
Molybdenum	Growth retardation (in animals)	None known
Phosphorus	Rickets, neuropathy	Calcium deficiency
Potassium	Muscle weakness, cardiac abnormalities	Heart block
Selenium	Cardiomyopathy, anemia, myositis	Nail and hair changes, garlic odor
Sodium	Hypotension	Edema
Sulfur	Growth failure	None known
Zinc	Growth failure, dermatitis, hypogeusia, hypogonadism, alopecia, impaired wound healing	Gastroenteritis

Growth Assessment

Anthropometric measurements are used to assess growth. If children are measured once, their "growth status" for age is assessed by comparing this measurement with the appropriate reference curve or table (see Table 25.3 and Appendix A). If children are measured more than once, their growth status for age can be tracked over time in 2 ways. When sequential measurements are plotted on a growth chart,

Table 25.3.
Growth Reference Data by Age Group

		Growth Reference Data[a] By Age Group		
Age Group	Citation, Web Link, Data Source	Assessment Tool	Details and Recommendations	Comments
Length/Stature, Weight, and Head Circumference Growth Charts				
Preterm	**Citation:** Olsen et al 2010[16] **Web link:** http://www.aap.org/sections/perinatal/PDF/GrowthCurves.pdf **Data source:** Large sample of US birth data (1998-2006), ethnically representative of US births, from Pediatrix Clinical Data Warehouse	Weight-for-age curves Length-for-age curves Head circumference-for-age curves	23-41 wk gestational age (GA)	• Gender-specific intrauterine (IU) growth curves • 3rd to 97th percentiles
	Citation: Fenton 2013[10] **Web link:** http://ucalgary.ca/fenton/2013chart Data source: For preterm data: Canadian live birth data 1994-1996,[11] Australian data 1991-1994,[25] Italian data,[24] Scottish data,[26] German data,[27] and US data[16]; two of these data sets were used to create length and head circumference for age curves[16,24] For post-term data: • CDC 2000 growth curves[28] or • WHO child growth standards curves[29]	Weight-for-age curves Length-for-age curves Head circumference-for-age curves	22-50 wk GA	• Gender-specific IU growth curves • 3rd to 97th percentiles

	Citations / Web links / Data source	Curves	Recommendation	Features
LBW VLBW	**Citations:** Guo et al 1997,[30] Guo et al 1996[31] **Web links:** http://www.ncbi.nlm.nih.gov/entrez/query.fcgi?cmd=Retrieve&db=PubMed&dopt=Citation&list_uids=3706184 http://www.ncbi.nlm.nih.gov/entrez/query.fcgi?cmd=Retrieve&db=PubMed&dopt=Citation&list_uids=8790129 **Data source:** Longitudinal data collected on LBW preterm infants born in the United States from the **Infant Health and Development Program (IHDP)**, a national collaborative randomized multicenter clinical trial	Weight-for-age curves Length-for-age curves Head circumference-for-age curves Weight-for-length curves	Full-term to 36 mo • **May be used along with IU growth curves**	• Gender-specific postnatal growth curves • Low birth weight (LBW) curves for birth weight <2.5 kg • Very low birth weight (VLBW) curves for birth weight <1.5 kg • 5th to 95th percentiles
0 to 24 mo	**Citations:** WHO Multicentre Growth Reference Study Group 2006[29], and 2007[37] and de Onis et al 2006[5] **Web link:** http://www.who.int/childgrowth/standards/en/ **Data source:** Cross-sectional and longitudinal data from the WHO Multicentre Growth Reference Study (MGRS), an international sample of healthy children with "optimal" conditions for growth (eg, breastfed)	Weight-for-age curves Length-for-age curves Head circumference-for-age curves Weight-for-length curves BMI-for-age curves	0 to 60 mo • **Recommended by CDC for children <24 mo** • **Weight-for-length recommended for children <24 mo**	• Gender-specific growth *standard* curves[b] • 3rd to 97th percentiles
2 to 20 y	**Citation:** Kuczmarski et al 2000[28] (CDC 2000 growth charts) **Web link:** http://www.cdc.gov/growthcharts/clinical_charts.htm **Data source:** Strategic sample of US children (1963-1994) based on multiple cross-sectional national survey data and longitudinal data from the Fels Research Institute	Stature-for-age curves Weight-for-age curves BMI-for-age curves Weight-for-length curves Head circumference-for-age curves	0 to 20 y **Recommended by CDC for 2-20 y** 0 to 36 mo **May be used for 24-36 mo**	• Gender specific growth reference curves • "Set 1": 5th to 95th percentiles • "Set 2": 3rd to 97th percentiles • Weight charts (weight-for-age, BMI-for-age, weight-for-length) excluded data collected from for children >6 y (1988 to 1994) because of the increase in obesity prevalence

Incremental Growth Charts

VI

Table 25.3. (continued)

Growth Reference Data by Age Group

Age Group	Growth Reference Data[a] By Age Group			
	Citation, Web Link, Data Source	Assessment Tool	Details and Recommendations	Comments
0 to 24 mo	**Citation:** WHO Multicentre Growth Reference Study Group2009[40] **Web link:** http://www.who.int/childgrowth/standards/en/ **Data source:** Cross-sectional and longitudinal data from the WHO Multicentre Growth Reference Study (MGRS), an international sample of healthy children with "optimal" conditions for growth (eg, breastfed)	Weight velocity tables Length velocity tables Head circumference velocity tables	0 to 24 mo	• Gender-specific growth *standard* tables[b] • Percentile and z-score tables • 0–12 mo: increments of 1 mo • 0–24 mo: increments of 2 to 6 mo • 0–60 days: increments of 1 to 2 wk • Gender-specific growth *standard* tables[b] • Percentile and z-score tables • 0–24 mo: increments of 2 to 6 mo • Gender-specific growth *standard* tables[b] • Percentile and z-score tables • 0–12 mo: increments of 2 and 3 mo • 0–24 mo: increments of 4 and 6 mo

Age	Citation / Web link / Data source	Measure	Age range	Notes
2 to 18 y	**Citation:** Baumgartner et al 1986[34] **Web link:** http://www.ncbi.nlm.nih.gov/entrez/query.fcgi?cmd=Retrieve&db=PubMed&dopt=Citation&list_uids=3706184 **Data source:** Longitudinal US data from the Fels Longitudinal Study (1929–1978)	Weight velocity tables	0 to 13 y 0 to 3 y	• Gender-specific reference tables • 3rd to 97th percentiles • 0–12 mo: measurements at birth, 1, 3, 6, 12 mo • 1–18 y: increments of 6 mo
	Citation: Tanner and Davies 1985[36] **Web link:** http://www.ncbi.nlm.nih.gov/entrez/query.fcgi?cmd=Retrieve&db=PubMed&dopt=Citation&list_uids=3875704 **Data source:** 1977 National Center for Health Statistics growth charts data[41] were combined with data from other longitudinal studies	Length/stature velocity tables Height and height velocity curves and tables	3 to ˜8 y 2 to approx. 14–19 y (depending on gender and stage of maturity)	• Gender-specific reference curves and tables • 3rd to 97th percentiles • Curves for early, middle and late maturers • Gender-specific growth velocity curves
	Citation: Berkey et al 1993[35] **Web link:** http://www.ncbi.nlm.nih.gov/pubmed?term=Berkey%20Dockery%201993 **Data source:** Longitudinal data from a sample of US children participating in the Six Cities Study (1974–1989)	Height velocity curves	7 to 18 y	• Ages 7 to 18 y • Race-specific • Curves for early, average and late maturers • 3rd to 97th percentiles

Other Anthropometric Measures

	Citation / Web link / Data source	Measure	Age range	Notes
	Citation: WHO Multicentre Growth Reference Study Group 2007[37] **Web link:** http://www.who.int/childgrowth/standards/en/ **Data source:** Cross-sectional and longitudinal data from the WHO Multicentre Growth Reference Study, an international sample of healthy children with "optimal" conditions for growth (eg, breast-fed)	Arm circumference-for-age tables	3 mo to 5 y	• Gender-specific growth *standard* curves[b] • Percentile and z-score curves and tables
	Citation: Addo and Himes 2010[38] **Web link:** http://www.ncbi.nlm.nih.gov/pubmed?term=Addo%20Himes%202010 **Data source:** Sample created to reproduce the sample used for the CDC 2000 BMI-for-age curves[28]	Triceps skinfold-for-age tables Triceps skinfold-for-age tables	1.5 to 20 y	• Gender-specific growth (or partly prescriptive) tables because of exclusion of potentially obese children (like CDC 2000 weight growth curves) • 3rd to 97th percentiles

a Unless otherwise indicated, the growth curves and tables included in this table are considered *reference* (or descriptive) data, because they describe growth of children who participated in a survey or convenience sample.

b The WHO child growth standards are considered *standard* (or prescriptive) curves and tables, because they describe growth of a sample of children selected for optimal growth patterns (healthy, well-nourished, breastfed infants).

VI

the growth trajectory or degree of "tracking" (ie, maintaining centile rank on the growth chart) can be evaluated. In addition, growth velocity can be assessed to determine whether their rate of growth is appropriate for age compared to growth velocity reference data (see Appendix A). However, the intervals between measurements should be comparable to the intervals used to generate the reference data for valid comparisons. Because the accuracy of a growth assessment relies on the accuracy of the anthropometric measurements, particular care should be taken to use the appropriate equipment and measurement techniques detailed below (see Assessment Tools for Anthropometric Measurements by Age Group).

It is also important to use the most appropriate reference growth curves and tables to evaluate anthropometric measurements for growth status determination. Several considerations affect the appropriateness of reference data. First, it should be clear whether a growth curve or table is "descriptive," reference data that describe growth in a population of children, or "prescriptive," a growth standard that defines an optimal growth pattern.[4] For example, the reference values for children birth to 2 years of age from the World Health Organization (WHO) Multicentre Growth Reference Study are based on a large, international sample of healthy, exclusively breastfed infants; therefore, the WHO reference data are considered prescriptive. Differences between the WHO growth charts and other infant growth charts are attributable, in part, to the different patterns of growth associated with different feeding modes.[5] Other important features of a reference curve are (1) whether the sample is of sufficient size to capture the variability in the population at all ages, (2) whether appropriate statistical techniques were used to generate percentile distributions; (3) whether secular trends (eg, improvements in health care, obesity epidemic) may affect the applicability of older or current reference curves; and (4) the child's age and gender. Cutoffs for identifying high-risk small- and large-for-age infants and children will vary among growth curves for these reasons. See Table 25.3 for a summary of reference data.

Weight, length or stature, and head circumference (up to approximately 3 years of age) are the most common anthropometric measurements. Including a measure of relative weight, such as weight-for-length or BMI helps provide a more comprehensive picture of growth and nutritional status. Other measurements, such as mid-upper arm circumference (MAC) and triceps skinfold thickness (TSF), also may be useful in the growth assessment of an infant or child.

Assessment Tools for Anthropometric Measurements by Age Group

Preterm Infants

Two types of growth curves are available for the assessment of preterm infant growth: intrauterine curves and postnatal curves. Intrauterine growth curves[6-17] are generally accepted as the best available tool for growth assessment in the neonatal intensive care unit (NICU) at birth and postnatally. These curves are created using cross-sectional birth data, meaning a different group of infants is measured *at birth* for each gestational age. As a result, intrauterine growth curves curves represent intrauterine or fetal growth, which is considered the goal for preterm infant growth. Using birth data of preterm infants as an indicator of intrauterine growth is not perfect, because these infants are born smaller than if they had remained in utero,[13,18,19] but there is no method to *directly* measure fetal weight while still in utero. Thus, this method remains the best available option.[20-22]

There are many examples of intrauterine growth curves, but only some include weight, length, and head circumference, as followed in the NICU.[8,10,12-14,16] Many of the newer intrauterine curves include only weight-for-age curves[6,7,9,11,15]; the lack of length- and head circumference-for-age curves limit the usefulness of these curves in the NICU. For former preterm infants, growth measurements are plotted using corrected age for up to the first 3 years of life.[23]

A recent set of intrauterine growth curves from Olsen et al[16] (Appendix A) offer a number of advantages for use in the United States compared with other intrauterine curves; in particular, these gender-specific curves are based on newer data (1998-2006) and a large US sample that represents the racial distribution of US births. The 2013 revision of the 2003 Fenton curves[10] (Appendix A) commonly used in NICUs today are now gender specific and are based on 6 published data sets for the intrauterine portion of the curves, one US[16] and 5 non-US (Canada,[11] Italy,[24] Australia,[25] Scotland,[26] and Germany[27]). Two of these data sets were used for the length and head circumference-for-age-curves.[16,25] Similar to the 2003 Fenton curves, the 2013 Fenton curves are connected and smoothed to the 2000 growth curves from the Centers for Disease Control and Prevention(CDC)[28] and now the WHO curves,[29] somewhat distorting the data.[10]

Postntatal growth curves[30,31] (Appendix A) were created using longitudinal data; one group of infants was followed over time and repeated measurements were obtained. As a result, postnatal curves illustrate *actual* growth (ie, descriptive curves) over time, not *ideal* growth (prescriptive curves) of preterm infants. Postnatal curves allow for the comparison of one preterm infant's growth to the growth of other preterm infants and, therefore, may serve as useful adjunct assessment tools to the intrauterine growth curves.

Currently, there are no reference data available for growth velocity, arm circumference, or triceps skinfold measurements for preterm infants. See Table 25.3 for a summary of reference data.

Infants and Toddlers (Full-Term to <24 mo)

In 2010, the CDC published a report detailing new recommendations for the use of the WHO Multicentre Growth Reference Study growth charts[29] (Appendix A) for children younger than 24 months (regardless of diet) in place of the currently used CDC 2000 growth charts.[28,32] These charts are available online (http://www.who.int/childgrowth/standards/en/) and include charts for weight-for-age, length-for-age, head circumference-for-age; weight-for-length (recommended for children ages 0-24 months) and BMI-for-age. The WHO growth charts are based on an international sample of healthy children (singleton and full-term at birth) living in "optimal" conditions to support growth (eg, breastfed, nonsmoking environment).[29,32] Thus, the WHO charts are growth *standard* curves (or prescriptive) versus the growth *reference* (or descriptive) CDC 2000 curves, which describe the size and growth of US children between 1963-1994 on the basis of a combination of cross-sectional national survey data and longitudinal data from the Fels Research Institute.[4,22,28,32] In contrast to the sample in the WHO Multicentre Growth Reference Study, the infants used to create the CDC 2000 growth curves were predominantly fed cow milk-based formula.

The WHO data for children younger than 24 months were a combination of longitudinal data (birth to 23 months) and cross-sectional data (birth data only for infants who did not meet the feeding and maternal nonsmoking criteria) collected between 1997 and 2003. The CDC and the American Academy of Pediatrics (AAP) recommend using the 2.3rd and 97.7th percentiles of the WHO (labeled as 2nd and 98th on the curves, or 2 standard deviations above and below the median) to identify children with potentially suboptimal growth in the first 24 months after birth.[32]

For clinicians, there are several important implications of converting from the CDC charts to the WHO charts in the United States.[32] First, the WHO charts have a steeper rise in weight from 0 to 3 months of age than do the CDC curves (attributed to the differences in growth of breastfed vs formula-fed infants), so more infants in this age range are identified as low weight-for-age. Secondly, the WHO charts have a slower rise in weight (for age and for length) than do the CDC charts starting at approximately 3 months and thereafter. Consequently, fewer 6- through 23-month-old children are identified as low weight-for-age, and fewer 0- through 23-month-old children are identified as low weight-for-length. Lastly, differences in length-for-age are small between the charts, so significant clinical differences are not expected. In summary, the different growth patterns of predominantly breastfed (WHO standard growth charts) and formula-fed infants (CDC 2000 growth charts) help to explain why a formula-fed infant plots low on the WHO charts within the first few months and then high (and cross percentiles) on the WHO charts at older ages.[32]

The WHO Child Growth Standards also provide norms for growth velocity (for weight, length, and head circumference; see Growth Velocity) in table format (Appendix A) and arm circumference-for-age and triceps skinfold-for-age (3 to 24 months) in both curve and table formats (Appendix A). See the sections on anthropometric measurement and clinical body composition for details on arm circumference and triceps skinfold, respectively. See Table 25.3 for a summary of reference anthropometric data.

Children (>24 months)

The CDC and the AAP recommend the continued use of the CDC 2000 growth charts (Appendix A) for children 2 to 20 years of age.[28,32] These are available online (https://www.cdc.gov/growthcharts) and include growth curves for weight-for-age, length/stature-for-age, BMI-for-age, weight-for-length (for use from 24 to 36 months of age, as needed) and head circumference-for-age (for use from 24 to 36 months of age, as needed). The CDC charts, published in 2000, are based on a series of large cross-sectional surveys conducted from 1963 to 1994. As a result, the CDC growth curves are reference growth curves and *describe* the growth in strategically sampled US children over this time period.[28] The weight-for-age, weight-for-length, and BMI-for-age curves excluded the data for children older than 6 years collected from 1988 to 1994 because of the increase in obesity prevalence during this time frame. Consequently, these 3 curves are partly prescriptive. Generally, the CDC 2000 curves allow for the comparison of one child's growth to that of a large reference population of other children.

Two sets of CDC 2000 growth charts are available for use (https://www.cdc.gov/growthcharts). Set 1 provides curves that span from the 5th to the 95th percentiles and are most commonly used in the clinical setting to classify and monitor over time the growth of healthy children; set 2 provides curves that span from the 3rd and 97th percentiles and are helpful in the growth assessment of children whose growth falls at the extremes.[33]

VI

Growth velocity reference data based on US children are available for children >24 months of age[34-36] (see Growth Velocity). The WHO Child Growth Standards provide norms for arm circumference-for-age and triceps skinfold-for-age for children up to 5 years of age.[37] Addo and Himes provide triceps skinfold-for-age norms for children 1.5 to 20 years of age[38] using US survey data. See the sections on anthropometric measurements and clinical body composition for details on arm circumference and triceps skinfold, respectively. See Table 25.3 for a summary of reference data.

Growth Velocity

Growth increments can be a sensitive indicator of nutritional status, because they reflect the recent state of the infant. Growth increments are determined as the change in weight (or length/height or head circumference) divided by the time interval. Growth increments are sensitive to the time interval between measurements, because growth occurs in as a series of intermittent small or large spurts,[39] which typically vary with age, gender, maturational status, and season. Comparison of a growth increment based on a longer or shorter interval than that used in the reference curve may overestimate or underestimate incremental growth status. In addition, the accuracy of growth increments is dependent on the accuracy and precision of the 2 measurements on which it is calculated, each with its own measurement error. Therefore, growth increments should be based on accurate growth assessments, obtained over appropriate time intervals, carefully calculated, and compared with appropriate reference values.

The newest set of reference data for growth velocity is available from the WHO (http://www.who.int/childgrowth/standards/en/). These growth standards are presented in table format for children 0 to 24 months of age (see Appendix A for selected tables). Weight growth velocity reference data are available in 1-mo increments (birth to 12 months of age), in 2- to 6-month increments (birth to 24 months of age) and in 1- and 2-week increments (birth to 60 days of age). Length growth velocity values are available in 2- to 6-month increments (birth to 24 months of age). Head circumference velocity values are available in 2- to 3-month increments (birth to 12 months of age) and in 4- to 6-month increments (birth to 24 months of age). Clinicians are encouraged to use the interval that most closely approximates the time passed between the child's measurements. Because of the variability in growth velocity over time as discussed previously, a growth assessment should always consider achieved growth (ie, size-for-age, as discussed earlier in this chapter) when interpreting growth velocity values.[40]

Growth velocity reference data based on US children are also available for older age groups (see Table 25.3). Baumgartner et al[34] published gender-specific weight and length/height velocity tables for children 0 to 18 years of age based on longitudinal measurements obtained in the Fels Longitudinal Study. Tanner and Davies[36] created height velocity curves and tables that are specific to gender and stage of maturity. They combined data from the US 1977 growth charts[41] with longitudinal data from other studies. Lastly, gender- and race-specific height velocity centiles are available from Berkey et al[35] for children 7 to 18 years of age based on data collected in a large US multi-center study conducted between 1974 and 1989.

Anthropometric Measurements

Length or Stature

Length or stature is the most useful indicator of linear growth status. Recumbent length is measured in infants and children younger than 2 years and in children 2 to 3 years of age who are unable to stand unsupported. Devices for measuring length and stature should be appropriately calibrated and accurate to 0.1 cm. Two people are required to accomplish this measurement. The measuring table or board should consist of a fixed headboard, a movable footboard, and a rule attached at one side. The infant should be positioned with the body flat and the midline centered on the board. Interfering hair adornments should be removed. One measurer should hold the crown of the infant's head firmly against the headboard with the external auditory meatus and the lower margin of the eye orbit aligned perpendicular to the table. The second measurer gently flattens the infant's knees to fully extend the legs and grips both ankles of the infant with one hand. The footboard is then guided gently to the feet such that the feet are positioned flat on the foot board in order to obtain the measurement. The recumbent length should be recorded to the nearest 0.1 cm.

Stature, or standing height, is measured in children older than 2 years. A wall-mounted device should be used with a head board that glides at a 90° angle to the wall. The use of measuring devices attached to beam balance scales is discouraged, because accurate measurement cannot be achieved. Measurements are made with the child's feet bare and interfering hair adornments removed. The child should stand erect, and if possible, with the heels, buttocks, shoulders, and head touching the measuring device, and the arms down and relaxed at his or her side. The heels should be as close together as possible with the feet at a 60-degree angle. The head should be positioned with the child looking ahead and the external auditory meatus and lower margin of the orbit aligned horizontally. Children should be told to make themselves "as tall as possible with their heels on the ground." Asking them to take a deep breath often helps to improve posture and stand as tall as possible. The head board is then gently glided to the top of the crown and stature is recorded to the nearest 0.1 cm.

For both length and stature, measurements are best obtained when the child is relaxed and cooperative. Accurate measurement is particularly important for calculating growth velocity. Reference values for length, stature, and growth velocity are shown in Appendix A. Reference values for length and stature are also available for preterm infants (Appendix A). See Table 25.3 for a summary of reference growth data.

When possible, the parents' stature should be obtained to determine the influence of genetics on growth. If only one parent is available, the maternal stature is more valuable for comparison. There are 2 approaches to estimating the influence of heredity on stature. The parent-specific adjustments for evaluation of recumbent length and stature of children[42] uses a table of values, whereby an adjustment value at each age is given for mid-parental height. The adjustment value is added to the measured height or length, and this value is plotted on the growth chart to obtain the parent-specific percentile. For example, because children of tall parents are generally tall for their age, a short child with tall parents would have a negative adjustment value and their "adjusted height" would be less than their measured height. A tall child with tall parents would have no adjustment to their actual height. The "adjusted height" can be plotted on a growth chart to separate the estimated genetic contribution from other factors, such as malnutrition or disease, which may affect height. In children with cystic fibrosis, parent-adjusted heights are more strongly associated with the child's lung function than unadjusted heights.[43] The alternative approach for children 2 to 9 years of age is to estimate the child's adult height based on the following formula[44]:

For boys: [father's height + (mother's height + 5 inches or 13 centimeters)] / 2

For girls: [mother's height + (father's height − 5 inches or 13 centimeters)] / 2

The estimated adult height is plotted on the growth chart to determine a target percentile. The child's current height percentile is compared with his or her target percentile as an estimate of genetic versus other factors influencing the child's growth status. Both the mid-parental height adjustment and the adult height prediction methods are based on studies of people of European origin, and it is unknown whether further adjustment is needed for other population ancestry groups. The mid-parental height adjustment is more difficult to use, because it requires the use of published tables that are age, sex, and height specific. However, this method accounts for the fact that the association between child's height and mid-parental height varies with age.

Estimating Length/Stature From Knee Height

For children who are unable to stand unsupported, such as those with severe cerebral palsy, spina bifida, and other conditions with which they are wheelchair bound or bedridden, stature can be estimated by the use of prediction equations based on lower leg length measurements. Lower leg length is measured from the heel to the superior surface of the knee. Prediction equations for stature are given in Table 25.4.

Table 25.4.
Prediction of Stature (cm) From Knee Height

Without Cerebral Palsy[43]			
Males	6-18 y	White	[Knee Height (cm) × 2.22] + 40.54
		African American	[Knee Height (cm) × 2.18] + 39.60
	19-60 y	White	[Knee Height (cm) × 1.88] + 71.85
		African American	[Knee Height (cm) × 1.79] + 73.42
Females	6-18 y	White	[Knee Height (cm) × 2.15] + 43.21
		African American	[Knee Height (cm) × 2.02] + 46.59
	19-60 y	White	[Knee Height (cm) × 1.87] − [Age (years) × 0.06] + 70.25
		African American	[Knee Height (cm) × 1.86] − [Age (years) × 0.06] + 68.10
With Cerebral Palsy[44]			
All	0 to 12 y	All	[Knee Height (cm) × 2.69] + 24.2

Two caveats of this approach are (1) there are differences in limb length relative to stature that cluster within population ancestry groups (people of Asian ancestry have shorter lower legs and people of African ancestry have longer legs relative to stature than those of European ancestry); and (2) nonambulatory children can have stunted growth of lower limbs.

Weight

Various types of scales (infant scales, beam-balance scales, and digital scales) are available to measure body weight. Scales need to be regularly calibrated to maintain accuracy. Scales should be zeroed before a measurement is obtained. Infants should be weighed with clothing and diaper removed; if this is not possible, the infant may be weighed in a clean diaper after the scale is zeroed with a clean diaper on it. Children should be weighed in light clothing or examination gowns with shoes removed. Reference data for body weight are included in Appendix A. Weight

VI

reference values for preterm infants are shown in Appendix A. Reference values for infant weight gain are now available (see Appendix A), but attention should be given to the time interval between measurements when using these reference charts (see Growth Velocity for details). See Table 25.3 for a summary of reference data.

Measures of Relative Weight

Weight relative to length/stature provides a more complete picture of an infant's or child's nutritional status than weight or length alone. It is useful for identifying children whose weight is appropriate for their age, yet their weight may be low or high relative to their length/stature. Likewise, for very short or tall children, relative weight is a good indicator of whether body weight is appropriate for size. The relationship between weight and length/stature changes as a function of age and sexual maturation. Weight-for-length measurement is recommended for full-term infants through 2 years of age. BMI is recommended for children 2 years and older. Ponderal index (weight/length^3) is a common measure of relative weight in preterm infants, although it is not routinely used; there is evidence to suggest that it may not be the most appropriate measure for all preterm infants,[45] and the most appropriate index has yet to be determined.[46]

Weight for Length

For infants, the relationship of weight to length can be used to differentiate stunted growth from wasting and is independent of age. Stunting frequently is constitutional but can also be caused by malnutrition, chronic illness, and genetic or endocrine abnormalities. Stunting typically results in a child who is small for age but has a body weight proportional to length. Wasting results from acute or subacute nutritional deprivation and can be caused by medical conditions, such as diarrhea or malabsorption, in which body weight is depleted out of proportion to length, resulting in a low weight-for-length/height. The current accepted index is the weight-for-length percentile or z-score based on the WHO Child Growth Standards growth charts (0 to 2 years of age). Reference values for weight in relation to length are shown in Appendix A. See Table 25.3 for a summary of reference data.

BMI

BMI (weight/height^2) is a good screening measure of adiposity in children (starting at 2 years of age) and adolescents (Appendix A; Table 25.3). BMI is calculated as weight in kg divided by the square of height in meters (kg/m^2). It can also be calculated by dividing the weight in lb by the square of height in inches, multiplied by 703 (lb/in^2 x 703). The calculated BMI is then plotted on the CDC 2000 BMI-for-age growth curve to determine the BMI-for-age percentile, which is used to categorize relative weight status. A BMI-for-age less than the 5th percentile is considered "underweight," the 5th to less than the 85th percentile is considered "healthy weight," the 85th to less than the 95th percentile is considered "overweight," and 95th percentile is considered "obese."[47] All children followed by a physician should have their BMI calculated and plotted periodically. If the child begins to cross percentile lines (upward) on the BMI-for-age chart, the family can be counseled early about prevention of obesity.[48]

Head Circumference

Head circumference is a proxy measure for brain growth and a useful screening tool for identification of hydrocephalus until approximately 3 years of age, when head growth slows. Head circumference is measured with a narrow and nonstretchable measuring tape with interfering hair adornments removed. The tape is positioned on the forehead just above the supraorbital ridges, and wrapped around the occiput so that the maximum circumference is obtained, keeping the tape level on both sides; it is a good practice to move the tape slightly up and down to ensure maximum circumference. The tape should have sufficient tension to press the hair against the skull, and head circumference is recorded to the nearest 0.1 cm. Reference values from birth to 3 years of age are shown in Appendix A. Reference values for preterm infants are shown in Appendix A. See Table 25.3 for a summary of reference data.

Mid-Arm Circumference

Mid-upper–arm circumference is an indicator of soft tissue growth in all ages. The right arm is measured at its mid-point using a flexible, nonstretchable tape measure. The upper arm midpoint is marked midway between the acromion (shoulder) and the olecranon (elbow) on the vertical axis of the upper arm between the lateral and medial surface of the arm with the arm bent at a right angle. For the circumference measurement, the arm should hang loosely at the side with the tape passed around the arm at the level marked and perpendicular to the long axis of the arm. The tape is positioned so that it touches but does not compress the skin or alter the contour of the arm. Reference values from the WHO for children 3 months to 5 years of age are presented as curves and tables in Appendix A. See Table 25.3 for a summary of reference data.

VI

Nutritional Assessment Through the Measurement of Body Composition

Body composition assessment, depending on the method used, can provide information about the fat, lean, and bone tissue compartments. Fat is an indicator of energy stores and varies with overnutrition and undernutrition. Lean mass is composed of organs and skeletal muscle and is representative of protein stores in the body. Like fat, protein can be used for energy, but all protein in the body is present as functional tissue, so its utilization potentially results in a decrease in the functional body mass. Bone is the primary reservoir for calcium, and adequate bone accretion during childhood is important for lifelong skeletal health. Many methods of measuring body composition exist; however, few are used clinically and some are not practical in infants and/or children because of safety, feasibility, and availability. Some methods offer easy measurement of fat and fat-free mass accompanied by reference data so they can enhance the surveillance of the nutritional status of children. However, body composition methods vary in underlying assumptions and are not standardized, so methods need to be selected with care, and results from different methods are not interchangeable. Most body composition methods are research tools; understanding them is important for interpreting the pediatric nutrition literature, so they are summarized below. A few body composition assessment methods are now more widely available for clinical application. These will be reviewed separately.

Research Body Composition Assessment Techniques

Hydrodensitometry

The oldest method of estimating the fat and fat-free mass compartments in the human body is hydrodensitometry, introduced in 1942 by Albert Behnke.[49] Hydrodensitometry, or underwater weighing, is based on Archimedes' principle, which observes that the weight of an object completely immersed in water, relative to its weight in air, is proportional to the weight of the volume of water displaced. Because 1 mL of water has a mass of 1 g, the difference between the mass in air and the mass under water (in g) is equivalent to the volume (in mL) of the object. Body density is then calculated as mass divided by volume. Corrections are needed for the volume of air in the lungs and intestines and for the density of air and water. With the assumption that the density of fat and the lean tissue are essentially constant, calculation of the proportion of each is possible when the density of the whole body is known. The Siri formula[50] is most widely used for estimating the proportion of fat in the body as follows:

Siri[50] % body fat = (4.95/Body Density − 4.50) × 100

Hydrodensitometry requires that the individual is capable of being completely submerged in water long enough to take the measurements. This is not feasible for younger children, infants, hospitalized patients, or individuals with cognitive or physical disabilities. Also, the method assumes a constant density of fat-free mass; however, the hydration of fat-free mass decreases and bone density increases through the course of childhood. This results in small errors in the estimation of fat-free mass and fat mass during childhood.[51] Newer methods using this principle with air rather than water displacement have been developed (see Air-Displacement Plethysmography).

Total Body Potassium

The body cell mass represents the fat-free intracellular space of the body. This is the most metabolically active cellular compartment of the body, because it includes organs and muscles.[52] Because potassium is located in the intracellular fluids, body cell mass can be estimated by measuring total body potassium in a specially designed scintillation chamber or whole-body potassium counter.[53,54] Potassium (^{40}K), a naturally occurring stable isotope in human tissue, occurs as a very small percentage (0.0118%) of the nonradioactive ^{39}K also present in the body. The whole-body potassium counter measures the gamma rays emitted by ^{40}K to determine whole-body content of ^{40}K. The method assumes a constant ratio of intracellular fluid to body cell mass, so body cell mass is estimated as: total body K (mmol) x 0.0083. This technique is noninvasive but not practical, because (1) it is not widely available and requires an entirely lead-shielded room; (2) requires isolation in a special chamber for 30 to 60 minutes; and (3) it is not sufficiently sensitive to measure infants or small children who have little lean body mass and relatively fewer radioactive disintegrations per unit of time than do adults.

Total Body Water

The nonfat compartment of the body is largely comprised of water, so determination of the body's water content can easily be used to estimate total body fat and fat-free mass.[55] Stable isotopes of water, deuterium (^{2}H), or oxygen 18 (O^{18}) are naturally occurring and can be consumed orally in small concentrations to determine the total body water space. Following collection of a baseline biological specimen, administration of a small oral dose of ^{2}H or O^{18}, an equilibration period of a few hours, and a subsequent specimen collection, total body water can be estimated based on the change in concentration of the isotope within a body fluid, such as serum, urine, or saliva. The method is safe, is noninvasive, and involves minimal participant burden and can be used in a variety of natural settings as well as hospitalized infants and children. However, analysis of specimens to determine isotopic concentration is primarily performed in research laboratories, so it is of little usefulness clinically. In adults, the water content of lean body mass is relatively constant (72.3%), but in infants and children, the hydration of lean tissues changes with age.[56,57] Lean tissue hydration also increases with obesity.[58] These factors influence the accuracy of total body water and body composition estimates in infants and children using this technique.

VI

Neutron Activation

In vivo neutron activation analysis is the technique used to measure the elemental composition of the body.[59] The human body comprises more than 60 elements. Just 4 elements constitute 95% of the body's composition: oxygen (65%), carbon (18%), hydrogen (10%), and nitrogen (3%). Other elements that contribute to the composition of the total body in proportions greater than 0.05% are: sodium, potassium, phosphorus, chlorine, calcium, magnesium, and sulfur. The neutron activation method involves a whole-body chamber within which the subject receives a low dose of neutron irradiation. The neutrons interact with body tissues to excite the targeted element, creating unstable isotopes that emit gamma radiation. A whole-body gamma radiation counter measures the energy emitted and the decay rate to determine the total quantity of the element in the body. The resulting information is used to understand the elemental composition of the body and can also be used to estimate other body compartments based on the known contribution of elements to target tissues. For example, total body nitrogen can be used to estimate lean body mass, and total calcium content can be used to estimate bone mass. This method is completely impractical for use in infants and children because of the risks involved and the very small number of neutron activation chambers available worldwide.

Imaging Technologies

Imaging methods, such as quantitative computed tomography (QCT) and magnetic resonance imaging (MRI), have created new opportunities for understanding the growth and development of body compartments. QCT is an x-ray based technique that relies on the attenuation characteristics of a tissue, determined by the tissue density and chemical composition, to determine the size and density of an organ or tissue compartment.[60] For example, QCT images of the mid-section can be used to determine vertebral trabecular density[61] or the cross-sectional area of subcutaneous and intra-abdominal fat.[62] MRI uses a powerful magnetic field combine with radio frequency pulses specific to hydrogen to generate signals that can be converted to detailed images of organs and tissues. MRI is safer to use than QCT, because it does not involve radiation exposure. It has been used to estimate the volume of intra-abdominal adipose tissue, as well as intermuscular adipose tissue, the size of skeletal muscles, and volume of internal organs.[63] Magnetic resonance spectroscopy is a further technological development that has led to breakthroughs in such areas as measurement of intramyocellular and intrahepatic lipid fractions.[64] Of note, both MRI and QCT are costly techniques that require cooperation. Sedation may be required for infants and children to complete these tests, making it undesirable for many research applications.

Clinical Assessment Tools for Body Composition Assessment

Skinfold Thickness Measurements

Total or regional body fat can be estimated using skinfold thickness, a technique that can be easily performed in the clinical setting or at the bedside. With proper training, this technique is safe, reasonably accurate, rapid and inexpensive. Skinfold thickness is determined using spring-loaded calipers at standardized measurement sites. The use of Holtain (Holtain, LTD, Cyrmych, UK) or Lange (Cambridge Instruments, Silver Spring, MD) calipers is recommended. Measurements are obtained on the right side, if possible. The triceps skinfold thickness is often measured, because it is an easily accessible site and is generally representative of energy status. When combined with an arm circumference measurement, mid-upper arm fat area and muscle area can be estimated.

To measure triceps skinfold thickness, the child should be upright with his or her right arm hanging down in a relaxed position. The fold of fat and skin is lifted away from the underlying triceps muscle at the same level of the mid-upper arm, where the arm circumference is measured (midway between the acromion and the olecranon with the arm bent at a right angle). While holding the tissue in place, the calipers are placed over the skinfold and released so that they exert a constant pressure on the subcutaneous fat fold. The reading should be taken 3 seconds after releasing the caliper's handles. The subscapular skinfold thickness is a measure of fat stores on the trunk of the body. It is obtained by lifting a skinfold on an inferior lateral diagonal below the inferior angle of the scapula. A strong advantage of these skinfold thickness measures is the availability of excellent pediatric reference data[37,38] (see Table 25.3). In addition, prediction equations to estimate total body fat using triceps and subscapular skinfold thickness can be used.[65] Additional equations have been published using 4 skinfold thickness measures—the triceps, biceps, subscapular, and suprailiac skinfolds.[66,67] The primary disadvantages of measuring skinfold thickness is the inability to get accurate measurements in obese individuals and the training required to get reproducible measurements.

Air-Displacement Plethysmography

A new, rapid, noninvasive method for measuring fat and fat-free mass of the total body in infants, children, and adults is air-displacement plethysmography.[68-70] The method measures the volume of air displaced by the body. The air displacement plethysmograph contains 2 chambers of known volume; 1 for the patient and the other for measuring changes in pressure as the diaphragm connecting the 2 chambers oscillates. These pressure changes are accurately measured, and displaced volume is determined by invoking Boyle's Law, which states that volume and pressure are inversely related. Corrections are made for lung volume and for

VI

noncompressible regions around the body, such as hair, and microconvection of air at the skin surface. Because the individual's weight is known and volume is measured, density can be calculated. Body density is then used to estimate the fat and fat-free mass compartments (as in hydrodensitometry). Two versions of this instrument exist at the present time; the Bod Pod (Life Measurement Inc, Concord, CA) is used to measure children and adults, and the Pea Pod is designed for infants weighing up to 8 kg. These instruments are more user-friendly than underwater weighing and can be more easily used in obese individuals than some other clinically available body composition methods. The primary limitations are: (1) it requires the individual to be sealed into a chamber, limiting its use in patients requiring electronic monitoring or continuous infusions; and (2) it involves assumptions about the hydration and mineral composition of fat-free mass.

Dual-Energy X-ray Absorptiometry

Dual-energy x-ray absorptiometry (DXA) is rapidly becoming the preferred method for body composition determination and can be used in infants, children, and adults. The technique uses very low-energy x-rays and measures the attenuation of the x-rays as they pass through tissues of different density.[71] For a given x-ray energy level, tissues such as fat, muscle, and bone have unique attenuation properties. The attenuation is a function of a constant specific to that tissue and the tissue mass. The use of 2 energy beams of different intensity allows for determination of 2 tissue compartments. As the x-ray beam passes over soft tissue regions, the respective masses of lean and fat tissues are determined. As the beam passes over regions that also include bone, the algorithm solves for bone versus soft tissue, assuming that the composition of soft tissue surrounding the bone is similar to the adjacent soft tissue of muscle and fat. In this manner, DXA is able to estimate the mass of lean, fat, and bone mineral from a whole-body DXA scan.[55,72]

Although DXA is widely used as a body composition assessment tool in children, it is not a well-validated technique. Differences between DXA manufacturers and changes in software specifications can have a significant impact on body fat measurements.[73,74] Comparisons of fat estimates by DXA to measurements of a 4-compartment model, an approach that combines total body water, bone mass, and body density measurements, show a systematic bias in pediatric samples such that fatness is overestimated in obese children.[75,76] The increased hydration and lower density of lean mass in obesity may account for this pattern. Because DXA model type and software specifications affect body composition results in children, DXA body composition should not be considered a "gold standard." Despite these limitations, the recent publication of reference values for lean body mass from the National Health and Nutrition Examination Survey[77] for children 8 years and older has the potential to increase the clinical utility of DXA body composition assessment.

DXA is more widely used for the assessment of bone mass and density. Total body and regional DXA scans of the lumbar spine, proximal femur, and forearm are commonly used to determine bone mineral density (BMD) in adults; total body less head and lumbar spine DXA scans are the preferred scan sites for children, although the lateral distal femur scan is an optimal site for children with contractures or metal implants that preclude other scan sites.[78] The spine provides an index of the density of trabecular bone, and the total body is largely cortical bone. In addition, total body scans can generate an estimate of total body calcium. Of note, BMD by DXA is not an authentic volumetric density measure, because DXA is a 2-dimensional imaging technique that is not capable of determining the thickness of bone. BMD by DXA is often referred to as areal-BMD, because it is based on bone mineral content (BMC) divided by bone area from the 2-dimensional projection. As children grow, BMC increases and bone size increases in 3 dimensions. As a consequence, age-related changes in areal-BMD are largely growth dependent and only partly reflect volumetric BMD changes.[79]

Abnormalities in bone mineral accretion can be attributable to a primary disorder, such as osteogenesis imperfecta, or to secondary disorders, such as preterm birth or diseases associated with inflammation, malabsorption, altered dietary intake, reduced physical activity, or use of medications affecting bone mineral metabolism, such as glucocorticoids.[80] In addition to calcium and vitamin D, other nutrients that may be associated with bone density include vitamin K, phosphorus, zinc, magnesium, and protein intake.[81,82] DXA has several advantages: it is safe (radiation exposure equivalent to background radiation), accurate, reproducible, rapid, and widely available. For children and adolescents, excellent reference data are now available for BMC, BMD,[83] and body composition.[77] Limitations of DXA are: (1) it cannot be performed in pregnant females or individuals with indwelling hardware within scan regions; (2) most DXA devices have an upper weight limit, so total body and spine scans cannot be acquired in very obese individuals; (3) it requires cooperation without movement for short time periods (depending on the scan); and (4) it assumes a constant tissue composition of fat, lean, and bone.

Bioelectrical Impedance Analysis

Bioelectrical impedance analysis (BIA) is a portable, inexpensive method of body composition that is often used in survey type research studies and is becoming somewhat popular in settings such as exercise programs. The method is based on the principle that electrical currents are conducted through the water and

VI

electrolytes in the body. The impedance to electrical flow is directly proportional to the amount of lean tissue present; prediction equations translate the measured resistance to estimates of fat and fat free mass. The prediction equations were developed by validation studies that compared BIA to measures of body composition derived from other techniques, such as hydrodensitometry and/or total body water measurement by isotope dilution in adults. The validity of the prediction equations is not always well established and may vary as a function of ethnicity,[84] obesity status,[85] age,[86] or health condition.[87]

BIAs come in several forms. The original devices used 4 electrodes, 2 placed on the hand and 2 placed on the foot. Eight electrode devices have also been used. Because these designs allow flexibility in the placement location of the electrodes, they can be used to assess total and appendicular body composition.[88] There are now foot-to-foot analyzers, hand-to-hand analyzers,[89] and a model that combines both.[90]

Small changes in body water, such as normal diurnal variation, appear to make significant differences in the estimate of lean body mass. For models using electrodes, proper placement of the source and detectors electrodes is critical and can be problematic in very small children. The changing water content and distribution of the lean body mass of growing children should cause the impedance to change progressively with age, making this method extremely difficult to calibrate for children.[56] Various modifications are being made to these instruments in an attempt to enhance their precision.

Multifrequency BIA and bioelectrical impedance spectroscopy operate on principles similar to single-frequency BIA. The difference resides in the frequencies. At low frequency (<5 kHz), the impedance to current flow is an index of extracellular water, because this frequency does not penetrate the cell membrane. At higher frequencies, the cell membrane no longer acts as a capacitor, and the intracellular water also conducts current, thereby reducing impedance at higher frequencies. Thus, total body water and extracellular water are estimated by impedance, and intracellular water is derived from these 2 measures. As with single-frequency BIA devices, prediction equations are needed to convert the measured impedance to body water and body composition estimates. Typically, these prediction equations are based on healthy individuals with normal nutritional status and may not be applicable to patients outside the age range, those with health conditions that affect fluid balance, or those at the extremes of nutritional status. They also fail to account for variability in the contribution of bone mass to fat-free mass. Thus, although promising, these methods are not yet sufficiently accurate for use in monitoring individual clinical patients but may be useful for studying group characteristics.[91]

Laboratory Assessment

The initial laboratory assessment of nutritional status includes the measurement of hematologic status and protein nutrition. The absence of anemia may not exclude nutritional deficiencies, such as iron, folate, and vitamin B_{12} deficiencies. Red blood cell size is valuable in the differential diagnosis of anemias. Albumin concentration is a better measure of protein nutrition than is serum globulin concentration, because its biologic half-life is shorter (approximately 20 days). A low albumin concentration occurs with malnutrition, in liver disease, or when albumin is lost from the body in large amounts, as in nephrosis, exudative enteropathy, burns, or surgical drains. The so-called visceral proteins synthesized by the liver (such as retinol-binding protein with a half-life of 12 hours, transthyretin [prealbumin] with a half-life of 1.9 days, and transferrin with a half-life of 8 days) have shorter half-lives than does albumin, and their concentrations are better indicators of shorter-term protein status (ie, anabolism or catabolism) than is the serum albumin concentration. Serum concentrations of essential amino acids may be lower than those of nonessential amino acids, and 3-methyl histidine excretion is increased during states of protein insufficiency. Other abnormalities of protein depletion include a decreased creatinine concentration and decreased hydroxyproline excretion. Values for protein status may or may not reflect the degree of nutritional deficiency. In simple starvation (marasmus), a tendency to maintain the circulatory pool of visceral proteins at the expense of somatic protein is evident. The blood urea nitrogen concentration tends to decrease during starvation; however, in patients in whom water intake is restricted, such as those with anorexia nervosa, the serum concentration may be elevated.

The serum sodium concentration is frequently decreased in malnutrition as the result of dilution, because total body water is physiologically increased during starvation. This value is seldom lower than 133 mEq/L, however. The dilution effect can also be seen with hematologic parameters, such as hematocrit and hemoglobin concentrations. Immunologic abnormalities, such as loss of delayed hypersensitivity, fewer T-lymphocytes, and changes in lymphocyte response to in vitro stimulation by phytohemagglutinin, are sometimes helpful clinical measurements of nutritional status.

Assays of specific nutrients can be helpful in the assessment of the nutritional status of an individual, but their usefulness is limited by their wide variation within normal groups and the lack of easy availability of many of the vitamin assays. Normal values for some of these biochemical measurements are shown in Table 25.5. Other vitamins, such as biotin and niacin, as well as essential fatty acids, can be measured, but these measurements are seldom clinically indicated. Assessment of the concentrations of minerals, such as calcium, magnesium, phosphorus, iodine, copper, and selenium, is readily available in most laboratories and sometimes is important to measure as part of the nutritional assessment.

VI

Table 25.5.
Normal Values: Biochemical Measurement of Specific Nutritional Parameters

		Normal Range	
	Age	Male	Female
Protein, Blood			
Serum albumin, g/dL[a]	Day 0-5	2.6-3.6	2.6-3.6
	Day 6-30	2.8-4.0	2.8-4.0
	1-6 mo	3.1-4.2	3.1-4.2
	7-11 mo	3.3-4.3	3.3-4.3
	1-3 y	3.5-4.6	3.5-4.6
	4-6 y	3.5-5.2	3.5-5.2
	7-19 y	3.7-5.6	3.7-5.6
	20+ y	3.5-5.0	3.5-5.0
Retinol-binding protein, mg/dL[b]		3.0-6.0	3.0-6.0
Blood urea nitrogen, mg/dL[a]	0-2 y	2.0-19.0	2.0-19.0
	3-12 y	5.0-17.0	5.0-17.0
	13-18 y	7.0-18.0	7.0-18.0
	19-20 y	8.0-21.0	8.0-21.0
	21+ y	9.0-20.0	7.0-17.0
Transferrin, mg/dL[a]		180-370	180-370
Prealbumin, mg/dL[a]	0-11 mo	6.0-21.0	6.0-21.0
	1-5 y	14.0-30.0	14.0-30.0
	6-9 y	15.0-33.0	15.0-33.0
	10-13 y	20.0-36.0	20.0-36.0
	14+ y	22.0-45.0	22.0-45.0
Protein, Urine			
Creatinine/height index		>0.9	>0.9
3-methyl histidine, nmol/mg creatinine[a]	Day 1-6	81-384	81-384
	Day 7-8 wk	75-430	75-430
	9 wk-12 mo	142-377	142-377
	13 mo-3 y	134-647	134-647
	4+ y	93-323	93-323
Creatinine (24-h), mg/dL[b]	0-2 y	NA	NA
	3-8 y	140-700	140-700
	9-12 y	300-1300	300-1300
	13-17 y	500-2300	400-1600
	18-50 y	1000-2500	700-1600
Hydroxyproline index		>2	>2
Vitamin A			
Serum or plasma retinol, µg/dL[b]	0-1 mo	18-50	18-50
	2 mo-12 y	20-50	20-50
	13 yr-17 y	26-70	26-70
	18+ y	30-120	30-120

		Normal Range	
	Age	Male	Female
Vitamin D			
25-OH-D, ng/mL[a] 1-25-OH$_2$-D, pg/mL[b]		>20 15-75	>20 15-75
Folic acid			
Serum folate, ng/mL[a]	0-1 y 2-3 y 4-6 y 7-9 y 10-12 y 13-17 y 18+ y	7.2-22.4 2.5-15.0 0.5-13.0 2.3-11.9 1.5-10.8 1.2-8.8 2.8-13.5	6.3-22.7 1.7-15.7 2.7-14.1 2.4-13.4 1.0-10.2 1.2-7.2 2.8-13.0
Red blood cell folate, ng/mL[b]		280-903	280-903
Vitamin K			
Prothrombin time, sec[a]	0-5 mo 6+ mo	NA 11.7-13.2	NA 11.7-13.2
Vitamin E			
Serum or plasma α-tocopherol, mg/L[a]	0-1 mo 2-5 mo 6-12 mo 2-12 y 13+ y	1.0-3.5 2.0-6.0 3.5-8.0 5.5-9.0 5.5-18.0	1.0-3.5 2.0-6.0 3.5-8.0 5.5-9.0 5.5-18.0
Vitamin C			
Plasma vitamin C, mg/dL[b]		0.4-2.0	0.4-2.0
Vitamin B$_{12}$			
Serum vitamin B$_{12}$, pg/mL[a]	0-1 y 2-3 y 4-6 y 7-9 y 10-12 y 13-17 y 18+ y	293-1208 264-1216 245-1078 271-1170 183-1088 214-865 199-732	228-1514 416-1209 313-1407 247-1174 197-1019 182-820 199-732
Iron			
Hematocrit, %[a]	Day 0 Day 1-29 1-2 mo 3-5 mo 6-12 mo 2-5 y 6-11 y 12-17 y 18+ y	42.0-60.0 45.0-65.0 31.0-55.0 29.0-41.0 33.0-39.0 34.0-40.0 35.0-45.0 37.0-49.0 41.0-52.0	42.0-60.0 45.0-65.0 31.0-55.0 29.0-41.0 33.0-39.0 34.0-40.0 35.0-45.0 36.0-46.0 36.0-46.0

VI

Table 25.5. *(continued)*

Normal Values: Biochemical Measurement of Specific Nutritional Parameters

		Normal Range	
	Age	Male	Female
Hemoglobin, g/dL[a]	Day 0	13.5-19.5	13.5-19.5
	Day 1-29	14.5-22.0	14.5-22.0
	1-2 mo	10.0-18.0	10.0-18.0
	3-5 mo	9.5-13.5	9.5-13.5
	6-12 mo	10.5-13.5	10.5-13.5
	2-5 y	11.5-13.5	11.5-13.5
	6-11 y	11.5-15.5	11.5-15.5
	12-17 y	13.0-16.0	12.0-16.0
	18+ y	13.5-17.0	12.0-16.0
Serum ferritin, ng/mL[b]	0-6 mo	6-400	6-430
	7-35 mo	12-57	12-60
	3-14 y	14-80	12-73
	15-19 y	20-155	12-90
	20-29 y	38-270	12-114
Serum iron, μg/dL[b]	0-6 wk	100-250	100-250
	7 wk-11 mo	40-100	40-100
	1 yr-10 y	50-120	50-120
	11+ y	50-170	30-160
Serum total iron binding capacity, μg/dL[b]	0-2 mo	59-175	59-175
	3 mo-17 y	250-400	250-400
	18+ y	240-450	240-450
Serum transferrin saturation, %[b]		20-50	20-50
Serum transferrin, mg/dL[a]		180-370	180-370
Erythrocyte porphyrin (whole blood), μg/dL[b]		0-35	0-35
Zinc			
Serum zinc, μg/dL[a]	0-16 y	66-144	66-144
	17+ y	75-291	65-256
Phosphorus			
Serum phosphate, mg/dL[a]	Day 0-11 mo	4.8-8.2	4.8-8.2
	1-3 y	3.8-6.5	3.8-6.5
	4-6 y	4.1-5.4	4.1-5.4
	7-11 y	3.7-5.6	3.7-5.6
	12-13 y	3.3-5.4	3.3-5.4
	14-15 y	2.9-5.4	2.9-5.4
	16-20 y	2.7-4.7	2.7-4.7
	21+ y	2.5-4.5	2.5-4.5

	Age	Normal Range Male	Normal Range Female
Calcium			
Serum total calcium, mg/dL[a]	Day 0	6.9-9.4	6.9-9.4
	Day 1-6	8.0-11.4	8.0-11.4
	Day 7-13	8.0-11.2	8.0-11.2
	Day 14-29	9.3-10.9	9.3-10.9
	1 mo	9.3-10.7	9.3-10.7
	2 mo	9.3-10.6	9.3-10.6
	3-4 mo	9.2-10.5	9.2-10.5
	5-11 mo	9.2-10.4	9.2-10.4
	1-3 y	8.7-9.8	8.7-9.8
	4-20 y	8.8-10.1	8.8-10.1
	21+ y	8.4-10.2	8.4-10.2
Serum ionized calcium, mmol/L[a]	Day 0	1.07-1.27	1.07-1.27
	Day 1-1 y	1.00-1.17	1.00-1.17
	2-4 y	1.21-1.37	1.21-1.37
	5-17 y	1.15-1.34	1.15-1.34
	18+ y	1.12-1.3	1.12-1.3
Magnesium			
Serum magnesium, mg/dL[a]	0-20 y	1.5-2.5	1.5-2.5
	21+ y	1.6-2.3	1.6-2.3
Copper			
Serum copper, μg/dL[b]	0-6 mo	20-70	20-70
	7 mo-18 y	90-190	90-190
	19+ y	70-140	80-155
Selenium			
Serum selenium, μg/L[b]		23-190	23-190

NA indicates not available.

[a] Laboratory values from the clinical laboratories at Children's Hospital of Philadelphia (2011).

[b] Laboratory values retrieved from ARUP laboratories at http://www.aruplab.com/ (June 27, 2011).

References

1. Fomon SM. *Nutritional Disorders of Children: Prevention, Screening, and Followup.* Bethesda, MD: Department of Health and Human Services; 1977. DHEW Publication No. HSA 77-5104

2. Gibson RS. Measuring food consumption of individuals. In: Gibson RS, ed. *Principles of Nutritional Assessment.* 2nd ed. New York, NY: Oxford University Press; 2005:41-64

3. Baker JP, Detsky AS, Wesson DE, et al. Nutritional assessment: a comparison of clinical judgement and objective measurements. *N Engl J Med.* 1982;306(16):969-972

4. Cameron N. The use and abuse of growth charts. In: Johnston FE, Zemel B, Eveleth PB, eds. *Human Growth in Context.* London, United Kingdom: Smith-Gordon; 1999:65-74

VI

5. de Onis M, Onyango AW, Borghi E, Garza C, Yang H, WHO Multicentre Growth Reference Study Group. Comparison of the World Health Organization (WHO) Child Growth Standards and the National Center for Health Statistics/WHO international growth reference: implications for child health programmes. *Public Health Nutrition*. 2006;9(7):942-947

6. Alexander GR, Himes JH, Kaufman RB, Mor J, Kogan M. A United States national reference for fetal growth. *Obstet Gynecol*. 1996;87(2):163-168

7. Arbuckle TE, Wilkins R, Sherman GJ. Birth weight percentiles by gestational age in Canada. *Obstet Gynecol*. 1993;81(1):39-48

8. Babson SG, Benda GI. Growth graphs for the clinical assessment of infants of varying gestational age. *J Pediatr*. 1976;89(5):814-820

9. Bonellie S, Chalmers J, Gray R, Greer I, Jarvis S, Williams C. Centile charts for birthweight for gestational age for Scottish singleton births. *BMC Pregnancy Childbirth*. 2008;8:5

10. Fenton TR, Kim JH. A systematic review and meta-analysis to revise the Fenton growth chart for preterm infants. *BMC Pediatr*. 2013;13:59

11. Kramer MS, Platt RW, Wen SW, et al. A new and improved population-based Canadian reference for birth weight for gestational age. *Pediatrics*. 2001;108(2):e35

12. Lubchenco LO, Hansman C, Boyd E. Intrauterine growth in length and head circumference as estimated from live births at gestational ages from 26 to 42 weeks. *Pediatrics*. 1966;37(3):403-408

13. Lubchenco LO, Hansman C, Dressler M, Boyd E. Intrauterine growth as estimated from liveborn birth-weight data at 24 to 42 weeks of gestation. *Pediatrics*. 1963;32:793-800

14. Niklasson A, Albertsson-Wikland K. Continuous growth reference from 24th week of gestation to 24 months by gender. *BMC Pediatr*. 2008;8:8

15. Oken E, Kleinman KP, Rich-Edwards J, Gillman MW. A nearly continuous measure of birth weight for gestational age using a United States national reference. *BMC Pediatr*. 2003;3:6

16. Olsen IE, Groveman SA, Lawson ML, Clark RH, Zemel BS. New intrauterine growth curves based on United States data. *Pediatrics*. 2010;125(2):e214-e224

17. Riddle WR, DonLevy SC, Qi XF, Giuse DA, Rosenbloom ST. Equations to support predictive automated postnatal growth curves for premature infants. *J Perinatol*. 2006;26(6):354-358

18. Bukowski R, Gahn D, Denning J, Saade G. Impairment of growth in fetuses destined to deliver preterm. *Am J Obstet Gynecol*. 2001;185(2):463-467

19. Doubilet PM, Benson CB, Wilkins-Haug L, Ringer S. Fetuses subsequently born premature are smaller than gestational age-matched fetuses not born premature. *J Ultrasound Med*. 2003;22(4):359-363

20. Ehrenkranz RA. Estimated fetal weights versus birth weights: should the reference intrauterine growth curves based on birth weights be retired? *Arch Dis Child Fetal Neonatal Ed*. 2007;92(3):161-162

21. Moyer-Mileur LJ. Anthropometric and laboratory assessment of very low birth weight infants: the most helpful measurements and why. *Semin Perinatol*. 2007;31(2):96-103

22. Rao SC, Tompkins J. Growth curves for preterm infants. *Early Hum Dev*. 2007;83(10):643-651

23. Engle WA. Age terminology during the perinatal period. *Pediatrics*. 2004;114(5):1362-1364

24. Bertino E, Spada E, Occhi L, et al. Neonatal anthropometric charts:the Italian neonatal study compared with other European studies. *J Pediatr Gastroenterol Nutr*. 2010;51(3):353-361

25. Roberts CL, Lancaster PA. Australian national birthweight percentiles by gestational age. *Med J Aust*. 1999;170(3):114-118

26. Bonellie S, Chalmers J, Gray R, Greer I, Jarvis S, William C. Centile charts for birthweight for gestational age for Scottish singleton births. *BMC Pregnancy Childbirth*. 2008;8:5

27. Voigt M, Guthman F, Hesse V, Gorlich Y, Straube S. Somatic classification of neonates based on birth weight, length, and head circumference: quantification of the effects of maternal BMI and smoking. *J Perinat Med*. 2011;39(3):291-297

28. Kuczmarski RJ, Ogden CL, Grummer-Strawn LM, et al. CDC growth charts: United States. *Adv Data*. 2000;(314):1-27

29. WHO Child Growth Standards based on length/height, weight and age. *Acta Paediatr Suppl*. 2006;450:76-85

30. Guo SS, Roche AF, Chumlea WC, Casey PH, Moore WM. Growth in weight, recumbent length, and head circumference for preterm low-birthweight infants during the first three years of life using gestation-adjusted ages. *Early Hum Dev*. 1997;47(3):305-325

31. Guo SS, Wholihan K, Roche AF, Chumlea WC, Casey PH. Weight-for-length reference data for preterm, low-birth-weight infants. *Arch Pediatr Adolesc Med*. 1996;150(9):964-970

32. Grummer-Strawn LM, Reinold C, Krebs NF. Use of World Health Organization and CDC growth charts for children aged 0-59 months in the United States. *MMWR Recomm Rep*. 2010;59(RR-9):1-15

33. Centers for Disease Control and Prevention. Clinical Growth Charts. Available at: http://www.cdc.gov/growthcharts/clinical_charts.htm#Summary. Accessed November 16, 2012

34. Baumgartner RN, Roche AF, Himes JH. Incremental growth tables: supplementary to previously published charts. *Am J Clin Nutr*. 1986;43(5):711-722

35. Berkey CS, Dockery DW, Wang X, Wypij D, Ferris B Jr. Longitudinal height velocity standards for U.S. adolescents. *Stat Med*. 1993;12(3-4):403-414

36. Tanner JM, Davies PS. Clinical longitudinal standards for height and height velocity for North American children. *J Pediatr*. 1985;107(3):317-329

37. World Health Organization Multicentre Growth Reference Study Group. WHO Child Growth Standards: Head circumference-for-age, arm circumference-for-age, triceps skinfold-for-age and subscapular skinfold-for-age: methods and development. Geneva, Switzerland: World Health Organization; 2007

38. Addo OY, Himes JH. Reference curves for triceps and subscapular skinfold thicknesses in US children and adolescents. *Am J Clin Nutr*. 2010;91(3):635-642

39. Lampl M, Thompson AL, Frongillo EA. Sex differences in the relationships among weight gain, subcutaneous skinfold tissue and saltatory length growth spurts in infancy. *Pediatr Res*. 2005;58(6):1238-1242

VI

40. World Health Organization Multicentre Growth Reference Study Group. WHO Child Growth Standards: Growth velocity based on weight, length and head circumference: methods and development. Geneva: World Health Organization; 2009

41. Hamill PV, Drizd TA, Johnson CL, Reed RB, Roche AF. NCHS growth curves for children birth-18 years. United States. *Vital Health Stat*. 1977;11(165):i-iv, 1-74

42. Himes JH, Roche AF, Thissen D, Moore WM. Parent-specific adjustments for evaluation of recumbent length and stature of children. *Pediatrics*. 1985;75(2):304-313

43. Chumlea WC, Guo SS, Steinbaugh ML. Prediction of stature from knee height for black and white adults and children with application to mobility-impaired or handicapped persons. *J Am Diet Assoc*. 1994;94(12):1385-1388

44. Stevenson RD. Use of segmental measures to estimate stature in children with cerebral palsy. *Arch Pediatr Adolesc Med*. 1995;149(6):658-662

45. Cole TJ, Henson GL, Tremble JM, Colley NV. Birthweight for length: ponderal index, body mass index or Benn index? *Ann Hum Biol*. 1997;24(4):289-298

46. Olsen IE, Lawson ML, Meinzen-Derr J, et al. Use of a body proportionality index for growth assessment of preterm infants. *J Pediatr*. 2009;154(4):486-491

47. Centers for Disease Control and Prevention. About BMI for Children and Teens. Available at: http://www.cdc.gov/healthyweight/assessing/bmi/childrens_bmi/about_childrens_bmi.html#How%20is%20BMI%20calculated. Accessed November 16, 2012

48. Krebs NF, Jacobson MS. Prevention of pediatric overweight and obesity. *Pediatrics*. 2003;112(2):424-430

49. Lohman TG. Skinfolds and body density and their relation to body fatness: a review. *Hum Biol*. 1981;53(2):181-225

50. Siri W. The gross composition of the body. In: Tobias C, Lawrence JH, ed. *Advances in Biological and Medical Physics*. New York, NY: Academic Press; 1956:239-280

51. Wells JC, Williams JE, Chomtho S, et al. Pediatric reference data for lean tissue properties: density and hydration from age 5 to 20 y. *Am J Clin Nutr*. 2010;91(3):610-618

52. Heymsfield S, Wang Z, Baumgartner RN, Ross R. Human body composition: advances in models and methods. *Annu Rev Nutr*. 1997;17:527-558

53. Forbes GB, Schultz F, Cafarelli C, Amirhakimi GH. Effects of body size on potassium-40 measurement in the whole body counter (tilt-chair technique). *Health Phys*. 1968;15(5):435-442

54. Remenchik AP, Miller CE, Kessler WV. Body composition estimates derived from potassium measurements. ANL-7461. *ANL Rep*. 1968:73-90

55. Ellis KJ. Human body composition: in vivo methods. *Physiol Rev*. 2000;80(2):649-680

56. Wells JC, Fuller NJ, Dewit O, Fewtrell MS, Elia M, Cole TJ. Four-component model of body composition in children: density and hydration of fat-free mass and comparison with simpler models. *Am J Clin Nutr*. 1999;69(5):904-912

57. Schoeller D. Hydrometry. In: Roche A, Heymsfield SB, Lohman TG, ed. *Human Body Composition*. Champaign, IL: Human Kinetics; 1996:25-43

58. Haroun D, Wells JC, Williams JE, Fuller NJ, Fewtrell MS, Lawson MS. Composition of the fat-free mass in obese and nonobese children: matched case-control analyses. *Int J Obes (Lond)*. 2005;29(1):29-36

59. Ellis K. Whole-body counting and neutron activation analysis. In: Roche AF, Lohman TG, eds. *Human Body Composition*. Champaign, IL: Human Kinetics; 1996:45-61

60. Heymsfield SB, Fulenwider T, Nordlinger B, Barlow R, Sones P, Kutner M. Accurate measurement of liver, kidney, and spleen volume and mass by computerized axial tomography. *Ann Intern Med*. 1979;90(2):185-187

61. Gilsanz V. Bone density in children: a review of the available techniques and indications. *Eur J Radiol*. 1998;26(2):177-182

62. Goran MI, Bergman RN, Gower BA. Influence of total vs. visceral fat on insulin action and secretion in African American and white children. *Obes Res*. 2001;9(8):423-431

63. Lee SY, Gallagher D. Assessment methods in human body composition. *Curr Opin Clin Nutr Metab Care*. 2008;11(5):566-572

64. Shen W, Liu H, Punyanitya M, Chen J, Heymsfield SB. Pediatric obesity phenotyping by magnetic resonance methods. *Curr Opin Clin Nutr Metab Care*. 2005;8(6):595-601

65. Slaughter MH, Lohman TG, Boileau RA, et al. Skinfold equations for estimation of body fatness in children and youth. *Hum Biol*. 1988;60(5):709-723

66. Brook CG. Determination of body composition of children from skinfold measurements. *Arch Dis Child*. 1971;46(246):182-184

67. Durnin J, Rahaman M. The assessment of the amount of fat in the human body from measurements of skinfold thickness. *Br J Nutr*. 1967;21:681-689.

68. Dempster P, Aitkens, S. A new air displacement method for the determination of human body composition. *Med Sci Sports Exerc*. 1995;27:1692-1697

69. Dewit O, Fuller NJ, Fewtrell MS, Elia M, Wells JC. Whole body air displacement plethysmography compared with hydrodensitometry for body composition analysis. *Arch Dis Child*. 2000;82(2):159-164

70. Fields DA, Gilchrist JM, Catalano PM, Gianni ML, Roggero PM, Mosca F. Longitudinal body composition data in exclusively breast-fed infants: a multicenter study. *Obesity (Silver Spring)*. 2011;19(9):1887-1891

71. Laskey MA. Dual-energy X-ray absorptiometry and body composition. *Nutrition*. 1996;12(1):45-51

72. Prentice A. Application of dual energy x-ray absorptiometry and related techniques to the assessment of bone and body composition. In: Davies PSW, editor. *Body Composition Techniques in Health and Disease. Society for the Study of Human Biology Symposium 36*. Cambridge, United Kingdom: Cambridge University Press; 1995:1-13

73. Shypailo RJ, Butte NF, Ellis KJ. DXA: can it be used as a criterion reference for body fat measurements in children? *Obesity (Silver Spring)*. 2008;16(2):457-462

74. Pearson D, Horton B, Green DJ. Cross Calibration of Hologic QDR2000 and GE Lunar Prodigy for whole body bone mineral density and body composition measurements. *J Clin Densitom*. 2011;14(3):294-301

75. Sopher AB, Thornton JC, Wang J, Pierson RN Jr, Heymsfield SB, Horlick M. Measurement of percentage of body fat in 411 children and adolescents: a comparison of dual-energy X-ray absorptiometry with a four-compartment model. *Pediatrics*. 2004;113(5):1285-1290

VI

76. Wells JC, Haroun D, Williams JE, Wilson C, Darch T, Viner RM, et al. Evaluation of DXA against the four-component model of body composition in obese children and adolescents aged 5-21 years. *Int J Obes (Lond)*. 2010;34(4):649-655

77. Kelly TL, Wilson KE, Heymsfield SB. Dual energy X-Ray absorptiometry body composition reference values from NHANES. *PLoS One*. 2009;4(9):e7038

78. Gordon CM, Bachrach LK, Carpenter TO, et al. Dual energy X-ray absorptiometry interpretation and reporting in children and adolescents: the 2007 ISCD Pediatric Official Positions. *J Clin Densitom*. 2008;11(1):43-58

79. Wren TA, Liu X, Pitukcheewanont P, Gilsanz V. Bone acquisition in healthy children and adolescents: comparisons of dual-energy x-ray absorptiometry and computed tomography measures. *J Clin Endocrinol Metab*. 2005;90(4):1925-1928

80. Leonard MB, Zemel BS. Current concepts in pediatric bone disease. *Pediatr Clin North Am*. 2002;49(1):143-173

81. Bounds W, Skinner J, Carruth BR, Ziegler P. The relationship of dietary and lifestyle factors to bone mineral indexes in children. *J Am Diet Assoc*. 2005;105(5):735-741

82. Jesudason D, Clifton P. The interaction between dietary protein and bone health. *J Bone Miner Metab*. 2011;29(1):1-14

83. Zemel BS, Kalkwarf HJ, Gilsanz V, et al. Revised reference curves for bone mineral content and areal bone mineral density according to age and sex for black and non-black children: results of the Bone Mineral Density in Childhood Study. *J Clin Endocrinol Metab*. 2011;96(10):3160-3169

84. Haroun D, Taylor SJ, Viner RM, Hayward RS, Darch TS, Eaton S, et al. Validation of bioelectrical impedance analysis in adolescents across different ethnic groups. *Obesity (Silver Spring)*. 2010;18(6):1252-1259

85. Sluyter JD, Schaaf D, Scragg RK, Plank LD. Prediction of fatness by standing 8-electrode bioimpedance: a multiethnic adolescent population. *Obesity (Silver Spring)*. 2010;18(1):183-9.

86. Clasey JL, Bradley KD, Bradley JW, Long DE, Griffith JR. A New BIA Equation Estimating the Body Composition of Young Children. *Obesity (Silver Spring)*. 2011;19(9):1813-1817

87. Puiman PJ, Francis P, Buntain H, Wainwright C, Masters B, Davies PS. Total body water in children with cystic fibrosis using bioelectrical impedance. *J Cyst Fibros*. 2004;3(4):243-247

88. Kriemler S, Puder J, Zahner L, Roth R, Braun-Fahrlander C, Bedogni G. Cross-validation of bioelectrical impedance analysis for the assessment of body composition in a representative sample of 6- to 13-year-old children. *Eur J Clin Nutr*. 2009;63(5):619-626

89. Erceg DN, Dieli-Conwright CM, Rossuello AE, Jensky NE, Sun S, Schroeder ET. The Stayhealthy bioelectrical impedance analyzer predicts body fat in children and adults. *Nutr Res*. 2010;30(5):297-304

90. Haroun D, Croker H, Viner RM, et al. Validation of BIA in obese children and adolescents and re-evaluation in a longitudinal study. *Obesity (Silver Spring)*. 2009;17(12):2245-2250

91. Buchholz AC, Bartok C, Schoeller DA. The validity of bioelectrical impedance models in clinical populations. *Nutr Clin Pract*. 2004;19(5):433-446

Chapter 26

Pediatric Feeding and Swallowing Disorders

Introduction

Children with pediatric dysphagia have feeding and/or swallowing difficulties and may be at risk of compromised health and nutrition. The prevalence of feeding and swallowing disorders in the general pediatric population varies from 25% to 45% and is much higher in children with developmental disabilities.[1] Failure to thrive, aspiration pneumonia, and food refusal are some of the common issues reported in children with feeding and swallowing disorders. The causes of these disorders include neurologic, respiratory, gastrointestinal, psychosocial, and anatomical disorders.[2-4] Thus, a multidisciplinary approach is important to provide optimal care for this population. This includes gastroenterology, nutrition, pulmonology, neurology, otolaryngology, speech-language pathology, occupational therapy, physical therapy, and psychology. An interdisciplinary team, such as a feeding team, is an excellent resource for children with complex feeding issues. Members of a feeding team may include a speech-language pathologist, dietitian, occupational therapist, psychologist, and nurse or physician. The role of the speech-language pathologist is to provide assessment and intervention for oral motor deficits, developmental feeding delays, and swallowing dysfunction. An occupational therapist may also intervene with feeding difficulties, especially for sensory-based feeding complications and fine motor difficulties.

When determining which services a child may require, it is important to distinguish between feeding and swallowing problems, because the assessment and management needs are different. A feeding disorder or difficulty refers to the oral management of food or liquids, including immature developmental feeding skills, oral/sensory aversion, selective eating, low appetite, and food refusal. A swallowing disorder, or dysphagia, generally refers to impairment of swallowing coordination, either structural or motor-based, that leads to risk of aspiration. Therefore, distinguishing between feeding and swallowing problems helps to guide appropriate assessment and intervention, such as a clinical feeding evaluation or an instrumental assessment of swallow function. The severity of the feeding and/or swallowing complication dictates what approach is required.

Differential Diagnosis of Feeding Versus Swallowing Disorders

A major feature that distinguishes swallowing issues from feeding difficulties is the concern for aspiration while swallowing and the subsequent potential for pulmonary complications. Also, children with swallowing issues or dysphagia frequently have either concomitant neurologic issues (eg, seizures, cerebral palsy) or a structural anomaly of the upper airway (eg, laryngeal cleft, tracheoesophageal fistula) that is the

VI

primary etiology disrupting swallow coordination.[3,4] Children with feeding difficulties more often present with gastrointestinal tract issues (gastroesophageal reflux [GER], food allergies, delayed gastric emptying), immature sensory systems, behavior dysregulation, or developmental delay. However, from simple observation, it can be difficult at times to differentiate between feeding and swallowing problems. For example, a parent may describe their child as choking when the child gags on food as it touches the tongue, in which case the issue may simply be an oral sensitivity to taste or food texture. Similarly, a child with immature chewing skills may incompletely chew the food or not control the food in the mouth and choke. Solid-food dysphagia (a swallowing disorder) is uncommon in children unless there are pharyngeal/esophageal motility issues, an airway mass, esophageal stenosis, or prior tracheoesophageal fistula repair. If the child can consume liquids and smooth foods without difficulty but chokes on textured foods, it is a feeding disorder, not a swallowing problem. Issues of drooling, behavioral feeding problems, long-term deprivation of oral feeding as infants, or abnormal posture (eg, hyperextension of the neck with scapular retraction and shoulder girdle elevation) are also risks for swallowing abnormalities.[5,6] Dysphagia should also be suspected in children who have diseases that have been associated with swallowing dysfunction. Fig 26.1 and 26.2 provide key differences between feeding and swallowing problems.

Fig 26.1.
Manifestations of a FEEDING problem

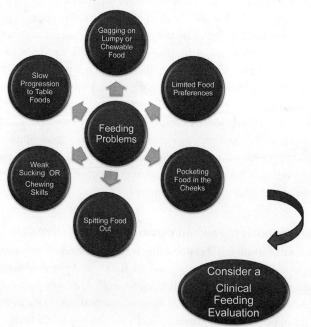

Fig 26.2.
Manifestations of a SWALLOWING problem

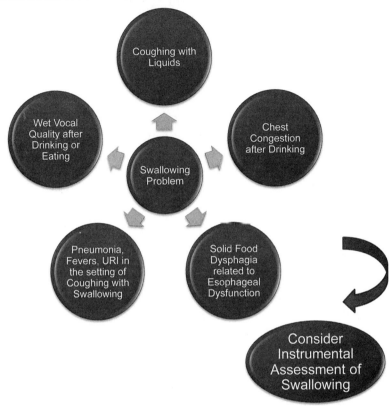

Feeding Disorders

Etiologies

Feeding disorders include oral stage issues that can be motor or sensory based.[7] Motor-based feeding problems can involve difficulty moving the food from the front to the back of the mouth before swallowing. For example, children with low muscle tone may have weak or uncoordinated tongue movements resulting in prolonged mealtimes or even choking with liquids, because food spills in the airway before the swallow has been initiated. Children with motor-based feeding problems may have difficulty chewing because of weak chewing muscles. Also, the child may present with developmental feeding delays, such as slow onset of chewing skills, related to lack of experience, or compromise from chronic illness. In contrast to motor-based swallowing problems, difficulties with eating can also stem from dysfunction with the sensory system. This includes difficulty integrating sensory

VI

information related to the taste and texture of food. It is not uncommon to find sensory-based feeding problems when there is a history of GER, significant food or formula allergies/sensitivities, delayed gastric emptying, or sensitivity to touch. A common feeding history may include difficulty transitioning to textured foods and gagging and vomiting either at the smell of foods or when the food is placed on the tongue. These children may also present with additional sensory problems, such as sensitivity to touch, loud noises, and light. Parents may also report the child not tolerating going barefoot on the carpet or grass, preferring not to be "messy" while eating, and severe discomfort from tags in their clothing or seams in their socks. Thus, these "sensitive" infants and children may have more pronounced reactions to reflux or bodily discomfort that results in feeding disruption. Neurologic-based sensory issues, as seen in autism spectrum disorders (ASDs), can result in long-term feeding issues, including high food selectivity and oral aversion behaviors.[8] Assessment scales, such as the Brief Autism Mealtime Behavior Inventory (BAMBI), can help guide observations and monitor outcomes when measuring progress in feeding intervention approaches.[9,10] Gastrointestinal tract issues occur frequently in ASDs.[11]

Symptoms

Parents often pose questions regarding whether or when their child's feeding issues will resolve. Once early GER and food allergy symptoms begin to subside by 1 to 2 years of age, feeding difficulties related to gastrointestinal tract issues generally begin to resolve as well. However, an unresolved issue is whether these otherwise healthy children establish normal eating habits. Lefton-Grief[12] reported on retrospective findings from an 8-year follow-up of 19 otherwise healthy children with early respiratory problems of unexplained etiology. Aspiration of liquids was found in approximately 58% of the cases, and the majority of these resolved at an average age of 3 years. Approximately 30% of the children had persistent coughing issues in grade school. Hawdon[13] reported persistent feeding issues for approximately 50% of 35 preterm infants with an average gestational age of 34 weeks as the babies reached 6 and 12 months of age. Certainly children with ongoing developmental disability and neurologic deficits may have lifelong feeding difficulties. However, this milder subgroup of persistent feeding problems may require attention as well. Some school programs are formally addressing feeding and swallowing issues within the school setting. Homer[14] describes the challenge of more medically fragile children attending school with feeding issues. School therapists, including speech pathologists and occupational and physical therapists, may be involved in feeding programs. In these programs, it is important to have systematic written documentation of feeding procedures and performance outcomes as well as education for staff or classroom aids to implement feeding techniques at meal or snack times.[14]

Educational guidelines, such as Free and Appropriate Public Education (FAPE) and the Individual with Disabilities Education Act (IDEA), require schools to provide these health-related services.

Management

Assessment is often performed by an interdisciplinary feeding team for complex feeding issues, especially when health is compromised, because there may be multiple medical issues of concern, including poor weight gain. With milder feeding issues that occur when the child is otherwise healthy but not progressing with age-expected feeding behaviors because of gagging or refusal, a single provider assessment with a feeding specialist/speech-language pathologist or occupational therapist will be sufficient. Interventions for sensory-based feeding issues can be a long process. Patel[15] has offered some feeding approaches. Children who exhibit frequent food packing or retaining textured foods in the mouth can have low food volume intake. A better volume and energy intake may be achieved by offering less-textured foods during meal times. Also, high-textured foods can increase oral aversion responses in children with high oral sensitivity. Thus, starting with low-textured foods and graduating texture as tolerated can be a better feeding approach. Children can also be overwhelmed with large amounts per spoon, so smaller spoonfuls can be better accepted. Praise and encouragement are a good model for shaping positive feeding behavior versus critical statements and negative reinforcement.[16,17]

Summary of Feeding Disorders

Etiologies: Developmental delay, lack of experience, chronic illness, ASDs, neuromuscular or craniofacial disorders, sensory integration disorder (SID), behavioral issues, food allergies, GER.

Symptoms: Difficulty chewing, drooling, food spilling from mouth, gagging and/or choking on chewable foods, prolonged time to finish meal or manage single bite, food refusal, poor progression with textures, selective eating/limited food repertoire, nausea/vomiting with smell of food, disrupted family dynamics, feeding best when partly asleep.

Management: Feeding or sensory treatment, single provider assessment with a feeding specialist, or multidisciplinary assessment and treatment that may include speech-language pathologist, occupational therapist, physical therapist, dietitian, nurse, pediatrician, social services professional, or specialty services, such as a neurologist, gastroenterologist, pulmonologist, otorhinolaryngologist, psychologist, or behavioral specialist.[18] Often, feeding teams have a core of these individuals, and additional referrals are made as needed. Adequate management of gastrointestinal

VI

tract symptoms can be critical for developmental or behavioral treatment approaches to be effective. Sometimes, reflux medications are discontinued too early, when mild symptoms persist, and eating regression can occur. Intensive, short-term multidisciplinary treatment options are available at primarily hospital-based venues for severe feeding issues, such as inability to wean from nonoral tube feeding or dysfunctional behavioral feeding dynamics that lend to persistent feeding difficulties.

Swallowing Disorders

Etiologies

Swallowing disorders involve pharyngeal and esophageal dysfunction that creates aspiration risks. Primary aspiration during the act of swallowing occurs when there is disruption of the complex pharyngeal stage of swallowing while the larynx is elevating, the vocal cords are closing to protect the airway, and the pharyngeal muscles are moving in a wave-like motion to move food into the esophagus. Vocal cord paralysis, especially bilateral paralysis, is an important cause of dysphagia and choking disorders, especially in the presence of other airway anomalies or neuromotor involvement. Abnormal muscle tone can also affect the muscles in the pharynx (pharyngeal constrictors), creating weak peristalsis, smooth muscle dysmotility, or muscle spasm, such as cricopharyngeal dysfunction. Medical problems that affect the respiratory system (eg, chronic lung disease [CLD], laryngo- or tracheomalacia, significant tachypnea) can also disrupt swallowing coordination and create risks of choking or even aspiration.[19] In addition, children with significant GER can develop reduced sensitivity in the hypopharynx from inflammation, which can result in compromise of swallow coordination. These motor- and sensory-based swallowing problems can lead to serious medical compromise. Therefore, further radiologic assessment may be performed with imaging techniques that examine the oral/pharyngeal stages of swallowing, such as videofluoroscopic swallowing studies or fiberoptic endoscopic examination of swallowing (FEES).[20-22]

Symptoms

Aerodigestive disorders occur frequently with swallowing issues. Airway problems that may affect swallowing include: vocal fold paralysis or paresis, significant subglottic stenosis, laryngomalacia, tracheoesophageal fistula, moderate to severe laryngeal clefts, neck or airway tumors such as a teratoma, or laryngeal inflammation with altered sensation. Such issues can create risks of laryngeal aspiration.[23] Digestive issues such as reflux more commonly lead to feeding problems with food refusal and gagging symptoms. GER can also be the cause of secondary aspiration, especially in the presence of reflux into the pharynx (laryngopharyngeal reflux), creating edema and reduced upper airway sensation with risk of silent secondary aspiration.[24] Upper airway issues and subsequent swallowing problems are more frequently managed with a team approach, such as airway or aerodigestive teams.[25] Such clinics may involve otolaryngology, pulmonology, gastroenterology, nursing, and speech-language pathology. Reasons for referral often include chronic cough, asthma, persistent pulmonary issues with unclear etiology, and upper airway anomalies. The most common swallowing complaints include chronic cough during drinking and gagging on chewable foods. Adverse consequences of feeding and swallowing issues include inadequate volume or caloric intake and subsequent inadequate growth. When chronic cough is reported, it may or may not be the result of a swallowing problem. Therefore, it is important to determine whether the cough occurs in tandem with the act of swallowing or is a delayed symptom after eating, such as with GER. Chronic cough is a frequent initial symptom of mild laryngeal cleft.[26,27] Chronic cough can also be unrelated to feeding, such as with asthma and upper airway irritation.

Aspiration pneumonia in children is another concerning symptom. Aspiration without pulmonary symptoms occurs in both healthy and disabled children and adults.[28-30] Several studies have shown that silent aspiration occurs in 20% to 30% of dysphagic adults,[29] although it does not necessarily result in pulmonary compromise. In a reported study of 43 infants referred for dysphagia, laryngeal penetration, aspiration, and nasal backflow occurred in almost half of the infants.[28] Interestingly, these symptoms generally emerged after multiple normal swallows, with an average of almost 1 minute from the onset of the first swallow. Laryngeal penetration and aspiration occurred most frequently from material pooled in the pyriform sinus (above the upper esophageal opening). In addition, unlike adults, the infants cleared laryngeal penetration during the swallow without coughing. Half of the infants developed 1 episode of pneumonia, but the correlation was not strong between the timing of the aspiration episode identified on the imaging study and the episodes of pneumonia. This led to the recommendation to evaluate at least 1 minute of swallowing performance when performing videofluoroscopic studies, because dysphagic episodes may not occur during the first several swallows.

When children experience aspiration while consuming thin liquids, a frequent recommendation is to substitute thickened fluids. This can lead to concerns for adequate hydration, especially when children refuse thickened liquids. Unfortunately, there are no randomized-controlled studies that have examined the safety of plain water consumption by children with thin liquid dysphagia and, thus, no current reliable guidelines on water consumption in children with thin liquid aspiration.[31]

Management
Evaluation of swallowing problems may include nasoendoscopy, bronchoscopy, Ph probe, videofluoroscopic swallow examination (or modified barium swallow

VI

[MBS]), and/or FEES. The gold standard for swallow assessment continues to be the MBS or VFSS. The radiation dose has been described as low and an acceptable risk, although concerns have been expressed with younger infants.[32] The MBS examination provides information on the dynamics of all 3 swallowing phases, presence/absence of aspiration, and pharyngeal function issues. If results of the MBS are negative but aspiration is suspected, a FEES can be helpful in detecting mild dysphagia issues, such as intermittent microaspiration, as sometimes seen with type I laryngeal clefts.[26] In addition, the FEES examination provides information on the anatomy of the upper airway, including vocal fold function, edema, or anatomic anomalies. Therefore, the FEES and MBS examinations can complement one another. Successful use of FEES with children can be age dependent for tolerance.

Summary of Swallowing Problems

Etiologies: respiratory, neuromuscular, anatomic (airway anomalies, pharyngeal or esophageal dysmotility, abnormal muscle tone, poor tongue control, laryngeal cleft, tracheoesophageal fistula, chronic lung disease, tachypnea)

Symptoms: choking associated with swallowing, especially on thin liquids; pneumonia; vocal quality change after swallowing; frequent upper respiratory infections

Management: Swallow assessment with MBS and/or FEES; medical management of GER, respiratory issues, and airway problems; and swallowing therapy when indicated with a speech-language pathologist. The World Health Organization has outlined 4 parameters to examine the effects of swallowing problems: (1) impairment of structure/function, (2) degree of limiting activity, (3) ability to participate in daily routines, and (4) the degree of distress to the child.[33] Progress in swallow function can be monitored across these parameters.

Evaluation of Pediatric Dysphagia

The complex nature of feeding and swallowing problems requires multidisciplinary involvement to address the multifaceted issues that affect the feeding and swallowing process. The evaluation process can involve both a clinical evaluation of feeding behavior as well as instrumental assessment when swallowing concerns are present. Clinical evaluations may include a feeding team to manage feeding concerns or an airway clinic for upper airway and swallowing concerns. Typically, children with selective eating or slow progression to age-appropriate foods may advance with maturation and not require comprehensive assessment. Or, if the feeding issue is isolated to developmental feeding skills or food texture progression, a feeding specialist alone may be sufficient, and a team approach may not be warranted. A comprehensive history and physical examination are important in the evaluation of the child with dysphagia; during this evaluation, emphasis should be placed on the feeding history and neurologic, pulmonary, and gastrointestinal tract function. Ethical dilemmas may arise when oral feeding negatively affects a child's nutrition or hydration status or compromises pulmonary health.[34] If a risk of aspiration or oropharyngeal stage dysfunction is suspected, then a videofluoroscopic or FEES examination is indicated to further assess the swallow function and safety for oral eating. This examination is generally conducted by a speech-language pathologist in conjunction with a pediatric radiologist. When significant dysphagia is present, the recommendation for nonoral feeding may be made. This decision requires thoughtful consideration by all providers as well as the family. Parents may hold the final decision with regard to withholding or altering how nutrition is delivered to their child.[34] If concerns arise related to feeding and growth for children with complex medical issues, a referral should be made to a multidisciplinary feeding team.[35,36] Core members of such a team usually include a speech-language pathologist or an occupational therapist; nurse, dietitian, and perhaps a gastroenterologist, developmental pediatrician, or physical therapist. Fig 26.3 and 26.4 provide referral guidelines for further evaluation of feeding and swallowing problems on the basis of the complexity of the feeding or swallowing problem. Despite these general guidelines, the referral process needs standards of care for consistency in management of dysphagia problems. Sheppard[37] supports early referral for children with developmental delay or medically complex issues that affect feeding and swallowing (see Fig 26.3, 26.4).

Fig 26.3.
Management of feeding problems from simple to complex

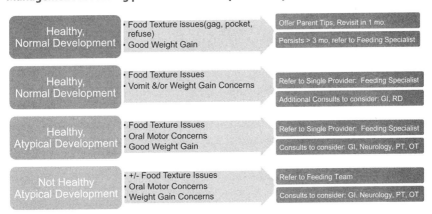

Fig 26.4.
Management of swallowing problems from mild to severe

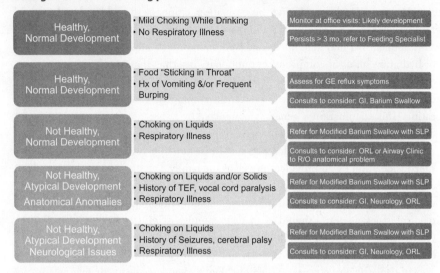

Clinical Evaluation

Clinical evaluation of pediatric feeding and swallowing involves assessment of how effectively the child performs the oral, pharyngeal, and esophageal phases of swallowing, along with several other factors.[19,28,38,39] The child's feeding history is important to the clinical evaluation. Elements of the history include: (1) how the child received nutrients and fluids; (2) the duration of nonoral nutrition; and (3) the child's ability to swallow effectively when first given oral feedings. Children who have been ill and have been fed by alternative methods have often not had normal oral experiences and, therefore, may not show interest in eating.

Once the medical status, medication use, and feeding history of the child have been ascertained, examination of the oral-peripheral structures is performed. In addition, respiratory status at baseline and during eating should be monitored along with developmental feeding skills. Observing how the child manages oral secretions provides information about swallowing function, airway protection, and oral-motor control. Swallow function can be screened with observation of secretion management, laryngeal movement, and vocal quality during and after swallowing. When problems with the pharyngeal or esophageal phase of the swallow are suspected and the reason is unclear, radiographic or instrumental evaluation is indicated.

Instrumental Evaluation of Dysphagia

Videofluoroscopy

Videofluoroscopy, or MBS, is the current procedure of choice for the assessment of children with swallowing disorders. The study is generally performed under the direction of a radiologist and a speech-language pathologist. During a swallow, the oral cavity, pharynx, and cervical esophagus are visualized first in the lateral view to assess aspiration; an antero-posterior view is later taken to study symmetry. Therapeutic techniques may be evaluated at this time to monitor their effectiveness. The study is videotaped or recorded digitally for later review.[40] In the detection of aspiration from the oral cavity, which is defined as the passage of food below the true vocal cords, videofluoroscopy is superior to bedside clinical assessment and has also effectively determined which patients are at risk of pneumonia.[40-42] Other radiologic methods to evaluate dysphagia include ultrasonography and scintigraphy.[43-46] Ultrasonography is a noninvasive approach that provides information about tongue, hyoid, and soft palate movement during swallowing but does not allow direct viewing of aspiration or penetration. Advancing technology in ultrasonography has allowed more detailed and effective swallow assessment for both oral stage function (eg, tongue dynamics) and pharyngeal swallowing development (eg, in utero).[47]

Pharyngeal Manometry

Pharyngeal manometry is the best method for evaluating pharyngeal and esophageal motor function. Manometry requires the transnasal insertion of a catheter housing a series of intraluminal pressure transducers.[48] In the evaluation of dysphagia, it is best used as a complementary diagnostic procedure to endoscopy, videofluoroscopy, or electromyography.[48,49] In children, manometry has been used mainly to investigate gastroesophageal reflux, esophageal motor, and pharyngeal motor disorders.

Fiberoptic Endoscopic Evaluation of Swallowing

Fiberoptic endoscopy has been used primarily in the evaluation of adults, for whom videofluoroscopy is unsuitable, but use is now increasing in the pediatric population. An endoscope is passed transnasally through the nasopharynx and hypopharynx and positioned just above the false vocal folds. This technique is particularly useful to directly assess laryngeal function for adduction and airway protection. Children with reflux and upper airway issues, in addition to swallowing disorders, can benefit from a FEES examination. Other indications for a FEES examination include assessment of possible anatomic contributing factors, assessment of pharyngeal or laryngeal sensitivity, and a risk of aspiration of even minute amounts of material.[21] Other reported advantages include detection of pooling in the

VI

pharynx and training the child to use compensatory swallowing techniques. The age of the child is a factor for tolerance of the procedure.[21-22,27]

Treatment

Treatment of pediatric feeding and swallowing disorders varies greatly depending on the symptoms, the cause of the problem, and the child's feeding history. However, treatment can generally be categorized into 6 areas: positioning, oral sensory normalization, modification of food consistency, swallowing maneuvers, adaptive feeding devices, and oral feeding exercises.[50,51] Providers of pediatric feeding therapy are typically speech-language pathologists or occupational therapists. Children with neuromotor disorders require secure positional support while maintaining head and spine alignment. Collaboration with the physical therapist and the feeding specialist for proper seating and positional needs can be helpful.[52] Children with motor impairment may also require simplification of food choices (smooth vs chewable foods), the use of swallow maneuvers for older children (eg, effortful swallow, breath hold, and cough after swallowing) and thickened liquids in cases of aspiration risk. Children with behavioral and sensory-related eating issues can benefit from regulation of sensory modulation, food texture modification, and fostering developmental feeding skills.[53] For example, children with a history of GER often respond well to high-alerting food flavors in their food, such as garlic, curry, lemon, or sweet and sour. In general, thinner consistencies (eg, thin liquids) are indicated for children with problems with bolus transport and children who are weak or fatigue easily. Thicker consistencies (eg, purees and soft solids) are indicated when oral containment of the bolus, poor tongue control, delayed swallow initiation, or decreased laryngeal closure during the swallow is the problem. Bottles and cups can be selected with varying flow rates as well.[37]

Behavioral Approaches

In addition to medical management concerns, family dynamics and mealtime routines also influence feeding success. Therefore, it is important to query parents about the way they are feeding their children. Force feeding, chasing a child from room to room, offering inappropriate textures, having prolonged mealtimes, or being a short-order cook for a child does not foster a positive or helpful feeding environment for children with feeding difficulties. Modifying the parent's approach to feeding can be a starting point when behavior dynamics are a component of feeding difficulties. Behavioral approaches may include following the child's lead, feeding the child when hunger signs begin, gaining the child's attention but not overarousing, and watching for the child's signals for satiation.[16] Also, some general rules to follow may include having a regular mealtime schedule, providing a neutral atmosphere with avoidance of force feeding, and offering small portions with solids first and fluids last. In the interim before achieving a normal eating pattern, parents are encouraged to maintain mealtime routines when possible, not to have the child "grazing" on food continuously, and to provide a high-energy diet to reduce episodes of forced feeding to meet energy intake goals. Table 26.1 provides a summary of parent tips for mealtime. Nutritional supplements can provide an entire meal for children who are averse to solid foods. An evaluation by a dietitian is critical when determining the child's energy and growth needs and the optimal nutrition plan to meet those needs.[54] Behavior-based feeding issues, including parent-child interaction difficulties, may require additional intervention with a child behavioral specialist who is familiar with feeding disorders.

Table 26.1.
Parent Tips for Successful Mealtimes

- Regular mealtime schedule when possible
- Avoid force feeding
- Present the meal in small parts so as not to overwhelm the child
- Avoid continuous grazing throughout the day; allow 2 to 3 hours between meals/snacks to build hunger
- Always have 1 favorite/preferred food at each meal
- Limit meals to 20-30 minutes
- Offer high-energy, easy-to-eat foods at meals and more challenging foods at snack times

Enteral Feeding: How it Affects the Feeding Process

When children require supplemental alternative nutrition for prolonged periods, gastrostomy tubes are preferred over nasogastric tubes to minimize oral aversion, discomfort with oral feeding, irritation of the upper aerodigestive tract, and increasing frequency of GER episodes.[55] For children with marked developmental disability or severe failure to thrive who require a gastrostomy tube, enteral feedings can lessen mealtime pressures on parents and support children's nutrition and growth. Energy needs that are not met at mealtimes can be given later by gastrostomy tube until the child is ready to begin weaning from the tube feedings. However, along with these benefits, parents of children who receive all their nutrition by enteral feedings experience other stressful situations, such as coping with a child who does not eat by mouth, social stigmata, and medical complications with tube function.[56] Nevertheless, it has been reported that families of children with developmental problems and feeding issues but are feeding by mouth, experienced stress that is equal to families of children who were totally dependent on a gastrostomy tube for feeding. Of concern are the children with frequent refusal of oral feeding but without oral motor or swallow dysfunction who require gastrostomy tube feedings for poor growth. These children are at risk of future

VI

difficulties when transitioning to full oral feeding. This is an area that requires further investigation for long-term implications.[57] Most health care professionals who treat patients with dysphagia believe that the best exercise for swallowing is swallowing. Thus, the goal for all children with dysphagia is safe eating, even if only in small amounts.

Weaning From Nonoral Feedings

The weaning process from nonoral feedings should be a slow and gradual process.[58] The approach requires attention to establishing adequate hunger cues, establishing adequate feeding and oral motor skills, maximizing caregiver interactions, and often, behavioral therapy.[59] Children who have received chronic tube feedings often miss critical transition periods for eating, such as beginning solid foods. Subsequently, these children can demonstrate significant oral aversion to eating, especially textured foods. It has been suggested that nonoral feeding during the first year of life adversely affects cortical development because of reduced input into the motor and sensory pathways between the oropharynx and cortex.[60] A methodical process to wean from tube feedings is required for children who meet the appropriate criteria.[57] One method is to first transition patients on continuous feedings to bolus feedings. Next, offer food by mouth before each daytime bolus feed to simulate a mealtime schedule. The eventual plan is to eliminate night-time tube feedings. As the child consumes more calories by mouth, then the tube feedings can be decreased accordingly. This process will be most successful when performed in conjunction with an oral sensory treatment program and under close monitoring by a dietitian and pediatrician. Assessment scales, such as the *Pediatric Assessment Scale for Severe Feeding Problems,* can be helpful to measure and monitor the tube-weaning process.[61] Currently, there are multiple approaches to the tube-weaning process, including intensive inpatient and outpatient hospital-based programs. Components to consider when selecting a weaning approach may include medical diagnosis, developmental feeding skill level, child temperament, duration and method of tube feeding, and family psychosocial dynamics.[57]

Dysphagia and the Preterm Infant

It has been reported that the longer feeding issues persist, the more likely it is that behavioral problems will occur. Frequently, practitioners find a continuum of organic versus functional feeding problems that cannot be easily separated. For example, sensory-based feeding problems have been associated with a history of nasogastric tube feeding and a history of aspiration or ventilation in first 6 months of life[62,63]; however, the study population was described as overrepresented by preterm infants with a gestational age of <34 weeks.

Overall, children born preterm or those who present with developmental delays are more likely to have persistent feeding issues.[2,4,13] In the setting of the neonatal intensive care unit, when infants have a guarded prognosis, decisions about oral feeding may be guided by ethical hospital policies and mandates, such as the Born-Alive Infants Protection Act (Pub L No. 107-207), which was passed by Congress in 2002. The Born-Alive Infants Protection Act requires that parents be informed and involved regarding decisions about their preterm child, but physicians are granted final decision making regarding life and death.[34] Up to 80% of this population may demonstrate feeding difficulties.[2] Gastrointestinal tract issues are most common, along with various accompanying problems, such as behavior/sensory issues, airway compromise, or oral-motor problems. Among extremely preterm infants, degree of prematurity, number of medical complications, and length of time that oxygen therapy was required are all risk factors for future motor- and sensory-based feeding complications.[10,64,65]

Assessment and Treatment Updates for Pediatric Dysphagia

- Trends persist to use short-term hunger for children younger than 3 years as a feeding intervention to resume hunger-satiation cycles, especially for children with prolonged supplemental tube feeding.[10,66]

- Children with symptoms similar to GER (eg, food refusal, oral aversion, vomiting, failure to thrive, eczema) who do not respond to medical therapy may be assessed for eosinophilic esophagitis. Asthma and food/environmental allergies are common in children with eosinophilic esophagitis.[67]

- Food allergies in children have been increasing the past 5 years.[68] Food allergies can create a tipping point or complicating factor for children with baseline feeding difficulties.

Conclusion

Dysphagia is commonly associated with certain pediatric disorders and can result in substantial morbidity. Further, the type of medical condition or developmental problems a child demonstrates can often be a strong predictor for specific feeding and swallowing symptoms.[63,69] Timely identification of pediatric feeding and swallowing disorders is important for initiating evaluation and treatment when indicated. This can prevent or reduce future medical and/or nutritional compromise for the at-risk child. Differentiating between feeding and swallowing problems helps to guide the proper evaluation and treatment approaches and streamline healthcare. Finally, a multidisciplinary team approach is the most effective means for managing

VI

complex pediatric feeding and swallowing problems for children in at-risk populations, whereas healthy, typically developing children with immature feeding skills, food texture aversion, vomiting, and/or gastrointestinal tract complications who present with weight gain issues may be managed with a feeding specialist only as a single provider. For the healthy child without weight gain concerns but slow progression to age level foods, time and simple parent tips may be the best approach.

References

1. Lefton-Greif MA, Arvedson JC. Pediatric feeding and swallowing disorders: state of health, population trends, and application of International Classification of Functioning, Disability, and Health. *Semin Speech Lang.* 2007;28(3):161-165

2. Manikam, R, Perman, JA. Pediatric feeding disorders. *J Clin Gastroenterol.* 2000;30(1):34-46

3. Burklow KA, Phelps AN, Schultz JR, McConnell K, Rudolph C. Classifying complex pediatric feeding disorders. *J Ped Gastroenterol Nutr.* 1998;27(2):143-147

4. Burklow KA, McGrath AM, Valerius KS, Rudolph C. Relationship between feeding difficulties, medical complexity, and gestational age. *Nutr Clin Pract.* 2002;17(6):373-378

5. Lespargot A, Langevin MF, Muller S, Guillemont S. Swallowing disturbances associated with drooling in cerebral-palsied children. *Dev Med Child Neurol.* 1993;35(4):298-304

6. Tuchman DN. Cough, choke, sputter: the evaluation of the child with dysfunctional swallowing. *Dysphagia.* 1989;3(3):111-116

7. Palmer MM, Heyman MB. Assessment and treatment of sensory-versus motor-based feeding problems in very young children. *Infants Young Child.* 1993;6(2):67-73

8. Whiteley P. Developmental, behavioural and somatic factors in pervasive developmental disorders: preliminary analysis. *Child Care Health Dev.* 2004;30(1):5-11

9. Lukens C, Linscheid TR. Development and validation of an inventory to assess mealtime behavior problems in children with autism. *J Autism Dev Disord.* 2008;38(2):342-352

10. Miller KC. Updates on pediatric feeding and swallowing. *Curr Opin Otolaryngol Head Neck Surg.* 2009;17(3):194-199

11. Horvath K, Papadimitriou JC, Rabsztyn A, et al. Gastrointestinal abnormalities in children with autistic disorder. *J Pediatr.* 1999;135(5):559-563

12. Lefton-Greif M. Long-term follow-up of oropharyngeal dysphagia in children without apparent risk factors [abstr]. Presented at the meeting of the Dysphagia Research Society, March 2006; Scottsdale, AZ

13. Hawdon JM, Beauregard N, Slattery J, Kennedy G. Identification of neonates at risk of developing feeding problems. *Dev Med Child Neurol.* 2000;42(4):235-239

14. Homer EM. An interdisciplinary team approach to providing dysphagia treatment in the schools. *Semin Speech Lang.* 2003;24(3):215-234

15. Patel MR, Piazza CC, Layer SA, Coleman R, Swartzwelder DM. A systematic evaluation of food textures to decrease packing and increase oral intake in children with pediatric feeding disorders. *J Appl Behav Anal.* 2005;38(1):89-100

16. Satter E. Feeding dynamics: helping children to eat well. *J Pediatric Health Care.* 1995;9(4):178-184

17. Satter E. *How to Get Your Kid to Eat…But Not Too Much.* Palo Alto, CA: Bull Publishing; 1987

18. Arvedon JC. Assessment of pediatric dysphagia and feeding disorders: clinical and instrumental assessments. *Dev Disabil Res Rev.* 2008;14(2):118-127

19. Miller CK, Willging JP. Advances in the evaluation and management of pediatric dysphagia. *Curr Opin Otolaryngol Head Neck Surg.* 2003;11(6):442-446

20. Sonies BC. Instrumental procedures for dysphagia diagnosis. *Semin Speech Lang.* 1991;12:185-198

21. Hartnick CJ, Hartley BE, Miller C, Willging P. Pediatric fiberoptic endoscopic evaluation of swallowing. *Ann Otol Rhinol Laryngol.* 2000;109(11):996-999

22. Leder SB, Karas DE. Fiberoptic endoscopic evaluation of swallowing in the pediatric population. *Laryngoscope.* 2000;110(7):1132-1136

23. Richter GT. Management of oropharyngeal dysphagia in the neurologically intact and developmentally normal child. *Curr Opin Otolaryngol Head Neck Surg.* 2010;18:554-563

24. Suskind D, Thompson D, Gulati M, et al. Improved infant swallowing after gastroesophageal disease treatment: function of improved laryngeal sensation? *Laryngoscope.* 2006;116:1397-1403

25. Wiatrak BJ, Hood J, Lackey P. Paediatric airway clinic: an 18 month experience. *J Otolaryngol.* 1997;26(3):149-154

26. Ashland J, Haver K, Hardy S, Hartnick CJ. Type I laryngeal clefts in children: dysphagia assessment and outcomes [abstr]. Presented at the meeting of the Dysphagia Research Society; March 2006; Scottsdale, AZ

27. Boseley ME, Ashland J, Hartnick CJ. The utility of the fiberoptic evaluation of swallowing (FEES) in diagnosing and treating children with type I laryngeal clefts. *Int J Pediatr Otorhinol.* 2006;70(2):339-343

28. Newman LA, Keckley C, Petersen MC, Hamner A. Swallowing function and medical diagnoses in infants suspected of dysphagia. *Pediatrics.* 2001;108(6):1-4

29. Ramsey D, Smithard D, Kalra L. Silent aspiration: what do we know? *Dysphagia.* 2005;20(3):218-225

30. Sheikh S, Allen E, Shell R, et al. Chronic aspiration without gastroesophageal reflux as a cause of chronic respiratory symptoms in neurologically normal infants. *Chest.* 2001;120(4):1190-1195

31. Weir K, McMahon S, Chang AB. Restriction of oral intake of water for aspiration lung disease in children. *Cochrane Database Syst Rev.* 2005;(4):CD005303

32. Weir K, McMahon S, Long G, et al. Radiation doses in children during modified barium swallow studies. *Pediatr Radiol.* 2007;37(3):283-290

33. Skeat J, Perry A. Outcome measurement in dysphagia: not so hard to swallow. *Dysphagia.* 2005;20(2):113-122

VI

34. Arvedson JC, Lefton-Greif MA. Ethical and legal challenges in feeding and swallow intervention for infants and children. *Semin Speech Lang*. 2007;28(3):232-238

35. Lane SL, Cloud HH. Feeding problems and intervention: an interdisciplinary approach. *Top Clin Nutr*. 1988;3(3):23-32

36. Lefton-Greif, MA, Arvedson, JC. Pediatric feeding/swallowing teams. *Semin Speech Lang*. 1997;18(1):5-11

37. Sheppard JJ. Case management challenges in pediatric dysphagia. *Dysphagia*. 2001;17(1):74

38. Darrow DH, Harley CM. Evaluation of swallowing disorders in children. *Otolaryngol Clin North Am*. 1998;31(3):405-418

39. Newman L. Optimal care patterns in pediatric patients with dysphagia. *Semin Speech Lang*. 2000;21(4):281-291

40. Arvedson JC, Lefton-Grief, MA. *Pediatric Videofluoroscopic Swallow Studies: A Professional Manual with Caregiver Guidelines*. Tucson, AZ: Therapy Skill Builders; 1998

41. Friedman B, Frazier JB. Deep laryngeal penetration as a predictor of aspiration. *Dysphagia*. 2000;15(3):153-158

42. Arvedson J, Rogers B, Buck G, Smart P, Msall M. Silent aspiration prominent in children with dysphagia. *Int J Ped Otorhinolaryngol*. 1994;28(2-3):173-181

43. Weber F, Woolridge MW, Baum JD. An ultrasonographic study of the organization of sucking and swallowing by newborn infants. *Dev Med Child Neurol*. 1986;28(1):19-24

44. Guillet J, Basse-Cathalinat B, Christopher E, et al. Routine studies of swallowed radionuclide transit in paediatrics: experience with 400 patients. *Eur J Nucl Med*. 1984;9(2):86-90

45. Muz J, Mathog RH, Rosen R, Miller PR, Borrero G. Detection and quantification of laryngotracheopulmonary aspiration with scintigraphy. *Laryngoscope*. 1987;97(10):1180-1185

46. Baikie G, South MJ, Reddihough DS, et al. Agreement of aspiration tests using barium videofluoroscopy, salivagram, and milk scan in children with cerebral palsy. *Dev Med Child Neurol*. 2005;47(2):86-93

47. Miller JL. Ultrasound and the aerodigestive system: the research past, the imaging present, and the clinical future [abstr]. Presented at the Dysphagia Research Society Annual Meeting; March 2006; Scottsdale, AZ

48. Feussner H, Kauer W, Siewert JR. The place of esophageal manometry in the diagnosis of dysphagia. *Dysphagia*. 1993;8(2):98-104

49. Elidan J, Shochina M, Gonen B, Gay I. Manometry and electromyography of the pharyngeal muscles in patients with dysphagia. *Arch Otolaryngol Head Neck Surg*. 1990;116:910-913

50. Rudolf, MC, Logan, S. What is the long-term outcome for children who fail to thrive? A systematic review. *Arch Dis Child*. 2005;90(9):925-931

51. Morris SE, Klein MD. *Prefeeding Skills: A Comprehensive Resource for Mealtime Development*. Tucson, AZ: Therapy Skill Builders; 2000

52. Redstone F, West JF. The importance of postural control for feeding. *Pediatr Nurs*. 2004;30(2):97-100

53. Field D, Garland M, Williams K. Correlates of specific childhood feeding problems. *J Paediatr Child Health*. 2003;39(4):299-304

54. Kovar A. Nutrition assessment and management in pediatric dysphagia. *Semin Speech Lang*. 1997;18(1):39-49

55. Bazyk S. Factors associated with the transition to oral feeding in infants fed by nasogastric tubes. *Am J Occup Ther*. 1990;44(12):1070-1079

56. Burklow KA, McGrath AM, Allred KE, Rudolph C. Parent perceptions of mealtime behaviors in children fed enterally. *Nutr Clin Pract*. 2002;17(5):291-295

57. Mason SJ, Harris G, Blissett J. Tube feeding in infancy: implications for the development of normal eating and drinking skills. *Dysphagia*. 2005;20(1):46-61

58. Palmer MM. Weaning from gastrostomy tube feeding: commentary on oral aversion. *Pediatr Nurs*. 1995;23(6):475-478

59. Benoit D, Wang EEL, Zlotkin SH. Discontinuation of enterostomy tube feeding by behavioral treatment in early childhood: a randomized controlled study. *J Pediatr*. 2000;137(4):498-503

60. Senez C, Guys JM, Mancini J, Paz Paredes A, Lena G, Choux M. Weaning children from tube to oral feeding. *Child Nerv Syst*. 1996;12(10):590-594

61. Crist W, Dobbelsteyn C, Brousseau AM, Napier-Phillips A. Pediatric assessment scale for severe feeding problems: validity and reliability of a new scale for tube-fed children. *Nutr Clin Pract*. 2004;19(4):403-408

62. Davies WH, Berlin KS, Sato AF, et al. Reconceptualizing feeding and feeding disorders in interpersonal context: the case for relational disorder. *J Fam Psychol*. 2006;20(3):409-417

63. Rommel N, De Meyer AM, Feenstra L, Veereman-Wauters G. The complexity of feeding problems in 700 infants and young children presenting to a tertiary care institution. *J Pediatr Gastroenterol Nutr*. 2003;37(1):75-84

64. Weiss MH. Dysphagia in infants and children. *Otolaryngol Clin North Am*. 1998;21(4):727-735

65. Poor M, Barlow S, Wang J, et al. Respiratory treatment history predicts suck pattern stability in preterm infants. *J Neonatal Nurs*. 2008;14:185-192

66. Kindermann A, Kneepkens CM, Stok A, van Dijk EM, Engels M, Douwes AC. Discontinuation of tube feedings in young children by hunger provocation. *J Pediatr Gastroenterol Nutr*. 2008;47(1):87-91

67. Putnam P. Eosinophilic esophagitis in children: clinical manifestations. *Gastroenterol Clin North Am*. 2008;37(2):369-338

68. Branum AM, Lukacs SL. Food allergy among U.S. children: trends in prevalence and hospitalizations. *NCHS Data Brief*. 2008;(10):1-8

69. Prasse J, Kikano G. An overview of pediatric dysphagia. *Clin Pediatr (Phila)*. 2009;48:247-251

VI

Chapter 27

Failure to Thrive

Introduction

Failure to thrive (FTT) is an imprecise, archaic term that refers to children whose growth is significantly lower than the norms for their age and gender.[1] Less pejorative terms, such as "growth faltering," have been suggested[2] but have never come into widespread clinical use. Traditionally, FTT was characterized as "organic failure to thrive," in which the child's growth failure was ascribed to a major medical illness, and "nonorganic failure to thrive," which was attributed primarily to psychological neglect or "maternal deprivation."[3] This simplistic dichotomous conceptualization of FTT is obsolete.[4] In all cases of "nonorganic" FTT and in many cases of "organic" FTT, it is recognized that the proximate cause of growth failure is malnutrition, whether primary or secondary.[4-6] Malnutrition not only jeopardizes the child's growth but also impairs immunocompetence and contributes to concurrent and long-term deficits in cognition and socioaffective competence.[7,8] The modern diagnosis and treatment of FTT focus on the assessment of and therapy for malnutrition and its complications and the contexts in which they occur.[1,4,6,8] The needs of each child who is not thriving should be assessed along 4 parameters—medical, nutritional, developmental, and social—and should include an assessment of the entire family. Before addressing the clinical care of any individual child and family, however, it is important to understand the ecologic context in which childhood malnutrition occurs in a resource-rich nation.

Ecologic Context

Poverty remains the most significant social risk factor for developing FTT, although not all children with FTT come from impoverished or food-insecure families. Conversely, many children without FTT experience food insecurity, defined as a household's inability to consistently provide all its members with enough food for an active and healthy life. Twenty-two percent of children younger than 6 years lived in food-insecure households in the United States in 2010.[9]

The cumulative effects of days and weeks of inadequate diets are reflected in higher rates of short stature among low-income children participating in various national and state surveys in the United States and the United Kingdom, with rates approaching 10% of children with heights below the National Center for Health Statistics (NCHS) 5th percentile norms in most settings.[10,11] Thus, children clinically identified as "failing to thrive" are drawn disproportionately from low-income families and represent the extreme end of a spectrum of nutritional

VI

deprivation of children in or near poverty that often goes unrecognized by health care providers in less obvious cases.[12]

By definition, the federal poverty level ($22 350 in the 48 contiguous states for a family of 4 in 2011) is set at 3 times the annual cost of a minimally nutritious diet represented by the United States Department of Agriculture (USDA) Thrifty Food Plan. In addition to an insufficient budget for food purchases, economically disadvantaged families often lack access to supermarkets and live in homes lacking adequate food-storage and food-preparation facilities.[9,13] National programs designed to protect the health and nutritional status of low-income children have not been adequately funded to meet the needs of many American children or may not be accessible to their families. For example, the USDA reports that only 66% of income eligible households across the nation received food stamps (known now as the Supplemental Nutrition Assistance Program [SNAP]) in 2007.[14] In fiscal year 2010, the maximum monthly food stamp allotment was $200/person in a 1-person household. Food stamp benefits vary across states, according to state budgets; in fiscal year 2010, the average amount of food stamps/SNAP per person/per month was $133.79 and per household/per month was $289.61.[15] Most families do not receive even this inadequate maximum benefit, so many families relying on the program routinely run out of food near the end of the month.[13] The USDA estimates that the Special Supplemental Nutrition Program for Women, Infants, and Children (WIC) reaches only 81% of all eligible women, and the Committee on National Statistics of the National Academies has stated that the actual number is "substantially lower" than USDA estimates.[16,17] WIC program food packages, although substantially revised in 2007 to meet guidelines of the American Academy of Pediatrics (AAP) and recommendations from the Institute of Medicine, are intended as only a supplement to the other food provided in the household and, thus, provide less than 100% of the Recommended Dietary Allowances (RDAs) for a number of nutrients.[16] For some children in certain age groups and many pregnant and postpartum mothers receiving WIC, the combination of WIC food and other food available in the household is insufficient to provide adequate nutrients.[16] Even with simultaneous participation in multiple programs (food stamps/SNAP, WIC, school meals), many low-income families are unable to obtain enough food to avoid frequent episodes of food insecurity and hunger and the chronic mild-to-moderate undernutrition that can ensue[13,18] (see also Chapter 51: Community Nutrition Services).

To minimize the temptation to scapegoat families in clinical assessment and intervention, it is important to recognize that FTT often reflects economic conditions and changes in social policy that are far beyond the control of individual parents or health care providers.[19] Children also fail to thrive in homes of all social classes, in cases of parent-child interactive disorders, feeding disorders of infancy and early childhood,[20] parental psychopathology, family dysfunction, organic pathology, or developmental impairment. The effect of such problems on children's health increases dramatically in the context of poverty; lack of economic means to provide adequate care for a child with increased or unusual nutritional requirements is often a major factor in the development of FTT.[9,13,19] Clinicians must always consider that FTT most often occurs in financial and social circumstances that would make it difficult for any parent to address successfully a child's physical and emotional needs. For this reason, true primary prevention of FTT, which is beyond the scope of this chapter, requires a concerted effort to reduce or eliminate family poverty and must include assessment of the family's psychosocial stresses.[13,16,19,21]

Medical Issues in Evaluation and Treatment

Family History

The assessment of FTT begins with a family history, focusing on issues such as consanguinity, recurrent miscarriage or stillbirth, developmental delay, atopy, human immunodeficiency virus (HIV) infection, alcoholism and other substance use, psychiatric diagnoses, and potentially growth-retarding familial conditions, such as cystic fibrosis, celiac disease, inflammatory bowel disease, or lactose intolerance (see also chapters related to each condition). The height of both parents should be ascertained, as well as their history of growth delay in childhood and timing of puberty. A familial pattern of short stature or constitutional delay of growth may obviate the need for extensive workup if the child is short but not underweight for height.[22] It is critical, however, to assess whether the parents themselves were malnourished as children, as is often the case among immigrant and low-income families. In such cases, the parents' stature does not provide an accurate indication of the child's genetic growth potential.[23] Moreover, an experience of severe childhood deprivation may influence the parents' caregiving practices.[24]

Perinatal Factors

After ascertaining family history, the medical assessment of a child who is not thriving should proceed to a detailed assessment of the child's prenatal and perinatal history by interview and, when possible, by review of neonatal records. This approach not only elucidates potential biological risks to growth but also may be helpful in identifying ongoing psychosocial risk factors that are concurrently influencing postnatal growth. Low birth weight is a major predictor of later referral for FTT. In several clinical series, 10% to 40% of children hospitalized for FTT without a major medical diagnosis had a birth weight less than 2500 g, compared with 7% to 8% of the general population.[4,25] In controlled studies of FTT that excluded infants with birth weights less than 2500 g from their definition of FTT, infants later diagnosed as FTT still had lower birth weights than those who grew normally.[26] To evaluate accurately the effects of perinatal risk factors on later growth, a detailed history should be obtained covering the issues summarized in Table 27.1. It is critical to ascertain not

VI

Table 27.1.
Pregnancy and Delivery

Mother's reproductive history
Age Gravidity/parity/abortions (spontaneous or induced), stillbirths History of pregnancy with identified patient

Conception planned or unplanned
    Difficulties with fertility
    Conceived while mother using contraception
    Was abortion considered?
Mother's nutritional status during pregnancy
    Weight at conception
    Pregnancy weight gain
    WIC
    Hyperemesis
Mother's health habits during pregnancy
    Cigarettes per day
    Alcohol
    Prescribed drug use (particularly anticonvulsants and antidepressants)
    Herbal, traditional, or over-the-counter remedies
    Illicit drug use
    X-rays
    Occupational exposure
Complications of pregnancy
    Infections/high fevers
    Bleeding
    Toxemia
    Violence or trauma
Labor and delivery

Vaginal or cesarean Anesthesia Maternal complications Neonatal status
Gestational age Apgar scores Birth weight, length, head circumference (parameters and percentiles for gestational age) Neonatal course

Mother and child separation
    Need for neonatal intensive care
    Duration of hospitalization for mother and child
Complications: jaundice, respiratory, central nervous system, sepsis, necrotizing enterocolitis
Early feeding difficulties
Transfusions
Eye examination
Hearing examination

only the child's birth weight but also gestational age, length, and head circumference at birth. Such data will identify prematurity as well as various patterns of intrauterine growth retardation that have prognostic implications for later growth.

Prematurity

Children born preterm may be inappropriately labeled as FTT if the percentiles used for assessing growth parameters are not corrected for gestational age by subtracting the number of weeks the child was preterm from the child's postnatal age at time of assessment. Earlier work suggested a statistically significant difference in growth percentiles will be found without such correction in head circumference until 18 months' postnatal age, in weight until 24 months' postnatal age, and in length until 40 months' postnatal age.[27] More recently, it has been recommended that from 42 weeks following birth, former preterm infant born as early as 23 weeks' gestation be plotted on the United Kingdom 2009 preterm growth charts. These have been adapted from the 2006 World Health Organization (WHO) growth standards and corrected for gestational age until 24 months' postnatal age. One should note that these charts are intended for use with English- and Scottish-born infants, and thus, the charts may not reflect the population represented in the WHO Multicentre Growth Reference Study (MGRS) sample (http://www.rcpch.ac.uk/growthcharts).[28] There is no definitive research to show when it is clinically appropriate to discontinue such corrections.[29] Even after correcting for gestational age, infants with very low birth weights (less than 1501 g) may remain smaller than infants born at term for at least the first 3 years of life.[30] In these children, the distribution of mean weight, height, and head circumference is shifted downward relative to the NCHS or WHO norms so that the proportion of children with attained weight or height below the anthropometric cut points for concern is increased.[30] A single study from the developing world suggests that, despite faster linear growth rates, even late preterm children (34-36 weeks' gestational age) are at increased risk of stunting compared with term peers, but wasting among late preterm infants was infrequent.[31] The rate of growth of formerly preterm infants, however, should approximate that of term infants of the same corrected age.[30,32] Moreover, weight for length should resemble that of the reference standard, despite somewhat lower fat stores.[33,34] Preterm and small-for-gestational-age infants with postnatal weight faltering are more likely to show persistent deficits in growth and in cognitive and academic achievement at 8 years of age than are children with similar birth histories whose growth does not falter, with the maximum incidence of growth faltering occurring between 8 and 12 months' corrected age.[29,35]

There is, as yet, no consensus as to which growth curves are optimal for monitoring the postnatal growth of very low birth weight infants (<1500 g).[34] Whatever

VI

the grow curve chosen, the optimal rates of growth for formerly preterm infants that maximize cognitive/developmental outcomes while minimizing risks in adulthood of insulin resistance, hypertension, and ischemic heart disease are not known.[29] In infants of European origin, catch-up growth seems partially to reflect social conditions, such that preterm infants of parents of higher social classes are less likely to show persistent height deficits than those of similar birth weight whose parents are less privileged,[36] highlighting the significant contribution of postnatal socioeconomic conditions to growth faltering. Thus, formerly preterm children who show depressed weight for length, a velocity of weight gain that is decelerating from the standard for corrected age, or growth that progressively deviates from a channel parallel to the growth standard should be assessed carefully for potentially correctable causes of growth faltering. The neurologic, gastrointestinal, and cardiorespiratory sequelae of prematurity, as well as the oral-motor discoordination and behavioral disorganization characteristic of some preterm infants, may all contribute to postnatal malnutrition. Growth difficulties should not be discounted in such children on the grounds that they were "born small."[29]

The most common iatrogenic cause of growth faltering in former preterm infants is a diet inappropriate for corrected as opposed to chronologic age. One common example of this is early discontinuation of the nutrient-dense formula the preterm infant is being fed or initiation of solid feedings at 6 months' postnatal age for an infant born at 28 weeks whose corrected age is only 3 months. Although there are no definitive guidelines, in general, preterm infants born before 34 weeks' gestation should receive a nutrient-dense "preterm infant formula" until they weigh at least 2000 g. Data are inconsistent as to whether the use of these formulas after infants reach 2 kg enhances weight gain length, head circumference, or developmental test scores to 18 months of age. Longer-term outcomes are not known.[37] Such enriched formulas are more expensive than term infant formulas and may be difficult for economically stressed families to afford unless the family receives a physician's prescription to receive WIC. In general, when indicated, these postdischarge formulas should be continued until at least 6 months' corrected age or until the baby's weight for length is maintained above the 25 percentile[38] (see also Chapter 5: Nutritional Needs of the Preterm Infant).

In addition to affecting the infant's behavior or physical growth potential directly, preterm birth and low birth weight also may act indirectly to increase the risk of growth failure by intensifying family stress, both during the long periods some infants spend in the neonatal intensive care unit and thereafter.

Small-for-Gestational-Age Infants

Weight and length at birth reflect both the duration and the rate of growth during gestation. Infants whose rate of intrauterine growth is depressed are at risk of postnatal growth failure, regardless of gestational age. Small-for-gestational-age (SGA) infants are conventionally defined as those with birth weight less than the 10th percentile for gestational age. The degree of risk of postnatal growth failure for SGA infants is not uniform, varying with both the cause of the small size and the pattern of relative deficit in length, weight, or head circumference at birth.

The best prognosis for postnatal growth pertains to SGA infants who are asymmetric—that is, whose weight at birth is disproportionately more depressed than their length or head circumference. Such infants are at risk for FTT because they are often behaviorally difficult.[39] With enhanced postnatal nutrition, however, they can manifest significant catch-up growth in the first 6 to 8 months of life so that later growth trajectories may be within the normal range.[39,40] For such infants, early identification of growth failure and intensive nutritional and environmental intervention is critical because the potential for catch-up growth to repair the intrauterine deficit is maximal in the first 6 months of life.[41] Again, it is not known what the optimal rate of weight gain is for these infants that will optimize cognitive development while not increasing later risk of obesity and insulin resistance, but close monitoring of weight gain and dietary practices is indicated.

SGA infants whose weight, length, and head circumference are proportionately depressed at birth (ie, "symmetric"), carry a relatively poor prognosis for later growth and development. A symmetric pattern should alert the clinician to the possibility of chromosomal abnormalities, intrauterine infections, or prenatal teratogen exposure. For this reason, symmetrically growth-retarded children should be carefully scrutinized for dysmorphic features that may suggest a "syndrome" diagnosis. Exposure to anticonvulsants, including hydantoin and valproate, may be associated with symmetrically depressed size and dysmorphic features.[42] Prenatal exposure to legal and illegal psychoactive substances during pregnancy often contributes to symmetric growth retardation at birth, but the prognostic implications for later growth, particularly somatic growth, are variable.[43]

Prenatal Exposure to Legal Psychoactive Substances and Later Growth

Although heavy use of caffeine prenatally is associated in some studies with depressed intrauterine growth, such use has no detectable effects on the later size of exposed infants.[44] Some investigators, but not all, have noted correlations between heavy cigarette exposure during pregnancy and statistically significant decrements in stature at school age, but the magnitude of the deficit (1 to 2 cm) is usually not large enough to trigger referral for FTT.[45,46] Postnatal use of fluoxetine in breast-feeding women was associated with some reduction in infant weight gain between 2 weeks and 6 months of age.[47] The effects of prenatal alcohol exposure are variable. Growth deficits persist from infancy to school age in children with dysmorphic features consistent with fetal alcohol syndrome and in children from lower-income (but not higher-income) families who were exposed prenatally to alcohol but are not dysmorphic.[46,48,49] Length and head circumference are more depressed than weight in such cases.[46]

Although fetal alcohol syndrome and, perhaps, fetal alcohol spectrum disorder constrain postneonatal growth, clinicians also must remain alert to potentially treatable postneonatal medical and psychosocial factors that may be preventing children with fetal alcohol syndrome or other intrauterine exposures from attaining even their limited growth potential. As with very low birth weight infants, children with fetal alcohol syndrome, in whom rate of growth deviates from their own previously established patterns, should be evaluated meticulously.[50,51] Neurologically based oral-motor difficulties are often associated with fetal alcohol syndrome and may limit caloric intake, unless gastrostomy tubes are placed.[51] Even more commonly, the poor weight gain of children with fetal alcohol syndrome who remain in the care of mothers with active untreated alcoholism may represent inadequate care and nutrition. Such children should not remain in conditions of profound deprivation on the grounds that they have fetal alcohol syndrome and cannot grow. Clinical experience shows that with appropriate nutritional, neurodevelopmental, and psychosocial intervention, children with fetal alcohol syndrome and fetal alcohol spectrum disorder can be brought into the normal range of weight for height but may remain short and microcephalic despite intervention.[52]

Prenatal Exposure to Illicit Psychoactive Substances and Later Growth

Until recently, the 3 most frequently used illicit drugs during pregnancy were marijuana, cocaine, and opiates. Concern is now also focusing on methamphetamine exposure during pregnancy. There are an increasing number of follow-up studies of the growth of infants exposed to marijuana, cocaine, or opiates beyond the neonatal period. Infants exposed to marijuana during pregnancy have been reported as having a decreased weight and length and sometimes head circumference, compared with unexposed newborn infants, presumably because smoking marijuana, like smoking tobacco, increases maternal carbon monoxide levels and decreases fetal oxygenation.[53-55] In one long-term follow-up study, of children at 6 years of age had decreased heights correlated with prenatal marijuana exposure.[55] However, in a similar study of prenatal marijuana exposure, children with a history of prenatal marijuana exposure had weights and lengths significantly greater than their nonexposed peers, even after controlling for confounding variables.[56] Therefore, it is unclear whether prenatal marijuana exposure is a biological risk factor for later FTT, and clinicians should not dismiss FTT in these children by attributing it to prenatal marijuana exposure.

Intrauterine cocaine exposure is independently associated with decrements in gestational age and with consistently lower birth weight, length, and head circumference.[54] At age 7 to 16 weeks, no difference was found in feeding behaviors between infants who were exposed prenatally to cocaine and those who were not exposed.[57] If levels of exposure to cigarettes and alcohol are not controlled statistically, researchers have noted small but statistically significant decrements in head circumference, and in one cohort, in weight, among children who were exposed to cocaine in utero and followed until 3 years of age.[58,59] However, in 2 studies that controlled statistically for the level of prenatal exposure to tobacco and alcohol, no incremental negative effect of prenatal cocaine exposure was noted on weight, height, or head circumference.[60,61] More recent studies with follow-up to school age are not consistent, with the majority showing no effect of prenatal cocaine exposure on weight and inconsistent effects on height.[62] Accelerated rates of postneonatal weight gain have been noted after prenatal cocaine exposure.[58,60,63] Therefore, clinicians should not accept prenatal exposure to cocaine as a sufficient explanation for postnatal failure to gain weight.

Intrauterine exposure to heroin or methadone also has been linked to depressed birth weight, length, and head circumference, but follow-up studies of the growth patterns of these infants are not entirely consistent. Wilson et al[64] reported that 3- to 6-year-old children with intrauterine exposure to heroin were smaller in all growth parameters than were nonexposed social class controls. In most studies, however, smaller head circumference but few differences in somatic growth were noted when opiate-exposed infants were compared with children of the same social class without opiate exposure.[65]

A single, large follow-up study of children up to 3 years of age with intrauterine methamphetamine exposure, found that, compared with similar unexposed children, those with intrauterine methamphetamine exposure were marginally shorter but did not differ in weight for age, weight for length, or head circumference.[66]

The quality of care the child is receiving at the time of referral also must be evaluated, because continued parental substance abuse may be contributing to concurrent nutritional deprivation of the child. Even though intrauterine exposure to psychoactive substances may cause a decrease in weight, length, and head circumference at birth, most such substances do not inhibit a child from showing postnatal somatic catch-up growth in response to adequate nutrition.[43] Heavy prenatal exposure to alcohol or opiates may be associated with relative microcephaly, and fetal alcohol syndrome is characterized by persistent short stature. However, intrauterine exposure to the most commonly used psychoactive substances may not entirely explain a child who is underweight for height or one whose growth progressively deviates from a previously established trajectory. Other medical and environmental factors must be assessed.

VI

Postnatal Medical Issues

Almost all severe and chronic childhood illnesses can cause growth failure. The mechanisms of such failure are multiple—enzymatic, metabolic, and endocrine in some cases—but also nutritional and psychosocial.[67,68] Chronic physical conditions that necessitate procedures, such as gastrostomy tube or nasogastric feedings, may impede the development of normal patterns of feeding (see also Chapter 24: Enteral Nutrition).

Hospitalization of children with FTT should not be regarded as a diagnostic test for chronic illness.[69] According to an old myth, environmentally deprived children ("nonorganic" FTT) grow in the hospital, whereas children with serious medical illnesses ("organic" FTT) do not. In fact, a positive growth response to hospitalization is a poor indicator of major organic illness, because both children with such illness and children with primary malnutrition will grow if given adequate caloric intake for their needs.[70] Chronically ill children who do well in the hospital usually have complex technical, psychosocial, and nutritional needs that can be met by multiple shifts of highly trained medical personnel but overwhelm parents who are not receiving adequate caregiving support at home. Conversely, unless the hospital provides specialized milieu therapy, usually not available in acute care wards, children with severe interactive feeding disorders or depression may deteriorate nutritionally in the hospital, because separation from primary attachment figures and interaction with multiple caregivers may exacerbate their affective and behavioral feeding difficulties. Children who are simply underfed do well either in the hospital or in any setting when adequate calories are offered. Thus, response to hospitalization, in itself, does not necessarily contribute to identifying the cause of FTT.

Whether in inpatient or outpatient settings, chronic illnesses severe enough to jeopardize weight gain usually can be suggested by a meticulous history and physical examination (Tables 27.2 and 27.3). The list of occult medical conditions presenting as FTT is relatively circumscribed, and often, these are identified during the review of systems (outlined in Table 27.2), focusing on infections, neurologic symptoms, and conditions that interfere with caloric intake, retention, or utilization. In reported series of children hospitalized for FTT of unknown origin, the most common previously undiagnosed conditions affect the gastrointestinal tract, including chronic nonspecific diarrhea, celiac disease, food allergies, gastroesophageal reflux, cystic fibrosis, and lactose intolerance.[3,71-73] Immigrant children, those who have recently traveled abroad, and children attending congregate child care or living in homeless shelters should be evaluated for giardiasis and enteric pathogens if they have gastrointestinal tract symptoms, such as anorexia, diarrhea, or abdominal pain, because these infections are treatable causes of depressed appetite, malabsorption, and growth failure.[74]

Table 27.2.
Child's Postnatal Health History

Immunizations
Allergies
Surgeries
Hospitalizations
Current medications
Midparental height
Consanguinity
Heritable conditions
Review of systems
Timing of onset of growth faltering
   Weight loss
   Diarrhea/vomiting
   Dysphagia
   Snoring, difficulty with tonsils or adenoids
   Recurring pneumonia, otitis, or sinusitis
   Painful teeth
   Loss of previously acquired milestones, seizures
   Thrush/recurrent monilial rash
   Atopic dermatitis, hives
   Hearing loss, visual impairment
   Acute life-threatening events
Pets
Travel
Passive tobacco exposure
Congregate child care

Outside the gastrointestinal system, clinicians should consider urinary tract infections and renal tubular acidosis as potentially clinically silent contributors to FTT. Subtle neurologic dysfunction manifested as fine motor and oral motor dysfunction also should be considered and evaluated by direct observation.[75] Poor appetite, observed sometimes as early as the first 6 weeks of life,[2] delayed or dysfunctional oral-motor development with unusually prolonged feedings,[76] and deficient signaling of needs during mealtimes may contribute to FTT by decreasing nutrient intake. Although children with autism spectrum disorders, as a group, may show early acceleration of somatic and head circumference growth,[77] the constipation and intense food selectivity that are more prevalent in children with autism than in typically developing children[78] may, in some cases, manifest as early FTT, even before the diagnosis of autism spectrum disorder can be made.[79]

Both overdiagnosis and underdiagnosis of "food allergy" or food sensitivities, such as lactose or gluten intolerance, can contribute to FTT. Only those reactions that are the consequence of an immune response to a food or food additive are clinically considered to be food allergies, which are a subgroup of adverse reactions to foods.[80]

VI

An exceedingly restrictive diet based on an imprecise or factitious diagnosis of food allergy may present as FTT. It is crucial that the cause of an apparent adverse reaction to a food be aggressively sought. Whereas negative skin tests are 95% accurate, positive tests are only 50% accurate and must be confirmed by history or a food challenge.[66] Conversely, 30% of atopic dermatitis in young children is triggered by food allergy, so evaluation for food allergy should be considered in any child with FTT and eczema, especially if the eczema persists in spite of optimal topical management or the child has a history of reaction after ingestion of a specific food.[80] Food allergy should also be considered even in the absence of atopic dermatitis, when young children present with otherwise unexplained reflux, nausea, vomiting, diarrhea, or irritability with food refusal and weight loss.[80] It may take as long as 14 days to see a clinical response to an elimination diet. A double-blind, placebo-controlled oral food challenge is the "gold standard" for food allergy diagnosis but is often not practical in primary care settings.[81] Skin or serum tests for immunoglobulin (Ig) E anti-food allergens are more commonly used in this setting. Because children often "outgrow" their adverse reaction to cow milk, soy, and egg white by 3 years of age, such evaluations should be repeated periodically so that the child's diet does not remain unnecessarily restricted[81] (see also Chapter 35: Food Allergy).

In addition to primary illnesses that may be associated with secondary malnutrition and growth failure, the clinician must be alert to the medical complications of primary malnutrition, particularly recurring infections and lead poisoning. Malnutrition severe enough to produce growth failure also impairs immunocompetence, particularly cell-mediated immunity and the production of complement and secretory IgA.[82,83] Recurring otitis media and gastrointestinal and respiratory tract illnesses are more common among children who fail to thrive than among well-nourished children of the same age.[11,84]

In recent years, the differential diagnosis of FTT with recurring infections has expanded to include HIV infection, usually acquired perinatally. Women in the United States of childbearing age acquire HIV primarily via heterosexual contact, making risk factors more difficult to discern. The diagnosis must also be ruled out in children of immigrants from areas where HIV is endemic. For information on HIV risk factors, refer to guidelines provided by the Centers for Disease Control and Prevention[85] (see also Chapter 40: HIV Infection).

Even among the majority who are not HIV infected, children who fail to thrive are often trapped in an infection-malnutrition cycle. With each illness, the child's appetite and nutrient intake decrease while nutrient requirements increase as a result of fever, diarrhea, and vomiting. In settings in which nutrient intake is already marginal, even when the child is well, cumulative nutritional deficits occur, leaving the child increasingly vulnerable to more severe and prolonged infections and even less adequate growth. Commonly, in developing countries and occasionally in resource-rich countries, malnourished children succumb to fulminating infections (see also Chapter 36: Nutrition and Immunity).

Elevated lead concentrations correlate with impaired growth, even in the 5- to 35-μg/dL range.[86] Here, too, a negative cycle develops. Nutritional deficiencies of iron and calcium enhance the absorption of lead and other heavy metals.[87] As lead concentrations increase, constipation, abdominal pain, and anorexia occur, leading to even less adequate dietary intake.[88] In one study, 16% of children with FTT had lead concentrations high enough to warrant chelation.[89]

Physical Examination and Laboratory Evaluation

The physical examination of the child who fails to thrive, summarized in Table 27.3, has 3 goals: (1) identification of chronic illness, (2) recognition of syndromes that alter growth, and (3) documentation of the effects of malnutrition. Some findings may be nonspecific and require elucidation by laboratory assessment; for example, hepatic enlargement may be seen with primary malnutrition, acquired immunodeficiency syndrome (AIDS), inborn errors of metabolism, or primary liver disease.

Table 27.3.
Physical Examination

Vital signs: blood pressure if over 2 y, temperature, pulse, respirations, oxygen saturation
Anthropometry (see Table 27.5)
General appearance: activity, affect, posture
Skin: hygiene, rashes, trauma (bruises, burns, scars)
Head: hair whorls, color and pluckability of hair, occipital alopecia, fontanel size and patency, frontal bossing, sutures, shape, facial dysmorphisms, philtrum
Eyes: ptosis, strabismus, fundoscopic examination where possible, palpebral fissures, conjunctival pallor, icterus, cataracts
Ears: external form, rotation, tympanic membranes
Mouth, nose, throat: thinness of lip, hydration, dental eruption and hygiene caries, glossitis, cheilosis, gum bleeding, marked tonsillar enlargement
Neck: hairline, masses, lymphadenopathy
Cardiovascular: evidence of congestive heart failure, cyanosis
Abdomen: protuberance, hepatosplenomegaly, masses
Genitalia: malformations, hygiene, trauma
Rectum: fissures, trauma, hemorrhoids
Extremities: edema, dysmorphisms, rachitic changes, nails and nail beds
Neurologic: cranial nerves, reflexes, tone, retention of primitive reflexes, quality of voluntary movement

Laboratory evaluation should be restrained and guided by history and the findings of the physical examination. For example, a child who has no symptoms of cardiorespiratory distress or heart murmur does not need an electrocardiogram or echocardiogram. Basic laboratory studies should be used to identify derangements caused by malnutrition and to rule out the common potentially occult diseases just described. All children should have a complete blood cell (CBC) count with differential, assessment of lead concentration, urinalysis, and tuberculin test if in a demographic risk group. Iron deficiency with or without anemia is a common finding. In cases in which the CBC count is unrevealing, measures of iron nutriture[90] may be considered. If the child does not respond promptly to nutritional intervention, a more detailed laboratory evaluation is warranted.[91] Blood urea nitrogen, creatinine and serum electrolytes, and urine pH not only rule out renal failure and renal tubular acidosis but are mandatory in children with recurrent or persistent vomiting or diarrhea, clinically obvious dehydration, or severe malnutrition, which is often associated with hypokalemia. In children with severe anthropometric deficits, it is useful to obtain serum albumin and prealbumin (transthyretin) concentrations to assess protein status and to determine serum alkaline phosphatase, calcium, and phosphorus concentrations. A decreased alkaline phosphatase concentration suggests zinc deficiency; an increased concentration, especially if associated with a decreased phosphorous concentration, is suggestive of rickets.[92] HIV testing, sweat tests, and stool assessments for *Giardia* organisms and other parasites should be performed in epidemiologically at-risk populations.[83] Serum IgA and anti-tissue transglutaminase antibodies screen for celiac disease.[93] Serum IgE testing for food allergies should be considered in children with FTT and atopic dermatitis as well as for those with a history of rash, urticaria, or recurring vomiting and diarrhea after ingestion of selected foods. In a child with FTT and vomiting not explained by food allergies and unresponsive to empiric management, radiographic or endoscopic studies may be indicated to rule out anatomic abnormalities, gastroesophageal reflux, and esophagitis, particularly among children with neurologic impairments and unexplained respiratory symptoms.[94] Children with unexplained vomiting, an enlarged liver, jaundice, or any suspicion of inborn errors of metabolism should also have liver functions evaluated.[91] If inborn errors of metabolism are suspected on the basis of the initial workup, referral to a subspecialist in metabolic disorders should be considered.[91]

For short children with weight proportionate to height, bone-age radiographic studies of the wrists and knees are helpful in discriminating those who are constitutionally short (bone age equals chronologic age and is greater than height age) from those with growth hormone or thyroid deficiencies or chronic malnutrition (bone age equals height age and is less than chronologic age). A child who has short stature and whose weight is lower on the growth chart than height does not have an endocrine cause for short stature and should be evaluated for FTT.

Careful physical examination will usually identify untreated dental cavities and abscesses that make eating and chewing painful and lead to inadequate caloric intake.[95] Large tonsils or a history of chronic snoring warrant ear, nose, and throat evaluation and possibly a sleep study, because tonsillar-adenoidal hypertrophy and sleep-disordered breathing may contribute to growth failure.[96] It is important to observe a child feeding, because subtle oral-motor difficulties may interfere with dietary intake in children with subclinical neurologic abnormalities.[75]

Medical Management

The pediatric health care provider should play an ongoing role in the management of children who fail to thrive. Children with FTT must be seen more frequently than is dictated by routine health management schedules to monitor their growth and development in response to interventions. Weekly to biweekly visits are often necessary at the beginning of diagnosis and treatment. Meticulous management of concurrent chronic illness is essential, enlisting and coordinating assessments in as many disciplines as necessary. Lead poisoning, if identified, should be treated according to standard protocols.

The health care provider must take an aggressive stance to interrupt the infection-malnutrition cycle. Because of the compromised immune status of malnourished children, children with FTT should receive all immunizations recommended by the AAP, even during supply shortages, if possible. The AAP immunization schedule is available online at http://www2.aap.org/immunization/.[97] Families should be instructed to seek care at the first signs of infection so that immediate workup and treatment are provided. Recurring otitis or sinusitis are indications for referral to an otolaryngologist. In addition, for each episode of acute illness, the clinician should provide specific instruction about appropriate diet during and after the illness to try to maintain and repair nutritional status. A child should never receive a clear liquid diet for more than 24 hours.[74]

Hospitalization is indicated for severely malnourished children, for children with serious intercurrent infections, for those whose safety is in question, or if the specialized coordination of disciplines or diagnostic procedures is necessary and can be assembled most efficiently inside the hospital. In many centers, the availability of interdisciplinary outpatient clinics for the diagnosis and management of FTT has greatly reduced the need for hospitalization.[98] Referral for specialized inpatient or outpatient assessment and care should be considered, however, for any child who has not responded to 2 or 3 months of intensive management in a primary care setting.

Nutritional Evaluation and Treatment

The major components of a nutritional history for a child who is failing to thrive are summarized in Table 27.4. The assessment should focus not only on current feeding practices, but also on the development of feeding since birth. Often, a child's growth failure is triggered by a shift in feeding practices. For example, the

VI

shift from soy formula to whole milk at 12 months of age, as mandated by the WIC program, may trigger FTT in a child with milk protein allergy.[99] In many children, feeding struggles and growth failure begin with the introduction of solid foods at 5 to 7 months of age. In some instances, the introduction of gluten-containing cereals triggers celiac disease and growth failure. Nutritional rickets occurs almost exclusively in breastfed infants who have not received vitamin D supplementation as recommended by the AAP.[100] Thus, comparison of the lifelong feeding history with the growth curve can provide diagnostic clues to the nutritional risk factors in FTT.

Table 27.4.
Nutritional Evaluation Protocol

Interview
Feeding history adjusted for age
   Breast- or formula-fed
   Age solids introduced
   Age switched to whole milk
   Food allergy or intolerance
   Vitamin or mineral supplements
Current feeding behaviors
   Difficulties with sucking, chewing, or swallowing
   Frequency of feeding
   Duration of feeding episodes
   Who feeds
   Where fed (alone or held, with or separate from family, lap or high chair)
   "Finickiness," negativism
   Perceived appetite
   Pica
Caregiver's nutrition knowledge
   Difficulties with English or literacy
   Adequacy of developmentally appropriate nutrition information
   Unusual dietary belief (religious or food fad constraints on permitted foods): are some foods perceived as dangerous?
Adequacy of financial resources for food purchase
   SNAP (formerly food stamps): how much/month for how many people
   WIC
   Adequacy of earned income
   Benefits: Transitional Aid to Needy Families (TANF), Supplemental Social Security Income (SSI) Unemployment Insurance
   Recent change in food budget (cuts or increases in benefits, new mouths to feed, job gain or loss)
   Family's knowledge of how to budget food purchasing
Material resources for food preparation and storage
   Refrigeration
   Cooking facilities
   Running water
   24-h dietary recall: was yesterday typical?
Food frequency

In assessing current feeding practices of the child who fails to thrive, the clinician should ascertain when, where, how, and by whom the child is fed as well as what the child is fed and why. Comprehensive assessment of feeding problems requires a combination of methods, such as structured interviews with primary caregivers and direct observation of the child's response to feeding in multiple situations. Breastfeeding difficulties should be managed by a pediatric health care provider with expertise in such issues, perhaps with input from a certified lactation consultant. Overdilution of formula is a readily treatable contributor to FTT in infancy.[101] A licensed clinician should elicit behavioral feeding problems (eg, spitting out food, tantrums during meals, food refusal) and determine how the parents have tried to manage the child's problems.[102] When language and literacy permit, caregivers may be asked to supply a few days of food-intake records. Ideally, the history should be supplemented by a home-based feeding observation that will elucidate not only interactive or mechanical feeding difficulties but also the material conditions of the home and family routines.[103]

Heptinstall et al[104] found that inconsistent timing of the presentation of meals and dysfunctional mealtime procedures, such as solitary meals without supervision, occurred more frequently in growth-deficient children than in normal controls. Common sources of difficulty in the timing of feedings include infrequent feedings (restricting a toddler to 3 meals a day), constant feedings (grazing), and lack of a consistent feeding schedule. Children are often fed in inappropriate settings, which may or may not be under the parents' control. For example, children in welfare motels or homeless shelters may have to be fed sitting on the floor or the bed because there is nowhere else to sit. Many parents can be encouraged to put the child in a high chair, when one is available, and not to position the child in front of the television or other distractions during feeding. A hammer-lock hold in a parent's lap is usually ineffective and uncomfortable for both parent and child. A home observation also will elucidate the affective tone of the feeding process and identify dysfunctional interactions, such as interrupting the feeding too often to clean the child, struggles over the child's efforts to feed independently, or inappropriate coaxing or threatening of the child. Efforts should be made to identify all the different caregivers (relatives, neighbors, siblings, child care providers, etc) involved in feeding the child to enlist these individuals in improving the child's nutritional intake.

In addition to how the child is fed, the clinician must ascertain what the child is fed and why. The family's level of nutritional knowledge and dietary beliefs should be assessed in conjunction with the family's exposure to diverse traditional and new media. Parents and children are continually bombarded with nutritional misinformation from television and other commercial sources, urging them to spend their scarce food resources on expensive heavily sweetened or salted foods of low nutritional quality. Television alone exposes young people to over 40 000 advertisements per year; this does not include advertising within programming, nor advertising on the Internet, within video games, or in other forms of marketing.[105] Certain groups of parents, particularly adolescents, and those who are intellectually limited or illiterate, are particularly likely to lack adequate information regarding nutritionally sound feeding practices. Immigrants are at risk unless they are able to obtain or prepare culturally appropriate foods. Any parent pressed for time may choose convenience over nutrition, regardless of income, education, or literacy level. Strict vegan or other highly restricted diets may also prove inadequate to support growth.[106] Parents seeking to prevent obesity or cardiovascular disease also may inadvertently cause their toddlers to fail to thrive by overzealous enforcement of a low-fat "prudent diet" appropriate for adults but not for growing children.[107] Restricted diets imposed because of actual or presumed food allergies or gluten intolerance often are not adequately supplemented with alternate sources of calories and micronutrients, with consequent nutritional deficiencies.[80]

As discussed in the introduction, the family's economic resources for food purchase, food storage, and food preparation must be tactfully ascertained. Finally, a 24-hour dietary recall and 7-day food frequency are essential in determining the quality and quantity of the child's diet. Common findings among children with FTT include excessive intake of juice, water, tea, coffee, or carbonated and sweetened beverages, including "sports drinks," which depress appetite but provide few nutrients. In addition, fruit juices high in fructose or sorbitol have been associated with malabsorption and osmotic diarrhea in some cases of FTT.[108] Low-income families may have particular difficulties in meeting the needs of children with increased nutritional needs (such as children born preterm or children with significant heart or lung disease) or those with medically restricted and, therefore, more expensive diets, as in the cases of multiple food allergies, lactose intolerance, or gluten-sensitive enteropathy.[109]

Anthropometric Assessment

Serial anthropometric assessments of weight, length/height, and head circumference are critical to the management of FTT. Initial measurements of the growth trajectory form the basis for triage and calculation of caloric needs (see subsequent discussion) and provide some prognostic information regarding later developmental potential. Frequent follow-up assessments also provide the clearest indication of the effectiveness of intervention.

Children referred for FTT must be measured in a standard fashion by trained personnel using the same scale and linear measuring instrument at each visit, according to published protocols for obtaining accurate and reproducible anthropometric measurements. Standardized protocols include the *National Health and Examination Survey (NHANES) Anthropometry Procedures Manual*[110] and the World Health Organization training video or procedural manual.[111] Infants should be weighed naked, and young children should wear underwear only. Once these measurements have been obtained, values must be plotted on the appropriate growth chart. Head circumference (which should be measured at each contact on every child younger than 3 years) should be plotted on the growth grid consistent with the one being used to plot somatic growth.

Before September 2010, the growth charts from the Centers for Disease Control and Prevention/National Center for Health Statistics (CDC/NCHS) from 2000 (www.cdc.gov/growthcharts/)[112] were recommended for children of all ages in the United States. In September 2010, the AAP and CDC published joint recommendations supporting continued used of the CDC/NCHS charts for children older than 2 years and supporting the use of WHO charts (www.who.int/childgrowth/standards/en) for all children younger than 2 years, regardless of breastfeeding status, ethnic origin, gestational age, or other factors. The joint publication encouraged continued research into the clinical implications of using these standards in US practice, particularly among low birth weight or preterm infants.[113]

Whether or not these standards are optimal for health promotion of US children is yet to be determined. The WHO charts and the CDC/NCHS charts appear similar at first glance; measurement practices are the same, and correction for prematurity has not changed. Clinicians accustomed to the CDC/NCHS charts will need to adapt to new percentiles that should trigger concern and further evaluation; rather than the 5th and 95th percentiles, the WHO standards use the 2.3rd and 97.7th percentiles (±2 standard deviations). When using the CDC/NCHS growth charts for children ages 2 through 19 years, clinicians should continue to use the 5th and 95th percentiles as upper and lower bounds for concern.

The clinical implications of the use of the WHO growth standards to determine those at risk of growth failure is an unresolved issue. The population studied for the WHO standard was optimally nourished, including exclusive breastfeeding for 4 to 6 months, and did not include children of the lowest socioeconomic status, whereas the CDC/NCHS data were derived from a random sample of the US population, which was largely not breastfed and included all socioeconomic strata.[112] Anthropometric characteristics of these 2 populations differ, which can lead to differences in classification for an individual child when plotted on the 2 graphs; for instance, there are certain children who will have low weight for age according to the CDC/NCHS charts but will be in the normal range on the WHO charts. Functional issues affecting the children in this "seam," including access to

VI

developmental intervention and benefit programs such as WIC, are currently being investigated.

The relationship of the child's weight and height to each other and to growth standards (WHO) or reference norms (CDC/NCHS) is used to identify both the chronicity and the severity of nutritional deficit (http://www.cdc.gov/growthcharts/).[112]

Weight for age, the most powerful predictor of mortality, provides a composite measure of past and present nutrition and growth, reflecting both current and previous insults.[114] When constitutional, endocrine, and genetic factors can be ruled out, decreased length or height for age is considered a manifestation of the cumulative effects of chronic malnutrition.[115] In contrast, decreased weight for height indicates acute and recent nutritional deprivation.[115] The trajectory leading to short stature is often not known to the clinician if a child presents for FTT without available documentation of previous measurements, so all possibilities must be considered. The CDC/NCHS norms provide weight-for-length/height graphs for children up to 6 years of age as well as body mass index (BMI) norms for children older than 2 years. The WHO standards use only BMI instead of weight-for length/height. Children at highest risk of mortality and morbidity are those for whom both weight for height or BMI and height for age are decreased, indicating acute malnutrition superimposed on a chronic problem.[115]

Most children with a diagnosis of FTT have weights or heights at or below the lower percentiles on the WHO or CDC/NCHS charts, so additional calculations are necessary to quantify the severity of nutritional risk. Historically, techniques devised by Waterlow (mild/moderate/severe acute and chronic malnutrition) and Gomez (degree of malnutrition) have been used to determine the severity of a child's FTT status. Criteria and calculations for both techniques are described in Table 27.5. Neither of these approaches have been tested using the WHO standards, which provide precalculated z-score indicators. Decisions regarding hospitalization for FTT may come down to clinical judgment, particularly when using the WHO charts. Children older than 2 years (thus, measured using CDC/NCHS growth references) with third-degree malnutrition (weight for age less than 60% of median, or weight for height less than 70% of median) are in acute danger of severe morbidity and possible mortality from their malnutrition and should be hospitalized, if possible. Calculating a patient's z-score, which is a standardized score using the standard deviation as the unit of measurement, will show how far from the population mean a child's parameters lie and will give a more accurate representation of how malnourished the child is in comparison to a healthy child of that gestational age. As can be seen see in the subsequent example, the z-score will change depending on whether a clinician uses the CDC/NCHS reference or the WHO growth standards.

Table 27.5.
Percent of Median Values as an Indicator of Severity of Nutritional Deficit

Grade of Malnutrition	Weight for Age	Height for Age	Weight for Height
Normal	90-110	>95	>90
First degree (mild)	75-89	90-94	80-90
Second degree (moderate)	60-74	85-89	70-79
Third degree (severe)	<60	<85	<70

The goal of nutritional intervention in FTT is to achieve "catch-up" growth, that is, growth at a faster-than-normal rate for age so that the child's relative deficit of body size is restored—that is, the child's length or weight is improving relative to the median (50th percentile) for his or her age or length.[116] If the child with an established growth deficit simply resumes growth at the normal rate for age, relative deficits persist compared with children of the same age who have always grown normally. To assess whether catch-up growth is occurring, the clinician must be aware of age-specific changes in normal growth rates, as summarized by Guo et al.[117] Median weight gain in the first 3 months of life is 26 to 31 g/day; from 3 to 6 months is 17 to 18 g/day; from 6 to 9 months is 12 to 13 g/day; from 9 to 12 months is 9 g/day; and from 12 months onward is 7 to 9 g/day. Pediatric nutritionists also frequently refer to adaptations of Fomon's catch-up growth parameters based on a 1982 body composition study, which include catch-up growth for preterm infants.[118] The generally accepted goal for catch-up growth is 2 to 3 times the average rate of weight gain for corrected age. Thus, a 1-year-old child who is gaining 30 g/day is showing excellent catch-up growth, whereas a 1-month-old infant who also is gaining 30 g/day is growing at only the normal rate for age and will not repair existing deficits. Rather, the 1-month-old infant should be gaining 60 to 90 g/day to catch up to his or her age group. The goal for catch-up growth must be continually revised as the child matures and gradually decreases as the child's weight for height approaches the target level. Such diligence ensures catch-up growth occurs without a child eventually becoming overweight later in childhood.

Principles of Nutritional Treatment

To achieve catch-up growth, the underweight child must receive nutrients in excess of the normal age-specific requirements of the RDAs for age.[119] RDA is used, as opposed to the umbrella-term Dietary Reference Intake (DRI), because RDA calculations are focused on an individual, and the DRI is a population-wide

VI

reference. One commonly used formula based on the RDA for weight age (age at which child's current weight would be 50th percentile) is[120]:

$$\text{kcal per kg required} = \frac{\text{RDA for weight age (kcal/kg)} \times \text{Ideal weight for height}}{\text{Actual weight}}$$

where "ideal" weight is the median weight for the patient's length/ height (as read from the appropriate WHO or CDC/NCHS weight for length/height curves).

For example, a 6.5-month-old term male infant with a weight of 6.1 kg and length of 64.5 cm has the following anthropometric measures according to the CDC/NCHS and WHO criteria.[121] Weight age is approximately 3 months in CDC/NCHS criteria and 2 months in WHO criteria. The z-scores only vary slightly in this child's case, but by either classification, a clinician would need to consider how to achieve catch-up growth. Because his RDA for calories for a weight age of 2 months is 108 kcal/kg/day and his ideal weight for his length (64.5 cm) according to WHO standards is 6.98 kg, his estimated caloric requirement for catch-up growth is (108 kcal/kg/day × 6.98 kg)/6.1 kg = 124 cal/kg/day. Similarly, because his RDA for protein is 2.2 g/kg/day, his protein requirement for catch-up growth is (2.2 × 6.98)/6.1 = 2.5 g/kg/day.

Case Example:
6.5-month-old male with a weight of 6.1kg and a length of 64.5cm, measured lying recumbent

Measurement	z-Score CDC/NCHS	Percentile by CDC/NCHS	z-Score 2006 WHO	Percentile by 2006 WHO
Weight/age	−2.52	0.6th	−2.58	0.5th
Length/age	−1.35	8.5th	−1.82	3.5th
Weight/length (CDC/NCHS) or BMI (WHO)	−1.96	2.5th	−1.98	2.4th

Nutritional rehabilitation must address the child's needs for micronutrients as well as calories and protein. Iron deficiency, with or without associated anemia, is seen in as many as one half of all children presenting with FTT.[1] Vitamin D deficiency/rickets also has been described.[92] Even among children whose micronutrient stores are adequate at initial presentation with FTT, the nutrient requirements from rapid tissue synthesis during catch-up growth may produce nutritional deficiencies. Whether or not zinc status can be measured, zinc supplementation should be provided to meet the RDA, but not in excess, because appropriate zinc supplementation has been shown to decrease the energy cost of weight gain.[122,123] A multivitamin supplement containing the RDA for all vitamins and for iron and zinc should, therefore, be prescribed routinely for children with FTT during nutritional rehabilitation, with additional supplementation of iron or vitamin D to therapeutic levels in children with iron deficiency or low serum vitamin D. Although once-a-day vitamin supplements help reduce pressure on caregivers to ensure that their child is receiving a completely balanced diet, it is important that clinicians continue to support healthy feeding practices, including the incorporation of fruits and vegetables. For example, a finicky eater may be persuaded to eat vegetables if mixed with cheese. Pediatric nutritionists can help caregivers and children develop eating habits not only to solve the acute nutrition issues but also to foster healthy eating practices for later in life.

In general, it is not possible for a child to eat twice the normal volume of food to obtain the nutrient levels necessary for catch-up growth. Instead, the child's usual diet must be fortified to increase nutrient density, for example, by providing formula of 24 to 30 kcal/oz rather than the standard 20 kcal/oz. Several prepackaged 30-kcal/oz preparations, both cow milk and soy based, for children 1 to 6 years of age are now commercially available.[116] However, care must be taken that these formulas are used as supplements in small doses after nutrient-dense meals rather than as meal replacements. Detailed protocols for other methods of dietary supplementation have been published elsewhere.[124] The participation of an experienced pediatric nutritionist is critical in developing a dietary regimen appropriate for each child.

The process of refeeding to promote catch-up growth must be undertaken with care in children with third- and severe second-degree malnutrition. If high food intakes are provided at the beginning of nutritional resuscitation, these children may develop a refeeding syndrome with vomiting, diarrhea, and circulatory decompensation.[125] To minimize these complications, such children should, for the first 7 to 10 days of treatment, be restricted to the normal dietary intake for age, offered as frequent small feedings. During a hospitalization, clinicians need to be aware that this may not coincide with cafeteria schedules and may require scheduling of additional feedings. Intake may then be gradually advanced over the next week to a diet that meets the calculated requirements for catch-up growth. Moderately and mildly malnourished children may be offered food ad libitum while calorie counts are maintained. Once a baseline of spontaneous intake is established, preferred foods may be enriched to bring dietary intake to catch-up levels.

Depending on the severity of the initial deficit, 2 days to 2 weeks may be required to initiate catch-up growth.[5] Less severely malnourished children who are not hospitalized should be monitored frequently as outpatients during this phase. Accelerated growth must then be maintained for 4 to 9 months to restore a child's weight for height.[5,116] Biweekly to monthly outpatient visits for weight checks, adjustment of diet, and treatment of intercurrent medical problems are essential during this period. Intake and rates of growth spontaneously decelerate toward normal levels for age as deficits are repleted. Because weight is restored more rapidly than height, caregivers may become alarmed that the child is becoming obese. They should be reassured that the catch-up growth in height lags behind that in weight by several months but that balance will occur if dietary treatment is gradually adjusted.[126] Although no firm guidelines exist, a criterion for discharge from a specialized outpatient program is often when the child is able to maintain weight for height above the 10th percentile and a normal rate of weight gain for age on at least 2 assessments, 1 month apart, on a normal diet for age (ie, the weight-for-height deficit is repaired and the child no longer requires an especially enriched diet to sustain normal growth).

Psychosocial Issues in Evaluation and Treatment

Intellectual Development

Children who experience prolonged malnutrition and/or chronic FTT appear to be at risk of intellectual deficits severe enough to affect their learning potential.[127,128] The severity of developmental impairments varies substantially, however, among preschool- and school-aged children with histories of early FTT.[129-133] Studies have underscored the central importance of a history of serious malnutrition as well as the quality of the home environment and educational experience in predicting the cognitive development of affected children in later life.[131,132,134-138]

Intellectual assessment can be a productive means of involving the parents of children with FTT in their child's treatment planning.[139] Observing their child's assessment helps parents to appreciate the nature of their children's intellectual strengths and difficulties. When parents have observed developmental testing, it is also easier and more productive to discuss the pattern of their child's intellectual strengths and difficulties with them. If parents are invited to discuss their child's development and participate in the evaluation, they are less defensive about the overall evaluative process.

In evaluating the child's development, the clinician should pay careful attention to the potential effects of the child's nutritional state on his or her response to test items. Infants who have experienced nutritional and/or stimulus deprivation are often withdrawn, which may severely limit their capacity to respond, at least initially.[140] For this reason, intellectual tests given early during the hospitalization, when the child is apathetic from undernutrition, may underestimate intellectual potential. Conducting the assessment soon after the hospital admission and repeating it once nutritional recovery is well underway (taking into account practice effects) should provide a more predictive estimate of intellectual potential than one assessment.[141] In addition, just as the child's progress in physical growth can be evaluated through the use of the growth grid, the child's intellectual progress can be monitored through the use of repeated assessments; however, assessment of the child's current intellectual level does not shed light on the causes of deficits or on developmental prognosis, with the exception that extremely low scores are more predictive than are those within the normal range.[142] Randomized intervention trials in the United States and abroad have demonstrated that nutrition interventions alone are not sufficient to minimize long-term developmental/behavioral sequelae of malnutrition, but weekly home-based developmental interventions sustained for several years in early childhood are associated with decreased academic and behavioral deficits into young adulthood.[143,144]

Socioemotional Development

Children with FTT are at risk of suboptimal socioemotional development. Although no one pattern of behavioral disturbance is associated with FTT, deficits in social responsiveness, affect, activity level, and avoidance of social contact have been noted by many observers.[145-147] Polan[148] found that children with FTT consistently demonstrated less positive affect in a range of situations than did normally growing children and that acute and chronic malnutrition were associated with heightened negative affect.

Because multiple areas of psychological development may be affected, a comprehensive assessment of several behavioral domains, including social responsiveness, affect, and response to feeding, is generally necessary for children with FTT.[149] A comprehensive assessment of the child's behavior and emotional development can be used to generate a profile of behavioral strengths and difficulties to guide treatment planning and evaluation of the child's progress. Ordinarily, one would expect improvement in the FTT child's social responsiveness and affect after nutritional treatment. Some children, however, continue to demonstrate significant deficits in responsiveness and/or problems in feeding that pose a salient burden to their caregivers and, hence, should be addressed in specialized intervention.

Assessment of the Family Environment

In addition to assessing the effects of FTT and associated risk factors on the child's psychological development, it also is necessary to assess aspects of the family environment (relationships, resources, and parent-child interaction) that would be expected to influence the child's response to medical and psychological intervention. Given the effects of parent-child relationships on child development, observations of the parents' interactions with the child in a range of situations (feeding, teaching the child a skill, or free play) provides a useful method of assessment.[150]

VI

The patterns of parent-child relationships associated with FTT are complex and heterogeneous.[102,151,152] Deficient or excessive but insensitive stimulation are some typical patterns; conflict and parental reinforcement of deviant behavior is another.[102] Several methods of assessment are available.[102,151]

One of the difficulties in assessing parent-child interaction in a hospital or clinic situation is that the child is removed from his or her home environment, and it is difficult to create a naturalistic setting for assessment. It may be possible, however, to use play or feeding situations to approximate important interactions. To make effective judgments about strengths and problem areas in parent-child relationships, clinicians must have extensive experience with a wide range of infants with FTT and their parents.

Intervention

The clinical management of FTT should be approached as a chronic condition requiring long-term, multidisciplinary follow-up, with exacerbations and remissions expected. Successful intervention requires active team involvement from the time of referral of a pediatric health care provider, a pediatric nutritionist, a social worker, and professionals with expertise in behavior, development, and family function. The initial focus of interdisciplinary management is assessment of the child and family for purposes of planning treatment. Subsequently, the focus concerns intervention and ongoing monitoring of the child's progress. In an optimal team approach, professionals interact frequently and directly with the family and with each other, ideally in the context of scheduled weekly to monthly clinic visits and periodic case conferences. In addition, regular home visits by one or several of these professionals are effective to gather diagnostic information and to provide ongoing support and guidance for the family.[4,153]

The first priority must be to stabilize the child's acute medical problems and nutritional deficits and to enhance, as much as possible, the material conditions of the home and family resources by helping parents to use federal feeding programs, referring to local emergency relief programs, and providing advocacy around housing, heat, and other survival issues. Certainly, medical care and nutritional resuscitation facilitate survival and physical growth but alone are not sufficient to deal with the developmental and emotional deficits that constitute the major long-term morbidity in children who have had malnutrition in early life. For this reason, it is often useful to distinguish between (1) a core intervention plan, which includes identification and treatment of the child's medical problems, nutritional treatment, advice to parents about nutrition, pediatric follow-up, and attempts to stabilize issues such as heating and housing; and (2) specialized interventions including referral to early intervention programs and preschools, which may provide developmental stimulation as well as parent training, family counseling, or behavioral treatment of feeding problems, which may be necessary to address specific problems.[141]

Once care of medical and nutritional problems has been initiated and is well in place, the assessment refocuses on the ongoing developmental needs of the child and the quality of interaction between family and child. Referral to early intervention or HeadStart programs is often indicated to enhance the child's level of cognitive development and to reduce the risk for developmental problems in later life.[144] Children who fail to thrive may be eligible on the basis of their deficits in growth and development for Supplemental Social Security Income (SSI) payments, which are frequently higher than those usually provided by Transitional Assistance to Needy Families (TANF). However, SSI standards for disability are strict and can be difficult to meet. Impoverished families should receive help in applying for these benefits. Moreover, whenever possible, services that supplement and structure the efforts of the primary caregiver, such as visiting nurses, trained homemakers, or respite day care, can be helpful and should be used. Various forms of mental health intervention, ranging from behavior modification of feeding problems to medication for a severely depressed parent to multigenerational family therapy, should be provided as indicated by the clinical assessment. Even after nutritional resuscitation has been achieved, families and children should be offered periodic reassessment as the child reaches school age to ensure early identification of behavioral or psycho-educational problems, which may require specialized educational services.

Indications for Protective Service Involvement

Although the AAP published in 2005 a clinical report "Failure to Thrive as a Manifestation of Child Neglect,"[154] it is important to recognize that abuse or neglect are clear precursors of FTT in a relatively small percentage of children. Many of the risk factors for neglect as a cause of FTT listed in the AAP report, including social isolation, lack of knowledge of normal growth and development, or parental psychopathology, are common psychosocial correlates of living in poverty—the overriding context that puts children at higher risk of developing FTT—and do not necessarily suggest neglect or abuse on the part of the child's caregivers. Nonetheless, practitioners inevitably encounter families of children with FTT who are both highly dysfunctional and resistant to recommended interventions. In a minority of children, FTT may result from diagnosable neglect by caregivers. One study found increased risk of subsequent involvement with protective services in children diagnosed with FTT in the first year of life.[155] Children with FTT who are also diagnosed by protective services as neglected have less optimal cognitive outcomes than those with FTT without a diagnosis of neglect.[156] For this reason, the clinician must clearly and carefully document the

VI

family's response to intervention as well as the child's physical, nutritional, and developmental progress.

Children with FTT who are referred to protective agencies fall into 2 broad categories: those whose safety, in the judgment of clinical personnel, requires placement away from their current caregivers, and those in less severe jeopardy, whose current caregivers require protective monitoring and support to obtain or comply with necessary services for the health and growth of the child. Placement of a child with FTT outside of the home should not be considered a routine diagnostic strategy but is the only safe intervention in certain situations, particularly when caregivers are out-of-control substance abusers, have inflicted injury on the child, have intentionally withheld available food from the child, or are profoundly psychiatrically or cognitively impaired and when no other competent caregivers are available within the existing family system.[156-159] School-aged children with psychosocial dwarfism (more recently termed "hyperphagic short stature") are systematically physically abused, often confined in small spaces, and given only periodic access to food and water. To this treatment, they often respond by binge eating when food is available and by developing bizarre behaviors, such as drinking from toilets. These children present as stunted and behaviorally disturbed with transient deficiencies of growth hormone. Unlike most infants with FTT, children with psychosocial dwarfism should immediately be treated by removal from the home or institution in which the maltreatment occurred.[155,160-162]

Placement outside the home must be undertaken with great care, because suboptimal foster care only worsens FTT.[162] Because children with FTT usually have multiple special needs requiring visits to many different professionals as well as specialized dietary, developmental, and medical management at home, foster parents must not be overburdened with the care of many other young or special needs children. Foster parents (whether professional or kinship) require the same intensive multidisciplinary support as biological parents to provide adequate care for a child who is failing to thrive. To avoid deterioration of the child with FTT who is placed in foster care, clinicians should meet face to face with prospective alternate caregivers and educate them regarding the child's dietary and behavioral regimen, medical problems, and emotional needs. Professional foster parents and kinship caregivers should have a WIC referral, appropriate nutritional supplements, child care equipment, and a health insurance card before children are placed in their homes. The professional or kinship foster family must be willing to commit to close cooperation with clinic visits and home-based treatment for the child who fails to thrive.

Protective service intervention without placement outside the home may be useful when the family is seriously noncompliant with health and nutritional care of the child, despite multiple efforts at voluntary outreach, and the child continues to grow poorly. Close communication between the protective agency and the health care providers may enhance parental adherence to recommendations. In addition, in some jurisdictions, the only way to obtain needed multidisciplinary services, such as home visits or developmentally appropriate child care, for a child who is failing to thrive, even from relatively compliant families, may be through a protective services referral. Ideally, such services should be available through other community agencies without the stigma of protective service involvement, but in today's fiscal climate, this is often not the case.

Conclusion

FTT is a chronic condition that is the final common pathway of the interaction of diverse medical, nutritional, developmental, and social stresses. Effective care is multidisciplinary, respectful of parents, and sustained beyond the time of acute nutritional and medical crises. Ultimately, the goal of sustained interdisciplinary management is a thriving child in a thriving family.

References

1. Bithoney WG, Rathbun JM. Failure to thrive. In: Levine M, Carey W, Crocker A, Gross R, eds. *Developmental-Behavioral Pediatrics*. Philadelphia, PA: WB Saunders; 1983:557-572

2. Wright CM, Parkinson KN, Drewett RF. How does maternal and child feeding behavior relate to weight gain and failure to thrive? Data from a prospective birth cohort. *Pediatrics*. 2006;117(4):1262-1269

3. Sills RH. Failure to thrive. The role of clinical and laboratory evaluation. *Am J Dis Child*. 1978;132(10):967-969

4. Frank DA, Zeisel SH. Failure to thrive. *Pediatr Clin North Am*. 1988;35(6):1187-1206

5. Casey PH, Arnold WC. Compensatory growth in infants with severe failure to thrive. *South Med J*. 1985;78(9):1057-1060

6. Whitten CF, Pettit MG, Fischhoff J. Evidence that growth failure from maternal deprivation is secondary to undereating. *JAMA*. 1969;209(11):1675-1682

7. Barrett DE, Frank DA. *The Effects of Undernutrition on Children's Behavior*. New York, NY: Gordon Breach; 1987

8. Drotar D, Robinson J. Developmental psychopathology of failure to thrive. In: Sameroff AJ, Lewis M, Miller SM, eds. *Handbook of Developmental Psychopathology*. 2nd ed. New York, NY: Kluwer Academic/Plenum; 2000:465-474

9. Coleman-Jensen, A, Nord M, Andrews M, Carlson S. Household Food Security in the United States in 2010. Washington, DC: US Department of Agriculture; 2011. Available at: http://www.ers.usda.gov/Publications/ERR125/ERR125.pdf. Accessed November 16, 2012

VI

10. Dowdney L, Skuse D, Morris K, Pickles A. Short normal children and environmental disadvantage: a longitudinal study of growth and cognitive development from 4 to 11 years. *J Child Psychol Psychiatry*. 1998;39(7):1017-1029

11. Mitchell WG, Gorrell RW, Greenberg RA. Failure-to-thrive: a study in a primary care setting. Epidemiology and follow-up. *Pediatrics*. 1980;65(5):971-977

12. Bithoney WG, Newberger EH. Child and family attributes of failure-to-thrive. *J Dev Behav Pediatr*. 1987;8(1):32-36

13. Wolkwitz K, Leftin J. *Characteristics of Food Stamp Households: Fiscal Year 2007*. Washington, DC: Mathematica Policy Research Inc; September 2008

14. Leftin J, Wolkwitz K. *Trends in Supplemental Nutrition Assistance Program Rates: 2000 to 2007*. Alexandria, VA: Mathematica Policy Research Inc; June 2009

15. US Department of Agriculture, Food and Nutrition Service. Supplemental Nutrition Assistance Program: Average Monthly Benefit Per Person. Available at: http://www.fns.usda.gov/pd/18SNAPavg$PP.htm. Accessed November 16, 2012

16. Institute of Medicine, Food and Nutrition Board. *WIC Food Packages: Time for a Change*. Washington, DC: National Academies Press; 2005

17. National Research Council. Estimating Eligibility and Participation for the WIC Program: Final Report. Washington, DC: National Academies Press; 2003

18. Thayer J, Murphy C, Cook JT, Ettinger de Cuba S, DaCosta R, Chilton M. *Coming Up Short: High Food Costs Outstrip Food Stamp A Benefits*. Boston, MA: Boston Medical Center; September 2008

19. Huston AC, McLoyd VC, Coll CG. Children and poverty: issues in contemporary research. *Child Dev*. 1994;65(2 Spec No):275-282

20. Nicholls D, Bryant-Waugh R. Eating disorders of infancy and childhood: definition, symptomatology, epidemiology, and comorbidity. *Child Adolesc Psychiatr Clin North Am*. 2009;18(1):17-30

21. Pearce DM. *When Wages Aren't Enough: Using the Self-Sufficiency Standard to Model the Impact of Child Care Subsidies on Wage Adequacy*. Swarthmore, PA: Pennsylavania Family Economic Self-Sufficiency Project and the Women's Association for Women's Alternatives Inc; 1998

22. Kaplowitz P, Webb J. Diagnostic evaluation of short children with height 3 SD or more below the mean. *Clin Pediatr (Phila)*. 1994;33(9):530-535

23. Frisancho AR, Cole PE, Klayman JE. Greater contribution to secular trend among offspring of short parents. *Hum Biol*. 1977;49(1):51-60

24. Fraiberg S, Adelson E, Shapiro V. Ghosts in the nursery. A psychoanalytic approach to the problems of impaired infant-mother relationships. *J Am Acad Child Psychiatry*. 1975;14(3):387-421

25. Martin JA, Kung HC, Mathews TJ, et al. Annual summary of vital statistics: 2006. *Pediatrics*. 2008;121(4):788-801

26. Pollitt E, Leibel R. Biological and social correlates of failure to thrive. In: Greene L, Johnson E, eds. *Social and Biological Predictions of Nutritional Status, Physical Growth, and Neurological Development*. New York, NY: Academic Press; 1980:173-200

27. Brandt I. Growth dynamics of low birthweight infants with emphasis on the prenatal period. In: Falkner F, Tanner J, eds. *Human Growth, Neurobiology and Nutrition*. 2nd ed. New York, NY: Plenum Press; 1986:415-486

28. Wright CM, Williams AF, Elliman D, et al. Using the new UK-WHO growth charts. *BMJ*. 2010;340:c1140

29. Casey PH. Growth of low birth weight preterm children. *Semin Perinatol*. 2008;32(1):20-27

30. Casey PH, Kraemer HC, Bernbaum J, Yogman MW, Sells JC. Growth status and growth rates of a varied sample of low birth weight, preterm infants: a longitudinal cohort from birth to three years of age. *J Pediatr*. 1991;119(4):599-605

31. Santos IS, Matijasevich A, Domingues MR, Barros AJ, Victora CG, Barros FC. Late preterm birth is a risk factor for growth faltering in early childhood: a cohort study. *BMC Pediatr*. 2009;9:71

32. Karniski W, Blair C, Vitucci JS. The illusion of catch-up growth in premature infants. Use of the growth index and age correction. *Am J Dis Child*. 1987;141(5):520-526

33. Georgieff MK, Mills MM, Zempel CE, Chang PN. Catch-up growth, muscle and fat accretion, and body proportionality of infants one year after newborn intensive care. *J Pediatr*. 1989;114(2):288-292

34. Sherry B, Mei Z, Grummer-Strawn L, Dietz WH. Evaluation of and recommendations for growth references for very low birth weight (< or =1500 grams) infants in the United States. *Pediatrics*. 2003;111(4 Pt 1):750-758

35. Casey PH, Whiteside-Mansell L, Barrett K, Bradley RH, Gargus R. Impact of prenatal and/or postnatal growth problems in low birth weight preterm infants on school-age outcomes: an 8-year longitudinal evaluation. *Pediatrics*. 2006;118(3):1078-1086

36. Teranishi H, Nakagawa H, Marmot M. Social class difference in catch up growth in a national British cohort. *Arch Dis Child*. 2001;84(3):218-221

37. McCormick FM, Henderson G, Fahey T, McGuire W. Multinutrient fortification of human breast milk for preterm infants following hospital discharge. *Cochrane Database Syst Rev*. 2010;(7):CD004866

38. American College of Chest Physicians, American Academy of Pediatrics. *ACCP/AAP Pediatric Pulmonary Medicine Board Review: 1st Edition*. Northbrook, IL: American College of Chest Physicians; 2010

39. Als H, Tronick E, Adamson L, Brazelton TB. The behavior of the full-term but underweight newborn infant. *Dev Med Child Neurol*. 1976;18(5):590-602

40. Villar J, Smeriglio V, Martorell R, Brown CH, Klein RE. Heterogeneous growth and mental development of intrauterine growth-retarded infants during the first 3 years of life. *Pediatrics*. 1984;74(5):783-791

41. Hediger ML, Overpeck MD, Maurer KR, Kuczmarski RJ, McGlynn A, Davis WW. Growth of infants and young children born small or large for gestational age: findings from the Third National Health and Nutrition Examination Survey. *Arch Pediatr Adolesc Med*. 1998;152(12):1225-1231

42. Hanson JW, Smith DW. The fetal hydantoin syndrome. *J Pediatr*. 1975;87(2):285-290

VI

43. Frank DA, Wong F. Effects of prenatal exposures to alcohol, tobacco, and other drugs. In: Kessler DB, Dawson P, eds. *Failure to Thrive and Pediatric Undernutrition: A Transdisciplinary Approach.* Baltimore, MD: Paul H. Brookes Publishing; 1999:275-280

44. Fried PA, O'Connell CM. A comparison of the effects of prenatal exposure to tobacco, alcohol, cannabis and caffeine on birth size and subsequent growth. *Neurotoxicol Teratol.* 1987;9(2):79-85

45. Lassen K, Oei TP. Effects of maternal cigarette smoking during pregnancy on long-term physical and cognitive parameters of child development. *Addict Behav.* 1998;23(5):635-653

46. Nordstrom-Klee B, Delaney-Black V, Covington C, Ager J, Sokol R. Growth from birth onwards of children prenatally exposed to drugs: a literature review. *Neurotoxicol Teratol.* 2002;24(4):481-488

47. Chambers CD, Anderson PO, Thomas RG, et al. Weight gain in infants breastfed by mothers who take fluoxetine. *Pediatrics.* 1999;104(5):e61

48. Coles CD, Brown RT, Smith IE, Platzman KA, Erickson S, Falek A. Effects of prenatal alcohol exposure at school age. I. Physical and cognitive development. *Neurotoxicol Teratol.* 1991;13(4):357-367

49. Fried PA, Watkinson B. 36- and 48-Month Neurobehavioral Follow-Up of Children Prenatally Exposed to Marijuana, Cigarettes, and Alcohol. *J Dev Behav Pediatr.* 1990;11(2):49-58

50. Hanson JW, Jones KL, Smith DW. Fetal alcohol syndrome. Experience with 41 patients. *JAMA.* 1976;235(14):1458-1460

51. Van Dyke DC, Mackay L, Ziaylek EN. Management of severe feeding dysfunction in children with fetal alcohol syndrome. *Clin Pediatr (Phila).* 1982;21(6):336-339

52. Klug MG, Burd L, Martsolf JT, Ebertowski M. Body mass index in fetal alcohol syndrome. *Neurotoxicol Teratol.* 2003;25(6):689-696

53. Frank DA, Bauchner H, Parker S, et al. Neonatal body proportionality and body composition after in utero exposure to cocaine and marijuana. *J Pediatr.* 1990;117(4):622-626

54. Zuckerman B, Frank DA, Hingson R, et al. Effects of maternal marijuana and cocaine use on fetal growth. *N Engl J Med.* 1989;320(12):762-768

55. Cornelius MD, Goldschmidt L, Day NL, Larkby C. Alcohol, tobacco and marijuana use among pregnant teenagers: 6-year follow-up of offspring growth effects. *Neurotoxicol Teratol.* 2002;24(6):703-710

56. Fried PA, Watkinson B, Gray R. Differential effects on cognitive functioning in 9- to 12-year olds prenatally exposed to cigarettes and marihuana. *Neurotoxicol Teratol.* 1998;20(3):293-306

57. Neuspiel DR, Hamel SC, Hochberg E, Greene J, Campbell D. Maternal cocaine use and infant behavior. *Neurotoxicol Teratol.* 1991;13(2):229-233

58. Chasnoff IJ, Griffith DR, Freier C, Murray J. Cocaine/polydrug use in pregnancy: two-year follow-up. *Pediatrics.* 1992;89(2):284-289

59. Hurt H, Brodsky NL, Betancourt L, Braitman LE, Malmud E, Giannetta J. Cocaine-exposed children: follow-up through 30 months. *J Dev Behav Pediatr.* 1995;16(1):29-35

60. Jacobson JL, Jacobson SW, Sokol RJ. Effects of prenatal exposure to alcohol, smoking, and illicit drugs on postpartum somatic growth. *Alcohol Clin Exp Res*. 1994;18(2):317-323

61. Richardson GA, Conroy ML, Day NL. Prenatal cocaine exposure: effects on the development of school-age children. *Neurotoxicol Teratol*. 1996;18(6):627-634

62. Ackerman JP, Riggins T, Black MM. A review of the effects of prenatal cocaine exposure among school-aged children. *Pediatrics*. 2010;125(3):554-565

63. Harsham J, Keller JH, Disbrow D. Growth patterns of infants exposed to cocaine and other drugs in utero. *J Am Diet Assoc*. 1994;94(9):999-1007

64. Wilson GS, McCreary R, Kean J, Baxter JC. The development of preschool children of heroin-addicted mothers: a controlled study. *Pediatrics*. 1979;63(1):135-141

65. Deren S. Children of substance abusers: a review of the literature. *J Subst Abuse Treat*. 1986;3(2):77-94

66. Zabaneh R, Smith LM, LaGasse LL, et al. The effects of prenatal methamphetamine exposure on childhood growth patterns from birth to three years of age. *Am J Perinatol*. 2012;29(3):203-210

67. Kappy MS. Regulation of growth in children with chronic illness. Therapeutic implications for the year 2000. *Am J Dis Child*. 1987;141(5):489-493

68. Phillip M, Hershkovitz E, Rosenblum H, et al. Serum insulin-like growth factors I and II are not affected by undernutrition in children with nonorganic failure to thrive. *Horm Res*. 1998;49(2):76-79

69. Fryer GE Jr. The efficacy of hospitalization of nonorganic failure-to-thrive children: a meta-analysis. *Child Abuse Negl*. 1988;12(3):375-381

70. Bithoney WG, McJunkin J, Michalek J, Egan H, Snyder J, Munier A. Prospective evaluation of weight gain in both nonorganic and organic failure-to-thrive children: an outpatient trial of a multidisciplinary team intervention strategy. *J Dev Behav Pediatr*. 1989;10(1):27-31

71. Berwick DM, Levy JC, Kleinerman R. Failure to thrive: diagnostic yield of hospitalisation. *Arch Dis Child*. 1982;57(5):347-351

72. Homer C, Ludwig S. Categorization of etiology of failure to thrive. *Am J Dis Child*. 1981;135(9):848-851

73. Fleisher DR. Comprehensive management of infants with gastroesophageal reflux and failure to thrive. *Curr Probl Pediatr*. 1995;25(8):247-253

74. Sullivan PB. Nutritional management of acute diarrhea. *Nutrition*. 1998;14(10):758-762

75. Reilly SM, Skuse DH, Wolke D, Stevenson J. Oral-motor dysfunction in children who fail to thrive: organic or non-organic? *Dev Med Child Neurol*. 1999;41(2):115-122

76. Mathisen B, Skuse D, Wolke D, Reilly S. Oral-motor dysfunction and failure to thrive among inner-city infants. *Dev Med Child Neurol*. 1989;31(3):293-302

77. Mraz KD, Green J, Dumont-Mathieu T, Makin S, Fein D. Correlates of head circumference growth in infants later diagnosed with autism spectrum disorders. *J Child Neurol*. 2007;22(6):700-713

78. Ibrahim SH, Voigt RG, Katusic SK, Weaver AL, Barbaresi WJ. Incidence of gastrointestinal symptoms in children with autism: a population-based study. *Pediatrics*. 2009;124(2):680-686

VI

79. Keen DV. Childhood autism, feeding problems and failure to thrive in early infancy. Seven case studies. *Eur Child Adolesc Psychiatry*. 2008;17(4):209-216

80. Boyce JA, Assa'ad A, Burks AW, et al. Guidelines for the Diagnosis and Management of Food Allergy in the United States: Summary of the NIAID-Sponsored Expert Panel Report. *J Allergy Clin Immunol*. 2010;126(6):1105-1118

81. Niggemann B, Sielaff B, Beyer K, Binder C, Wahn U. Outcome of double-blind, placebo-controlled food challenge tests in 107 children with atopic dermatitis. *Clin Exp Allergy*. 1999;29(1):91-96

82. Chevalier P, Sevilla R, Sejas E, Zalles L, Belmonte G, Parent G. Immune recovery of malnourished children takes longer than nutritional recovery: implications for treatment and discharge. *J Trop Pediatr*. 1998;44(5):304-307

83. American Academy of Pediatrics. *Red Book: 2012 Report of the Committee on Infectious Diseases*. Pickering LK, Baker CJ, Kimberlin DW, Long SS, eds. 29th ed. Elk Grove Village, IL: American Academy of Pediatrics; 2012

84. Cunningham-Rundles S, McNeeley DF, Moon A. Mechanisms of nutrient modulation of the immune response. *J Allergy Clin Immunol*. 2005;115(6):1119-1128

85. Centers for Disease Control and Prevention. Mother-to-Child (Perinatal) HIV Transmission and Prevention. Available at: http://www.cdc.gov/hiv/topics/perinatal/resources/factsheets/perinatal.htm. Accessed November 16, 2012

86. Schwartz J, Angle C, Pitcher H. Relationship between childhood blood lead levels and stature. *Pediatrics*. 1986;77(3):281-288

87. Mahaffey KR, Annest JL, Roberts J, Murphy RS. National estimates of blood lead levels: United States, 1976-1980: association with selected demographic and socioeconomic factors. *N Engl J Med*. 1982;307(10):573-579

88. Centers for Disease Control and Prevention. *Preventing Lead Poisoning in Young Children*. Atlanta, GA: Centers for Disease Control and Prevention; 2004

89. Bithoney WG. Elevated lead levels in children with nonorganic failure to thrive. *Pediatrics*. 1986;78(5):891-895

90. Baker RD; Greer FR; Committee on Nutrition American Academy of Pediatrics. Diagnosis and prevention of iron deficiency and iron-deficiency anemia in infants and young children (0-3 years of age). *Pediatrics*. 2010;126(5):1040-1050

91. Ficicioglu C, An Haack K. Failure to thrive: when to suspect inborn errors of metabolism. *Pediatrics*. 2009;124(3):972-979

92. Bergstrom WH. Twenty ways to get rickets in the 1990s. *Contemp Pediatr*. 1991;8:88-106

93. Catassi C, Fasano A. Celiac disease as a cause of growth retardation in childhood. *Curr Opin Pediatr*. 2004;16(4):445-449

94. Rudolph CD, Mazur LJ, Liptak GS, et al. Guidelines for evaluation and treatment of gastroesophageal reflux in infants and children: recommendations of the North American Society for Pediatric Gastroenterology and Nutrition. *J Pediatr Gastroenterol Nutr*. 2001;32(Suppl 2):S1-S31

95. Acs G, Shulman R, Ng MW, Chussid S. The effect of dental rehabilitation on the body weight of children with early childhood caries. *Pediatr Dent*. 1999;21(2):109-113

96. American College of Chest Physicians, American Academy of Pediatrics. *ACCP/AAP Pediatric Pulmonary Medicine Board Review: 1st Edition.* Northbrook, IL: American College of Chest Physicians; 2010.

97. American Academy of Pediatrics. Immunization. Available at: http://www.aap.org/immunization/izschedule.html. Accessed November 16, 2012

98. Peterson KE, Washington J, Rathbun JM. Team management of failure to thrive. *J Am Diet Assoc.* 1984;84(7):810-815

99. Zeiger RS, Sampson HA, Bock SA, et al. Soy allergy in infants and children with IgE-associated cow's milk allergy. *J Pediatr.* 1999;134(5):614-622

100. Wagner CL, Greer FR; American Academy of Pediatrics, Committee on Nutrition. Prevention of rickets and vitamin D deficiency in infants, children, and adolescents. *Pediatrics.* 2008;122(5):1142-1152

101. McJunkin JE, Bithoney WG, McCormick MC. Errors in formula concentration in an outpatient population. *J Pediatr.* 1987;111(6 Pt 1):848-850

102. Linscheid TR, Rasnake LK. Behavioral approaches to the treatment of failure to thrive. In: Drotar D, ed. *New Directions in Failure to Thrive: Implications for Research and Practice.* New York, NY: Plenum Press; 1985:279-294

103. Pollitt E. Failure to thrive: socioeconomic, dietary intake and mother-child interaction data. *Fed Proc.* 1975;34(7):1593-1597

104. Heptinstall E, Puckering C, Skuse D, Start K, Zur-Szpiro S, Dowdney L. Nutrition and mealtime behaviour in families of growth-retarded children. *Hum Nutr Appl Nutr.* 1987;41(6):390-402

105. Strasburger VC; American Academy of Pediatrics, Committee on Communications. Children, adolescents, and advertising. *Pediatrics.* 2006;118(6):2563-2569

106. Zmora E, Gorodischer R, Bar-Ziv J. Multiple nutritional deficiencies in infants from a strict vegetarian community. *Am J Dis Child.* 1979;133(2):141-144

107. Pugliese MT, Weyman-Daum M, Moses N, Lifshitz F. Parental health beliefs as a cause of nonorganic failure to thrive. *Pediatrics.* 1987;80(2):175-182

108. American Academy of Pediatrics, Committee on Nutrition. The use and misuse of fruit juice in pediatrics. *Pediatrics.* 2001;107(5):1210-1213

109. Maldonado J, Gil A, Narbona E, Molina JA. Special formulas in infant nutrition: a review. *Early Hum Dev.* 1998;53(Suppl):S23-32

110. National Health and Nutrition Examination Survey (NHANES). *Anthropometry Procedures Manual.* Atlanta, GA: Centers for Disease Control and Prevention; 2007

111. World Health Organization. The Training Course on Child Growth Assessment. Available at: http://www.who.int/childgrowth/training/en/. Available at: November 16, 2012

112. Centers for Disease Control and Prevention. CDC Growth Charts. Available at: http://www.cdc.gov/growthcharts/. Accessed November 16, 2012

113. Centers for Disease Control and Prevention. Use of World Health Organization and CDC growth charts for children aged 0-59 months in the United States. *MMWR Recomm Rep.* 2010;59(RR-9):1-15

114. Kielmann AA, McCord C. Weight-for-age as an index of risk of death in children. *Lancet.* 1978;1(8076):1247-1250

VI

115. Waterlow JC. Classification and definition of protein-calorie malnutrition. *Br Med J.* 1972;3(5826):566-569

116. Morales E, Craig LD, MacLean WC Jr. Dietary management of malnourished children with a new enteral feeding. *J Am Diet Assoc.* 1991;91(10):1233-1238

117. Guo SM, Roche AF, Fomon SJ, et al. Reference data on gains in weight and length during the first two years of life. *J Pediatr.* 1991;119(3):355-362

118. Fomon SJ, Haschke F, Ziegler EE, Nelson SE. Body composition of reference children from birth to age 10 years. *Am J Clin Nutr.* 1982;35(5 Suppl):1169-1175

119. Murphy SP, Barr SI. Practice paper of the American Dietetic Association: using the Dietary Reference Intakes. *J Am Diet Assoc.* 2011;111(5):762-770

120. Samour PQ, Helm KK. *Handbook of Pediatric Nutrition.* 3rd ed. Sudbury, MA: Jones & Bartlett Learning; 2005

121. World Health Organization. WHO Anthro (version 3.2.2, January 2011) and macros. Available at: http://www.who.int/childgrowth/software/en. Accessed November 16, 2012

122. Doherty CP, Sarkar MA, Shakur MS, Ling SC, Elton RA, Cutting WA. Zinc and rehabilitation from severe protein-energy malnutrition: higher-dose regimens are associated with increased mortality. *Am J Clin Nutr.* 1998;68(3):742-748

123. Black MM. Zinc deficiency and child development. *Am J Clin Nutr.* 1998;68(2 Suppl):464S-469S

124. Rathbun JM, Peterson KE. Nutrition in failure to thrive. In: Grand R, Sutphen J, Dietz W, eds. *Pediatric Nutrition: Theory and Practice.* Boston, MA: Butterworths; 1987

125. Waterlow J. Treatment of children with malnutrition and diarrhoea. *Lancet.* 1999;354(9185):1142

126. Black MM, Krishnakumar A. Predicting longitudinal growth curves of height and weight using ecological factors for children with and without early growth deficiency. *J Nutr.* 1999;129(2S Suppl):539S-543S

127. Galler JR, Ramsey F, Solimano G, Lowell WE, Mason E. The influence of early malnutrition on subsequent behavioral development. I. Degree of impairment in intellectual performance. *J Am Acad Child Psychiatry.* 1983;22(1):8-15

128. Silver J, DiLorenzo P, Zukoski M, Ross PE, Amster BJ, Schlegel D. Starting young: improving the health and developmental outcomes of infants and toddlers in the child welfare system. *Child Welfare.* 1999;78(1):148-165

129. Drewett RF, Corbett SS, Wright CM. Cognitive and educational attainments at school age of children who failed to thrive in infancy: a population-based study. *J Child Psychol Psychiatry.* 1999;40(4):551-561

130. Galler JR, Ramsey F, Solimano G. The influence of early malnutrition on subsequent behavioral development III. Learning disabilities as a sequel to malnutrition. *Pediatr Res.* 1984;18(4):309-313

131. Galler JR, Ramsey F, Solimano G. A follow-up study of the effects of early malnutrition on subsequent development. II. Fine motor skills in adolescence. *Pediatr Res.* 1985;19(6):524-527

132. Mendez MA, Adair LS. Severity and timing of stunting in the first two years of life affect performance on cognitive tests in late childhood. *J Nutr*. 1999;129(8):1555-1562

133. Skuse D, Pickles A, Wolke D, Reilly S. Postnatal growth and mental development: evidence for a "sensitive period." *J Child Psychol Psychiatry*. 1994;35(3):521-545

134. Black MM, Hutcheson JJ, Dubowitz H, Berenson-Howard J. Parenting style and developmental status among children with nonorganic failure to thrive. *J Pediatr Psychol*. 1994;19(6):689-707

135. Drotar D, Eckerle D. The family environment in nonorganic failure to thrive: a controlled study. *J Pediatr Psychol*. 1989;14(2):245-257

136. Galler JR, Ramsey F, Solimano G. Influence of early malnutrition on subsequent behavioral development. V. Child's behavior at home. *J Am Acad Child Psychiatry*. 1985;24(1):58-64

137. McKay H, Sinisterra L, McKay A, Gomez H, Lloreda P. Improving cognitive ability in chronically deprived children. *Science*. 1978;200(4339):270-278

138. Zeskind PS, Ramey CT. Fetal malnutrition: an experimental study of its consequences on infant development in two caregiving environments. *Child Dev*. 1978;49(4):1155-1162

139. Drotar D, Wilson F, Sturm LA. Parent intervention in failure to thrive. In: Schaefer C, Briesmeister J, eds. *Handbook of Parent Training: Parents as Cotherapists for Children's Behavioral Problems*. New York, NY: Wiley; 1989:364-391

140. Dobbing J. Infant nutrition and later achievement. *Nutr Rev*. 1984;42(1):1-7

141. Drotar D, Sturm LA. Psychological assessment and intervention with failure to thrive infants and their families. In: Olson M, Mullins L, Gillman P, eds. *Sourcebook of Pediatric Psychology*. Baltimore, MD: Johns Hopkins Press; 1994:26-41

142. VanderVeer B, Schweid E. Infant assessment: stability of mental functioning in young retarded children. *Am J Ment Defic*. 1974;79(1):1-4

143. Black MM, Dubowitz H, Krishnakumar A, Starr RH Jr. Early intervention and recovery among children with failure to thrive: follow-up at age 8. *Pediatrics*. 2007;120(1):59-69

144. Walker SP, Chang SM, Vera-Hernandez M, Grantham-McGregor S. Early childhood stimulation benefits adult competence and reduces violent behavior. *Pediatrics*. 2011;127(5):849-857

145. Drotar D, Sturm L. Personality development, problem solving, and behavior problems among preschool children with early histories of nonorganic failure-to-thrive: a controlled study. *J Dev Behav Pediatr*. 1992;13(4):266-273

146. Powell GF, Low J. Behavior in nonorganic failure to thrive. *J Dev Behav Pediatr*. 1983;4(1):26-33

147. Ramey CT, Yeates KO, Short EJ. The plasticity of intellectual development: insights from preventive intervention. *Child Dev*. 1984;55(5):1913-1925

148. Polan HJ, Leon A, Kaplan MD, Kessler DB, Stern DN, Ward MJ. Disturbances of affect expression in failure-to-thrive. *J Am Acad Child Adolesc Psychiatry*. 1991;30(6):897-903

149. Wolke D, Skuse D, Mathisen B. Behavioral style in failure-to-thrive infants: a preliminary communication. *J Pediatr Psychol*. 1990;15(2):237-254

150. Polan HJ, Ward MJ. Role of the mother's touch in failure to thrive: a preliminary investigation. *J Am Acad Child Adolesc Psychiatry*. 1994;33(8):1098-1105

VI

151. Casey PH. Failure to thrive: a reconceptualization. *J Dev Behav Pediatr.* 1983;4(1):63-66
152. Ramey CT, Hieger L, Klisz D. Synchronous reinforcement of vocal responses in failure-to-thrive infants. *Child Dev.* 1972;43(4):1449-1455
153. Black MM, Dubowitz H, Hutcheson J, Berenson-Howard J, Starr RH Jr. A randomized clinical trial of home intervention for children with failure to thrive. *Pediatrics.* 1995;95(6):807-814
154. Block RW, Krebs NF, American Academy of Pediatrics Committee on Child Abuse and Neglect, American Academy of Pediatrics Committee on Nutrition. Failure to thrive as a manifestation of child neglect. *Pediatrics.* 2005;116(5):1234-1237
155. Skuse DH, Gill D, Reilly S, Wolke D, Lynch MA. Failure to thrive and the risk of child abuse: a prospective population survey. *J Med Screen.* 1995;2(3):145-149
156. Mackner LM, Starr RH Jr, Black MM. The cumulative effect of neglect and failure to thrive on cognitive functioning. *Child Abuse Negl.* 1997;21(7):691-700
157. Bullard DM Jr, Glaser HH, Heagarty MC, Pivchik EC. Failure to thrive in the "neglected" child. *Am J Orthopsychiatry.* 1967;37(4):680-690
158. Goldson E, Cadol RV, Fitch MJ, Umlauf HJ Jr. Nonaccidental trauma and failure to thrive. *Am J Dis Child.* 1976;130(5):490-492
159. Koel BS. Failure to thrive and fatal injury as a continuum. *Am J Dis Child.* 1969;118(4):565-567
160. Gilmour J, Skuse D. A case-comparison study of the characteristics of children with a short stature syndrome induced by stress (Hyperphagic Short Stature) and a consecutive series of unaffected "stressed" children. *J Child Psychol Psychiatry.* 1999;40(6):969-978
161. Krieger I. Food restriction as a form of child abuse in ten cases of psychosocial deprivation dwarfism. *Clin Pediatr (Phila).* 1974;13(2):127-133
162. Wyatt DT, Simms MD, Horwitz SM. Widespread growth retardation and variable growth recovery in foster children in the first year after initial placement. *Arch Pediatr Adolesc Med.* 1997;151(8):813-816

Chapter 28

Chronic Diarrheal Disease

Introduction and Pathophysiology

Infants and children with chronic or persistent diarrhea continue to pose a significant medical challenge. Aggressive oral rehydration programs have reduced the frequency of hospitalization and death from acute diarrhea and have begun to demonstrate an influence on the morbidity and mortality from chronic diarrhea in developing countries.[1] Despite these advancements, the World Health Organization (WHO) has estimated that approximately 13% of all childhood deaths worldwide are caused by diarrheal diseases, 50% of which are chronic diarrheal illnesses.[2]

The WHO defines persistent diarrhea as "diarrheal episodes of presumed infectious etiology that begin acutely but last at least 14 days."[3] Although patients or their parents often assess the presence of diarrhea by reporting stool consistency and frequency, one can more scientifically define diarrhea as stool volume greater than 10 g/kg/day in infants and toddlers and greater than 200 g/day in older children.[4] However, diarrhea should not be defined solely by stool weight. Some healthy adolescents and adults may have up to 300 g of formed stool/day without any complaints.[5]

The etiologies of chronic diarrhea can be divided by pathophysiology into 4 often overlapping mechanisms. The first is osmotic diarrhea, secondary to the failure to absorb a luminal solute resulting in secretion of fluids and net water retention across an osmotic gradient, producing increased fluid losses. This can result from either congenital or acquired disease and is most evident in the failure to absorb a carbohydrate, such as lactose. Other carbohydrates may be malabsorbed either because of disaccharidase deficiencies or because the absorptive capacity of the intestine for that sugar may be overwhelmed by excessive consumption (eg, fructose and sorbitol).[6] Such excessive intake may be seen in young children drinking fruit juices. Disaccharidase deficiencies, such as lactose deficiency, are rarely congenital and more often are a result of gut mucosal injury secondary to some process later in infancy, such as enteritis.[4] By definition, the diarrhea ceases with elimination of the offending solute from the diet.

The second form, secretory diarrhea, occurs when there is a net secretion of electrolyte and fluid from the intestine relative to the degree of absorption. Endogenous substances, often called "secretagogues," induce fluid and electrolyte secretion into the lumen even in the absence of an osmotic gradient. Typically, secretagogues affect ion transport in the large and small bowel both by inhibiting sodium and chloride absorption and by stimulating chloride secretion via cystic fibrosis transmembrane regulator (CFTR) activation. Examples include multiple

VI

congenital disorders with identified genetic mutations that affect gut epithelial ion transport.[7] This form of diarrhea persists even with cessation of oral intake.

The third form of chronic diarrhea results from intestinal dysmotility. Children with this form usually have intact absorptive ability even in the face of rapid transit. Intestinal transit time is decreased, the time allowed for absorption is minimized, and fluid is retained within the lumen. High-amplitude propagated contractions (HAPCs) have been found to be more frequent in patients with diarrhea-predominant irritable bowel syndrome (IBS-D), commonly diagnosed in adolescents.[8] The most common example of this form of diarrhea presents in the first few years of life as "toddler's diarrhea" or chronic nonspecific diarrhea. Changes in small intestinal motility also have been implicated in the cause of chronic nonspecific diarrhea.[9]

The fourth pathophysiologic form of diarrhea is inflammatory diarrhea. This often encompasses components of all of the prior 3 forms as well. The etiologies range from acute viral enteritis to chronic villus or colonic inflammation from celiac disease to inflammatory bowel disease (IBD). Increased enteric loss of protein, mucus, and blood may also be noted in the stool.

Evaluation of the Infant and Child With Persistent Diarrhea

History and Physical Examination

It is very important initially to define the character of the diarrhea using criteria such as frequency, volume, duration, characteristics of the stool, and relationship to feeding or dietary intake. A prospective 3- to 5-day history of dietary intake, stool pattern, and associated symptoms is very helpful. Also important is the presence or absence of abdominal pain, weight loss, rash, fatigue, vomiting, joint aches, or oral ulcers among other extraintestinal symptoms. Important historical components include family history, cultural influences on feeding, travel, and preschool exposures.

The physical examination begins with the documentation of weight, height, and head circumference, plotted on a standardized reference growth chart. The examination should focus on evidence of chronic disease and nutrient deficiency, such as rickets in vitamin D deficiency, abdominal distension with loss of subcutaneous tissue in cases of malabsorption in celiac disease, or perianal dermatitis in zinc deficiency. The physical examination should include a rectal examination.

Examination of Stool Sample

Confirmation of the cause of persistent diarrhea requires evaluation of a fresh stool sample.[10] This begins with the macroscopic inspection of the stool for consistency and color. The stool should be tested for the presence of blood and polymorphonuclear leukocytes. The presence of leukocytes is expected with invasive bacterial disease and inflammatory colitis and argues against viral or malabsorptive diarrheas. Techniques for analysis of the stool for malabsorbed fat using Sudan black stains are available in clinical laboratories but are too cumbersome and dependent on an experienced observer for routine office use. Unabsorbed carbohydrates in the stool can be detected by reagent tablets for reducing sugars or test-tape analysis for glucose. Breastfed healthy infants will often have traces of reducing sugar in the stool. Sucrose is not a reducing sugar; thus, stool samples from infants who are fed sucrose-containing formulas will need to be hydrolyzed with hydrochloric acid solution and heated before testing for reducing sugars.

Analysis of the stool for electrolyte content and osmolarity may be helpful in distinguishing osmotic from a secretory diarrhea. Osmotic diarrhea is usually present if the osmolar gap (stool osmolarity − 2[stool sodium + stool potassium]) is >50, and secretory diarrhea needs to be strongly considered if the gap is lower. Alternatively, if the patient is stable and well hydrated or receiving intravenous fluids, food and drink can be withheld for 24 hours to determine whether the volume of the diarrhea is affected. In purely secretory diarrhea, a liquid stool output continues, even when the patient is not consuming any food or drink orally. The measurement of stool volume and electrolytes also allows documentation of the child's ongoing electrolyte needs and the effect of malabsorbed carbohydrates in the feedings. Suspected loss of protein from the mucosal surface can be confirmed by determining the fecal content of alpha-1-antitrypsin, a large molecular weight serum protein that is resistant to proteolytic degradation in the gastrointestinal tract.

To exclude ongoing infection as a contributing factor to persistent diarrhea, it is appropriate to culture the stool for enteric pathogens. Bacterial infections from organisms such as *Yersinia* species, *Escherichia coli*, and *Salmonella* species may develop into chronic illness and can be evaluated for by routine stool culture. Additionally, some stool cultures may include testing for diarrhea-causing *Aeromonas* species and *Plesiomonas* species. *Clostridium difficile* toxin assay should be performed, especially in the setting of recent antibiotic use. Antigen detection for *Giardia* species and *Cryptosporidium* species is more sensitive and specific than routine microscopy-based "ova and parasite" examinations and, therefore, may be helpful if these infections are suspected.[11] Diarrhea caused by viruses does not usually have a duration of more than 14 days and more typically has a duration of 2 days (eg, Norwalk-like virus) to 11 days (enteric adenoviruses).[10] However, rotavirus may cause diarrhea lasting up to 20 days and may be diagnosed by stool tests.[12]

For children with diarrhea in the context of failure to thrive (FTT) or suspected steatorrhea, a formal documentation of quantitative fecal fat can be performed on a 72-hour collection of stool. This is coupled with a 4-day history of dietary fat

VI

intake, which is optimized to be >30 g/day in infants and >50 g/day in school-aged children. A coefficient of fat malabsorption more than 5% is generally abnormal after early infancy (15% fat malabsorption may be normal in early infancy). Additionally, one can measure the amount of elastase in the stool, which gives an indication of exocrine pancreatic function, with low fecal elastase suggesting pancreatic insufficiency.

Sweat Test

The analysis of sweat sodium and/or chloride by iontophoresis should be performed in all infants and toddlers with growth failure and diarrhea as well as any child with suspected or documented steatorrhea to rule out cystic fibrosis. A genotypic analysis for the known mutations in cystic fibrosis can also be performed on a sample of blood (and in most states is part of the newborn screening process). The nutritional support of children with cystic fibrosis is discussed in detail in Chapter 48.

Screening Laboratory Blood Studies

An analysis of blood or serum constituents is individualized according to the clinical situation and degree of concern for malabsorption, malnutrition, and inflammatory disease. A routine complete blood cell count with indices addresses issues of anemia as well as iron, vitamin B_{12}, and folate sufficiency. An elevated platelet count may indicate vitamin E deficiency or inflammation, because platelets are acute phase reactants. Characteristic alterations of red cell morphology are seen in abetalipoproteinemia. Erythrocyte sedimentation rate and C-reactive protein support inflammation but are nonspecific.

Serum immunoglobulins are measured specifically, with special emphasis on immunoglobulin (Ig) A. To screen for celiac disease, the specific IgA anti-tissue transglutaminase antibody has replaced the role of less specific anti-gliadin antibodies. Elevated tissue transglutaminase IgA antibody has a high specificity for celiac disease of greater than 95% and a sensitivity of up to 96%, but a low total serum IgA level may result in a false-negative test result.[13] Low serum albumin and prealbumin concentrations reflect low dietary protein intake.

Serum calcium, phosphorus, and alkaline phosphatase concentrations should be determined, along with concentrations of one or more of the fat-soluble vitamins—A, D, E, and K—if fat malabsorption or deficiency is suspected. Serum vasoactive intestinal peptide (VIP) and/or urinary concentrations of the catecholamines homovanilmandelic and vanilmandelic acids should be obtained when diarrhea appears to be secretory.

Imaging

The value of radiologic studies for the evaluation of chronic diarrhea is limited. A plain film of the abdomen may reveal constipation, dilated blind loops of bowel, or calcifications of the biliary or pancreatic system. Oral contrast studies and computed tomography scans with contrast are routine for the evaluation of inflammatory bowel disease, identifying, in particular, areas of small bowel disease not viewable by endoscopy. Magnetic resonance enterography has been recognized also as an important imaging modality in IBD, because it may demonstrate intestinal inflammation without exposure to radiation.[14]

Breath Hydrogen Analysis

The hydrogen breath test is a noninvasive test that can be used to examine for carbohydrate malabsorption. The test requires commensal hydrogen-producing enteric bacterial flora and generally is not valid after recent antibiotic use. When an oral carbohydrate is given, it is either digested and absorbed normally or it reaches the bacterial flora (normally found in the cecum and colon) intact and is fermented to produce hydrogen gas that is absorbed and excreted in the breath. Analysis of breath hydrogen that reveals an increase of >20 ppm from the fasting baseline suggests carbohydrate malabsorption or bacterial overgrowth. The test is performed with oral lactose (for lactase deficiency), sucrose (for sucrase-isomaltase deficiency), or lactulose (for small-bowel bacterial overgrowth).

Endoscopic Procedures

When persistent diarrhea appears to be related to an inflammatory process of the small bowel or colon, invasive endoscopic visualization of the bowel with biopsy is indicated. Endoscopy may reveal duodenal villous blunting and intraepithelial lymphocytes in celiac disease or evidence of ileal or colonic inflammation in infectious colitis or IBD. Small bowel biopsy during endoscopy also may show evidence of duodenitis in parasitic infections. Routine staining of tissue samples may be supplemented by electron microscopy, which might reveal microvillus inclusion disease, or biochemical analysis of the biopsy sample, which might reveal the lack of a disaccharidase.

Differential Diagnosis of Chronic Diarrhea

A review of the many disorders capable of inducing persistent or chronic diarrhea is beyond the scope of this chapter. In Table 28.1, the major conditions are listed as either commonly associated with normal growth or those expected to be complicated by growth failure or failure to thrive. Inappropriate nutritional

VI

Table 28.1.
Chronic Diarrhea in Childhood

Diarrhea Without Failure to Thrive
Chronic nonspecific (toddler's) diarrhea Dietary-induced diarrhea • Excessive juice, tea • Prolonged low-fat diet • Disaccharide intolerance: lactose, sucrose Persistent enteritis • Parasitic: *Giardia* species, *Strongyloides* species, *Cryptosporidium* species, *Cyclospora* species • Immunodeficient: IgA deficiency, human immunodeficiency virus infection • Small-bowel bacterial overgrowth Factitious diarrhea • Laxative abuse • Encopresis • Munchausen by proxy Secretory diarrhea • Neural crest tumors • Congenital chloride diarrhea • Congenital sodium diarrhea
Diarrhea With Failure to Thrive

Pancreatic insufficiency
• Cystic fibrosis
• Shwachman-Diamond syndrome
Disorders of lipid digestion, absorption, or transport
• Primary bile acid (micelle) deficiency
• Abetalipoproteinemia
• Intestinal lymphangiectasia
• Chylomicron retention disease
Disorders of the mucosal villus
• Congenital
  – Microvillus inclusion disease
  – Tufting disease
• Reduced mucosal surface area
  – Short-bowel syndrome
  – Malnutrition
  – Ischemic, radiation enteropathy
  – Graft-versus-host disease
Disorders of ion transport
  Congenital chloride diarrhea
  Glucose-galactose malabsorption
  Congenital sodium diarrhea
  Absence of enteric hormones
  Congenital bile-acid diarrhea
  Congenital lactase deficiency

- Inflammatory villus injury
  - Postgastroenteritis diarrhea with malabsorption
  - Acute infectious diarrhea
  - Celiac disease
  - Dietary protein induced enteropathy: milk, soy, egg, fish
  - Allergic eosinophilic gastroenteropathy
  - Autoimmune enteritis
  - Crohn's disease
  - Blind loop/pseudo-obstruction
  - Whipple enteropathy
  - Intractable diarrhea

---

management of any of these disorders, however, can lead to weight loss and growth failure.[15]

Diarrhea Without Failure to Thrive

Chronic Nonspecific (Toddler's) Diarrhea

This is the most common form of persistent diarrhea in the first 3 years of life.[16] It may begin acutely before 1 year of age but settles into a pattern of 2 to 5 loose to watery stools daily. Typically, patients pass stools only during waking hours, often beginning with a large formed or semiformed stool after awakening. As the day progresses, stools become more watery and smaller in volume. Transit time of enteral contents may be especially short, and parents frequently describe undigested food remnants in the stool. Although some affected children describe mild abdominal discomfort, most appear healthy and maintain a normal appetite and activity level.[17,18] Multiple dietary manipulations may produce transient improvement but usually contribute to the problem by removing higher-fat foods and increasing ingestion of fruit juices ("juiceorrhea"). This is especially true with the intake of high sorbitol-containing noncitrus juices, such as prune, pear, cherry, or apple juices. The American Academy of Pediatrics (AAP) policy statement on the use and misuse of fruit juices discourages fruit juice in infants younger than 6 months and recommends against the use of fruit juice in the treatment of dehydration or the management of diarrhea.[19]

By definition, children with chronic nonspecific diarrhea are clinically well, maintaining weight and height, with normal intestinal digestive and absorptive ability. Toddlers will do best on a normal diet that includes 30% to 40% of calories from fat and less than 4 to 6 oz of juice per day. Diarrhea often resolves with the

VI

acquisition of successful bowel toilet training, which allows greater duration of rectal retention.

Disaccharide Intolerance

Lactose is a major dietary constituent for most children, because it is the primary carbohydrate of all mammalian milks other than the sea lion. Lactose is both a major source of energy and a facilitator for the intestinal absorption of calcium, magnesium, and manganese. It is digested by an intestinal mucosal brush-border disaccharidase—lactase—to glucose and galactose. Lactase activity decreases, in many species, under genetic control, after weaning. Approximately 70% of the world's adult population has primary acquired lactase deficiency. Age of onset varies among populations, with one fifth of Hispanic, Asian, and black children becoming lactose intolerant before 5 years of age. White children typically do not lose lactase function until after 5 years of age and often much later, during later teen years or beyond.[20] Molecular studies have elucidated differences in messenger RNA expression among races that might explain population-based variations in lactase activity.[21] Congenital lactase deficiency is exceedingly rare, and only a handful of cases have been published in the literature.[20]

As lactase activity decreases, dietary lactose is incompletely digested and induces an osmotic secretion of electrolytes and fluid in the distal small bowel. As the lactose reaches the bacterial flora of the distal bowel, it is fermented to hydrogen, methane, and carbon dioxide. This allows the diagnosis by breath hydrogen and methane analysis and also contributes to the child's sense of discomfort from gas and increased flatus. The fermentation of lactose also produces volatile fatty acids that are absorbed across the colonic epithelium as an energy source.

The first step in the treatment of lactose malabsorption involves eliminating lactose from the diet to determine whether symptoms resolve. A gradual reintroduction of lactose-containing foods can help determine the threshold for tolerance of lactose in the diet. Lactose-reduced milks are commonly available, as are lactase tablets, which are taken before ingesting lactose-containing foods. A number of probiotics to enhance lactose tolerance are under investigation, but none have demonstrated reproducible beneficial effects on symptoms. The heating and fermentation of many cheeses reduce lactose content, and yogurt is also lower in lactose than fluid milk. The major risk of lactose-restricted diets is the reduction in dietary calcium intake, particularly in the age group of 9 to 18 years, when desired daily intakes of 1300 mg of calcium are difficult to achieve in the absence of dairy products in the diet.

Infants with diarrhea on sucrose or glucose polymer-containing formulas may have congenital sucrase-isomaltase deficiency. This diagnosis is confirmed by sucrose breath hydrogen testing, and sucrase deficiency can be treated with a baker's yeast (*Saccharomyces cerevisiae*) processed to a high content of a yeast invertase that cleaves

AAP

What the AAP Says About Lactose[20]

1. Lactose intolerance is a common cause of abdominal pain in older children and teenagers.

2. Lactose intolerance attributable to primary lactase deficiency is uncommon before 2 to 3 years of age in all populations; when lactose malabsorption becomes apparent before 2 to 3 years of age, other etiologies must be sought.

3. Evaluation for lactose intolerance can be achieved relatively easily by dietary elimination and challenge. More formal testing is usually noninvasive, typically with fecal pH in the presence of watery diarrhea and hydrogen breath testing.

4. If lactose-free diets are used for treatment of lactose intolerance, the diets should include a good source of calcium and/or calcium supplementation to meet daily recommended intakes.

5. Treatment of lactose intolerance by elimination of milk and other dairy products is not usually necessary given newer approaches to lactose intolerance, including use of partially digested products (such as yogurts, cheeses, products containing *Lactobacillus acidophilus*, and pretreated milks). Evidence that avoidance of dairy products may lead to inadequate calcium intake and consequent suboptimal bone mineralization makes these important as alternatives to milk. Dairy products remain principle sources of protein and other nutrients that are essential for growth in children.

Heyman MB; American Academy of Pediatrics, Committee on Nutrition, Lactose intolerance in infants, children, and adolescents. *Pediatrics*. 2006;118(3):1279-1286

sucrose. In normal children, sucrase-isomaltase activity reaches near-adult levels by 1 month of age and is highly resistant to mucosal injury.[22]

Infectious Colitis and Enteritis

Salmonella species is one of the most common causes of laboratory-confirmed cases of foodborne intestinal disease reported to the Centers for Disease Control and Prevention each year.[23] The infection is usually contracted from exposure to food of animal origin related to poultry, eggs, beef, and dairy products. Nontyphoidal *Salmonella* organisms typically cause gastroenteritis with diarrhea, abdominal cramping, and fever. *Salmonella* organisms are generally detected in routine stool culture for up to 5 weeks but may be excreted in stool for >1 year in 5% of patients.[24] Antibiotic therapy for uncomplicated nontyphoidal *Salmonella* serotypes is not indicated, because it does not shorten the disease duration and may prolong the duration of excretion of

VI

bacteria in the stool.[25] Antibiotics are appropriate, however, in infants younger than 3 months of age or with immunosuppressive diseases, given the increased risk for invasive disease (bacteremia, osteomyelitis, abscess, meningitis) in these populations.[23]

Yersinia enterocolitica and *Yersinia pseudotuberculosis* may cause chronic diarrhea but less commonly than *Salmonella* organisms in US children. Infection typically occurs via exposure to food products, specifically pork (major *Yersinia* reservoir) and dairy products. Diarrheal stool may contain blood, mucus, and leukocytes, and symptoms may mirror appendicitis or ileal Crohn's disease because of inflammation of the terminal ileum. The efficacy of antibiotics in treating uncomplicated *Yersinia* has not been established.[26]

Other causes of bacterial chronic diarrhea include *Escherichia coli*, *Campylobacter* species, *Aeromonas* species, and *Plesiomonas* species. Enteropathogenic *E coli* (EPEC) is a leading cause of chronic diarrhea in developing countries, sometimes associated with fever, abdominal pain, and vomiting.[27] EPEC is one type of *E coli* infection for which antibiotic therapy has been shown to reduce morbidity and mortality in uncomplicated diarrheal disease.[28] Persistent bloody diarrhea with abdominal pain should raise suspicion for enterohemorrhagic *E coli* (EHEC), particularly because EHEC may result in hemolytic-uremic syndrome, a potentially dangerous complication. *Campylobacter* infection often originates from poultry and may cause diarrhea for only 4 to 5 days, but relapses are common. *Aeromonas* species, long considered a normal commensal organism, has recently been shown to cause secretory diarrhea with up to 20 watery stools/day. Symptoms are persistent in approximately one third of patients. Antibiotics do not seem to be helpful in uncomplicated *Campylobacter* and *Aeromonas* infections. *Plesiomonas* species can be found in fish, shellfish, cats, and dogs; also causes secretory diarrhea; and has a course that may be shortened by antibiotic therapy.[29]

The protozoa *Giardia intestinalis* and *Cryptosporidium* species may affect immunocompetent as well as immunodeficient children and adolescents. Both infections may affect the duodenum and upper small bowel, leading to mild villous blunting, disaccharidase deficiency, and resultant osmotic and secretory diarrhea. Malabsorption of fat, protein, and carbohydrates may occur, worsening diarrhea. Both infections are linked to contaminated water and may be associated with child care centers, exposure to wild animals, or recent travel to developing countries. Symptomatic giardiasis should be treated even in immunocompetent children. *Cryptosporidium* infection generally does not need to be treated unless the patient is immunocompromised. Nutritional support is particularly important during such cases of enteritis.

Small-Bowel Bacterial Overgrowth

Bacterial overgrowth has been recognized as a cause of persistent diarrhea and abdominal discomfort, especially in children younger than 2 years.[30] The diagnosis is established by a breath hydrogen test using lactulose as the carbohydrate; because there is no mucosal enzyme for lactulose hydrolysis, it is fermented by the bacteria in the proximal small bowel and in the large intestine. Thus, both an early and late rise of breath hydrogen after ingestion may indicate bacterial overgrowth in the small intestine. As well, a high fasting breath hydrogen level (>20 ppm) suggests bacterial overgrowth. Treatment with a brief course of an antibiotic agent, such as metronidazole or the nonabsorbable rifaximin, often followed by the use of a probiotic, may be effective in relieving symptoms.[30,31]

Irritable Bowel Syndrome

The symptoms of IBS often start in adolescence. The history often suggests the diagnosis, with abdominal pain relieved with defecation and an associated change in stool frequency without evidence of a structural or metabolic abnormality. These patients do not have rectal bleeding, anemia, weight loss, or fever. Celiac disease should be ruled out. Treatment is often challenging. Antispasmodic agents, tricyclic antidepressants, and selective serotonin-reuptake inhibitors may improve symptoms. Some probiotics have been useful in adult and pediatric IBS, but results are not consistent.[32] One randomized-control trial in children with IBS showed no effect of *Lactobacillus rhamnosus GG* over placebo in the relief of pain.[33]

Diarrhea With Failure to Thrive

Postgastroenteritis Diarrhea With Malabsorption/Intractable Diarrhea of Infancy

Persistent diarrhea after an acute episode of infectious diarrhea (intractable diarrhea of infancy [IDI]) remains a major clinical issue in developing countries but has decreased drastically in the resource-rich nations with the increased attention paid to the nutritional management of the child with acute diarrhea. This disorder is unique compared with chronic nonspecific diarrhea, because in IDI, there is weight loss associated with malabsorption and histologic evidence of enteropathy. Small-bowel biopsies reveal patchy villus atrophy with increased inflammatory infiltrates, featuring intraepithelial lymphocytes with increased plasma cells and macrophages in the lamina propria and adherent bacteria on the mucosal surface.[34] Nutrient malabsorption may occur in the jejunum and ileum. Disaccharide intolerance is common, contributing to osmotic diarrhea and increased fluid needs.

The characteristics most commonly associated with IDI include young age, relative malnutrition, and an altered immune response.[15] In developing countries, lack of breastfeeding is a major risk factor. Infants younger than 6 months are particularly susceptible. The diagnosis of IDI is based on the practitioner's awareness and the exclusion of alternative explanations. Intestinal biopsy should be deferred until the infant fails to respond to nutritional intervention with a lactose-free, sucrose-free diet with medium chain triglycerides. Although a subgroup will

VI

require amino acid-based or elemental diets, most can be managed on traditional diets or mixed protein diets.[35,36] Breastfeeding of infants is encouraged when possible. Both macronutrient and micronutrient deficiencies may occur from reduced intake and increased fecal loss. Total caloric needs for enteric recovery and catch-up growth often exceed 120 kcal/kg/day.

Enteric feedings are encouraged, either by continuous tube feeding or frequent small-volume bolus feedings. Initial caloric intake is attempted at 50 to 75 kcal/kg per day, increasing over 5 to 7 days to 130 to 150 kcal/kg/day. Protein is initiated at 1 to 2 g/kg/day, increasing to 3 to 4 g/kg/day as energy intake is maximized. The requirement for potassium, calcium, phosphorus, magnesium, and trace minerals is usually increased and must be monitored closely in severely affected infants. Although renal and cardiac function are usually normal, rapid changes in fluid and electrolyte intake must be monitored closely. Aggressive refeeding may rarely precipitate acute pancreatitis.

To prevent IDI, AAP recommendations for managing acute gastroenteritis should be followed: avoiding formula dilution and promoting early feeding that reduces intestinal permeability and illness duration and improves nutritional outcomes.[37] Dietary protein and fat are important in recovery, but simple carbohydrates should be minimized. Highly restricted carbohydrate-based diets are unnecessary and nutritionally suboptimal.

Celiac Disease (Gluten-Sensitive Enteropathy)

Celiac disease is an immune-mediated enteropathy that occurs with gluten ingestion in a genetically susceptible individual. With its prevalence in adults and children approaching 1% worldwide, celiac disease has become a more commonly diagnosed disorder.[38] Oat proteins are generally tolerated, although this remains somewhat controversial. The protein-induced injury triggers a release of tissue transglutaminase, a highly specific endomysial antigen. The IgA antibody to this transglutaminase is detected in serum of affected children and serves as a highly specific screening test. The diagnosis is confirmed by small-bowel biopsy, obtained by esophagogastroduodenoscopy. Treatment is by complete elimination of foods containing wheat (gluten), barley, and rye. Gluten-free foods are now readily marketed, and parents of children with celiac disease are instructed to read the labels of processed foods carefully. Anti-tissue transglutaminase antibody testing is repeated 6 to 8 months after the start of the gluten-free diet, and a decrease in serum concentrations is usually seen if the patient is adhering to the diet. The risk of developing celiac disease is even higher in children with diabetes, Williams syndrome, trisomy 21, and thyroid-related autoimmune disorders.

Short-Bowel Syndrome (See Also Chapter 47)

Short-bowel syndrome is the consequence of massive small bowel resection and the resulting severe nutrient malabsorption that occurs with loss of mucosal surface area. It is seen after surgical intervention for long-segment necrotizing enterocolitis, midgut volvulus, acute ischemic injury, small-bowel aganglionosis, gastroschisis, and diffuse Crohn's disease of the small bowel. The best prognosis is for children in whom the duodenum, distal ileum, and ileocecal valve can be preserved.

In the initial postoperative period following loss of a significant length of small bowel, total parenteral nutrition is universally used. The early initiation of enteral feedings maximizes the enteric hormonal stimulation and adaptation of the residual bowel by elongation, hypertrophy, and reduction in peristaltic rate.

The greatest potential for recovery is in infancy. The normal absorptive surface area at birth is approximately 950 cm^2, increasing to 7500 cm^2 in the adult. As noted, enteral feedings are begun as soon as possible to minimize the mucosal atrophy that occurs with prolonged total parenteral nutrition. Initial feedings usually contain protein as a hydrolysate or amino acids, lipid with a combination of medium-chain and long-chain triglycerides, and carbohydrate as glucose polymer. As with postgastroenteritis malabsorption, calories are gradually increased by 5 to 15 kcal/kg/day by intragastric infusion to full oral intake.

Inflammatory Bowel Disease

The nutritional consequences of diffuse small bowel inflammatory bowel disease (Crohn's disease) can be devastating. Affected children present with abdominal pain and diarrhea that is minimized by reduced energy intake. Combined with increased enteric loss of protein, zinc, and blood across the inflamed mucosa, the result is weight loss, reduced growth rate, delayed puberty, and anemia unresponsive to dietary iron. This is further complicated when active disease occurs during puberty, when nutritional needs for growth are increased, and by the use of anti-inflammatory and growth-inhibiting corticosteroid therapy. For further discussion of nutritional support in patients with inflammatory bowel disease, see Chapter 44.

Allergic Enteropathy

Allergic enteropathy, or eosinophilic enteropathy, associated with FTT, vomiting, and diarrhea, should be distinguished from allergic colitis occurring in otherwise healthy and thriving infants. As in allergic colitis, allergic enteropathy is induced by food proteins, with the most common being cow milk and soy proteins. In allergic enteropathy, however, there is small-intestinal mucosal damage resulting in malabsorption of protein, carbohydrate, and fat. When severe, vomiting and/or diarrhea may lead to lethargy, dehydration, and hypotension (often mimicking sepsis). Alternatively, this may present at 1 year of age, when breastfeeding is discontinued and the ingestion of cow milk is begun. The enteropathy resolves with elimination of

VI

the responsible protein, most often cow milk or soy. Protein hydrolysate and sometimes amino acid-based formulas are used as nutritional sources for these children.

Probiotics and Chronic Diarrhea

Probiotics, as defined by the Food and Agriculture Organization of the United Nations, are live microorganisms that confer a beneficial health effect on the host when administered in adequate amounts. Although probiotics have been shown to be of benefit in the management of acute diarrheal disorders, especially secondary to rotavirus, their advantage in chronic diarrhea is more variable, depending on the probiotic and the disease entity. Few randomized-controlled trials have been performed in children. Two principal findings in such trials have been the successful use of probiotics in treating acute viral gastroenteritis (mostly rotavirus) in healthy children and in preventing antibiotic-associated diarrhea in healthy children. There is some evidence that probiotics prevent necrotizing enterocolitis in very low birth weight infants, but probiotic strains and doses vary between studies. There has been no clear and reproducible success in treating pediatric ulcerative colitis or Crohn disease with probiotics. *L rhamnosus GG* and *Saccharomyces boulardii* have been effective in severe, recurrent *C difficile* diarrhea, and some probiotics have shown efficacy in the management of IBS and in bacterial overgrowth syndromes.[39]

Summary

Chronic diarrhea in childhood can result from many different causes that often must be defined before definitive treatment can be initiated. Particular attention should be paid to growth measurements to distinguish between chronic diarrhea with or without associated "failure to thrive." Understanding the 4 basic pathophysiologic mechanisms of diarrhea—osmotic, secretory, inflammatory, and intestinal dysmotility—may also aid in making a diagnosis. Nutrition support is the mainstay of treatment in children with an undefined cause of chronic diarrhea. Throughout the evaluation process, appropriate nutrition must be provided to meet the child's needs, either enterally or parentally if necessary, to facilitate healing and good health.

References

1. Victora CG, Bryce J, Fontaine O, Monasch R. Reducing deaths from diarrhoea through oral rehydration therapy. *Bull World Health Organ*. 2000;78(10):1246-1255

2. Abba K, Sinfield R, Hart CA, Garner P. Pathogens associated with persistent diarrhoea in children in low and middle income countries: systematic review. *BMC Infect Dis*. 2009;9:88

3. Snyder JD, Merson MH. The magnitude of the global problem of acute diarrhoeal disease: a review of active surveillance data. *Bull World Health Organ*. 1982;60(4):605-613

4. Vanderhoof JA. Chronic diarrhea. *Pediatr Rev*. 1998;19(12):418-422

5. Wenzl HH, Fine KD, Schiller LR, Fordtran JS. Determinants of decreased fecal consistency in patients with diarrhea. *Gastroenterology*. 1995;108(6):1729-1738

6. Gibson PR, Newnham E, Barrett JS, Shepherd SJ, Muir JG. Review article: fructose malabsorption and the bigger picture. *Aliment Pharmacol Ther*. 2007;25(4):349-363

7. Binder HJ. Causes of chronic diarrhea. *N Engl J Med*. 2006;355(3):236-239

8. Spiller R. Role of motility in chronic diarrhoea. *Neurogastroenterol Motil*. 2006;18(12):1045-1055

9. Fenton TR, Harries JT, Milla PJ. Disordered small intestinal motility: a rational basis for toddlers' diarrhoea. *Gut*. 1983;24(10):897-903

10. Keating JP. Chronic diarrhea. *Pediatr Rev*. 2005;26(1):5-14

11. Bruijnesteijn van Coppenraet LE, Wallinga JA, Ruijs GJ, Bruins MJ, Verweij JJ. Parasitological diagnosis combining an internally controlled real-time PCR assay for the detection of four protozoa in stool samples with a testing algorithm for microscopy. *Clin Microbiol Infect*. 2009;15(9):869-874

12. Valencia-Mendoza A, Bertozzi SM, Gutierrez JP, Itzler R. Cost-effectiveness of introducing a rotavirus vaccine in developing countries: the case of Mexico. *BMC Infect Dis*. 2008;8:103

13. Rostom A, Murray JA, Kagnoff MF. American Gastroenterological Association (AGA) Institute technical review on the diagnosis and management of celiac disease. *Gastroenterology*. 2006;131(6):1981-2002

14. Paolantonio P, Ferrari R, Vecchietti F, Cucchiara S, Laghi A. Current status of MR imaging in the evaluation of IBD in a pediatric population of patients. *Eur J Radiol*. 2009;69(3):418-424

15. Bhutta ZA, Hendricks KM. Nutritional management of persistent diarrhea in childhood: a perspective from the developing world. *J Pediatr Gastroenterol Nutr*. 1996;22(1):17-37

16. Cohen SA, Hendricks KM, Eastham EJ, Mathis RK, Walker WA. Chronic nonspecific diarrhea. A complication of dietary fat restriction. *Am J Dis Child*. 1979;133(5):490-492

17. Kneepkens CM, Hoekstra JH. Chronic nonspecific diarrhea of childhood: pathophysiology and management. *Pediatr Clin North Am*. 1996;43(2):375-390

18. Kleinman RE. Chronic nonspecific diarrhea of childhood. *Nestle Nutr Workshop Ser Pediatr Program*. 2005;56:73-79

19. American Academy of Pediatrics. Where We Stand: Fruit Juice. Elk Grove Village, IL: American Academy of Pediatrics; 2011. Available at: http://www.healthychildren.org/English/healthy-living/nutrition/Pages/Where-We-Stand-Fruit-Juice.aspx. Accessed November 16, 2012

20. Heyman MB; American Academy of Pediatrics, Committee on Nutrition. Lactose intolerance in infants, children, and adolescents. *Pediatrics*. 2006;118(3):1279-1286

21. Wang Y, Harvey CB, Hollox EJ, et al. The genetically programmed down-regulation of lactase in children. *Gastroenterology*. 1998;114:1230-1236

22. Treem WR. Clinical heterogeneity in congenital sucrase-isomaltase deficiency. *J Pediatr*. 1996;128(6):727-729

VI

23. American Academy of Pediatrics, Committee on Infectious Diseases. *Salmonella* infections. In: Pickering LK, Baker CJ, Kimberlin DW, Long SS, eds. *Red Book: 2012 Report of the Committee on Infectious Diseases*. 29th ed. Elk Grove Village, IL: American Academy of Pediatrics; 2009:635-640

24. Buchwald DS, Blaser MJ. A review of human salmonellosis: II. Duration of excretion following infection with nontyphi *Salmonella*. *Rev Infect Dis*. 1984;6(3):345-356

25. Barber DA, Miller GY, McNamara PE. Models of antimicrobial resistance and foodborne illness: examining assumptions and practical applications. *J Food Prot*. 2003;66(4):700-709

26. American Academy of Pediatrics, Committee on Infectious Diseases. *Yersinia enterocolitica* and *Yersinia pseudotuberculosis* infections. In: Pickering LK, Baker CJ, Kimberlin DW, Long SS, eds. *Red Book: 2012 Report of the Committee on Infectious Diseases*. 29th ed. Elk Grove Village, IL: American Academy of Pediatrics; 2009:795-797

27. Fagundes-Neto U, Scaletsky IC. The gut at war: the consequences of enteropathogenic *Escherichia coli* infection as a factor of diarrhea and malnutrition. *Sao Paulo Med J*. 2000;118(1):21-29

28. Nelson JD. Duration of neomycin for enteropathogenic *Escherichia coli* diarrheal disease: a comparative study of 113 cases. *Pediatrics*. 1971;48(2):248-258

29. Kain KC, Kelly MT. Clinical features, epidemiology, and treatment of *Plesiomonas shigelloides* diarrhea. *J Clin Microbiol*. 1989;27(5):998-1001

30. Singh VV, Toskes PP. Small bowel bacterial overgrowth: presentation, diagnosis, and treatment. *Curr Treat Options Gastroenterol*. 2004;7(1):19-28

31. Lauritano EC, Gabrielli M, Lupascu A, et al. Rifaximin dose-finding study for the treatment of small intestinal bacterial overgrowth. *Aliment Pharmacol Ther*. 2005;22:31-35

32. Kligler B, Hanaway P, Cohrssen A. Probiotics in children. *Pediatr Clin North Am*. 2007;54(6):949-967

33. Bausserman M, Michail S. The use of *Lactobacillus GG* in irritable bowel syndrome in children: a double-blind randomized control trial. *J Pediatr*. 2005;147(2):197-201

34. Shiner M, Putman M, Nichols VN, Nichols BL. Pathogenesis of small-intestinal mucosal lesions in chronic diarrhea of infancy: I. A light microscopic study. *J Pediatr. Gastroenterol Nutr*. 1990;11(4):455-463

35. Kleinman RE, Galeano NF, Ghishan F, Lebenthal E, Sutphen J, Ulshen MH. Nutritional management of chronic diarrhea and/or malabsorption. *J Pediatr Gastroenterol Nutr*. 1989;9(4):407-415

36. Bhatnagar S, Bhan MK, Singh KD, Saxena SK, Shariff M. Efficacy of milk-based diets in persistent diarrhea: a randomized, controlled trial. *Pediatrics*. 1996;98(6 Pt 1):1122-1126

37. King CK, Glass R, Bresee JS, Duggan C. Managing acute gastroenteritis among children: oral rehydration, maintenance, and nutritional therapy. *MMWR Recomm Rep*. 2003;52(RR-16):1-16

38. Green PH, Cellier C. Celiac disease. *N Engl J Med*. 2007;357:1731-1743

39. Thomas DW, Greer FR; American Academy of Pediatrics, Committee on Nutrition, Section on Gastroenterology, Hepatology, and Nutrition. Probiotics and prebiotics in pediatrics. *Pediatrics*. 2010;126(6):1217-1231

Chapter 29

Oral Therapy for Acute Diarrhea

Introduction

Diarrheal illness and accompanying acute dehydration remains a major cause of childhood deaths in the world, resulting in an estimated almost 2 million deaths annually.[1,2] Reduction of the morbidity and mortality from diarrhea through the use of oral rehydration salts (ORS) solutions continues to be a major goal of the United Nations Children's Fund (UNICEF) and the World Health Organization (WHO) as one of the major strategies for saving children's lives.[1,3,4] Because of its simplicity, great effectiveness, and low cost, ORS solution is an ideal treatment for use in the developing world and in industrialized nations.[3-5] In developing countries, ORS solution has played a major role in reducing the estimated number of deaths from diarrhea in children younger than 5 years by more than half.[1,6,7] Although the death rate from diarrheal illness in resource-rich countries like the United States is low, diarrheal illness still accounts for a substantial proportion of preventable childhood deaths and a large proportion of the morbidity and the expense associated with pediatric care.[8] For example, in the United States alone, approximately 150 000 to 200 000 children younger than 5 years are admitted each year for treatment of acute gastroenteritis, and as many as 16 million episodes of diarrheal illness occur in this age group.[9]

Physiologic Principles

The physiologic basis of ORS solution is, at the same time, simple and extraordinarily elegant. A combination of sodium with simple organic molecules, such as glucose, in the lumen of the small intestine can promote the absorption of water.[10] This system, discovered and characterized in the 1960s,[11] is now referred to as the glucose-sodium cotransport system.[10,12] Molecular details of the system are now reasonably well understood. In the cotransport mechanism, a single molecule of glucose or other simple organic substrate is transported across the luminal membrane of the villus crypt cells of the small intestine.[10,12] In concert with the transport of a glucose molecule, a sodium molecule is also brought from the luminal side of the membrane to the interior of the cell. This sodium ion is subsequently transferred into the adjacent capillaries and, thus, into the circulation. Water follows the movement of sodium along a concentration gradient, with the net result being absorption of sodium and water. The earliest clinical studies of solutions that take advantage of the cotransport system were performed in patients with cholera.[13] We now know that the glucose-sodium cotransport system remains intact in virtually all kinds of infectious diarrhea. This fact makes oral therapy appropriate for use in any kind of enteric

VI

infection in which dehydration is an end result.[5,10] The other components of ORS solution include potassium and chloride to replace stool losses and base, usually in the form of citrate, to replace stool losses and to combat acidosis.[10,12]

Many fluids that have traditionally been recommended for the treatment of diarrhea and dehydration are inappropriate, are nonphysiologic, and may worsen the condition.[4,5,10] For example, juices such as apple or white grape juice have a high osmolality related to their high sugar content and contain virtually no sodium and very little potassium, thus increasing the risk of hyponatremia. Table 29.1 lists the composition of some currently available rehydration solutions. Some of the frequently used inappropriate fluids are listed for comparison. Particular attention should be paid to the osmolality of the fluids. In general, solutions with osmolality lower than serum (approximately 310 mOsm/L) make the most effective ORS solutions if the ratio of glucose to sodium is maintained near one.[10,14] Solutions containing less sodium than the standard WHO/UNICEF formulation and having glucose to sodium ratios of approximately 3 have also proven effective in maintaining hydration in noncholera diarrhea.[6]

Table 29.1.

Composition of Fluids Frequently Used in Oral Rehydration Compared With Fluids Not Recommended for Oral Rehydration

Solution	Glucose/ CHO, g/L	Sodium, mEq/L	HCO_3^-, MEq/L	Potassium mEq/L	Osmolality, mmol/L	CHO/ Sodium
Pedialyte[b] (Abbott Laboratories)	25	45	30	20	250	3.1
Enfalyte (Mead Johnson)	30	50	34	25	200	
Pediatric Electrolyte[c] (Nutramax)	25	45	20	30	250	3.1
WHO ORS, 2002[d] (reduced osmolarity)	13.5	75	10†	20	245	1.0
WHO ORS, 1975, (original formulation)	20	90	10†	20	311	1.2
Cola[a]	126	2	13	0.1	750	1944
Apple juice[a]	125	3	0	32	730	1278
Gatorade[a]	45	20	3	3	330	62.5

CHO indicates carbohydrate; HCO_3^-, bicarbonate; and WHO, World Health Organization

[a] Cola, juice, and Gatorade are shown for comparison only; they are not recommended for use (as is the case for energy drinks, vitamin waters, gelatin desserts, and other fluids that do not contain glucose and sodium in appropriate concentrations).

[b] Mainly for maintenance therapy; may be used for rehydration therapy in mildly dehydrated patients.

[c] This formulation is supplied to many retail establishments to which they apply their company name.

[d] Best for rehydration therapy; may be used during the maintenance phase with adequate access to free water in the form of human milk, infant formula, or diluted juices.

The Search for a More Effective ORS

Although ORS solution has an impressive record of success, it remains underutilized.[1,4,5,15] Perhaps the most important factor limiting the use of ORS solution has been the lack of antidiarrheal properties.[5] The original ORS solutions were very effective at replacing fluid and electrolyte losses but had no effect on the volume or duration of diarrhea.[1,4,10,14]

The initial efforts to create ORS solutions that would decrease stool volume and output focused on the addition of other sodium cotransport molecules, such as the amino acids glycine, alanine, and glutamine.[3,10,16] However, these solutions proved to be no more effective than ORS solution, were more expensive, and had some potentially dangerous adverse effects.[3,17] At about the same time, studies of complex carbohydrates (starches) from cereals were undertaken. Starches do not contribute significantly to the osmotic content of the solution and yield individual glucose molecules at the brush border of the small intestine.[10] This allows the delivery of large numbers of glucose molecules to the cotransport system without causing osmotic diarrhea. Numerous studies demonstrated that cereal-based ORS solutions can reduce the volume of stools and the duration of diarrheal illness, though not necessarily in the case of noncholera diarrhea.[18,19] These solutions have not had a major effect, because the precooked dry cereal forms were more expensive than standard ORS solutions, and the home-cooked cereal forms were time-consuming to prepare and required often-expensive cooking fuel. In addition, when cereal-based solutions were compared with the combination of glucose-based solutions and the early reinstitution of feeding, the differences between the 2 approaches disappeared, so that cereal-based ORS solutions have not replaced the easier-to-prepare glucose ORS solution.[18,20]

The search for more effective oral rehydration solutions was greatly aided by the discovery that reduced osmolarity glucose-electrolyte solutions can result in improved water and electrolyte transport from the intestinal lumen.[3,21] This discovery led to series of studies that have demonstrated that reduced-osmolarity ORS solutions are more effective in replacing fluid and electrolyte losses compared with the standard WHO ORS solution.[14,22] Reduced-osmolarity ORS solutions have not been shown to decrease stool volume or duration of diarrhea. However, a meta-analysis of clinical trials in children in developing countries showed that these solutions resulted in less need for supplemental intravenous fluids, less vomiting, and a slight reduction in stool output compared with the standard WHO ORS.[23] On the basis of these findings, WHO and UNICEF have recommended that a single reduced-osmolarity ORS be used to treat all cases of diarrhea.[24] The main concern raised about the reduced-osmolarity ORS solutions is that they would lead to hyponatremia, especially when used for treatment of patients with high-purging

VI

diarrheas, like cholera, because the sodium content is only about two thirds that of the standard WHO ORS.[25] Data from the initial trials indicate that hyponatremia occurs more commonly with these solutions, but symptomatic hyponatremia has been very uncommon.[3,24]

Zinc Supplementation

Zinc supplementation during acute and chronic noncholera diarrhea has been shown to reduce diarrhea duration and stool frequency and decrease reoccurrence of symptoms for 2 to 3 months.[26,27] The WHO now recommends zinc supplementation (20 mg/day for 10-14 days for children 6 months and older, 10 mg/day for children younger than 6 months) in combination with ORS solution for children with acute diarrhea.[28]

Early, Appropriate Feeding

For more than 20 years, clinicians have recognized that return to an age-appropriate and healthy diet early in the course of diarrheal illness is superior to the outdated practice of "resting the gut" by providing only clear liquids or dilute milks.[5,10,29] Appropriate feeding is the component of oral therapy that has the potential for the greatest impact on stool volume and duration.[4,5] In addition, the appetite of the infant and child is generally better maintained, and intestinal repair can occur.[5]

Successful feeding trials have been carried out using human milk, dilute or full-strength animal milk or animal milk formulas, dilute and full-strength lactose-free formulas, and mixed diets of staple foods with milk.[5,29,30] Data from multiple studies support the use of lactose-containing milks during diarrhea, especially if given with complex carbohydrates.[31] In general, the change to a lactose-free formula should be made only if the stool output increases on a milk-based diet.[55] Semisolid and solid foods that have proven to be effective in controlled trials include rice, wheat, peas, potatoes, chicken, and eggs.[5,29]

Oral Therapy for Diarrhea

In addition to the use of a physiologically sound ORS solution and early, appropriate feeding, effective oral therapy requires a thoughtful parental education component. When possible, explaining to the parent that the child's diarrhea is likely to continue, regardless of therapy, for 3 to 7 days can be extremely helpful. Parents who understand that hydration is the primary concern, not the duration of the diarrheal stool, will generally be more comfortable managing the child's illness at home. By emphasizing to the parents that ORS solution replaces fluid and electrolyte losses but does not stop diarrhea, less disappointment and discouragement should develop. A positive approach to teaching parents includes pointing out the degree of control that parents retain when the child receives ORS solution compared with the loss of that control that results when intravenous solutions are used. In addition, parents are often reassured to know that ORS solution is less painful, has fewer complications, and is just as effective as intravenous therapy.[32] Finally, most parents greatly desire to feed their child, particularly when the child appears to be hungry and thirsty, and this should be encouraged. The following management guidelines are based on the severity of the child's condition.[4,5]

Children With Diarrhea and No Dehydration

If no dehydration develops, which is the case in the great majority of diarrhea cases in the United States, continued age-appropriate feeding is the only therapy required.[4] Nonweaned infants should receive human milk or continue use of regular formula. Formula does not require dilution if the diarrhea remains mild. If a diluted formula is used, the concentration should be increased rapidly if the diarrhea does not worsen. Weaned infants and children should have their regular nutritionally balanced diet continued, emphasizing complex carbohydrates (such as rice, wheat, and potatoes), meats (especially chicken), and the child's regular milk or formula. Diets high in simple sugars and fats should be avoided.[4,5] The "BRATT" diet (bananas, rice, applesauce, tea, and toast) should be avoided, because it is not a balanced diet and is low in energy.[5]

Children With Mild or Moderate Dehydration

After dehydration is corrected (Table 29.2), appropriate feeding is begun, using the guidelines in the previous paragraph. The most convenient method for carrying out rehydration is to divide the total volume deficit by 4 and aim to deliver this volume of fluid during each of the 4 hours of the rehydration phase. A teaspoon or 5-mL syringe can be used for the initial administration of fluid, especially if the child is vomiting. The parent is instructed to administer at least 1 teaspoon (5 mL) of solution each minute. Having a clock with a sweep second hand available is useful. Although this rate of fluid delivery may appear slow, 5 mL per minute results in an hourly intake of 300 mL. In a 10-kg infant, this is equivalent to 30 mL/kg. Children larger than 15 to 20 kg can receive 2 teaspoons, or 10 mL, per minute and achieve a similar volume of fluid intake. In general, this rate of fluid administration is more than adequate to replace the entire calculated volume deficit within a 4-hour period.

VI

Table 29.2.
Fluid Therapy Chart

Degree of Dehydration	Signs	Fluids	Feeding
Mild[a]	Slightly dry mucous membranes, increased thirst	ORS, 50-60 mL/kg[b]	Breastfeeding, undiluted lactose-free formula, full-strength cow milk, or lactose-containing formula
Moderate	Sunken eyes, sunken fontanelle, loss of skin turgor, dry mucous membranes	ORS, 80-100 mL/kg[b]	Same as above
Severe	Signs of moderate dehydration plus one or more of the following: rapid thready pulse, cyanosis, rapid breathing, delayed capillary refill time, lethargy, coma	Intravenous or intraosseous isotonic fluids (0.9% saline solution or lactated Ringer solution), 40 mL/kg per hour until pulse and state of consciousness return to normal, then 50-100 mL/kg of ORS based on remaining degree of dehydration[c]	Begin after clinically improved and ORS has started

[a] If no signs of dehydration are present, rehydration phase may be omitted. Proceed with maintenance therapy and replacement of ongoing losses.

[b] First 4 hours, repeat until no signs of dehydration remain. Replace ongoing stool losses and vomitus with oral rehydration solution (ORS), 10 mL/kg for each diarrheal stool and 5 mL/kg for each episode of vomiting.

[c] While parenteral access is being sought, nasogastric infusion of ORS may be begun at 30 mL/kg per hour, provided airway protective reflexes remain intact.

During rehydration, the volume of stool and emesis should be carefully recorded and added to the hourly quantity of fluid to be administered. After 1 or 2 hours of successful rehydration using a syringe or teaspoon, most infants and children will be able to take the fluid ad libitum. On rare occasions, a child will not cooperate in taking the solution from a syringe (this is most often the case with toddlers) or may be too exhausted to remain awake during the administration of fluid. In these cases and after carefully establishing that airway protective reflexes are intact, a soft 5F polymeric silicone nasogastric tube may be placed into the lumen of the stomach. The ORS solution may then be administered via the nasogastric tube at approximately 5 to 10 mL/kg per minute. This method has been widely used in the developing world and has also proved quite successful in industrialized countries.

Children With Severe Dehydration

Children with severe dehydration, which is a shock or a near shock-like condition, should be treated as an emergency.[4,5] A large-bore catheter should be used for the infusion of lactated Ringer solution, normal saline solution, or similar solution, and boluses of 20 to 40 mL/kg should be administered until signs of shock resolve. Fluid and electrolyte resuscitation may require more than 1 intravenous site, and the use of alternate access sites, including venous cutdown, femoral vein, or interosseous locations, may be needed. As the level of consciousness improves, oral rehydration therapy can be instituted. Hydration status must be frequently reassessed to monitor the effectiveness of the therapy. When rehydration is complete, feeding is continued as described for children without dehydration.

Common Concerns About ORS Solutions in the United States

Refusal to Take ORS

One of the most common complaints about ORS solutions from children and their parents in the United States is the salty taste.[15] However, children who are dehydrated rarely refuse ORS solution, because they usually crave salt and water. By recognizing that ORS solution may not be required in children with mild diarrhea and no dehydration, the problem of refusal could be greatly reduced.[5] Methods to try to increase ORS intake have included the use of flavoring in ORS solutions, which does not alter the composition of fluid and electrolytes but improves taste.[5] Flavored ORS solutions are now the most popular forms of ORS sold in North America. Another effective technique to increase intake is to freeze the ORS solution in an ice-pop form.

Vomiting

Vomiting, which is commonly associated with acute diarrhea, can make oral rehydration therapy more challenging, but almost all children with vomiting can be treated successfully with ORS solution.[2,4,5,22] Correction of fluid and electrolyte deficits with balanced electrolyte ORS solution can help speed recovery from vomiting. As vomiting decreases, ORS solution can be given in larger volumes. A precautionary note must be made about vomiting, which can be evidence of bowel obstruction. For this reason, efforts should be made to eliminate the possible diagnosis of bowel obstruction on a clinical basis before proceeding with ORS solution. In a patient who may have an obstructive or other acute process, immediate vascular access must be gained, a surgical consultation must be obtained, and the child should be kept without oral fluids or food.

VI

Hypernatremia

ORS solutions were originally developed to treat dehydration resulting from cholera, in which stool losses of sodium are substantial. In resource-rich countries like the United States, concerns have been expressed about the risk of hypernatremia with the use of solutions containing 90 mEq/L of sodium in infants and children whose diarrhea results from noncholera organisms.[4,5,15] In the presence of mature, functioning kidneys, the earlier 90-mEq sodium solution and newer 75-mEq sodium solution are both safe and extremely effective in children with a wide range of initial serum sodium concentrations and are effective treatments for hypernatremia.[4,5] In contrast, when solutions with little sodium, such as juices, sodas, or water (Table 29.1) are used, the risk of hyponatremia is very real.[4,5] Of greater importance than the sodium concentration is the ratio of sodium to glucose (or other cotransport molecule), which should be close to one.[3,5,10]

Failure of Therapy

Failure of ORS solution occurs when the net output over a 4- to 8-hour period exceeds net intake or when clinical indicators of dehydration are worsening rather than improving. Before determining that ORS solution has failed in a child, a review of the treatment guidelines should be made with the parents or other caregiver. Often, treatment failures and unnecessary intravenous line placement can result from lack of understanding or failure to encourage staff or parents to continue to administer ORS solution.

References

1. Black RE, Morris SS, Bryce J. Where and why are 10 million children dying every year? *Lancet*. 2003;361(9376):2226-2234

2. Boschi-Pinto C, Velebit L, Shibuya K. Estimating child mortality due to diarrhoea in developing countries. *Bull World Health Organ*. 2008;86(9):710-717

3. Duggan C, Fontaine O, Pierce NF, et al. Scientific rationale for a change in the composition of oral rehydration solution. *JAMA*. 2004;291(21):2628-2631

4. King CK, Glass R, Bresee JS, Duggan C. Managing acute gastroenteritis among children: oral rehydration, maintenance, and nutritional therapy. *MMWR Recomm Rep*. 2003;52(RR-16):1-16

5. American Academy of Pediatrics, Provisional Committee on Quality Improvement, Subcommittee on Acute Gastroenteritis. Practice parameter: the management of acute gastroenteritis in young children. *Pediatrics*. 1996;97(3):424-435

6. Parashar UD, Hummelman EG, Bresee JS, Miller MA, Glass RI. Global illness and deaths caused by rotavirus disease in children. *Emerg Infect Dis*. 2003;9(5):565-572

7. Snyder JD, Merson MH. The magnitude of the global problem of acute diarrhoeal disease: a review of active surveillance data. *Bull World Health Organ*. 1982;60(4):605-613

8. Fischer TK, Viboud C, Prashar U, et al. Hospitalizations and deaths from diarrhea and rotavirus among children <5 years of age in the United States, 1993-2003. *J Infect Dis.* 2007;195(8):1117-1125

9. Glass RI, Lew JF, Gangarosa RE, LeBaron CW, Ho MS. Estimates of morbidity and mortality rates for diarrheal diseases in American children. *J Pediatr.* 1991;118(4 Pt 2):S27-S33

10. Hirschhorn N, Greenough WB III. Progress in oral rehydration therapy. *Sci Am.* 1991;264(5):50-56

11. Sladen GE, Dawson AM. Interrelationships between the absorptions of glucose, sodium and water by the normal human jejunum. *Clin Sci.* 1969;36(1):119-132

12. Field M. Intestinal ion transport and the pathophysiology of diarrhea. *J Clin Invest.* 2003;111(7):931-943

13. Hirschhorn N. The treatment of acute diarrhea in children. An historical and physiological perspective. *Am J Clin Nutr.* 1980;33(3):637-663

14. CHOICE Study Group. Multicenter, randomized, double-blind clinical trial to evaluate the efficacy and safety of a reduced osmolarity oral rehydration salts solution in children with acute watery diarrhea. *Pediatrics.* 2001;107(4):613-618

15. Avery ME, Snyder JD. Oral therapy for acute diarrhea. The underused simple solution. *N Engl J Med.* 1990;323(13):891-894

16. Bhan MK, Mahalanabis D, Fontaine O, Pierce NF. Clinical trials of improved oral rehydration salt formulations: a review. *Bull World Health Organ.* 1994;72(6):945-955

17. Santosham M, Burns BA, Reid R, et al. Glycine-based oral rehydration solution: reassessment of safety and efficacy. *J Pediatr.* 1986;109(5):795-801

18. Gore SM, Fontaine O, Pierce NF. Impact of rice based oral rehydration solution on stool output and duration of diarrhoea: meta-analysis of 13 clinical trials. *BMJ.* 1992;304(6822):287-291

19. Fontaine O, Gore SM, Pierce NF. Rice-based oral rehydration solution for treating diarrhoea. *Cochrane Database Syst Rev.* 2000;(2):CD001264

20. Fayad IM, Hashem M, Duggan C, et al. Comparative efficacy of rice-based and glucose-based oral rehydration salts plus early reintroduction of food. *Lancet.* 1993;342(8874):772-775

21. Thillainayagam AV, Hunt JB, Farthing MJ. Enhancing clinical efficacy of oral rehydration therapy: is low osmolality the key? *Gastroenterology.* 1998;114(1):197-210

22. Santosham M, Fayad I, Abu Zikri M, et al. A double-blind clinical trial comparing World Health Organization oral rehydration solution with a reduced osmolarity solution containing equal amounts of sodium and glucose. *J Pediatr.* 1996;128(1):45-51

23. Hahn S, Kim Y, Garner P. Reduced osmolarity oral rehydration solution for treating dehydration due to diarrhoea in children: systematic review. *BMJ.* 2001;323(7304):81-85

24. World Health Organization. Reduced Osmolarity Oral Rehydration Salts (ORS). New York, NY: UNICEF House; July 18, 2001

25. Nalin DR, Hirschhorn N, Greenough W, 3rd, Fuchs GJ, Cash RA. Clinical concerns about reduced-osmolarity oral rehydration solution. *JAMA.* 2004;291(21):2632-2635

VI

26. Bhatnagar S, Bahl R, Sharma PK, Kumar GT, Saxena SK, Bhan MK. Zinc with oral rehydration therapy reduces stool output and duration of diarrhea in hospitalized children: a randomized controlled trial. *J Pediatr Gastroenterol Nutr*. 2004;38(1):34-40

27. Lukacik M, Thomas RL, Aranda JV. A meta-analysis of the effects of oral zinc in the treatment of acute and persistent diarrhea. *Pediatrics*. 2008;121(2):326-336

28. World Health Organizaiton and United Nations Children's Fund. Clinical management of acute diarrhoea. Geneva, Switzerland/New York, NY: World Health Organizaiton and United Nations Children's Fund; 2004

29. Brown KH. Dietary management of acute childhood diarrhea: optimal timing of feeding and appropriate use of milks and mixed diets. *J Pediatr*. 1991;118(4 Pt 2):S92-S8

30. Brown KH. Appropriate diets for the rehabilitation of malnourished children in the community setting. *Acta Paediatr Scand Suppl*. 1991;374:151-159

31. Brown KH, Peerson JM, Fontaine O. Use of nonhuman milks in the dietary management of young children with acute diarrhea: a meta-analysis of clinical trials. *Pediatrics*. 1994;93(1):17-27

32. Hartling L, Bellemare S, Wiebe N, Russell K, Klassen TP, Craig W. Oral versus intravenous rehydration for treating dehydration due to gastroenteritis in children. *Cochrane Database Syst Rev*. 2006;(3):CD004390

Chapter 30

Inborn Errors of Metabolism

Definitions

Metabolism may be defined as the sum of chemical processes through which food is converted into smaller molecules and energy. An inborn error of metabolism (IEM), therefore, may be defined as an inherited defect in the structure or function of a key protein in a metabolic pathway. These diseases involve processes of energy production; the anabolism and catabolism of fats, carbohydrates, or amino acids; the synthesis and degradation of complex macromolecules; the transport of substances across cell membranes; and the detoxification of cellular wastes. The spectrum of cardinal features, age of clinically apparent symptoms, morbidity, mortality, and types of currently used therapies vary widely across this diverse group of disorders.

Inheritance

Each individual IEM occurs only rarely, with population incidences ranging from 1:2500 births for hemochromatosis to only a few single case reports of other disorders. Collectively, the total incidence of IEMs in the population is approximately 1:1000 births. Many IEMs are known or considered to be autosomal-recessive diseases attributable to single-gene defects encoded by nuclear DNA. A few IEMs are inherited in an autosomal-dominant pattern, and a small fraction are X-linked disorders, exhibiting a more severe phenotype in hemizygous males than in heterozygous females. Still other IEMs are attributable to alterations in the mitochondrial DNA and are inherited only through a maternal lineage.

Newborn Screening for IEMs

Although a few IEMs, such as fructokinase deficiency (essential fructosuria), do not cause any clinical disease, the vast majority of IEMs cause organ dysfunction. With some disorders, signs and symptoms may not be present in the immediate neonatal period, although deleterious compounds are accumulating in the brain, other organs, and body fluids. Because recognition of the disease and early institution of therapy can significantly alter the morbidity and mortality of these initially occult disorders, screening tests have been developed. The American College of Medical Genetics advocates neonatal screening for 29 core conditions in the United States, including aminoacidopathies such as phenylketonuria, several disorders of fatty acid oxidation or organic acid metabolism, galactosemia, biotinidase deficiency, hypo-thyroidism, congenital adrenal hyperplasia, and hemoglobinopathies,[1] and as of July 2011, all states are fully compliant with this recommendation. Many states also screen for other secondary conditions for which evidence of screening efficacy is less compelling. The National Newborn Screening Resource Center (http://genes-r-us.uthscsa.edu) maintains an up-to-date database listing the disorders currently tested for in each individual state. The American Academy of Pediatrics has published 2 technical reports regarding newborn screening, which include fact sheets on a number of metabolic disorders (biotinidase deficiency, tyrosinemia, phenylketon-uria, medium-chain acyl-CoA dehydrogenase [MCAD] deficiency, maple syrup urine disease, homocystinuria, and galactosemia).[2,3] Key elements to a successful screening program are rapid transit of specimens to the newborn screening labora-tory, timely specimen testing and identification of abnormal results, notification of health care providers, follow-up with a definitive confirmatory assay, and the initiation of effective treatment to be carried out in consultation with a multidisci-plinary center specializing in IEM therapy. Patients with abnormal results, especially when the disease in question may have acute manifestations, should be referred promptly to a metabolic disease center that can further evaluate the potential disorder. If the patient is at risk of acute or severe illness, immediate consultation with a physician specializing in metabolic disorders by telephone for diagnosis and treatment options is advised. Precise and early diagnosis is essential so that effective therapies can be instituted safely and the family receives proper counseling. Recommendations for dealing with newborn screening results in the primary care setting have been published by the American Academy of Pediatrics in a clinical report.[4]

Signs and Symptoms of IEMs

IEMs should be suspected whenever a newborn infant has an acute catastrophic illness following a period of normal behavior and feeding or when a child of any age has unexplained lethargy or coma, recurrent seizures, persistent or recurrent vomiting, jaundice, failure to thrive, unusual body odor, developmental delay, hyperammonemia, hypoglycemia, metabolic acidosis, or a family history of recurrent illness or unexplained deaths in siblings. The steps and timing of the evaluation are tempered, in part, by the acuity of the problem and by the presentation. Algorithms for evaluation of patients with these signs and symp-toms have been published.[5,6] If an IEM is suspected, early consultation with a metabolic specialist for advice regarding the appropriate diagnostic evaluation is advised.

Emergency Therapy of Suspected IEM

Once an IEM is diagnosed, or in the case of infants in an acutely decompensated state, as soon as the suspicion of such a disorder is entertained, therapy should be instituted. After appropriate blood, urine, and cerebrospinal fluid samples have been obtained for diagnostic evaluation but prior to a definitive diagnosis being made, immediate nonspecific therapy should include restriction of dietary protein and fat intake with vigorous administration of intravenous fluids. Although this initial approach is not ideal for every known IEM, it is appropriate for the most common IEMs, which are usually the result of urea cycle defects or abnormalities of amino or organic acid metabolism. The key to acute nonspecific therapy is the reversal of catabolism and the promotion of anabolism. Intravenous fluids should contain at least 10% dextrose and be given at double the usual maintenance rate to provide energy and to promote urinary excretion of toxic metabolites. Severe acidosis (pH <7.1) should be treated with sodium bicarbonate infusion. Hyperammonemia, if not immediately responsive to intravenous fluid therapy, should be treated by hemodialysis. Insulin infusions have been used to prevent hyperglycemia and promote anabolism when giving large amounts of glucose for metabolic decompensation in such disorders as maple syrup urine disease, disorders of fatty acid oxidation, and organic acidemias.[7] Enteral feedings will also promote anabolism and may be safely given if the protein content is restricted to 0.5 g/kg/day and the fat content to less than 30% of total energy intake. Multivitamins should also be provided in this situation.

Once the diagnosis of a specific IEM has been made, therapy should be tailored to the specific disorder. Therapy for IEM is rapidly evolving, and specialists in metabolic disease and contemporary medical literature should be consulted for new advances. Therapy for any inherited metabolic disease is based on the pathophysiologic effects of the disease. For many IEMs attributable to a single-enzyme defect, disease-associated pathology is caused by accumulation of an immediate or remote precursor of the impaired reaction. The accumulated substrate may have direct toxic effects or may secondarily impair other critical biochemical reactions. For instance, the accumulation of phenylalanine in phenylalanine hydroxylase deficiency is the primary cause of the pathology associated with untreated phenylketonuria (PKU). For other disorders, symptoms may be caused by a deficiency of a critical reaction product. Finally, the substrate of the deficient reaction may be converted to an alternative product via little-used pathways. These secondary metabolites may, in themselves, be toxic. For example, succinylacetone, a product of alternative metabolism of fumarylacetoacetic acid, accumulates in the disease tyrosinemia type I, inhibits certain steps in heme synthesis, and causes symptoms

VI

mimicking porphyria. Disease-specific therapy may, therefore, include attempts to limit the accumulation of substrate, enhance the excretion of toxic substrate or secondary metabolites, restore the supply of an essential product, or inhibit alternative metabolism of the substrate. Other therapeutic approaches may include stabilization of the impaired enzyme to improve residual activity, replacement of deficient enzymatic cofactors, induction of enzyme production, enzyme replacement, or even correcting the defect at the level of the abnormal gene (gene therapy).

Nutritional Therapy Using Synthetic Medical Foods

Manipulation of precursors and limitation of substrates that lead to toxic metabolites form a major portion of the available therapies for many IEMs. Disorders that involve the intermediary metabolism of protein, carbohydrate, or lipids are most responsive to treatment with medical nutritional therapy. In the specialized diets designed for IEMs, the intake of precursor nutrients is severely limited, balancing the normal nutritional requirements for these nutrients against their potential toxicities. The necessary restriction of normal food is associated with significant risk for iatrogenic nutritional deficiency. For example, the elimination of dairy products, as is necessary in the treatment of galactosemia and for many disorders of amino acid and organic acid metabolism, is associated with risk of calcium deficiency and consequent osteoporosis. Furthermore, dietary protein or fat restriction is associated with risks of iron-deficiency anemia, vitamin B_{12} deficiency, and deficiency of essential polyunsaturated fatty acids. Commercially available medical foods (Table 30.1 and Appendix N) for the treatment of IEMs support normal growth and development by supplying a complete complement of dietary macro- and micronutrients required in the context of restricted intake of normal foods. For IEMs requiring dietary protein restriction, a variety of low-protein food products (pastas, breads, baking mixes, etc) that mimic normal foodstuffs are available to improve the palatability and appeal of the restricted diet. However, all medical foods are, by design, nutritionally incomplete and, therefore, are not to be used without the guidance of trained specialists. Purchase of these products from their manufacturers typically requires physician authorization.

Table 30.1.
Select Inborn Errors of Metabolism Treated With Commercially Available Medical Foods

IEM	Modify or Restrict	Vitamin or Cofactor Responsive	Other Therapies
Phenylketonuria	Phenylalanine	<1% of cases due to biopterin synthetic defect and require biopterin supplementation; sapropterin dihydrochloride treatment lowers blood phenylalanine in an additional 20% to 40% of PKU patients	Supplemental tyrosine or other large neutral amino acids
Tyrosinemia type I	Phenylalanine, tyrosine, methionine	No	NTBC – a 4-hydroxyphenyl-pyruvate dioxygenase inhibitor
Tyrosinemia type II	Phenylalanine, tyrosine	No	
Maple syrup urine disease	Leucine, valine, isoleucine	Some cases are thiamine responsive	
Isovaleric acidemia	Leucine	No	Supplemental carnitine and glycine
Methylmalonic acidemia	Isoleucine, valine, methionine, threonine	Some cases due to defect in cobalamin metabolism	Supplemental carnitine
Propionic acidemia	Isoleucine, valine, methionine, threonine	Possible role for biotin	Supplemental carnitine
Homocystinuria	Methionine	50% pyridoxine responsive	Supplemental folate, betaine
Ornithine transcarbamylase deficiency	Protein	No	Supplemental citrulline, benzoate, phenylacetate, phenylbutyrate
Citrullinemia	Protein	No	Supplemental arginine, benzoate, phenylacetate, phenylbutyrate
Glutaric aciduria type I	Lysine, tryptophan	Possible role for riboflavin	Supplemental carnitine

VI

Medical foods are therapeutic agents specifically designed for the treatment of IEMs, not unlike prescription pharmaceuticals. These medical foods are quite expensive, with the wholesale cost of disease-specific infant medical formulas up to 2.5 times the retail cost of regular infant formula and the cost of low-protein food products 2 to 8 times the retail price of typical foodstuffs. However, insurance reimbursement for medical foods in the United States is inconsistent and creates significant financial hardship for those who do not benefit from coverage stipulated by state legislative mandate or support through Medicaid. All 50 states practice newborn screening for as many as 40 different disorders, yet as of 2011, only 38 states have mandated insurance coverage for medical foods in the treatment of these disorders. Additionally, these mandates vary in their scope with differences in the specific disorders covered, the types of food included in the coverage, and age restrictions. Several medical professional organizations, including the American Academy of Pediatrics, have endorsed reimbursement for medical foods and low-protein products, yet barriers to treatment coverage remain.[8] Federal legislation that would require uniform national insurance coverage for the treatment of screenable disorders has been proposed.

Education of the family and patient regarding the pathophysiology of the disorder and the rationale for dietary therapy is essential. Families must be taught to prepare medical formulas and implement a feeding schedule, design daily menus, and track the intake of protein, fat, or carbohydrate, depending on the specific disorder. Family support and ongoing clinical supervision of therapy adherence are critical components of effective implementation of these complex regimens. There is little room for spontaneity with this type of therapeutic food lifestyle. Restaurants are generally not an option as a source of a complete meal. The constant need to count dietary macronutrient content and the lack of any preprepared "fast food" meal options are challenging to any family's commitment to dietary treatment.

For some IEMs, families must also be taught to recognize the signs and symptoms of impending metabolic decompensation and to institute emergency procedures, including the administration of a generally more restrictive "sick" diet. The successful implementation of a satisfactory diet during a period of relative health does not ensure that the diet is appropriate during periods of metabolic decompensation. The increased metabolic stress of even minor illness associated with increased energy requirements and increased catabolism of endogenous energy sources frequently necessitate further restriction or even elimination of dietary protein intake in individuals with an aminoacidopathies or organic acidemias. Families must be encouraged to contact health care providers during these minor illnesses, because the additionally restricted diet is nutritionally incomplete and may not be adequate to prevent further metabolic derangement. Illnesses that would normally be manageable at home in typical children may trigger the need for hospitalization in patients with an IEM. Intravenous hydration, nutrition, and in some IEMs, administration of special medications play major roles in correcting the acutely decompensated state.

Other Nutritional Therapies

Some IEMs are or may be vitamin or cofactor responsive. Cofactor supplementation may be an adjunct to therapy with medical foods for some of the IEMs listed in Table 30.1. For other IEMs, cofactor administration may be the mainstay of treatment. Cofactor dependency can be determined empirically through controlled trials of vitamin supplementation with monitoring of laboratory studies and clinical response. For instance, a subset of individuals with PKU (20%-40% of patients, depending on the specific population) respond to treatment with sapropterin dihydrochloride, a synthetic version of tetrahydrobiopterin cofactor.[9] Oral sapropterin is administered daily over 4 to 6 weeks while dietary phenylalanine intake is kept relatively constant; a substantial and sustained decrease in blood phenylalanine concentration measured weekly indicates sapropterin responsiveness. For some IEMs, such as maple syrup urine disease, cofactor dependency may be assessed through in vitro assays of enzyme function in the presence and absence of cofactor. The goal of cofactor therapy may be to stabilize a poorly functional enzyme, to overcome a block in cofactor binding, or to correct a block in cofactor metabolism that results in secondary metabolic derangement.

Therapy for other select IEMs is presented in Table 30.2. The treatment of several of these IEM is based on dietary avoidance of substrate, but for these disorders, dietary supplement with synthetic medical food is not required. For instance, the treatment of galactosemia includes avoidance of dietary galactose, which is primarily found as lactose (milk sugar) in dairy products. In infancy, this dietary restriction is easy to accomplish, because the affected infant may be fed lactose-free soy-based formula. As the child ages, however, avoidance of dairy products, especially in baked goods and processed foods, is more difficult. Parents and patients must be taught to read food labels and to contact manufacturers of prepared foods to determine whether food stuffs contain galactose. They should assume that all new foods contain galactose until proven otherwise and should be encouraged to seek other hidden sources of galactose in over-the-counter and prescription medications.

Table 30.2.
Therapy of Other Select IEMs

IEM	Modify or Restrict	Vitamin or Cofactor Responsive	Other Therapies
Biotinidase	None	Biotin	
Familial hypophos-phatemic rickets	None	1,25-dihydroxy-vitamin D	Phosphorus
Acrodermatitis enteropathica	None	Zinc	
Pyruvate dehydrogenase deficiency	Low-carbohydrate, high-fat diet	Possibly thiamine responsive	Alkali therapy
Galactosemia (transferase deficiency)	Galactose, lactose		Lactose-free infant formula
Glycogen storage diseases	Lactose, fructose, sucrose		Frequent feedings, complex starches, high-protein diet
Fructosemia (fructose-1,6-bisphosphatase or aldolase deficiency)	Fructose		Frequent glucose feedings in bisphosphatase deficiency
Medium-chain acyl-CoA dehydrogenase deficiency	Dietary fat	Riboflavin	Avoid fasting, supplemental carnitine
Long-chain fatty acid oxidation disorders	Dietary long-chain fatty acids		Avoid fasting, supplement with medium-chain triglyceride oil
Barth syndrome (X-linked 3-methyl-glutaconic aciduria	None	Pantothenic acid	
Cystinosis	None	None	Cysteamine, phosphate, potassium, vitamin D, alkali
Alcaptonuria	None	Vitamin C	
Alpha-aminoadipic semialdehyde dehydrogenase deficiency (pyridoxine responsive epilepsy)		Pyridoxine	
Cerebral folate deficiency	None	Folinic acid	
Creatine synthesis disorders	None	Creatine	
Thiamine-responsive megaloblastic anemia syndrome	None	Thiamine	

Fructose ingestion must be strictly avoided by individuals with either hereditary fructose intolerance or fructose 1,6-bisphosphatase deficiency. Ingestion of fruits, fruit juices, or any food product sweetened with fructose-containing sweetener (eg, high-fructose corn syrup in baked goods and soda) can trigger potentially life-threatening episodes of abdominal pain, vomiting, metabolic acidosis, and electrolyte disturbance. Individuals with fructose 1,6-bisphosphatase deficiency are also intolerant of fasting, because this enzyme participates in gluconeogenesis. In mannose phosphate isomerase deficiency (congenital disorder of glycosylation type 1b), a rare disease that impairs glycosylation of cellular proteins and lipids, potentially fatal liver dysfunction is completely prevented by addition of mannose to the diet.

In type 1 glycogen storage disease, glycogenolysis during fasting is impaired, because glucose-6-phosphate cannot be converted to glucose. Consumption of nonglucose carbohydrates (fructose, galactose) leads to excessive glycogen storage or shunting through alternative pathways to form lactate, uric acid, or triglycerides. Frequent feedings during infancy, overnight enteral tube feedings, and after 1 year of age, the administration of uncooked cornstarch as a slowly released source of glucose are key to the prevention of hypoglycemia and preservation of liver function. In other forms of glycogen storage disease involving the liver, gluconeogenesis is intact. Amino acids can serve as precursors for endogenous glucose production, and a high-protein diet (3 g/kg per day) is recommended.

In MCAD deficiency, the most common disorder of fatty acid oxidation in white people, prevention of fasting eliminates the body's need to metabolize fat for energy, reduces the accumulation of toxic partially oxidized fatty acids, and reduces the risk of hypoglycemia. Infants with disorders of long-chain fatty acid oxidation, such as very long-chain acyl-coenzyme A dehydrogenase deficiency or trifunctional protein deficiency, and others are more sensitive to fasting, with associated hypoglycemia, metabolic acidosis, liver dysfunction, or cardiomyopathy. Dietary long-chain fatty acid intake must be restricted; supplementation with medium-chain triglyceride oil provides a fuel source that bypasses the block in fatty acid oxidation.[10]

Prevention of micronutrient deficiencies is another important aspect of nutritional therapy for IEMs. These deficiencies may be direct effects of certain IEMs or may be a consequence of dietary restrictions. For instance, the elimination of dairy products in low-protein diets or in the therapy of galactosemia increases risk of calcium deficiency and osteoporosis. The lack of meat in low-protein diets also raises the risk of iron-deficiency anemia and vitamin B_{12} deficiency. Zinc and selenium deficiencies are also potential problems in organic acidemias. Severe dietary fat restriction for disorders of fatty acid metabolism or the administration of nutritionally incomplete synthetic medical foods may lead to deficiencies of

VI

essential polyunsaturated fatty acids. Multivitamin preparations with minerals should be prescribed to all patients on altered diets who are not receiving most of their nutrition from vitamin-fortified medical foods. All patients on nutritional therapy must be periodically assessed for micronutrient deficiencies.

Other Therapeutic Modalities

Nutritional therapy, although important, is only one modality used for many of the disorders of metabolism. Pharmacologic agents, such as alkali to reduce metabolic acidosis, benzoate and phenylacetate to provide alternative metabolic sinks and to enhance alternative pathways for ammonia excretion in urea cycle disorders, vitamin D and phosphorus supplementation in hypophosphatemic rickets, and cysteamine to enhance cellular cystine release in the lysosomal storage disease cystinosis, form another class of therapies. Ascorbic acid (vitamin C) administration greatly reduces the potential for degenerative arthritis in alcaptonuria. A rare form of congenital megaloblastic anemia is completely corrected with thiamine supplementation. Treatment with pyridoxine or folinic acid is critical to the prevention of convulsions in alpha-aminoadipic semialdehyde dehydrogenase deficiency (formerly known as pyridoxine responsive epilepsy) or cerebral folate deficiency, respectively. Rare disorders of creatine synthesis present with seizures, abnormal involuntary movements, and expressive speech delay; creatine supplementation may improve symptoms dramatically.

For a few disorders, enzyme replacement therapies are available. In cystic fibrosis, exogenous digestive enzymes are given as enteral supplements to replace the deficient secretion of the exocrine pancreas. In Gaucher disease, a lysosomal storage disease, repetitive intravenous infusions of purified enzyme is used to gradually reduce the amount of stored glucocerebroside, reversing some of the pathophysiologic changes and improving the quality of life. Similar enzyme-replacement strategies are now clinically available for a variety of lysosomal storage diseases including Pompe disease, Fabry disease, and several mucopolysaccharidoses.

Organ transplantation has been attempted in several IEMs. The most common transplanted organs are bone marrow and liver. Bone marrow or stem cell transplantation has been used in many lysosomal storage disorders, such as the mucopolysaccharidoses, in attempts to provide a tissue that is capable of metabolizing the stored material. The efficacy of this therapy is highest when the procedure is carried out in young children (typically younger than 2 years) in disorders associated with accumulation of storage material in brain because of the inability of donor hematopoietic cells to penetrate into brain in older children. Liver transplantation has been performed in tyrosinemia type I to prevent hepatocellular carcinoma, a known complication of the disease, and to correct the primary defect. With the use of nitisinone, liver transplantation is now required only for a minority of patients with tyrosinemia, although lifelong monitoring for hepatocellular carcinoma is recommended. Fewer than 5% of children placed on nitisinone before 2 years of age will develop hepatocellular carcinoma.[11] Liver transplantation has also been used to successfully to cure urea cycle disorders,[12] maple syrup urine disease, and some organic acidemias. Thus, a successful graft may have a profound effect on the health of an individual with an IEM. The infusion of hepatocytes into the portal vein for engraftment into liver may also hold promise as a treatment for many liver enzyme deficiencies, such as urea cycle disorders.[13]

Permanent replacement of the mutant gene with the correct DNA sequence in the somatic cells of an individual with an IEM is a very attractive potential future treatment modality. Several research centers around the world are actively investigating gene therapy as a treatment for a wide variety of IEMs. Using contemporary DNA transfer methods, achieving stable, physiologically significant gene expression continues to be the major limiting factor in clinical gene therapy trials. Issues of treatment toxicity using certain gene transfer technologies have also slowed the progress of moving gene therapy from the lab to the clinical bedside. However, recent success using gene therapy to treat hemophilia,[14] inherited immunodeficiencies,[15] congenital retinopathies,[16] and X-linked adrenoleukodystrophy[17] in humans has provided renewed promise that gene therapy may be a viable treatment option for treatment of IEMs in the future.

Conclusion

Regardless of the specific therapy plan, successful treatment of IEMs requires a multidisciplinary approach to include the expertise of the metabolic physician, clinic nurse, nutritionist, genetic counselor, and social worker backed up by a full complement of medical specialists and ancillary services. Education of the family, genetic counseling, and family support are all essential components. Genetic counseling teaches the family about the risks associated with future pregnancies and demystifies the concepts of defective genes being passed from asymptomatic carrier to affected child. The availability and implications of prenatal diagnosis for IEMs are also explained. Heterozygote detection and the ethical issues of sharing that information within a family or with future mates are other issues that may be addressed by counseling. Support for the family needs to ensure availability of coping mechanisms for dealing with a member who may have significant restrictions in developmental capacity or who has extraordinary needs for care. Educational goals include the successful implementation of the diet and the need for immediate intervention during metabolic crises.

VI

Nutritional therapies will continue to be the cornerstone of treatment for most IEMs in the foreseeable future. The lessons learned with several IEMs, especially PKU, emphasize the need for lifelong therapy in all these disorders. The necessity of "diet for life" has been affirmed by a National Institutes of Health Consensus Development Conference on the treatment of PKU.[18] This necessity, therefore, requires a long-term commitment from parents, patient, and health care providers to implement and maintain the appropriate dietary therapy. The needs of an individual for energy, protein, and cofactors change with age and body mass. Therapeutic diets must be established and reevaluated at regular intervals to allow for the most normal growth and development possible. The adequacy of nutritional therapy must be assessed periodically through combinations of diet diary review, food list recollection, anthropometric measurement, and laboratory testing. Cooperation of the patient, family, and the metabolic clinic as a dedicated team throughout the life of the patient is essential for successful treatment of IEMs.

AAP

It is the position of the American Academy of Pediatrics that reimbursement should be mandatory for special medical foods that are used in the treatment of any inherited metabolic disorder. This includes but is not limited to disorders of carbohydrate metabolism, lipid metabolism, vitamin metabolism, mineral metabolism, or amino acid and nitrogen metabolism.

American Academy of Pediatrics, Committee on Nutrition. Reimbursement for foods for special dietary use. *Pediatrics.* 2003;111(5 Pt 1):1117-1119

References

1. Newborn screening: toward a uniform screening panel and system. *Genet Med.* 2006;8(Suppl 1):1S-252S

2. Kaye CI, Accurso F, La Franchi S, et al. Newborn screening fact sheets. *Pediatrics.* 2006;118(3):e934-e963

3. Kaye CI, Accurso F, La Franchi S, et al. Introduction to the newborn screening fact sheets. *Pediatrics.* 2006;118(3):1304-1312

4. American Academy of Pediatrics, Newborn Screening Authoring Committee. Newborn screening expands: recommendations for pediatricians and medical homes— implications for the system. *Pediatrics.* 2008;121(1):192-217

5. Saudubray JM, Charpentier C. Clinical phenotypes: diagnosis/algorithms. In: Valle D, Beaudet AL, Vogelstein B, Kinzler KW, Antonarakis SE, Ballabio A, eds. *The Online Metabolic and Molecular Bases of Inherited Disease.* New York, NY: McGraw-Hill; 2011:1327-1403

6. Gilbert-Barness E, Barness LA. Approach to diagnosis of metabolic diseases. In: Natick MA, ed. *Metabolic Disease. Foundations of Clinical Management, Genetics, and Pathology.* Vol 1. Eaton Publishing; 2000:1-14

7. Prietsch V, Lindner M, Zschocke J, Nyhan WL, Hoffmann GF. Emergency management of inherited metabolic diseases. *J Inherit Metab Dis.* 2002;25(7):531-546

8. American Academy of Pediatrics, Committee on Nutrition. Reimbursement for foods for special dietary use. *Pediatrics.* 2003;111(5 Pt 1):1117-1119

9. Levy H, Burton B, Cederbaum S, Scriver C. Recommendations for evaluation of responsiveness to tetrahydrobiopterin (BH(4)) in phenylketonuria and its use in treatment. *Mol Genet Metab.* 2007;92(4):287-291

10. Gillingham MB, Scott B, Elliott D, Harding CO. Metabolic control during exercise with and without medium-chain triglycerides (MCT) in children with long-chain 3-hydroxy acyl-CoA dehydrogenase (LCHAD) or trifunctional protein (TFP) deficiency. *Mol Genet Metab.* 2006;89(1-2):58-63

11. Holme E, Lindstedt S. Nontransplant treatment of tyrosinemia. *Clin Liver Dis.* Nov 2000;4(4):805-814

12. Leonard JV, McKiernan PJ. The role of liver transplantation in urea cycle disorders. *Mol Genet Metab.* 2004;81(Suppl 1):S74-S78

13. Meyburg J, Das AM, Hoerster F, et al. One liver for four children: first clinical series of liver cell transplantation for severe neonatal urea cycle defects. *Transplantation.* 2009;87(5):636-641

14. Nathwani AC, Tuddenham EG, Rangarajan S, et al. Adenovirus-associated virus vector-mediated gene transfer in hemophilia B. *N Engl J Med.* 2011;365(25):2357-2365

15. Hacein-Bey-Abina S, Hauer J, Lim A, et al. Efficacy of gene therapy for X-linked severe combined immunodeficiency. *N Engl J Med.* 2010;363(4):355-364

16. Simonelli F, Maguire AM, Testa F, et al. Gene therapy for Leber's congenital amaurosis is safe and effective through 1.5 years after vector administration. *Molecular Ther.* 2010;18(3):643-650

17. Cartier N, Hacein-Bey-Abina S, Bartholomae CC, et al. Hematopoietic stem cell gene therapy with a lentiviral vector in X-linked adrenoleukodystrophy. *Science.* 2009;326(5954):818-823

18. National Institutes of Health Consensus Development Conference Statement. Phenylketonuria: screening and management, October 16-18, 2000. *Pediatrics.* 2001;108(4):972-982

VI

Chapter 31

Nutrition Therapy for Children and Adolescents With Type 1 and Type 2 Diabetes Mellitus

Introduction

From the initial descriptions of diabetes mellitus dating back more than 2000 years ago, nutritional therapy has and continues to remain a therapeutic cornerstone. Within the past century, tremendous progress has been made in understanding the pathophysiology of the disease, hormonal therapy, and comorbidities observed in patients with diabetes mellitus. These advances have played an integral role in shaping current nutrition recommendations for both children and adults with diabetes mellitus. Providing guidance on appropriate dietary intake for children with type 1 or type 2 diabetes is an essential component to any successful diabetes program. The following discussion reviews the most accepted and evidenced-based practices for nutritional management of pediatric diabetes mellitus.

Background

Type 1 Diabetes Mellitus

Type 1 diabetes mellitus (T1DM) is an autoimmune disorder that results in the destruction of pancreatic beta cells and eventual insulin deficiency. T1DM affects approximately 1 in 500 individuals in the United States, but the incidence of the disease is slowly increasing in the United States and worldwide.[1] Individuals with T1DM are dependent on insulin to avoid acute and chronic complications of the disease.

Since the discovery of insulin in 1922, management of diabetes mellitus has rapidly and steadily evolved. Prior to the availability of insulin, therapy for diabetes mellitus primarily consisted of severely restricting the intake of carbohydrate in the diet, but the disease was most often fatal in early life. Once technology improved enough to isolate and purify insulin derived from animals (mainly pigs and cows), insulin therapy became the mainstay of treatment. Still, availability and allergic responses limited treatment. Insulin is now produced using recombinant DNA technology, providing a plentiful supply of a bioequivalent form of human insulin that essentially eliminates the risks of allergic reactions that occurred with the use of animal derived insulin. Forms of insulin that varied in their onset and duration of action were designed by substituting amino acids within the insulin peptide that effectively changed the bioavailability of the insulin protein once in the subcutaneous tissue. As newer insulins arrived, nutritional therapies and meal plans were designed around the use of these insulins to best fit the lifestyle of the individual patient. Insulin pump therapy further revolutionized insulin delivery and provided greater flexibility in meal planning.

VI

Current nutritional management for patients with T1DM is centered on having an understanding of the nutritional composition of foods, particularly carbohydrates, in order to use present-day insulins effectively. The general goal is for these patients to consume well-balanced diets that promote a healthy weight, provide essential vitamins and minerals, and reduce risks of future cardiovascular disease.

Type 2 Diabetes Mellitus

The incidence of type 2 diabetes mellitus (T2DM) in children has become more frequent over the past 2 decades, mirroring the increase in pediatric obesity observed globally. T2DM now accounts for the majority of new cases of diabetes among American Indian/Alaska Native, African-American, and Hispanic adolescents in the United States, with an overall prevalence of approximately 1 in 1000 adolescents.[2] Pediatric T2DM, similar to adult T2DM, encompasses a spectrum of disease that begins with insulin resistance. Insulin resistance is driven by the cascade of metabolic derangements stemming from increased visceral adiposity in a genetically at-risk population. As insulin resistance increases, progressive stress on beta cell secretory capacity to maintain normoglycemia occurs. Disordered glucose metabolism occurs in individuals who experience some degree of beta cell failure, which eventually may progress to hyperglycemia consistent with T2DM.

Similar to children with T1DM, an understanding of nutrition is a critical component of disease management in pediatric patients with T2DM. Strategies that promote a healthy weight by improving diet quality, reducing empty-calorie carbohydrates, and enhancing insulin sensitivity through physical activity are cornerstones of nutritional therapy. Although a number of pharmaceutical agents that improve glycemic control through a variety of mechanisms are approved for use in adults, only metformin, a biguanide that enhances insulin sensitivity, is approved for use in children. Insulin therapy is also frequently required in children (and adults) requiring a working knowledge of carbohydrate content in foods.

Reducing Risks of Microvascular and Macrovascular Complications

Present-day glycemic targets and glycosylated hemoglobin (HbA1c) goals for children and adults emerged primarily from the Diabetes Care and Complications Trial (DCCT) and its follow-up study, the Epidemiology of Diabetes Intervention and Complications (EDIC) trial. These studies demonstrated that intensive insulin administration to maintain normoglycemia rather than the prior standard of care (2 injections per day) was superior with respect to improving glycemic control, lowering HbA1c concentrations, and decreasing risks of both micro- and macrovascular complications.[3,4] In children, achieving these tight glycemic goals must be balanced with avoiding hypoglycemic events, especially in younger children, in whom the effects of hypoglycemia can be potentially more deleterious to their neurocognitive development.

General Principles for Nutritional Management of Children With Diabetes Mellitus

The primary goals of treatment for all forms of pediatric diabetes mellitus remain: (1) maintaining glucose concentrations in as physiologically a normal range as possible; (2) minimizing episodes of hypoglycemia and; (3) allowing for normal growth and development, both physically and emotionally. To achieve these goals, current nutrition recommendations for children and adolescents with diabetes mellitus are rooted in the same principles as those established for all healthy children and adolescents without diabetes. Individualized meal plans should emphasize a wide variety of healthy food choices to meet the recommended nutrient intakes for essential vitamins and minerals, energy, and fiber and to provide for normal growth and development.[5-7] Strategies for nutrition therapy may be based on individual, cultural, and family needs. Examples of such interventions include reducing energy and fat intake, carbohydrate counting, simplified meal plans, healthy food choices, individualized meal planning strategies, exchange lists, insulin-to-carbohydrate ratios, physical activity, and behavioral strategies. Nutrition recommendations should be practical and comprehensible to families and patients, and the relationship between food and blood glucose should be emphasized. Cultural and traditional food practices, food preferences, family eating schedules, economic considerations, school and child care menus, willingness to change, and physical activity patterns should be taken into consideration when working with patients and families. A summary of general guidelines is provided in Table 31.1.

Table 31.1.
General Nutrition Recommendations for Children With Diabetes Mellitus[5]

- Consultation with a dietitian to develop/discuss the medical nutrition plan is encouraged, as part of initial team education and on referral, as needed; generally requires a series of sessions over the initial 3 months after diagnosis, then at least annually, with young children requiring more frequent reevaluations
- Evaluate height, weight, BMI, and nutrition plan annually
- Energy intake should be adequate for growth and restricted if a child becomes overweight

Beyond the standard nutrition guidelines for healthy children, evidence-based nutrition therapy has emerged as a critical component in the management of diabetes in children and adolescents.[8,9] Nutrition therapy should balance blood glucose goals while avoiding hypoglycemia and should promote a healthy lipid profile and blood pressure.[10] Achieving adequate control of blood glucose is likewise essential for normal growth and development.[11] Strategies to reduce calories should be implemented if the child becomes overweight. Energy needs can be evaluated by tracking weight gain, body mass index (BMI), and growth patterns on pediatric growth charts from the Centers for Disease Control and Prevention (CDC).[12]

VI

Nutritional Deficits Among Children With Diabetes Mellitus

Despite current guidelines and food availability, American children with diabetes mellitus have significant deficits in several aspects of their dietary intake. In a recent analysis of the SEARCH study, only a minority of children with either type 1 or type 2 diabetes mellitus met daily requirements for recommended intake of vitamin C, vitamin E, calcium, and fiber. In addition, less than 15% met guidelines for reducing total and saturated fat to <30% and 10%, respectively, of their daily caloric intake.[13] Vitamin D deficiency is more common among children with T1DM[14] and in obese children with insulin resistance.[15] The prevalence of overweight among children with T1DM appears to be increasing, as 22.6% of children with T1DM were categorized as overweight (BMI, 85%-95%) compared with only 16.1% of a matched control population.[16] Overweight among this population of patients with diabetes mellitus may suggest disordered eating,[17] which can affect glycemic control. These data highlight the importance of emphasizing a global, healthy approach to nutrition, focusing on the quality of food, not just the quantity.

Guidelines For Nutritional Medical Management of T1DM

Evidence-based Nutrition Principles and Recommendations for T1DM

Nutrition therapy for T1DM should be based on available evidence and current standards of medical care. The American Diabetes Association (ADA) publishes clinical practice recommendations annually that include nutrition therapy, in addition to position statements.[10,18] The American Academy of Nutrition and Dietetics has compiled a vast evidence analysis library for medical nutrition therapy for type 1 and type 2 diabetes mellitus.[19] Recommendations for macro- and micronutrients and other pertinent nutrition therapy for children with T1DM are summarized in Table 31.2.

Table 31.2.
Specific Recommendations for Management of T1DM in Children[8,10]

> - The mix of dietary carbohydrate, protein, and fat may be adjusted to meet the metabolic goals and individual preferences of the person with diabetes mellitus, but in general, daily energy intake should be targeted to include 50% to 55% carbohydrate, 10% to 15% protein, and 30% to 35% fat.
> - Monitoring carbohydrate, whether by carbohydrate counting, choices, or experience-based estimation, remains a key strategy in achieving glycemic control.
> - For individuals with diabetes, the use of the glycemic index and glycemic load may provide a modest additional benefit for glycemic control over that observed when total carbohydrate is considered alone.
> - Saturated fat intake should be <7% of total calories.
> - Reducing intake of trans–fatty acids lowers low-density lipoprotein and increases high-density lipoprotein; therefore, intake of trans–fatty acids should be minimized.
> - Routine supplementation with antioxidants, such as vitamins E and C and beta-carotene, is not advised because of lack of evidence of efficacy and concerns related to long-term safety.
> - Individualized meal planning should include optimization of food choices to meet RDA/DRI for all micronutrients.

Individual Nutrient Considerations

Carbohydrate

Total carbohydrate intake and available insulin are the primary determinants of postprandial glucose concentrations. Therefore, matching insulin to carbohydrate intake to obtain target postprandial blood glucose control is recommended. Given the flexibility in current management strategies (ie, basal-bolus insulin therapy), it is also important to monitor carbohydrate quality to avoid excess energy intake from "empty" calorie carbohydrates (eg, nondiet soda, juice, sweets, snacks). The Recommended Dietary Allowance (RDA)/Dietary Reference Intake (DRI) for carbohydrate for infants 0 to 6 months of age is 60 g, for infants 7 to 12 months of age is 95 g, and for children and adolescents is 130 g. Diets that contain less than 130 g of carbohydrate for children older than 1 year may not provide adequate glucose as fuel for the central nervous system without relying on gluconeogenesis from ingested protein and fat. Low-carbohydrate diets also restrict intake of essential nutrients, energy, and fiber from carbohydrates found in whole grains, fruits, vegetables, dried peas and beans, legumes, nuts and seeds, and low-fat milk and yogurt.[6,9,10,18,19]

Sucrose

Intake of up to 35% of calories from sucrose (glucose + fructose), or table sugar, has not been shown to have a negative effect on glycemic response or HbA1c outcomes in children and adolescents when compared with isocaloric, lower-sucrose diets.[20-22] Foods containing sucrose may be substituted for other carbohydrates in the meal plan or, if consumed in addition to the meal plan, covered with insulin. Sucrose-containing foods typically provide additional calories from fats and are frequently devoid of essential nutrients. Nutrition therapy strategies should focus on consuming these foods in moderation in the context of a healthy well-balanced diet.[9,10,18,19]

Protein

In individuals with T1DM (and T2DM) with normal renal function, protein intake is based on the RDA for all children and adolescents. Nutrition therapy should emphasize lean protein sources that are low in saturated fat, such as fish, lean cuts of meat, low-fat dairy products, and legumes.[8] Typical protein intakes in children in the United States have minimal effects on blood glucose and lipid concentrations and insulin concentrations (in patients with endogenous insulin secretion). Protein should not be used to treat hypoglycemia or prevent hypoglycemia overnight. In patients with microalbuminuria, a reduction of protein to 0.8 to 1.0 g/kg of body weight/day may slow the progression of nephropathy.[10] Overt nephropathy necessitates reduction of protein to 0.8 g/kg/day.[6,9,10,18,19]

VI

Fat

Because of the increased risk of cardiovascular disease in people with T1DM, nutrition therapy also emphasizes a diet low in saturated fat, as outlined by the National Cholesterol Education Program and the American Heart Association, for all children and adolescents. These guidelines include reductions in trans-fatty acids, saturated fats, and total dietary cholesterol along with interventions to reduce blood pressure (ie, low-sodium diets). Less than 7% of daily caloric intake should come from saturated fat, dietary cholesterol should amount to <200 mg/day, and intake of trans-fatty acids should be minimized. Saturated fatty acids are found in fatty and processed meats, butter, lard, shortening, hydrogenated fats, coconut, palm and palm kernel oils, cocoa butter, and high-fat dairy products. Added trans-fatty acids are primarily found in stick margarine and processed and commercially prepared foods. Dietary cholesterol is only found in foods of animal origin.

Healthier fats, including monounsaturated and polyunsaturated fats, are the favored sources of dietary fats in patients with diabetes because of their relative cardioprotective profile compared with saturated fats and trans-fatty acids.[9] Sources of mono- and polyunsaturated fats include olive, canola, and peanut oils; olives; nuts; seeds; avocados; and soft-tub or spray margarines. In addition, omega-3 fatty acids, specifically eicosapentaenoic acid (EPA) and docosahexaenoic acid (DHA), have emerged as important dietary adjuncts for individuals at risk of cardiovascular disease and in adults who have already experienced a cardiovascular event. Omega-3 fatty acids have moderate effects on lowering triglycerides, with more modest lowering effects on low-density lipoprotein (LPL) cholesterol, blood pressure, and platelet aggregation in people without diabetes mellitus.[23] Randomized-controlled trials have demonstrated a reduction in further cardiovascular events in adult patients with preexisting coronary artery disease.[24,25] In adults with diabetes mellitus, no consistent effect on glycemic control has been demonstrated with omega-3 fatty acid supplementation, but beneficial effects on lipid profiles have been shown.[26] No similar data currently exist for children. The American Heart Association currently recommends marine-derived omega-3 fatty acids as a dietary adjunct to aid in the reduction of serum triglycerides,[27] which can safely be used in children with diabetes and hypertriglyceridemia. Eating 2 or more servings of fish per week (with the exception of commercially fried fish filets) is recommended to provide an excellent source of omega-3 polyunsaturated fatty acids. Other potent marine sources of omega-3 polyunsaturated fatty acids are salmon, albacore tuna, herring, sardines, mackerel, trout, and anchovies. Omega-3 polyunsaturated fatty acids can also be found in flax seeds and oil, various nuts, and canola and soybean oil, although larger amounts of these plant-derived sources are needed to achieve the same lipid-lowering effect as marine-derived sources.[28,29]

Micronutrients

Several individual micronutrients have previously been proposed as potential adjunctive therapies in patients with diabetes. Chromium supplementation in adults with diabetes mellitus has not consistently demonstrated a glycemic benefit and/or has been limited by small study populations and study design.[30,31] Additional concerns regarding potential toxicity associated with chromium supplementation should preclude its routine use, especially in the pediatric population. Routine supplementation of antioxidants, vitamins E and C, and beta carotene cannot be recommended because of a lack of evidence for benefit and concerns regarding long-term safety.[8,18] Low serum 25-hydroxyvitamin D concentrations are globally associated with children and adolescents with T1DM,[14,32,33] although no-cause-and-effect relationship has been demonstrated. Vitamin D screening and supplementation should, therefore, be considered in children and adolescents with T1DM, and they should be meeting the RDA of 600 IU vitamin D per day. In summary, there is no clear evidence of benefit from vitamin or mineral supplementation in people with diabetes mellitus (compared with the general population) that do not have underlying deficiencies.[9] Supplementation with micronutrients is not necessary if a well-balanced, healthy diet is consumed.

Sodium

In some people with normal blood pressure as well as those with hypertension, a reduction in sodium lowers blood pressure. Current sodium intake guidelines for healthy children and adolescents are the same as for the general, nonhypertensive population (less than 2300 mg/day). For individuals with hypertension, a reduction to 1500 mg/day of sodium is recommended. The majority of the sodium in the American diet today comes from processed and convenience foods, restaurant meals, and fast foods. Using fresh or frozen ingredients or low- or no-sodium packaged foods in preparing meals is a way to decrease sodium in the diet.[6,9,10,18,19]

Nutritive and Nonnutritive Sweeteners

Nutritive and nonnutritive sweeteners are considered to be safe for use by children with diabetes mellitus when consumed within the daily intake levels established by the Food and Drug Administration (FDA). Nutritive sweeteners approved by the FDA include sugar alcohols (polyols), erythritol, isomaltose, lactitol, maltitol, mannitol, sorbitol, xylitol, tagatose, and hydrogenated starch hydrolysates. These sweeteners contain approximately 2 kcal/g, which is half the calories of nutritive sweeteners, such as sucrose. Subtraction of half the sugar alcohol grams from the total carbohydrate in grams is advised when reading food labels and calculating the total carbohydrate from the Nutrition Facts Panel. Sugar alcohols may cause diarrhea, especially in children.

VI

Six nonnutritive sweeteners have been approved by the FDA for use in the United States: acesulfame potassium, aspartame, neotame, saccharin, sucralose, and stevia. The safety of all of these sweeteners has been rigorously evaluated and confirmed, and they may be consumed by children and adolescents with diabetes mellitus and women during pregnancy. Stevia, a naturally occurring, nonnutritive sweetener derived from plants is the latest nonnutritive sweetener to receive approval and has been approved as generally recognized as safe (GRAS); however, no acceptable daily intake (ADI) has been established for stevia. An ADI has been approved for all other nonnutritive sweeteners by the FDA. Consumption of nonnutritive sweeteners does not increase blood glucose concentration or affect insulin response in adults, although no similar data is available in children. Because foods containing nonnutritive sweeteners may still contain carbohydrates (and calories), careful reading of food labels is always recommended.[9,10,18,19]

Fiber

The recommended fiber intake for children with diabetes is based on the DRI for all children and adolescents: 14 g/1000 kcal, or approximately 19 to 38 g of fiber/ day. High-fiber diets (60 g/day) have been demonstrated to decrease postprandial glucose concentrations among adolescents with T1DM.[34] Practically, however, consumption of fiber in this range is difficult to achieve, and typical fiber intakes up to 24 g/day have not been shown to have beneficial effects on blood glucose concentration.[9] Dietary fiber is found in whole grains, fruits, vegetables, dried peas, beans, and legumes, nuts, and seeds. Soluble fiber sources should be emphasized, because studies in people without diabetes show that diets high in total and soluble fiber (7-13 g) can reduce total cholesterol by 2% to 3% and LDL cholesterol up to 7%.[6,9,10,18,19] Potent sources of soluble fiber include oatmeal, oat cereal, lentils, apples, oranges, pears, oat bran, strawberries, nuts, flaxseeds, beans, dried peas, blueberries, psyllium, cucumbers, celery, and carrots.

Carbohydrate Counting Basics, Reading Food Labels

Carbohydrate counting has become increasingly common as insulin regimens have become more flexible, allowing patients to base their rapid-acting insulin dose on the amount of carbohydrates consumed. Counting carbohydrates gives children and adolescents flexibility in food choices as well as freedom to adjust their eating schedule according to individual circumstances and preferences. Pertinent family members and care providers should also be acquainted with this approach to maintain euglycemia. As children grow older and become more independent, it should not be assumed that they understand how to count carbohydrates, because typically family members have always done this for them. Frequent visits with a registered dietitian can help them to learn to count carbohydrates on their own as well as to reinforce basic principles in follow up visits. It is also imperative that healthy diets are maintained and assessed periodically, as focusing exclusively on carbohydrates can lead to diets that are high in fat and deficient in many nutrients.

Carbohydrates are primarily classified as "sugars" (previously referred to as simple sugars) and "starches" (previously referred to as complex carbohydrates). Most foods contain carbohydrates. Those most commonly considered to have significant amounts of carbohydrates include grains (bread, rice, pasta, and cereal); fruits (fresh, canned, and dried fruit and fruit juice); starchy vegetables (potatoes, corn, peas, and winter squash); milk and yogurt; dried peas and beans and legumes; desserts; sweetened drinks; and snack foods.

There are 2 methods to count carbohydrates: counting *grams* of carbohydrate as listed on food labels or a simplified method commonly referred to as carbohydrate *choices, units,* or *exchanges.* One carbohydrate choice/unit/exchange equals 12 to 15 g of total carbohydrates. To calculate carbohydrate choices/units/exchanges, divide the grams of total carbohydrates by 15 to determine how many carbohydrate units are in the food. There are many education materials with food lists showing either method that patients can use when counting carbohydrates. Counting in carbohydrate grams is advantageous when utilizing intensive insulin regimens with multiple daily injections or an insulin pump as it allows for better precision with the insulin dose. Using other methods of meal planning, specifically the "exchange food lists" also incorporate carbohydrate counting. Each of these methods can be successfully used to manage the carbohydrate load in diabetes mellitus, with no clear advantage of one over the other.[35]

When reading a food label for carbohydrates, it is important to emphasize 2 points: the *serving size* in household measures and the *total carbohydrate* in grams. The grams of sugar in food are included in the total carbohydrate and need not be counted separately. In Fig 31.1, the serving size is ½ cup and the total carbohydrate is 13 g. If a patient needed 1 unit of rapid-acting insulin per 15 g of carbohydrate, he or she would use this information to help determine the insulin dose, which would be approximately 1 unit of rapid-acting insulin for 1 serving (1/2 cup) of this food item. Dietary fiber is not digestible and does not affect blood glucose unless large quantities are consumed. If a food item has more than 5 g of fiber, half of the total fiber can be subtracted from the grams of total carbohydrates to calculate the grams of carbohydrates in the item. Practically speaking, very few foods consumed in the typical American diet are high enough in fiber to make this adjustment. The serving size is also commonly underestimated, overlooked, or ignored, because many children or teenagers may not pay attention to the amount of food they are eating and, therefore, will underdose insulin. Frequent follow-up visits and reinforcement of these issues are helpful. Additionally, assisting caregivers as well as

VI

patients to learn how to interpret the other information on the food label can help them to make healthier food selections. A list of common food items and their associated carbohydrate content are outlined in Table 31.3.

Fig. 31.1
Reading a food label for carbohydrates

Nutrition Facts

Serving Size ½ cup (114g)
Servings Per Container 4

Amount Per Serving

Calories 90   Calories from Fat 30

	% Daily Value*
Total Fat 3g	**5%**
Saturated Fat 0g	**0%**
Cholesterol 0mg	**0%**
Sodium 300mg	**13%**
Total Carbohydrate 13g	**4%**
Dietary Fiber 3g	**12%**
Sugars 3g	
Protein 3g	

Vitamin A 80%	•	Vitamin C 60%
Calcium 4%	•	Iron 4%

*Percent Daily Values are based on a 2,000 calorie diet. Your daily values may be higher or lower depending on your caloric needs:

	Calories:	2,000	2,500
Total Fat	Less than	65g	80g
Sat Fat	Less than	20g	25g
Cholesterol	Less than	300mg	300mg
Sodiuum	Less than	2,400mg	2,400mg
Total Carbohydrate		300g	375g
Dietary Fiber		25g	30g

Calories per gram:
Fat 9 • Carbohydrate 4 • Protein 4

Table 31.3.
Amount of Carbohydrates in Typical Food Groups/Items

One carbohydrate unit or choice or exchange = 15 g of total carbohydrate
Starches: 15 g carbohydrate equals:
One slice bread or dinner roll (whole wheat, rye, white, or pumpernickel)
One 6-inch tortilla, chapati, roti or injera bread
One waffle or pancake (the size of a slice of bread)
1/4 large bagel
1/2 English muffin, pita, hot dog bun, hamburger bun or naan bread
1/2 cup cooked cereal or 3/4 cup most dry cereals
One small egg roll or spring roll, one medium meat samosa, or 1/2 vegetable samosa
One 4-inch rice or corn patty (baked)
1/3 cup cooked rice or pasta (wheat, egg or rice noodles)
1/2 cup cooked mung bean or chow mein noodles
1/2 cup cooked peas, corn, sweet potato, white potato, taro, plantains or legumes (dried beans, peas or lentils, including dal or chole)
1 cup winter squash
31 (3/4 oz) pretzels sticks
18 (1 oz) potato chips or tortilla chips
3 cups popped popcorn
4 to 6 crackers
Fruit: 15 g carbohydrate equals:
One small fresh fruit (the size of a tennis ball)
1/2 cup mango, 1 cup papaya, or 1/2 grapefruit
1/2 cup canned fruit (packed in its own juice)
1/2 cup orange juice or apple juice
1/3 cup grape, cranberry or prune juice
1 cup melon or berries
17 small grapes
¼ cup dried fruit
2 tablespoons raisins or craisins
3 dried figs

VI

Table 31.3. *(continued)*
Amount of Carbohydrates in Typical Food Groups/Items

One carbohydrate unit or choice or exchange = 15 g of total carbohydrate
Milk: 12-15 g carbohydrate equals:
1 cup (8 oz) fat-free or low-fat milk or buttermilk
1 cup fat-free yogurt (plain)
6-8 oz light yogurt
1 cup (8 oz) soymilk
Nonstarchy vegetables: 15 g carbohydrate equals:
1 ½ cups most vegetables (except potato, peas, corn, squash) such as:
Green beans
Broccoli
Carrots
Cauliflower
Tomatoes
Cucumber
Celery
Asparagus
Cabbage and green leafy vegetables
Zucchini
Note: 1 cup lettuce or raw spinach equals 1 g of carbohydrate
Other: 15 g carbohydrate equals:
2-inch square of cake or brownie
2 small cookies
2 fortune cookies
1/2 cup ice cream or frozen yogurt
1/2 cup sherbet or sorbet
1/4 cup rice pudding or *kheer*
1 tablespoon syrup, molasses, jam, jelly, sugar, or honey
1 tablespoon sweet-and-sour sauce

Glycemic Index and Glycemic Load

Although the primary determinants of postprandial glucose response are total amount of carbohydrates consumed and available insulin, a number of other factors may influence the glycemic response to food. These factors include the type of sugar (glucose, fructose, sucrose, lactose), type of starch (amylase, amylopectin, resistant starch), cooking and food processing (degree of starch gelatinization, particle size, cellular form), food form, and other food components such as fat and natural substances (lectins, phytates, tannins, and starch-protein and starch-lipid combinations) that can slow digestion.

The glycemic index (GI) has been proposed as a tool to account for the relative differences of various carbohydrates on postprandial plasma glucose concentrations. The GI for a particular carbohydrate is calculated by comparing the relative area under the 2-hour postprandial glucose curve of 50 g of the proposed digestible carbohydrate to 50 g of a reference food, either glucose or white bread. Pure glucose is the standard comparative carbohydrate, with a GI of 100. The GI, therefore, ranks carbohydrates on a scale from 0 to100 according to the extent to which they increase blood glucose concentrations after eating. It is important to note that the GI does not measure how rapidly blood glucose increases. Low-GI foods are defined as less than 55, moderate-GI foods are 55-70, and high-GI foods are greater than 70. Foods containing little or no carbohydrate (such as meat, poultry, fish, eggs, cheese, fats and oils, wine, beer, spirits, and most non-starchy vegetables) do not have a GI. The glycemic load (GL) takes into consideration the amount of carbohydrate in the portion actually consumed. The GL is calculated by multiplying the GI by the grams of total carbohydrate in the portion eaten, divided by 100. A GL of less than 10 is low, 11 to 19 is intermediate, and 20 or more is high. Examples of the GI and GL for various foods can be found in Table 31.4.

The use of the GI as a means of controlling postprandial blood glucose or weight is controversial as foods are rarely consumed alone. In addition, selecting foods according to their GI is not necessarily an indicator of healthy food choices. Addition of fat or protein with carbohydrate may further reduce the postprandial glycemic increase because of delayed gastric emptying. The GI of foods can also be lowered by adding or substituting sugars, especially fructose and sugar alcohols. Pre- and postprandial blood glucose testing can help evaluate the use of the GI for each individual.

Several studies have evaluated the use of a GI-specific diet and its effect on glycemic outcomes and diet composition. Children with T1DM who consume a low-GI meal plan do not appear to have more limited food choices or a worse macronutrient diet composition compared with children who follow a traditional carbohydrate exchange diet.[37,38] Gilbertson et al studied 104 children with T1DM

Table 31.4.
Carbohydrate, Glycemic Index, and Glycemic Load Examples[36]

Food	Carb (g)	GI	GL
1 oz white bread	16	71	11
1 oz whole wheat bread	14	74	10
½ cup mashed potato	20	71	14
½ cup carrots	8	47	4
½ cup corn	16	55	9
Apple-small	16	40	6
1 cup apple juice	30	44	13
Orange-small	12	47	6
1 cup regular soda	26	63	16
1 cup skim milk	13	37	5
½ cup lentils	20	29	6
4 tablespoons peanuts	7	13	1
1 cup rice	42	72	30
1 cup spaghetti	46	39	18
1 cup macaroni and cheese	51	64	33
1 oz potato chips	18	57	10
2 teaspoons sugar	10	65	7
1 large banana	25	51	13
2.5 oz banana cake	46	47	17
¾ cup sugar coated cornflakes	26	55	14
1 cup oatmeal	26	55	14
3 oz chocolate cake/frosting	52	38	20
1 regular chocolate bar	31	42	13

over a 12-month period, comparing a moderate-GI diet (GI, 65-70) versus a standard carbohydrate-counting group. At the end of the 12-month period, participants following the low-GI diet experienced a significantly lower HbA1c (8.15 vs 8.6) without increasing the risk of hypoglycemia.[37] Rovner et al examined the effect of a low-GI diet (mean GI, 34 ± 6) versus typical diets (mean GI, 57 ± 6) in 23 children with T1DM who served as their own controls. Blood glucose concentration was measured using continuous glucose monitoring systems for 1 day on each diet. Mean daytime blood glucose concentrations were lower, fat intakes were less, and fiber intakes were greater on the low-GI day compared with the typical diet, without differences in calorie, carbohydrate, or protein intake.[39] Nansel et al studied 20 children with T1DM on intensive insulin therapy using continuous glucose monitoring for 1 day comparing a low-GI diet (GI, 40) versus a moderate-GI diet (GI, 64). Significantly lower overall daytime mean blood glucose concentrations and less time spent at concentrations >180 mg/dL was observed in the low-GI diet. No differences between groups for daytime or night-time hypoglycemia (blood glucose <70 mg/dL) or low blood glucose index values were observed.[40] Ryan et al studied 22 children with T1DM on intensive insulin therapy to quantify the effects of a low-GI meal on postprandial glucose excursions (PPGE) and to determine optimal insulin therapy. High-GI breakfasts (GI, 84) versus low-GI breakfasts (GI, 48) were consumed over 4 days with equal macronutrient content. Both meals were consumed using both regular and rapid-acting insulin on different occasions and monitoring occurred via continuous glucose monitoring systems. PPGE was found to be significantly lower for the low-GI meal compared with the high-GI meal when preprandial rapid acting insulin was used.[41]

Each of these studies evaluating the effect of low-GI diets in children and adolescents with T1DM has been difficult to interpret, given the inter and intra-variability among individuals and study groups, along with inconsistent definitions of GI used.[42,43] A meta-analysis from 2003 concluded that use of a low-GI diet results in a modest but significant reduction in medium-term glycemic control.[44] However, to this point, governing bodies have not adopted routine use of the GI nor promoted a low-GI index diet. The American Academy of Nutrition and Dietetics guidelines state: "Use of the glycemic index as a method of meal planning shows conflicting evidence of the effectiveness of this method. Studies comparing high- vs. low-GI diets report mixed effects on HbA1c levels. These studies are complicated by differing definitions of high-GI or low-GI diets or quartiles, as well as possible confounding dietary factors."[9] The American Diabetes Association *2011 Standards of Medical Care* made the following statement regarding the glycemic index in people with diabetes: "For individuals with diabetes, the use of the glycemic index and glycemic load may provide a modest additional benefit for glycemic control over that observed when total carbohydrate is considered alone."[10]

Hypoglycemia

Hypoglycemia in children with diabetes mellitus, defined as a blood glucose concentration less than 70 mg/dL, may result from a combination of excess insulin administration, decreased food intake, or increased physical activity. Hypoglycemia should always be treated immediately, and patients and family members need to be educated on signs and symptoms of low blood glucose concentration as well as appropriate treatment. Patients with diabetes mellitus should always carry a source of carbohydrate with them when away from home to treat hypoglycemia in

VI

addition to their blood glucose meter. The goal of treatment is to achieve rapid normalization of blood glucose without consuming excess carbohydrate and resultant rebound hyperglycemia.

Hypoglycemia should be treated with an appropriate amount of carbohydrate to increase blood glucose concentrations to a safe range in approximately 10 to 15 minutes. Glucose or sucrose is the preferred treatment; fructose is less desirable.[45] As a rule of thumb, 15 g of carbohydrate will increase the blood glucose approximately 30 mg/dL. Blood glucose measurement should be repeated 15 minutes after treatment, and more carbohydrate should be consumed if it remains low. Once blood glucose concentration returns to normal, a meal or snack may be consumed to prevent recurrence of hypoglycemia, especially if continued physical activity is expected. A proposed treatment algorithm for hypoglycemia is listed in Table 31.5.

Table 31.5.
Treatment of Hypoglycemia[10]

1. Test blood glucose
2. If blood glucose is 51 mg/dL to 70 mg/dL, eat or drink 15-20 g of carbohydrate. If blood glucose is less than 50 mg/dL, eat or drink 30 g of carbohydrate. Each of the following equals 15 g of carbohydrate: – 3 to 4 glucose tablets – 1/2 cup (4 oz) regular soft drink (soft drink with sugar) or fruit juice – 1 small box of raisins – 1 cup (8 oz) skim milk – 1 tablespoon of honey or sugar – 1 small tube (15 g) of glucose gel
3. Wait 15 minutes before eating anything else. Then, retest blood glucose.
4. Repeat these steps until blood glucose is between 70 mg/dL and 100 mg/dL. It should be at least 100 mg/dL if: • the individual is going to drive. • the individual is going to exercise—this includes housework, yard work, running, jumping, or other physical activity. • the next meal is more than an hour away.

Carbohydrate Adjustments for Exercise and/or Increased Physical Activity in Patients With T1DM

Exercise recommendations for children with T1DM are the same as for other children, but they must take precautionary measures to avoid either hyperglycemia or hypoglycemia during or after exercise. For most children, a decrease in insulin administration or the consumption of extra carbohydrate may be necessary to avoid hypoglycemia during or after exercise. The increased use of insulin pump therapy and peakless insulins has improved convenience in reducing insulin administration. A discussion of insulin lowering strategies (eg, use of temporary basal rates) in anticipation of exercise is beyond the scope of this chapter.

For managing exercise strictly with dietary changes, the type, duration, and intensity of exercise, as well as the initial blood glucose concentration, will dictate the amount of carbohydrate required. Patients should be instructed to monitor their blood glucose before, during, and after exercise to establish patterns. New sports or activities frequently may result in different blood glucose patterns, and therefore, more frequent monitoring is recommended once again until patterns are established. A general starting guideline is to consume 15 g of carbohydrate for every 30 to 60 minutes of physical activity (Table 31.6).

Table 31.6.
Guidelines for Carbohydrate Intake When Exercising to Prevent Low Blood Glucose (from the American Diabetic Association)[46]

Duration of Exercise	Exercise Intensity	Grams of Carbohydrate Needed Prior to Exercise		
		Blood Glucose < 90 mg/dL	Blood Glucose 90-150 mg/dL	Blood Glucose 150-250 mg/dL
15-30 min	Mild	15	0-15	0
	Moderate	15	15	0-15
	Hard	15	15	0-15
30-60 min	Mild	15-30	15-30	0-15
	Moderate	15-45	15-30	15
	Hard	30-45	15-30	15-30
60-90 min	Mild	15-45	15-45	15-30
	Moderate	30-45	30-45	30-45
	Hard	30-60	30-45	30-45
>90 min	Mild, moderate, or hard	Follow guidelines for 60-90 min of activity. Check blood glucose and consume 15 g of carbohydrate for every 30 min of exercise		

Meal Planning Strategies Using Intensive Insulin Therapy Versus Fixed Insulin Doses in T1DM

Intensive insulin therapy is defined as multiple daily injections or continuous subcutaneous insulin infusion (insulin pump therapy). The basal-bolus approach consists of a once- or twice-daily long-acting insulin given as background or basal insulin, while frequent doses of rapid-acting insulin are given throughout the day to correct hyperglycemia and to "cover" dietary carbohydrates. Use of such flexible insulin plans allows people with diabetes mellitus freedom to eat normally and not according to their insulin action time. In children and adolescents, this method provides them with a more normal approach to eating and can help improve quality of life.[47] The use of carbohydrate counting works very well with intensive insulin therapy. Families and patients and other caregivers should all be instructed on carbohydrate counting, and follow-up visits are necessary as children become more independent and may try to count carbohydrates on their own. Meal and snack insulin doses should be adjusted to match carbohydrate intake, which is referred to as an insulin-to-carbohydrate ratio. Overall quality of the child's diet as well as protein and fat content must not be overlooked when using this approach, because excessive energy intake will lead to weight gain.

Comprehensive nutrition education and counseling by the health care team on the relationship between food and blood glucose concentration, interpretation of blood glucose patterns, and nutrition-related insulin adjustment is important for optimal care. Registered dietitians should follow up with patients at least annually for reinforcement of basic carbohydrate counting, especially if they experience deterioration in glycemic control, as well as healthy eating review. Initial studies in patients with T1DM who adjusted their mealtime insulin to match their planned carbohydrate intake had improved glycemic control.[47,48] A prospective observational study in Australia in patients with T1DM and T2DM taught to use insulin-to-carbohydrate ratios reported improvements in average HbA1c at 1 year.[49]

Fixed Insulin Doses
Fixed insulin doses may also be used in intensive diabetes management, but carbohydrate amounts must also be fixed and distributed throughout the day to optimize glycemic control and avoid hypoglycemia.[50-52] Similar to basal bolus therapy, this strategy also relies on matching carbohydrate intake to insulin administration to effectively maintain glucose concentrations in a normal range while avoiding hypoglycemia.

Therapy For T2DM and Prediabetes
Therapeutic data from children with T2DM, compared with those from children with T1DM, are far more limited, but the same principles (lifestyle modification in conjunction with pharmacologic intervention) have been adopted.[53,54[1]] AAP recommendations for management of T2DM are shown in the text box. Dietary modification, as part of a lifestyle modification program, has been shown to be an effective means of decreasing BMI, markers of insulin resistance, and other metabolic abnormalities (dyslipidemia, hypertension) commonly observed in obese children without T2DM.[55,56] Children meeting diagnostic criteria for T2DM should be treated with metformin as a first-line pharmacologic agent (with or

without insulin) along with adopting lifestyle modifications, including dietary changes and increased physical activity.[54] Although still considered a critical component of treatment in pediatric T2DM, metformin is superior to lifestyle modification alone in achieving adequate glycemic control and minimizing lost patients to follow-up.[54] In a recent multicenter trial of treatment options for T2DM in adolescents, the combined intervention of metformin with an intensive lifestyle intervention program was not superior to metformin alone with respect to the rate of progression to glycemic failure (HbA1c >8% or inability to wean from insulin).[57] At this time, however, it remains accepted that attention to lifestyle modification, including dietary changes, should remain an important, adjunctive component of therapy for T2DM.

AAP

AAP Recommends for Treatment of Diabetes Mellitus Type 2[54]

1. Clinicians must ensure that insulin therapy is initiated for children and adolescents with TD2DM who are ketotic or in diabetic ketoacidosis and in whom the distinction between T1DM and T2DM is unclear; and, in usual cases should initiate insulin therapy for patients:
   a. who have random venous or plasma blood glucose concentrations ≥250mg/dL; or
   b. whose HbA1c is > 9%
2. In all instances, clinicians should initiate a lifestyle modification program, including nutrition and physical activity, and start metformin as first-line therapy for children and adolescents at the time of diagnosis of TD2DM.
3. The committee suggests that clinicians monitor HBA1c concentrations every 3 months and intensify treatment if treatment goals for blood glucose and HbA1c concentrations are not being met.
4. The committee suggests that clinicians advise patients to monitor finger–stick blood glucose concentrations in those who
   a. are taking inulin or other medications with a risk of hypoglycemia; or
   b. are initiating or changing their diabetes treatment goals; or
   c. have not met treatment goals; or
   d. have intercurrent illness
5. The committee suggests that clinicians incorporate the Academy of Nutrition and Dietetics *Pediatric Weight Management Evidence Based Nutrition Practice Guidelines* in the nutrition counseling of patients with T2DM both at the time of diagnosis and as part of ongoing management.
6. The committee suggests that clinicians encourage children and adolescents with T2DM to engage in moderate-to-vigorous exercise for at least 60 minutes daily and to limit nonacademic screen time to less than 2 hours per day.

VI

Given the strong association of obesity[16] and insulin resistance as inherent risk factors for pediatric T2DM, recommendations are aimed at weight loss and increased physical activity to improve insulin sensitivity. The goals of management are to (1) achieve normoglycemia and HbA1c targets; (2) achieve appropriate weight and normal linear growth; and (3) reduce comorbidities (dyslipidemia, hypertension) that are frequently present.[8,19]

Dietary modifications in all forms of pediatric diabetes, but particularly T2DM, should be a family-based effort[58] and should focus on reductions in total and saturated fat intake, increasing fiber intake, and targeting calorie intake goals that result in a healthy BMI. Similar to recommendations for children with exogenous obesity, juices and other sugar-based soft drinks should be eliminated and replaced with lower-energy beverages. Scheduled meal times with the entire family are integral to establishing healthy eating behaviors. Parents should serve as models for healthy eating behavior and oversee portion sizes for their children in conjunction with guidance from a dietitian. Increased energy expenditure through physical activities that are enjoyable for the child promotes improved insulin sensitivity and is needed, in combination with dietary changes, to achieve weight loss. Specific recommendations from an expert committee on therapy in pediatric obesity can also be applied to the pediatric T2DM population (Table 31.7).

Table 31.7.
Evidence-Based Initial Lifestyle Interventions to Treat Pediatric Obesity[57]

• Eliminate sugar-sweetened beverages
• Increase intake of water or skim milk
• Eat a healthy breakfast daily
• Strive for 5 total fruits and vegetables daily at a minimum
• Set short-term attainable goals for incremental changes
• Eat family meals together as much as possible
• Limit eating out at restaurants, particularly fast food
• Limit portion sizes
• Encourage consumption of skim and low-fat milk in place of whole milk and increase consumption of calcium

Special Situations and Chronic Diseases Associated With Diabetes Mellitus in Children

Nutrition Management in the School and Child Care Setting for Children Requiring Insulin

Children and adolescents with diabetes mellitus need assistance with managing their blood glucose concentrations at school and in child care. School nurses play a critical role, along with other school personnel, in assisting and supervising blood glucose monitoring, insulin administration, treatment of hypoglycemia, and meal plans.

Federal laws that protect children with diabetes mellitus include Section 504 of the Rehabilitation Act of 1973 (Pub L No. 93-112) and the Individuals with Disabilities Education Act (Pub L No. 108-446 [originally the Education for All Handicapped Children Act of 1975, Pub L No. 94-142]) and the Americans with Disabilities Act (Pub L No. 101-336). Diabetes mellitus is considered to be a disability under these laws; therefore, it is illegal for schools and/or child care centers to discriminate against children with diabetes mellitus. Any school that receives federal funding or any facility considered open to the public must reasonably accommodate the special needs of children with diabetes mellitus. Federal law requires an individualized assessment for any child with diabetes mellitus. The required accommodations should be documented in a written plan developed under the applicable federal law, such as a Section 504 Plan or individualized education plan (IEP). An individualized diabetes medical management plan (DMMP) should be developed by the student's diabetes health care team with input from the parent or guardian. The DMMP should address the information about the student's meal/snack schedule. For young children, instructions should be given for when food is provided during school parties and other activities.[60]

Celiac Disease

Celiac disease is an autoimmune disorder that occurs more frequently in individuals with preexisting T1DM. Approximately 1% to 16% of people with T1DM have celiac disease, compared with 0.3% to 1% in the general population.[61,62] Care providers who work in diabetes care must be well versed on the intricacies of the gluten-free diet and celiac disease in relation to its influence on nutritional status and metabolic control in children and adolescents with diabetes mellitus. Frequent visits with patients and families as well as other caregivers are necessary to ensure comprehension because of the complexity of the gluten-free diet. Children with celiac disease who carefully follow a well-balanced, healthy gluten-free diet have the same nutrition requirements as other children once the intestinal mucosa is healed. Consultation with a registered dietitian experienced in managing both diabetes and celiac disease is strongly recommended.[10] A discussion of celiac disease is found in Chapter 28, but principles of screening and treatment are outlined in Table 31.8.

VI

Table 31.8.
Recommendations for Screening and Treatment of Screening and Treatment of Celiac Disease in Children With T1DM

- Children with T1DM should be screened for celiac disease by measuring tissue transglutaminase or antiendomysial antibodies, with documentation of normal total serum immunoglobulin (Ig) A concentrations soon after the diagnosis of diabetes.
- Testing should be repeated in children with growth failure, failure to gain weight, weight loss, diarrhea, flatulence, abdominal pain, or signs of malabsorption or in children with frequent unexplained hypoglycemia or deterioration in glycemic control
- Children with positive antibodies should be referred to a gastroenterologist for evaluation with endoscopy and biopsy
- Children with biopsy-confirmed celiac disease should be placed on a gluten-free diet and have consultation with a dietitian experienced in managing both diabetes and celiac disease

Nutrition Recommendations for Cystic Fibrosis-Related Diabetes Mellitus in Children and Adolescents

Cystic fibrosis-related diabetes (CFRD) has become the most common comorbidity in people with cystic fibrosis as the population ages. CFRD occurs in approximately 20% of adolescents with cystic fibrosis, with an incidence of approximately 3% per year beginning in the teenage years, but has been observed at all ages, including infants.[63] The etiology of diabetes in cystic fibrosis is not related to either T1DM or T2DM; however, there are some shared similarities.[64] Nutrition therapy for CFRD differs significantly from that for T1DM and T2DM.[65]

There are many critical differences in nutrition recommendations for CFRD that must be understood to ensure survival in these individuals, specifically with regard to energy, fat, protein, sodium, and supplemental vitamins and minerals. Adequate energy intake to maintain the recommended BMI for children and adolescents is critical for health and survival.[66] The diagnosis of CFRD does not change the usual cystic fibrosis nutrition recommendations. Normalization of blood glucose concentration is essential to optimize nutrient metabolism and to improve BMI and lean body mass.[67] Energy intake should almost never be restricted. The high-energy eating pattern does not replace the need for healthy, nutrient-dense food intake, and most people with cystic fibrosis will need routine vitamin and mineral supplementation because of malabsorption. Appetite can be highly variable from day to day in people with cystic fibrosis, necessitating the use of oral high-energy supplements and/or enteral tube feedings to meet energy requirements in many patients.[68] For these reasons, meal plans are not practical. The use of carbohydrate counting and insulin-to-carbohydrate ratios in conjunction with the cystic fibrosis eating pattern to guide insulin therapy are essential to optimize blood glucose control.[65] Insulin regimens can be individualized to allow for adequate glycemic control for frequent meals or enteral feedings overnight.

The risk of hypoglycemia in CFRD is no different from insulin-treated patients with T1DM or T2DM. Absorption of fat-free carbohydrates is not compromised, because patients with cystic fibrosis are able to secrete amylase in their saliva.[68] Therefore, low blood glucose concentrations should be treated with fat-free carbohydrate sources that do not require pancreatic enzyme replacement.

Eating Disorders With Diabetes in Children and Adolescents

Eating disorders are common among adolescents with T1DM and negatively affect glycemic control.[69] Bulimia is the most common eating disorder in females with T1DM, with insulin omission (diabulimia) used as an additional method to lose weight. Diabetes and eating disorders both involve attention to food and weight, and therefore, it is not uncommon for patients to use their diabetes to conceal the eating disorder. The combination of diabetes mellitus and an eating disorder (diabetic ketoacidosis, electrolyte disturbances, cardiac conduction abnormalities, edema) can be serious or even fatal; therefore, timely identification and appropriate treatment is imperative.[70] Ideally, patients diagnosed with both diabetes mellitus and an eating disorder will be referred to a team of providers who are comfortable treating both diseases and are knowledgeable regarding diabetes management, given the differences that may exist between the treatment approaches.[71] A diabetes-specific screening tool for youth with eating disorders and T1DM has been developed and should be used if eating disorders are suspected.[17]

Summary/Conclusion

Treatment of diabetes mellitus is a complex task, integrating multiple factors, but ultimately is centered on the approach to nutrition. Although a focus on careful carbohydrate counting is integral to insulin delivery and glycemic control for patients with T1DM, many of the other fundamental principles of nutrition management are applicable to children with either T1DM or T2DM. A team approach, capitalizing on the expertise of pediatric dietitians, psychologists, nurses, and physicians can best assist children and their families overcome challenges in their care and reach their therapeutic goals. Table 31.9 provides additional educational resources for care providers, patients, and families.

VI

Table 31.9.
Resources for Nutrition Education

Academy of Nutrition and Dietetics	http://www.eatright.org/Shop/ *Choose Your Foods: Exchange Lists for Diabetes* (English and Spanish versions) *Eating Healthy with Diabetes: Easy Reading Guide* *Advanced Carbohydrate Counting*
American Diabetes Association	http://www.shopdiabetes.org/Categories/8-Diabetes-Books.aspx *The Complete Guide to Carbohydrate Counting*, 3rd ed *Diabetes Carbohydrate and Fat Gram Guide*, 4th ed *Diabetic Carb-Smart Essentials* *ADA Guide to Healthy Restaurant Eating*, 4th ed *Diabetic Meal Planning Essentials*
Diabetes and Celiac Disease	Diabetes and Celiac Disease: http://www.gluten.net/Diabetes%20CD%2006-2011.pdf Counting Gluten Free Carbohydrates: http://www.csaceliacs.info/files.jsp?file_id511
Cystic Fibrosis Related Diabetes	*Managing Cystic Fibrosis-Related Diabetes (CFRD): An Instruction Guide for Patients and Families.* 5th ed: http://www.cff.org/UploadedFiles/LivingWithCF/StayingHealthy/Diet/Diabetes/CFRD-Manual-5th-edition.pdf
US Department of Agriculture National Nutrient Database for Standard Reference	http://www.nal.usda.gov/fnic/foodcomp/search/
National Institute of Diabetes and Digestive and Kidney Diseases (NIDDK)	http://diabetes.niddk.nih.gov/dm/pubs/eating_ez/index.aspx

References

1. Liese AD, D'Agostino RB Jr, Hamman RF, et al. The burden of diabetes mellitus among US youth: prevalence estimates from the SEARCH for Diabetes in Youth Study. *Pediatrics.* 2006;118(4):1510-1518

2. Dabelea D, Bell RA, D'Agostino RB Jr, et al; Writing Group for the SEARCH for Diabetes in Youth Study Group. Incidence of diabetes in youth in the United States. *JAMA.* 2007;297(24):2716-2724

3. The Diabetes Control and Complications Trial Research Group. The effect of intensive treatment of diabetes on the development and progression of long-term complications in insulin-dependent diabetes mellitus. *N Engl J Med.* 1993;329(14):977-986

4. Nathan DM, Cleary PA, Backlund JY, et al; Diabetes Control and Complications Trial/Epidemiology of Diabetes Interventions and Complications (DCCT/EDIC) Study Research Group. Intensive diabetes treatment and cardiovascular disease in patients with type 1 diabetes. *N Engl J Med.* 2005;353(25):2643-2653

5. Silverstein J, Klingensmith G, Copeland K, et al. Care of children and adolescents with type 1 diabetes: a statement of the American Diabetes Association. *Diabetes Care.* 2005;28(1):186-212

6. Institute of Medicine, Food and Nutrition Board. *Dietary Reference Intakes: The Essential Guide to Nutrient Requirements.* Otten JJ, Meyers LD, eds. Washington, DC: National Academies Press; 2006

7. Institute of Medicine, Food and Nutrition Board. Dietary Reference Intakes for Vitamin D and Calcium. Ross C, Yaktine AL, Del Valle HB, eds. Washington, DC: National Academies Press; 2011

8. Smar, C, Aslander-van Vliet E, Waldron S. Nutritional management in children and adolescents with diabetes. *Pediatr Diabetes.* 2009;10(Suppl 12):100-117

9. Franz MJ, Powers MA, Leontos C, et al. The evidence for medical nutrition therapy for type 1 and type 2 diabetes in adults. *J Am Diet Assoc.* 2010;110(12):1852-1889

10. American Diabetes Association. Standards of medical care in diabetes—2011. *Diabetes Care.* 2011;34(Suppl 1):S11-S61

11. Wise JE, Kolb EL, Sauder SE. Effect of glycemic control on growth velocity in children with IDDM. *Diabetes Care.* 1992;15(7):826-830

12. Centers for Disease Control and Prevention. Clinical Growth Charts. Available at: http://www.cdc.gov/growthcharts/clinical_charts.htm. Accessed December 3, 2012

13. Mayer-Davis EJ, Nichols M, Liese AD, et al. Dietary intake among youth with diabetes: the SEARCH for Diabetes in Youth Study. *J Am Diet Assoc.* 2006;106(5):689-697

14. Svoren BM, Volkening LK, Wood JR, Laffel LM. Significant vitamin D deficiency in youth with type 1 diabetes mellitus. *J Pediatr.* 2009;154(1):132-134

15. Kelly A, Brooks LJ, Dougherty S, Carlow DC, Zemel BS. A cross-sectional study of vitamin D and insulin resistance in children. *Arch Dis Child.* 2011;96(5):447-452

16. Liu LL, Lawrence JM, Davis C, et al. Prevalence of overweight and obesity in youth with diabetes in USA: the SEARCH for Diabetes in Youth study. *Pediatr Diabetes.* 2010;11(1):4-11

17. Markowitz JT, Butler DA, Volkening LK, Antisdel JE, Anderson BJ, Laffel LM. Brief screening tool for disordered eating in diabetes: internal consistency and external validity in a contemporary sample of pediatric patients with type 1 diabetes. *Diabetes Care.* 2009;33(3):495-500

18. American Diabetes Association; Bantle JP, Wylie-Rosett J, Albright AL, et al. Nutrition recommendations and interventions for diabetes: a position statement of the American Diabetes Association. *Diabetes Care.* 2008;31(Suppl 1):S61-S78

19. American Diabetes Association. Diabetes Type 1 and 2 Evidence Project. Available at: http://www.adaevidencelibrary.com/topic.cfm?cat=1615. Accessed December 3, 2012

20. Loghmani E, Rickard K, Washburne L, Vandagriff J, Fineberg N, Golden M. Glycemic response to sucrose-containing mixed meals in diets of children of with insulin-dependent diabetes mellitus. *J Pediatr.* 1991;119(4):531-537

21. Schwingshandl J, Rippel S, Unterluggauer M, Borkenstein M. Effect of the introduction of dietary sucrose on metabolic control in children and adolescents with type I diabetes. *Acta Diabetol.* 1994;31(4):205-209

VI

22. Rickard KA, Cleveland JL, Loghmani ES, Fineberg NS, Freidenberg GR. Similar glycemic responses to high versus moderate sucrose-containing foods in test meals for adolescents with type 1 diabetes and fasting euglycemia. *J Am Diet Assoc.* 2001;101(10):1202-1205

23. Kris-Etherton PM, Harris WS, Appel LJ. Fish consumption, fish oil, omega-3 fatty acids, and cardiovascular disease. *Circulation.* 2002;106(21):2747-2757

24. Dietary supplementation with n-3 polyunsaturated fatty acids and vitamin E after myocardial infarction: results of the GISSI-Prevenzione trial. Gruppo Italiano per lo Studio della Sopravvivenza nell'Infarto miocardico. *Lancet.* 1999;354(9177):447-455

25. Burr ML, Fehily AM, Gilbert JF, et al. Effects of changes in fat, fish, and fibre intakes on death and myocardial reinfarction: diet and reinfarction trial (DART). *Lancet.* 1989;2(8666):757-761

26. De Caterina R, Madonna R, Bertolotto A, Schmidt EB. n-3 fatty acids in the treatment of diabetic patients: biological rationale and clinical data. *Diabetes Care.* 2007;30(4):1012-1026

27. Miller M, Stone NJ, Ballantyne C, et al; American Heart Association Clinical Lipidology, Thrombosis, and Prevention Committee of the Council on Nutrition, Physical Activity, and Metabolism; Council on Arteriosclerosis, Thrombosis and Vascular Biology; Council on Cardiovascular Nursing; Council on the Kidney in Cardiovascular Disease. Triglycerides and cardiovascular disease: a scientific statement from the American Heart Association. *Circulation.* 2011;123(20):2292-2333

28. Prasad K. Flaxseed and cardiovascular health. *J Cardiovasc Pharmacol.* 2009;54(5):369-377

29. Saremi A, Arora R. The utility of omega-3 fatty acids in cardiovascular disease. Am J Ther. 2009;16(5):421-436

30. Althuis MD, Jordan NE, Ludington EA, Wittes JT. Glucose and insulin responses to dietary chromium supplements: a meta-analysis. *Am J Clin Nutr.* 2002;76(1):148-155

31. Balk EM, Tatsioni A, Lichtenstein AH, Lau J, Pittas AG. Effect of chromium supplementation on glucose metabolism and lipids: a systematic review of randomized controlled trials. *Diabetes Care.* 2007;30(8):2154-2163

32. Janner M, Ballinari P, Mullis PE, Flück CE. High prevalence of vitamin D deficiency in children and adolescents with type 1 diabetes. *Swiss Med Wkly.* 2010;140:w13091

33. Borkar VV, Devidayal VS, Bhalla AK. Low levels of vitamin D in North Indian children with newly diagnosed type 1 diabetes. *Pediatr Diabetes.* 2010;11(5):345-450

34. Kinmonth AL, Angus RM, Jenkins PA, Smith MA, Baum JD. Whole foods and increased dietary fibre improve blood glucose control in diabetic children. *Arch Dis Child.* 1982;57(3):187-194

35. Smart CE, Ross K, Edge JA, King BR, McElduff P, Collins CE. Can children with Type 1 diabetes and their caregivers estimate the carbohydrate content of meals and snacks? *Diabetes Med.* 2010;27(3):348-353

36. University of Sydney. Search for the Glycemic Index. Available at: www.glycemicindex.com. Accessed December 3, 2012

37. Gilbertson HR, Brand-Miller JC, Thorburn AW, Evans S, Chondros P, Werther GA. The effect of flexible low glycemic index dietary advice versus measured carbohydrate exchange diets on glycemic control in children with type 1 diabetes. *Diabetes Care*. 2001;24(7):1137-1143

38. Gilbertson HR, Thorburn AW, Brand-Miller JC, Chondros P, Werther GA. Effect of low-glycemic-index dietary advice on dietary quality and food choice in children with type 1 diabetes. *Am J Clin Nutr*. 2003;77(1):83-90

39. Rovner AJ, Nansel TR, Gellar L. The effect of a low-glycemic diet vs a standard diet on blood glucose levels and macronutrient intake in children with type 1 diabetes. *J Am Diet Assoc*. 2009;109(2):303-307

40. Nansel TR, Gellar L, McGill A. Effect of varying glycemic index meals on blood glucose control assessed with continuous glucose monitoring in youth with type 1 diabetes on basal-bolus insulin regimens. *Diabetes Care*. 2008;31(4):695-697

41. Ryan RL, King BR, Anderson DG, Attia JR, Collins CE, Smart CE. Influence of and optimal insulin therapy for a low-glycemic index meal in children with type 1 diabetes receiving intensive insulin therapy. *Diabetes Care*. 2008;31(8):1485-1490

42. Vega-Lopez S, Ausman LM, Griffith JL, Lichtenstein AH. Interindividual variability and intra-individual reproducibility of glycemic index values for commercial white bread. *Diabetes Care*. 2007;30(6):1412-1417

43. Pi-Sunyer FX. Glycemic index and disease. *Am J Clin Nutr*. 2002;76(1):290S-298S

44. Brand-Miller J, Hayne S, Petocz P, Colagiuri S. Low-glycemic index diets in the management of diabetes: a meta-analysis of randomized controlled trials. *Diabetes Care*. 2003;26(8):2261-2267

45. Husband AC, Crawford S, McCoy LA, Pacaud D. The effectiveness of glucose, sucrose, and fructose in treating hypoglycemia in children with type 1 diabetes. *Pediatr Diabetes*. 2010;11(3):154-158

46. Franz M. Nutrition, physical activity, and diabetes. In: Devlin JT, Schneider SH, Kriska A, eds. *Handbook of Exercise in Diabetes*. Alexandria, VA: American Diabetes Association; 2002:321-337

47. DAFNE Study Group. Training in flexible, intensive insulin management to enable dietary freedom in people with type 1 diabetes: dose adjustment for normal eating (DAFNE) randomised controlled trial. *BMJ*. 2002;325(7367):746

48. The Diabetes Control and Complications Trial Research Group. The effect of intensive treatment of diabetes on the development and progression of long-term complications in insulin-dependent diabetes mellitus. *N Engl J Med*. 1993;329(14):977-986

49. Lowe J, Linjawi S, Mensch M, James K, Attia J. Flexible eating and flexible insulin dosing in patients with diabetes: Results of an intensive self-management course. *Diabetes Res Clin Pract*. 2008;80(3):439-443

50. Wolever TM, Hamad S, Chiasson JL, et al. Day-to-day consistency in amount and source of carbohydrate intake associated with improved blood glucose control in type 1 diabetes. *J Am Coll Nutr*. 1999;18(3):242-247

51. Boden G, Sargrad K, Homko C, Mozzoli M, Stein TP. Effect of a low-carbohydrate diet on appetite, blood glucose levels, and insulin resistance in obese patients with type 2 diabetes. *Ann Intern Med*. 2005;142(6):403-411

VI

52. Nielsen JV, Jonsson E, Ivarsson A. A low carbohydrate diet in type 1 diabetes: clinical experience—a brief report. *Ups J Med Sci*. 2005;110(3):267-273

53. Rosenbloom AL, Silverstein JH, Amemiya S, Zeitler P, Klingensmith GJ; International Society for Pediatric and Adolescent Diabetes. ISPAD Clinical Practice Consensus Guidelines 2006-2007. Type 2 diabetes mellitus in the child and adolescent. *Pediatr Diabetes*. 2008;9(5):512-526

54. Copeland KC, Silverstein J, Moore KR, et al. Management of newly diagnosed type 2 diabetes mellitus (T2DM) in children and adolescents. *Pediatrics*. 2013;131(2):364-382

55. Chen AK, Roberts CK, Barnard RJ. Effect of a short-term diet and exercise intervention on metabolic syndrome in overweight children. *Metabolism*. 2006;55(7):871-878

56. Monzavi R, Dreimane D, Geffner ME, et al. Improvement in risk factors for metabolic syndrome and insulin resistance in overweight youth who are treated with lifestyle intervention. *Pediatrics*. 2006;117(6):e1111-e1118

57. TODAY Study Group. A Clinical Trial to Maintain Glycemic Control in Youth with Type 2 Diabetes. *New Engl J of Med*. 2012; 366: (2247-2256).

58. Wrotniak BH, Epstein LH, Paluch RA, Roemmich JN. Parent weight change as a predictor of child weight change in family-based behavioral obesity treatment. *Arch Pediatr Adolesc Med*. 2004;158(4):342-347

59. Barlow SE; Expert Committee. Expert committee recommendations regarding the prevention, assessment, and treatment of child and adolescent overweight and obesity: summary report. *Pediatrics*. 2007;120(Suppl 4):S164-S192

60. American Diabetes Association. Diabetes care in the school and day care setting. *Diabetes Care*. 2011;33(Suppl 1):S70-S74

61. Holmes GK. Screening for coeliac disease in type 1 diabetes. *Arch Dis Child*. 2002;87(6):495-498

62. Rewers M, Liu E, Simmons J, Redondo MJ, Hoffenberg EJ. Celiac disease associated with type 1 diabetes mellitus. *Endocrinol Metab Clin North Am*. 2004;33(1):197-214

63. Moran A, et al. Cystic fibrosis-related diabetes: current trends in prevalence, incidence, and mortality. *Diabetes Care*. 2009;32(9):1626-1631

64. Moran A, Doherty L, Wang X, Thomas W. Abnormal glucose metabolism in cystic fibrosis. *J Pediatr*. 1998;133(1):10-17

65. Moran A, Brunzell C, Cohen RC, et al. Clinical care guidelines for cystic fibrosis-related diabetes: a position statement of the American Diabetes Association and a clinical practice guideline of the Cystic Fibrosis Foundation, endorsed by the Pediatric Endocrine Society. *Diabetes Care*. 2010;33(12):2697-2708

66. Stallings VA, Stark LJ, Robinson KA, Feranchak AP, Quinton H; Clinical Practice Guidelines on Growth and Nutrition Subcommittee; Ad Hoc Working Group. Evidence-based practice recommendations for nutrition-related management of children and adults with cystic fibrosis and pancreatic insufficiency: results of a systematic review. *J Am Diet Assoc*. 2008;108(5):832-839

67. Moran A, Pekow P, Grover P, et al; Cystic Fibrosis Related Diabetes Therapy Study Group. Insulin therapy to improve BMI in cystic fibrosis-related diabetes without fasting hyperglycemia: results of the cystic fibrosis related diabetes therapy trial. *Diabetes Care*. 2009;32(10):1783-1788

68. Borowitz D, Baker RD, Stallings V. Consensus report on nutrition for pediatric patients with cystic fibrosis. *J Pediatr Gastroenterol Nutr*. 2002;35(3):246-259

69. Neumark-Sztainer D, Patterson J, Mellin A, et al. Weight control practices and disordered eating behaviors among adolescent females and males with type 1 diabetes: associations with sociodemographics, weight concerns, familial factors, and metabolic outcomes. *Diabetes Care*. 2002;25(8):1289-1296

70. Colton P, Rodin G, Bergenstal R, Parkin C. Eating disorders and diabetes: introduction and overview. *Diabetes Spectrum*. 2009;22(3):138-142

71. Criego A, Crow S, Goebel-Fabbri AE, Kendall D, Parkin C. Eating disorders and diabetes: screening and detection. *Diabetes Spectrum*. 2009;22(3):143-146

VI

Chapter 32

Hypoglycemia in Infants and Children

Introduction and Definition of Hypoglycemia

Hypoglycemia is a surrogate marker for harmfully low levels of energy in the central nervous system (CNS). However, the degree and duration of low plasma glucose that can cause CNS damage in infants and children are uncertain. Important determinants of CNS energy sufficiency include the efficiency of the transport of glucose into the brain, the need of brain cells for energy, and the availability of alternative energy sources. Serum glucose concentrations do not accurately measure any of these processes.[1] This is particularly important in hyperinsulinism, because there is diminished availability of alternative substrates for the brain. Glucose is transported from the circulation across the blood-brain barrier, and such transport may vary depending on the availability and efficiency of specific glucose transporters. GLUT-1 is the major transporter of glucose across the blood-brain barrier, but other transporters are important for the entry of glucose into neurons and glial cells.[2] A rare genetic exemplar is that children with a defective copy of one GLUT-1 gene may have severe symptomatic CNS glucose deficiency with normal circulating serum glucose concentrations.[3] Energy utilization in the CNS varies depending on the activation state of neural tissues. Seizure activity, for instance, rapidly depletes neurons of energy even when peripheral plasma glucose concentration is normal.[4] Alternative substrates, such as ketones, lactate, and perhaps, free fatty acids and amino acids, also support the energy needs of the brain.[1,5,6] These substrates circulate in the plasma in concentrations that are dependent on the metabolic state of the child and, in general, cross the blood-brain barrier assisted by specific transporters.[7] Because of the potential differences in glucose transport to the brain, the utilization rate by neural tissues, and the availability of alternative energy substrates, plasma glucose concentration is not a precise measure of CNS cellular energy supply.

Variation in measurement of circulating glucose can further confound this problem. Early studies used whole blood glucose measures. Human red blood cell concentrations of glucose are about half those of plasma. Therefore, measures of whole blood glucose are 10% to 15% lower than the plasma or serum glucose measurement commonly obtained in automated analyzers. If the hematocrit concentration is higher than adult norms, as occurs in ill neonates, whole blood glucose measures may be even lower. In addition, blood samples obtained for the assay of glucose must be maintained on ice, analyzed rapidly, and/or protected from glycolysis by the addition of fluoride. Glycolytic degradation of glucose is more rapid in the neonate than in adult blood and can markedly decrease measured blood glucose in unprotected samples stored at room temperature.[8]

VI

Acceptable plasma glucose concentrations in the neonate may be defined statistically or by examination of acute or chronic outcomes. A systematic review of this issue suggests that no adequate data exist to define the concentration of peripheral glucose in the neonate that is associated with a poor developmental outcome.[9] However, there is a reasonable correlation among these statistical, epidemiologic, and acute experimental approaches, which gives some assurance that for most infants, plasma glucose concentrations commonly accepted as normal are clinically sound. Lower limits in term newborn infants have been defined epidemiologically as a plasma glucose concentration less than 45 mg/dL (2.5 mmol/L) in the first 48 hours.[10,11] A plasma glucose concentration less than 47 mg/dL (2.6 mmol/L) was the lower limit of normal for venous cord blood in term newborn infants.[12] A plasma glucose concentration less than 47 mg/dL (2.6 mmol/L) was associated with abnormal auditory evoked responses in older infants.[13] In preterm neonates, blood glucose concentrations below 30 to 45 mg/dL (1.67–2.5 mmol/L) were associated with a compensatory increase in cerebral blood flow, suggesting the neonate is stressed even without clinical symptoms.[14] In addition, a single plasma glucose concentration less than 47 mg/dL (2.6 mmol/L) in newborn infants was associated with a worse neurodevelopmental outcome at 18 months of age.[15] In another study, recurrent neonatal hypoglycemia in preterm neonates who were small for gestational age correlated better with poor neurodevelopmental outcomes at 5 years of age than did the severity of a single episode.[16] In adults, hypoglycemic symptoms are generally reported below plasma glucose concentrations of 60 mg/dL (3.3 mmol/L),[17,18] and this number is often taken as the lower limit of normal in children and adolescents. However, the set-point for physiologic counter-regulation seems higher in children than in adults.[19]

Operational thresholds for neonates (plasma glucose concentrations at which clinical interventions should be considered) were determined by a consensus conference and were based on available data (Table 32.1).[20] Participants in the consensus conference determined that routine monitoring of plasma glucose concentration is not necessary in a term infant with a normal pregnancy and delivery. However, low plasma glucose concentrations were considered sufficient for intervention if measured because of symptoms of hypoglycemia or risk factors for hypoglycemia.[12] Previous data suggesting that preterm infants have lower plasma glucose concentrations were felt to reflect deficient nutritional management. The same operational thresholds were, therefore, suggested for term and preterm neonates. A more recent consensus from the American Academy of Pediatrics has suggested similar guidelines.[21] Nonetheless, children with hyperinsulinism or fatty acid oxidation disorders should be maintained at blood glucose concentrations of 70 mg/dL or greater, because they are almost entirely dependent on CNS glucose transport for brain energy. Identifying these children is immensely important, because they are at risk of CNS damage at levels of blood glucose considered "normal" in newborn infants in the first 24 to 48 hours of life.

Table 32.1.
Operational Thresholds for Hypoglycemia in Neonates, Including Preterm Infants[a]

- A plasma glucose <45 mg/dL (2.5 mmol/L) and symptoms of hypoglycemia
- A plasma glucose <36 mg/dL (2.0 mmol/L) in a neonate with risk factors[b]
- A plasma glucose <60 mg/dL (3.3 mmol/L) in a neonate with persistent hyperinsulinemic hypoglycemia

[a] Breastfed term infants were not included; it was believed that they may tolerate lower plasma glucose concentrations, because they have more ketogenesis and higher ketone levels than formula-fed infants. A bedside glucose meter result should be confirmed with a serum sample.

[b] Risk factors include: those associated with maternal metabolism (intrapartum administration of glucose, terbutaline, ritodrine, propanolol, oral hypoglycemic agents, infant of a diabetic mother); those associated with neonatal problems (perinatal hypoxia-ischemia, infection, hypothermia, hyperviscosity, erythroblastosis fetalis, congenital cardiac disease, prematurity); intrauterine growth restriction; hyperinsulinism; endocrine disorders; and inborn errors of metabolism.

Clinical Manifestations of Hypoglycemia

Signs and symptoms of hypoglycemia can be broadly divided into those resulting from neuroglycopenia and those from adrenergic responses to hypoglycemia. The early signs of hypoglycemia are usually adrenergic and include sweating, weakness, tachycardia, tremor, hunger, paresthesias, pallor, anxiety or nervousness, nausea, and palpitations. Prolonged hypoglycemia may lead to more symptoms of neuroglycopenia, including lethargy, dizziness, irritability, mental confusion, behavior that is out of character, blurred vision, difficulty speaking, loss of coordination, and in its extreme, seizures, coma, and death. These signs and symptoms are less obvious or absent in infants and young children. The nonspecific signs of hypoglycemia in newborn and young infants may be manifested by irritability, jitteriness, feeding difficulties, lethargy, apnea, cyanosis, bradycardia, tachypnea, abnormal cry, hypothermia, hypotonia, apathy, and seizures. These signs are not specific for hypoglycemia and are also the early manifestations of other severe newborn disorders (sepsis, congenital heart disease, ventricular hemorrhage, respiratory distress syndrome and aspiration). With repeated or prolonged episodes of hypoglycemia, the threshold for autonomic symptoms decreases compared with the neuroglycopenic symptoms. As a result, the infant develops severe hypoglycemia with little or no warning, a condition termed "hypoglycemia unawareness."[22]

VI

Etiology of Hypoglycemia

Neonates

In newborn infants, the differential diagnosis of hypoglycemia initially can be guided but not limited by birth weight (Table 32.2). If the newborn infant remains hypoglycemic after the first 48 hours of life, then causes of prolonged neonatal

Table 32.2.

Causes of Hypoglycemia in Newborn Infants

Small for gestational age (SGA)   Primary failure to produce and store glycogen

Appropriate for gestational age (AGA)
   Endocrine deficiency:
   • Hypopituitarism/growth hormone deficiency
   • Cortisol/adrenocorticotropic hormone (ACTH) deficiency
   • ACTH unresponsiveness
   Increased rate of glucose utilization:
   • Perinatal stress/hypoxia
   • Cold stress
   • Sepsis
   Depletion of glycogen stores in congenital heart failure/congenital heart disease
   Inborn errors of carbohydrate, protein, and lipid metabolism
   Hyperinsulinism attributable to:
   • Alloimmune hemolytic disease of the newborn after exchange transfusion
   • Perinatal asphyxia
   • Maternal intrapartum treatment with glucose or with antihyperglycemia agents, such as sulfonylureas
   • Malposition of an umbilical catheter

Large for gestational age (LGA): hyperinsulinism
   Infant of a diabetic mother
   Beckwith-Wiedemann syndrome
      AKT2 activating mutation leading to upregulated insulin action
   Gene mutations causing congenital hyperinsulinism
      (Persistent hyperinsulinemic hypoglycemia of infancy [PHHI])[a]
   • SUR1 (sulphonylurea receptor type 1) inactivating gene mutation
   • KIR 6.2 (inward-rectifying potassium channel) inactivating gene mutation
   • SCHAD (short-chain L-3-hydroxyacyl-CoA dehydrogenase enzyme) inactivating gene mutation
   • GK (glucokinase) activating gene mutation
   • GDH (glutamate dehydrogenase) activating gene mutation
   • HNF4A (hepatocyte nuclear factor 4 alpha gene) inactivating gene mutation
   • MCT1 (monocarboxylate transporter 1) activating gene mutation
   • SLC16A1 gene (solute carrier family 16, member 1)
   • UCP2 gene (uncoupling protein 2)

[a] Because these disorders can be of variable severity and may not always present at birth, they are not invariably associated with fetal overgrowth.

hypoglycemia, such as perinatal stress-induced hyperinsulinism or hypopituitarism, and causes of permanent neonatal hypoglycemia, such as congenital hyperinsulinism or inborn errors of metabolism, should be considered.[23]

Children

The most common cause of hypoglycemia in children is insulin-induced hypoglycemia in individuals with type 1 diabetes mellitus. In other children, hypoglycemia can be categorized as ketotic fasting hypoglycemia, hypoketotic fasting hypoglycemia, or reactive or postprandial hypoglycemia. Postprandial hypoglycemia in young children is usually a result of fundoplication procedures, but in adolescents, it may be associated with obesity and high-carbohydrate eating habits (Table 32.3). This categorization generally aids in diagnosis but should not limit clinical judgment. Mild reactive hypoglycemia is common in the otherwise healthy adolescent population and is not considered a disease.

Evaluation of Hypoglycemia

Neonates

The history and physical examination are often revealing. Gestational age and birth weight; maternal health, including history of diabetes or glucose intolerance; and medications may guide diagnosis, prognosis, and therapy. Most hypoglycemic infants who are large for gestational age are hyperinsulinemic, although a recently described rare disorder of macrosomia and localized overgrowth with severe hypoglycemia and low insulin levels has been traced to an activating mutation in the molecular pathway that controls insulin effects.[24] Most hyperinsulinemic babies are born to women with diabetes, and the hypoglycemia and hyperinsulinemia are of relatively short duration (24 hours to a few days).[25] Other rare transient causes of hyperinsulinism include Beckwith-Wiedemann syndrome, characterized by macrosomia, large tongue, omphalocele/umbilical hernia, visceromegaly, and horizontal grooves on ear lobes.[26] Persistent hyperinsulinism and hypoglycemia require careful genetic and physiologic evaluation and management planning. Genetic hyperinsulinism because of mutations in genes controlling insulin release, including beta-cell potassium channels, glucokinase, and glutamate dehydrogenase genes, must always be considered, although it is rare (1:50 000 children, except in inbred populations). These disorders require immediate intervention and continued and definitive therapy. Most infants born preterm or small for gestational age are unable to produce enough glucose through glycogenolysis and gluconeogenesis to meet the needs of their relatively large brains. These babies usually will respond with increased glucose when sufficient fat is included in their diet to alter the hepatocellular ratio of nicotinamide adenine dinucleotide (NAD) to reduced nicotinamide

VI

Table 32.3.

Causes of Hypoglycemia in Children

Ketotic Fasting Hypoglycemia
Accelerated starvation ("ketotic hypoglycemia")
Endocrine deficiencies: growth hormone (GH), ACTH/cortisol, hypopituitarism (ACTH/cortisol and GH)
Metabolic defects:
    Disorders of carbohydrate metabolism:
        Glycogen synthase deficiency
        Type III glycogen storage disease (amylo-1,6-glucosidase deficiency)
        Type VI glycogen storage disease (phosphorylase deficiency)
        Type IX glycogen storage disease (phosphorylase kinase deficiency)
        Defects in gluconeogenesis: pyruvate carboxylase deficiency, PEPCK deficiency, fructose 1-6-biphosphatase deficiency
    Disorders of protein metabolism (organic acidemias) examples:
        Maple syrup urine disease (branched-chain ketoacid decarboxylase deficiency)
        Methylmalonic acidemia
Miscellaneous:
    Salicylate intoxication
    Reye syndrome
    Ethanol intoxication
    Malaria
    Diarrhea
    Malnutrition
    Jamaican vomiting sickness (ingestion of unripe ackee)

Hypoketotic Fasting Hypoglycemia
    Glycogen storage disease type 1 (glucose-6-phosphatase deficiency)
    Tyrosinemia
    Disorders of fatty oxidation and ketone synthesis:
        Carnitine transport and metabolism
        Beta-oxidation cycle
        Electron transfer
        HMG-CoA synthase or lyase deficiency
    IGF-1, IGF-2 excess
    Insulinoma
    Sulfonylurea or other insulin secretagogue ingestion
    Exogenous insulin administration
    Persistent hyperinsulinemic hypoglycemia of infancy (PHHI) (See Table 32.2)

Reactive or Postprandial Hypoglycemia:
    "Metabolic dumping syndrome"
    Galactosemia
    Fructose intolerance (fructose-1-phosphate aldolase deficiency)

PEPCK indicates phosphoenolpyruvate carboxykinase; HMG, 3-hydroxy-3-methylglutaryl

IGF, insulin-like growth factor.

adenine dinucleotide (NADH) in favor of gluconeogenesis.[27] However, some of these infants may also have prolonged hyperinsulinism, and the etiology is, as yet, unclear.[28] Normal-weight babies are most likely to have an endocrine deficiency disorder or an inborn error of carbohydrate or fatty acid metabolism. Prolonged neonatal jaundice, microphallus in a boy, or facial midline anomalies might suggest hypopituitarism. Hepatomegaly might suggest a genetic disorder of glycogen synthesis or release. Metabolic disorders may present in the immediate neonatal period or somewhat later. Those that cause acidosis may manifest as hyperventilation that is misdiagnosed as pneumonia or reactive airway disease or may be misdiagnosed as overwhelming sepsis in the first months of life. A history of unusual odors may be a clue in maple syrup urine disease, isovaleric acidemia, 3-methylcrotonyl coenzyme A carboxylase deficiency, and glutaric acidemia type II. Many states now perform neonatal screening for these disorders so that diagnosis is made early, often before the infants are symptomatic.

Children

Birth weight, history of neonatal complications, age of onset, and frequency of symptoms can aid in diagnosis. Symptoms of hypoglycemia at birth or during the neonatal period might point to hypopituitarism or hyperinsulinism; prolonged neonatal jaundice might suggest cortisol and/or thyroid deficiency. The temporal relationship of symptoms to food intake may aid in diagnosis. Hypoglycemia that occurs within about 2 hours of eating is considered reactive. It may be observed in dumping syndrome, which is more common after a fundoplication, in obese individuals with overactive insulin response to carbohydrate, and very rarely in individuals with galactosemia or hereditary fructose intolerance. The specific content of feedings and relationship to onset of symptoms as well as food intolerance or aversion may guide the diagnosis, as may the usual laboratory evaluation. Early dumping syndrome, which occurs within 60 minutes of feeding, is characterized by postprandial irritability, diaphoresis, abdominal pain, and diarrhea. Late dumping syndrome presents with hypoglycemia 1 to 4 hours after the feeding and may present without other systemic symptoms.[29]

Symptomatic hypoglycemia that appears approximately 4 hours after eating more commonly occurs in defects of glycogenolysis or in hyperinsulinism. Hypoglycemia that occurs 10 to 12 hours after feedings suggests a defect of gluconeogenesis or fatty acid oxidation but may also represent hyperinsulinism.

A potential drug exposure should be sought in all children with hypoglycemia. Insulin, hypoglycemic agents, and alcohol are often implicated. Erratic episodes of hypoglycemia may be a warning of Munchausen syndrome by proxy.[30]

VI

Findings from the physical examination suggestive of growth hormone deficiency or hypopituitarism are short stature or growth failure, microphallus, midline defects (cleft lip and palate, single central incisor), and optic nerve hypoplasia (in septo-optic dysplasia). Hepatomegaly is usually present in glycogen storage diseases, disorders of gluconeogenesis, galactosemia, hereditary fructose intolerance, disorders of fatty acid oxidation and carnitine metabolism, and tyrosinemia type 1. Increased pigmentation may be present in Addison disease. Disorders of fatty acid oxidation may cause cardiomyopathy.

Laboratory Investigation of Unexplained Hypoglycemia

Glucose meters for self-plasma glucose monitoring are calibrated to normal blood or plasma glucose ranges and adult ranges for hypoglycemia (50 mg/dL or less plasma glucose). Readings may be influenced by hematocrit, because meters are calibrated to read plasma glucose within an adult range of hematocrit, and plasma glucose concentration is higher than whole blood glucose concentration.

Even the best meters are not consistently reliable at low blood glucose concentrations. Hence, a glucose meter value below 45 mg/dL should be confirmed by a laboratory glucose value. If appropriate additional laboratory studies are obtained at the same time, this laboratory plasma glucose value may serve as a "critical" or diagnostic sample. It may be necessary to perform a monitored fast of 8 to 24 hours, depending on the age of the child. Fasting may induce cerebral edema in a child with a fatty acid oxidation defect. This should be ruled out before performing the fast by determination of nonfasting plasma acylcarnitines and urinary acylglycines.[31] Table 32.4 outlines the protocol, which can be used for the monitored fasting evaluation, and lists the laboratory tests to send with the "critical blood sample." Although still in the research phase, continuous interstitial glucose monitoring could be used to detect episodes of asymptomatic hypoglycemia.[32]

Differential Diagnosis of Hypoglycemia

Neonates

Hyperinsulinism

In the neonate, the diagnostic challenge is to ensure that the child does not have persistent hyperinsulinism. This disorder carries a worse prognosis than other causes of hypoglycemia for several reasons. First, high insulin concentrations will make alternative brain fuels like ketones, lactate, and free fatty acids unavailable so that the need of the CNS for glucose will be greater than in other types of hypoglycemia.[33,34] Second, at least one of the disorders associated with hyperinsulinism

Table 32.4.
Monitored Fasting for Evaluation of Hypoglycemia

If blood glucose reaches 45 mg/dL or less, obtain the following studies in the appropriate tube for your laboratory:
Glucose Insulin C-peptide IGF-1[a] IGF-2[a] Beta-hydroxybutyrate Free fatty acids Cortisol Growth Hormone Lactate-free flowing blood Pyruvate-free flowing blood Carnitine and acylcarnitine panel[a] Free T_4 and TSH[a] Urine sample for organic acids and amino acids[a]

Before starting the monitored fast, confirm that appropriate blood tubes are ready and labeled for these tests; some must be obtained on ice and in special tubes. After sending the blood sample, administer 30 µg/kg of glucagon intravenously or subcutaneously, and obtain blood for glucose concentration at 10, 15, 20, and 30 minutes. If the blood glucose has not increased with glucagon, administer 2 mL/kg of 25% glucose intravenously and feed or treat with a continuous glucose infusion as possible.

T_4 indicates thyroxine; TSH, thyroid-stimulating factor.

[a] These tests do not need to be drawn during the hypoglycemic event.

(glutamate dehydrogenase-activating mutations leading to hyperinsulinemia and hyperammonemia) involves metabolic pathways common to the brain so that the underlying disorder may separately interfere with neuronal function and development.[35] Last, hypoglycemia from hyperinsulinism is often quite difficult to control, requiring large quantities of glucose (>10-12 mg/kg/minute, intravenously) and additional therapeutic agents, such as diazoxide and octreotide, which have their own toxicities.[33,36] In many children, either partial or total pancreatectomy is necessary for control of blood glucose concentration. The decision about surgery and the type of surgery requires sophisticated techniques to assess the etiology of the hyperinsulinism and the nature of the pancreatic involvement. Once congenital hyperinsulinism is confirmed or suspected, transfer to a specialist is prudent. Diagnosis should be suspected if the need for glucose is greater than 10 to 12 mg/kg per minute and the child's hypoglycemia is not relieved by physiologic cortisol supplementation. Plasma insulin concentration must be determined at the same time as the glucose concentration. Insulin concentrations obtained at the time of hypoglycemia are generally higher than anticipated for hypoglycemia (>2 µU/mL), but many assays designed to measure adult insulin concentrations will not be able

VI

to detect concentrations this low and will report no measurable insulin in plasma, even in infants suffering from hyperinsulinism.

Other Etiologies of Hypoglycemia

Cortisol deficiency can be difficult to diagnose in neonates who often do not respond to hypoglycemia with elevations in cortisol but can respond to adrenocorticotropic hormone (ACTH) testing. However, treatment with cortisol should rapidly ameliorate the hypoglycemia. The underlying etiology is usually panhypopituitarism. Absence of ketonemia is indicative of hyperinsulinism, except in rare disorders of ketogenesis or in congenital hypopituitarism in many cases. Neonates have a high renal threshold for ketones and may have normal ketogenesis with hypoglycemia without measurable ketonuria.[37] Ketonuria in a newborn infant with hypoglycemia suggests either glycogen storage disease type III or rare genetic organic acidemias. Urinary organic acid determination is critical to determine the presence of abnormal ketoacids. If available, the rapid bedside meter and strip method for checking serum levels of beta-hydroxybutyrate can be diagnostically useful.

Children

The laboratory differential diagnosis can be initially guided by the presence or absence of ketonuria or ketonemia.

Ketotic Hypoglycemia

Ketoacids in normal fasting individuals include beta-hydroxybutyrate, measured in plasma with specific reagent strips and a meter or (preferred) by a reference laboratory, and acetoacetate, measured in urine as "ketones" on a test strip. Acetoacetate is quite labile and will not persist in a stored plasma sample unless handled very carefully, but beta-hydroxybutyrate is more stable. In the presence of adequate ketosis, if the urine organic acids do not show an abnormal diagnostic pattern and there is no hepatomegaly, the following diagnoses should be considered: accelerated starvation, growth hormone or cortisol deficiency, and glycogen synthase deficiency. "Accelerated starvation" (previously termed ketotic hypoglycemia) is a diagnosis of exclusion and should be made when the other causes of ketotic hypoglycemia have been ruled out. Children with this disorder are typically underweight for height. Hypoglycemia usually occurs after 12 to 24 hours of fasting and is associated with a normal metabolic response to hypoglycemia with ketonuria, low plasma alanine concentration, normal lactate and pyruvate concentrations, suppressed insulin, and elevated growth hormone and cortisol concentrations. The response to glucagon administration is blunted at the time of hypoglycemia, because hepatic and other glycogen stores have been used for energy.[38]

The presence of a large liver should point to the diagnosis of glycogen storage disease and disorders of gluconeogenesis. The diagnosis of glycogen synthase deficiency can be confirmed at the molecular level after an oral glucose tolerance test demonstrates initial hyperglycemia, followed by hypoglycemia at 3 to 4 hours.[39] The urine organic or amino acid pattern should give the diagnosis in the case of disorders of organic acid or amino acid metabolism. A plasma cortisol concentration less than 10 μg/dL during hypoglycemia suggests cortisol/ACTH deficiency. A low plasma growth hormone concentration should raise suspicion of growth hormone deficiency/hypopituitarism, but low growth hormone and cortisol levels are sometimes found in normal individuals following persistent or frequent hypoglycemia.

Hypoketotic Hypoglycemia

Insulin should be undetectable during hypoglycemia. In hyperinsulinism, insulin inhibits ketone production and lipolysis, and ketone and free fatty acid concentrations are inappropriately low during hypoglycemia. The plasma insulin concentration will be inappropriately high during hypoglycemia (>2 μU/mL). A positive response to glucagon (30 μg/kg, subcutaneously or intravenously) with an increment in plasma glucose of at least 30 mg/dL (1.7 mmol/L), despite severe hypoglycemia, is also diagnostic of hyperinsulinism.[40] However, some children with hyperinsulinism have required a larger dose of glucagon (up to 1 mg) to elicit significant glycogenolysis. Typically, the intravenous glucose rate required to maintain normoglycemia is 2 to 4 times greater than the glucose production rate (6-8 mg/kg/minute in a newborn infant, 4-6 mg/kg/minute in a slightly older child, and 1-2 mg/kg/minute in an adult). The reason for the differences in glucose production rate is evident in Fig 32.1, which demonstrates that to maintain euglycemia, glucose production rate must equal glucose utilization rate. As the relative brain size compared with body weight decreases with age, the relative glucose utilization rate per kg of body weight also decreases.[41]

In hyperinsulinism, plasma cortisol and growth hormone concentrations may be normal or inappropriately low if the hypoglycemia occurs gradually or is recurrent (blunted counter-regulatory response). A low C-peptide concentration associated with elevated insulin concentrations suggests exogenous insulin administration.

Imaging of the pancreas with computerized axial tomography or ultrasonography is very rarely sensitive enough to identify an insulinoma and cannot visualize focal adenomatous hyperplasia or diffuse beta-cell hyperplasia. The type and location of the pancreatic lesion (diffuse versus focal) can be determined by preoperative pancreatic catheterization and intraoperative histopathologic studies, which should be performed at a center experienced in these studies. Mutational analysis can be helpful in the diagnosis of focal hyperinsulinism and in defining a

VI

Fig 32.1

Total glucose rate of disappearance (Rd) (mmol/min) as a function of body weight from infancy to adulthood (n = 141; body weights range from 0.6 to 94 kg). The data points represent mean values for subjects with brain sizes in kg of 0.14 (0.070-0.20); 0.37 (0.22-0.40); 0.44 (0.40-0.57); 0.0, 1.2, 1.3, and 1.4, respectively. Reproduced with permission from Haymond MW, Sunehag A. Controlling the sugar bowl. Regulation of glucose homeostasis in children. *Endocrinol Metab Clin North Am.* **1999;28(4):663-694.**

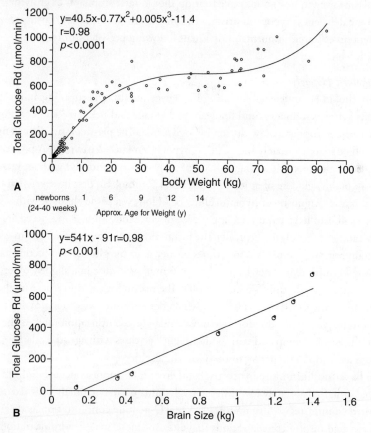

$y = 40.5x - 0.77x^2 + 0.005x^3 - 11.4$
$r = 0.98$
$p < 0.0001$

$y = 541x - 91 \quad r = 0.98$
$p < 0.001$

genetic etiology. Preoperative positron emission tomography (PET) using ^{18}F dihydroxyphenylalanine (DOPA) as a marker has proved very useful in localization and in making this diagnostic distinction but is presently available at only a few specialized centers.[34,42]

If the plasma insulin concentration is adequately suppressed with hypoketotic hypoglycemia, a fatty acid oxidation defect should be suspected. A diagnostic pattern is often seen in the concentrations of urine organic acids and acylglycine and plasma acylcarnitine.[31]

Treatment of Hypoglycemia

Infants and Young Children

A pragmatic management plan is not based on outcome measures but depends on the clinical picture, including laboratory-determined plasma glucose concentration and signs and symptoms.

If the plasma glucose concentration is between 35 and 45 mg/dL (1.9-2.5 mmol/L) and the neonate is able to feed, then breastfeeding or formula feeding or 5% dextrose administration by nipple is appropriate. If the neonate is very symptomatic and unable to feed, intravenous glucose with 5% to 12.5% dextrose at a rate of 4 to 6 mg/kg/minute[-1] should be initiated. If the plasma glucose concentration is between 25 and 34 mg/dL (1.4-1.9 mmol/L), intravenous glucose with 5% to 12.5% dextrose at a rate of 6 to 8 mg/kg/minute[-1] should be started regardless of symptoms, and oral feedings should be allowed as tolerated.[21,43]

If the plasma glucose concentration is less than 25 mg/dL (1.4 mmol/L), it is appropriate to administer a minibolus of 2 mL/kg of 10% dextrose (200 mg/kg) over 5 to 10 minutes, followed by an infusion rate of 6 to 8 mg/kg/minute[-1]. It has been argued that a minibolus given over 1 minute could cause hyperosmolar cerebral edema, because it exceeds glucose uptake capacity and might, if the dose is large enough, induce excessive insulin secretion, worsening the hypoglycemia.[44-46] The glucose infusion rate can be calculated with the following formula:

$$\text{glucose (mg/kg/min}^{-1}) = (\%\text{glucose in solution} \times 10) \times$$
$$(\text{rate of infusion per hour}) / (60 \times \text{weight [kg]})$$

The glucose concentration should be monitored every 30 minutes. Therapy should be intensified if hypoglycemia is not corrected by the initial measures. Maintenance of blood glucose at greater than 60 to 70 mg/dL is reasonable for neuroprotection, although no outcome data support this consensus approach. The glucose infusion rate should be increased to achieve euglycemia with the minimal concentration of glucose required. Infusion rates greater than 15 mg/kg/minute[-1] should be given by a central venous catheter, except in emergency situations. The

VI

glucose infusion rate should be gradually reduced rather than abruptly terminated to avoid reactive hypoglycemia.

If euglycemia is not maintained with a dextrose infusion rate above 15 mg/kg/minute^{-1}, the use of corticosteroids should be considered. Although it will not be effective in hyperinsulinism, hydrocortisone administered at a dose of 5 mg/kg/day, intravenously or orally, divided every 12 hours, or prednisone administered at a dose of 1 to 2 mg/kg/day, orally, as a temporizing measure can be useful. Gradual decrease should be attempted once euglycemia is achieved. Glucagon may be given in a dose of 30 μg/kg at the time of hypoglycemia to assess glycogenolysis. A response of more than 30 mg/dL at 30 minutes is confirmatory of hyperinsulinism.[40] Sometimes a higher dose of glucagon (up to 1 mg) is necessary to elicit glycogenolysis, even in infants with hyperinsulinism.

The consensus aim for neuroprotection, although there are no supportive outcome data, should be to maintain plasma glucose concentrations above 70 mg/dL (3.9 mmol/L) in infants and young children with persistent hyperinsulinism or other disorders in which alternative brain energy substrates are not available. This may require glucose infusion rates of higher than 20 mg/kg/minute^{-1}, in addition to frequent enteral feedings. A central venous catheter and a nasogastric tube or a gastrostomy tube may be necessary. Pharmacologic agents should be added to normalize the carbohydrate intake and decrease insulin secretion.[33,34,36] Diazoxide (10-20 mg/kg per day in 2-3 divided oral doses) with added chlorothiazide or furosemide if the patient is edematous (7-10 mg/kg per day in 2 divided oral doses) are recommended for the initial treatment. The response is variable depending on the underlying etiology of the hyperinsulinism. If the response is suboptimal or the adverse effects of fluid retention and cardiac failure from diazoxide are significant, nifedipine could be the next choice in management, at a dose of 0.25 to 2.5 mg/kg/day, orally, divided every 8 hours. A very limited number of hyperinsulinemic young children have responded to nifedipine, but this drug is not often effective. Monitoring of blood pressure is mandatory. Second-line agents given by infusion or injection include octreotide, which is a somatostatin analogue, and glucagon. Both can cause tachyphylaxis at high doses. They should be used when the orally administered drugs have not been effective and if the infant or young child remains glucose-infusion dependent. Some argue to use both concurrently, because glucagon may stimulate insulin secretion. Glucagon has specific benefit in neonates who are hyperinsulinemic and may be infused at a rate of approximately 5 to 10 μg/kg/hour. This may be a useful adjunct as a child is being prepared for management in an experienced referral center. Prolonged glucagon usage in this manner could be associated with proteolysis and skin rashes as seen in the glucagonoma syndrome. Octreotide can be given at a rate of 5 to 20 μg/kg/day in an intravenous or subcutaneous infusion. If octreotide is effective as an infusion, it can be converted to a chronic parenteral therapy, administered by subcutaneous injection 3 times a day.

As mentioned, tachyphylaxis often occurs, preventing it from being used chronically. In addition, it has been associated with necrotizing enterocolitis.

The criteria for successful medical management of hyperinsulinism are a feeding regimen acceptable to the family with normal plasma glucose concentrations after reasonable periods of fasting (at least 6 hours in newborn infants, 8 hours for slightly older infants). Failure of pharmacologic therapy in a period of a few days to weeks should lead to surgical treatment with either a localized or a near-total (95%-99%) pancreatectomy.[33,34] Recurrent hypoglycemia is to be avoided as much as possible because of its long-term deleterious effects on neurologic functioning.

Older Children

Acute hypoglycemia associated with a mismatch between insulin administration and insulin need in children with diabetes mellitus should be treated on the basis of the severity of hypoglycemia. If the child is alert and able to drink or eat safely, treatment with 10 to 20 g of rapidly available carbohydrate in the form of fruit juice, sweetened drink, candy, or specially prepared glucose tablets is adequate for initial therapy. The response usually lasts less than 2 hours, so it should be followed by a mixed snack containing carbohydrate, fat, and protein or a scheduled meal. In children who require the assistance of another person to treat hypoglycemia, gel preparations of carbohydrate are available that can be administered orally and are effective as long as swallowing is preserved. Buccal absorption of carbohydrate is minimal. Children who are unable to eat or drink by mouth or are comatose or seizing should immediately receive a subcutaneous or intramuscular injection of glucagon of 0.02 to 0.03 mg/kg to a maximum of 1 mg. Families should be taught how much glucagon to prepare and administer for such emergencies, and the dosage should be changed as the child gains weight. Children respond within 15 minutes and then should be encouraged to eat, because the effect of the glucagon is relatively short lived, and nausea and vomiting are common adverse effects of both hypoglycemia and glucagon administration.

In the emergency department or hospital, regardless of the cause of hypoglycemia, if the child is unable to drink or eat, after critical blood samples are obtained, 25% dextrose (2-3 mL/kg) should be administered intravenously. This should be followed by a continued infusion of 10% dextrose initially, at a rate of 6 to 8 mg/kg/minute^{-1}, to avoid rebound hypoglycemia and maintain normoglycemia. The plasma glucose concentration should be monitored, and the infusion rate should be adjusted to maintain a concentration above 80 mg/dL (4.5 mmol/L). Children with

VI

hyperinsulinism will require higher rates of infusion. Long-term treatment is similar to that in the neonate (see previous section).

In disorders of fatty acid oxidation, a glucose infusion rate of 10 mg/kg/minute[-1], by stimulating insulin release and inhibiting lipolysis, reverses the acute metabolic disorder.[31] Long-term treatment of endocrine deficiency disorders and genetic metabolic disorders should be specific for the disorder.

Treatment and prevention of ketotic hypoglycemia, or "accelerated starvation," consists of educating parents to avoid prolonged periods of fasting and offer a bedtime snack consisting of both carbohydrate and protein. During an intercurrent illness, carbohydrate-rich drinks should be given at frequent intervals. Parents are instructed to test urine or blood for ketones. Ketonuria and ketonemia precedes hypoglycemia by several hours.

Frequent feedings with glucose protect children with types 1 and 3 glycogen storage diseases from hypoglycemia and reduces hepatomegaly. Intermittent or continuous glucose can be provided during the day, and continuous glucose can be provided during the night by a nasogastric or gastrostomy tube. After 6 to 8 months of age, the infantile gut has matured to the point that it can digest uncooked cornstarch. Feedings of uncooked starch (1.75-2.5 g) can be given intermittently, because it is slowly absorbed into the circulation, acting like a continuous source of glucose. It is given in water or artificially flavored drinks. Carbohydrate sources should only be glucose or glucose polymers. Blood glucose monitoring allows the creation of a successful feeding regimen.[47] Uncooked cornstarch at bedtime may help to prevent hypoglycemia in other groups of children, including children receiving insulin for diabetes.[48]

Children with metabolic dumping syndrome causing reactive hypoglycemia can be treated with an alpha-glucosidase inhibitor like acarbose (12.5-50 mg) before each feeding to slow carbohydrate absorption.[29]

Hereditary fructose intolerance is treated with elimination of fructose and sucrose. Fructose 1,6-diphosphatase deficiency is treated by elimination of fructose and sucrose and avoidance of prolonged fasting. During intercurrent illness, intravenous glucose may be necessary to arrest catabolism. Galactosemia is treated by elimination of galactose from the diet.

Summary

Hypoglycemia is the result of an alteration in the metabolic and hormonal interrelationships that balance glucose absorption, release, and production with glucose utilization. Symptomatic hypoglycemia is caused by decreased CNS energy levels (neuroglycopenia) and is reflected somewhat imperfectly in measures of blood sugar. It is the health care professional's task to recognize the signs and symptoms of hypoglycemia, document hypoglycemia with laboratory test results, and obtain appropriate studies to identify the etiology. Initial symptomatic treatment of hypoglycemia will preserve brain function, but long-term management depends on identification of the cause of the energy imbalance.

References

1. McCall A. Cerebral glucose metabolism in diabetes mellitus. *Eur J Pharmacol.* 2004;490(1-3):147-158

2. McEwen B, Reagan L. Glucose transporter expression in the central nervous system: relationship to synaptic function. *Eur J Pharmacol.* 2004;490(1-3):13-24

3. Wang D, Pascual JM, Yang H, et al. Glut-1 deficiency syndrome:clinical and therapeutic aspects. *Ann Neurol.* 2005;57(1):111-118

4. Fujikawa D, Vannucci RC, Dwyer BE, Wasterlain CG. Generalized seizures deplete brain energy reserves in normoxemic newborn monkeys. *Brain Res.* 1988;454(1-2):51-59

5. Settergren G, Lindblad BS, Persson B. Cerebral blood flow and exchange of oxygen, glucose, ketone bodies, lactate, pyruvate and amino acids in infants. *Acta Paediatr Scand.* 1976;65(3):343-353

6. Vannucci R, Vannucci S. Hypoglycemic brain injury. *Semin Neonatol.* 2001;6(2):147-155

7. Mason G, et al. Increased brain monocarboxylic acid transport and utilization in type 1 diabetes. *Diabetes.* 2006;55(4):929-934

8. Cornblath M, Schwartz R. *Disorders of Carbohydrate Metabolism in Infancy.* Chicago, IL: Year Book Medical Publishers Inc; 1991

9. Boluyt N, van Kempen A, Offringa M. Neurodevelopment after neonatal hypoglycemia: a systematic review and design of an optimal future study. *Pediatrics.* 2006;117(6):2231-2243

10. Heck LJ, Erenberg A. Serum glucose levels in term neonates during the first 48 hours of life. *J Pediatr.* 1987;110(1):119-122

11. Srinivasan G, Pildes RS, Cattamanchi G, Voora S, Lilien LD. Plasma glucose values in normal neonates: a new look. *J Pediatr.* 1986;109(1):114-117

12. Hawdon JM, Ward Platt MP, Aynsley-Green A. Patterns of metabolic adaptation for preterm and term infants in the first neonatal week. *Arch Dis Child.* 1992;67(4 Spec No):357-365

13. Koh TH, Aynsley-Green A, Tarbit M, Eyre JA. Neural dysfunction during hypoglycaemia. *Arch Dis Child.* 1988;63(11):1353-1358

14. Pryds O, Christensen N, Friis-Hansen B. Increased cerebral blood flow and plasma epinephrine in hypoglycemic, preterm neonates. *Pediatrics.* 1990;85(2):172-176

15. Lucas A, Morley R, Cole TJ. Adverse neurodevelopmental outcome of moderate neonatal hypoglycaemia. *BMJ.* 1988;297(6659):1304-1308

16. Duvanel CB, Fawer CL, Cotting J, Hohlfeld P, Matthieu JM. Long-term effects of neonatal hypoglycemia on brain growth and psychomotor development in small-for-gestational-age preterm infants. *J Pediatr.* 1999;134(4):492-498

VI

17. Schwartz NS, Clutter WE, Shah SD, Cryer PE. Glycemic thresholds for activation of glucose counterregulatory systems are higher than the threshold for symptoms. *J Clin Invest*. 1987;79(3):777-781

18. Mitrakou A, Ryan C, Veneman T, et al. Hierarchy of glycemic thresholds for counterregulatory hormone secretion, symptoms, and cerebral dysfunction. *Am J Physiol*. 1991;260(1 Pt 1):e67-e74

19. Jones T, Boulware SD, Kraemer DT, Caprio S, Sherwin RS, Tamborlane WV. Independent effects of youth and poor diabetes control on responses to hypoglycemia in children. *Diabetes*. 1991;40(3):358-363

20. Cornblath M, Hawdon JM, Williams AF, et al. Controversies regarding definition of neonatal hypoglycemia: suggested operational thresholds. *Pediatrics*. 2000;105(5):1141-1145

21. Adamkin DH; American Academy of Pediatrics, Committee on Fetus and Newborn. Clinical report: postnatal glucose homeostasis in late-preterm and term infants. *Pediatrics*. 2011;127(3):575-578

22. Cryer P. Mechanisms of hypoglycemia-associated autonomic failure and its component syndromes in diabetes. *Diabetes*. 2005;54(12):3592-3601

23. De Leon DD, Stanley CA. Mechanisms of eisease: advances in diagnosis and treatment of hyperinsulinism in neonates. *Nat Clin Pract Endocrinol Metab*. 2007;3(1):57-68

24. Hussain K, Challis B, Rocha N, et al. An activating mutation of AKT2 and human hypoglycemia. *Science*. 2011;334(6055):474

25. Nold J, Georgieff M. Infants of diabetic mothers. *Pediatr Clin North Am*. 2004;51(3):619-637

26. Shuman C, et al. Beckwith-Wiedemann syndrome. In: Pagon RA, Bird TD, Dolan CR, Stephens K, eds. *GeneReviews*. Seattle, WA: University of Washington; 2000. Updated 2010

27. Sabel K, Olegård R, Mellander M, Hildingsson K. Interrelation between fatty acid oxidation and control of gluconeogenic substrates in small-for-gestatinal-age (SGA) infants with hypoglycemia and normoglycemia. *Acta Paediatr Scand*. 1982;71(1):53-61

28. Hoe F, et al. Clinical features and insulin regulation in infants with a syndrome of prolonged neonatal hyperinsulinism. *J Pediatr*. 2006;148(2):207-212

29. Ng DD, Ferry RJ Jr, Kelly A, Weinzimer SA, Stanley CA, Katz LE. Acarbose treatment of postprandial hypoglycemia in children after Nissen fundoplication. *J Pediatr*. 2001;139(6):877-879

30. de Lonlay P, Giurgea I, Sempoux C, et al. Dominantly inherited hyperinsulinaemic hypoglycaemia. *J Inherit Metab Dis*. 2005;28(3):267-276

31. Vianey-Liaud C, Divry P, Gregersen N, Mathieu M. The inborn errors of mitochondrial fatty acid oxidation. *J Inherit Metab Dis*. 1987;10(Suppl 1):159-200

32. Harris DL, Battin MR, Weston PJ, Harding JE. Continuous glucose monitoring in newborn babies at risk of hypoglycemia. *J Pediatr*. 2010;157(2):198.e1-202.e1

33. Arnoux J-B, Verkarre V, Saint-Martin C. Congenital hyperinsulinism: current trends in diagnosis and therapy. *Orphanet J Rare Dis*. 2011;6:63

34. Aynsley-Green A, Hussain K, Hall J, et al. Practical management of hyperinsulinism in infancy. *Arch Dis Child Fetal Neonatal Ed*. 2000;82(2):F98-F107

35. Raisen D, Brooks-Kayal A, Steinkrauss L, Tennekoon GI, Stanley CA, Kelly A. Central nervous system hyperexcitability associated with glutamate dehydrogenase gain of function mutations. *J Pediatr*. 2005;146(3):388-394

36. Hussain K, Aynsley-Green A, Stanley C. Medications used in the treatment of hypoglycemia due to congenital hyperinsulinism of infancy (HI). *Pediatr Endocrinol Rev*. 2004;2(Suppl 1):163-167

37. Warshaw J, Curry E. Comparison of serum carnitine and ketone body concentrations in breast- and formula-fed newborn infants. *J Pediatr*. 1980;97(1):122-125

38. Bodamer OA, Hussein K, Morris AA, et al. Glucose and leucine kinetics in idiopathic ketotic hypoglycemia. *Arch Dis Child*. 2006;91(6):483-486

39. Bachrach B, Weinstein DA, Orho-Melander M, Burgess A, Wolfsdorf JI. Glycogen synthase deficiency (glycogen storage disease type 0) presenting with hyperglycemia and glycosuria: report of three new mutations. *J Pediatr*. 2002;140(6):781-783

40. Finegold D, Stanley C, Baker L. Glycemic response to glucagon during fasting hypoglycemia: an aid in the diagnosis of hyperinsulinism. *J Pediatr*. 1980;96(2):257-259

41. Haymond MW, Sunehag AL. Controlling the sugar bowl. Regulation of glucose homeostasis in children. *Endocrinol Metab Clin North Am*. 1999;28(4):663-694

42. Hussain K, Seppänen M, Näntö-Salonen K, et al. The diagnosis of ectopic focal hyperinsulinism of infancy with (^{18}F)-dopa positron emission tomography. *J Clin Endocrinol Metab*. 2006;91(8):2839-2842

43. Cornblath M. *Risk Management Techniques in Perinatal and Neonatal Practice*. Donn SM, Fisher CW, eds. Armonk, NY: Futura; 1996

44. Cowett R, Farrag H. Neonatal glucose metabolism. In: *Principles of Perinatal-Neonatal Metabolism*. Cowett R, ed. New York, NY: Springer-Verlag; 1998:683-722

45. Farrag RM. Hypoglycemia in the newborn, including infant of a diabetic mother. In: Lifshitz F, ed. *Pediatric Endocrinology*. New York, NY: Marcel Dekker; 2003:541-574

46. Mehta A. Prevention and management of neonatal hypoglycaemia. *Arch Dis Child Fetal Neonatal Ed*. 1994;70(1):F54-F59

47. Wolfsdorf JI, Crigler JF Jr. Cornstarch regimens for nocturnal treatment of young adults with type 1 glycogen storage disease. *Am J Clin Nutr*. 1997;65(5):1507-1511

48. Kaufman FR, Devgan S. Use of uncooked cornstarch to avert nocturnal hypoglycemia in children and adolescents with type 1 diabetes. *J Diabetes Complications*. 1996;10(2):84-87

VI

Chapter 33

Hyperlipidemia

Introduction

Coronary artery disease and blood cholesterol levels are statistically related. Although the incidence of coronary artery disease is now declining in the United States, it remains the leading cause of death in adults in the United States and most resource-rich countries. The familial occurrence of coronary heart disease has been known since the 19th century; however, the familial risk factors have been delineated only in recent decades. The Framingham study[1] and subsequent studies have identified the following risk factors for coronary heart disease:

1. Family history
2. Male gender
3. Elevated serum total cholesterol level
4. Reduced level of high-density lipoprotein (HDL)-cholesterol
5. Elevated level of low density lipoprotein (LDL)-cholesterol
6. Elevated level of triglycerides
7. Hypertension
8. Cigarette smoking
9. Diabetes mellitus
10. Lack of physical activity

Not all investigators agree that an elevated level of plasma triglycerides is an independent risk factor for coronary heart disease. Although a direct correlation is evident in univariate analysis, this effect is lost when the influences of obesity, diabetes mellitus, total cholesterol, and HDL-cholesterol are removed.[1]

In 1992 and again most recently in 2008, the American Academy of Pediatrics (AAP) endorsed the findings and recommendations of the Expert Panel on Blood Cholesterol in Children and Adolescents of the National Cholesterol Education Program (NCEP).[2-4] The NCEP found that:

1. Certain inborn or acquired diseases accompanied by hypercholesterolemia are associated with premature atherosclerosis.
2. Serum cholesterol levels are higher than usual in people with coronary heart disease.
3. People with high serum cholesterol levels develop coronary heart disease more often and at a younger age than those with normal levels.

VI

4. The mortality rate from coronary heart disease in different countries varies in relation to the average blood cholesterol values (and with dietary fat and animal protein intake).

5. Experimentally induced hypercholesterolemia in animals is associated with atherosclerotic deposits.

6. Atherosclerotic plaques contain lipids similar in composition to those in the blood.

Evidence that atherosclerosis begins in childhood includes the following:

1. In autopsies of black and white males and females between 15 and 19 years old, the coronary arteries showed fatty streaks in 71% to 83% and raised atherosclerotic lesions in 7% to 22%.[5]

2. When bodies of US soldiers who died at a mean age of 22 years were examined, 77% of those from the Korean Conflict[6] and 45% of those from the Vietnam War[7] had evidence of coronary vessel atherosclerosis.

3. US adolescents who died of nonatherosclerotic causes show atherosclerotic changes of a magnitude directly related to postmortem LDL-cholesterol plus very low-density lipoprotein (VLDL)-cholesterol levels and inversely related to HDL-cholesterol levels.[8]

4. Clustering of risk factors results in increased atherosclerotic burden in adolescents and young adults.[9]

Lipoproteins

Lipoproteins are necessary to make fats soluble so they can be transported in the plasma. All lipoproteins contain an outer polar layer of phospholipid, unesterified cholesterol, and protein (called apoprotein). The inner, nonpolar core contains cholesterol ester and triglyceride in varying proportions. The types of lipoproteins are:

1. Chylomicrons, which are formed from dietary fat and enter the plasma via the thoracic duct. Chylomicrons are removed from the blood by the activity of lipoprotein lipase (LPL) with the fatty acids, stored in adipose tissue as triglyceride, or catabolized by the liver. They do not form other lipoproteins.

2. VLDLs (also called prelipoproteins), which are formed from dietary glucose and nonesterified fatty acids in the liver and are then secreted into the plasma. The outer surface of VLDLs contains apoproteins B-100 and E. The LPL on capillary endothelium of adipose tissue and cardiac and skeletal muscle partially metabolizes the VLDLs to nonesterified fatty acids for storage or for energy, leaving a remnant. The apoprotein E allows the remnant to be taken up by the

liver. Several types of hyperlipoproteinemia have been identified.[10]

3. LDL-cholesterol, which is formed in the liver from VLDL remnants containing apoprotein B-100; LDL-cholesterol is an important source of cholesterol for peripheral tissues. An important step in the regulation of cholesterol metabolism is the attachment of LDL-cholesterol to receptor sites on cell surfaces.

4. HDL-cholesterol, which is secreted by the liver and small intestine and is important in helping to remove cholesterol from cells (high levels are protective; low levels are a strong risk factor for coronary heart disease).

Types of Hyperlipidemia

The hereditary types of hyperlipidemias are sometimes difficult to distinguish from the hyperlipidemias related to diabetes and other conditions, but an attempt should be made to do so by family studies and other tests.[10,11]

Type I

Type I hyperlipoproteinemia is found in children and is usually associated with pancreatitis and abdominal pain. The triglycerides in this disorder are primarily chylomicron triglycerides. The activity of LPL-cholesterol is diminished or absent. This enzyme is responsible for hydrolysis and removal of chylomicrons from the blood. Thus, the pathophysiologic mechanism is decreased triglyceride catabolism. Type I hyperlipoproteinemia is relatively rare; it may occur secondarily in children with lupus erythematosus, pancreatitis, or immunologic disorders.

Type II-a

Type II-a hyperlipoproteinemia, which consists of elevation of the level of serum total cholesterol and LDL-cholesterol, is probably the most common of the 5 lipoprotein disorders to manifest in childhood. The homozygous form occurs in 1 in 1 million individuals and can be seen during the first year of life, and the differential diagnosis can be made on the basis of the following:

1. Serum cholesterol higher than 12.95 mmol/L (500 mg/dL)
2. Concentrations of LDL-cholesterol approximately twice that of heterozygotes in the same kindred
3. Both parents with elevated serum cholesterol levels
4. Xanthomas appearing before the age of 10 years
5. Vascular disease before the age of 20 years
6. Exclusion of clinically similar secondary hyperlipidemias

In the heterozygous condition, which occurs in 1 in 500 individuals, usually no skin xanthomas are present, and the serum cholesterol level is lower than 12.95 mmol/L (500 mg/dL); yet, these individuals have a definite predisposition to

VI

coronary heart disease during early adulthood. The basic metabolic defect is a lack of functional LDL receptors on the cell membrane, with 3 different classes of mutations.[12] As a result of the LDL not attaching to the cell membrane, cholesterol is not released to suppress the rate-limiting enzyme in cholesterol synthesis, hydroxymethylglutaryl-coenzyme A (CoA) reductase.

Type II-b

Type II-b hyperlipoproteinemia, which includes familial combined hyperlipidemia, consists of elevated triglyceride and total cholesterol levels, with concomitant increased LDL-cholesterol and VLDL-cholesterol. This is the third most frequent of the types with the onset during childhood, but the situation often is confusing, because the parents may have other types of hyperlipoproteinemia and because of the variations in the cholesterol and triglyceride levels caused by changes in diet and exercise.

Type III

Type III hyperlipoproteinemia, "floating beta," with the LDL having an abnormal density and consisting of an abnormal protein, is rare. The onset is usually after the age of 20 years. The basic defect is thought to be in the conversion of VLDL to LDL (abnormal remnant catabolism) because of an abnormal apoprotein E. Increased remnants, VLDL, chylomicrons, and apoprotein E are all present. Xanthomas may occur, and early coronary and peripheral vascular diseases have been reported.

Type IV

Type IV hyperlipoproteinemia, "familial hypertriglyceridemia," is associated with elevated levels of serum triglycerides and is the second most common of the disorders found in children, although the elevation in level of serum triglycerides may not occur in some patients until a later age. This condition is a monogenic autosomally inherited disorder. It involves an increase in production and secretion of triglyceride-rich VLDL.

Elevated triglyceride levels can occur in relation to other factors, such as infrequent exercise, stress, an inadequate period of fasting before obtaining blood samples, diabetes, and obesity. Establishing that the patient has the genetic disease and excluding another cause for the elevation is important. This is best accomplished by studying parents and other family members as well as the patient.

Type V

Type V hyperlipoproteinemia is rare in childhood and is associated with increased triglyceride levels related to increased chylomicrons and increased VLDL-cholesterol. This condition may be primarily hereditary or it may be secondary to diabetes, nephrotic syndrome, or hypothyroidism. The onset may be similar to that of type I, although it occurs in adulthood rather than childhood.

Prevention of Atherosclerosis and Prudent Lifestyle and Diet

In 1983, 1986, 1992, 1998, and 2008,[2,3,13,14] the AAP made recommendations about the risks of atherosclerosis and the avoidance of those risks. Of these, avoidance of smoking, increased physical activity, and treatment of hypertension and diabetes are emphasized. After 1 year of age, it was recommended that a varied diet be consumed to best ensure nutritional adequacy. Decreased consumption of saturated fats, cholesterol, and sodium (Appendix P) and increased intake of monounsaturated and polyunsaturated fats were recommended. No restriction of fat or cholesterol intake was recommended for infants younger than 2 years, because this is a period of rapid growth and neurologic development with high energy requirements. However, in the 2008 recommendations, the AAP noted that when there was a concern about obesity or a family history of cardiovascular disease, reduced-fat milk could be considered, starting at 12 months of age.[3] Early recognition and treatment of obesity and hypertension, a regular exercise program, and counseling about the dangers of smoking were recommended for all children older than 2 years. It is recommended that less than 10% of calories in the diet come from saturated fat. The optimal total fat intake was suggested to be approximately 30% of calories for children older than 2 years.

Some studies have shown safety in decreasing fat intakes in infants.[15] Approximately 50% of the calories in the diet of the exclusively breastfed infant comes from the fat content of the milk. As solids are introduced during the first and second years of life, the percentage of calories in the diet contributed by fat may decrease. At age 2 to 3 years, if only 30% of total calories are derived from fat, for some infants, the protein content would have to provide 15% or more of calories for the diet to meet the recommended dietary allowances for minerals. Early childhood, therefore, should be considered a transition period during which the fat and cholesterol content of the diet should gradually decrease to the recommended amounts. Particular care should be taken to avoid excessive intake of total calories, which may lead to obesity. Care should also be taken to avoid excessive restriction of calories and fat in the diet, which can result in failure to thrive. The consumption of lower-fat dairy products and lean meats; critical sources of protein, iron, and calcium; and grains, cereals, fruits, and vegetables should be encouraged in this transition period, starting at 1 year of age and throughout childhood and adolescence (see Appendix Q).

The NCEP Expert Panel on Blood Cholesterol Levels in Children and Adolescents and the AAP offer the following specific recommendations for the population older than 2 years[3,4]:

1. Nutritional adequacy should be achieved by eating a wide variety of foods.
2. Energy (calories) should be adequate to support growth and to reach or maintain desirable body weight and avoid obesity development.
3. The following intake pattern is recommended: saturated fatty acids, less than 10% of total energy intake (serum cholesterol appears most responsive to dietary saturated fatty acids); total fat, averaged over several days, no less than 20% of total calories and no more than 30% of calories; and dietary cholesterol, less than 300 mg/day.

Carbohydrate content of the diet should be 55% to 60% of the calories, of which the majority should be complex carbohydrates. Fiber is an important dietary constituent that can affect blood cholesterol levels. Current recommendations for fiber intake in children range from 0.5 g/kg to approximately 12 g/1000 kcal. Protein should provide 10% to 15% of dietary calories. This diet is similar to the diet recommended by the American Heart Association for moderate reduction of serum cholesterol levels. Similarly composed diets may also be useful in controlling obesity.

Screening for Hyperlipidemia

The AAP had endorsed an individualized approach to screening and treating children (older than 2 years) and adolescents whose risk of developing coronary vascular disease as adults can be identified through family history. However, it should be noted that screening on the basis of family history has been shown to miss many children with elevated total and LDL-cholesterol levels.[16] Many children with the most elevated LDL-cholesterol and the highest risk of early cardiovascular disease have a genetic dyslipidemia. Unfortunately, the family history is often unobtainable or incomplete. This has led to the recommendation for universal screening for children 9 to 11 years of age (before the pubertal changes in lipids and lipoproteins) by the National Heart Lung and Blood Institute and the National Lipid Association.[17,18] This approach is directed at the identification of children with heterozygous familial hypercholesterolemia, which occurs in 1 in 400 to 500 live births.

A nonfasting, non–HDL-cholesterol level should be used to evaluate a child's lipid status by 9 to 11 years of age and before the onset of puberty. This is determined by subtracting the HDL-cholesterol from the total cholesterol and has been found to be a useful risk indicator in adults and children.[17] If the non–HDL-cholesterol is ≥145 mg/dL, then a fasting lipid panel should be obtained. Fig 33.1 presents an algorithm for screening and initiating therapy.

Fig 33.1.

Classification, education, and follow-up based on LDL-cholesterol (LDL-C) from National Cholesterol Education Program [NCEP][4]). To convert mg/dL to mmol/L, multiply by 0.02586.

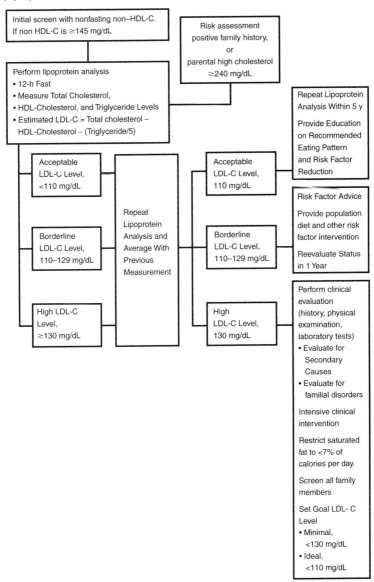

Initial screen with nonfasting non–HDL-C.
If non HDL-C is ≥145 mg/dL

Risk assessment
positive family history,
or
parental high cholesterol
≥240 mg/dL

Perform lipoprotein analysis
• 12-h Fast
• Measure Total Cholesterol,
• HDL-Cholesterol, and Triglyceride Levels
• Estimated LDL-C = Total cholesterol –
  HDL-Cholesterol – (Triglyceride/5)

Acceptable
LDL-C Level,
<110 mg/dL

Repeat
Lipoprotein
Analysis and
Average With
Previous
Measurement

Acceptable
LDL-C Level,
110 mg/dL

Borderline
LDL-C Level,
110–129 mg/dL

Borderline
LDL-C Level,
110–129 mg/dL

High LDL-C
Level,
≥130 mg/dL

High
LDL-C Level,
130 mg/dL

Repeat Lipoprotein
Analysis Within 5 y

Provide Education
on Recommended
Eating Pattern
and Risk Factor
Reduction

Risk Factor Advice

Provide population
diet and other risk
factor intervention

Reevaluate Status
in 1 Year

Perform clinical
evaluation
(history, physical
examination,
laboratory tests)
• Evaluate for
  Secondary
  Causes
• Evaluate for
  familial disorders

Intensive clinical
intervention

Restrict saturated
fat to <7% of
calories per day.

Screen all family
members

Set Goal LDL- C
Level
• Minimal,
  <130 mg/dL
• Ideal,
  <110 mg/dL

VI

In a fasting lipid profile, levels of total cholesterol, HDL-cholesterol, and triglycerides are determined; the LDL-cholesterol level is estimated from these. In some laboratories, LDL-cholesterol can be measured directly. Non–HDL-cholesterol can be a useful screening measurement. It can be measured without the patient fasting and is calculated by subtracting the HDL-cholesterol from the total cholesterol. Interpretations are given in Table 33.1 for children and adolescents. Appropriate examinations or tests for secondary causes of hypercholesterolemia should be performed (Table 33.2) before treatment.

Table 33.1.
Interpretation of Cholesterol Levels for Children and Adolescents[a]

Term	Total Cholesterol, mg/dL	LDL Cholesterol, mg/dL	HDL Cholesterol, mg/dL	Non–HDL-Cholesterol, mg/dL	Triglycerides, mg/dL
Acceptable	<170	<110	>45	<120	<90
Borderline	170–199	110–129	40–44	120–144	90–129
High	>200	>130	(Low) <40	≥145	≥130

[a] From National Cholesterol Education Program (NCFP).[4] To convert g/dL to mmol/L, multiply by 0.02586.

Table 33.2.
Causes of Secondary Hypercholesterolemia

Exogenous Drugs Oral contraceptives, corticosteroids, isotretinoin (Accutane), thiazides, anticonvulsants, beta-blockers, anabolic steroids Alcohol Obesity	**Storage Diseases** Glycogen storage diseases Sphingolipidoses **Obstructive Liver Diseases** Biliary atresia Biliary cirrhosis
Endocrine and Metabolic Hypothyroidism Diabetes mellitus Lipodystrophy Pregnancy Idiopathic hypercalcemia	**Chronic Renal Diseases** Nephrotic syndrome **Others** Anorexia nervosa Progeria Collagen vascular disease Klinefelter syndrome

Treatment

Therapy should be initiated after the diagnosis of hyperlipidemia is confirmed by 2 separate blood tests performed at least 2 weeks apart. Dietary therapy is the first mode of treatment in almost all instances, whether or not elevations are attributable to a genetic cause. A 3-day diet record is extremely helpful for suggesting changes; this record should be as typical as possible of the child's usual intake, including both weekdays and weekend days. Consultation with a dietitian or nutritionist is very helpful.

The population diet (Table 33.3) suggests an average intake of saturated fatty acids less than 10% of total calories, total fat 20% to 30% of calories, and cholesterol less than 300 mg/day. The polyunsaturated fatty acids constitute up to 10% and the monounsaturated fatty acids 10% to 15% of the total calories. The 2010 Dietary Guidelines for Americans can be a useful guide to a healthful diet for children and adolescents.[19]

Table 33.3.
Serving Sizes in Food Groups

Bread, Cereal, Rice, and Pasta Group (Grains Group)—Whole Grain and Refined
• 1 slice bread • About 1 cup of ready-to-eat cereal • 1 cup of cooked cereal, rice, or pasta
Vegetable Group
• 1 cup raw, leafy vegetables • 1/2 cup of other vegetables—cooked or raw • 1 cup vegetable juice
Fruit Group
• 1 medium apple, banana, orange, pear • 1 cup chopped, cooked, or canned fruit • 1 cup fruit juice
Milk, Yogurt, and Cheese Group (Milk Group)
• 2 cups fat free milk or yogurt • 1 oz of natural cheese (such as cheddar) • 2 oz of processed cheese (such as American)
Meat, Poultry, Fish, Dry Beans, Eggs, and Nuts Group (Meat and Beans Group)
• 2–3 oz of cooked lean meat, poultry, or fish • 1/2 cup of cooked dry beans or 1/2 cup of tofu counts as 1 oz of lean meat • 2 oz of soy burger or 1 egg counts as 1 oz of lean meat • 2 tbsp of peanut butter or 1/3 cup of nuts counts as 1 oz of meat

Table 33.4.
Diets for Control of Cholesterol

Nutrient	Recommended Intake	
	Population Diet	**More Restrictive Diet**
Total fat	Average of no more than 30% of total calories and no less than 20%	Same as step I diet
Saturated fatty acids	Less than 10% of total calories	Less than 7% of total calories
Polyunsaturated fatty acids	Up to 10% of total calories	Same as step I diet
Monounsaturated fatty acids	Remaining dietary fat calories	Same as step I diet
Cholesterol	Less than 300 mg/day	Less than 200 mg/day
Carbohydrates	About 55% of total calories	Same as step I diet
Protein	About 15% of total calories	Same as step I diet
Calories	To promote growth and development	Same as step I diet

Adapted from National Cholesterol Education Program (NCEP) and AAP Committee on Nutrition.[3,4]

Avoidance of smoking, the value of exercise, attaining weight appropriate for age and body build, and correction of or treatments for other risk factors are also emphasized. If, after 3 months of diet intervention, desired lipid levels are not achieved, a more restrictive diet is initiated. Intake of saturated fatty acids is reduced to approximately 7% of the caloric intake and intake of cholesterol is reduced to less than 200 mg/day. Dietary fat must be even further restricted in patients with type I hyperlipoproteinemia to achieve lower plasma triglyceride concentrations.

The NCEP Panel for Children and Adolescents and the AAP recommend that after an adequate trial of diet therapy has been completed (6 months to 1 year), drug therapy should be considered in children 10 years or older under the following conditions:

1. If LDL cholesterol remains greater than 4.9 mmol/L (190 mg/dL); or
2. If LDL cholesterol remains greater than 4.1 mmol/L (160 mg/dL) *and* there is a positive family history of cardiovascular disease before age 55 years; *or* 2 or more other risk factors for cardiovascular disease are present.

The optimal goal of drug therapy is to achieve an LDL-cholesterol level to approach 2.85 mmol/L (110 mg/dL). In some circumstances, however, a target of 130 mg/dL for LDL-cholesterol may be appropriate. Drugs recommended for children and adolescents include the bile acid sequestrants. Bile acid sequestrants have been shown to be safe and effective.[20] However, these drugs are often difficult for adolescents to take, which may result in low adherence.[21] Hydroxymethylglutaryl-CoA reductase inhibitors (statins) are also recommended for use in children and adolescents, because clinical trials of these agents in children have now been completed. Several short-term studies of the use of hydroxymethylglutaryl-CoA reductase inhibitors in adolescents have shown their efficacy, acceptability, and safety.[21-26] However, because the long-term effects of these drugs have not been tested, careful monitoring of liver function and the assessment of the presence of myositis should be performed throughout childhood and adolescence. Myositis is a rare complication of statin use in adolescents, but it is quite important to monitor, because it may progress to rhabdomyolysis, which can result in fatality. In addition, ezetimibe, which blocks cholesterol absorption in the gastrointestinal tract, can also be used in children and adolescents.[20] However, ezetimibe has not been extensively studied in pediatric patients and is not approved by the Food and Drug Administration for pediatric patients. Niacin is not generally recommended for use in children because of adverse effects, including flushing.

Table 33.5.

Number of Servings From Each of the Food Groups That Should Be Taken for the Step I Diet*

FOOD GROUPS	Children 2 to 6 y, Women, Some Older Adults (About 1600 kcal)	Older Children, Teen Girls, Active Women, Most Men (About 2200 kcal)	Teen Boys, Active Men (About 2800 kcal)
Bread, cereal, rice, and pasta group (grains group)—especially whole grain	6	9	11
Vegetable group	3	4	5
Fruit group	2 or 3	2 or 3	2 or 3
Meat, poultry, fish, dry beans, eggs, and nut groups, (meat and beans group—preferably lean or low fat)	2, for a total of 5 oz	2, for a total of 6 oz	3, for a total of 7 oz

* Based on Dietary Guidelines for Americans 2010. US Department of Agriculture, US Department of Health and Human Services. Available at: http://health.gov/dietaryguidelines/

VI

References

1. Kannel WB, Castelli WP, Gordon T. Cholesterol in the prediction of atherosclerotic disease. New perspectives based on the Framingham study. *Ann Intern Med.* 1979;90(1):85–91

2. American Academy of Pediatrics, Committee on Nutrition. Statement on cholesterol. *Pediatrics.* 1992;90(3):469–473

3. Daniels SR, Greer FR; American Academy of Pediatrics, Committee on Nutrition. Lipid screening and cardiovascular health in childhood. *Pediatrics.* 2008;122(1):198-208

4. National Cholesterol Education Program (NCEP): highlights of the report of the Expert Panel on Blood Cholesterol Levels in Children and Adolescents. *Pediatrics.* 1992;89(3):495–501

5. Strong JP, McGill HC Jr. The pediatric aspects of atherosclerosis. *J Atherosclerosis Res.* 1969;9(3):251–265

6. Enos WF Jr, Beyer JC, Holmes RH. Pathogenesis of coronary disease in American soldiers killed in Korea. *JAMA.* 1955;158(11):912–914

7. McNamara JJ, Molot MA, Stremple JF, Cutting RT. Coronary artery disease in combat casualties in Vietnam. *JAMA.* 1971;216(7):1185–1187

8. Strong JP, Malcom GT, McMahan CA, et al. Prevalence and extent of atherosclerosis in adolescents and young adults: implications for prevention from the Pathobiological Determinants of Atherosclerosis in Youth Study. *JAMA.* 1999;281(8):727–735

9. Berenson GS, Srinivasan SR, Bao W, Newman WP 3rd, Tracy RE, Wattigney WA. Association between multiple cardiovascular risk factors and atherosclerosis in children and young adults. The Bogalusa Heart Study. *N Engl J Med.* 1998;338(23):1650-1656

10. Fredrickson DS, Goldstein JL, Brown MS. The familial hyperlipoproteinemias. In: Stanbury JB, Wyngaarden JB, Fredrickson DS, eds. *The Metabolic Basis of Inherited Disease.* 4th ed. New York, NY: McGraw-Hill Book Co; 1978:604–655

11. Havel RJ, Kane JP. Introduction: structure and metabolism of plasma lipoproteins. In: Scriver CR, Beaudet AL, Sly WS, Valle D, eds. *The Metabolic Basis of Inherited Disease.* Vol 1. 6th ed. New York, NY: McGraw-Hill Book Co; 1989:1129–1138

12. Goldstein JL, Brown MS. The LDL receptor defect in familial hypercholesterolemia. Implications for pathogenesis and therapy. *Med Clin North Am.* 1982;66(2):335–362

13. American Academy of Pediatrics, Committee on Nutrition. Toward a prudent diet for children. *Pediatrics.* 1983;71:78–80

14. American Academy of Pediatrics, Committee on Nutrition. Prudent life-style for children: dietary fat and cholesterol. *Pediatrics.* 1986;78:521–525

15. Simell O, Niinikoski H, Viikari J, Rask-Nissila L, Tammi A, Ronnemaa T. Cardiovascular disease risk factors in young children in the STRIP baby project. *Ann Med.* 1999;31(Suppl 1):55–61

16. Ritchie SK, Murphy ECS, Ice C, Cottrell LA, Minor V, Elliott E, Neal W. Universal versus targeted blood cholesterol screening among youth: the CARDIAC Project. *Pediatrics.* 2010;126(2):260-265

17. National Heart, Lung, and Blood Institute Expert Panel. Integrated guidelines for cardiovascular health and risk reduction in children and adolescents. *Pediatrics.* 2011;128(Suppl 5):S213-S256

18. Daniels SR, Gidding SS, de Ferranti SD. Pediatric aspects of familial hypercholesterolemias: recommendations from the National Lipid Association Expert Panel on Familial Hypercholesterolemia. *J Clin Lipidol.* 2011;5(3 Suppl):S30-S37

19. US Department of Agriculture, US Department of Health and Human Services. *Dietary Guidelines for Americans, 2012.* 7th ed. Washington, DC: US Government Printing Office; December 2010

20. Stein EA, Marais AD, Szamosi T, et al. Colesevelam hydrochloride: efficacy and safety in pediatric subjects with heterozygous familial hypercholesterolemia. *J Pediatr.* 2010;156(2):231-236.e1-e3

21. McCrindle BW, Urbina EM, Dennison BA, et al; American Heart Association, Atherosclerosis, Hypertension, and Obesity in Youth Committee; American Heart Association, Council of Cardiovascular Disease in the Young, Council on Cardiovascular Nursing. *Circulation.* 2007;115(14):1948-1967

22. Stein EA, Illingworth DR, Kwiterovich PO Jr, et al. Efficacy and safety of lovastatin in adolescent males with heterozygous familial hypercholesterolemia: a randomized controlled trial. *JAMA.* 1999;281(2):137–144

23. McCrindle BW, Ose L, Marais AD. Efficacy and safety of atorvastatin in children and adolescents with familial hypercholesterolemia or severe hyperlipidemia: a multicenter, randomized, placebo-controlled trial. *J Pediatr.* 2003;143(1):74-80

24. deJongh S, Ose L, Szamosi T, et al; Simvastatin in Children Study Group. Department of Vascular Medicine, Emma Children's Hospital, Academic Medical Center, University of Amsterdam, Amsterdam, The Netherlands. Efficacy and safety of statin therapy in children with familial hypercholesterolemia: a randomized, double-blind, placebo-controlled trial with simvastatin. *Circulation.* 2002;106(17):2231-2237

25. McCrindle BW, Ose L, Marais AD. Efficacy and safety of atorvastatin in children and adolescents with familial hypercholesterolemia or severe hyperlipidemia: a multicenter, randomized, placebo-controlled trial. *J Pediatr.* 2003;143(1):74-80

26. Wiegman A, Hutten BA, de Groot E, et al. Efficacy and safety of statin therapy in children with familial hypercholesterolemia: a randomized controlled trial. *JAMA.* 2004;292(3):331-337

VI

Chapter 34

Pediatric Obesity

Introduction

Pediatric obesity has been on the rise since 1963, peaking in 2007 and 2008. In 2007-2008, 16.9% of children from 2 to 19 years of age had body mass index (BMI) greater than the 97th percentile, and 9.5% of infants and toddlers were at or above the 95th percentile for weight for length. The prevalence of obesity did not change in 2009-2010.[1] Given the burden of pediatric obesity on child health as well as associated health care costs, it has been recognized as an urgent public health priority.[2,3] Understanding the pathophysiology of obesity is important to appreciate the complexity of the dysregulation of energy balance, the mechanisms driving hunger and satiety, and the gene-environment interaction (epigenetic) driving the epidemic. It is also important to understand the role of excess adiposity, ectopic fat, and adipocyte dysfunction in the development of obesity-related comorbidities. Obesity prevention is aimed at optimizing energy balance to support healthy growth and development without accumulation of excess adipose tissue. Once energy balance is altered toward fat accumulation, treatment is directed at identifying and reversing factors that contribute to energy excess and optimizing factors that contribute to energy expenditure. An awareness of the complexity of the dysregulation of energy balance is crucial to devising prevention and treatment strategies. It is also important in understanding why the results of treatment remain modest and why prevention of pediatric obesity is of primary importance.

Adipose Tissue: An Organ

Obesity may be defined functionally as a maladaptive increase in adipose tissue. Adipose tissue is the major organ system involved in energy regulation and accounts for up to 25% of body weight in a person of normal weight.[4] White adipose tissue is also an important secretory organ that has roles in immune response, blood pressure control, hemostasis, bone mass, and thyroid and reproductive functions through synthesis of secreted hormones called adipokines.[5] It also functions as an insulating and structural element in the body. Excess accumulation of white adipose tissue results in obesity, and products of the increased visceral storage depot drain directly into the portal system, exacerbating obesity-related metabolic comorbidities. In addition to increased adiposity, when children become obese, ectopic fat deposition occurs, with accumulation of triglycerides within nonadipose tissue, such as the liver, muscles, pancreas, and heart. This compromises organ structure and function.[6] Both brown and white adipocytes are derived from fibroblasts. Brown adipose tissue is found only in mammals, and its primary function is to produce heat by nonshivering thermogenesis.[7] White adipose tissue is made up of both adipocytes (25%-60%) and nonadipocytes, including fibroblastic preadipocytes, endothelial cells, mast cells, and macrophages.[8] Adipocytes are key regulators of energy balance. Other factors important for energy balance are genetics, physical activity, nutrition, and environmental and behavior influences. Environmental and behavior influences include the state of overall health, medication use, composition of intestinal microflora,[9] and psychological/emotional factors that influence food intake and energy expenditure. All of these factors are operative in the overall energy balance equation.[10]

Pathophysiology

Energy Balance

The accumulation of stored energy (fat) is caused by intake in excess of energy expenditure. A small excess of energy intake relative to expenditure will, over time, lead to a gradual but substantial increase in body weight. For example, an individual increasing daily energy intake by 150 kcal above daily energy expenditure would consume an excess of 55 000 kcal per year and could gain approximately 15 pounds per year. Despite the potentially large effects of small imbalances in energy intake versus expenditure, complex integrated control mechanisms ensure that adults maintain a relatively constant body weight, and most children tend to grow steadily along individualized weight percentiles for age, with little conscious effort to regulate energy intake or expenditure.[11] In addition, the high rate of recidivism to previous levels of adiposity after a period of weight loss in obese children and adults and the tendency for individuals to maintain a relatively stable body weight over long periods of time despite wide variations in caloric intake, provide empirical evidence that body weight is regulated and that energy intake and expenditure are not independent processes but are regulated by complex interlocking control mechanisms.[12] However, data generated from studies of energy homeostasis in adults must be applied cautiously to children. Unlike adults, children accrue both fat mass and fat-free mass as they grow, and the magnitude and composition of this weight gain is more age and gender dependent. A simplified overview of this complex system controlling energy balance is shown in Fig 34.1, illustrating the interaction of the hypothalamus, brainstem, gut hormones, and adipose tissue that regulate body weight and energy intake and expenditure. Input to the hypothalamus from energy stores and hunger signals are integrated with efferent output regarding feeding behavior, satiety, insulin secretion, and autonomic regulation of adipocytokines, including leptin secreted by adipose tissue. These molecules directly or indirectly affect the hypothalamus, from which outflow tracts affect energy expenditure.

Fig 34.1.
Overweight trends in children and adolescents. Reproduced with permission from Suzuki K, Jayasena CN, Bloom SR. The gut hormones in appetite regulation. *J Obes.* 2011;2011:528401. Epub 2011 Sep 22.

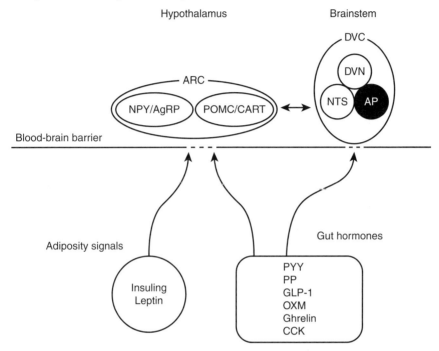

Diagram summarizing the major signaling pathways that converge on the hypothalamus and brainstem to regulate food intake. ARC, arcuate nucleus; NPY/AgRP, neuropeptide Y and agouti-related peptide; POMC/CART, proopiomelanocortin and cocaine- and amphetamine-regulated transcript; DVC, dorsal vagal complex; DVN, the dorsal motor nucleus of vagus; NTS, the nucleus of the tractus solitarius; AP, area postrema; GLP-1, glucagon-like peptide-1; CCK, cholecystokinin; PP, pancreatic polypeptide; PYY, peptide YY; OXM, oxyntomodulin. Reprinted with permission from Suzuki K, Jayasena CN, Bloom SR. The gut hormones in appetite regulation. *J Obes.* 2011;2011:528401. Epub 2011 Sep 22.

Hypothalamus and Energy Homeostasis

Within the hypothalamus, the arcuate nucleus (ARC) responds to signals regarding energy stores from the gut, adipose tissue, pancreas, and other parts of the nervous system by increasing or decreasing the expression of the potent orexigens and anorexigens (Fig 34.1). Orexigenic peptides that increase food intake and decrease energy expenditure include neuropeptide Y (NPY) and agouti-related peptide (AGRP). Anorexigenic peptides that decrease food intake and reduce body weight include pro-opiomelanocortin (POMC) and cocaine- and amphetamine-related transcript (CART).[13,14] Gut hormones, such as cholecystokinin (CCK), ghrelin, and

VI

peptide YY (PYY), and vagal nerve signals also input information at the hypothalamic level to regulate hunger and satiety.[14] The ARC interacts with the brainstem via the dorsal vagus complex (DVC) that includes the dorsal vagal motor nucleus (DVN [receives signals from visceral organs via the vasovagal reflex]), the nucleus tractus solitarius (NTS [taste, afferent signals from visceral organs]), and the area postrema (AP), which is outside the blood-brain barrier and receives physiologic signals from molecules/hormones in the blood (controls nausea and vomiting; Fig 34.1).

In addition, central alpha-adrenergic stimulation results in increased food intake and decreased energy expenditure (orexiant effect), whereas beta-adrenergic and dopaminergic stimulation have anorexiant effects and increase energy expenditure. Peripheral alpha-adrenergic stimulation inhibits lipolysis, whereas peripheral beta-adrenergic stimulation is lipolytic.[15,16]

Leptin is secreted from adipose tissue and provides a signal linking fat mass to food intake and energy expenditure (Fig 34.2). Leptin binds to cells in the ARC of the hypothalamus to effect the expression of POMC,[17] producing alpha-, beta-, and gamma-melanocyte–stimulating hormones. These peptides signal target neurons in the lateral hypothalamus that express the melanocortin receptors MC3R and MC4R, which results in a decrease in food intake and increase in energy expenditure.[18] Insulin inhibits release of free fatty acids from adipocytes. In obesity, adipose tissue becomes resistant to insulin, and release of free fatty acids (FFAs) increases. This increase in FFAs is associated with the development of insulin resistance in peripheral muscle and liver.[19]

Gut peptides (Fig 34.1 and 34.2) play an important role in both long- and short-term energy regulation.[20,21] Peptide YY (PYY) is produced in the distal gut and increases for several hours after a meal to reduce appetite.[22] Pancreatic polypeptide (PP) is increased after a meal secondary to vagal stimulation and release of cholecystokinin (CCK) and reduces food intake.[23] Glucagon-like peptide 1 (GLP-1) is produced in the ileum in response to ingested carbohydrates and fat. It stimulates the islet cells in the pancreas to secrete insulin and has been shown to reduce appetite and body weight.[24] Oxyntomodulin (OXM) has been shown to reduce food intake and body weight[25] and to improve glucose homeostasis. OXM increases after gastric bypass surgery.[26] OXM is secreted postprandially by the gut endocrine cells (L-cells) in the small intestine together with GLP-1 and PYY. Ghrelin is a peptide produced by the gastric mucosal X/A-like cells of the gastric fundus.[27] Ghrelin stimulates NPY and AGRP in the ARC, causing increased food intake and reduced energy expenditure, and is suppressed by eating (Fig 34.1).[28,29] There is some evidence that anticipating a meal can enhance ghrelin suppression after a meal, indicating a possible cognitive link in peptide secretion.[30] CCK is released in the blood as a result of the presence of fat or protein in the duodenum and suppresses appetite by delaying gastric emptying.[31]

Fig 34.2.
The role of the hypothalamus in systems regulating energy homeostatis. Adapted with permission from Korner J, Aronne LJ. The emerging science of body weight regulation and its impact on obesity treatment. *J Clin Invest.* 2003;111(5):565-570

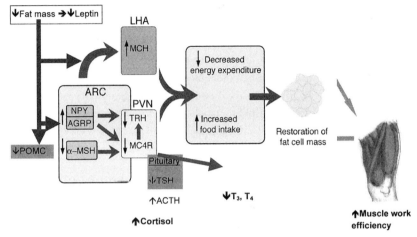

LHA indicates lateral hypothalamus area; MCH, melanin-concentrating hormone; POMC, proopiomelanocortin; ARC, arcuate nucleus; NPY, neuropeptide Y; AGRP, agouti-related peptide; α-MSH, alpha melanocyte-stimulating hormone; PVN, paraventricularis nucleus; TRH, thyrotropin-releasing hormone; MC4R, melanocortin-4 receptor; TSH, thyroid-stimulating hormone; T3, triiodothyronine; T4, thyroxine. Schematic of model of effects of weight loss on hypothalamic neuropeptides, neuroendocrine function, autonomic function, and energy homeostasis. Decreased leptin leads to decreased POMC, increased NPY, and increased MCH. Decreased POMC leads to decreased α-MSH, decreasing pro-TRH release with resultant declines in pituitary TSH release and circulating concentration of thyroid hormones, and β-EP, disinhibiting CRF release and increasing pituitary ACTH and adrenal cortisol production. CRF has also been shown to have an anorexiant effect when administered directly into the hypothalamus. Increased NPY and AGRP expression and decreased α-MSH lead to decreased activation of melanocortin receptors. Increased MCH inhibits SNS outflow and sensitivity. The net result of these leptin-mediated actions in the hypothalamus are decreased sympathetic nervous system tone and hypothalamus-pituitary-thyroid axis activation, increased hypothalamus-pituitary-adrenal axis activation, decreased energy expenditure, and increased hunger.

Adapted with permission from Korner J, Aronne LJ. The emerging science of body weight regulation and its impact on obesity treatment. *J Clin Invest.* 2003;111(5):565-570

There is also an emerging link between gut microbiota and obesity, and some of the proposed mechanisms for this include increased energy production from dietary constituents, modification in gut PYY and glucagon-like peptide secretion, and alteration of intestinal barrier permeability.[32]

Role of Inflammation
Adipocytes produce inflammatory cytokines and acute-phase proteins, and obesity can be considered a low-grade inflammatory state.[33] Macrophages migrate into

adipose tissue, and tumor necrosis factor-alpha secreted by adipocytes stimulates the production of monocyte chemoattractant protein.[34] Inflammatory factors have been found in children with obesity as young as 3 years of age.[35]

Lifestyle intervention has shown reductions in low-grade inflammation and macrophage infiltration in adipose tissue and in reduction of inflammatory cytokines.[36,37] Increased inflammatory cytokine production and inflammation occur in nonalcoholic fatty liver disease and nonalcoholic steatohepatitis[38] and in skeletal muscle in obesity.[39] Proinflammatory cytokines are produced in the hypothalamus in animals fed diets high in calories and dietary fat, causing resistance to both insulin and leptin.[40] In addition, adipokines produced by the adipocytes play a role in regulation of blood pressure, lipid metabolism, hemostasis, appetite and energy balance, immunity, insulin sensitivity, and angiogenesis.[41]

Genetics

Genetic differences in predisposition to obesity or excess fat storage clearly exist. In a study of monozygotic twins with regulated physical activity and overfed by precise amounts, differences in body weight, body composition, and body fat variation were threefold greater *between* twin pairs than *among* twin pairs, indicating that components of energy balance are under strong genetic influence.[42]

Body weight is a polygenic trait and is highly heritable, with estimates of genetic contribution to BMI ranging from 64% to 84% and to body fatness and fat distribution ranging from 30% to 70%.[43] However, lifestyle factors, such as diet, physical activity, stress, and sleep cycles may modify DNA expression through DNA methylation and histone acetylation (epigenetic changes). These changes, once made, are lifelong and heritable, and this has important implications for prevention of obesity through early intervention.[44]

Recent studies have also identified significant genetic influences on resting metabolic rate, feeding behavior, food preferences, and changes in energy expenditure that occur in response to overfeeding.[45] The *FTO* gene mutations are associated with increased total and fat dietary intake[46,47] as well as with diminished satiety and/or increased feeling of hunger in children.[48] The *FTO* gene is located on chromosome 16 and codes for the obesity-associated protein. *MC4R* gene mutations (see Fig 34.2) in children are also associated with increased feeling of hunger, increased snacking, decreased satiety, and increased total energy, fat, and protein intakes and are the most common single gene mutation associated with obesity in childhood, although this accounts for only small percentage of individuals with a BMI >35.[49-51]

The monogenic forms of obesity illustrate the pivotal role of genetics in the control of body weight and are listed in Table 34.1.[52,53] These syndromes with obesity must be differentiated from the more common polygenic form of obesity.

Table 34.1

Human Single Gene Mutations[a] Associated With Obesity

Syndrome	Chromosome	Phenotype
Prader-Willi	15q11–q13 (uniparental maternal disomy)	Short stature, small hands and feet, mental retardation, neonatal hypotonia, failure to thrive, cryptorchidism, almond-shaped eyes, and fi sh-like mouth.
Alström	2p13 (autosomal recessive)	Childhood blindness attributable to retinal degeneration, nerve deafness, acanthosis nigricans, chronic nephropathy, primary hypogonadism in males only, type 2 diabetes mellitus, infantile obesity that may diminish in adulthood. This gene has been cloned.
Bardet-Biedl	11q13,16q21, 3p12–13, 15q22–23, 2q31, 20p12, 4q27 (2 mutations), 14q32	At least 8 different forms of varying severity. Most common phenotypes are retinitis pigmentosa, mental retardation, polydactyly, hypothalamic hypogonadism, rarely glucose intolerance, deafness, and cystic renal disease. Known genes are in pathway(s) affecting ciliary motor function.
Borjeson-Forssman-Lehmann	Xq26 (X-linked dominant)	Truncal obesity, mental retardation, coarse facies, microcephaly, short stature, gynecomastia. Infants show poor feeding, hypotonia, failure to thrive, large ears, and hypogonadism. Females may be asymptomatic because of selective lyonization of carrier X-chromosome.
Carpenter	unknown (autosomal recessive)	Acrocephaly, syndactyly, polydactyly, congenital heart disease, mental retardation, hypogonadism (males only), obesity, umbilical hernia, and bony abnormalities.
Cohen	8q22–q23 (autosomal recessive)	Mental retardation, microcephaly, short stature, dysmorphic facies.
Prohormone convertase	5q15–q21 (autosomal recessive)	Abnormal glucose homeostasis, hypogonadotropic hypogonadism, hypocortisolism, and elevated plasma proinsulin.
Beckwith-Wiedemann	11p15.5 (autosomal recessive)	Hyperinsulinism, hypoglycemia, neonatal hemihypertrophy, intolerance of fasting.
Nesidioblastosis	11p15.1 (autosomal recessive or dominant)	Hyperinsulinism, hypoglycemia, intolerance of fasting This gene has been cloned.
Pseudohypo-parathyroidism (type IA)	20q13.2 (autosomal recessive)	Mental retardation, short stature, short metacarpals and metatarsals, short thick neck, round facies, subcutaneous calcifi cations, increased frequency of other endocrinopathies (hypothyroidism, hypogonadism).

(continued)

VI

Leptin	7q31.3 (autosomal recessive)	Hypometabolic rate, hyperphagia, pubertal delay, infertility, impaired glucose tolerance attributable to leptin defi ciency.
Leptin receptor	1p31–p32 (autosomal recessive)	Hypometabolic rate, hyperphagia, pubertal delay attributable to deranged leptin signal transduction.
POMC	2p23.3 (autosomal recessive)	Red hair, hyperphagia, adrenal insuffi ciency attributable to impaired POMC production in individuals unable to make POMC.
Melanocortin-4 receptor defects	multiple autosomal recessive and dominant mutations	Obesity, tall stature, increased bone density, eating disorders

[a] The primary physiological sites of the derangements in some of the human mutations can be seen in Fig. 34.2.

Assessment

Although direct assessment of adiposity can be accomplished using hydrodensitometry (underwater weighing), air displacement plethysmography, or dual-energy x-ray absorptiometry, these are primarily research tools. In clinical practice, BMI (weight [kg]/[height {m^2}]) is used as a surrogate measure of adiposity that correlates well with direct measures of body fatness within a population.[54,55] Current definitions of overweight and obesity are based on population norms from the National Health and Nutrition Examination Survey I (NHANES I), which were determined before the current obesity epidemic began. Children between 2 and 18 years of age with a BMI between the 85th and 95th percentile for age and gender based on NHANES I (1971-1974) data are categorized as "overweight." Children 2 to 18 years of age with a BMI greater than the 95th percentile or BMI >30 kg/m^2 (whichever is smaller) are categorized as "obese."[56]

For children from birth to 2 years of age, the weight-for-recumbent length percentiles are appropriate for evaluating weight relative to linear growth, but the term obese generally should not be applied to children this young. Weight-for-length greater than the 95th percentile is termed overweight.[56] The Centers for Disease Control and Prevention (CDC) and American Academy of Pediatrics (AAP) recommend using the World Health Organization (WHO) growth charts released in 2006 for weight, length, and weight for length for children younger than 2 years.[57] The WHO growth charts for 0 to 2 years of age also include BMI charts, but these are not recommended for routine use at this time (see Chapter 25: Nutritional Assessment, and Appendix A).

BMI may be calculated directly as kg/m^2 or, if measured in pounds and inches, calculated [weight (in pounds)/[height (in inches)]2] × 703. BMI calculators are available at http://apps.nccd.cdc.gov/dnpabmi/. BMI percentile may be found by plotting BMI for age on the BMI graph[58] (see Appendix A).

Although the use of WHO or CDC growth charts are recommended for all children, there is some evidence to suggest that differences in body composition by race and ethnicity exist. Adipose tissue has its own growth curve, and calculations based on skinfold measurements illustrate the gender dimorphism in adiposity. Boys and girls have similar growth patterns until 9 years of age, with percentage of body fat peaking for boys at 11 years of age but continuing to increase for girls throughout adolescence. Median percentage of body fat at 18 years of age for boys is 17.0% and for girls is 27.8%.[59]

African-American children have somewhat less fat, and Hispanic and Southeast Asian children have a higher percentage of body fat than do white children at the same BMI.[60-65] It should also be noted that body fat distribution at any given level of body fatness may constitute an independent risk factor for adiposity-related morbidity.[66,67]

Measurement of skinfold thickness has been a standard method of nutritional assessment. Skinfold measurements correlate with total body fat lipid levels, blood pressure, plasma glucose and insulin levels as well as insulin resistance, and indicators of inflammation.[68-71] However, because it is difficult to produce reliable and reproducible measurements and there are no reference standards or criteria for treatment, the AAP does not recommend measurement of skinfold thicknesses for routine clinical use.[56]

Measurements of waist circumference provide a better estimate of visceral adiposity in children than does BMI.[56] Waist circumference can also predict insulin resistance, blood pressure, and lipid levels[72-75] but may be no better than BMI measurements for this purpose.[76] The AAP currently does not recommend routine used of waist circumference in the office setting until more clinical experience with its use is available.[56]

Epidemiology of Pediatric Obesity

The rising trend in pediatric obesity from 1963 to 2008 is shown in Fig 34.3. In 2007-2008, 31.7% of children 2 to 19 years of age were above the 85th percentile for BMI (classified as overweight), 16.9% were above the 95th percentile (classified as obese), and 11.9% were above the 97th percentile.[77] This high prevalence of obesity is also seen at very young ages, as 9.5% of infants and toddlers were at or above the 95th percentile for weight for length.[77] The newest data from 2009-2010 reveal that the prevalence of obesity in children and adolescents was 16.9%—unchanged from 2007-2008.[1] The prevalence of childhood overweight and obesity mirrors that of adult obesity and is highest in the southeastern region of the United States (Fig 34.4). However, within states, individual counties have dramatically different obesity prevalences, highlighting the importance of community environments (Fig 34.5).

VI

Fig 34.3.
Trends in childhood obesity, 1963-2008

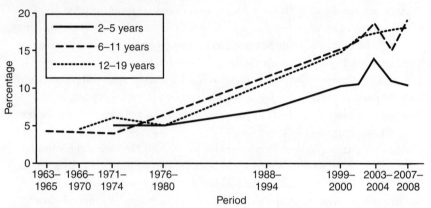

Centers for Disease Control and Prevention. CDC Grand Rounds: childhood obesity in the United States. *MMWR Morb Mortal Wkly Rep.* 2011;60(2):42-46

Fig 34.4.
2007 rates of overweight and obese children

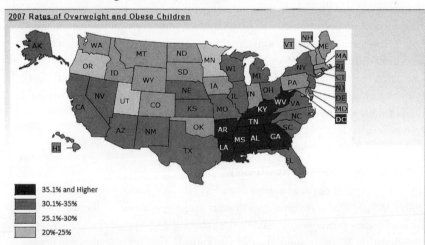

* Obesity is defined as body mass index (BMI) at or above the 95th percentile of the 2000 Centers for Disease Control and Prevention BMI-for-age growth charts. Children with BMI between the 85th and 95th percentile are classified as overweight. BMI is calculated as weight in kilograms divided by the square of height in meters. Children age 10-17 are included in this data.

Reprinted from National Conference of State Legislatures. Available at: http://www.ncsl.org/?tabid=13877.

Fig 34.5.

Geographic Patterns Among Low-Income, Preschool-Aged Children 2006–2008

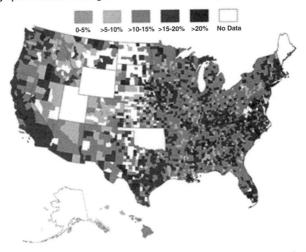

Reprinted from American Obesity Treatment Association. Available at: http://www.americanobesity.org/childhoodObesity.htm

Influence of the Life Cycle on Pediatric Obesity

Before 2 Years of Age

As noted previously, 9.5% of infants and toddlers are overweight for length.[1,77] The concept of the childhood onset of adult disease points to the importance of disease prevention from the preconceptual period throughout pregnancy and early infancy and into childhood. Thus, the fetal period and the first 2 years of life may be critical periods for the programming of obesity and related behaviors. The long-term impacts of both under- and overnutrition in the prenatal period on pediatric obesity have been well described.

Prenatal Undernutrition

Barker originally proposed that the intrauterine environment could affect an individual's later risk of disease.[78] This hypothesis was based on epidemiologic studies of the birth weights of adults with cardiovascular disease.[78] Ravelli et al also examined adults conceived during the Dutch "Winter Hunger," of 1944-1945 and compared their long-term health to those conceived before or after the famine.[79,80] They determined that the prevalence of impaired glucose tolerance was highest in infants with low birth weights who were in utero while mothers were exposed to the famine during the last 2 trimesters of pregnancy. These studies suggested that there is environmental programming in the prenatal period for disease risk in humans.

VI

Maternal risk factors during pregnancy are particularly highlighted as precursors of later disease. Maternal obesity is one of the strongest and best predictors of childhood obesity.[81] Diabetes in pregnancy results in increased risk of childhood obesity and diabetes,[82] as does maternal smoking.[83] Epigenetic mechanisms may be responsible for the ability of the intrauterine environment to affect phenotypic outcomes.[84] Low birth weight (small for gestational age or preterm birth) can also be a marker of increased risk of later obesity, insulin resistance, type 2 diabetes mellitus, hypertension, and cardiovascular disease.[85,86] Hypothesized mechanisms for the association of low birth weight and increased metabolic and cardiovascular disease risk have included the "thrifty phenotype," postnatal accelerated or catch-up growth, oxidative stress, prenatal hypoxia, placental dysfunction, and epigenetic changes.[87] Rapid postnatal weight gain of underweight infants can also increase this risk.[88,89]

In the thrifty phenotype hypothesis, intrauterine undernutrition results in endocrine changes, such as increased insulin resistance, that would tend to divert a limited nutrient supply to nourish the fetal heart and brain at the expense of somatic growth, a life-saving adaptation to limitations of the intrauterine environment. This is accomplished by permanently reducing the number and functional capacity of islet cells. If the fetus is subsequently born into a world of abundance, the increased insulin resistance increases the risk of obesity and type 2 diabetes mellitus, because the child is unable to adapt to the higher glucose levels[89-91] (Fig 34.6). Oxidative stress[92] and prenatal hypoxia[93] have also been advanced as possible mechanisms for creating insulin resistance in low birth weight infants. These associations of low birth weight with type 2 diabetes mellitus and impaired glucose tolerance have been reported in adults through the seventh and eighth decades of life.[94-96]

Prenatal Overnutrition

Macrosomia at birth, indicative of fetal over nutrition, is associated with increased deposition of body fat in childhood and increased risk of obesity[97-99] and the metabolic syndrome.[100] The infant of a mother with diabetes is a model for the influences of fetal over nutrition on postnatal adiposity. Exposure of the fetus to high ambient glucose concentrations stimulates fetal hyperinsulinism, increases fat deposition, and results in macrosomia. This alters the developing neuroendocrine system in a manner that favors deposition of stored calories as fat as well as insulin resistance.[101] In studies controlled for the effects of maternal adiposity, being an infant of a mother with diabetes is still associated with an increased risk of obesity, independent of pre- and perigravid maternal adiposity.[102-104]

Epigenetic change may be the link between an adverse intrauterine environment and chronic disease states, such as obesity, later in life. Animal studies have demonstrated transmission to the next generation of programmed phenotypes of diabetes based on maternal gestational diabetes.[105]

Fig 34.6.
Reprinted with permission from Hales CN, Barker DJ. The thrifty phenotype hypothesis. *Br Med Bull.* 2001;60:5–20

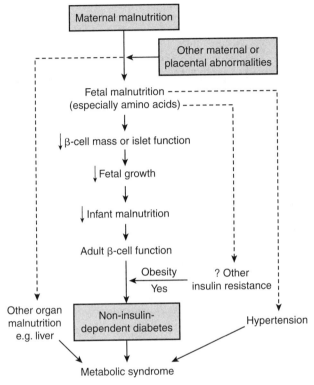

Newborn/Infancy

Infant weight gain has shown a positive association with subsequent obesity.[106-108] Upward crossing of 2 weight-for-length percentiles on the CDC 2000 growth curves in the first 6 months of life is associated with the highest prevalence of obesity 5 and 10 years later.[106] There is one report of feeding infants with formula containing a lower amount of protein that resulted in slower weight gain and lower weight status at 24 months of age.[109] However, long-term follow-up is needed to see if the effect on weight is sustained.

Many observational studies suggest an increased risk of obesity in children who have been formula fed compared with those who have been breastfed.[110] Exclusively breastfed children have been found to have lower mean BMI z-scores than children who were never breastfed, and this may be explained in part by weight gain in infancy.[111] However, any casual association based on these observational studies is unclear. At least 3 studies of siblings who were discordant for breastfeeding status

VI

have been performed.[112-114] Two concluded that formula feeding increased the risk of obesity, and the third did not find any association. A recent study found that breastfeeding was associated with reduced obesity at 3 years of age compared with formula feeding (7% vs 13%, respectively) and that the sum of triceps and subscapular skinfolds was increased for formula-fed infants. In that study, breastfeeding was also associated with delayed introduction of solid foods; 8% of breastfeeding mothers introduced solid foods before 4 months of age, compared with 33% of formula-feeding mothers. In addition, 17% of breastfed infants started solid food after 6 months of age, compared with 9% of formula fed infants.[115]

Toddler/Preschool Years

Obesity in the young child is associated with significant risk of adult obesity. In one study, more than 50% of obese 3- to 6-year olds became obese adults.[116] Accelerated weight gain in preschool children has been associated with higher baseline fat intakes and inappropriately large portion sizes.[117] For children 2 to 3 years of age between the 85th and 95th percentiles for BMI, as little as 1 extra sweetened drink a day (eg, juice, soda, fruit drink) doubled their risk of having a BMI greater than the 95th percentile in the following year.[118] At 5 to 6 years of age, body fatness normally declines to a minimum, a point called adiposity rebound (AR), before increasing again until the onset of adolescence. AR before 5 years of age is associated with an increased risk of adult obesity.[119]

In a study of TV time, children as young as 3 years watched an average of 1.7 hours/day. For each 1-hour increase in viewing, they had increased intake of sugar-sweetened beverages, fast food, red and processed meat, total energy intake, and percentage of energy from trans–fatty acids. Increased TV time was also associated with lower fruit and vegetable, calcium, and fiber intakes.[120]

Parental obesity is the major predictor of overweight and obesity in this age group. In addition to the strong genetic influence, poor lifestyle choices by parents have a negative influence on the nutrition and activity level of the child. In a large nationally representative sample of 4-year-olds, obesity prevalence was reduced from 24.5% to 14.3% in households in which the following routines were maintained: (1) eating the evening meal (dinner) as a family 6 to 7 times/week; (2) obtaining >10.5 hours of night-time sleep/day; and (3) limiting screen/viewing time (television/video/DVD) to 2 hours or less/day.[121] Preschool children with active parents are more likely to be active than those with sedentary parents, and a low level of physical activity in this age group has been associated with increased subcutaneous fat by first grade.[122] The type of child care can also influence BMI. A toddler cared for in someone else's home is more likely to have a higher BMI than a child cared for in a center or in their own home by someone other than their parent.[123]

School Age

School age is also a period when many eating, physical activity, and sedentary habits are established or reinforced. The effect of parental and family behavior on child behavior remains significant. However, entering school can result in increased exposure to additional obesity risk factors. Exposure to foods competing with school lunches begins in elementary school and escalates through high school. Vending machines can be found in 17% of elementary schools, and up to 37% of school fundraisers use high-calorie, nutrient-poor foods.[124] Sugar-sweetened beverages can add to total energy consumption and enhance weight gain,[125] and juice consumption of more than 12 oz/day has also been linked to overweight.[126] The AAP recommends that children 7 to 18 years of age should limit their juice consumption to 8 to 12 oz/day, and children 6 years and younger should limit juice to 4 to 6 oz/day.[127]

Many children eat both breakfast and lunch at school. School breakfast and lunch choices may be limited in elementary school. In its 2010 report *School Meals: Building Blocks for Healthy Children*, the Institute of Medicine recommends that the US Department of Agriculture (USDA) adopt standards for menu planning, including: increasing the amount and variety of fruits, vegetables, and whole grains, setting a minimum and maximum level of calories, and focusing more on reducing saturated fat and sodium.[128] Mid-morning snacks are often encouraged, and after-school programs usually provide a snack. This means that the majority of a school-aged child's calorie intake may occur outside the home, and parents may be unaware of the quality or quantity of the food consumed. In a study of 8- to 10-year-old African-American girls, greater low-fat food preparation at home was related to lower consumption of total fat.[129] Access to screen time is an issue, and snacking increases with hours of television watched, and this effect is magnified in families with one or both parents who are overweight.[130]

Adolescence

During adolescence, parents continue to be responsible to supply a healthy food environment, but adolescents make their own specific choices of food. There is a normal increase in insulin resistance at the onset of puberty, peaking at mid–puberty, coinciding with peak height velocity and decreasing to almost prepubertal levels by the completion of puberty. Insulin resistance and BMI are strongly correlated throughout puberty.[131] Obesity increases the risk of insulin resistance and impaired glucose tolerance, a precursor of type 2 diabetes mellitus.[132] In one study, up to 21% of obese adolescents had impaired glucose tolerance,[133] and in another, impaired glucose tolerance was identified in 35% of adolescents with both obesity and a positive family history of type 2 diabetes mellitus.[134] Elevated BMI in

VI

adolescence, even with normalization of weight as an adult, had an independent association with the onset of coronary artery disease in young adulthood (30 years of age).[135]

Although 60 minutes of exercise is recommended on 5 days/week, only 35.8% of high school students met these goals in 2005. Girls, older adolescents, minority adolescents, and disadvantaged teenagers are less likely to meet this baseline requirement.[136] Healthy People 2010 set a goal of 75% for the proportion of adolescents who watch television for fewer than 2 hours/day, but a report in 2007 revealed that adolescents averaged about 20 hours/week.[137] Adolescents with obesity have been found to have limited exercise tolerance because of the greater oxygen demand of their excess body mass. Exercise recommendations for these adolescents should be tailored to allow for activities that can be sustained without fatigue caused by lactate accumulation.[138]

Comorbidities of Obesity

Obesity adversely affects every organ system. Obesity in childhood constitutes a risk factor for adiposity-related adult morbidity and mortality, even if childhood obesity does not persist. In 40- to 50-year follow-up studies of obese and lean adolescents, adolescent obesity was a powerful predictor of mortality, cardiovascular disease, colorectal cancer, gout, and arthritis irrespective of body fatness at the time that the morbidity was diagnosed.[139] Adiposity-related morbidities, such as hyperlipidemia, which are evident in childhood, track well into adulthood,[140] as do the precursors of coronary artery disease, including elevated circulating concentrations of inflammatory markers and hypertension.[141] Childhood obesity can be thought of as an accelerator of adult diseases. Obese children and adolescents experience comorbidities including type 2 diabetes mellitus, hypertension, dyslipidemia, obstructive sleep apnea, and nonalcoholic steatohepatitis (NASH), which had previously been seen predominantly in adults. In addition, obesity in childhood can result in serious orthopedic problems, such as slipped capital femoral epiphysis (SCFE) and Blount disease. These comorbidities give urgency to the need to institute prevention and early intervention as well as diagnosis and treatment of pediatric obesity.[141]

Complications of obesity can be life threatening. Obesity-related emergencies include diabetic ketoacidosis, pulmonary embolism, cardiomyopathy of obesity ,and hyperglycemic hyperosmolar state (HHS).[142] Type 2 diabetes mellitus can present with HHS. Symptoms may be nonspecific, such as vomiting, abdominal pain, dizziness, weakness, polyuria and polydipsia with severe dehydration, weight loss, and diarrhea. If unrecognized, patients may develop hyperosmolar nonketotic coma and die.[142] Diagnostic criteria for HHS include a plasma glucose concentration of greater than 600 mg/dL, total serum carbon dioxide concentration of greater than 15 mmol/L, minimal ketonuria and ketonemia, an effective serum osmolality of greater than 320 mOsm/kg, and stupor or coma.[142]

Pulmonary embolism may occur. The risk factors for pulmonary embolism include obesity, obesity-hypoventilation syndrome, obstructive sleep apnea syndrome, and coagulation disorder. Symptoms include dyspnea, chest pain, decreased blood oxygen concentration, and hemoptysis.[143] Pulmonary embolism has been reported as a complication of gastric bypass in adolescence.[144]

Congestive heart failure resulting from obesity has been seen in morbidly obese adolescents and is thought to result from high metabolic activity of excessive fat, which increases total blood volume and cardiac output and leads to left ventricular dysfunction. Pulmonary hypertension caused by upper airway obstruction can also occur. Signs and symptoms of cardiac failure should point to this diagnosis.[143,145]

Other comorbidities that require attention and action include idiopathic intracranial hypertension (IIH), SCFE, Blount disease, obstructive sleep apnea syndrome, NASH, cholelithiasis, polycystic ovarian syndrome (PCOS), and type 2 diabetes mellitus.

IIH is defined as increased intracranial pressure with papilledema and normal cerebrospinal fluid in the absence of ventricular enlargement. IIH has been associated with obesity but may also occur in children with normal weight.[146,147] The presentation may range from an incidental finding of papilledema on funduscopic examination to headaches, vomiting, blurred vision, or diplopia. Loss of peripheral visual fields and reduction in visual acuity may be present at diagnosis.[148] Neck, shoulder, and back pain have also been reported.[148] Treatment of IIH includes acetazolamide, ventriculo-peritoneal shunt in severe cases, and weight loss.[147,149] IIH is a diagnosis of exclusion after other causes of increased intracranial pressure are eliminated.[143]

SCFE is a slipping of the femoral epiphysis through the zone of hypertrophic cartilage cells, which are under the influence of gonadal hormones and growth hormone.[150] Fifty to 70% of patients with SCFE are obese.[151] Patients can present with a limp or complaints of groin, thigh, or knee pain. Hips should be examined, and radiographs of both hips should be obtained, because bilateral slips occur in 20% of cases. Medial and posterior displacement of the femoral epiphysis is seen through the growth plate relative to the femoral neck.[152] Treatment is surgical pinning of the hip.[143]

The diagnosis of Blount disease involves the identification of bowing of the tibia and femur. This can affect one or both knees. This condition results from the overgrowth of the medial aspect of the proximal tibial metaphysis. Obesity has been reported in two thirds of patients with Blount disease,[153] and the risk of Blount disease is increased by vitamin D deficiency.[154] Treatment requires surgical correction and weight loss.

VI

Obstructive sleep apnea syndrome is commonly associated with obesity. This syndrome is defined as a disorder of breathing during sleep characterized by prolonged partial upper airway obstruction or intermittent complete obstruction that disrupts normal ventilation during sleep and normal sleep patterns.[155] Symptoms can include night-time awakening, restless sleep, difficulty awakening in the morning, daytime sleepiness, napping, enuresis, decreased concentration and memory, and poor school performance.[156] Night-time polysomnography is the diagnostic procedure of choice to make this diagnosis. If left untreated, children can have pulmonary hypertension, systemic hypertension, and right-sided heart failure.[155] Weight gain, hypertrophy of the tonsils and adenoids, and intercurrent upper respiratory infections can provoke symptoms.

Nonalcoholic steatohepatitis is suspected when elevated liver enzymes are found in the context of fatty liver identified by ultrasonography or other imaging techniques in the absence of other causes of liver disease. Twenty to 25% of obese children have been found to have evidence of steatohepatitis.[157] The definitive diagnosis is by liver biopsy in which evidence of inflammatory infiltrates and fibrosis can be seen. Nonalcoholic steatohepatitis can progress to cirrhosis and end-stage liver disease.[158] Weight loss reduces fatty infiltration and may decrease fibrosis.

Risk of cholelithiasis is higher for people of Hispanic ethnicity and increases with BMI.[159] Cholelithiasis symptoms in children include abdominal pain and tenderness, with diagnosis made by ultrasonography and appropriate laboratory studies.

PCOS can occur in obese adolescents and is characterized by insulin resistance in the presence of elevated androgens. Clinical signs and symptoms include oligomenorrhea or amenorrhea, hirsutism, acne, polycystic ovaries, and obesity. There is some evidence that girls with premature adrenarche are at risk of PCOS.[160]

Type 2 diabetes mellitus occurs in obese adolescents when the diagnosis of hyperglycemia is made in the presence of insulin resistance and an elevated insulin level. Type 2 diabetes mellitus can present with HHS, diabetic ketoacidosis, or symptoms of polyuria, polydipsia, and weight loss. Diagnosis can also be made based on symptoms of hyperglycemia, such as abdominal pain, vomiting, dizziness, weakness, or more subtle polydipsia and polyuria, in an obese patient.[143]

Metabolic syndrome is a cluster of conditions characterized by insulin resistance observed in adults. The components include obesity, elevated blood pressure, elevated triglyceride levels, decreased high-density lipoprotein cholesterol, increased low-density lipoprotein cholesterol, and impaired glucose tolerance.[143] Obese children may have all or some of these findings, although it is not clear whether metabolic syndrome exists as a stable syndrome in childhood.

Prevention of Childhood Obesity

Although community, family, and individual change is crucial in obesity prevention and treatment, the interaction of the complex array of factors that result in either healthy or unhealthy weight can be illustrated by the ecologic model of predictors of childhood overweight in Fig 34.7. This model can serve as a tool for identifying partners and highlighting opportunities for change and can be used in a 360-degree assessment for an individual child/family or community. Recommendations for obesity prevention and treatment can be found in the 2007 AAP expert committee report[161] and updated in the 2013 clinical report "Prevention of Pediatric Obesity: The Role of Pediatric Practice."[162]

The 2012 Institute of Medicine Report *Accelerating Progress in Obesity Prevention: Solving the Weight of the Nation* established 5 goals for obesity prevention for the United States and emphasized the importance of obesity prevention in the pediatric population.[163] Goal one is to make physical activity an integral and routine part of daily life and includes a recommendation to adopt physical activity requirements for licensed child care providers. Goal two is to create food and beverage environments that ensure that healthy food and beverage options are the routine and easy choice and includes a recommendation to increase the availability of lower-calorie and healthier food and

Fig 34.7.
Ecological model of predictors of childhood overweight. Reprinted with permission from Davison KK, Birch LL. Childhood overweight: a contextual model and recommendations for future research. *Obes Review.* **2001;2(3):159-171.**

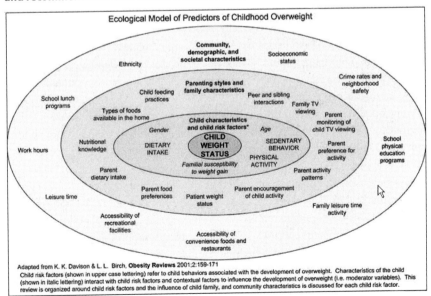

beverage options for children in restaurants. Goal three is to transform messages about physical activity and specifically recommends implementation of common standards for marketing foods and beverages to children and adolescents. Goal four is to expand the role of health care providers, insurers, and employers and recommends that standards or practice include routine screening of BMI, counseling, and behavioral interventions for children and adolescents. Goal five is to make schools a national focal point for obesity prevention. Schools should be required to provide quality physical education and opportunities for physical activity. There should be strong nutritional standards for all foods and beverages sold or provided in schools. Thus, prevention of childhood obesity remains a public health priority, because obesity is the most prevalent chronic health condition in the pediatric population. Although, as noted in the report, many constituents of the society need to be mobilized to address this problem, pediatric primary care practice has a unique role to play and is an integral part of the solution.

To address obesity prevention effectively in clinical practice, pediatricians should become familiar with the complex and interconnected factors that lead to excessive weight gain. They should understand how these factors converge in a developmental fashion and how they create important periods for preventive intervention. By better understanding the environmental determinants of obesity, including those that they cannot control, pediatric practitioners can improve their ability to provide recommendations that are relevant to their patients and their families.

Most prevention strategies that can be used in pediatric practice have not been rigorously tested through scientific research. However, preliminary evidence, indirect evidence, and inferences from other settings provide clues to recommend evidence-informed approaches, especially those with low risk for a negative health effect or with other known health benefits. Although the prevention messages are similar for all, counseling should be tailored to the child's developmental stage as well as the socioeconomic, cultural, and psychological characteristics of families.

Pediatric practice is critical in identifying children who are early on the path to become obese by calculating BMI and plotting it on percentile charts at every health care visit. These children can also be identified through the nutrition, sedentary, and physical activities questions that are part of the *Bright Futures* templates as well as through family history.

Education and advice alone are likely to be ineffective in most cases for obesity prevention. Pediatricians should, therefore, become familiar with other forms of interventions as they apply to obesity prevention, such as behavior modification techniques, environment control approaches, or the promotion of improved parenting skills. They should also become familiar with the resources available in the area they are serving so that they are better suited to help each individual family.

There is no evidence for health benefits and some evidence for negative health effects of sweetened beverages (sodas, ice teas, sport drinks, juice drinks). Therefore, health-promotion efforts should aim at removing all sweetened beverages from children's diets. The ideal beverage for children at all meals and during the day is water, whereas low-fat or fat-free, preferably unflavored, milk also has an important place in the diet of children beginning at 12 months of age. Fruit juice (100% only) should not be used before 1 year of age and should limited after that. Eating fruit should be encouraged over consumption of fruit juice.

Promotion of a diet rich in foods with low caloric density (vegetables, fruits, whole grain, low-fat dairy products, lean meats, lean fish, legumes) and poor in foods with high caloric density (fat-rich meats, fried foods, baked goods, sweets, cheeses, oil-based sauces) is likely to contribute to the prevention of obesity (see Appendix Q).

All forms of sedentary entertainment, including watching television and newer forms of electronic entertainment or communications, should be excluded for infants and children up to 2 years of age and limited to 2 hours/day in children 2 years and older. Promotion of active play, lifestyle, family-based, or sport-based moderate to vigorous physical activity for a total of 60 minute per day on most days is likely to contribute to the prevention of obesity.

Prevention of childhood obesity should start by promoting healthy maternal weight beginning in the prenatal period, smoking cessation before pregnancy, appropriate gestational weight gain and diet, breastfeeding and appropriate weight gain in infancy, transition to healthier foods with weaning, elimination of sedentary entertainment, active play for physical activity, and parental role modeling of healthy dietary and physical activity behaviors.

The AAP has recommended a staged approach to prevention and treatment of pediatric obesity including the following elements: prevention at the office level, prevention at the community level, structured weight management, comprehensive weight management, and tertiary care/hospital management of obesity and comorbidities.

Prevention—Primary Care Provider

Universal attention to age-appropriate healthy nutrition and activity should be part of every child's primary care. The AAP Clinical Decision Support 10 chart[161] recommends using the following pneumonic:

5 **Eat at least 5 servings of fruits and vegetables each day**

2 **Limit screen time unrelated to school to 2 hours or less each day**

1 **Hour or more of moderate to vigorous physical activity every day and 20 minutes of vigorous activity at least 2 times/week**

0 **Sweetened beverages; use water and low-fat milk instead of sugar sweetened drinks**

VI

Additional preventive measures should be taken with children with a BMI between the 85th and 94th percentiles. In addition to the prevention message earlier, families should be encouraged to: (1) eat a daily breakfast; (2) limit meals outside the home; (3) have family meals 5 to 6 times/week; (4) allow the child to self-regulate at meals without overly restrictive behavior.

The goal should be weight maintenance with subsequent growth resulting in a decreased BMI. Follow-up visits should occur monthly. After 3 to 6 months, if there is no improvement in BMI/weight, move to the next stage.

Prevention: Community

Community factors that can be improved to decrease the prevalence of obesity through various measures to improve the environment include: (1) improving access to healthy foods by increasing availability of and safe access to supermarkets; (2) encouraging farmers markets to accept SNAP (Supplemental Nutrition Assistance Program, formerly known as Food Stamps) and food coupons from the Special Supplemental Nutrition Program for Women Infants, and Children (WIC); (3), creating incentives for corner markets and vendors to carry healthier foods; and (4) increasing availability of healthier foods at public venues. Strategies to limit unhealthy foods in communities by limiting fast food outlets and restricting availability of unhealthy foods at public venues should be implemented. Communities can influence point-of-purchase decision making by incentivizing restaurants to provide healthier food options, requiring menu labeling (nutrition information including calories), smaller portion sizes, lower fat and salt content of foods, increasing access to safe drinking water to replace sugar-sweetened beverages, and encouraging family-friendly and healthy vending machine policies. Communities can also promote healthier eating using media campaigns, and consider tax strategies that discourage consumption of energy-dense but nutrient-poor foods.

Physical activity in the community can be promoted by building and maintaining infrastructure for safe indoor and outdoor activity, improving access to safe recreational facilities, creating and promoting youth athletic leagues, encouraging walking and biking, and reducing transit fares.

Schools are important locations where improvements in healthy eating and activity can occur by implementing the recently issued USDA rules for healthier school meals that follow the Dietary Guidelines for Americans 2010, which include reducing the availability of competitive energy–dense, nutrient-poor foods sold in schools (including fundraisers) and providing healthier vending machine food and drink choices. Physical education opportunities should be increased and active recess should be promoted. Physical activity should be incorporated into the school day and in after-school programs.

Pediatricians are in a unique position to influence healthy behaviors of families and patients in the community. Physicians' offices can support healthy eating among the office staff and provide guides to sources of healthy foods in the community. Vending in hospitals and clinic sites can include healthier snacks and menu labeling. Healthy eating and physical activity can be promoted in the office with posters, brochures, and health-related magazines. TV and video can be limited in waiting rooms, and families can be provided with resources for after school/family activities to try at home. Physicians can institute employee wellness programs in their practices; encourage physical activity for employees, patients, and families through events; and provide lists of community activities for family participation. More in-depth strategies and examples to carry out community intervention can be found on the AAP obesity Web site under the heading Policy Tool at http://www2.aap.org/obesity/community_5.html

Treatment of Pediatric Obesity[161,162]

Structured Weight Management (Primary Care Provider With Appropriate Training)

Structured weight management is for children for whom prevention was not successful, for children with a BMI from the 85th through 94th percentile, and for children with BMI greater than the 95th percentile. Counseling should build on all previous messages and include (1) a plan for utilization of a balanced macronutrient diet emphasizing a low amount of energy-dense foods; (2) increased structured daily meals and snacks; (3) supervised active play of at least 60 minutes/day; (4) screen time limited to 1 hour or less/day; and (5) increased monitoring (screen time, physical activity, dietary intake, restaurant logs) by provider, patients, and family.

The goal is weight maintenance, resulting in a decreasing BMI as age increases and increasing weight loss, not to exceed 1 lb (0.5 kg) per month in children 2 to 11 years of age, or an average of 2 lb (1.0 kg) per week in older overweight/obese children and adolescents. Follow-up visits should occur monthly, and if no improvement in BMI is observed after 3 to 6 months, the patient should be advanced to a more comprehensive, multidisciplinary, intervention.

Comprehensive Multidisciplinary Intervention—Weight Management Clinic With Multidisciplinary Team (Expert Committee)

Intervention built on previous stages and includes (1) structured behavioral modification program, including food and activity monitoring and development of short-term diet and physical activity goals; and (2) involvement of primary caregivers/families for behavioral modification in children younger than 12 years and training of primary caregivers/families for all children. Goals are weight maintenance or gradual weight loss until BMI reaches less than the 85th percentile, not to

VI

exceed 1 lb (0.5 kg) per month in children 2 to 5 years of age or 2 lb (1.0 kg) per week in older obese children and adolescents.

Tertiary Care Interventions—Hospital Based With Expertise in Childhood Obesity for Selected Patients

This intervention is recommended for children with BMI greater than the 95th percentile with significant comorbidities unsuccessful with previous stages and children with BMI greater than the 99th percentile who have shown no improvement under comprehensive multidisciplinary intervention. It is especially relevant to children demonstrating 1 or more comorbidities associated with obesity. This intervention involves a multidisciplinary team with expertise in childhood obesity, operating under a designated protocol; continued diet and activity counseling; consideration of possible additions as meal replacements; very low-calorie diet; medication; and surgery.

The expert committee also recommended techniques such as motivational interviewing and/or brief focused negotiation to help families and patients increase motivation and confidence that they can accomplish lifestyle change.[161] Cognitive behavioral therapy has also been used in treatment of childhood obesity with promising results.[164]

For every child, a detailed history and physical examination should be performed to assess each child for current obesity-related morbidities and for birth history or family history that suggests risk of such morbidities. Anthropometric data should be plotted on height and weight velocity charts as well as standard curves for BMI.

Treatment Strategies

The time required to significantly reduce adiposity can be estimated to be 1 year during normally rapid weight gain periods, such as adolescence, and 2 years during periods of slower weight gain. One to 2 years of weight maintenance will reduce excess weight-for-height by approximately 20% in a growing child.

If gradual statural growth into the child's weight is not possible because child is already obese by adult standards (ie, body mass is so great that BMI will still be greater than the 85th percentile, even if weight remains stable until adult stature is achieved), then a weight-loss regimen, as outlined later, should be considered.

Therapeutic weight reduction is usually indicated for the child with evidence of current adiposity-related morbidity. Studies of compliance with weight-reduction plans have emphasized the importance of a family-oriented approach. Any therapeutic regimen should involve the entire family as well as the child's school. Frequent physical examination of the child and monitoring of school performance should be included.

Dietary Intervention

Recommendations for changes in diet should never be presented in a negative manner. The emphasis should be on healthy eating and the value of good nutrition, and, if at all possible, the child and the entire family should follow the same nutritional plan. This allows the parents to provide a healthy nutritional environment for the whole family, reduce food triggers, and allow for positive role modeling. If appropriate, the significance of any evident reduction in morbidity (eg, lowering of blood pressure or cholesterol) can be reinforced. Reasonable goals in the form of behavioral change that are achievable by the next visit should be set jointly with provider, family, and child. The diet should contain the recommended amounts of protein, essential fatty acids, vitamins, and minerals and should be low in saturated fats.[165] The USDA Web site www.Choosemyplate.gov can provide families with food group information, tips, and recipes to use at home. Parents and adult caregivers should understand the important role they play in the development of proper eating habits in their children. Parents' food preferences, the quantities and variety of foods in the home, and the parents' eating behavior and physical activity patterns all determine how supportive the home environment is to the child.

Weight reduction will occur only if energy expenditure exceeds energy intake in a consistent manner. A 300- to 400-kcal/day energy deficit should result in weight loss of approximately 1 lb (0.5 kg) per week. This can be determined by assessing dietary history or as calculated on the basis of a formula relating anthropometry to energy expenditure (eg, the Harris-Benedict equation).[166] A reduction in soft drinks/soda, sports drinks, or juice could accomplish this goal, as could reduction in eating fast food. Weight reduction, per se, causes decreased energy expenditure. This phenomenon, plus the ongoing loss of metabolic mass, necessitates periodic downward adjustments of energy intake to sustain ongoing weight loss unless there is ongoing increase in aerobic activity and increase in lean body mass.

Activity/Exercise

Exercise will promote increased muscle mass, thereby raising total metabolic rate, and reduce visceral adipose tissue mass, which may independently lower the risk of hyperlipidemia and diabetes mellitus. However, the energy cost of even vigorous exercise is low when compared with the calorie content of many foods and snacks. For example, walking at 3 miles/hour for 1 hour consumes approximately 200 kcal, approximately the same amount contained in a 1¾-oz bag of potato chips. Food should not be used as an incentive to exercise. Clinicians should encourage children to participate in organized or individual sports (stressing participation, not watching from the bench) and advocate for better community- and school-based activity programs.

VI

Television, Screen Time

Food constitutes the most heavily advertised product on children's television in the United States. Adiposity was significantly correlated with time spent watching television but not with time spent watching videos,[167] suggesting that the bulk of the positive association of television watching and adiposity is attributable to the fact that approximately 60% of advertising that is devoted to food.[168]

Bariatric Surgery

Although still relatively uncommon, bariatric surgery has been increasing in adolescents in the last few years as the only method that has proven effective to date to treat subjects with a BMI greater than 50. The most common laparoscopic bariatric procedures are Roux-en-Y gastric bypass surgery (GB), adjustable gastric banding (LAGB), and sleeve gastrectomy (SG). There is extensive experience with adult gastric bypass surgery. Briefly, a 15- to 30-mL gastric pouch is created surgically, just below the gastroesophageal junction, and is then anastomosed to the jejunum. The least invasive and most reversible procedure is an adjustable gastric banding, in which a prosthetic band with an adjustable inner diameter is placed around the proximal stomach, restricting food entry to the volume of a small proximal gastric pouch. The band is connected to a subcutaneous port into which saline can be injected to alter the inner diameter of the band, thus requiring close follow-up with a physician and perhaps resulting in earlier detection of any complications. Sleeve gastrectomy is the newest bariatric procedure in which the goal is to reduce the stomach to about 25% of its original size by surgical removal of a large portion of the stomach following the major curve. The open edges are then attached together to form a sleeve or tube with a banana shape.

It is appropriate to consider bariatric surgery in some extremely obese adolescents with serious morbidity in whom all other interventions have failed, with the caveat that long-term follow-up and monitoring is needed. Agreed on criteria for pediatric bariatric surgery include the following[169,170]:

1. The adolescent has attained Tanner stage 4 or 5 pubertal development and final or near-final adult height.
2. The adolescent is severely obese (BMI $\geq$40) with serious obesity-related comorbidities or have a BMI of $\geq$50 with less severe comorbidities.
3. Severe obesity and comorbidities persist despite a formal program of lifestyle modification and weight management, with or without a trial of pharmacotherapy.
4. The adolescent demonstrates commitment to comprehensive medical and psychologic evaluation before and after surgery and demonstrates the ability to adhere to the principles of healthy dietary and activity habits.

5. Psychological evaluation confirms the stability and competence of the family unit.

6. The female adolescent agrees to avoid pregnancy for at least 1 year.

7. There is access to an experienced surgeon in a medical center employing a team capable of long-term follow-up of the metabolic and psychosocial needs of the patient and family, and the institution is either participating in a study of the outcome of bariatric surgery or sharing data.

Current expert opinion recommendations for guidelines and criteria needed to deliver safe and effective bariatric surgical specialty care to adolescents have been published.[171] In a 2012 preliminary report from the annual meeting of the Society of American Gastrointestinal and Endoscopic Surgeons, discharge data from the University Health System Consortium was accessed during a 45-month period from October 2007 to June 2011.[172] All adolescent patients (13 to 18 years of age) with the assorted diagnosis of obesity undergoing laparoscopic surgery (LAGB, SG, and GB) were evaluated. The report included data on 416 adolescent patients during this period. At the same time, 59 490 adult bariatric surgeries were performed. In the adolescents, 182 patients underwent LAGB, 46 underwent SG, and 188 patients underwent GB. During this 4-year period, there was an increasing trend for SG: 3, 8, 15, and 20 cases/year. LAGB showed a decreasing trend, and GB remained stable. Identified comorbidities included hypertension (25.7%), chronic pulmonary disease (21.8%), depression (16.1%), diabetes (15.4%), liver disease (11.3%), and hypothyroidism (6%). The individual and summative morbidity and mortality rates for these procedures was zero. Compared with adult bariatric surgery, the length of stay and overall costs were decreased significantly in the adolescent patients, and intensive care unit admission rate (8.68% vs 6.91%; $P = .19$) and 30-day readmission rate (1.23 % vs 1.98%; $P = .34$) were comparable in adolescent bariatric surgery.[172]

As more adolescents are undergoing bariatric surgery, pediatricians may be seeing either immediate or late-onset surgical complications. Early complication of gastric bypass can include bleeding, bowel perforation, deep vein thrombosis, pulmonary embolism, dehydration, dysphagia, nausea/vomiting, dumping syndrome, small bowel obstruction, anastomotic leak, peritonitis, anastomotic stricture, and abdominal adhesions. Late complications can include cholecystitis, dysphagia, gastroesophageal reflux, incisional hernia, malnutrition, pancreatitis, ulcers, renal calculi, internal hernia, and small bowel obstruction. Protein deficiency can also occur and include hair loss, edema, hypoalbuminemia, anemia, and fatigue. Vitamin and mineral deficiencies may also occur and include vitamin B_{12}, folic acid, iron, and fat-soluble vitamin deficiencies. Complications of gastric banding

VI

can include intraoperative conversion to open gastrostomy, hemorrhage, port infection, stomal obstruction, perforation, late mechanical dysfunction, hiatal hernia, erosion, and band or port slippage.[173,174]

All adolescent patients who undergo bariatric surgery should be monitored for their lifetime, given the fact that long-term effects of bariatric surgery in younger, reproductively active populations have not been well characterized. Further studies are also needed to evaluate the long-term data regarding long-term weight loss, late complications, and mortality.

Pharmacotherapy

Orlistat (Xenical [Roche Pharmaceuticals, Nutley, NJ]) is the only drug approved by the Food and Drug Administration for weight loss for the pediatric age group, specifically in children older than 12 years. The mechanism of action is by decreasing intestinal lipase activity, which results in decreased hydrolysis of dietary fat and, thus, allows approximately 30% of the fat ingested to pass through the gut undigested.[175] The most common adverse effects are loose stools, flatulence, and oily discharge, leading to soiling of underwear. Inhibition of pancreatic lipase also causes loss of fat-soluble vitamins (A, D, E, and K) in the stool, and vitamin supplementation is recommended.[176,177] Studies have shown small weight loss effects, and use needs to be combined with a structured weight-management program.[178] The use of lipase inhibitors has not been well studied in adolescents. Initial studies of lipase inhibitors as part of weight-reduction therapy in obese adolescents have reported that all patients experienced some gastrointestinal adverse effects and that 1 in 3 found them intolerable.[179] Lipase-inhibitor therapy in adolescents provoked significant reductions in circulating concentrations of vitamin D, even when they were provided with vitamin supplements.[180] Because of the possible effects of impaired vitamin D absorption on the extensive bone mineralization that occurs in adolescence, the use of any therapy that inhibits such absorption should be thoroughly investigated before it is prescribed for teenagers.

Overview of Therapeutic Options

Long-term studies of weight-reduced children and adults have shown that 80% to 90% return to their previous weight percentiles. Weight loss maintenance is difficult for reasons noted in the pathophysiology section of this chapter. Obese children and their families must recognize that maintenance of a reduced degree of body fatness requires change that will need to become incorporated into the child's and family's life. Diets extremely low in calorie content or with unusual distributions of calories as fat, protein, and carbohydrate may precipitate cardiac arrhythmias, severe electrolyte disturbances, or other morbidities. As many as 80% of children using unsupervised diets obtained from popular magazines have been found to suffer from weakness, headaches, fatigue, nausea, constipation, nervousness, dizziness, poor concentration, dysmenorrhea, and/or fainting. Children on a supervised diet must also be closely monitored for treatment-associated psychological morbidities. Bariatric surgery is the last resort for some extremely obese adolescents with serious morbidity in whom all other interventions have failed.

Therapeutic intervention should emphasize the need for participation of the entire family and lifelong attention to, and benefits of, a healthy lifestyle as well as ongoing positive reinforcement and family and community support.

Resources

- We Can! (contains dietary recommendations, physical activity recommendations, monitoring tools)
  http://wecan.nhlbi.nih.gov/
- Dietary Guidelines for Americans (provides dietary recommendations for children above the age of two years and adults)
  http://www.cnpp.usda.gov/dietaryguidelines.htm
- Choose My Plate (contains dietary recommendations to the public based on Dietary Guidelines for Americans)
  http://www.choosemyplate.gov/
- BAM! (contains dietary recommendations, physical activity recommendations, monitoring tools)
  http://www.bam.gov/
- Let's Move! and AAP (contains dietary recommendations, physical activity recommendations and prescription, tips to change home environment)
  http://www.letsmove.gov/
  http://www2.aap.org/obesity/whitehouse/index.html
  http://www2.aap.org/obesity/
- Exercise is Medicine (contains recommendations for physicians to include physical activity prescription as part of their practice)
  http://www.exerciseismedicine.org/physicians.htm
- Healthychildren.org (contains dietary recommendations, physical activity recommendations, tips to change home environment, parenting skills advices)
  http://www.healthychildren.org/
- WebMD (contains interactive content for children, teens, and parents)
  www.fit.webmd.com

VI

- Mindless eating (contains tips to change home environment)
  http://www.mindlesseating.org/
- Calorie King (online and book to calculate calorie-content of foods)
  http://www.calorieking.com/
- Which Helmet for Which Activity?
  http://www.cpsc.gov/CPSCPUB/PUBS/349.pdf
- Protect the Ones You Love: Child Injuries are Preventable
  http://www.cdc.gov/safechild/Sports_Injuries/index.html

References

1. Ogden CL, Carroll MD, Bit BK, et al. Prevalence of obesity trends in body mass index among US children and adolescents, 1999-2010. *JAMA*. 2012;307(5):483-490
2. Institute of Medicine, Food and Nutrition Board. *Preventing Obesity: Health in the Balance*. Washington, DC: National Academies Press; 2005
3. Kumanyika SK, Obarsanek E, Stettler N, et al. Population-based prevention of obesity; the needs for comprehensive promotion of healthful eating, physical activity, and energy balance: a scientific statement from American Heart Association Council on Epidemiology and Prevention, Interdisciplinary Committee for Prevention. *Circulation*. 2008;118(4):428-464
4. Rosen ED, Spiegelman BM. Adipocytes as regulators of energy balance and glucose homeostatsis. *Nature*. 2006;444(7121):847-853
5. Trayhurn P. Endocrine and signaling role of adipose tissue: new perspectives on fat. *Acta Physiol Scand*. 2005;184(4):285–293
6. Lettner A, Roden M. Ectopic fat and insulin resistance. *Curr Diab Rep*. 2008;8(3):185-191
7. Cannon B, Nedergarard J. Brown adipose tissue; function and physiological significance. *Physiol Rev*. 2004;84(1):277-359
8. Divoux A, Tordjman J, Lacasa D, et al. Fibrosis in human adipose tissue: composition, distribution, and link with lipid metabolism and fat mass loss. *Diabetes*. 2010;59(11):2817-2825
9. Vael C, Verhulst SL, Nelen V, Goossens H, Desager KN. Intestinal microflora and body mass index during the first three years of life: an observational study. *Gut Pathog*. 2011;3(1):8
10. Rosen E, Spiegelman B. Adipocytes as regulators of energy balance and glucose homeostasis 2. *Nature*. 2006;444(7121):847–853
11. American Academy of Pediatrics. Pediatric obesity. In: Kleinman RE, ed. *Pediatric Nutrition Handbook*. Elk Grove Village IL: American Academy of Pediatrics; 2009:733-782
12. Spiegelman BM, Flier JS. Obesity and the regulation of energy balance. *Cell*. 2001;104(4):531-543
13. Andino LM, Ryder DJ, Shapiro A, et al. POMC overexpression in the ventral tegmental area ameliorates dietary obesity. *J Endocrinol*. 2011;210(2):199-207

14. Korner J, Leibel RL. To eat or not to eat how the gut talks to the brain. *N Engl J Med*. 2003;349(10):926-927

15. Wellman P. Modulation of eating by central catecholamine systems. *Curr Drug Targets*. 2005;6:191-199

16. Saper C, Chou T, Elmquist J. The need to feed: homeostatic and hedonic control of eating. *Neuron*. 2002;36:199-211

17. Baker M, Gaukrodger N, Mayosi BM, et al. Association between common polymorphisms of the proopiomelanocortin gene and body fat distribution; a family study. *Diabetes*. 2005;54(8):2492-249

18. Yeo GS, Farooqi IS, Challis BG, Jackson RS, O'Rahilly S. The role of melanocortin signaling in the control of body weight: evidence from human and murine genetic models. *QJM*. 2000;93(1):7–14

19. Kovacs P, Stumvoll M. Fatty acids and insulin resistance in muscle and liver. *Best Pract Res Clin Endocrinol Metab*. 2005;19(4):625-635

20. Small CJ, Bloom SR. Gut hormones and the control of appetite. *Trends Endocrinol Metab*. 2004;15(6):259-263

21. Strader AD, Woods SC. Gastrointestinal hormones and food intake. *Gastroenterology*. 2005;128(1):175-191

22. Batterham RL, Cowley MA, Small CJ, et al. Gut hormone PYY3-36 physiologically inhibits food intake. *Nature*. 2002;418(6898):650-654

23. Howarth FC, Al Kitbi MK, Hameed RS, Adeghate E. Pancreatic peptides in young and elderly Zucker type 2 diabetic fatty rats. *JOP*. 2011;12(6):567-573

24. Zander M, Madsbad S, Madsen JL, Holst JJ. Effect of 6 week course of glucagon like peptide 1 on glycemic control, insulin sensitivity, and beta cell function in type 2 diabetes a parallel group study. *Lancet*. 2002;359(9309):824-830

25. Wynne K, Park AJ, Small CJ, et al. Subcutaneous oxyntomodulin reduces body weight in overweight and obese subjects: a double-blind, randomized, controlled trial. *Diabetes*. 2005;54(8):2390–2395

26. Laferrère B, Swerdlow N, Bawa B, et al. Rise of oxyntomodulin in response to oral glucose after gastric bypass surgery in patients with type 2 diabetes. *J Clin Endocrinol Metab*. 2010;95(8):4072-4076

27. Ariyasu H, Takaya K, Tagami T, et al. Stomach is a major source of circulating ghrelin, and feeding state determines plasma ghrelin-like immunoreactivity levels in humans. *J Clin Endocrinol Metab*. 2001;86(10):4753–4758

28. Schwarz NA, Rigby BR, La Bounty P, Shelmadine B, Bowden RG. A review of weight control strategies and their effects on the regulation of hormonal balance. *J Nutr Metab*. 2011;2011:237932. Epub 2011 Jul 28

29. Koliaki C, Kokkinos A, Tentolouris N, et al. The effect of ingested macronutrients on postprandial ghrelin response: a critical review of existing literature data. *Int J Pept*. 2010;2010. pii: 710852

30. Ott V, Friedrich M, Zemlin J, et al. Meal anticipation potentiates postprandial ghrelin suppression in humans. *Psychoneuroendocrinology*. 2012;37(7):1096-1100. Epub November 16, 2011

VI

31. Kisseleff HR, Carretta JC, Geleibter A, et al. Cholecystekinin and stomach distension combine to reduce food intake in humans. *Am J Physiol Reg Interg Comp Physiol*. 2003;285(5):R992-R998

32. Musso G, Gambino R, Cassader M. Obesity, diabetes, and gut microbiota: the hygiene hypothesis expanded? *Diabetes Care*. 2010;33(10):2277–2284

33. Lumeng CN, Saltiel AR. Inflammatory links between obesity and metabolic disease. *J Clin Invest*. 2011;121(6):2111-2117

34. Wellen KE, Hotamisligil GS. Obesity-induced inflammatory changes in adipose tissue. *J Clin Invest*. 2003;112(12):1785-1788

35. Skinner AC, Steiner MJ, Henderson FW, et al. Multiple markers of inflammation and weight status: cross-sectional analyses throughout childhood. *Pediatrics*. 2010;125(4):e801-e809

36. Bruun JM, Helge JW, Richelsen B, et al. Diet and exercise reduce low grade inflammation and macrophage infiltration in adipose tissue but not in skeletal muscle in severely obese subjects. *Am J Physiol Endocrinol Metab*. 2006;290(5):e961-e967

37. Balagopal P, George D, Patton N, et al. Lifestyle-only intervention attenuates the inflammatory state associated with obesity: a randomized controlled study in adolescents. *J Pediatr*. 2005;146(3):342-348

38. Fabbrini E, Magkos F, Mohammed BS, et al. Intrahepatic fat, not visceral fat, is linked with metabolic complications of obesity. *Proc Natl Acad Sci U S A*. 2009;106(36):15430-15435

39. Saghizadeh M, Ong JM, Garvey WT, et al. The expression of TNF alpha by human muscle. Relationship to insulin resistance. *J Clin Invest*. 1996;97(4):1111–1116

40. Thaler JP, Schwartz MW. Minireview: inflammation and obesity pathogenesis: the hypothalamus heats up. *Endocrinology*. 2010;151(9):4109-4115

41. Tryahurn P, Wood IS. Adipokines; inflammation and the pleiotrophic role of white adipose tissue. *Br J Nutr*. 2004;92(3):347-355

42. Bouchard C, Tremblay A, Despres JP, et al. The response to long-term overfeeding in identical twins. *N Engl J Med*. 1990;322(21):1477-1482

43. Stunkard AJ, Foch TT, Hrubec Z. A twin study of human obesity. *JAMA*. 1986;256(1):51-54

44. Alegría-Torres JA, Baccarelli A, Bollati V. Epigenetics and lifestyle. *Epigenomics*. 2011;3(3):267-277

45. Choquet H, Meyre D. Genetics of obesity: what have we learned? *Curr Genomics*. 2011;12(3):169-179

46. Cecil JE, Tavendale R, Watt P, et al. An obesity-associated FTO gene variant and increased energy intake in children. *N Engl J Med*. 2008;359(24):2558–2566

47. Timpson NJ, Emmett PM, Frayling TM, et al. The fat mass- and obesity-associated locus and dietary intake in children. *Am J Clin Nutr*. 2008;88(4):971–978

48. Wardle J, Carnell S, Haworth CM, et al. Obesity associated genetic variation in FTO is associated with diminished satiety. *J Clin Endocrinol Metab*. 2008;93(9):3640–3643

49. Stutzmann F, Cauchi S, Durand E, et al. Common genetic variation near MC4R is associated with eating behaviour patterns in European populations. *Int J Obes (Lond)*. 2009;33(3):373–378

50. Valladares M, Dominguez-Vasquez P, Obregon AM, et al. Melanocortin-4 receptor gene variants in Chilean families: association with childhood obesity and eating behavior. *Nutr Neurosci*. 2010;13(2):71–78

51. Qi L, Kraft P, Hunter DJ, et al. The common obesity variant near MC4R gene is associated with higher intakes of total energy and dietary fat, weight change and diabetes risk in women. *Hum Mol Genet*. 2008;17(22):3502–3508

52. Chung WK, Leibel RL. Molecular physiology of syndromic obesities in humans. *Trends Endocrinol Metab*. 2005;16(6):267-272

53. Perrone L, Marzuillo P, Grandone A, del Giudice EM. Chromosome 16p11.2 deletions: another piece in the genetic puzzle of childhood obesity. *Ital J Pediatr*. 2010;36:43

54. Pietrobelli A, Faith MS, Allison DB, et al. Body mass index as a measure of adiposity among children and adolescents: a validation study. *J Pediatr*. 1998;132(2):204-210

55. Reilly JJ, Dorosty AR, Emmett PM. Identification of the obese child: adequacy of the body mass index for clinical practice and epidemiology. Avon Longitudinal Study of Pregnancy and Childhood Study Team. *Int J Obes Relat Metab Disord*. 2000;24(12):1623-1627

56. Krebs N, Himes J, Jacobson D, Nicklas TA, Guilday P, Styne D. Assessment of child and adolescent overweight and obesity. *Pediatrics*. 2007;120(Suppl 4):S193-S228

57. Centers for Disease Control and Prevention. Use of World Health Organization and CDC growth charts for children aged 0–59 months in the United States. *MMWR Recomm Rep*. 2010;59(RR-09):1-15

58. Centers for Disease Control and Prevention, National Center for Health Statistics. Clinical Growth Charts. Available at: http://www.cdc.gov/growthcharts/clinical_charts.htm. Accessed December 12, 2012

59. Laurson KR, Eisenmann JC, Welk GJ. Body fat percentile curves for U.S. children and adolescents. *Am J Prev Med*. 2011;41(4 Suppl 2):S87-S92

60. Ellis KJ, Abrams SA, Wong WW. Monitoring childhood obesity: assessment of the weight/height index. *Am J Epidemiol*.1999;150(9):939–946

61. Ehtisham S, Crabtree N, Clark P, et al. Ethnic differences in insulin resistance and body composition in United Kingdom adolescents. *J Clin Endocrinol Metab*. 2005;90(7):3963–3969

62. Wang J, Thornton JC, Burastero S, et al. Comparisons for body mass index and body fat percent among Puerto Ricans, blacks, whites and Asians living in the New York City area. *Obes Res*. 1996;4(4):377–384

63. Sisson SB, Katzmarzyk PT, Srinivasan SR, et al. Ethnic differences in subcutaneous adiposity and waist girth in children and adolescents. *Obesity (Silver Spring)*. 2009;17(11):2075-2081

64. Liu A, Byrne NM, Kagawa M, et al. Ethnic difference in the relationship between body mass index and percentage body fat among Asian children from different backgrounds. *Br J Nutr*. 2011;106(9):1390-1397

VI

65. Borrud LG, Flegal KM, Looker AC, et al. Body composition data for individuals 8 years of age and older: U.S. population, 1999-2004. *Vital Health Stat 11*. 2010 Apr;(250):1-87

66. Bjorntorp P. Classification of obese patients and complications related to the distribution of surplus fat. *Am J Clin Nutr*. 1987;45(5 Suppl):1120-1125

67. Bjorntorp P. Possible mechanisms relating fat distribution and metabolism. In: Bouchard C, Johnston FE, eds. *Fat Distribution During Growth and Later Health Outcomes*. New York, NY: Alan R. Liss Inc; 1988:175-191

67. Bjorntorp P. Possible mechanisms relating fat distribution and metabolism. In: Bouchard C, Johnston FE, eds. *Fat Distribution During Growth and Later Health Outcomes*. New York, NY: Alan R. Liss Inc; 1988:175-191

68. Chu NF, Rimm EB, Wang DJ, Liou HS, Shieh SM. Relationship between anthropometric variables and lipid levels among school children: the Taipei Children Heart Study. *Int J Obes Relat Metab Disord*. 1998;22(1):66-72

69. Hansen SE, Hasselstrøm H, Grønfeldt V, Froberg K, Andersen LB. Cardiovascular disease risk factors in 6–7-year-old Danish children: the Copenhagen School Child Intervention Study. *Prev Med*. 2005;40(6):740-746

70. Moran A, Jacobs DR Jr, Steinberger J, et al. Insulin resistance during puberty: results from clamp studies in 357 children. *Diabetes*. 1999;48(10):2039-2044

71. Sikram NK, Misra A, Pandey RM, et al. Adiponectin, insulin resistance, and C-reactive protein in postpubertal Asian Indian adolescents. *Metabolism*. 2004;53(10):1336-1341

72. Brambelia P, Bedogni G, Moreno LA, et al. Cross validation of anthropometry against magnetic resonance imaging for the assessment of visceral and subcutaneous adipose tissue in children. *Int J Obes (Lond)*. 2006;30(1):23-30

73. Lee S, Bacha F, Gungor N, et al. Waist circumference is an independent predictor of insulin resistance in black and white youths. *J Pediatr*. 2006;148(2):188-194

74. Maffeis C, Pietrobelli A, Grezzani A, Provera S, Tatò L. Waist circumference and cardiovascular risk factors in prepuberal children. *Obes Res*. 2001;9(3):179-187

75. Savva SC, Tornaritis M, Savva ME, et al. Waist circumference and waist to height ratio are better predictors of cardiovascular disease risk factors in children than body mass index. *Int J Obes Relat Metab Disord*. 2000;24(11):1453-1458

76. Kotlyarevska K, Wolfgram P, Lee JM. Is waist circumference a better predictor of insulin resistance than body mass index in U.S. adolescents? *J Adolesc Health*. 2011;49(3):330-333

77. Ogden CL, Carroll MD, Curtin LR, Lamb MM, Flegal KM. Prevalence of high body mass index in US children and adolescents, 2007-2008. *JAMA*. 2010 ;303(3):242-9

78. Barker DJ, Hales CN, Fall CH, Osmond C, Phipps K, Clark PM. Type 2 (non-insulin-dependent) diabetes mellitus, hypertension and hyperlipidaemia (syndrome X): relation to reduced fetal growth. *Diabetologia*. 1993;36(1):62–67

79. Ravelli AC, van der Meullen JH, Osmond C, Barker DJ, Bleker OP. Infant feeding and adult glucose tolerance, lipid profile, blood pressure, and obesity. *Arch Dis Child*. 2000;82(3):248-252

80. Ravelli AC, van der Meulen JH, Michels RP, et al. Glucose tolerance in adults after prenatal exposure to famine. *Lancet*. 1998;351(9097):173-177

81. Parsons TJ, Power C, Logan S, et al. Childhood predictors of adult obesity: a systematic review. *Int J Obes Relat Metab Disord*. 1999;23(Suppl 8):S1-S107

82. Crume TL, Ogden L, Daniels S, Hamman RF, Norris JM, Dabelea D. The impact of in utero exposure to diabetes on childhood body mass index growth trajectories: the EPOCH study. *J Pediatr*. 2011;158(6):941-946

83. Pryor LE, Tremblay RE, Boivin M, et al. Developmental trajectories of body mass index in early childhood and their risk factors: an 8-year longitudinal study. *Arch Pediatr Adolesc Med*. 2011;165(10):906-912

84. Godfrey KM, Sheppard A, Gluckman PD, et al. Epigenetic gene promoter methylation at birth is associated with child's later adiposity. *Diabetes*. 2011;60(5):1528-1534

85. Barker D, Eriksson J, Forsen T, et al. Fetal origins of adult disease: strength of effects and biological basis. *Int J Epidemiol*. 2002;31(6):1235-1239

86. Barker D, Osmond C, Forsen T, et al. Trajectories of growth among children who have coronary events as adults. *N Engl J Med*. 2005;353(17):1802-1809

87. Luo Z, Xiao L, Nuyt A. Mechanisms of developmental programming of the metabolic syndrome and related disorders. *World J Diabetes*. 2010;1(3):89-98

88. Bhargava S, Sachdev H, Fall C, et al. Relation of serial changes in childhood body mass index to impaired glucose tolerance in young adulthood. *N Engl J Med*. 2004;350(9):865-875

89. Cianfarani S, Germani D, Branca F. Low birthweight and adult insulin resistance: the "catch-up growth" hypothesis. *Arch Dis Child Fetal Neonatal Ed*. 1991;81(1):F71-F73

90. Hales CN, Barker DJ. Type 2 (non-insulin-dependent) diabetes mellitus: the thrifty phenotype hypothesis. *Diabetologia*. 1992;35(7):595-601

91. Lucas A. Programming by early nutrition: an experimental approach. *J Nutr*. 1998;128(2 Suppl):401S-406S

92. Luo ZC, Fraser WD, Julien P, et al. Tracing the origins of "fetal origins" of adult diseases: programming by oxidative stress? *Med Hypotheses*. 2006;66(1):38-44

93. Zhang L. Prenatal hypoxia and cardiac programming. *J Soc Gynecol Investig*. 2005;12(1):2-13

94. Rich-Edwards JW, Colditz GA, Stampfer MJ, et al. Birthweight and the risk for type II diabetes mellitus in adult women. *Ann Intern Med*. 1999;130(4 Pt 1):278-284

95. Phillips DI, Barker DJ, Hales CN, Hirst S, Osmond C. Thinness at birth and insulin resistance in adult life. *Diabetologia*. 1994;37(2):150-154

96. Hales C, Barker D, Clark PM, et al. Fetal and infant growth and impaired glucose tolerance at age 64. *BMJ*. 1991;303(6809):1019-1022

97. Schaefer-Graf UM, Pawliczak J, Passow D, et al. Birth weight and parental BMI predict overweight in children from mothers with gestational diabetes. *Diabetes Care*. 2005;28(7):1734-1740

98. Vohr BR, McGarvey ST. Growth patterns of large-for-gestational-age and appropriate-for-gestational-age infants of gestational diabetic mothers and control mothers at age 1 year. *Diabetes Care*. 1997;20(7):1066-1072

99. Gillman MW, Rifas-Shiman R, Berkey CS, et al. Maternal gestational diabetes, birth weight, and adolescent obesity. *Pediatrics*. 2003;111(3):e221-e226

VI

100. Boney CM, Verma A, Tucker R, et al. Metabolic syndrome in childhood: association with birth weight, maternal obesity, and gestational diabetes mellitus. *Pediatrics*. 2005;115(3):e290-e296

101. Pettitt DJ, Baird HR, Aleck KA, et al. Excessive obesity in offspring of Pima Indian women with diabetes during pregnancy. *N Engl J Med*. 1983;308(5):242-245

102. Plagemann A. Perinatal programming and functional teratogenesis: impact on body weight regulation and obesity. *Physiol Behav*. 2005;86(5):661-668

103. Pettitt DJ, Knowler WC, Bennett PH, Aleck KA, Baird HR. Obesity in offspring of diabetic Pima Indian women despite normal birth weight. *Diabetes Care*. 1987;10(1):76-80

104. Pettitt DJ, Aleck KA, Baird HR, Carraher MJ, Bennett PH, Knowler WC. Congenital susceptibility to NIDDM. Role of intrauterine environment. *Diabetes*. 1988;37(5):622-628

105. Pinney SE, Simmons RA. Metabolic programming, epigenetics, and gestational diabetes mellitus. *Curr Diab Rep*. 2012;12(1):67-74

106. Taveras EM, Rifas-Shiman SL, Sherry B, et al. Crossing growth percentiles in infancy and risk of obesity in childhood. *Arch Pediatr Adolesc Med*. 2011;165(11):993-998

107. Ong KK, Loos RJ. Rapid infancy weight gain and subsequent obesity: systemic reviews and hopeful suggestions. *Acta Paediatr*. 2006;95(8):904-908

108. Druet C, Stettler N, Sharp S, et al. Prediction of childhood obesity by infancy weight gain: an individual-level meta-analysis. *Paediatr Perinat Epidemiol*. 2012;26(1):19-26

109. Koletzko B, von Kries R, Closa R, et al. Lower protein in infant formula is associated with lower weight gain up to age 2 y: a randomized clinical trial. *Am J Clin Nutr*. 2009;89(6):1836-1845

110. Owen CG, Martin RM, Whincup PH, et al. Effect of infant feeding on the risk of obesity across the life course: a quantitative review of published evidence. *Pediatrics*. 2005;115(5):1367-1377

111. Van Rossem L, Taveras E, Gillman M, et al. Is the association of breastfeeding with child obesity explained by infant weight change? *Int J Pediatr Obesity*. 2011;6(2-2):e415-e422

112. Nelson MC, Gordon-Larsen P, Adair LS. Are adolescents who were breast-fed less likely to be overweight? Analyses of sibling pairs to reduce confounding. *Epidemiology*. 2005;16(2):247-253

113. Metzger MW, McDade TW. Breastfeeding as obesity prevention in the United States: a sibling difference model. *Am J Hum Biol*. 2010;22(3):291-296

114. Gillman MW, Rifas-Shiman SL, Berkey CS, et al. Breast-feeding and overweight in adolescence: within-family analysis [corrected]. *Epidemiology*. 2006;17(1):112-114

115. Huh SY, Rifas-Shiman SL, Taveras EM, Oken E, Gillman MW. Timing of solid food introduction and risk of obesity in preschool-aged children. *Pediatrics*. 2011;127(3):e544-e551

116. Whitaker RC, Wright JA, Pepe MS, Seidel KD, Dietz WH. Predicting obesity in young adulthood from childhood and parental obesity. *N Engl J Med*. 1997;337(13):869–873

117. Orlet Fisher J, Rolls BJ, Birch LL. Children's bite size and intake of an entrée are greater with large portions than with age-appropriate or self-selected portions. *Am J Clin Nutr*. 2003;77(5):1164–1170

118. Welsh JA, Cogswell ME, Rogers S, et al. Overweight among low-income preschool children associated with the consumption of sweet drinks: Missouri, 1999-2002. *Pediatrics*. 2005;115(2):e223–e229

119. Whitaker RC, Pepe MS, Wright JA, Seidel KD, Dietz WH. Early adiposity rebound and the risk of adult obesity. *Pediatrics*. 1998;101(3):e5-e8

120. Miller SA, Taveras EM, Rifas-Shiman SL, et al. Association between television viewing and poor diet quality in young children. *Int J Pediatr Obes*. 2008;3(3):168-176

121. Anderson SE, Whitaker RC. Household routines and obesity in US preschool-aged children. *Pediatrics*. 2010;125(3):420-8

122. Moore LL, Lombardi DA, White MJ, et al. Influence of parents' physical activity levels on activity levels of young children. *J Pediatr*. 1991;118(2):215–219

123. Benjamin S, Rifas-Shiman S, Taveras E, et al. Early child care and adiposity at ages 1 and 3 years. *Pediatrics*. 2009;124(2):555-562

124. Finkelstein DM, Hill EL, Whitaker RC. 2008. The third school nutrition and dietary assessment study (SNDAIII). School food environments and policies in US public schools. *Pediatrics*. 2008;122(1):e251-e259

125. Berkey CS, Rockett HR, Field AE, et al. Sugar-added beverages and adolescent weight change. *Obes Res*. 2004;12(5):778-788

126. Dennison BA, Rockwell HL, Baker SL. Excess fruit juice consumption by preschool-aged children is associated with short stature and obesity. *Pediatrics*. 1997;99(1):15-22

127. American Academy of Pediatrics, Committee on Nutrition. The use and misuse of fruit juice in pediatrics. *Pediatrics*. 2001;107(5):1210-1213

128. Institute of Medicine, Food and Nutrition Board. *Building Blocks for Healthy Children*. Washington, DC: National Academies Press; 2010

129. Cullen KW, Baranowski T, Klesges LM, et al. Anthropometric, parental, and psychosocial correlates of dietary intake of African-American girls. *Obes Res*. 2004;12(Suppl):20S-31S

130. Francis LA, Lee Y, Birsch LL. Parental weight status and girls' television viewing, snacking, and body mass indexes. *Obes Res*. 2003;11(1):143-151

131. Moran A, Jacobs DR, Steinberger J, et al. Insulin resistance during puberty. Results from clamp studies in 357 children. *Diabetes*. 1999;48(10):2039-2044

132. Li C, Ford ES, Zhao G, Mokdad AH. Prevalence of pre-diabetes and its association with clustering of cardiometabolic risk factors and hyperinsulinemia among US adolescents: NHANES 2005–2006. *Diabetes Care*. 2009;32(2):342-347

133. Sinha R, Fisch G, Teague B, et al. Prevalence of impaired glucose tolerance among children and adolescents with marked obesity. *N Engl J Med*. 2002;346(11):802–810

134. Wiegand S, Maikowski U, Blankenstein O, Biebermann H, Tarnow P, Grüters A. Type 2 diabetes and impaired glucose tolerance in European children and adolescents with obesity—a problem that is no longer restricted to minority groups. *Eur J Endocrinol*. 2004;151(2):199–206

135. Tirosh A, Shai I, Afek A, et al. Adolescent BMI trajectory and risk of diabetes versus coronary disease. *N Engl J Med*. 2011;364(14):1315-1325

VI

136. US Department of Health and Human Services. *Physical Activity Guidelines Advisory Committee Report 2008*. Washington, DC: US Department of Health and Human Services; 2008

137. Boone JE, Gordon-Larsen P, Adair LS, Popkin BM. Screen time and physical activity during adolescence: longitudinal effects of obesity in young adulthood. *Int J Behav Nutr Phys Act*. 2007;4:26

138. Norman AC, Drinkard B, McDuffie JR, et al. Influence of excess adiposity on exercise fitness and performance in overweight children and adolescents. *Pediatrics*. 2005;115(6):e690–e696

139. Must A, Jacques PF, Dallal GE, Bajema CJ, Dietz WH. Long-term morbidity and mortality of overweight adolescents. A follow-up of the Harvard Growth Study of 1922 to 1935. *N Engl J Med*. 1992;327(19):1350-1355

140. Webber LS, Srinivasan SR, Wattigneyy WA, Berenson GS. Tracking of serum lipids and lipoproteins from childhood to adulthood. The Bogalusa Heart Study. *Am J Epidemiol*. 1991;133(9):884-899

141. Field AE, Cook NR, Gillman MW. Weight status in childhood as a predictor of becoming overweight or hypertensive in early adulthood. *Obes Res*. 2005;13(1):163-169

142. Morales AE, Rosenbloom AL. Death caused by hyperglycemic hyperosmolar state at the onset of type 2 diabetes. *J Pediatr*. 2004;144(2):270-273

143. Hassink S. Pediatric *Obesity: Prevention, Intervention, and Treatment Strategies for Primary Care*. Elk Grove Village, IL: American Academy of Pediatrics; 2006

144. Sugerman HJ, Sugerman EL, DeMaria EJ, et al. Bariatric surgery for severely obese adolescents. *J Gastrointest Surg*. 2003;7(1):102-108

145. Alpert MA. Obesity cardiomyopathy: pathophysiology and evolution of the clinical syndrome. *Am J Med Sci*. 2001;321(4):225-236

146. Scott IU, Siatkowski RM, Eneyni M, et al. Idiopathic intracranial hypertension in children and adolescents. *Am J Ophthalmol*. 1997;124:253-255

147. Faz G, Butler IJ, Koenig MK. Incidence of papilledema and obesity in children diagnosed with idiopathic "benign" intracranial hypertension: case series and review. *J Child Neurol*. 2010;25(11):1389-1392

148. Lessell S. Pediatric pseudotumor cerebri (idiopathic intracranial hypertension). *Surv Ophthalmol*. 1992;37(3):155-166

149. Distelmaier F, Sengler U, Messing-Juenger M, et al. Pseudotumor cerebri as an important differential diagnosis of papilledema in children. *Brain Dev*. 2006;28:190-195

150. Kempers MJ, Noordam C, Rouwe CW, et al. Can GnRH-agonist treatment cause slipped capital femoral epiphysis? *J Pediatr Endocrinol Metab*. 2001;14(6):729-734

151. Wilcox PG, Weiner DS, Leighley B. Maturation factors in slipped capital femoral epiphysis. *J Pediatr Orthop*. 1988;8(2):196-200

152. Busch MT, Morrissy RT. Slipped capital femoral epiphysis. *Orthop Clin North Am*. 1987;18(4):637-647

153. Dietz WH, Gross WL, Kirkpatrick JA. Blount disease (tibia vara): another skeletal disorder associated with childhood obesity. *J Pediatr*. 1982;101(5):735-737

154. Montgomery CO, Young KL, Austen M, et al. Increased risk of Blount disease in obese children and adolescents with vitamin D deficiency. *J Pediatr Orthop*. 2010;30(8):879-882

155. Marcus CL, Brooks LJ, Ward SD, et al; Technical report: diagnosis and management of childhood obstructive sleep apnea syndrome. *Pediatrics*. 2012;130(3):e714-e755

156. Gozal D. Sleep-disordered breathing and school performance in children. *Pediatrics*. 1998;102(3 Pt 1):616-620

157. Tazawa Y, Noguchi H, Nishinomiya F, Takada G. Serum alanine aminotransferases activity in obese children. *Acta Paediatr*. 1997;86(3):238-241

158. Harrison SA, Diehl AM. Fat and the liver—a molecular overview. *Semin Gastrointest Dis*. 2002;13(1):3-6

159. Mehta S, Lopez ME, Chumpitazi BP, et al. Clinical characteristics and risk factors for symptomatic pediatric gallbladder disease. *Pediatrics*. 2012;129(1):e82-e88

160. Ibanez L, Dimartino-Nardi J, Potau N, et al. Premature adrenarche—normal variant or forerunner of adult disease? *Endocr Rev*. 2000;21(6):671-696

161. Barlow SE; Expert Committee. Expert committee recommendations regarding the prevention, assessment, and treatment of child and adolescent overweight and obesity: summary report. *Pediatrics*. 2007;120(Suppl 4):S164-S192

162. Daniels SR, Hassink SG; American Academy of Pediatrics, Committee on Nutrition. Prevention of pediatric obesity: the role of the pediatric practice. *Pediatrics*. In press

163. Institute of Medicine. *Accelerating Progress in Obesity Prevention. Solving the Weight of the Nation*. Washington, DC: National Academies Press; 2012

164. Moens E, Braet C, Van Winckel M. An 8-year follow-up of treated obese children: children's, process and parental predictors of successful outcome. *Behav Res Ther*. 2010;48(7):626-633

165. American Heart Association, Nutrition Committee. Diet and lifestyle recommendations revision 2006: a scientific statement from the American Heart Association Nutrition Committee. *Circulation*. 2006;114(1):82-96

166. Roza AM, Shizgal HM. The Harris Benedict equation reevaluated: resting energy requirements and the body cell mass. *Am J Clin Nutr*. 1984;40(1):168-182

167. Hernandez B, Gortmaker SL, Colditz GA, et al. Association of obesity with physical activity, television programs and other forms of video viewing among children in Mexico city. *Int J Obes Relat Metab Disord*. 1999;23(8):845-854

168. Borzekowski DL, Robinson TN. The 30-second effect: an experiment revealing the impact of television commercials on food preferences of preschoolers. *J Am Diet Assoc*. 2001;101(1):42-46

169. August GP, Caprio S, Fennoy I, et al. Prevention and treatment of pediatric obesity; an Endocrine Society clinical practice guideline based on expert opinion. *J Clin Endocrinol Metab*. 2008;93(12):4576-4599

170. Inge TH, Krebs NF, Garcia VF, et al. Bariatric surgery for severely overweight adolescents: concerns and recommendations. *Pediatrics*. 2004;114:217-223

171. Michalsky M, Kramer RE, Fullmer MA, et al. Developing criteria for pediatric/adolescent bariatric surgery programs. *Pediatrics*. 2011;128(Suppl 2):S65-S70

VI

172. Pallati P, Simorov A, Meyer A, et al. Trends in adolescent bariatric surgery evaluated by UHC database collection. Presented at the SAGES 2012 Annual Meeting. Available at: http://thesagesmeeting.org/trends-in-adolescent-bariatric-surgery-evaluated-by-uhc-database-collection/. Accessed December 12, 2012

173. Zitsman JL, Fennoy I, Witt MA, Schauben J, Devlin M, Bessler M. Laparoscopic adjustable gastric banding in adolescents: short-term results. *J Pediatr Surg*. 2011;46(1):157-162

174. Decker GA, Swain JM, Crowell MD, Scolapio JS. Gastrointestinal and nutritional complications after bariatric surgery. *Am J Gastroenterol*. 2007;102(11):2571-2580

175. Sjöström L, Rissanen A, Andersen T, et al. Randomised placebo-controlled trial of orlistat for weight loss and prevention of weight regain in obese patients. *The Lancet*. 1998;352(9123):167-172

176. Finer N, James WP, Kopelman PG, Lean ME, Williams G. One-year treatment of obesity: a randomized, double-blind, placebo-controlled, multicentre study of orlistat, a gastrointestinal lipase inhibitor. *Int J Obes Relat Metab Disord*. 2000;24(3):306-313

177. Hill JO, Hauptman J, Anderson JW, et al. Orlistat, a lipase inhibitor, for weight maintenance after conventional dieting: a 1-y study. *Am J Clin Nutr*. 1999;69(6):1108-1116

178. Butryn ML, Wadden TA, Rukstalis MR, et al. Maintenance of weight loss in adolescents: current status and future directions. *J Obes*. 2010;2010:789280. Epub Jan 2, 2011. doi: 10.1155/2010/789280

179. Ozkan B, Bereket A, Turan S, Keskin S. Addition of orlistat to conventional treatment in adolescents with severe obesity. *Eur J Pediatr*. 2004;163(12):738-741

180. McDuffie JR, Calis KA, Booth SL, et al. Effects of orlistat on fat-soluble vitamins in obese adolescents. *Pharmacotherapy*. 2002;22(7):814-822

Chapter 35

Food Allergy

Adverse reactions to foods may result from immunologic (*food allergy*) and nonimmunologic responses.[1] Food allergy has recently been defined by an expert panel as an "adverse health effect arising from a specific immune response that occurs reproducibly on exposure to a given food."[2] Food allergy affects 4% to 8% of children in the United States, although rates of parent-perceived allergies are significantly higher.[3-5] It is not clear whether the discordance of self-perceived allergy compared with true allergy is the result of lay perceptions regarding any adverse response to a food being an "allergy," or simply incorrect self-diagnosis, but the discordance indicates the need for a physician diagnosis to avoid unnecessary dietary avoidance. Food allergies can be severe and potentially fatal,[6] also indicating the need for careful diagnostic assessments and appropriate education regarding allergen avoidance and treatment of reactions.

There are a number of adverse reactions to foods that are not allergies. Toxins or pharmacologically active components of the diet account for a number of nonimmune adverse reactions, such as food poisoning. Food intolerance is another adverse reaction not involving the immune system. A common example is lactose intolerance caused by lactase insufficiency. Symptoms include abdominal discomfort, bloating, and loose stools from a reduced ability to digest lactose. Examples of adverse reactions to foods are shown in Table 35.1. This chapter focuses on food allergies. Although celiac disease involves an immune response to gluten, it is not generally considered among food allergies and is not discussed in this chapter (see Chapter 28).

Table 35.1.
Examples of Adverse Reactions to Foods

Intolerance
Lactose intolerance (from lactase deficiency)
Caffeine (jitteriness)
Tyramine in aged cheeses (migraine)
Toxins
Bacterial food poisoning (*Staphylococcus aureus, Salmonella* species, *Clostridium botulinum,* etc)
Scombroid (from spoilage of dark-meat fish, may mimic allergy)
Food allergy (immune responses)
IgE-mediated
Non–IgE-associated
Mixed IgE/non-IgE (eosinophilic gastrointestinal disease, atopic dermatitis)
Neurologic and psychological/psychiatric
Auriculotemporal syndrome (facial flush with salivation)
Gustatory rhinitis (rhinorrhea from spicy foods)
Anorexia nervosa and food aversions

VI

Pathophysiology

Immune responses to foods are a normal phenomenon resulting in oral tolerance.[7] Normal responses include the production of immunoglobulin (Ig) G antibodies directed at food proteins. In contrast, aberrant immune responses to food proteins can result in food allergies. It is conceptually and diagnostically helpful to consider food-allergic disorders by immunopathology among those that are or are not associated with detectable food-specific IgE antibodies. Disorders with an acute onset of symptoms following ingestion are typically mediated by IgE antibodies. Food-specific IgE antibodies bind to high-affinity IgE receptors on tissue mast cells and blood basophils, a state termed *sensitization*. Reexposure to the food proteins results in binding and cross-linking of allergen-specific IgE antibodies, initiating signal transduction pathways that result in the release of mediators, such as histamine. The release of mediators then results in symptoms that may affect the skin, gastrointestinal tract, respiratory tract, and cardiovascular system. Another group of food-allergic disorders affecting primarily the gastrointestinal tract, such as food protein-induced enteropathy and food protein-induced enterocolitis, are subacute or chronic and are mediated primarily by T lymphocytes. Atopic dermatitis and eosinophilic gastrointestinal disorders are a third group of chronic disorders that may be associated with food allergies and are variably associated with detectable IgE antibody (IgE associated/cell-mediated disorders).

Food Allergens

Most relevant food allergens are water-soluble glycoproteins that are 10 to 70 kD in size and relatively stable to heat, acid, and proteases. The foods accounting for most significant allergic reactions are cow milk, egg, peanut, tree nuts (ie, cashew, walnut, hazel, Brazil, etc), fish, Crustacean shellfish, wheat, and soy. However, more than 170 foods are described to have caused allergic reactions in some individuals, and seeds, such as sesame seeds, appear to represent emerging potent allergens. Certain fruits and vegetables typically cause mild reactions, such as oral pruritus, presumably because the causal proteins are labile and do not enter the bloodstream intact after digestion. Sensitivity to these proteins is most often the result of initial reactivity to homologous proteins in pollens (pollen-food related syndrome). For example, a protein in Birch pollen is homologous with a protein in raw apple. Heating the apple denatures this protein, so affected children can tolerate apple juice or sauce without symptoms.

Although many botanically related proteins share regions of homology and may show cross-reactivity on allergy testing, clinical evidence of cross-reactivity is not as common.[8] For example, peanut is a legume, and most people with peanut allergy have IgE antibodies that recognize proteins in other legumes, such as peas and string beans. This phenomenon leads to positive allergy test results for these other legumes.

However, 95% of children with peanut allergy tolerate most other beans. The rate of clinically relevant cross-reactivity varies by food, with high rates of allergy among fish and shellfish (>50%) and low rates of cross-reactivity among grains (<20%). There is no significant cross-reactivity between finned fish and shellfish. Although many children with peanut or tree nut allergy may be allergic to multiple related foods, this is not a consistent finding. A child may be allergic, for example, to cashew and pistachio but not to other tree nuts. Some physicians suggest avoidance of food "families" to avoid misidentification or cross-contact of allergens that could result in reactions; for example, some may suggest avoiding all tree nuts if there is an allergy to any. Some tree nuts have homologous proteins, such as walnut with pecan, cashew with pistachio, and hazelnut with almond.

Allergic reactions to food additives, such as colors or preservatives, are uncommon. Food additives derived from natural sources contain proteins that may trigger allergic reactions.[9] These include colors derived from paprika, seeds (annatto), and insects (carmine/cochineal). Chemical additives are not likely to cause IgE-associated allergic reactions, but some may cause adverse reactions, including symptoms that are allergy-like, or may invoke immune responses. Tartrazine (yellow #5) is a synthetic color that has been extensively investigated because of concerns that it may trigger hives, allergic reactions, and asthma. However, well-conducted studies have generally not validated these concerns. Like tartrazine, many other synthetic colors have not been proven to cause allergic reactions; however, some of these chemicals have rarely been associated with rashes. Sulfites can, in sensitive people, induce asthma and very rarely cause more significant allergic-like responses.

Prevalence

Food allergy is estimated to affect 4% to 8% of children and appears to be increasing in prevalence.[3-5] A study from the Centers for Disease Control and Prevention (CDC) reporting the results of the National Health Interview Survey suggested an 18% increase in prevalence from 1997-2007.[3] Studies of peanut allergy in children suggest almost a tripling in prevalence in just over a decade,[10] with multiple studies worldwide indicating that more than 1% of school-aged children are affected.[11-14] The reasons for the increase remain unclear, but theories include changes in food processing, timing of introduction of foods (either too early in infancy or too late in childhood), alterations in other components of the diet, such as fats or vitamins, and the "hygiene hypothesis" that lack of farm living and control of infection has resulted in immune dysregulation.[15,16] Genetic risk factors for food allergy include a family or personal history of atopic disorders (asthma, atopic dermatitis, allergic rhinitis, food allergy).

VI

Clinical Disorders

The clinical manifestations of food allergy are diverse and result from underlying immune mechanisms, and their effects on particular target organs. Food allergy may present as an acute reaction with a sudden onset of stereotypical symptoms, such as hives or respiratory compromise; as an increase in chronic symptoms, such as exacerbation of atopic dermatitis; or as a chronic disease in which recognition of symptom patterns suggests a food allergy. Specific disorders are summarized by pathophysiology in Table 35.2.

Table 35.2.
Clinical Disorders Associated With Food Allergy According to Pathophysiology

IMMUNOPATHOLOGY/DISORDER
IgE antibody-associated
Urticaria/angioedema Oral allergy syndrome (pollen-related) Anaphylaxis Food-associated, exercise-induced anaphylaxis Onset of isolated symptoms (wheeze, abdominal pain, vomiting, etc)
IgE antibody-associated/cell-mediated, chronic
Atopic dermatitis Eosinophilic gastroenteropathies
Non-IgE–associated
Dietary protein enterocolitis Dietary protein proctitis Dietary protein enteropathy Contact dermatitis Pulmonary hemosiderosis

IgE-Mediated Food Allergies

IgE-mediated food-allergic reactions typically occur within minutes and rarely beyond an hour following ingestion of a triggering food. The organ system/systems affected and the specific symptoms additionally define these reactions. *Urticaria* and/or *angioedema*, pruritus, and flushing are common skin manifestation of food allergy, either alone or in combination with other symptoms. *Contact urticaria* describes lesions that occur at the site of direct contact with the food that may not induce a reaction when ingested.

Pollen-food syndrome (oral allergy syndrome) is a form of allergy confined primarily to direct contact with raw fruits and vegetables in the oropharynx.[17] Initial sensitization to pollen proteins may result in symptoms when homologous proteins in particular fruits/vegetables are ingested, as described previously. This type of allergy is probably the most common of all food allergies and requires exposure to pollen seasons to develop.[4]

Symptoms are usually limited to the oropharynx with pruritus and mild angioedema, but progression to a systemic reaction may occur. Causal proteins are presumably heat-labile, because cooking the food typically abolishes reactions.

Although chronic asthma and allergic rhinitis are not typically solely attributable to food allergy, the same symptoms may accompany systemic food-allergic reactions.[2] Inhalation of airborne allergenic food proteins may also induce respiratory reactions when stable proteins become aerosolized during cooking or processing, such as boiling milk.

Food-induced anaphylaxis is a serious systemic allergic reaction that is rapid in onset and may cause death.[18] Symptoms vary and may affect any combination of organ systems among the skin, respiratory tract, gastrointestinal tract, and cardiovascular system. Symptoms may include an aura of "impending doom." Life-threatening symptoms include laryngeal edema, severe asthma, and cardiovascular compromise. Serum tryptase elevation is often not detected during food-associated anaphylaxis. Reactions may follow a biphasic course, with initial symptoms waning and recurrence of severe symptoms 1 to 2 hours later or longer. Fatal reactions appear to be more common in teenagers and young adults, possibly because of risk-taking behaviors. Victims typically have a diagnosed food allergy and asthma and delay treatment with epinephrine despite significant symptoms during a reaction.[6] *Food-associated, exercise-induced anaphylaxis* is a syndrome in which anaphylaxis only occurs if exercise follows ingestion of a causal food that is otherwise tolerated.

Mixed IgE/Non-IgE–Associated Food Allergies (Atopic Dermatitis/Eosinophilic Gastrointestinal Disease)

Studies using double-blind, placebo-controlled oral food challenges show that approximately 1 in 3 young children with moderate to severe *atopic dermatitis* has a food allergy.[19] There is controversy about the role of foods in the chronic rash.[2] There is agreement that children with moderate to severe atopic dermatitis are at increased risk of having immediate-type food-allergic reactions. When there is food-responsive dermatitis, studies reveal that food-specific IgE antibody is usually detectable to the trigger foods.[20] However, food-responsive disease has also been documented in children without IgE detectable to the causal food; therefore, cell-mediated mechanisms are likely involved.[20] Because of the chronic nature of the disorder and its waxing and waning course, it is difficult to associate symptoms with particular foods by history. Studies in children identify that more than 90% of reactions are attributed to "major" allergens, including milk, egg, wheat, and soy.[21]

Allergic eosinophilic esophagitis/gastroenteritis is a group of disorders characterized by eosinophilic inflammation in the gastrointestinal tract. Symptoms overlap those of other gastrointestinal disorders and may include dysphagia, vomiting, diarrhea, and malabsorption. Almost all children are food responsive, although it may be difficult to identify the offending food, and implicated foods may or may not be associated with evidence of IgE antibody.[22]

Non-IgE–Mediated Disorders

These disorders may also affect various target organs.[2,23] In regard to skin manifestations, contact dermatitis, a type IV hypersensitivity response, may occur from contact with foods. A rare pulmonary disorder affecting infants, Heiner syndrome or milk-induced pulmonary hemosiderosis, is associated with precipitating (IgG) antibodies to cow milk. Symptoms include anemia, pulmonary infiltrates, recurrent pneumonia, and growth failure, which resolve with milk elimination.

Several non-IgE mediated disorders of the gastrointestinal tract affect primarily infants.[24] *Food protein-induced proctocolitis* is characterized by mucous and blood in stools. Patients are usually breastfed infants, and the bleeding usually resolves with maternal exclusion of cow milk. The infant is otherwise well. Foods other than milk are sometimes implicated. Empiric dietary exclusion is commonly instituted. If rectal biopsy is performed, eosinophilic inflammation is observed. The disorder is not associated with detectable IgE antibody to milk and typically resolves by 1 year of age.[25] Infants with *food protein-induced enteropathy* experience diarrhea, poor growth, and edema attributable to hypoproteinemia caused by malabsorption when ingesting the causal food. A dramatic form of non-IgE mediated gastrointestinal food allergy is *food protein-induced enterocolitis syndrome*. The onset is usually in infancy and is characterized by a symptom complex of profuse vomiting and heme positive diarrhea, failure to thrive, and potentially dehydration and shock during chronic ingestion of the causal protein.[26] These infants also may develop acidemia and methemoglobinemia and present with symptoms mimicking sepsis, including an elevated peripheral polymophonuclear leukocyte count. Cow milk and soy are most often responsible, but grains, such as rice and oat, and poultry are increasingly recognized triggers.[27] Among those with reactions to cow milk, there is an increased risk of reactions to soy. Ingestion of the causal protein after resolution of symptoms may lead to a delayed (about 2 hours) recurrence of symptoms that may be severe and include shock. Resolution of the allergy usually occurs in 2 to 3 years, but readministration of the causal protein can trigger severe reactions and is typically undertaken under controlled settings with an intravenous line in place to administer steroids and hydration.

Diagnosis

The clinical evaluation of an adverse reaction to food requires a careful history and physical examination to determine the type of adverse response, whether potentially IgE or non-IgE associated.[2] Important factors to consider include the types of symptoms, the chronicity, reproducibility, and alternative explanations for symptoms. If symptoms indicate a nonimmune etiology, additional evaluation can be directed to the specific suspicion. For example, lactose intolerance may be confirmed through breath hydrogen testing. For chronic disorders, such as atopic dermatitis and eosinophilic gastroenteritis, the identification of suspect foods is difficult, because food is ingested throughout the day and symptoms are often chronic with a waxing and waning course. Symptom diaries are helpful but rarely diagnostic. In addition, individuals with these disorders often sensitized to multiple foods, many of which may not be causing illness. Care in selecting and interpreting the tests is paramount, and consideration of the previously reviewed epidemiology and pathophysiology of food allergies is helpful for test selection and interpretation.

Following a history, tests for food-specific IgE antibodies may be performed. The test modalities include skin prick tests, performed using a probe to introduce food protein to the superficial skin layer, or serum tests. The tests have similar performance characteristics. They are generally very sensitive (~75%-95%) and modestly specific (~30%-60%).[1] Skin prick tests are used on rash-free skin while the patient is avoiding antihistamines; intradermal skin tests should not be used. Although commercial extracts are available for performing skin prick tests for many foods, fresh extracts, particularly when testing fruits and vegetables for which proteins are prone to degradation, may be more sensitive. If IgE antibody specific for the food protein is present, a wheal and flare will occur that is compared to positive (histamine) and negative (saline) controls. The skin prick test is available to allergists and has advantages of immediate results and low cost.

A more widely available test is a serum test for food-specific IgE antibodies. There are 3 commercial manufacturers of the test[28]; results between them vary, probably because the reagents have slight differences in the proteins displayed.[29] Previous generation tests used radioactivity (radioallergosorbent test [RAST]), but these assays are no longer used.

A positive skin prick test or serum IgE test result merely indicates that food-specific IgE is present, a state termed *sensitization*. Sensitization does not confirm an allergy.[2] Increasingly larger wheal diameters or increasing concentrations of IgE antibodies are associated with increasingly higher probability that the test reflects clinical allergy. In a limited number of studies of a few foods in infants and/or children, diagnostic values associated with very high (≥95%) predictive values for reactions have been determined, although not universally confirmed.[1,30-32]

Food-specific IgE may be detected despite tolerance of a food or may remain detectable but typically declines as a food allergy resolves. Obtaining "panels" of food allergy tests without consideration of history is not a good practice, because numerous irrelevant positive results may result, creating confusion and anxiety. History is key for test selection and interpretation. Food-specific IgE test results are expected to be negative when the pathophysiology of the response is consistent with non-IgE–mediated reactions. However, acute anaphylactic reactions may also

VI

occasionally occur despite a negative test result,[33,34] so caution is needed when evaluating a patient with a convincing history but a negative test result. Neither the size of the skin prick test reaction nor concentration of IgE in serum usefully predicts the type or severity of reaction. The atopy patch test, which is performed by placing the food allergen on the skin under occlusion for 48 hours and assessing for a delayed rash at 24 to 72 hours, shows some promise for diagnosing non-IgE–mediated disorders, but more studies are needed to determine utility.[1] There are other tests that have been touted for the diagnosis of food allergy but have never been found useful in blinded studies. These tests, which are not recommended, include measurement of IgG_4 antibody, provocation-neutralization (drops placed under the tongue or injected to diagnose and treat various symptoms), and applied kinesiology (muscle strength testing).[2] A clinical report from the American Academy of Pediatrics (AAP) on the topic of allergy testing emphasized the benefits and limitations of the tests, and provides additional recommendations as summarized in the text box.[35]

AAP

Summary of IgE Test Characteristics and Limitations

- Treatment decisions for infants and children with allergy should be made on the basis of the appropriate diagnosis and identification of causative allergens, which may be identified through directed specific IgE testing.
- Allergy tests for specific IgE must be selected and interpreted in the context of a clinical presentation; test relevance may vary according to the patient's age, allergen exposure, and performance characteristics of the test.
- Positive specific IgE test results indicate sensitization, which is not equivalent to clinical allergy. Large panels of indiscriminately performed screening tests may, therefore, provide misleading information.
- Tests for specific IgE may be influenced by cross-reactive proteins that may or may not have clinical relevance to disease.
- Increasingly higher levels of specific IgE (higher concentrations on serum tests or skin prick test wheal size) generally correlate with an increased risk of clinical allergy.
- Specific IgE test results typically do not reflect severity of allergies.
- Tests for allergen-specific IgG antibodies are not helpful for diagnosing allergies.
- Consultation with a board-certified allergist-immunologist should be considered, because test limitations often warrant additional evaluation to confirm the role of specific allergens.

Sicherer SH, Wood RA; American Academy of Pediatrics, Section on Allergy and Immunology. Allergy testing in childhood: using allergen-specific IgE tests. *Pediatrics*. 2012;129(1):193-197[35]

For evaluation of chronic diseases, such as atopic dermatitis and eosinophilic esophagitis, improvement of symptoms during dietary elimination of suspected foods provides presumptive evidence of causality. Elimination diets can be undertaken by removing foods suspected to be causing symptoms, removing all but a selected group of foods that are rarely allergenic (oligoantigenic diet), or giving an elemental diet consisting only of a hypoallergenic extensively hydrolyzed formula or a nonallergenic amino acid-based formula. The elemental diet provides the most definitive trial, but is difficult for children and teenagers to follow. The type of elimination diet selected will depend on *a priori* reasoning concerning offending foods based on history and epidemiology, and, when appropriate, the results of tests for IgE antibody. The length of trial depends on the type of symptoms, but 1 to 6 weeks is usually the range required. A dietitian may be needed to ensure nutritional sufficiency of trial diets. For breastfed infants, maternal dietary elimination is required. When a food to which IgE has been demonstrated is removed from the diet during a chronic disorder, it is possible for reintroduction to induce severe reactions.[36] Thus, guidance from an allergist is prudent.

When history and IgE testing have not confirmed an allergy, or when the development of tolerance is suspected, an oral food challenge may be required to confirm clinical allergy.[1,2] An oral food challenge is performed by feeding gradually increasing amounts of the suspected food under medical observation.[37] Oral food challenges are performed either openly, where the patient and physician know the food being tested is being ingested, or blinded by camouflaging the food in a carrier food. The double-blind placebo-controlled food challenge is least prone to bias and is considered the "gold standard." Briefly, this format of oral food challenge has a third party develop 2 feedings that are identical in taste/texture but only one has the test allergen. The oral food challenge is randomized such that true or placebo doses are given, for example on separate days, and the patient and observer are not aware of the content. The oral food challenge can be used to evaluate any type of adverse response. For non-IgE-mediated reactions, the oral food challenge is usually the only means of diagnosis. Feeding tests, particularly in IgE-mediated reactions and enterocolitis syndrome, can induce severe reactions. The supervising clinician, usually an allergist, must have medications and supplies for resuscitation immediately available to manage reactions. Negative challenges should always be followed by a supervised open feeding of a relevant portion of the tested food in its commonly prepared state. More details about undertaking oral food challenges are provided in a recent report.[37]

Treatment

Dietary Avoidance

The mainstay of treatment is avoidance of the food and preparation for treatment in the event of an accidental ingestion leading to an allergic reaction. Most

VI

formula-fed infants who are allergic to standard cow milk formulas will tolerate a formula labeled "hypoallergenic" for infants with milk allergy (eg, an extensively hydrolyzed, casein-based formula). If the infant is reactive to these cow milk-derived formulas, an amino acid-based formula should be tolerated. Alternatively, a soy-based formula may be selected, because it is usually tolerated among infants with IgE-mediated cow milk allergy, although soy may present a higher risk for infants with enterocolitis syndrome. Foods in the maternal diet may trigger reactions in highly sensitive breastfed infants who are allergic to the particular food allergen. Therefore, maternal avoidance of the allergen may be required.

For children on limited diets, nutritional counseling and growth monitoring is recommended.[2] In the United States, labeling laws (see Chapter 52) require plain English disclosure of the "major" food allergens—milk, egg, wheat, soy, peanut, tree nuts, fish, and shellfish. The specific type of food is required to be named for categorical types (eg, cod, shrimp, walnut). Currently, additional potent allergens, such as sesame, are not included in the laws. Advisory labels (ie, "may contain peanut") are not regulated, are increasingly common, and reflect variable risks.[38,39] Strict avoidance, therefore, requires avoidance of products with advisory labeling. Cross-contamination and errors in restaurants are an additional obstacle, so it is imperative that individuals notify and discuss their allergy with restaurant personnel, who may need some coaching about situations in which foods may become contaminated with allergens, such as in fryers, shared bowls, cutting boards, etc.[40,41] For children, dietary management in schools can be difficult, because food sharing, school projects using foods, parties, lack of on-site medical personnel, and other issues arise.[42] Ingestion, rather than skin or air exposure, is the primary concern for avoidance,[43] although attention should be paid to avoid fumes of allergens (eg, boiling milk, steaming shellfish) and, for adolescents, passionate kissing when a partner recently consumed the allergen.[44]

Although strict avoidance is generally advised, there is a growing body of literature indicating that, in some cases, this may not be necessary.[45] Approximately 70% of children with allergic reactions to milk products or egg can tolerate these foods when they are heated extensively—for example, baked into muffins or breads.[46-48] It is presumed that heating these particular foods results in conformational changes in the proteins, allowing ingestion for people with a milder form of the allergy, probably a phenotype that is also more likely to resolve the allergy. Adding such foods to the diet can improve quality of life and nutrition, but the effect on the natural course of allergy is not well studied. Early evidence suggests that immune responses to the addition of these foods are similar to those seen during successful active immunotherapy—for example, an increase in food-specific IgG antibodies is noted, and some suppression of IgE responses is also observed, and there is some indication of accelerated tolerance.[49] However, caution is advised with this approach, because some children experience anaphylaxis to the heated products.

Medical Management

In the event of an allergic reaction, antihistamines may be required to reduce itching and rash. However, for children experiencing more severe symptoms of anaphylaxis with respiratory and/or cardiovascular symptoms, additional therapies are required.[2] Self-injectable epinephrine should be prescribed for those at risk of anaphylaxis, as described in national guidelines and an AAP clinical report, as summarized in the text box.[2,50] There are no adequate fixed-dose autoinjectors for children weighing less than 15 kg, and physicians may consider alternatives, such as ampule/syringe, particularly for infants younger than 10 kg, although administration in this form is problematic. It is essential to periodically review the indications and technique of administration of self-injectable epinephrine. Patients must be instructed that following the administration of the medications and prompt transportation to an emergency facility (ie, ambulance) should be sought with prolonged observation (>4 hours), because recurrence of severe symptoms is possible. Individuals with potential shock should remain prone with legs raised; rising upright without proper treatment has rarely been reported to result in death as a result of "empty ventricle syndrome."[51] Patients should obtain medical jewelry identifying their allergy and be reminded to update expired epinephrine injectors. An important component of the school or camp management of food allergy is to have a clear written emergency plan in place, medications readily available, and school personnel trained in recognizing and treating reactions.[52] Teenagers are at special risk of fatal reactions,[6] probably because of risk-taking behaviors.[53] It is, therefore, important to encourage education of the affected teenager, school staff, and his or her friends about the allergy and when to treat with epinephrine.[52]

AAP

Candidates for Prescription of Self-Injectable Epinephrine and Dosing

Self-injectable epinephrine should be prescribed for children with:
  Prior systemic allergic reactions
  Food allergy and asthma
  Food allergy to peanut, tree nut, fish, or shellfish (and considered for any IgE-mediated food allergy)
Dosing of fixed dose epinephrine auto-injectors (0.15 or 0.3 mg)(see Boyce et al[2] and the AAP clinical report[50] for additional discussion)
  Children weighing <25 kg: 0.15 mg auto-injector
  Children weighing ≥25 kg: 0.3 mg auto-injector
Epinephrine solution (1:1000): 0.01 mg/kg, maximum 0.5 mg, intramuscularly
      Sicherer SH, Simons FE; American Academy of Pediatrics, Section on Allergy and Immunology. Self-injectable epinephrine for first-aid management of anaphylaxis. *Pediatrics.* 2007;119(3):638-646

VI

The emotional toll of living with food allergy should not be minimized. Various studies have identified a serious effect on quality of life as well as increased anxiety.[54-58] Children with food allergies may be subjected to bullying as well.[59] Therefore, discussion of the psychosocial factors involved with management, ensuring that families are coping appropriately and not overly isolating themselves, and considering mental health referral are important components of management.

Natural History

Most children (approximately 85%) lose their sensitivity to most allergenic foods (egg, milk, wheat, soy) within the first 3 to 5 years of life.[60] Recent studies from a referral center indicate that the rate of resolution may be slowing, but is still usually achieved prior to adolescence.[61,62] In contrast, allergy to peanut, tree nuts, and seafood is rarely lost. Approximately 20% of peanut-allergic children younger than 2 years and 5% to 10% of those with tree nut allergy may achieve tolerance by school age.[63,64] Tolerance is typically determined by repeated testing, with reduced food-specific IgE antibodies possibly indicating resolution, and with physician-supervised oral food challenges.

Prevention

Early approaches for prevention of food allergy focused on having infants avoid allergenic foods.[65] This approach was based partly on studies demonstrating that infants ingesting hypoallergenic forms of cow milk formula had less atopic dermatitis than those randomized to whole protein cow milk.[66] However, extensive delays in introducing potentially allergenic foods from otherwise well but "at risk" infants, based on their family history of atopy, have not been well studied. Concerns have arisen that such delays may not be preventive. In fact, there are studies suggesting that delayed ingestion may allow more time for sensitization by routes such as skin or respiratory exposure, while mechanisms of oral tolerance are circumvented during a lack of ingestion. This concept has support in the observation that ingestion of peanut by family members is associated with a child's peanut allergy,[67] whereas maternal ingestion was not, or that use of peanut-containing skin creams was a risk factor for peanut allergy in young children.[68] Recent guidelines suggest a beneficial role for exclusive breastfeeding of infants at "high risk" of developing atopic disease (eg, infants with a parent or sibling with an atopic disease) for the first 3 to 6 months of life and for avoiding supplementation with cow milk or soy formulas in favor of hypoallergenic formulas if breastfeeding is not possible, but no additional dietary restrictions.[69] Some conflicting studies have maintained this as a very active area of investigation.[70] Primary prevention must be distinguished from secondary prevention; once a child has demonstrated allergies, for example to milk, there is an increased risk there will be or are concomitant food allergies to foods such as egg or peanut.[71] An AAP clinical report on atopic disease is summarized in the text box.

AAP

Atopy Prevention Through Diet

- There is lack of evidence that maternal dietary restrictions during pregnancy play a significant role in the prevention of atopic disease.
- Antigen avoidance during lactation does not prevent atopic disease, with the possible exception of atopic eczema, although more data are needed.
- For infants at high risk of atopic disease, exclusive breastfeeding for at least 4 months compared with feeding intact cow milk protein formula decreases the cumulative incidence of atopic dermatitis and cow milk allergy in the first 2 years of life.
- There is evidence that exclusive breastfeeding for at least 3 months protects against wheezing in early life, but evidence of long-term protection against asthma is lacking.
- In studies of infants at high risk of developing atopic disease who are not breastfed exclusively for 4 to 6 months or are formula fed, there is modest evidence that atopic dermatitis may be delayed or prevented by the use of extensively or partially hydrolyzed formulas, compared with cow milk formula, in early childhood. Not all formulas have the same protective benefit. Extensively hydrolyzed formulas may be more effective than partially hydrolyzed ones. The higher cost of the hydrolyzed formulas must be considered.
- There is no convincing evidence for the use of soy-based infant formula for the purpose of allergy prevention.
- Although solid foods should not be introduced before 4 to 6 months of age, there is no current convincing evidence that delaying their introduction beyond this period has a significant protective effect on the development of atopic disease.

From Greer FR, Sicherer SH, Burks AW; American Academy of Pediatrics, Committee on Nutrition and Section on Allergy and Immunology. Effects of early nutritional interventions on the development of atopic disease in infants and children: the role of maternal dietary restriction, breastfeeding, timing of introduction of complementary foods, and hydrolyzed formulas. *Pediatrics*. 2008;121(1):183-191[69]

Summary

Food allergy is common and appears to be increasing. An accurate diagnosis of food allergy requires rational use of the available diagnostic tests, relying heavily on clinical history for test selection and interpretation and recognizing that a physician-supervised oral food challenge is often required. Current management requires avoidance and reactionary treatment in the event of symptoms. However, studies are underway for improved therapies using strategies such as immunotherapy, anti-IgE antibodies, and others that may provide more definitive therapy in the future.[72]

VI

References

1. Chapman JA, Bernstein IL, Lee RE, Oppenheimer J, Nicklas RA, Portnoy, JM, et al. Food allergy: a practice parameter. *Ann Allergy Asthma Immunol*. 2006;96(3 Suppl 2):S1-68

2. Boyce JA, Assa'ad A, Burks AW, Jones SM, Sampson HA, Wood RA et al. Guidelines for the diagnosis and management of food allergy in the United States: report of the NIAID-sponsored expert panel. *J Allergy Clin Immunol*. 2010;126(6 Suppl):S1-58

3. Branum AM, Lukacs SL. Food allergy among children in the United States. *Pediatrics*. 2009;124(6):1549-1555

4. Sicherer SH. Epidemiology of food allergy. *J Allergy Clin Immunol*. 2011;127(3):594-602

5. Gupta RS, Springston EE, Warrier MJ, et al. The prevalence, severity, and distribution of childhood food allergy in the United States. *Pediatrics*. 2011;128(1):e9-e17

6. Bock SA, Munoz-Furlong A, Sampson HA. Further fatalities caused by anaphylactic reactions to food, 2001-2006. *J Allergy Clin Immunol*. 2007;119(4):1016-1018

7. Vickery BP, Scurlock AM, Jones SM, Burks AW. Mechanisms of immune tolerance relevant to food allergy. *J Allergy Clin Immunol*. 2011;127(3):576-584

8. Sicherer SH. Clinical implications of cross-reactive food allergens. *J Allergy Clin Immunol*. 2001;108(6):881-890

9. Simon RA. Adverse reactions to food additives. *Curr Allergy Asthma Rep*. 2003;3(1):62-66

10. Sicherer SH, Muñoz-Furlong A, Godbold JH, Sampson HA. US prevalence of self-reported peanut, tree nut, and sesame allergy: 11-year follow-up. *J Allergy Clin Immunol*. 2010;125(6):1322-1326

11. Ben Shoshan M, Kagan RS, Alizadehfar R, Joseph L, Turnbull E, St Pierre Y et al. Is the prevalence of peanut allergy increasing? A 5-year follow-up study in children in Montreal. *J Allergy Clin Immunol*. 2009;123(4):783-788

12. Hourihane JO, Aiken R, Briggs R, Gudgeon LA, Grimshaw KE, Dunngalvin A et al. The impact of government advice to pregnant mothers regarding peanut avoidance on the prevalence of peanut allergy in United Kingdom children at school entry. *J Allergy Clin Immunol*. 2007;119(5):1197-1202

13. Liu AH, Jaramillo R, Sicherer SH, Wood RA, Bock SA, Burks AW et al. National prevalence and risk factors for food allergy and relationship to asthma: results from the National Health and Nutrition Examination Survey 2005-2006. *J Allergy Clin Immunol*. 2010;126(4):798-806

14. Nicolaou N, Poorafshar M, Murray C, Simpson A, Winell H, Kerry G et al. Allergy or tolerance in children sensitized to peanut: prevalence and differentiation using component-resolved diagnostics. *J Allergy Clin Immunol*. 2010;125(1):191-197

15. Lack G. Epidemiologic risks for food allergy. *J Allergy Clin Immunol*. 2008;121(6):1331-1336

16. Sicherer SH, Sampson HA. Peanut allergy: emerging concepts and approaches for an apparent epidemic. *J Allergy Clin Immunol*. 2007;120(3):491-503

17. Ortolani C, Ispano M, Pastorello E, Bigi A, Ansaloni R. The oral allergy syndrome. *Ann Allergy*. 1988;61(6 Pt 2):47-52

18. Sampson HA, Munoz-Furlong A, Campbell RL, Adkinson NF, Jr., Bock SA, Branum A et al. Second symposium on the definition and management of anaphylaxis: Summary report-Second National Institute of Allergy and Infectious Disease/Food Allergy and Anaphylaxis Network symposium. *J Allergy Clin Immunol*. 2006;117(2):391-397

19. Sicherer SH, Sampson HA. Food hypersensitivity and atopic dermatitis: pathophysiology, epidemiology, diagnosis, and management. *J Allergy Clin Immunol*. 1999;104(3 Pt 2):S114-S122

20. Mehl A, Rolinck-Werninghaus C, Staden U, Verstege A, Wahn U, Beyer K et al. The atopy patch test in the diagnostic workup of suspected food-related symptoms in children. *J Allergy Clin Immunol*. 2006;118(4):923-929

21. Ellman LK, Chatchatee P, Sicherer SH, Sampson HA. Food hypersensitivity in two groups of children and young adults with atopic dermatitis evaluated a decade apart. *Pediatr Allergy Immunol*. 2002;13(4):295-298

22. Liacouras CA, Furuta GT, Hirano I, Atkins D, Attwood SE, Bonis PA et al. Eosinophilic esophagitis: Updated consensus recommendations for children and adults. *J Allergy Clin Immunol*, 2011 [epub ahead of print]

23. Sicherer SH, Sampson HA. Food allergy. *J Allergy Clin Immunol*. 2010;125(2 Suppl 2):S116-S125

24. Sampson HA, Sicherer SH, Birnbaum AH. AGA Technical Review on the Evaluation of Food Allergy in Gastrointestinal Disorders. *Gastroenterology*. 2001;120(4):1026-1040

25. Ravelli A, Villanacci V, Chiappa S, Bolognini S, Manenti S, Fuoti M. Dietary protein-induced proctocolitis in childhood. *Am J Gastroenterol*. 2008;103(10):2605-2612

26. Sicherer SH. Food protein-induced enterocolitis syndrome: case presentations and management lessons. *J Allergy Clin Immunol*. 2005;115(1):149-156

27. Nowak-Wegrzyn A, Sampson HA, Wood RA, Sicherer SH. Food protein-induced enterocolitis syndrome caused by solid food proteins. *Pediatrics*. 2003;111(4 Pt 1):829-835

28. Hamilton RG, Williams PB. Human IgE antibody serology: a primer for the practicing North American allergist/immunologist. *J Allergy Clin Immunol*. 2010;126(1):33-38

29. Wang J, Godbold JH, Sampson HA. Correlation of serum allergy (IgE) tests performed by different assay systems. *J Allergy Clin Immunol*. 2008;121(5):1219-1224

30. Sporik R, Hill DJ, Hosking CS. Specificity of allergen skin testing in predicting positive open food challenges to milk, egg and peanut in children. *Clin Exp Allergy*. 2000;30(11):1541-1546

31. Sampson HA. Utility of food-specific IgE concentrations in predicting symptomatic food allergy. *J Allergy Clin Immunol*. 2001;107(5):891-896

32. Sicherer SH, Sampson HA. 9. Food allergy. *J Allergy Clin Immunol*. 2006;117(2 Suppl Mini-Primer):S470-S475

33. Leduc V, Moneret-Vautrin DA, Tzen JT, Morisset M, Guerin L, Kanny G. Identification of oleosins as major allergens in sesame seed allergic patients. *Allergy*. 2006;61(3):349-356

34. Hauswirth DW, Burks AW. Banana anaphylaxis with a negative commercial skin test. *J Allergy Clin Immunol*. 2005;115(3):632-633

VI

35. Sicherer SH, Wood RA; American Academy of Pediatrics, Section on Allergy and Immunology. Allergy testing in childhood: using allergen-specific IgE tests. *Pediatrics*. 2012;129(1):193-197

36. David TJ. Anaphylactic shock during elimination diets for severe atopic dermatitis. *Arch Dis Child*. 1984;59:983-986

37. Nowak-Wegrzyn A, Assa'ad AH, Bahna SL, Bock SA, Sicherer SH, Teuber SS. Work Group report: oral food challenge testing. *J Allergy Clin Immunol*. 2009;123(6 Suppl):S365-S383

38. Pieretti MM, Chung D, Pacenza R, Slotkin T, Sicherer SH. Audit of manufactured products: use of allergen advisory labels and identification of labeling ambiguities. *J Allergy Clin Immunol*. 2009;124(2):337-341

39. Ford LS, Taylor SL, Pacenza R, Niemann LM, Lambrecht DM, Sicherer SH. Food allergen advisory labeling and product contamination with egg, milk, and peanut. *J Allergy Clin Immunol*. 2010;126(2):384-385

40. Ahuja R, Sicherer SH. Food-allergy management from the perspective of restaurant and food establishment personnel. *Ann Allergy Asthma Immunol*. 2007;98(4):344-348

41. Furlong TJ, DeSimone J, Sicherer SH. Peanut and tree nut allergic reactions in restaurants and other food establishments. *J Allergy Clin Immunol*. 2001;108(5 Part 1):867-870

42. Young MC, Munoz-Furlong A, Sicherer SH. Management of food allergies in schools: a perspective for allergists. *J Allergy Clin Immunol*. 2009;124(2):175-182

43. Simonte SJ, Ma S, Mofidi S, Sicherer SH. Relevance of casual contact with peanut butter in children with peanut allergy. *J Allergy Clin Immunol*. 2003;112(1):180-182

44. Maloney JM, Chapman MD, Sicherer SH. Peanut allergen exposure through saliva: assessment and interventions to reduce exposure. *J Allergy Clin Immunol*. 2006;118(3):719-724

45. Kim JS, Sicherer S. Should avoidance of foods be strict in prevention and treatment of food allergy? *Curr Opin Allergy Clin Immunol*. 2010;10(3):252-257

46. Lemon-Mule H, Sampson HA, Sicherer SH, Shreffler WG, Noone S, Nowak-Wegrzyn A. Immunologic changes in children with egg allergy ingesting extensively heated egg. *J Allergy Clin Immunol*. 2008;122(5):977-983

47. Nowak-Wegrzyn A, Bloom KA, Sicherer SH et al. Tolerance to extensively heated milk in children with cow milk allergy. *J Allergy Clin Immunol*. 2008;122(2):342-347

48. Wang J, Lin J, Bardina L, Goldis M, Nowak-Wegrzyn A, Shreffler WG et al. Correlation of IgE/IgG4 milk epitopes and affinity of milk-specific IgE antibodies with different phenotypes of clinical milk allergy. *J Allergy Clin Immunol*. 2010;125(3):695-702

49. Kim JS, Nowak-Wegrzyn A, Sicherer SH, Noone S, Moshier EL, Sampson HA. Dietary baked milk accelerates the resolution of cow milk allergy in children. *J Allergy Clin Immunol*. 2011 [epub ahead of print]

50. Sicherer SH, Simons FE; American Academy of Pediatrics, Section on Allergy and Immunology. Self-injectable epinephrine for first-aid management of anaphylaxis. *Pediatrics*. 2007;119(3):638-646

51. Pumphrey RS. Fatal posture in anaphylactic shock. *J Allergy Clin Immunol*. 2003;112(2):451-452

52. Sicherer SH, Mahr T; American Academy of Pediatrics, Section on Allergy and Immunology. Management of food allergy in the school setting. *Pediatrics.* 2010;126(6):1232-1239

53. Sampson MA, Muñoz-Furlong A, Sicherer SH. Risk-taking and coping strategies of adolescents and young adults with food allergy. *J Allergy Clin Immunol.* 2006;117(6):1440-1445

54. Flokstra-de Blok BM, Dunngalvin A, Vlieg-Boerstra BJ, Oude Elberink JN, Duiverman EJ, Hourihane JO et al. Development and validation of the self-administered Food Allergy Quality of Life Questionnaire for adolescents. *J Allergy Clin Immunol.* 2008;122(1):139-144

55. King RM, Knibb RC, Hourihane JO. Impact of peanut allergy on quality of life, stress and anxiety in the family. *Allergy.* 2009;64(3):461-468

56. Cummings AJ, Knibb RC, Erlewyn-Lajeunesse M, King RM, Roberts G, Lucas JS. Management of nut allergy influences quality of life and anxiety in children and their mothers. *Pediatr Allergy Immunol.* 2010;21(4 Pt 1):586-594

57. Resnick ES, Pieretti MM, Maloney J, Noone S, Munoz-Furlong A, Sicherer SH. Development of a questionnaire to measure quality of life in adolescents with food allergy: the FAQL-teen. *Ann Allergy Asthma Immunol.* 2010;105(5):364-368

58. Cohen BL, Noone S, Muñoz-Furlong A, Sicherer SH. Development of a questionnaire to measure quality of life in families with a child with food allergy. *J Allergy Clin Immunol.* 2004;114(5):1159-1163

59. Lieberman JA, Weiss C, Furlong TJ, Sicherer M, Sicherer SH. Bullying among pediatric patients with food allergy. *Ann Allergy Asthma Immunol.* 2010;105(4):282-286

60. Wood RA. The natural history of food allergy. *Pediatrics.* 2003;111(6 pt 3):1631-1637

61. Skripak JM, Matsui EC, Mudd K, Wood RA. The natural history of IgE-mediated cow milk allergy. *J Allergy Clin Immunol.* 2007;120(5):1172-1177

62. Savage JH, Matsui EC, Skripak JM, Wood RA. The natural history of egg allergy. *J Allergy Clin Immunol.* 2007;120(6):1413-1417

63. Fleischer DM, Conover-Walker MK, Christie L, Burks AW, Wood RA. The natural progression of peanut allergy: Resolution and the possibility of recurrence. *J Allergy Clin Immunol.* 2003;112(1):183-189

64. Fleischer DM, Conover-Walker MK, Matsui EC, Wood RA. The natural history of tree nut allergy. *J Allergy Clin Immunol.* 2005;116(5):1087-1093

65. American Academy of Pediatrics. Committee on Nutrition. Hypoallergenic infant formulas. *Pediatrics.* 2000;106(2 Pt 1):346-349

66. von Berg A, Filipiak-Pittroff B, Kramer U, et al. Preventive effect of hydrolyzed infant formulas persists until age 6 years: long-term results from the German Infant Nutritional Intervention Study (GINI). *J Allergy Clin Immunol.* 2008;121(6):1442-1447

67. Fox AT, Sasieni P, Du TG, Syed H, Lack G. Household peanut consumption as a risk factor for the development of peanut allergy. *J Allergy Clin Immunol.* 2009;123(2):417-423

68. Lack G, Fox D, Northstone K, Golding J. Factors associated with the development of peanut allergy in childhood. *N Engl J Med.* 2003;348(11):977-985

VI

69. Greer FR, Sicherer SH, Burks AW; American Academy of Pediatrics, Committee on Nutrition and Section on Allergy and Immunology. Effects of early nutritional interventions on the development of atopic disease in infants and children: the role of maternal dietary restriction, breastfeeding, timing of introduction of complementary foods, and hydrolyzed formulas. *Pediatrics*. 2008;121(1):183-191

70. Sicherer SH, Wood RA, Stablein D, Lindblad R, Burks AW, Liu AH et al. Maternal consumption of peanut during pregnancy is associated with peanut sensitization in atopic infants. *J Allergy Clin Immunol*. 2010;126(6):1191-1197

71. Sicherer SH, Wood RA, Stablein D, Burks AW, Liu AH, Jones SM et al. Immunologic features of infants with milk or egg allergy enrolled in an observational study (Consortium of Food Allergy Research) of food allergy. *J Allergy Clin Immunol*. 2010;125(5):1077-1083

72. Sicherer SH, Sampson HA. Food allergy: recent advances in pathophysiology and treatment. *Annu Rev Med*. 2009;60:261-277

Chapter 36

Nutrition and Immunity

Introduction

Nutrients play integral roles in the development and function of the immune system. The keystones of an effective immune response are rapid cellular proliferation and early synthesis of regulatory and/or protective proteins, all of which require a ready supply of nutrients as substrates, cofactors, and structural components. Therefore, insufficiency of one or more essential nutrients is potentially rate limiting in the development and maintenance of immune responses. Similarly, inflammation and other immune responses alter a person's nutritional status through sequestration of minerals (eg, iron and zinc), impaired absorption, increased nutrient loss, or altered nutrient utilization. Although the effects of the immune system on nutritional status are important during inflammation and other acute disease states, this discussion focuses on the role of nutrition in immune system development and effects of primary nutrient deficiencies on immune responses.

Nutrient-immune interactions are of special concern in infants and children because of the increased vulnerability of the developing immune system. Early in life, systemic humoral immunity is strongly dependent on maternal immunoglobulin (Ig) G acquired transplacentally, and specific mucosal immunity relies, to a great extent, on secretory IgA supplied via breastfeeding. This reliance on maternal factors is attributable to the paucity of production of those immunoglobulin isotypes during early infancy, the decreased repertoire of antibody binding specificities during that period, and the slow development of antibody responses to polysaccharide antigens during the first 2 to 3 years of age.[1] Adult concentrations of serum IgM and IgG do not develop until 4 to 6 years of age.[2] The thymus and other immune tissues continue to grow and develop through puberty. Thus, definitions of "normal" immune status and responses depend on a child's age and stage of development. Factors such as prematurity or low birth weight will further delay the development of the immune system.

To appreciate the importance to the child of nutrient-immune interactions, the ontogeny of the immune system must be considered in the context of the child's overall growth and development. Periods of rapid growth velocity increase the demands of muscle, organ, and other tissues on the available nutrient pool. If there is an insufficient supply of any nutrient, growth retardation and/or other functional deficits will occur. In some cases (eg, "catch-up" growth), nutrient repletion will promote nearly full recovery from a prior insult. In other cases (eg, cognitive development), moderate to severe nutritional insults early in life may overcome the system's plasticity and recovery may not be possible.

VI

In the case of the immune system, the degree and reversibility of an immune defect depends on the timing, duration, severity, and type of nutritional insufficiency. Early and/or severe nutrient deficiencies appear to cause long-lasting effects on the immune system. Thymic involution and reduced immune responsiveness occur during moderate to severe general undernutrition and various single nutrient deficiencies. Even after nutritional supplementation, immune responsiveness may not recover fully in previously malnourished children. Animal studies indicate that severe nutrient deficiencies during early development, especially in utero and in the preweaning period, may result in lifelong and even perhaps transgenerational immune deficiencies.[3] For example, in the prenatal zinc deficiency mouse model, immune deficits appears to carry over to the second and third generation.[4] Thus, in the growing child with nutrient deficiencies, the combination of increased nutrient demands and a rapidly developing immune system provide great potential for permanent adverse outcomes.

Nutritional status influences the immune system at different levels. Subclinical or frank deficiencies of some micronutrients (see Micronutrients and Immunity section in this chapter) reduce the circulating levels and functional capacities of key immune cells and proteins. Other micronutrient deficiencies, including essential fatty acids, folate, zinc, and vitamin A, cause mucosal lesions or reduce mucosal integrity, thus increasing susceptibility to infections. The most severe outcomes occur among children in developing nations, where severe, combined nutrient deficiencies adversely affect many parts of the immune system. This review focuses on nutrient-immune interactions likely to be encountered among children in the United States or other resource-rich countries.

Early Nutritional-Immunologic System Interactions

Current research amply documents the influence of early nutrition on (1) immunologic responses, (2) the immediate risks to infectious diseases, and (3) possibly, the risks to immune-related conditions expressed in later life stages. These influences have played major roles in the formulation of recommendations for the nutritional management of infants. Recognition of these influences comes principally from studies of infants fed human milk or synthetic formulas.[5,6]

Beyond the well-recognized nutritional roles of the major organic macronutrients (proteins, carbohydrates, and lipids), the macronutrients in human milk also play functional roles related to the infant's immune competence and ontogenic stage of development. These immunologic roles are expressed either actively (ie, by modulating the infant's ability to respond to an immunologic challenge) or passively (ie, attenuating or preventing infection without altering the infant's immunologic development or ability to respond to a specific challenge).[7]

Several proteins in human milk have the potential to modulate specific and/or nonspecific immune responses before their degradation to amino acids and the subsequent fulfillment of the classical metabolic roles associated with dietary proteins. Among the 2 most frequently studied examples of proteins with this characteristic are secretory IgA and lactoferrin. Although breastfeeding's general protective roles against infection are well documented, the only specific human milk component clinically proven to be protective is secretory IgA. Its efficacy against *Vibrio cholerae* O antigen and enterotoxin, *Campylobacter* species, and enterotoxin-producing *Escherichia coli* has been documented by various investigators.[8] Secretory IgA provides passive protection, presumably by neutralizing pathogens and their toxins and interfering with their adherence to the infant's gastrointestinal and upper respiratory tracts.

Human milk secretory IgA, however, also may provide a mechanism for active protection. The identification of anti-idiotypic antibodies in milk suggests that human milk may aid the infant's production of the corresponding idiotypic antibody.[8] Secretion of anti-idiotypic antibodies and excretion in milk of potential pathogens, such as cytomegalovirus, concomitantly with the secretion of corresponding neutralizing antibodies may serve as important natural immunization strategies in early infancy.[9]

Other human milk proteins, such as cytokines, may influence the infant's immune system through alternative mechanisms. The identification in human milk of substantial amounts of immunomodulating cytokines, including those that are ordinarily proinflammatory (eg, tumor necrosis factor-alpha, interleukin [IL]-1, IL-6]),[10–13] anti-inflammatory (eg, transforming growth factor-beta and IL-10),[14,15] colony stimulating (eg, granulocyte-colony stimulating factor and macrophage colony-stimulating factor),[16,17] chemotactic (IL-8),[18] and others[19] raises the possibility of roles for human milk cytokines in leukocyte development, mobilization, and activation; the regulation of cytokine production; the expression of class I and class II histocompatibility antigens; the up-regulation of secretory component production by epithelial cells; and the production of IgA dimers required for the assembly of secretory IgA in the recipient infant. Furthermore, hormones and growth factors such as prolactin, transforming growth factor-beta and insulin-like growth factor-1 (IGF-1) are components of human milk that contribute to intestinal development and, thus, directly or indirectly to mucosal immunity.[20]

The earlier demonstrations of urinary excretion of intact and large fragments of lactoferrin by preterm infants fed human milk[21,22] and their maternal origin[23] raise the possibility of the postnatal uptake of other intact or biologically active fragments of immunoregulatory molecules of maternal origin by the infant at this and other developmental stages. The roles that these and other immunoregulatory

VI

components and antigenic exposure play in determining disparate antibody responses to immunization and to differences in "baseline" serum immunoglobulin concentrations between breastfed and formula-fed infants remain unclear.[24]

Lactoferrin's strong iron-binding capacity is a well-described example of a "nonspecific" immune modulating activity of a major human milk protein. This capacity presumably limits the availability to potentially pathogenic enteric flora of an essential mineral in the infant's gastrointestinal lumen by competing effectively with bacterial enterochelins for iron.[25] This competition limits the growth of iron-dependent pathogens in the infant's gastrointestinal lumen. Lactoferrin also appears to modulate inflammatory responses by influencing macrophage responses. Lactoferrin also is able to kill certain bacterial and fungal pathogens by the membrane damaging effect of a peptide C (lactoferrin-H) located near the terminus of the lactoferrin molecule.

Anti-inflammatory capacity is not unique to lactoferrin. It is shared by several of the antimicrobial agents and other factors in human milk.[26] Beyond its actions as a single agent, lactoferrin also acts with secretory IgA to mutually enhance each other's antibacterial efficacy.[24]

Although infants rely on carbohydrates as a key energy source, human milk carbohydrates also serve immune-related roles. Oligosaccharides and more complex glycoproteins and glycolipids serve as receptor analogs that interfere with the adherence of pathogens, such as pneumococci and *Haemophilus influenzae,* and of enterotoxins, such as those of *V cholerae* and *E coli,* to epithelial cells.[27] These molecules may account partially for human milk's protection against gastroenteritis, respiratory infections, and possibly otitis media.[8]

Similarly, lipids provide essential fatty acids for structuring membranes, serving as an important energy source and contributing to the infant's immunologic responses. The precursor role of essential fatty acids in the synthesis of functional components, such as prostaglandins, and the antiviral and antibacterial properties of the shorter-chain fatty acids, such as lauric acid, are examples of the immunologically related functions of dietary lipids. Certain products from the hydrolysis of human lipids lyse enveloped viruses.[28] The human fat globule membrane and its mucin component's ability to bind s-fimbriated *E coli* suggest another potential protective property of the milk's lipid fraction.[29]

Human milk also plays another important role. The normal development of the gastrointestinal tract is subdivided into 4 phases.[30] In the first phase, the infants' intestinal microflora resemble maternal flora and those of the surroundings encountered by infants during birth and the immediate postnatal period. Maternal intestinal flora is a source of colonization in the neonatal intestine. However, the vertical transmission of *E coli* strains from mother to infant during delivery is generally reported to be less than 50% in either resource-rich or developing countries.[31,32] Transfer of enterobacteria other than *E coli* from mother to infant occurs infrequently, but horizontal transfer of enterobacteria, including *E coli,* occurs between neonates in the nursery.[33] The second phase is affected significantly by whether infants are breastfed or formula fed. Although there is some inconsistency among published studies, presumably because of methodologic differences, generally, initial similarities between the floras of breastfed and formula-fed infants on day 7 of postnatal life diminish substantially by day 30, especially in developing countries. Breastfed infants have less enterococci and clostridia in their flora than do formula-fed infants, and breastfed infants have more staphylococci and at younger ages.[34] Generally, breastfed infants have fewer *Klebsiella, Enterobacter*, and *Citrobacter* organisms in their flora, and the strains of *E coli* found in the flora differ between feeding groups. For example, P-fimbriated *E coli* are less common and type 1-fimbriated *E coli* are more common in the flora of breastfed infants than in the flora of formula-fed infants. P-fimbriae is the virulence factor most often associated with urinary tract infections.[34] Previous reports of highly marked differences between breastfed and formula-fed infants in the bifidobacteria content of their flora have not been confirmed for unexplained reasons by more recent investigations.[34] The third phase relates to the period following the initial introduction of solid foods. During this period, enterococci, bacteroides, clostridia, anaerobic streptococci, and other bacteria increase in the breastfed infants' flora. Less marked changes occur in the flora of formula-fed infants.[29] In the fourth phase (the time following the introduction of an adult diet), although the intestinal flora of infants remains distinct from that of adults, the flora increasingly resemble adult patterns.

The short-term benefits of these nutritional-immunologic interactions are clear.[5,35] The frequency in breastfed infants of gastrointestinal infections is lower in resource-rich and developing populations. Also, even when rates of infections are similar among breastfed and nonbreastfed infants, the duration and severity of infection often are less for breastfed infants. Attenuation of clinical responses has been reported for both gastrointestinal (eg, rotavirus infection) and respiratory tract infections (eg, respiratory syncytial virus infections). Such positive outcomes become progressively more significant as the frequency and severity of microbial challenges rise.

Increasing evidence shows that microbe-host interactions at specific times of prenatal host immune development influence future immune responses in maintaining health and development of immune-mediated diseases; thus, maternal exposure to microbes and the subsequent colonization of the neonatal intestine affect immune responses of the infant, possibly into adulthood.[36] Neonatal intesti-

VI

nal colonization is influenced by whether delivery is vaginal or by cesarean section, whether the infant is breastfed or formula fed, and the use of antibiotics.

The possibility that the antimicrobial, anti-inflammatory, and immunoregulatory components in human milk have longer-lasting effects on the infant's immune system and the effects of breastfeeding on the development of allergic diseases remain controversial. If breastfeeding prevents certain allergic disorders, it is unclear whether those positive outcomes are attributable to delays in the introduction of potentially allergenic foods, immunoregulatory components in human milk, or the balance among specific nutrients. For example, Wright and Bolton[37] reported a significantly greater proportion of linoleic acid and a smaller proportion of dihomo-gamma-linolenic acid in the human milk lipid fraction of mothers of infants with atopic eczema compared with controls.

In addition, there is evidence that some breastfed infants become sensitized to certain maternally ingested foods by the passage of those food antigens into human milk.[38] The topic is, however, controversial, because some of these same dietary proteins may be detected in human milk from mothers whose infants are asymptomatic, and one of the major suspected dietary allergens, bovine beta-lactoglobulin, immunologically cross-reacts with a fragment of human beta-casein.[39] Therefore, the diagnosis of allergic reactions in the breastfed infant attributable to food allergens passed via breastfeeding depends on tedious dietary elimination/oral provocation procedures in the lactating woman. The management of such problems requires either a cessation of breastfeeding or a long-term elimination of the food allergen from the maternal diet, and severely atopic infants may require support by a pediatric allergist. Current evidence indicates that breastfeeding for at least the first 4 months compared with formula feeding prevents or delays atopic disease, but there is no evidence to support maternal dietary restriction during pregnancy nor to delay introduction of solid foods beyond 4 to 6 months[40] (see also Chapter 35: Food Sensitivity).

The length of time infants are breastfed and the timing of the introduction of complementary foods and cow milk may have an effect on the occurrence of islet autoimmunity and later development of type 1 diabetes mellitus, particularly those at higher risk by HLA genotype and family history of type 1 diabetes mellitus.[41,42] Norris et al[41] reported that when cereals were introduced while children at risk of developing type 1 diabetes mellitus were breastfed, the risk of islet autoimmunity was reduced independent of the age when cereal was introduced, and there was no association between exposure to cow milk through formula or other dairy products and the risk of islet autoimmunity. More recently, the Trial to Reduce type 1 diabetes mellitus in the Genetically at Risk (TRIGR) Study Group found that for at-risk children, weaning to a highly hydrolyzed formula during infancy was associated with fewer signs of islet autoimmunity up to 10 years of age.[42]

Maternal diet can effect epigenetic heritable changes in gene expression potential that may be transgenerational and have a role in neonatal development and occurrence of disease even into adulthood.[43] Epigenetic nutritional and environmental factors are certain to be an important focus of research.

Preterm and Low Birth Weight Infants

Interactions between nutritional status and immune system function in infants of low birth weight, because of prematurity and/or intrauterine growth retardation, have not been studied systematically. Therefore, these interactions are difficult to describe beyond the qualitative assessment of immune function deficiencies that are imposed by preterm birth[44] (eg, decreased placental transfer of maternal IgG to the fetus, developmental delays in many components of the immune system, and/or intrauterine growth retardation) and are also linked inextricably to inadequate micronutrient status in low birth weight infants. Premature separation from the mother prevents the normal transfer of nutrients with key immunologic roles, because the transfer of nutrients, such as iron and zinc, occurs mostly in the third trimester. The vitamin status (eg, vitamin A) of low birth weight infants also is impaired. The inadequate nutrient transfer to the fetus that often accompanies growth retardation may be attributable to maternal nutrient deficiency states and/or secondary to impaired placental perfusion. In either case, the postnatal unavailability of adequate nutrient stores likely interferes with functions described in the nutrient-specific sections of this discussion. Schlesinger and Uauy[45] have reviewed potential nutrient-immune interactions in low birth weight infants.

Micronutrients and Immunity

Primary nutrient deficiencies are seen rarely in children in the United States, with the exception of iron deficiency. On the other hand, aberrant diets lacking key nutrients (eg, ascorbic acid[46]), certain medical conditions (eg, fat malabsorption, acrodermatitis enteropathica), and lifestyle choices (eg, vegan or macrobiotic diets) can induce moderate or severe nutrient deficiencies that may influence immune competence. Even in mild cases of nutrient deficiency, concern has been raised that immunologic effects of nutrient deficiency may precede the appearance of classic nutritional deficiency sequelae. Unfortunately, the bulk of scientific literature on nutritional deficiency and immune competence is based largely on data from severely malnourished individuals, cell culture experiments, animal models, and clinical trials with adult or elderly subjects. The greatest caution must be taken in extrapolating suggestive data from animals or adults into recommendations for children.

VI

Conversely, a number of vitamins, minerals, and other dietary ingredients are marketed and sold in the United States for their putative immune system-enhancing properties. Given the high rates of common infectious diseases (eg, cold, flu) among young children, parents may choose to use such supplements. A population survey found that half of all mothers gave vitamin supplements to their preadolescents.[47] Thus, pediatricians often are challenged by the need to be familiar with the scientific evidence about individual nutrients and other dietary supplement ingredients.

Iron

Iron deficiency is the most prevalent micronutrient deficiency among children in the United States, with a prevalence of 14% in children 1 to 2 years of age, 4% in children 3 to 5 years of age, and 9% of girls 12 to 19 years of age,[48] with the higher prevalence being higher among certain at-risk groups like Mexican Americans.[49] Iron deficiency is associated with an altered cytokine profile, an increase in cells expressing interferon-alpha, a decrease in proportion of cells expressing IL-4, and impaired lymphocyte proliferation and delayed-type hypersensitivity responses with relative preservation of humeral immunity.[50] Studies in France[51] and the United States[52] demonstrated that iron supplementation of children of low socioeconomic status who are iron deficient can normalize blood T-lymphocyte counts, delayed-type hypersensitivity skin responses, or in vitro IL-2 production, but the clinical consequences are unknown. Depriving microbial pathogens of iron to affect growth and virulence is a feature of the innate immune system; thus, there may be adverse consequences to iron supplementation in parts of the world with a high prevalence of infection with pathogens, such as malaria and tuberculosis.[50] A small placebo-controlled trial among 6- to 36-month-old children in Togo, West Africa (n = 163) found no change in infectious disease incidence after 6 months of iron supplementation.[53] Iron supplementation of iron-replete children is not known to improve immune function further, and increased availability of elemental iron in the gut has the potential to promote the growth and survival of pathogenic organisms.[54] Also, high-dose supplementation with iron alone can interfere with zinc absorption and, therefore, exacerbate zinc deficiency.[55] (Chapter 19: Iron)

Zinc

Moderate or severe zinc deficiency can impair both lymphocyte and phagocyte cell function in humans,[56] but this degree of zinc deficiency is encountered rarely in the United States. In developing countries, zinc supplementation reduces infectious disease morbidity, especially respiratory tract and diarrheal diseases, among infants and preschool children.[57-59] In a randomized, placebo-controlled trial of more than 1700 cases of acute diarrhea in Nepalese children, zinc supplementation reduced the duration of diarrhea and was not enhanced or dependent on concomitant vitamin A supplementation.[60] Zinc supplements have been used to modify the immune status of institutionalized elderly people[61] or as high-dose oral lozenges to treat the common cold in adults,[62] but there is no direct evidence that zinc supplementation may benefit zinc-replete children. Furthermore, there is a risk of zinc supplements impairing copper absorption at daily intakes greater than 7 mg for children younger than 3 years, 12 mg for children 4 to 8 years of age, or 23 mg for children 9 to 13 years of age[63] (see Chapter 20: Trace Elements).

Vitamin A

In developing countries, vitamin A supplementation of deficient children reduces overall mortality[64,65] and morbidity from diarrhea,[66] measles,[67] and possibly other diseases.[68] Vitamin A-deficient experimental animals have impaired T-lymphocyte responses to mitogens and antigens, reduced natural killer cell activity, and decreased production of interferon.[69] However, there is no direct evidence that vitamin A supplementation benefits the immune system of vitamin A-replete children. Daily intakes of retinol greater than 600 μg for children younger than 3 years, 900 μg for children 4 to 8 years of age, or 1700 μg for children 9 to 13 years of age[63] should be avoided to reduce the risk of vitamin A toxicity. This form of toxicity is not seen when vitamin A is supplied by provitamin A carotenoids (eg, alpha-carotene, beta-carotene) (see Chapter 21.I: Fat-Soluble Vitamins).

Vitamin D

The 2 active metabolites of vitamin D are $25\text{-}OH\text{-}D_3$, the measure of nutritional sufficiency, and $1,25\text{-}(OH)_2\text{-}D_3$, important in bone integrity and immune regulation.[70] Skin exposure to ultraviolet-B radiation is the main source of vitamin D_3 in humans by the conversion of 7-hydroxycholesterol to previtamin D_3 followed by metabolism in the liver to $25\text{-}OH\text{-}D_3$ and hydroxylation in the kidney to $1,25\text{-}(OH)_2\text{-}D_3$[70,71]; however, exposure to ultraviolet radiation is affected by latitude, skin pigmentation, clothing, and skin protection. Vitamin D as a natural ingredient in food is limited but may be provided as an additive to dairy products or as a supplement.

Vitamin D_3 has significant effects on both innate and acquired immunity.[71] Vitamin D_3 enhances monocyte differentiation into macrophages but impairs monocyte differentiation into dendritic cells, yet it enhances a tolerogenic phenotype and function of dendritic cells.[72] Vitamin D_3 down-regulates expression of tol-like receptors[73] and induces production of antimicrobial peptides in vitro by monocytes and dendritic cells, thus, enhancing microbial killing.[74]

The effects of vitamin D_3 on acquired immunity are also significant and complex. Vitamin D_3 increases Treg cell differentiation, decreases TH1 and TH17

VI

cell differentiation, and affects specific cytokines leading to decreased homing to lymph nodes, plasma cell development, antibody secretion and memory B cell differentiation.[71]

Increased awareness of the importance of vitamin D sufficiency in preventing osteomalacia, osteoporosis, and rickets as well as an important role in immunity and preventing autoimmune disease has led to recommendations by the American Academy of Pediatrics (AAP) to provide an intake of at least 400 IU/day of vitamin D to infants, children, and adolescents.[70] More recently, the Institute of Medicine recommended 600 IU/day for children at least 1 year of age, and some have suggested that even higher levels of vitamin D are required to maintain sufficiency.[72]

Vitamin E

Although high-dose vitamin E supplements can improve immune function in healthy elderly subjects,[73] it is unclear whether they are effective in children. Vitamin E supplements did not affect tetanus antibody titers in 2-month-old infants[74] or neutrophil function in preterm infants.[75] On the other hand, smaller increases in vitamin E intake may serve the child's overall nutritional adequacy, because few children in the United States consume the recommended amounts of vitamin E[76] (see Chapter 21.I: Fat-Soluble Vitamins).

Vitamin C

Vitamin C is commonly believed to benefit the immune system largely because Nobel laureate Linus Pauling advocated high-dose vitamin C to prevent the common cold.[77] A comprehensive meta-analysis indicates that high-dose vitamin C (1 g or more daily) does not reduce the incidence of the common cold, but it may slightly reduce the duration of the infection.[78] Five of the 11 studies evaluated in this meta-analysis were conducted in children, and the results in this subset were consistent with the overall finding. Few studies have addressed the role of vitamin C more generally in the immune system, although neutrophils are known to maintain high concentrations of the vitamin in vivo,[79] and vitamin C may inactivate histamine chemically.[80] Overall, it is unclear whether high-dose vitamin C supplements have any general immunologic benefit for pediatric populations (see Chapter 21.II: Water-Soluble Vitamins).

B Vitamins

Moderate to severe deficiencies of vitamin B_6,[81,82] vitamin B_{12},[83,84] pantothenic acid,[85,86] folate,[87] or biotin[88,89] suppress immune responses in adult humans and/or animal models. Biotin and pantothenic acid are nearly ubiquitous in the US diet,[90] and deficiency only occurs in unusual circumstances. Vitamin B_{12} deficiency may occur in breastfed infants of vegan mothers (who consume no animal products)[91] or, theoretically, in vegan children who do not consume a supplemental source of vitamin B_{12}. Much less information is available on the effects of B-vitamin supplements on immune responses, although a few preliminary studies indicate that pharmacological intakes of riboflavin[92] or vitamin B_6[93-95] can affect immunologic parameters. B-vitamin deficiency or supplementation studies have not been conducted in children, and the clinical relevance of these findings for the pediatric population is unknown (see Chapter 21.II: Water-Soluble Vitamins).

Nucleotides

Nucleotides (components of RNA and DNA) are found in human milk at concentrations ranging from 189 to 70 µmol/L.[96] Currently, nucleotides are added to several infant formulas in the United States. The mechanism by which dietary nucleotides may modify immune function is unknown,[97] although mouse-model studies indicate they may augment Th1-biased immune responses.[98,99] Studies in human infants have reported that adding nucleotides to infant formula increases natural killer cell activity, IL-2 production by monocytes, serum IgM and IgA concentrations, and serum antibody titers to food antigens.[100-102] The clinical relevance of these changes is unknown. Two studies have reported more clinically specific endpoints. One study showed higher antibody titers to *H influenzae* type b vaccine in treated infants,[103] and another study reported a reduced duration and frequency of diarrheal disease in a group of children of low socioeconomic status.[104] Such data are promising, but additional studies are needed to understand the mechanism of action, confirm clinical endpoints, and monitor the long-term effects of adding nucleotides to infant formula.

Long-Chain Polyunsaturated Fatty Acids

Human milk fat contains 0.10% to 0.35% docosahexaenoic acid (DHA) and 0.30% to 0.65% arachidonic acid (ARA), depending on the mother's polyunsaturated fatty acid intake.[105] Term infant formulas now also contain DHA and ARA.[106] Both DHA and ARA may contribute to visual acuity and cognitive development,[107,108] but their effects on infant immune function is not understood well. ARA is the precursor for prostaglandins and leukotrienes that regulate normal inflammatory processes.[109,110] In vivo, DHA feeding can inhibit both inflammation responses and T-lymphocyte signaling in animal models and adult humans.[111,112] A study of full-term infants at low risk of atopic disease fed formula supplemented with DHA and ARA had higher ex vivo lymphocyte production of TNF-alpha and interferon-alpha to stimulation with beta-lactoglobulin and soy protein compared with infants fed human milk or formula not supplemented with DHA and ARA.[113] The presumption is that the enhanced TH-1 response promotes the development of tolerance to food proteins. Infant data related to these responses are limited and difficult to interpret. Observational studies indicate that mothers of atopic infants

VI

have lower concentrations of DHA and ARA in their milk compared with mothers of nonatopic infants.[114,115] On the other hand, Field et al[116] found that preterm infants fed formula with DHA and ARA had more mature CD4+ T-lymphocytes with higher ex vivo IL-10 production (indicating a potential bias toward antibody and atopic responses) than infants fed formula without DHA and ARA. Additional studies are needed to determine whether DHA and ARA can have clinically significant effects on in vivo inflammation, immune responses, mucosal immune system development, or long-term immunocompetence.

Probiotics

Probiotics are live microorganisms that, in sufficient quantity, promote health by altering the intestinal microflora of the host to compete with the colonization of pathogenic bacteria or generate metabolic byproducts that enhance intestinal mucosal immune protection. Yogurt and certain other milk-based products contain *Lactobacillus* or *Bifidobacterium* species. These and other bacterial probiotics, such as *E coli* Nissle 1917, *Streptococcus salivarius* subspecies *thermophilus*, and the yeast *Saccharomyces boulardii*, may be added to foods or administered as supplements.

Several studies have investigated the use of probiotics in the prevention of acute gastrointestinal tract infections.[117] Modest benefit has been shown using probiotics to decrease the frequency and duration of diarrheal illness in infants[118] and children.[119] There is also evidence from randomized clinical trials that probiotics, specifically *Lactobacillus rhamnosus* GG, when given early in the course of acute infectious diarrhea, can reduce the number of diarrheal stools and duration by 1 day.[117,120] Probiotics can be used in association with antibiotics to decrease the incidence of antibiotic-associated diarrhea, but there is a lack of evidence for their use in treatment of antibiotic-associated diarrhea.[117,120]

Summary

Adequate nutrition is necessary for proper development and function of a child's immune system. Both human milk and synthetic formula can provide adequate nutrition, but human milk is clearly best for infants, because it provides unique components proven to protect and stimulate the developing immune system and contributes positively to growth and development in other ways. In older children, immune function appears to be preserved except in the most severe micronutrient deficiencies. The use of high-dose nutrient supplements and other dietary components to stimulate immune function in otherwise well-nourished children is controversial. Overall, considerably more research is needed to better understand how the maturation and function of the immune system interacts with the changing nutrient requirements of growth.

References

1. Adderson EE, Johnston JM, Shackerford PG, Carroll WL. Development of the human antibody repertoire. *Pediatr Res.* 1992;32(3):257–263

2. Burgio GR, Ugazio AG, Notarangelo LD. Immunology of the neonate. *Curr Opin Immunol.* 1989-1990;2(5):770–777

3. Gershwin ME, Beach RS, Hurley LS. Nutritional factors and immune ontogeny. In: *Nutrition and Immunity.* Orlando, FL: Academic Press Inc; 1985:99–127

4. Beach RS, Gershwin ME, Hurley LS. Gestational zinc deprivation in mice: persistence of immunodeficiency for three generations. *Science.* 1982;218(4571):469–471

5. Institute of Medicine. *Nutrition During Lactation.* Washington, DC: National Academies Press; 1991

6. Stevens S. Maturation of the immune system in breast-fed and bottle-fed infants. In: Cunningham-Rundles S, ed. *Nutrient Modulation of the Immune Response.* New York, NY: Marcel-Dekker Inc; 1993:301–318

7. Garza C, Schanler RJ, Butte NF, Motil KJ. Special properties of human milk. *Clin Perinatol.* 1987;14(1):11 32

8. Hanson LA, Adlerberth I, Carlsson BUM, et al. Human milk antibodies and their importance for the infant. In: Cunningham-Ruddles S, ed. *Nutrient Modulation of the Immune Response.* New York, NY: Marcel Dekker Inc; 1993:525–532

9. Peckham CS, Johnson C, Ades A, Pearl K, Chin KS. Early acquisition of cytomegalovirus infection. *Arch Dis Child.* 1987;62(8):780–785

10. Rudloff HE, Schmalstieg FC Jr, Mushtaha AA, Palkowetz KH, Liu SK, Goldman AS. Tumor necrosis factor-alpha in human milk. *Pediatr Res.* 1992;31(1):29–33

11. Munoz C, Endres S, van der Meer J, Schlesinger L, Arevalo M, Dinarello C. Interleukin-1 beta in human colostrum. *Res Immunol.* 1990;141(6):505–513

12. Saito S, Maruyama M, Kato Y, Moriyama I, Ichijo M. Detection of IL-6 in human milk and its involvement in IgA production. *J Reprod Immunol.* 1991;20(3):267–276

13. Rudloff HE, Schmalstieg FC, Palkowetz KH, Paszkiewicz EJ, Goldman AS. Interleukin-6 in human milk. *J Reprod Immunol.* 1993;23(1):13–20

14. Okada M, Ohmura E, Kamiya Y, et al. Transforming growth factor (TGF)-alpha in human milk. *Life Sci.* 1991;48(12):1151–1156

15. Garofalo R, Chheda S, Mei F, et al. Interleukin-10 in human milk. *Pediatr Res.* 1995;37(4 Pt 1):444–449

16. Gilmore WS, McKelvey-Martin VJ, Rutherford S, et al. Human milk contains granulocyte colony stimulating factor. *Eur J Clin Nutr.* 1994;48(3):222–224

17. Hara T, Irie K, Saito S, et al. Identification of macrophage colony-stimulating factor in human milk and mammary gland epithelial cells. *Pediatr Res.* 1995;37(4 Pt 1):437–443

18. Palkowetz KH, Royer CL, Garofalo R, Rudloff HE, Schmalstieg FC Jr, Goldman AS. Production of interleukin-6 and interleukin-8 by human mammary gland epithelial cells. *J Reprod Immunol.* 1994;26(1):57–64

19. Garofalo RP, Goldman AS. Cytokines, chemokines, and colony-stimulating factors in human milk: the 1997 update. *Biol Neonate.* 1998;74(2):134–142

VI

20. Donovan SM. Role of human milk components in gastrointestinal development: current knowledge and future needs. *J Pediatr.* 2006;149(5):S49-S61

21. Goldblum RM, Schanler RJ, Garza C, Goldman AS. Human milk feeding enhances the urinary excretion of immunologic factors in low birth weight infants. *Pediatr Res.* 1989;25(2):184–188

22. Goldman AS, Garza C, Schanler RJ, Goldblum RM. Molecular forms of lactoferrin in stool and urine from infants fed human milk. *Pediatr Res.* 1990;27(3):252–255

23. Hutchens TW, Henry JF, Yip TT, et al. Origin of intact lactoferrin and its DNA-binding fragments found in the urine of human milk-fed preterm infants. Evaluation by stable isotopic enrichment. *Pediatr Res.* 1991;29(3):243–250

24. Stephens S, Dolby JM, Montreuil J, Spik G. Differences in inhibition of the growth of commensal and enteropathogenic strains of *Escherichia coli* by lactotransferrin and secretory immunoglobulin A isolated from human milk. *Immunology.* 1980;41(3):597–603

25. Griffiths E, Humphreys J. Bacteriostatic effect of human milk and bovine colostrum on *Escherichia coli*: importance of bicarbonate. *Infect Immun.* 1977;15(2):396–401

26. Goldman AS, Thorpe LW, Goldblum RM, Hanson LA. Anti-inflammatory properties of human milk. *Acta Paediatr Scand.* 1986;75(5):689–695

27. Newburg DS. Oligosaccharides and glycoconjugates in human milk: their role in host defense. *J Mammary Gland Biol Neoplasia.* 1996;1(3):271–283

28. Isaacs CE, Thormar H. The role of milk-derived antimicrobial lipids as antiviral and antibacterial agents. *Adv Exp Med Biol.* 1991;310:159–165

29. Schroten H, Hanisch FG, Plogmann R, et al. Inhibition of adhesion of S-fimbriated Escherichia coli to buccal epithelial cells by human milk fat globule membrane components: a novel aspect of the protective function of mucins in the nonimmunoglobulin fraction. *Infect Immun.* 1992;60(7):2893–2899

30. Orrhage K, Nord CE. Factors controlling the bacterial colonization of the intestine in breastfed infants. *Acta Paediatr Suppl.* 1999;88(430):47–57

31. Gothefors L, Carlsson B, Ahlstedt S, Hanson LA, Winberg J. Influence of maternal gut flora and colostral and cord serum antibodies on presence of *Escherichia coli* in faeces of the newborn infant. *Acta Paediatr Scand.* 1976;65(2):225-232

32. Adlerberth I. Bacterial adherence and intestinal colonization in newborn infants [thesis]. Göteborg, Sweden: Göteborg University; 1996

33. Fryklund B. Epidemiology of enterobacteria and risk factors for invasive Gram-negative bacterial infection in neonatal special-care units [thesis]. Stokholm: Stockholm University; 1994

34. Wold AE, Adlerberth I. Breast feeding and the intestinal microflora of the infant— implications for protection against infectious diseases. *Adv Exp Med Biol.* 2000;478:77–93

35. Kramer MS, Chalmers B, Hodnett ED, et al. Promotion of Breastfeeding Intervention Trial (PROBIT): a randomized trial in the Republic of Belarus. *JAMA.* 2001;285(4):413–420

36. Kaplan JL, Shi HN, Walker WA. The role of microbes in developmental immunologic programming. *Pediatr Res.* 2011;69(6):465-472

37. Wright S, Bolton C. Breast milk fatty acids in mothers of children with atopic eczema. *Br J Nutr*. 1989;62(3):693–697

38. Goldman AS. Association of atopic diseases with breast-feeding: food allergens, fatty acids, and evolution. *J Pediatr*. 1999;134(1):5–7

39. Conti A, Giuffrida MG, Napolitano L, et al. Identification of the human beta-casein C-terminal fragments that specifically bind to purified antibodies to bovine beta-lactoglobulin. *J Nutr Biochem*. 2000;11(6):332–337

40. Greer FR, Sicherer FR, Burks AW; American Academy of Pediatrics, Committee on Nutrition and Section on Allergy and Immunology. Effects of early nutritional interventions on the development of atopic disease in infants and children: the role of maternal dietary restriction, breastfeeding, timing of introduction of complementary foods, and hydrolyzed formulas. *Pediatrics*. 2008;121(1):183-191

41. Norris JM, Barriga K, Klingensmith G, et al. Timing of initial cereal exposure in infancy and risk of islet autoimmunity. *JAMA*. 2003;290(13):1713-1720

42. Knip M, Virtanen SM, Seppä K, et al. Dietary intervention in infancy and later signs of beta-cell autoimmunity. *N Engl J Med*. 2010;363(20):1900-1908

43. Waterland RA, Michels KB. Epigenetic epidemiology of the developmental origins hypothesis. *Annu Rev Nutr*. 2007;27:363-388

44. Goldman AS. Back to basics: host responses to infection. *Pediatr Rev*. 2000;21(10):342–349

45. Schlesinger L, Uauy R. Nutrition and neonatal immune function. *Semin Perinatol*. 1991;15(6):469–477

46. Tamura Y, Welch DC, Zic JA, Cooper WO, Stein SM, Hummell DS. Scurvy presenting as painful gait with bruising in a young boy. *Arch Pediatr Adolesc Med*. 2000;154(7):732–735

47. Roche Vitamins. *Vitamin Consumption in the US*. Parsippany, NJ: Roche Vitamins Inc; 2000

48. Cogswell ME, Looker AC, Pfeiffer CM, et al. Assessment of iron deficiency in US preschool children and non-pregnant females of childbearing age: National Health and Nutrition Examination Survey 2003-2006. *Am J Clin Nutr*. 2009;89(5):1334-1342

49. Frith-Terhune AL, Cogswell ME, Khan LK, Will JC, Ramakrishnan U. Iron deficiency anemia: higher prevalence in Mexican American than in non-Hispanic white females in the third National Health and Nutrition Examination Survey, 1988–1994. *Am J Clin Nutr*. 2000;72(4):963–968

50. Cherayil BJ. Iron and immunity: immunological consequences of iron deficiency and overload. *Arch Immunol Ther Exp*. 2010;58(6):407-415

51. Thibault H, Galan P, Selz F, et al. The immune response in iron-deficient young children: effect of iron supplementation on cell-mediated immunity. *Eur J Pediatr*. 1993;152(2):120–124

52. Krantman HJ, Young SR, Ank BJ, O'Donnell CM, Rachelefsky GS, Stiehm ER. Immune function in pure iron deficiency. *Am J Dis Child*. 1982;136(9):840–844

53. Berger J, Dyck JL, Galan P, et al. Effect of daily iron supplementation on iron status, cell-mediated immunity, and incidence of infections in 6–36 month old Togolese children. *Eur J Clin Nutr*. 2000;54(1):29–35

VI

54. Kent S, Weinberg ED, Stuart-Macadam P. The etiology of the anemia of chronic disease and infection. *J Clin Epidemiol*. 1994;47(1):23–33

55. Couzy F, Keen C, Gershwin ME, Mareschi JP. Nutritional implications of the interactions between minerals. *Prog Food Nutr Sci*. 1993;17(1):65–87

56. Shankar AH, Prasad AS. Zinc and immune function: the biological basis of altered resistance to infection. *Am J Clin Nutr*. 1998;68(Suppl 2):447S–463S

57. Sazawal S, Black RE, Bhan MK, Bhandari N, Sinha A, Jalla S. Zinc supplementation in young children with acute diarrhea in India. *N Engl J Med*. 1995;333(13):839–844

58. Rosado JL, Lopez P, Munoz E, Martinez H, Allen LH. Zinc supplementation reduced morbidity, but neither zinc nor iron supplementation affected growth or body composition of Mexican preschoolers. *Am J Clin Nutr*. 1997;65(1):13–19

59. Sazawal S, Black RE, Jalla S, Mazumdar S, Sinha A, Bhan MK. Zinc supplementation reduces the incidence of acute lower respiratory infections in infants and preschool children: a double-blind, controlled trial. *Pediatrics*. 1998;102(1 Pt 1):1–5

60. Strand TA, Chandyo RK, Bahl R, et al. Effectiveness and efficacy of zinc for the treatment of acute diarrhea in young children. *Pediatrics*. 2002;109(5):898-903

61. Girodon F, Galan P, Monget AL, et al. Impact of trace elements and vitamin supplementation on immunity and infections in institutionalized elderly patients: a randomized controlled trial. MIN. VIT. AOX. geriatric network. *Arch Intern Med*. 1999;159(7):748–754

62. Mossad SB, Macknin ML, Medendorp SV, Mason P. Zinc gluconate lozenges for treating the common cold. A randomized, double-blind, placebo-controlled study. *Ann Intern Med*. 1996;125(2):81–88

63. Institute of Medicine. *Dietary Reference Intakes for Vitamin A, Vitamin K, Arsenic, Boron, Chromium, Copper, Iodine, Iron, Manganese, Molybdenum, Nickel, Silicon, Vanadium, and Zinc*. Washington, DC: National Academies Press; 2001

64. West KP Jr, Pokhrel RP, Katz J, et al. Efficacy of vitamin A in reducing preschool child mortality in Nepal. *Lancet*. 1991;338(8759):67–71

65. Rahmathullah L, Underwood BA, Thulasiraj RD, et al. Reduced mortality among children in southern India receiving a small weekly dose of vitamin A. *N Engl J Med*. 1990;323(14):929–935

66. Glasziou PP, Mackerras DE. Vitamin A supplementation in infectious diseases: a meta-analysis. *BMJ*. 1993;306(6874):366–370

67. Hussey GD, Klein M. A randomized, controlled trial of vitamin A in children with severe measles. *N Engl J Med*. 1990;323(3):160–164

68. Shankar AH, Genton B, Semba RD, et al. Effect of vitamin A supplementation on morbidity due to *Plasmodium falciparum* in young children in Papua New Guinea: a randomised trial. *Lancet*. 1999;354(9174):203–209

69. Scrimshaw NS, SanGiovanni JP. Synergism of nutrition, infection, and immunity: an overview. *Am J Clin Nutr*. 1997;66(2):464S–477S

70. Wagner CL, Greer FR; American Academy of Pediatrics, Section on Breasfeeding and Committee on Nutrition. Prevention of rickets and vitamin D deficiency in infants, children, and adolescents. *Pediatrics*. 2008;122(5):1142-1152

71. Hart PH, Gorman S, Finlay-Jones JJ. Modulation of the immune system by UV radiation: more than just the effects of vitamin D? *Nature Rev Immunol.* 2011;11(9):584-596

72. Pramyothin P, Holick MF. Vitamin D supplementation: guidelines and evidence for subclinical deficiency. *Curr Opin Gastroenterol.* 2012;28(2):139-150

73. Meydani SN, Meydani M, Blumberg JB, et al. Vitamin E supplementation and in vivo immune response in healthy elderly subjects. A randomized controlled trial. *JAMA.* 1997;277(17):1380–1386

74. Kutukculer N, Akil T, Egemen A, et al. Adequate immune response to tetanus toxoid and failure of vitamin A and E supplementation to enhance antibody response in healthy children. *Vaccine.* 2000;18(26):2979–2984

75. Mino M. Clinical uses and abuses of vitamin E in children. *Proc Soc Exp Biol Med.* 1992;200(2):266–270

76. US Department of Agriculture-Agricultural Research Service. *Food and Nutrient Intakes by Children 1994–96, 1998.* Table Set 17. Available at: http://www.ars.usda.gov/SP2UserFiles/Place/12355000/pdf/scs_all.PDF. Accessed December 18, 2012

77. Pauling L. The significance of the evidence about ascorbic acid and the common cold. *Proc Natl Acad Sci U S A.* 1971;68(11):2678–2681

78. Douglas RM, Chalker EB, Treacy B. Vitamin C for preventing and treating the common cold. *Cochrane Database Syst Rev.* 2000;(2):CD000980

79. Muggli R. Vitamin C and phagocytes. In: Cunningham-Rundles S, ed. *Nutrient Modulation of the Immune Response.* New York, NY: Marcel-Dekker; 1993:75–90

80. Johnston CS. The antihistamine action of ascorbic acid. *Subcell Biochem.* 1996;25:189–213

81. Frydas S, Reale M, Vacalis D, et al. IgG, IgG1 and IgM response in *Trichinella spiralis*-infected mice treated with 4-deoxypyridoxine or fed a Vitamin B6-deficient diet. *Mol Cell Biochem.* 1999;194(1-2):47–52

82. Rall LC, Meydani SN. Vitamin B6 and immune competence. *Nutr Rev.* 1993;51(8):217–225

83. Tamura J, Kubota K, Murakami H, et al. Immunomodulation by vitamin B12: augmentation of CD8+ T lymphocytes and natural killer (NK) cell activity in vitamin B12-deficient patients by methyl-B12 treatment. *Clin Exp Immunol.* 1999;116(1):28–32

84. Fata FT, Herzlich BC, Schiffman G, Ast AL. Impaired antibody responses to pneumococcal polysaccharide in elderly patients with low serum vitamin B12 levels. *Ann Intern Med.* 1996;124(3):299–304

85. Hodges RE, Bean WB, Ohlson MA, Bleiler RE. Factors affecting human antibody response. IV. pyridoxine deficiency. *Am J Clin Nutr.* 1962;11:180–186

86. Hodges RE, Bean WB, Ohlson MA, Bleiler RE. Factors affecting human antibody response. V. combined deficiencies of pantothenic acid and pyridoxine. *Am J Clin Nutr.* 1962;11:187–199

87. Dhur A, Galan P, Hercberg S. Folate status and the immune system. *Prog Food Nutr Sci.* 1991;15(1-2):43–60

88. Baez-Saldana A, Diaz G, Espinoza B, Ortega E. Biotin deficiency induces changes in subpopulations of spleen lymphocytes in mice. *Am J Clin Nutr.* 1998;67(3):431–437

VI

89. Rabin BS. Inhibition of experimentally induced autoimmunity in rats by biotin deficiency. *J Nutrition*. 1983;113(11):2316–2322

90. Institute of Medicine. *Dietary Reference Intakes for Thiamin, Riboflavin, Niacin, Vitamin B6, Folate, Vitamin B12, Pantothenic Acid, Biotin, and Choline*. Washington, DC: National Academies Press; 1998

91. Specker BL, Black A, Allen L, Morrow F. Vitamin B12: low milk concentrations are related to low serum concentrations in vegetarian women and to methylmalonic aciduria in their infants. *Am J Clin Nutr*. 1990;52(6):1073–1076

92. Araki S, Suzuki M, Fujimoto M, Kimura M. Enhancement of resistance to bacterial infection in mice by vitamin B2. *J Vet Med Sci*. 1995;57(4):599–602

93. Gebhard KJ, Gridley DS, Stickney DR, Shulz TD. Enhancement of immune status by high levels of dietary vitamin B6 without growth inhibition of human malignant melanoma in athymic nude mice. *Nutr Cancer*. 1990;14(1):15–26

94. Talbott MC, Miller LT, Kerkvliet NI. Pyridoxine supplementation: effect on lymphocyte responses in elderly persons. *Am J Clin Nutr*. 1987;46(4):659–664

95. Debes SA, Kirksey A. Influence of dietary pyridoxine on selected immune capacities of rat dams and pups. *J Nutr*. 1979;109(5):744–759

96. Motil KJ. Infant feeding: a critical look at infant formulas. *Curr Opin Pediatr*. 2000;12(5):469–476

97. Grimble GK, Westwood OM. Nucleotides as immunomodulators in clinical nutrition. *Curr Opin Clin Nutr Metab Care*. 2001;4(1):57–64

98. Jyonouchi H, Sun S, Abiru T, Winship T, Kuchan MJ. Dietary nucleotides modulate antigen-specific type 1 and type 2 T-cell responses in young C57Bl/6 mice. *Nutrition*. 2000;16(6):442–446

99. Nagafuchi S, Hachimura S, Totsuka M, et al. Dietary nucleotides can up-regulate antigen-specific Th1 immune responses and suppress antigen-specific IgE responses in mice. *Int Arch Allergy Immunol*. 2000;122(1-3):33–41

100. Carver JD, Pimentel B, Cox WI, Barness LA. Dietary nucleotide effects upon immune function in infants. *Pediatrics*. 1991;88(2):359–363

101. Martinez-Augustin O, Boza JJ, Del Pino JI, Lucena J, Martinez-Valverde A, Gil A. Dietary nucleotides might influence the humoral immune response against cow's milk proteins in preterm neonates. *Biol Neonate*. 1997;71(4):215–223

102. Navarro J, Maldonado J, Narbona E, et al. Influence of dietary nucleotides on plasma immunoglobulin levels and lymphocyte subsets of preterm infants. *Biofactors*. 1999;10(1):67–76

103. Pickering LK, Granoff DM, Erickson JR, et al. Modulation of the immune system by human milk and infant formula containing nucleotides. *Pediatrics*. 1998;101(2):242–249

104. Brunser O, Espinoza J, Araya M, Cruchet S, Gil A. Effect of dietary nucleotide supplementation on diarrhoeal disease in infants. *Acta Paediatr*. 1994;83(2):188–191

105. Jensen RG, Bitman J, Carlson SE, Couch SC, Hamosh M, Newburg DS. Milk lipids: human milk lipids. In: Jensen RG, ed. *Handbook of Milk Composition*. San Diego, CA: Academic Press; 1995:495–576

106. Food and Drug Administration, Office of Premarket Approval. Agency response letter GRAS notice GRN 000041. May 17, 2001. Available at: http://www.fda.gov/Food/FoodIngredientsPackaging/GenerallyRecognizedasSafeGRAS/GRASListings/ucm154126.htm. Accessed December 18, 2012

107. SanGiovanni JP, Berkey CS, Dwyer JT, Colditz GA. Dietary essential fatty acids, long-chain polyunsaturated fatty acids, and visual resolution acuity in healthy fullterm infants: a systematic review. *Early Hum Dev*. 2000;57(3):165–188

108. Gibson RA, Makrides M. The role of long chain polyunsaturated fatty acids (LCPUFA) in neonatal nutrition. *Acta Paediatr*. 1998;87(10):1017–1022

109. Griffiths RJ. Prostaglandins and inflammation. In: Gallin JI, Snyderman R, eds. *Inflammation: Basic Principles and Clinical Correlates*. 3rd ed. Philadelphia, PA: Lippincott Williams and Wilkins; 1999:349–360

110. Penrose JF, Austen F, Lam BK. Leukotrienes: biosynthetic pathways, release, and receptor-mediated actions with relevance to disease states. In: Gallin JI, Snyderman R, eds. *Inflammation: Basic Principles and Clinical Correlates*. 3rd ed. Philadelphia, PA: Lippincott Williams and Wilkins; 1999:361–372

111. Calder PC. N-3 polyunsaturated fatty acids, inflammation and immunity: pouring oil on troubled waters or another fishy tale? *Nutr Res*. 2001;21(1-2):309–341

112. McMurray DN, Jolly CA, Chapkin RS. Effects of dietary n-3 fatty acids on T cell activation and T cell receptor-mediated signaling in a murine model. *J Infect Dis*. 2000;182(Suppl 1):S103–S107

113. Field CJ, van Aerde JE, Robinson LE, Clandinin MT. Feeding a formula supplemented with long chain polyunsaturated fatty acids modifies the "ex vivo" cytokine responses to food proteins in infants at low risk for allergy. *Pediatr Res*. 2008;64(4):411-417

114. Duchen K, Casas R, Fageras-Bottcher M, Yu G, Björkstén B. Human milk polyunsaturated long-chain fatty acids and secretory immunoglobulin A antibodies and early childhood allergy. *Pediatr Allergy Immunol*. 2000;11(1):29–39

115. Businco L, Ioppi M, Morse NL, Nisini R, Wright S. Breast milk from mothers of children with newly developed atopic eczema has low levels of long chain polyunsaturated fatty acids. *J Allergy Clin Immunol*. 1993;91(6):1134–1139

116. Field CJ, Thomson CA, Van Aerde JE, et al. Lower proportion of CD45RO+ cells and deficient interleukin-10 production by formula-fed infants, compared with human-fed, is corrected with supplementation of long-chain polyunsaturated fatty acids. *J Pediatr Gastroenterol Nutr*. 2000;31(3):291–299

117. Thomas DW, Greer FR; American Academy of Pediatrics, Committee on Nutrition, Section on Gastroenterology, Hepatology, and Nutrition. Probiotics and prebiotics in pediatrics. *Pediatrics*. 2010;126(6):1217-1231

118. Weizman Z, Asli G, Alsheikh A. Effect of a probiotic infant formula on infections in child care centers: comparison of two probiotic agents. *Pediatrics*. 2005;115(1):5-9

119. Pedone CA, Arnaud CC, Postaire ER, Bouley CF, Reinert P. Multicentric study of the effect of milk fermented by *Lactobacillus casei* on the incidence of diarrhoea. *Int J Clin Pract*. 2005;54(9):568-571

120. Allen SJ, Okoko B, Martinez E, Gregorio G, Dans LF. Probiotics for treating infectious diarrhoea. *Cochrane Database Syst Rev*. 2004;(2):CD003048

VI

Chapter 37

Nutritional Support for Children With Developmental Disabilities

Introduction

Feeding difficulties and poor growth are well-recognized problems in children with neurologic impairment. In the care of such patients, monitoring of nutritional status and provision of adequate nutrition are essential. Despite the well-documented growth abnormalities in this population, the exact causes remain unclear. Both nutritional and nonnutritional factors may contribute to linear growth failure. In patients with moderate to severe cerebral palsy (CP), poor nutritional status is associated with increased health care utilization and limitation in social activities for both the child and the parents.[1] With appropriate nutritional support, weight, height, skinfold thickness, mid-arm circumference, body mass index (BMI), weight-for-age z-scores, and weight-for-height z-scores improve.[2] Improvement of nutritional status also enhances quality of life and well-being by decreasing irritability and spasticity, increasing resistance to infections, and promoting the healing of decubitus ulcers.[3-5] Nutritional repletion can also improve lower esophageal sphincter tone and gastroesophageal reflux.[6,7]

Promotion of growth and well-being must be an integral part of medical management. Because of the numerous factors that need to be considered, nutritional intervention is best accomplished by a multidisciplinary team involving dieticians, speech-language and occupational therapists, psychologists, physicians, and nurses.[8]

Growth Abnormalities in Children With Neurologic Impairment

Prevalence

Children with developmental disabilities are at high risk of malnutrition. They are often in a poor nutritional state, exhibiting marked linear growth failure, poor weight gain, and decreased lean body mass and fat stores.[9-13] The true prevalence of malnutrition in this population is not known, but a significant proportion of patients with neurologic impairment are shorter and lighter than the reference standard, and the discrepancies increase as they grow older.[14] The growth and nutritional status of children with spastic quadriplegia is generally more severely affected, but 30% of children with diplegia or hemiplegia also exhibit signs of malnutrition, with decreased weight and triceps skin fold thickness, and 23% are stunted.[10] A small proportion of patients with CP (8%–16%) are overweight. The

VI

proportion of overweight patients seems to be increasing, perhaps because of the increased use of gastrostomy tube feedings.[15]

Growth Standards

There are specific growth charts for patients with chromosomal abnormalities, but the population of patients with CP is heterogeneous, and their growth is affected by numerous factors. Thus, developing appropriate growth charts for them is difficult. The first set of growth charts for patients with quadriplegic CP were published by Krick et al in 1996.[14] A more recent set of growth charts, developed by Day et al, describes the growth of patients with CP divided in 5 groups according to their functional level and their ability to self-feed.[16] Stevenson et al also evaluated growth of children with CP based on their level on the Gross Motor Function Classification System (GMFCS) but did not publish their charts for clinical use.[17] It is important to remember that growth charts for patients with CP are descriptive (how a group of patients grew) and are not intended to be prescriptive (how they should grow).

To obtain cerebral palsy growth charts:
www.kennedykrieger.org
www.lifeexpectancy.com/articles/growthcharts.shtml

Pathophysiology

In children with neurologic impairment, inappropriate intake, oral motor dysfunction, increased losses, and abnormal energy expenditure clearly affect growth[18-24] and may increase the risk of specific nutrient deficiencies.[25] In patients with CP, height and weight z-scores are highly correlated, suggesting that nutritional factors indeed play a role in linear growth failure. However, height z-score may also decline with advancing age independently of weight z-score, suggesting that nonnutritional factors also contribute to linear growth failure.[13,26] The severity of neurologic disease correlates with an increased risk of growth failure, because height z-score is significantly lower in children with seizures, those who are nonambulatory, and those with spastic quadriplegia.[13] Linear growth of children with diplegia or hemiplegia is less affected than linear growth of those with spastic quadriplegia.[10] In children with spastic hemiplegia, significantly smaller measures of breadth and length on the affected side suggest the influence of the neurologic disease on growth,[26] and skeletal maturation is slower on the affected side.[27] Endocrine factors may be important, because statural growth of patients with CP seems to plateau at puberty instead of showing the pubertal growth spurt.[17] Patterns of growth hormone and insulin-like growth factor-1 secretion are similar to those of unaffected children, but levels are significantly lower in girls with CP. Boys show a similar although nonsignificant trend.[28] Immobility and lack of weight-bearing activity may also have an effect on growth. Environmental factors, such as the child's living situation, also have an effect on nutritional status.[29]

Children with CP spontaneously consume fewer calories than age-matched controls.[23,30-32] The major nutritional deficit seems to be quantitative rather than qualitative.[23] Inadequate energy intake is a major factor contributing to malnutrition, because aggressive nutritional supplementation using nasogastric or gastrostomy tube feedings improves growth[3-5,12,33] but is often introduced too late.[15] The first year of life and the adolescent growth spurt are the 2 periods during which children with neurologic impairment are most vulnerable, because their energy intake cannot adapt to support increased needs associated with rapid growth.

Because of their poor oral and fine motor skills, more than half of children with neurologic impairment are totally dependent on a caregiver for feedings.[34] Because they are often unable to communicate hunger and satiety, the caregiver controls intake. It has been shown that the caregiver often overestimates energy intake and time spent feeding the child.[31,34] The task of feeding such a child is difficult and time consuming, and inadequate intake may ensue.[30] On the other hand, it is possible to overfeed a child with CP; therefore, careful monitoring of growth is important, especially after initiating tube feedings, to avoid the deleterious effects of obesity.

Feeding difficulties are common in children with neurologic impairment.[34,35] Problems such as poor suck, vomiting, gagging, and choking are often reported as the first indication of a problem with the child, and in 60% of patients, severe feeding problems preceded the diagnosis of CP.[30,34] One study found oral-motor dysfunction in more than 90% of children with CP; 57% had sucking problems, 38% had swallowing problems, and 80% had been fed nonorally on at least 1 occasion in the first year of life.[34] Sucking and swallowing difficulties, inadequate lip closure, drooling, and a persistent extrusion reflex make oral feedings difficult. Feeding efficiency in patients with severe CP is far below normal, as it may take them 2 to 12 times longer than healthy control subjects to swallow pureed food and up to 15 times longer to chew and swallow solid food.[36] Mealtime becomes very frustrating and time-consuming for the caregiver and for the patient. Prolonged feeding time (more than 3 hours/day) was reported by 28% of parents of children with neurologic impairment.[22] On average, mothers of children with disabilities spend 3.3 hours a day feeding their child, compared with 0.8 hours per day spent by mothers of children without disabilities.[37] Even longer mealtimes do not compensate for the child's feeding impairment, and as a consequence, energy intake

VI

is often insufficient.[36] In addition, some children may experience significant hypoxemia during feedings because of silent aspiration.[38]

Oral motor dysfunction is a major factor in the pathogenesis of malnutrition in patients with CP, because oral intake, weight, height, and weight-for-height z-scores are significantly lower in patients with oral-motor dysfunction than in patients without.[18-24] Persistent, severe feeding difficulties are associated with poor growth and can identify children who will benefit from gastrostomy tube feeding.[20,21] In addition to decreased intake, excessive losses may occur from spillage because of poor hand-to-mouth coordination or inadequate swallowing. Abnormal gastric motility and gastroesophageal reflux (GER) are frequently encountered in patients with neurologic impairment. GER may contribute to increased loss of nutrients because of frequent emesis.[39-41]

Resting energy expenditure (REE) is generally reduced in children with neurologic impairment.[31,42-44] When measured by indirect calorimetry, REE in patients with spastic quadriplegic CP is significantly less than in healthy age-matched controls or from those calculated from World Health Organization (WHO) equations based on weight, age, and gender.[42] Calculation of total energy needs based on WHO standards for healthy children (1.5 to 1.6 × **calculated** REE) overestimates energy requirements in children with CP (1.1 × **measured** REE). Total Energy Expenditure (TEE) is lower in children with neurologic impairment who have a gastrostomy tube, who are more severely affected, and who have seizures.[45]

Muscle tone (hypotonicity, spasticity, and athetosis) and activity level (bedridden, moderately active, ambulatory) will influence energy needs. Patients who are ambulatory or who have athetosis have higher energy needs to achieve normal and catch up growth.[46] Energy needs also may be increased during infections, such as aspiration pneumonia.

Osteopenia is very common in children with neurologic impairment, and pathologic bone fractures may affect as many as 26% of children with CP.[47,48] Fractures often heal poorly, increasing the need for medical care and diminishing the child's quality of life. Inadequate intake of calcium, phosphorus, and vitamin D; malnutrition; use of anticonvulsants (particularly valproic acid); lack of weight-bearing activity and lack of sun exposure contribute to poor bone mineralization.[32,44,49-55] Anticonvulsants interfere with vitamin D metabolism by increasing its conversion to inactive metabolites and have been shown to be associated with osteomalacia in patients after prolonged treatment.[52,53] Ambulatory status is also important in the pathogenesis of osteopenia.[55,56] Low weight-for-age z-score is a strong predictor of low bone mineral density.[54] Measuring bone mineral density using bone densitometry may be difficult in some patients with skeletal deformities, patients with involuntary movements, or patients who cannot cooperate for densitometry studies. Bone quantitative ultrasonography may be an alternative method in such situations.[57] Supplemental vitamin D should be given to patients with neurologic impairment, especially if they are receiving anticonvulsants, lack exposure to sunlight, or are nonambulatory.[53] In a small controlled trial, bisphosphonates increased bone mineral density in children with CP by 89% over 18 months.[58] Bisphosphonates also decreased fracture rate in this population.[59]

Assessment

Assessment of the child with neurologic impairment should include medical, nutritional, and growth history as well as a family and social history. A physical examination, including anthropometric measurements, should be performed. Meal observations and appropriate investigation will complete the evaluation.

It is useful to evaluate the child's gross motor function using the 5-level GMFCS. This standardized system classifies patients with neurologic impairment in 5 functional levels.[60] Caloric needs, energy expenditure, and ability to self-feed are different according to the patient's GMFCS level[45] (see Table 37.1).

Table 37.1.
Gross Motor Function Classification System (GMFCS)

I	Walks without limitation
II	Walks with limitation
III	Walks using a handheld mobility device
IV	Self-mobility with limitation; may use powered wheelchair
V	Transported in a manual wheelchair

Medical History

Assessment of health status must include knowledge of the underlying disease to better understand its natural history. Some patients have a static condition with little or no potential for improvement, whereas others have a degenerative disease and some have reversible temporary neurologic impairment. The duration, severity, and prognosis of neurologic impairment will influence the type of nutritional intervention required by the patient.

The review of systems should focus on respiratory and gastrointestinal tract symptoms, because they influence the type of nutritional intervention required by the child. Chronic respiratory problems and recurrent pneumonias may be attributable to aspiration from GER or swallowing dysfunction. Frequent emesis and food refusal are suggestive of GER and esophagitis. Constipation is frequently seen in children with neurologic impairment and may be exacerbated by insufficient fluid and fiber intake.

It is important to review the medications used by the patient. Among the medications commonly used by children with neurologic impairment are anticonvulsants that may affect consciousness level, appetite, and vitamin D metabolism. Intrathecal baclofen (a derivative of gamma-aminobutyric acid) therapy has been shown to reduce muscle spasticity and, therefore, decrease REE in patients with CP, leading to increased weight gain.[61,62] Physicians must be able to appropriately intervene in this situation to avoid excessive weight gain. Use of laxatives, prokinetics, and H-2 blockers or proton-pump inhibitors reflects the presence of gastrointestinal tract problems.

Nutritional and Growth History

The nutritional history must review all aspects of the feeding process, including the child's appetite and ability to self-feed, the efficiency of the feeding process with different textures, and the time required to feed the child.

An appropriate evaluation of oral motor skills and swallowing function, including adequacy of lip closure, drooling, spilling, extrusion reflex, incoordination, gagging, and delayed swallowing must be performed, because oral motor impairment is a major factor leading to malnutrition.[18-23] Choking and coughing during meals are suggestive of aspiration, and fatigue progressing during meals may result from aspiration-induced hypoxia.[38] The amount of time spent feeding the child should be estimated. Sixty percent of patients with CP are totally dependent on a caregiver for their intake.[34] For the caregiver, often the parent, too much time spent around meals may impair the parent-child relationship and take time away from other activities. It is also important to assess the parental perception of mealtime, because it is often perceived as a stressful and not enjoyable experience.[22,30] Parents are under constant pressure to adequately feed their child to ensure sufficient weight gain.[63]

Keeping in mind that parental report often overestimates intake, a review of a typical day's food intake or a full 3-day food record will help assessing caloric intake but also adequacy of fiber, vitamin, and mineral intake. Food refusal or a recent change in feeding pattern may be indicative of an underlying problem.

A careful review of the entire growth pattern is important. Birth weight and length and subsequent available height, weight, and head circumference measurements should be plotted on growth charts to evaluate growth trajectory and to detect changes in growth patterns, such as weight loss, abnormal weight gain, or growth faltering. Infants with CP who had a low birth weight are at greater nutritional risk.

Family History

The height of the biological parents should be recorded to estimate the patient's genetic potential for linear growth.

Social History

The social situation, including the child's school and therapy schedule, the family environment, the presence of siblings, the parents' work schedule, medical insurance, and available home care must be considered. The amount of care required by a child with neurologic impairment has a great effect on the family's social life and financial situation, the parents' work, and the patient's siblings. Nutritional intervention should be well planned and integrated into the family's routine and environment as efficiently as possible.

Growth Assessment

Weight and length or height must be obtained at every visit and should be as accurate as possible, always using the same technique and equipment. Weight should be measured on the same scale every time with the child wearing little or no clothing. If the child is unable to stand, a bed scale or a chair scale should be available. Length should be obtained supine in children younger than 2 years or in older children who are unable to stand. Standing height should be obtained when possible. Head circumference must also be measured for children younger than 3 years but may be of limited use in children with brain damage.

Reliable length measurements may be difficult to obtain in children with severe contractures, spasms, scoliosis, or poor cooperation. For these patients, alternative techniques, such as knee height (KH), upper arm length (UAL), or lower leg length (LLL) may be used to assess body length.[64,65] The right side is measured unless the patient is hemiplegic, in which case the less affected side is used. UAL is usually less compromised than LLL in patients with CP[11] (see Table 37.2).

Table 37.2.
Alternative Length Measurements

Age Group	Measure	Method
Children <2 y	UAL	Distance between the top of the shoulder and the bottom of the elbow with joints at a right angle, obtained with a measuring tape
	LLL	Distance between the top of the knee to the sole of the heel with both joints at a right angle, obtained with a measuring tape
Children >2 y	UAL	Distance between the acromion and the head of the radius obtained with an anthropometer
	LLL	Distance between the superomedial border of the tibia and the inferior border of the medial malleolus with the child sitting, one leg crossed horizontally across the other, obtained with a measuring tape
All ages	KH	Distance between the proximal edge of the patella and the bottom of the heel with both the knee and the ankle at 90°, obtained with an anthropometer

VI

Once segmental measurements have been obtained, they can be compared with standards[65] or used to calculate an estimated stature. KH is the easiest measurement to obtain and has been shown to reliably correlate with recumbent length in patients with CP[64] (Table 37.3).

Table 37.3.
Calculated Stature Based on Knee Height or Upper Arm Length

Equation	Stature (S) in cm	Standard Error of Estimate
CP, birth to 12 years (Stevenson[66])	$S = (4.35 \times UAL) + 21.8$ $S = (2.69 \times KH) + 24.2$	1.7 1.1
Normal children, 6 to 18 y (Chumlea[67]) Boys: white black Girls: white black	 $S = (2.22 \times KH) + 40.54$ $S = (2.18 \times KH) + 39.60$ $S = (2.15 \times KH) + 43.21$ $S = (2.02 \times KH) + 46.59$	 4.21 4.58 3.90 4.39

Mid-arm circumference combined with triceps skinfold thickness are useful to estimate upper arm muscle and fat. Measurements should be obtained by the same observer every time to improve reliability. Triceps skin fold thickness is more sensitive than weight-for-height z-score to identify malnourished patients. A triceps skin fold value <10th percentile identified 96% of malnourished children, whereas weight-for-height <10th percentile failed to identify 45% of children with depleted fat stores.[68] Reference values may be found at http://www.ncbi.nlm.nih.gov/.

Subscapular skin fold may be less affected than triceps skin fold in malnourished patients with neurologic impairment (85% vs 60% of healthy controls).[9] This pattern of retention of truncal fat is often seen in malnutrition. Although widely available, anthropometric measures such as skinfold thickness and arm circumference do not perform well in predicting percentage of body fat in patients with neurologic impairment.[69] BMI tends to underestimate body fat in patients with low lean body mass.[69]

Physical Examination

Physical examination will reveal signs of malnutrition and may show signs of specific nutrient deficiencies. The skin examination may reveal pallor, edema, petechiae, decubitus ulcers, or rashes. Cheilitis, smooth tongue, or gingival bleeding can be seen. The chest should be examined to detect abnormal breath sounds, suggesting lung disease resulting from chronic aspiration, and abdominal examination may reveal signs of constipation. Assessment of muscle tone and activity level will help determine energy needs. Skeletal deformities, such as scoliosis and contractures, should be noted, because they may interfere with adequate positioning during meals or with the placement of a percutaneous gastrostomy tube.

Meal Observation

Observation of a meal, preferably in the house environment, provides important information with regard to positioning, food intake and spillage, aspiration, and parent-child interaction during meals. Poor positioning is often observed even when an adequately adapted seat has been provided.[30] Mealtime can be a stressful time for the caregiver, and the parent-child interaction during the meal may be poor.[30] Monitoring of oxygen saturation during the meal may help detect hypoxemia.

Laboratory Evaluation

In general, laboratory evaluation adds very little to the clinical evaluation of nutritional status. Selected blood tests may be useful to assess specific conditions when clinically suspected. Serum albumin and prealbumin concentrations reflect nutritional adequacy in the previous month and week, respectively. However, in a study involving patients with CP, albumin and prealbumin concentrations were rarely below normal and showed little correlation with nutritional status.[70] Therefore, normal values may lead to a false sense of security when assessing these children. A complete blood cell count and appropriate iron studies will detect iron deficiency and iron-deficiency anemia that may occur with inadequate iron intake or chronic blood loss from reflux esophagitis. Serum electrolyte and blood urea nitrogen (BUN) may help assess hydration status, but BUN may not be reliable because of significantly decreased muscle mass. Vitamin D and serum calcium, phosphorus, and alkaline phosphatase concentrations should be measured, especially in patients taking anticonvulsants. Parathyroid hormone measurement and bone densitometry may be performed if necessary. Low levels of vitamin D are often seen in patients with motor disability.[32] Evidence of micronutrient status in patients with CP is limited. Low levels of folate, zinc, selenium, alpha-tocopherol, vitamin B_6, and ferritin have been reported. These deficiencies can often be suspected on the basis of nutritional history.[25]

Specific Investigation

Special investigations may be warranted, according to the medical history, the physical examination findings, and the intervention plan.

Videofluoroscopy evaluates the efficiency of the swallowing process using liquids and different food textures (see Chapter 26: Pediatric Dysphagia). It provides a better assessment of the risk of aspiration, especially in patients who aspirate without the typical history of coughing and choking. The videofluoroscopic study should be performed in a setting that mimics the conditions in which the child is fed at home, because positioning and length of the meal modify the risk of

VI

aspiration. Results of the videofluoroscopy may help in adapting the patient's diet to decrease the risk of aspiration.

An upper gastrointestinal tract series is useful to detect anatomic abnormalities that may affect food intake or cause emesis, such as peptic stricture, hiatal hernia, malrotation, or superior mesenteric artery syndrome but should not be used for diagnosing GER. In a patient with severe scoliosis, the stomach is often abnormally located in the thorax, and an upper gastrointestinal tract series should be performed before placement of a percutaneous gastrostomy tube to determine the position of the stomach.

Although the diagnosis of GER can be made clinically in most instances, a 24-hour esophageal pH monitoring study may help uncover subclinical reflux in patients with food refusal or chronic respiratory symptoms. It is especially important if a gastrostomy is considered to evaluate the need for an antireflux procedure. Gastric emptying scans can help determine the presence of delayed gastric emptying and possible aspiration from reflux.

Nutritional Intervention

After a careful evaluation of nutritional status, feeding abilities, medical comorbidities, and social situation, an intervention plan taking into account the patient's unique needs is determined by a multidisciplinary team. The team initiates nutritional therapy and should also provide continuous support and periodic reevaluation of the patient's condition and nutritional status.

Early intervention is important, because the best response to nutritional repletion is seen in children with the shortest duration between the neurologic insult and institution of nutritional therapy.[5] Children with neurologic impairment who had a gastrostomy tube placed in the first year of life were more likely to exceed the fifth percentile for weight and height for age.[12]

Nutritional Requirements

Energy needs and nutrient requirements are difficult to determine in the heterogeneous population of children with developmental disabilities. Body composition, muscle tone, and physical activity are different from those of unaffected children. Defining energy needs is very important in children who are unable to communicate hunger and satiety. Dietary Reference Intakes (DRIs) for age are based on healthy individuals and may overestimate the needs of children with neurologic impairment. Energy needs can be estimated using REE. For healthy children, REE is **calculated** with the WHO, Schofield, or Harris-Benedict equations based on age, gender, weight, and height. However, these equations are not adequate to estimate the energy needs of children with neurologic impairment.[42,71-73] Ideally, the patient's

REE should be **measured** to individualize caloric needs. The caloric requirements of children with spastic quadriplegic CP are usually 1.1 × **measured** REE.[42] Newer methods, such as bioelectrical impedance analysis (BIA), may help determine body composition more accurately and help to better predict energy expenditure.[45,74]

Because measuring REE is difficult in most clinical settings, predictive models to determine energy needs have been developed using anthropometric measurements. For example, height has been used to estimate caloric needs. Children without motor dysfunction required 14.7 kcal/cm, ambulatory patients with motor dysfunction required 13.9 kcal/cm, and nonambulatory patients with motor dysfunction required 11.1 kcal/cm.[75]

A formula using basal metabolic rate (BMR) that takes into consideration muscle tone, activity level, and growth factors has been developed to calculate energy needs in children with severe CP.[76]

Calories (kcal/day) = (BMR × muscle tone factor x activity factor) + growth factor.

Where:

- BMR (kcal/day) = body surface area (m²) × standard metabolic rate (kcal/m²/h) × 24 h

- muscle tone factor: 0.9 if decreased, 1.0 if normal, 1.1 if increased

- activity factor: 1.15 if bedridden, 1.2 if dependent, 1.25 if crawling, 1.3 if ambulatory

- growth factor: 5 kcal/g of desired weight gain

Nevertheless, the best way to evaluate the adequacy of nutritional therapy is to monitor the response in terms of weight gain. Calorie intake should be readjusted accordingly. This is particularly important after initiation of tube feedings, because excessive weight gain may occur.[12]

Goal of Nutritional Intervention

Forcing the weight-for-height z-score to or above zero in children with quadriplegic CP may lead to excessive body fat accumulation.[33] Ideally, body weight for children whose activity level is normal should be on the 50th percentile on the weight-for-height chart. If the patient is wheelchair bound but able to accomplish independent transfers, weight-for-height should approximate that of the 25th percentile, if the patient is bedridden, the 10th percentile is sufficient for adequate nutrition but low enough to facilitate the care and mobilization of the child. An exception should be made for patients younger than 3 years (chronologic or height age), for whom weight-for-height should be between the 25th and the 50th percentile, independent of activity level.[76]

VI

Source of Nutrients

The choice of formula depends on the age of the patient, the presence of any specific nutrient deficiencies or medical problems, and caloric requirements. Before 1 year of age, infant formula is preferred. The formula may be concentrated to increase calories in patients with high calorie needs and to reduce the volume in those with feeding intolerance (see Appendix C).

Supplements of carbohydrates or lipids may be used to increase caloric density or to change the composition of the diet (Table 37.4). Carbohydrates may be added in the form of glucose polymers. Lipid can be supplied as long- or medium-chain triglycerides (MCTs), are energy dense, and have little influence on osmolality but may aggravate delayed gastric emptying. MCT oil is absorbed without the need for chylomicron formation but does not contain essential fatty acids.

Table 37.4.
Calorie Concentrations of Modular Nutrients

Modular Nutrients		
Carbohydrate		
Polycose powder	glucose polymer	23 kcal/tablespoon
Moducal	maltodextrin	30 kcal/tablespoon
Fat		
Microlipid	safflower oil emulsion	4.5 kcal/mL
MCT oil	coconut oil	7.7 kcal/mL

Precautions should be taken to avoid preparation errors. By concentrating the formula, the renal solute load (RSL) increases and the amount of free water decreases. RSL should not exceed 250 mOsm/L and can be estimated as follows: RSL (mOsm) = [protein (g) × 4] + [Na (mEq) + K (mEq) + Cl (mEq)].

When supplements are used to modify the calorie content, the final composition of the diet must be determined to ensure that the final diet provides 35% to 65% of calories as carbohydrates, 7% to 16% of calories as protein, and 30% to 55% of calories as fat. If more than 55% of calories are fat, ketosis may develop. Excess carbohydrate may overwhelm absorption capacity and cause diarrhea, and protein intakes exceeding 5 g/kg/day may cause azotemia.

After 1 year of age, a pediatric 1-kcal/mL (30-kcal/oz) formula is generally used. Pediatric formulas have a higher vitamin and mineral content and should be used to prevent vitamin D, phosphorus, calcium, and iron deficiencies.[44] Adult formulas should be avoided in children with neurologic impairment, because their calorie-to-nutrient ratio may be inappropriate in children with low energy needs and may lead to micronutrient deficiencies. In some patients with low energy needs, a low-calorie

(0.75 cal/mL), nutrient-dense formula may be useful.[77] High-energy formulas (1.5 or 2 cal/mL) are sometimes necessary in patients who do not tolerate large volumes, but these require careful monitoring of hydration status, because a relatively small volume of formula or a concentrated formula may not provide an adequate amount of free water. A fiber-containing formula may improve constipation. In children with neurologic impairment with gastroesophageal reflux, some studies have shown that a whey-based formula was better tolerated than casein-based formula, and its use was associated with faster gastric emptying. Amino-acid based formulas may also be useful in these children.[78-81]

Route of Enteral Feedings

In patients with adequate oral motor skill and low risk of aspiration, oral intake may be maintained. It is often necessary to increase the caloric density of the food and to add oral supplements to provide sufficient energy intake. Food consistency should be adjusted according to the swallowing function study. Thickening agents may be added to liquids and purees. An occupational therapist can provide adapted utensils and adequate positioning during meals. Oral feeding therapy may improve oral feeding skills but have led to limited results in promoting feeding efficiency or weight gain.[82,83]

In view of the daily commitment and effort required to feed the child orally, everyday reality must be considered. Some caregivers spend a considerable amount of time feeding the child with disappointing results in terms of weight gain. In patients who require an excessive amount of time to ingest sufficient calories and/or are unable to maintain adequate weight gain, oral intake may be supplemented with tube feedings.

The decision to initiate tube feedings is often difficult for parents. Tube feedings may be perceived by them as a failure, and they may feel guilty about not being able to feed their child.[63] Parents are often reluctant to agree to tube feedings, because they think that their child will lose the ability to eat by mouth.[84] Therefore, unless there is a medical contraindication to feed the child orally, parents should be involved in the decision-making process. The decision to initiate tube feedings should be made with the parents with the goal of improving their quality of life as well as the child's. In children with severe neurologic impairment, most parents (90%) considered that tube feedings, despite frequent minor complications, improved their quality of life.[85] Enteral nutrition often improves the patients' nutritional status dramatically.[3,5,12] Tube-fed children with CP have significantly higher weight-for-height z-scores than do orally fed children with CP.[33]

The decision to initiate tube feedings does not preclude maintaining oral intake. Without the stress of having to provide sufficient calories orally, eating may become

VI

an enjoyable activity. However, patients with significant oral motor dysfunction and high risk of aspiration should be tube fed exclusively.

Method of Tube Feeding

Nasogastric Tube Feedings

Nasogastric tube feedings are minimally invasive. They may be attempted initially in some patients but should not be used for long-term nutrition support. The nasogastric tube is unaesthetic and uncomfortable and is easily dislodged. A short trial of nasogastric feedings is often helpful to determine the patient's tolerance to gastric feedings or to improve nutritional status before a more permanent solution is elected.

Nasojejunal Tube Feedings

Nasojejunal tube feedings are preferred in patients with significant gastroesophageal reflux who do not tolerate nasogastric tube feedings. Nasojejunal tubes can be inserted in the stomach and allowed to migrate into the small intestine with or without the help of prokinetics.[86,87] Other techniques, such as pH probe[88,89] or fluoroscopic technique, have largely been replaced by endoscopic placement. Nasojejunal tube feedings should not be used on a long-term basis.

Gastrostomy Tube Feedings

If long-term enteral nutrition is required (>3 months), placement of a gastrostomy tube is preferred. Although evidence-based literature evaluating risks versus benefits associated with gastrostomy tube feedings is lacking,[90-92] there are many potential advantages associated with a gastrostomy tube. Patients fed by gastrostomy tube have less drooling, secretions, vomiting, and constipation. Their weight gain improves without increasing the amount of calories given, probably because spillage is reduced.[93] Almost all indicators of nutritional status improve. Weight-for-age and weight-for-height z-scores improve, and height increases but not height-for-age z-score. Body fat, total body protein, and bone mineral content (BMC) increase but not BMC z-score.[15,94,95] Gastrostomy tube feedings are unlikely to reverse muscle wasting caused by disuse atrophy, and weight gain is mainly through fat deposition.[33] Patients must be closely monitored to avoid excessive weight gain after gastrostomy tube feedings are initiated.[96] The presence of a gastrostomy tube seems to relieve the stress associated with feedings[22,63] and improves quality of life for the caregivers.[97] Even though most parents were initially resistant to the procedure, perceiving it as unnatural or as an additional disability, they reported improvement in their child's health after placement of the gastrostomy tube.[98,99] Gastrostomy tube feedings do not seem to increase respiratory morbidity in children with CP and may decrease the number of chest infections.[2,100]

The gastrostomy tube can be placed surgically or percutaneously using radiologic or endoscopic techniques. The choice between a surgical and a percutaneous gastrostomy tube placement will depend on the presence or absence of GER requiring antireflux procedure and on the existence of contraindication(s) to percutaneous placement. The percutaneous endoscopic gastrostomy (PEG) is a simple technique that requires brief anesthesia or conscious sedation, involves minimal postoperative discomfort, and can be used within 6 hours of placement. In some patients with severe scoliosis, the stomach may not be accessible percutaneously, which precludes a PEG. Other contraindications to PEG placement include the presence of ascites, hepatomegaly or splenomegaly, portal hypertension, and in some cases, prior abdominal surgery. Bowel perforation, pneumoperitoneum, peritonitis, gastrocolic fistulas, bleeding, exacerbation of GER, and local infections may occur with PEG placement. The rate of major complications (requiring surgery) following PEG placement is 2% to 17.5% in the pediatric population.[101-103] Minor complications (infection, granulation tissue formation, leakage from the stoma, or tube dysfunction) occur in 4% to 22%.[102,103] GER after PEG placement occurred in 25% to 27% of patients without prior clinical symptoms, and 17% of patients required an antireflux procedure (ARP).[104,105] Among those with preexisting clinical reflux, 18.5% subsequently required an ARP or a gastrojejunal tube.[105] Preoperative oesophageal pH monitoring for evaluation of GER should be considered, because 5% of patients with neurologic impairment with a normal pre-PEG pH probe study eventually required an ARP versus 29% if the study was abnormal.[101] Even in patients with mild to moderate reflux, a PEG remains a good option. If reflux intensifies after the procedure, medical treatment should be attempted before considering an ARP.

In patients with severe gastroesophageal reflux, a surgical gastrostomy with an ARP should be considered. The patient must be evaluated carefully, because ARP failures, postoperative complications, and need for reintervention are more common in patients with neurologic impairments than in those without. In patients with neurologic impairment, the failure rate of an ARP is between 19% and 28%, and the incidence of major complications, between 10% and 33%.[106-108] Surgical complications of the ARP include prolonged ileus, intussusception, bleeding, bowel perforation, wound infection or dehiscence, wrap herniation, tight wrap, and pneumonia. Furthermore, the ARP (Nissen procedure) may induce myoelectrical disturbances and inappropriate activation of the emetic reflex, inducing postoperative retching.[109] Patients with neurologic impairment are particularly at risk of developing dumping and gas bloat syndrome after an ARP. A careful evaluation of gastric emptying is necessary to identify patients who require a pyloroplasty in conjunction with ARP. There is no role for prophylactic ARP in patients with no prior reflux.

Surgical gastrostomy tube placement alone should be reserved for patients with contraindications to percutaneous gastrostomy tube placement or in patients whose stomach cannot be accessed percutaneously. Postgastrostomy reflux occurs more frequently with surgical gastrostomy than with PEG. Sixty-six percent of patients with normal pH probe studies prior to surgical gastrostomy tube placement had a positive study after the procedure.[110] In patients with neurologic impairment without reflux undergoing a surgical gastrostomy tube placement, between 14% and 44% developed reflux, and 14% to 33% subsequently required an ARP.[111,112]

Gastrojejunostomy Tube Feedings

Percutaneously placed gastrojejunal feeding tubes may be a reasonable alternative to gastrostomy tubes and an ARP for some patients.[113-115] They can be used for patients with reflux who are not good candidates for prolonged anaesthesia or patients with recurrence of reflux after an ARP. The gastrojejunal tube does not treat GER, and the patient will continue to require medication. A percutaneously placed gastrojejunal tube carries less risk of major complications in patients with neurologic impairment than a Nissen procedure with a surgically placed gastrostomy tube (11.8% vs 33.3%) but a higher risk of minor complications (44.1% vs 6.6%). Most of the minor complications associated with the gastrojejunal tube relate to tube malfunction.[115]

Method of Administration of Tube Feedings

The preferred mode of administration is bolus feeding. Bolus feedings physiologically mimic meals and are more convenient in ambulatory patients. Initially, continuous infusions at night may be required in combination with daytime boluses for patients with poor nutritional status and high energy needs. Subsequent change to daytime boluses may be attempted if tolerated. Some patients with reflux or delayed gastric emptying may not tolerate boluses and may require long-term continuous feeds. When the child requires transpyloric gastrojejunal feedings, a continuous infusion is necessary.

Approach to Feeding Intolerance

Vomiting and feeding intolerance occurs commonly after tube feedings are initiated. Although the nasogastric or gastrostomy tubes are frequently blamed, feeding intolerance may be the result of the major changes in the diet occurring with the initiation of tube feedings in terms of texture (mostly purees to liquid) and in terms of volume. A conservative approach should be favored. In the absence of intercurrent infections and anatomic problems, the feeding regimen should be reevaluated. Changing the feeding schedule from boluses to continuous feeds, decreasing the rate of infusion or concentrating the formula to decrease the volume may improve tolerance. The addition of pectin to the formula may help decrease reflux, vomiting, and respiratory symptoms in patients with CP.[116] Medical treatment of reflux with acid-suppressing therapy and/or prokinetics should be considered. If feeding intolerance persists, an ARP may be needed.

Ethical Considerations

With advances in medicine, children with developmental disabilities are surviving longer and are often cared for at home by their parents. There is increasing awareness that improving nutritional status improves their health and quality of life. Nutritional intervention should be carefully planned and discussed with the family. The decision to initiate tube feedings and, most of all, to have a gastrostomy tube placed, is often difficult.[98] Medical and parental opinions may be different, and parental concerns should not be overlooked. Parents may think of tube feedings as a failure from their part to adequately feed their child and to care for their child altogether. They may see this as burden or as further evidence of their child's disease.[117] Nutritional intervention is more than improving nutritional status. It should be viewed as a tool to improve the patient's and the parent's quality of life as well.

Conclusion

Children with neurologic disabilities often experience growth retardation, variable energy requirements, and abnormal body composition. One of the basic components of care for these patients, therefore, is provision of adequate nutrition. Medical management of these patients must include careful monitoring of their nutritional status, and early, multidisciplinary nutritional intervention is essential to promote appropriate growth and well-being. It is important to provide continuous support to the families of children with developmental disabilities with and without feeding problems to ensure the success of nutritional therapy.

References

1. Samson-Fang L, Fung E, Stallings VA, et al. Relationship of nutritional status to health and societal participation in children with cerebral palsy. *J Pediatr*. 2002;141(5):637-643
2. Soylu OB, Unalp A, Uran N, et al. Effect of nutritional support in children with spastic quadriplegia. *Pediatr Neurol*. 2008;39:330-334
3. Patrick J, Boland M, Stoski D, Murray GE. Rapid correction of wasting in children with cerebral palsy. *Dev Med Child Neurol*. 1986;28(6):734-739

VI

4. Shapiro BK, Green P, Krick J, Allen D, Capute AJ. Growth of severely impaired children: neurological versus nutritional factors. *Dev Med Child Neurol*. 1986;28(6):729-733

5. Sanders KD, Cox K, Cannon R, et al. Growth response to enteral feeding by children with cerebral palsy. *JPEN: J Parenter Enteral Nutr*. 1990;14(1):23-26

6. Lewis D, Khoshoo V, Pencharz PB, Golladay ES. Impact of nutritional rehabilitation on gastroesophageal reflux in neurologically impaired children. *J Pediatr Surg*. 1994;29(2):167-170

7. Campanozzi A, Capano G, Miele E, et al. Impact of malnutrition on gastrointestinal disorders and gross motor abilities in children with cerebral palsy. *Brain Dev*. 2007;29(1):25-29

8. Wodarski LA. An interdisciplinary nutrition assessment and intervention protocol for children with disabilities. *J Am Diet Assoc*. 1990;90(11):1563-1568

9. Stallings VA, Charney EB, Davies JC, Cronk CE. Nutrition-related growth failure of children with quadriplegic cerebral palsy. *Dev Med Child Neurol*. 1993;35(2):126-138

10. Stallings VA, Charney EB, Davies JC, Cronk CE. Nutritional status and growth of children with diplegic or hemiplegic cerebral palsy. *Dev Med Child Neurol*. 1993;35(11):997-1006

11. Stallings VA, Cronk CE, Zemel BS, Charney EB. Body composition in children with spastic quadriplegic cerebral palsy. *J Pediatr*. 1995;126(5 Pt 1):833-839

12. Rempel GR, Colwell SO, Nelson RP. Growth in children with cerebral palsy fed via gastrostomy. *Pediatrics*. 1988;82(6):857-862

13. Stevenson RD, Hayes RP, Cater LV, Blackman JA. Clinical correlates of linear growth in children with cerebral palsy. *Dev Med Child Neurol*. 1994;36(2):135-142

14. Krick J, Murphy-Miller P, Zeger S, Wright E. Pattern of growth in children with cerebral palsy. *J Am Diet Assoc*. 1996;96(7):680-685

15. Dahlseng MO, Finbraten AK, Juliusson PB, Skranes J, Andersen G, Vik T. Feeding problems, growth and nutritional status in children with cerebral palsy. *Acta Paediatr*. 2012;101(1):92-98

16. Day SM, Strauss DJ, Vachon PJ, Rosenbloom L, Shavelle RM, Wu YW. Growth patterns in a population of children and adolescents with cerebral palsy. *Dev Med Child Neurol*. 2007;49(3):167-171

17. Stevenson RD, Conaway M, Chumlea WC, et al. Growth and health in children with moderate-to-severe cerebral palsy. *Pediatrics*. 2006;118(3):1010-1018

18. Krick J, Van Duyn M. The relationship between oral-motor involvement and growth: a pilot study in a pediatric population with cerebral palsy. *J Am Diet Assoc*. 1984;84(5):555-559

19. Thommessen M, Heiberg A, Kase BF, Larsen S, Riis G. Feeding problems, height and weight in different groups of disabled children. *Acta Paediatr Scand*. 1991;80(5):527-533

20. Motion S, Northstone K, Emond A, Stucke S, Golding J. Early feeding problems in children with cerebral palsy: weight and neurodevelopmental outcomes. *Dev Med Child Neurol*. 2002;44(1):40-43

21. Troughton KEV, Hill AE. Relation between objectively measured feeding competence and nutrition in children with cerebral palsy. *Dev Med Child Neurol*. 2001;43(3):187-190

22. Sullivan PB, Lambert B, Rose M, Ford-Adams M, Johnson A, Griffiths P. Prevalence and severity of feeding and nutritional problems in children with neurological impairement: Oxford feeding study. *Dev Med Child Neurol.* 2000;42(10):674-680

23. Sullivan PB, Juszczak E, Lambert BR, Rose M, Ford-Adams ME, Johnson A. Impact of feeding problems on nutritional intake and growth: Oxford feeding study II. *Dev Med Child Neurol.* 2002;44(7):461-467

24. Fung EB, Samson-Fang L, Stallings VA, et al. Feeding dysfunction is associated with poor growth and health status in children with cerebral palsy. *J Am Diet Assoc.* 2002;102(3):361-373

25. Hillesund E, Skranes J, Trygg KU, Bohmer T. Micronutrient status in children with cerebral palsy. *Acta Paediatr.* 2007;96(8):1195-1198

26. Stevenson RD, Roberts KD, Vogtle L. The effect of non-nutritional factors on growth in cerebral palsy. *Dev Med Child Neurol.* 1995;37(2):124-130

27. Roberts CD, Vogtle L, Stevenson RD. Effect of hemiplegia on skeletal maturation. *J Pediatr.* 1994;125(5 Pt 1):824-828

28. Kuperminc MN, Gurka MJ, Houlihan CM, et al. Puberty, statural growth, and growth hormone release in children with cerebral palsy. *J Pediatr Rehabil Med.* 2009;2(2):131-141

29. Henderson RC, Grossberg RI, Matuszewski J, et al. Growth and nutritional status in residential center versus home-living children and adolescents with quadriplegic cerebral palsy. *J Pediatr.* 2007;151(2):161-166

30. Reilly S, Skuse D. Characteristics and management of feeding problems of young children with cerebral palsy. *Dev Med Child Neurol.* 1992;34(5):379-388

31. Stallings VA, Zemel BS, Davies JC, Cronk CE, Charney EB. Energy expenditure of children and adolescents with severe disabilities: a cerebral palsy model. *Am J Clin Nutr.* 1996;64(4):627-634

32. Kilpinen-Loisa P, Pihko H, Vesander U, Paganus A, Ritanen U, Makitie O. Insufficient energy and nutrient intake in children with motor disability. *Acta Paediatr.* 2009;98(8):1329-1333

33. Kong CK, Wong HS. Weight-for-height values and limb anthropometric composition of tube-fed children with quadriplegic cerebral palsy. *Pediatrics.* 2005;116(6):e839-e845

34. Reilly S, Skuse D, Poblete X. Prevalence of feeding problems and oral motor dysfunction in children with cerebral palsy: a community survey. *J Pediatr.* 1996;129(6):877-882

35. Dahl M, Thommessen M, Rasmussen M, Selberg T. Feeding and nutritional characteristics in children with moderate or severe cerebral palsy. *Acta Paediatr.* 1996;85(6):697-701

36. Gisel EG, Patrick J. Identification of children with cerebral palsy unable to maintain a normal nutritional state. *Lancet.* 1988;1(8580):283-286

37. Johnson CB, Deitz JC. Time use of mothers with preschool children: a pilot study. *Am J Occup Ther.* 1985;39(9):578-583

38. Rogers BT, Arvedson J, Msall M, Demerath RR. Hypoxemia during oral feedings of children with severe cerebral palsy. *Dev Med Child Neurol.* 1993;35(1):3-10

VI

39. Sondheimer JM, Morris BA. Gastroesophageal reflux among severely retarded children. 5. *J Pediatr*. 1979;94(5):710-714

40. Ravelli AM, Milla PJ. Vomiting and gastroesophageal motor activity in children with disorders of the central nervous system. *J Pediatr Gastroenterol Nutr*. 1998;26(1):56-63

41. Zangen T, Ciarla C, Zangen S, et al. Gastrointestinal motility and sensory abnormalities may contribute to food refusal in medically fragile toddlers. *J Pediatr Gastroenterol Nutr*. 2003;37(3):287-293

42. Azcue MP, Zello GA, Levy LD, Pencharz PB. Energy expenditure and body composition in children with spastic quadriplegic cerebral palsy. *J Pediatr*. 1996;129(6):870-876

43. Bandini LG, Schoeller DA, Fukagawa NK, Wykes LJ, Dietz WH. Body composition and energy expenditure in adolescents with cerebral palsy or myelodysplasia. *Pediatr Res*. 1991;29(1):70-77

44. Fried MD, Pencharz PB. Energy and nutrient intakes of children with spastic quadriplegia. *J Pediatr*. 1991;119(1):947-949

45. Rieken R, van Goudoever JB, Schierbeek H, et al. Measuring body composition and energy expenditure in children with severe neurologic impairment and intellectual disability. *Am J Clin Nutr*. 2011;94(3):759-766

46. Rose J, Gamble JG, Burgos A, Medeiros J, Haskell WL. Energy expenditure index of walking for normal children and for children with cerebral palsy. *Dev Med Child Neurol*. 1990;32(4):333-340

47. Brunner R, Doderlein L. Pathological fractures in patients with cerebral palsy. *J Pediatr Orthop B*. 1996;5(4):232-238

48. Henderson RC, Lark RK, Gurka MJ, et al. Bone density and metabolism in children and adolescents with moderate to severe cerebral palsy. *Pediatrics*. 2002;110(1 Pt 1):e5

49. Duncan B, Barton LL, Lloyd J, Marks-Katz M. Dietary considerations in osteopenia in tube-fed nonambulatory children with cerebral palsy. *Clin Pediatr (Phila)*. 1999;38(3):133-137

50. Henderson RC, Lin PP, Greene WB. Bone-mineral density in children and adolescents who have spastic cerebral palsy. *J Bone Joint Surg*. 1995;77(11):1671-1681

51. Morijiri Y, Sato T. Factors causing rickets in institutionalised handicapped children on anticonvulsant therapy. *Arch Dis Child*. 1981;56(6):446-449

52. Tolman KG, Jubiz W, Sannella JJ, Madsen JA, Belsey RE, Goldsmith RS, Freston JW. Osteomalacia associated with anticonvulsant drug therapy in mentally retarded children. *Pediatrics*. 1975;56(1):45-50

53. Bischof F, Basu D, Pettifor JM. Pathological long-bone fractures in residents with cerebral palsy in a long-term care facility in South Africa. *Dev Med Child Neurol*. 2002;44(2):119-122

54. Henderson RC, Kairalla J, Abbas A, Stevenson RD. Predicting low bone density in children and young adults with quadriplegic cerebral palsy. *Dev Med Child Neurol*. 2004;46(6):416-419

55. Baer MT, Kozlowski BW, Blyler EM, Trahms CM, Taylor ML, Hogan MP. Vitamin D, calcium, and bone status in children with developmental delay in relation to anticonvulsant use and ambulatory status. *Am J Clin Nutr*. 1997;65(4):1042-1051

56. Chad KE, McKay HA, Zello GA, Bailey DA, Faulkner RA, Snyder RE. Body composition in nutritionally adequate ambulatory and non-ambulatory children with cerebral palsy and a healthy reference group. *Dev Med Child Neurol.* 2000;42(5):334-339

57. Hartman C, Brik R, Tamir A, Merrick J, Shamir R. Bone quantitative ultrasound and nutritional status in severely handicapped institutionalized children and adolescents. *Clin Nutr.* 2004;23(1):89-98

58. Henderson RC, Lark RK, Kecskemethy HH, Miller F, Harcke HT, Bachrach SJ. Biphosphonates to treat osteopenia in children with quadriplegic cerebral palsy: A randomized, placebo-controlled clinical trial. *J Pediatr.* 2002;141(5):644-651

59. Bachrach SJ, Kecskemethy HH, Harcke HT, Hossain J. Decreased fracture incidence after 1 year of pamidronate treatment in children with spastic quadriplegic cerebral palsy. *Dev Med Child Neurol.* 2010;52(9):837-842

60. Palisano R, Rosenbaum P, Walter S, Russell D, Wood E, Galuppi B. Development and reliability of a system to classify gross motor function in children with cerebral palsy. *Dev Med Child Neurol.* 1997;39(4):214-223

61. Liu LF, Moyer-Mileur L, Gooch J, Samson-Fang L. The contribution of tone to resting energy expenditure in children with moderate to severe cerebral palsy: evaluation utilizing intrathecal baclofen injection. *J Pediatr Rehabil Med.* 2008;1(2):163-167

62. McCoy AA, Fox MA, Schaubel DE, Ayyangar RN. Weight gain in children with hypertonia of cerebral origin receiving intrathecal baclofen therapy. *Arch Phys Med Rehabil.* 2006;87(11):1503-1508

63. Sleigh G. Mothers' voice: a qualitative study on feeding children with cerebral palsy. *Child Care Health Dev.* 2005;31(4):373-383

64. Hogan SE. Knee height as a predictor of recumbent length for individuals with mobility-impaired cerebral palsy. *J Am Coll Nutr.* 1999;18(2):201-205

65. Spender QW, Cronk CE, Charney EB, Stallings VA. Assessment of linear growth of children with cerebral palsy: use of alternative measures to height or length. *Dev Med Child Neurol.* 1989;31(2):206-214

66. Stevenson RD. Use of segmental measures to estimate stature in children with cerebral palsy. *Arch Pediatr Adolesc Med.* 1995;149(6):658-662

67. Chumlea WC, Guo SS, Steinbaugh ML. Prediction of stature from knee height for black and white adults and children with application to mobility-impaired or handicapped persons. *J Am Diet Assoc.* 1994;94(12):1385-1388

68. Samson-Fang LJ, Stevenson RD. Identification of malnutrition in children with cerebral palsy: poor performance of weight for height centiles. *Dev Med Child Neurol.* 2000;42(3):162-168

69. Kuperminc MN, Gurka MJ, Bennis JA, et al. Anthropometric measures: poor predictors of body fat in children with moderate to severe cerebral palsy. *Dev Med Child Neurol.* 2010;52(9):824-830

70. Lark RK, Williams CL, Stadler D, et al. Serum prealbumin and albumin concentrations do not reflect nutritional state in children with cerebral palsy. *J Pediatr.* 2005;147(5):695-697

VI

71. Dickerson RN, Brown RO, Gervasio JG, Hak EB, Hak LJ, Williams JE. Measured energy expenditure of tube-fed patients with severe neurodevelopmental disabilities. *J Am Coll Nutr*. 1999;18(1):61-68

72. Dickerson RN, Brown RO, Hanna DL, Williams JE. Validation of a new method for estimating resting energy expenditure of non-ambulatory tube-fed patients with severe neurodevelopmental disabilities. *Nutrition*. 2002;18(7-8):578-582

73. Bandini LG, Puelzl-Quinn H, Morelli JA, Fukagawa NK. Estimation of energy requirements in persons with severe central nervous system impairment. *J Pediatr*. 1995;126(5 Pt 1):828-832

74. Liu LF, Roberts R, Moyer-Mileur L, Samson-Fang L. Determination of body composition in children with cerebral palsy: bioelectrical impedance analysis and anthropometry vs dual-energy x-ray absorptiometry. *J Am Diet Assoc*. 2005;105(5):794-797

75. Culley WJ, Thomas OM. Caloric requirements of mentally retarded children with and without motor dysfunction. *J Pediatr*. 1969;75(3):380-384

76. Krick J, Murphy PE, Markham JF, Shapiro BK. A proposed formula for calculating energy needs of children with cerebral palsy. *Dev Med Child Neurol*. 1992;34(6):481-487

77. Vernon-Roberts A, Wells J, Grant H, Alder N, Vadamalayan B, Eltumi M, Sullivan PB. Gastrostomy feeding in cerebral palsy: enough and no more. *Dev Med Child Neurol*. 2010;52(12):1099-1105

78. Fried MD, Khoshoo V, Secker DJ, Gilday DL, Ash JM, Pencharz PB. Decrease in gastric emptying time and episodes of regurgitation in children with spastic quadriplegia fed a whey-based formula. *J Pediatr*. 1992;120(4 Pt 1):569-572

79. Khoshoo V, Zembo M, King A, Dhar M, Reifen R, Pencharz P. Incidence of gastroesophageal reflux with whey- and casein- based formulas in infants and children with severe neurological impairment. *J Pediatr Gastroenterol Nutr*. 1996;22(1):48-55

80. Miele E, Staiano A, Tozzi A, Auricchio R, Paparo F, Troncone R. Clinical response to amino acid-based formula in neurologically impaired children with refractory esophagitis. *J Pediatr Gastroenterol Nutr*. 2002;35(3):314-319

81. Lightdale J, Gremse DA; American Academy of Pediatrics, Section on Gastroenterology, Hepatology, and Nutrition. Gastroesophageal reflux: management guidelines for the pediatrician. *Pediatrics*. 2013;131(5):e1684-e1695

82. Gisel EG, Applegate-Ferrante T, Benson JE, Bosma JF. Effect of oral sensorimotor treatment on measures of growth, eating efficiency and aspiration in the dysphagic child with cerebral palsy. *Dev Med Child Neurol*. 1995;37(6):528-543

83. Gisel EG. Effect of oral sensorimotor treatment on measures of growth and efficiency of eating in the moderately eating-impaired child with cerebral palsy. *Dysphagia*. 1996;11(1):48-58

84. Corwin DS, Isaacs JS, Georgeson KE, Bartolucci AA, Cloud HH, Craig CB. Weight and length increases in children after gastrostomy placement. *J Am Diet Assoc*. 1996;96(9):874-879

85. Smith SW, Camfield C, Camfield P. Living with cerebral palsy and tube feedings: a population-based follow-up study. *J Pediatr*. 1999;135(3):307-310

86. Taylor B, Schallom L. Bedside small bowel feeding tube placement in critically ill patients utilizing a dietician/nurse approach. *Nutr Clin Pract*. 2001;16:258-262

87. Kalliafas S, Choban PS, Ziegler D, Drago S, Flancbaum L. Erythromycin facilitates postpyloric placement of nasoduodenal feeding tubes in intensive care unit patients: randomized, double-blinded, placebo-controlled trial. *JPEN J Parenter Enteral Nutr.* 2004;20(6):385-388

88. Dimand RJ, Veereman-Waters G, Braner DA. Bedside placement of pH-guided transpyloric small bowel feeding tubes in critically ill infants and small children. *JPEN J Parenter Enteral Nutr.* 1997;21(2):112-114

89. Krafte-Jacobs B, Persinger M, Carver J, Moore L, Brilli R. Rapid placement of transpyloric feeding tubes: a comparison of pH-assisted and standard insertion techniques in children. *Pediatrics.* 1996;98(2 Pt 1):242-248

90. Sleigh G, Sullivan PB, Thomas AG. Gastrostomy feeding versus oral feeding alone for children with cerebral palsy. *Cochrane Database Syst Rev.* 2004;(2):CD003943

91. Sleigh G, Brocklehurst P. Gastrostomy feeding in cerebral palsy: a systematic review. *Arch Dis Child.* 2004;89(6):534-539

92. Samson-Fang L, Butler C, O'Donnell M. Effects of gastrostomy feeding in children with cerebral palsy: an AACPDM evidence report. *Dev Med Child Neurol.* 2003;45(6):415-426

93. Craig GM, Carr LJ, Cass H, et al. Medical, surgical, and health outcomes of gastrostomy feeding. *Dev Med Child Neurol.* 2006;48(5):353-360

94. Sullivan PB, Juszczak E, Bachlet AM, et al. Gastrostomy tube feeding in children with cerebral palsy: a prospective, longitudinal study. *Dev Med Child Neurol.* 2005;47(2):77-85

95. Arrowsmith F, Allen J, Gaskin K, Somerville H, Clarke S, O'Loughlin E. The effect of gastrostomy tube feeding on body protein and bone mineralization in children with quadriplegic cerebral palsy. *Dev Med Child Neurol.* 2010;52(11):1043-1047

96. Sullivan PB, Alder N, Bachlet AM, et al. Gastrostomy feeding in cerebral palsy: too much of a good thing? *Dev Med Child Neurol.* 2006;48(11):877-882

97. Sullivan PB, Juszczak E, Bachlet AM, et al. Impact of gastrostomy tube feeding on the quality of life of carers of children with cerebral palsy. *Dev Med Child Neurol.* 2004;46(12):796-800

98. Petersen MC, Kedia S, Davis P, Newman L, Temple C. Eating and feeding are not the same: caregivers' perceptions of gastrostomy feeding for children with cerebral palsy. *Dev Med Child Neurol.* 2006;48(9):713-717

99. Mahant S, Friedman JN, Connolly B, Goia C, Macarthur C. Tube feeding and quality of life in children with severe neurological impairment. *Arch Dis Child.* 2009;94(9):668-673

100. Sullivan PB, Morrice JS, Vernon-Roberts A, Grant H, Eltumi M, Thomas AG. Does gastrostomy tube feeding in children with cerebral palsy increase the risk of respiratory morbidity? *Arch Dis Child.* 2006;91(6):478-482

101. Sulaeman E, Udall JN, Brown RF, et al. Gastroesophageal reflux and Nissen fundoplication following percutaneous endoscopic gastrostomy in children. *J Pediatr Gastroenterol Nutr.* 1998;26(3):269-273

102. Khattak IU, Kimber C, Kiely EM, Spitz L. Percutaneous endoscopic gastrostomy in paediatric practice: complications and outcome. *J Pediatr Surg.* 1998;33(1):67-72

VI

103. Behrens R, Lang T, Muschweck H, Richter T, Hofbeck M. Percutaneous endoscopic gastrostomy in children and adolescents. *J Pediatr Gastroenterol Nutr*. 1997;25(5):487-491

104. Heine RG, Reddihough DS, Catto-Smith AG. Gastro-oesophageal reflux and feeding problems after gastrostomy in children with severe neurological impairment. *Dev Med Child Neurol*. 1995;37(4):320-329

105. Isch JA, Rescorla FJ, Scherer LR, West KW, Grosfeld JL. The development of gastroesophageal reflux after percutaneous endoscopic gastrostomy. *J Pediatr Surg*. 1997;32(2):321-322

106. Pearl RH, Robie DK, Ein SH, et al. Complications of gastroesophageal antireflux surgery in neurologically impaired versus neurologically normal children. *J Pediatr Surg*. 1990;25(11):1169-1173

107. Smith CD, Othersen HBJ, Gogan NJ, Walker JD. Nissen fundoplication in children with profound neurologic disability. *Ann Surg*. 1992;215(6):654-658

108. Spitz L, Roth K, Kiely EM, Brereton RJ, Drake DP, Milla PJ. Operation for gastro-oesophageal reflux associated with severe mental retardation. *Arch Dis Child*. 1993;68(3):347-351

109. Richards CA, Andrews PL, Spitz L, Milla PJ. Nissen fundoplication may induce gastric myoelectrical disturbance in children. *J Pediatr Surg*. 1998;33(12):1801-1805

110. Jolley SG, Smith EI, Tunell WP. Protective antireflux operation with feeding gastrostomy. Experience with children. *Ann Surg*. 1985;201(6):736-740

111. Langer JC, Wesson DE, Ein SH, Filler RM, Shandling B, Superina RA, Papa M. Feeding gastrostomy in neurologically impaired children: is an antireflux procedure necessary? *J Pediatr Gastroenterol Nutr*. 1988;7(6):837-841

112. Wheatley MJ, Wesley JR, Tkach DM, Coran AG. Long-term follow-up of brain-damaged children requiring feeding gastrostomy: should an antireflux procedure always be performed? *J Pediatr Surg*. 1991;26(3):301-304

113. Wales PW, Diamond IR, Dutta S, Muraca S, Chait P, Connoly B, Langer JC. Fundoplication and gastrostomy versus image-guided gastrojejunal tube for enteral feedings in neurologically impaired children with gastroesophageal reflux. *J Pediatr Surg*. 2002;37(3):407-412

114. Peters JM, Simpson P, Tolia V. Experience with gastrojejunal feeding tubes in children. *Am J Gastroenterol*. 1997;92(3):476-480

115. Albanese CT, Towbin RB, Ulman I, Lewis J, Smith SD. Percutaneous gastrojejunostomy versus Nissen fundoplication for enteral feeding of the neurologically impaired child with gastroesophageal reflux. *J Pediatr*. 1993;123(3):371-375

116. Miyazawa R, Tomomasa T, Kaneko H, Arakawa H, Shimizu N, Morikawa A. Effects of pectin liquid on gastroesophageal reflux disease in children with cerebral palsy. *BMC Gastroenterol*. 2008;8:11

117. Craig GM, Scambler G, Spitz L. Why parents of children with neurodevelopmental disabilities requiring gastrostomy feeding need more support. *Dev Med Child Neurol*. 2003;45(3):183-188

Chapter 38

Nutrition of Children Who Are Critically Ill

Introduction

Provision of optimal nutrition therapy is a critical aspect of care for critically ill infants and children. The goal of nutrition therapy is to meet both macronutrient and micronutrient requirements and to preserve lean body mass during the catabolic phase of the stress response to illness. The stress of a variety of critical illnesses, such as trauma, sepsis, surgery, or burns, places significant metabolic demands on the patient. Failure to accurately estimate and meet these demands can result in nutritional deterioration during illness.[1] Critically ill children have a high incidence of malnutrition on admission to the pediatric intensive care unit (PICU) and low metabolic reserves.[2] Furthermore, accurate estimation and bedside delivery of nutrient needs is often challenging in the PICU environment. As a result, the task of meeting the energy and protein needs during this period is difficult, and both underfeeding and overfeeding have been documented with deleterious consequences.[1,3-5] A sound understanding of the metabolic response to stress and awareness of the challenges to nutrient provision will help in the provision of optimal nutrition during critical illness. Prevention of nutritional deficiencies during critical illness must be prioritized in the PICU to achieve optimal nutritional and other clinical outcomes.

Malnutrition and Metabolic Reserves

Because the characteristics of critical illnesses are varied, valid assessment of nutritional status of PICU patients can be difficult.[6] Commonly used anthropometric techniques may be inaccurate because of fluid shifts and capillary leak that are inherent to the acute phases of many illnesses. The routine weighing and measuring of height (and, thus, body mass index) of a critically ill child may be impeded by the severity of illness. Standard biochemical measures of visceral protein and micronutrient concentrations are also altered during critical illness. Hence, the true incidence of malnutrition in the PICU may be unknown, although reports suggest that more than 25% of children in the PICU are already malnourished on admission.[7] Critical illness imposes the risk of further nutritional deterioration, with failure to estimate energy expenditure accurately and inadequate substrate delivery at the bedside.[8-11]

The body composition of healthy infants and children differs from adults, with limited resources of protein and lipids available during periods of stress.[12,13] The breakdown of protein is a principle feature of the metabolic stress response, making free amino acids available for anti-inflammatory and tissue healing pathways. This adaptive response, while sustaining an individual during acute stress, may cause significant lean body mass depletion during prolonged or chronic stress responses. Thus, infants and children are particularly at risk of the deleterious effects of protein imbalance from protracted catabolic stress. Providing optimal macronutrients requires an understanding of the characteristic features of macronutrient metabolism during critical illness.

Protein Metabolism

Critical illness is characterized by high protein turnover, with continuous protein degradation and decreased synthesis.[14] This adaptive response allows a large amount of amino acids to be available in the free amino acid pool. Free amino acids are redistributed away from skeletal muscle for tissue repair, wound healing and participation in inflammatory response pathways. In addition, the carbon skeleton is conscripted via the gluconeogenetic pathway to provide glucose for various organs. Protein turnover is increased in the acute phase of critical illness, and its contribution to the amino acid pool far outweighs that of dietary protein intake. The reprioritization of amino acids is manifested by a marked increase in the circulation of acute-phase proteins (such as C-reactive protein, fibrinogen, alpha-1-antitrypsin, haptoglobin) and decrease in liver-derived visceral proteins (such as albumin and retinol-binding protein). Overall, protein breakdown during critical illness exceeds protein synthesis and sets the stage for a negative protein (nitrogen) balance. Unlike in starvation, the provision of dietary glucose during critical illness does not suppress the protein breakdown, nor does it decrease endogenous gluconeogenesis, often resulting in hyperglycemia. A protracted response with ongoing protein turnover that is not matched by concomitant adequate protein intake, can result in a steady loss of lean body mass.[15] The likelihood of morbidity rises as muscle loss is not restricted to skeletal muscle but may involve cardiac and diaphragmatic muscles with resultant cardiopulmonary insufficiency. Optimal protein intake helps restore protein balance by enhancing protein synthesis, while having no effect on protein degradation.[12] Provision of optimal protein intake during critical illness is perhaps the most important aspect of nutrition therapy in this population. The use of specific amino acid solutions for specific groups of critically ill children remains investigational at this time. In addition, the role of hormonal and other interventions to reduce the severity of protein degradation during critical illness has not been adequately studied in the general PICU population.[16]

Carbohydrate and Lipid Metabolism

Once protein needs have been determined, the next step in devising the nutrition support plan involves a rational partitioning of carbohydrate and lipids as energy sources. The metabolism of carbohydrates during critical illness is characterized by the increase in glucose production as described previously. Gluconeogenesis ensures that there is an energy source for glucose-dependent organs, such as brain, erythrocytes, and renal medulla. The provision of glucose in the diet does not stop gluconeogenesis, and the concomitant decrease in glucose utilization from insulin insensitivity during critical illness results in hyperglycemia.[17] Stress hyperglycemia was long held as benign and an incidental feature of the acute response to illness. However, recent reports suggest an association between high serum glucose concentrations and poor outcomes during critical illness.[18-20] The role of the tight glycemic control (TGC) strategy, aimed at using insulin to prevent hyperglycemia in critically ill children, is currently being investigated in multicenter trials. Safe glycemic control in children involves attention to the risk of hypoglycemia, which remains the principal hurdle to insulin therapy for TGC.[21] In a large randomized control trial of TGC, more than 6000 critically ill adults were randomized to intensive glucose control (target blood glucose concentration, 80-108 mg/dL) using insulin or conventional glucose control (target blood glucose concentration, 108 mg/dL or less). The intensive glucose control group had a significantly higher incidence of hypoglycemia and mortality.[22] Although the results of this trial have generated considerable discussions regarding the wisdom of this strategy, the unacceptable incidence of hypoglycemia in the treatment arm has required future investigators to focus on the safe implementation of TGC. Newer modalities of blood glucose monitoring and sophisticated algorithms for insulin delivery may allow safe glycemic control to be undertaken in the future.[23] Until then, prudent glycemic control is generally practiced at individual centers, although the triggers for insulin use in the PICU remain widely variable.[24]

In contrast, the incidence of overfeeding during critical illness might be under-recognized in critically ill children.[4] Inaccurate estimation of the true energy needs, overestimation of the energy demands of the metabolic stress response, and failure to regularly follow weight all contribute to unintended overfeeding in this population. Overfeeding, especially with a predominantly carbohydrate-based diet, results in the excess glucose being synthesized to fat and presents an additional carbon dioxide burden to the individual.[25,26] In critically ill children with respiratory insufficiency, this might increase or prolong the needs for mechanical ventilation. Respiratory quotient, defined as the ratio of carbon dioxide production to oxygen consumption, can be measured by indirect calorimetry and is much higher in cases in which excess glucose is provided with concomitant fat synthesis.[27] On the other

VI

hand, excess dietary lipids are stored as triglycerides and do not increase the carbon dioxide burden. Thus, a mixed-fuel system, in which lipids account for 30% to 40% of total energy needs, is commonly employed in the PICU.

Energy Requirement During Critical Illness

Energy needs during critical illness might be related to the nature and severity of insult. The metabolic stress response was once thought to be associated with a significant energy burden on the host.[28] Indeed, patients with burn injury exhibit a hypermetabolic response, with energy expenditure that is elevated for several weeks after the initial insult.[29] Underfeeding during this hypermetabolic phase results in nutritional deterioration—in particular, loss of lean body mass—when protein intake is also limited. A variety of equations are used to estimate basal energy requirements and prescribe the daily energy allotment for children in the PICU population.[30,31] These equations, based on age, gender, and weight, are derived from healthy population data. Hence, estimates of energy expenditure from these equations are frequently inaccurate in the PICU population.[32] In addition, a variety of stress factors contribute to the equation for the estimated energy requirement, to account for the perceived energy cost of certain conditions, such as fever. Unfortunately, the actual delivery of energy at the bedside may fall far short of the prescribed amount. Failure to deliver the prescribed energy over a period of time results in cumulative energy imbalance with anthropometric deteriorations that eventually result in poor outcomes.[15,33]

In contrast, a variety of factors in critically ill children might actually decrease total energy expenditure. Lack of physical activity, temperature management in modern PICUs, modern anesthesia and pain-management strategies, and ventilatory support all contribute to the reduction in overall energy expenditure during critical illness. In recent years, newborn infants undergoing uncomplicated major surgery have only a transient 20% increase in energy expenditure that returns to baseline levels within 12 hours.[34] Newborn infants extubated after surgery for closure of large ventricular septal defects or soon after ligation of patent ductus arteriosus have resting energy expenditures that are lower than expected and almost resemble those of healthy infants at baseline.[35-37] Using a stable isotopic technique, the mean energy expenditures of critically ill neonates receiving extracorporeal membrane oxygenation (ECMO) support were similar to age- and diet-matched nonstressed controls.[38] Thus, the muted or transient increase in energy expenditure following a variety of stresses may result in an overestimation of the energy cost using the equations for estimating energy requirements in the critically ill population. As a result, unintended overfeeding is likely prevalent in the PICU and, like underfeeding, poses significant risks.[4,33] If overfeeding is sustained, especially in patients receiving parenteral nutrition with a high percentage of calories from carbohydrates, there is a significant carbon dioxide load on the patient. In children with chronic respiratory insufficiency, this could result in poorer outcomes, including prolonged ventilator dependence and PICU length of stay. Other deleterious effects of overfeeding include increased triglyceride concentrations, hyperglycemia, and hepatotoxicity.

Micronutrients

There has been a renewed interest in providing certain micronutrients with antioxidant properties during critical illness. To maintain homeostasis, a complex system of selected enzymes, cofactors (selenium, zinc, iron, and manganese), sulfhydryl group donors (glutathione), and vitamins (E and C) form a defense system that counters the oxidant stress seen in the acute phase of injury or illness. Critically ill patients may have deficiencies of micronutrients in the early phase of illness, as vitamins and trace elements are redistributed from the central circulation to tissues, and fluid losses from wounds, exudates, and third spacing might disturb micronutrient balance.[39,40] The stores of enzyme cofactors, vitamins, and trace elements decrease rapidly after injury and may remain at subnormal levels for weeks. There is an association between low endogenous antioxidant stores and an increase in free radical generation, augmented systemic inflammatory response, cell injury, and increased morbidity and mortality in critically ill people.[41] Recently, there has been increased interest in the role of vitamin D as an antioxidant. Serum concentrations of vitamin D in children with severe burns may be decreased for months after burn injury.[42] Indeed, low vitamin D concentrations have been reported in the general population in many geographic areas, especially those in the northern hemisphere.[43,44] The significance of the association of low serum vitamin D concentrations with outcomes and the role of supplementation during critical illness remains to be determined.

The concept of early micronutrient supplementation to prevent the development of acute deficiency to rectify the oxidant-antioxidant balance and to reduce oxidative-mediated injuries to organs has been investigated in recent trials in critically ill adults.[45] The role of micronutrients in the critically ill child is currently being investigated.[46]

Immunonutrition

In 1996, Bone and colleagues discussed the importance of a fine balance between the inflammatory and compensatory anti-inflammatory responses in an individual challenged with an injury or infection.[47] This highly coordinated biphasic inflammatory response is aimed at mounting an effective defense while keeping the proinflammatory response under control. Hence, it is thought that immunomodulation might play a significant role in the nature of the response to an infectious insult and affect outcomes in critically ill children. Immune-enhancing diets (IEDs) have been available for many years. An increasing number of studies in adult patients have examined the effect of IEDs in variety of illnesses, for their role in affecting outcomes. However, meta-analyses of such adult studies have provided conflicting results because of deficiencies in study design and the heterogeneity of IED formulations used in heterogeneous patient populations.[48] The commercially available diets for adults vary greatly and the role of individual compounds is impossible to interpret. The immunomodulating effects of individual compounds are dose dependent, and mixtures of different immunomodulating nutrients are likely to have synergistic as well as antagonistic effects. Although meta-analyses have failed to show any effect of decreasing mortality, adults who received enteral immunonutrition had a decreased incidence of nosocomial infections and decreased length of hospital stay compared with patients who received a standard enteral formula.[48] Although no conclusive data on the beneficial effects of IEDs have been established, glutamine, antioxidants, and fish oils are among the nutrients with the promise of beneficial effects in selected patient groups. At this time, the role of IEDs in critically ill children remains unknown.

Nutrient Delivery in the PICU – Challenges

The enteral route of feeding is preferred in children with a functioning gastrointestinal tract. The benefits of enteral nutrition include preservation of intestinal mucosal integrity, enhanced mucosal immunity, and reduction in parenteral nutrition use with its associated complications and risk of infections (see Chapter 24: Enteral Nutrition). Patients deprived of enteral nutrients rapidly develop adverse intestinal mucosal changes, including reduced crypt depth and villus height.[49] Overall, enteral nutrition is relatively more physiologic, safer, and more cost-effective compared with parenteral nutrition. However, establishing and maintaining enteral nutrition intake in critically ill children often conflicts with therapeutic and diagnostic interventions in the PICU. Furthermore, some patients do not tolerate enteral nutrition or are at risk of mucosal ischemia or pulmonary aspiration after enteral feeding. The benefits of enteral nutrition must be balanced against the risks in these children. Parenteral nutrition has been used to achieve nutritional goals as a supplement to enteral nutrition in children who do not tolerate full enteral nutrition.

A variety of barriers impede the optimal delivery for enteral nutrition at the bedside in critically ill children.[9,10] As a result, a large number of patients in the

PICU experience interruptions to or delays in initiating enteral nutrition. A majority of these events are related to conflicts with other procedures that require fasting, intolerance of enteral nutrition, or perceived contraindications to enteral nutrition. Prospective audits of nutritional practices suggest that a number of opportunities to initiate and sustain enteral nutrition are frequently overlooked in the PICU population because of lack of a uniform feeding strategy or myths regarding the safety of enteral nutrition in specific scenarios.

Summary

Nutrition therapy is an important aspect of critical care. Critically ill children are at risk of nutritional deterioration during acute illness, and careful attention to their metabolic state will allow prescription of optimal macronutrients and micronutrients during their PICU stay. The advantages of enteral nutrition are well documented. Awareness of the many challenges to nutrient delivery in the PICU will allow nutrition goals to be achieved and may improve clinical outcomes in this population. Nutrition therapy in the PICU must be recognized as a clinical and research priority.

References

1. Hulst J, Joosten K, Zimmermann L, et al. Malnutrition in critically ill children: from admission to 6 months after discharge. *Clin Nutr.* 2004;23(2):223-232
2. Pollack MM, Ruttimann UE, Wiley JS. Nutritional depletions in critically ill children: associations with physiologic instability and increased quantity of care. *JPEN J Parenter Enteral Nutr.* 1985;9(3):309-313
3. Chwals WJ. Overfeeding the critically ill child: fact or fantasy? *New Horiz.* 1994;2(2):147-155
4. Mehta NM, Bechard LJ, Dolan M, et al. Energy imbalance and the risk of overfeeding in critically ill children. *Pediatr Crit Care Med.* 2011;12(4):398-405
5. Mehta NM, Bechard LJ, Leavitt K, et al. Severe weight loss and hypermetabolic paroxysmal dysautonomia following hypoxic ischemic brain injury: the role of indirect calorimetry in the intensive care unit. *JPEN J Parenter Enteral Nutr.* 2008;32(3):281-284
6. Leite HP, Isatugo MK, Sawaki L, Fisberg M. Anthropometric nutritional assessment of critically ill hospitalized children. *Rev Paul Med.* 1993;111(1):309-313
7. Pollack MM, Wiley JS, Kanter R, et al. Malnutrition in critically ill infants and children. *JPEN J Parenter Enteral Nutr.* 1982;6(1):20-24
8. Mehta NM, Duggan CP. Nutritional deficiencies during critical illness. *Pediatr Clin North Am.* 2009;56(5):1143-1160
9. Mehta NM, McAleer D, Hamilton S, et al. Challenges to optimal enteral nutrition in a multidisciplinary pediatric intensive care unit. *JPEN J Parenter Enteral Nutr.* 2010;34(1):38-45

VI

10. Rogers EJ, Gilbertson HR, Heine RG, et al. Barriers to adequate nutrition in critically ill children. *Nutrition*. 2003;19(10):865-868

11. Taylor RM, Cheeseman P, Preedy V, et al. Can energy expenditure be predicted in critically ill children? *Pediatr Crit Care Med*. 2003;4(2):176-180

12. Duffy B, Pencharz P. The effects of surgery on the nitrogen metabolism of parenterally fed human neonates. *Pediatr Res*. 1986;20(1):32-35

13. Fomon SJ, Haschke F, Ziegler EE, et al. Body composition of reference children from birth to age 10 years. *Am J Clin Nutr*. 1982;35(5 Suppl):1169-1175

14. Mehta N, Jaksic T. The critically ill child. In: Duggan W, ed. *Nutrition in Pediatrics*. Hamilton, Ontario: BC Decker Inc; 2008:663-673

15. Hulst JM, Joosten KF, Tibboel D, et al. Causes and consequences of inadequate substrate supply to pediatric ICU patients. *Curr Opin Clin Nutr Metab Care*. 2006;9(3):297-303

16. Herndon DN, Hart DW, Wolf SE, et al. Reversal of catabolism by beta-blockade after severe burns. *N Engl J Med*. 2001;345(17):1223-1229

17. Long CL, Kinney JM, Geiger JW. Nonsuppressability of gluconeogenesis by glucose in septic patients. *Metabolism*. 1976;25(2):193-201

18. Branco RG, Garcia PC, Piva JP, et al. Glucose level and risk of mortality in pediatric septic shock. *Pediatr Crit Care Med*. 2005;6(4):470-472

19. Krinsley JS. Association between hyperglycemia and increased hospital mortality in a heterogeneous population of critically ill patients. *Mayo Clin Proc*. 2003;78(12):1471-1478

20. Laird AM, Miller PR, Kilgo PD, et al. Relationship of early hyperglycemia to mortality in trauma patients. *J Trauma*. 2004;56(5):1058-1062

21. Selig PM, Popek V, Peebles KM. Minimizing hypoglycemia in the wake of a tight glycemic control protocol in hospitalized patients. *J Nurs Care Qual*. 2010;25(3):255-260

22. Finfer S, Heritier S. The NICE-SUGAR (Normoglycaemia in Intensive Care Evaluation and Survival Using Glucose Algorithm Regulation) Study: statistical analysis plan. *Crit Care Resusc*. 2009;11(1):46-57

23. Steil GM, Langer M, Jaeger K, Alexander J, Gaies M, Agus MS. Value of continuous glucose monitoring for minimizing severe hypoglycemia during tight glycemic control. *Pediatr Crit Care Med*. 2011;12(6):643-648

24. Hirshberg E, Lacroix J, Sward K, et al. Blood glucose control in critically ill adults and children: a survey on stated practice. *Chest*. 2008;133(6):1328-1335

25. Alaedeen DI, Walsh MC, Chwals WJ. Total parenteral nutrition-associated hyperglycemia correlates with prolonged mechanical ventilation and hospital stay in septic infants. *J Pediatr Surg*. 2006;41(1):239-244

26. Askanazi J, Rosenbaum SH, Hyman AI, et al. Respiratory changes induced by the large glucose loads of total parenteral nutrition. *JAMA*. 1980;243(14):1444-1447

27. Long CL, Spencer JL, Kinney JM, et al. Carbohydrate metabolism in normal man and effect of glucose infusion. *J Appl Physiol*. 1971;31(1):102-109

28. Cuthbertson D. Intensive-care-metabolic response to injury. *Br J Surg*. 1970;57(10):718-721

29. Suman OE, Mlcak RP, Chinkes DL, et al. Resting energy expenditure in severely burned children: analysis of agreement between indirect calorimetry and prediction equations using the Bland-Altman method. *Burns*. 2006;32(3):335-342

30. Schofield WN. Predicting basal metabolic rate, new standards and review of previous work. *Hum Nutr Clin Nutr*. 1985;39(Suppl 1):5-41

31. World Health Organization. Energy and protein requirements. Report of a joint FAO/WHO/UNU Expert Consultation. *World Health Organ Tech Rep Ser*. 1985;724:1-206

32. Hardy CM, Dwyer J, Snelling LK, et al. Pitfalls in predicting resting energy requirements in critically ill children: a comparison of predictive methods to indirect calorimetry. *Nutr Clin Pract*. 2002;17(3):182-189

33. Mehta NM, Bechard LJ, Leavitt K, et al. Cumulative energy imbalance in the pediatric intensive care unit: role of targeted indirect calorimetry. *JPEN J Parenter Enteral Nutr*. 2009;33(3):336-344

34. Jones MO, Pierro A, Hammond P, et al. The metabolic response to operative stress in infants. *J Pediatr Surg*. 1993;28(10):1258-1262

35. Shew SB, Beckett PR, Keshen TH, et al. Validation of a [13C]bicarbonate tracer technique to measure neonatal energy expenditure. *Pediatr Res*. 2000;47(6):787-791

36. Shew SB, Keshen TH, Glass NL, et al. Ligation of a patent ductus arteriosus under fentanyl anesthesia improves protein metabolism in premature neonates. *J Pediatr Surg*. 2000;35(9):1277-1281

37. Ackerman IL, Karn CA, Denne SC, et al. Total but not resting energy expenditure is increased in infants with ventricular septal defects. *Pediatrics*. 1998;102(5):1172-1177

38. Shew SB, Keshen TH, Jahoor F, et al. The determinants of protein catabolism in neonates on extracorporeal membrane oxygenation. *J Pediatr Surg*. 1999;34(7):1086-1090

39. Galloway P, McMillan DC, Sattar N. Effect of the inflammatory response on trace element and vitamin status. *Ann Clin Biochem*. 2000;37(3):289-297

40. Maehira F, Luyo GA, Miyagi I, et al. Alterations of serum selenium concentrations in the acute phase of pathological conditions. *Clin Chim Acta*. 2002;316(1-2):137-146

41. Goode HF, Cowley HC, Walker BE, et al. Decreased antioxidant status and increased lipid peroxidation in patients with septic shock and secondary organ dysfunction. *Crit Care Med*. 1995;23(4):646-651

42. Gottschlich MM, Mayes T, Khoury J, et al. Hypovitaminosis D in acutely injured pediatric burn patients. *J Am Diet Assoc*. 2004;104(6):931-941

43. Gordon CM, DePeter KC, Feldman HA, et al. Prevalence of vitamin D deficiency among healthy adolescents. *Arch Pediatr Adolesc Med*. 2004;158(6):531-537

44. Gordon CM, Feldman HA, Sinclair L, et al. Prevalence of vitamin D deficiency among healthy infants and toddlers. *Arch Pediatr Adolesc Med*. 2008;162(6):505-512

45. Heyland DK, Dhaliwal R, Day AG, et al. REducing Deaths due to OXidative Stress (The REDOXS Study): rationale and study design for a randomized trial of glutamine and antioxidant supplementation in critically-ill patients. *Proc Nutr Soc*. 2006;65(3):250-263

46. Carcillo J, Holubkov R, Dean JM, et al. Rationale and design of the pediatric critical illness stress-induced immune suppression (CRISIS) prevention trial. *JPEN J Parenter Enteral Nutr*. 2009;33(4):368-374

VI

47. Bone RC, Grodzin CJ, Balk RA. Sepsis: a new hypothesis for pathogenesis of the disease process. *Chest*. 1997;112(1):235-243

48. Heyland DK, Novak F, Drover JW, et al. Should immunonutrition become routine in critically ill patients? A systematic review of the evidence. *JAMA*. 2001;286(8):944-953

49. Hernandez G, Velasco N, Wainstein C, et al. Gut mucosal atrophy after a short enteral fasting period in critically ill patients. *J Crit Care*. 1999;14(2):73-77

Chapter 39

Nutritional Support of Pediatric Patients With Eating Disorders

Introduction

Eating disorders are psychiatric illnesses defined by behavioral, cognitive, emotional, and physical criteria. The hallmarks of an eating disorder are severe disturbances in eating behavior and in the experience of the body that are associated with psychological distress, functional impairment, and often physical complications. The current *Diagnostic and Statistical Manual of Mental Disorders, Fourth Edition Text Revision (DSM-IV-TR)*[1] recognizes 3 eating disorders: anorexia nervosa (AN), bulimia nervosa (BN), and eating disorder not otherwise specified (EDNOS). The *DSM-IV-TR* provides specific diagnostic criteria for AN and BN; EDNOS is defined by clinically significant eating disorder symptoms that do not meet criteria for either AN or BN and may include subthreshold presentations that resemble AN or BN but fall short by one or more criteria as well as binge eating disorder. Although eating disorders most often occur in females, approximately 10% of patients with AN or BN are male, and the prevalence of eating disorders may be increasing in male, minority, and younger populations. Often, eating disorder symptoms first appear in childhood or early adolescence, and frank disorders typically have onset in middle or late adolescence or early adulthood. Lifetime prevalence estimates of eating disorders in individuals of all ages range from approximately 1% for AN to 1% to 4% for BN[1]; one recent epidemiologic study of adolescents reported lifetime prevalence rates of 0.3% for AN, 0.9% for BN, and 1.6% for one type of EDNOS (binge eating disorder), and rates of the full range of EDNOS are likely even higher.[2] Further, all prevalence rates reported may be underestimates, because eating disorders often go unrecognized, and individuals may be reluctant to acknowledge symptoms or seek treatment because of shame and fear of stigmatization. Early detection and intervention are critical and can lead to improved outcomes.[3]

Clinical research has focused on AN and BN, although EDNOS is the most common diagnosis in outpatient clinical settings. Children and adolescents, in particular, often do not meet full criteria for AN or BN, because they may present with failure to gain weight adequately rather than marked weight loss, or they may minimize or deny body image dissatisfaction or overvaluation of weight/shape, for example. Therefore, current *DSM-IV-TR* descriptions may not fully capture eating disorders in younger populations and often result in the diagnosis of EDNOS,

VI

which is clinically significant but heterogeneous and, therefore, conveys limited specific information. Because of the potential long-term effects of eating disorders on physical and emotional growth, clinicians should lower the threshold for intervention in children and adolescents. Indeed, it is crucial that pediatricians recognize that the medical and psychological complications of EDNOS can parallel those of AN or BN.

Given the predominance of empirical information available on AN and BN, this chapter focuses on nutritional considerations for patients with these primary eating disorders but also provides commentary on how and when modifications may be appropriate for individuals with EDNOS. The goals of this chapter are to provide clinicians working with children and adolescents with practical information regarding the assessment and treatment of eating disorders and, in particular, the assessment and treatment of the common problems that occur related to nutrition and health in these complex disorders.

Clinical Features

Anorexia Nervosa

Diagnostic Criteria

AN is characterized in the *DSM-IV-TR* by persistent low body weight, marked fear of weight gain, disturbance in the way that body image is experienced (eg, believing one is fat even though underweight), and amenorrhea in females (see Table 39.1). The forthcoming *Diagnostic and Statistical Manual of Mental Disorders, Fifth Edition (DSM-5)*, includes a slightly broadened definition of AN, and these proposed revisions are also presented in Table 39.1. Although current criteria provide a guideline for defining low body weight as less than 85% of that expected for age and gender, this threshold is often applied literally. *DSM-5* is expected to remove this guideline and instead suggest a more loosely defined weight criterion of less than the minimum expectation for age and gender. When working with children and adolescents, clinicians should review growth charts to ascertain historic growth trajectory to determine whether weight and height have "fallen off" the expected curve for the individual patient. Further, the amenorrhea criterion is likely to be eliminated in the *DSM-5*.

Table 39.1.
Diagnostic Criteria for Anorexia Nervosa

Criterion	DSM-IV-TR (2000)	Proposed for DSM-5 (2013)
Body weight	Refusal to maintain a body weight more than 85% of expected for height and age; failure to gain weight during a period of growth with body weight less than 85% expected for height and age.	Restriction of energy intake relative to requirements leading to a markedly low body weight (less than that minimally expected for age and height).
Menstruation	In postmenarchal females, the absence of three consecutive menstrual cycles (hormonally induced menstruation is excluded).	This criterion is likely to be deleted.
Fear of weight gain	Even though underweight, an intense fear of gaining weight or becoming fat.	Intense fear of gaining weight or becoming fat, or persistent behavior that interferes with weight gain, even though at a significantly low weight.
Body image	Disturbance in the way one's body weight or shape is experienced; denial of the seriousness of low body weight; an undue influence of body weight or shape on self-evaluation.	No change from DSM-IV-TR (slight wording change: "… persistent lack of recognition of the seriousness of current low body weight").

Individuals with AN achieve low weight through dietary restriction and often engage in excessive physical activity and manifest strict food rules. Although all individuals with AN are restricting intake to below nutritional needs, a subset periodically engage in binge eating and/or purging. DSM-IV-TR specifies 2 subtypes of AN: restricting type and binge/purge type. Whereas individuals with the restricting type may appear constricted in affect and personality, those with the binge-eating/purging type may be more likely to have comorbid impulsivity, including substance use disorders, cluster B personality disorders, mood lability, and suicidality. Additionally, those with binge/purge type AN may develop more severe medical complications, because binge/purge behaviors compound their low weight.

Associated Signs and Medical Complications
Psychologically, individuals with AN often present with severe body image distortion; preoccupation with weight, shape, and eating; restricted or negative affect; and limited insight into illness. They may be perfectionistic, obsessive, interpersonally insecure, and unsure of their own identity. Further, they often experience intrapersonal conflict around maturation, sexual development, separation, and individuation. Notably, AN has the highest mortality rate for any mental disorder; suicide and cardiac complications are the leading causes of death.

In individuals with AN, most systems are affected as weight loss becomes pronounced (see Table 39.2). Physical signs include bradycardia, hypotension, lanugo, alopecia, and edema. Those who self-induce vomiting may exhibit dental erosion and dorsal surface hand lesions. Laboratory findings could include electrolyte abnormalities, in particular hypokalemia. Gastrointestinal complications, such as constipation, delayed gastric motility, and delayed gastric emptying, are common. High concentrations of blood urea nitrogen may reflect renal abnormalities resulting from dehydration. Polyuria related to an abnormality in vasopressin secretion may also develop. Approximately 20% of patients experience peripheral edema, usually during refeeding. Mild anemia, leukopenia, and thrombocytopenia are often observed but typically reverse with refeeding. Neurologic abnormalities may include reduced gray matter volumes and increased sulcal cerebrospinal fluid volumes that persist after recovery.

Table 39.2.

Associated Signs and Medical Complications of Anorexia Nervosa

System	Features
Cardiac	Bradycardia, orthostatic hypotension, arrhythmia, mitral valve prolapse/murmur; decreased left ventricular forces, prolonged QT interval corrected for heart rate, increased vagal tone, pericardial effusion, congestive heart failure
Endocrine and metabolic	Amenorrhea, hypothyroidism, delayed puberty, arrested growth, hypothermia, osteopenia or osteoporosis, euthyroid sick syndrome, electrolyte disturbances, decreased serum testosterone or estradiol, hypercholesterolemia, hypercortisolism
Skeletal	Fractures due to bone mineralization loss, low bone mineral density
Breasts	Breast atrophy
Dermatologic	Cheilosis, acrocyanosis, hypercarotenemia, alopecia, xerosis, acne, lanugo, pallor
Oral/dental	Enamel erosion and gum recession; swelling of the parotid gland; salivary gland hypertrophy; elevated serum amylase levels; halitosis
Gastrointestinal	Palpable stool secondary to constipation, rectal prolapse, scaphoid abdomen; esophagitis; chest pain, dyspepsia; gastroesophageal reflux disease; esophageal rupture; hiatal hernias; irritable bowel syndrome; melanosis coli; atonic or cathartic colon
Pulmonary	Pneumothorax or aspiration secondary to vomiting, pulmonary edema during refeeding
Neurologic and mental status	Neurocognitive deficit, diminished muscle strength, peripheral neuropathy, movement disorder
Hematologic	Anemia, leukopenia, thrombocytopenia
Renal	Increased blood urea nitrogen, calculi

Electrocardiographic abnormalities (eg, low voltage, bradycardia, T-wave inversions, ST segment depression, and arrhythmias) are common and often normalize with refeeding. Some cardiac problems, including prolonged corrected QT intervals, myocardial damage, and arrhythmias secondary to electrolyte imbalances, may be fatal. Amenorrhea secondary to starvation-induced hypogonadism, hypothyroidism, reduction of growth hormones (insulin-like growth factor), and decreased serum leptin concentration are all among the endocrine sequelae.[4] The likelihood of these complications increases in adolescents who reach a lower percent of ideal body weight. Although many medical complications resolve when the adolescent achieves weight restoration, bone mineral density (BMD) loss resulting from hypothalamic amenorrhea in female patients or low testosterone in male patients does not necessarily resolve with weight gain. Reductions in BMD tend to occur at multiple skeletal sites in most with anorexia nervosa, leading to osteopenia and osteoporosis.[5] Although estrogen deficiency is an important cause of low BMD, administration of estrogen as an oral estrogen-progesterone combination pill is not effective in increasing BMD in women or girls with AN. In contrast, physiologic estrogen administration as replacement doses with transdermal estrogen or as small incremental doses of oral estrogen to mimic the early pubertal rise in estrogen does increase BMD in adolescent girls with AN when compared with placebo. However, bone accrual rates remain lower than in normal-weight controls, likely because other hormonal deficits are not addressed by estrogen replacement alone in the absence of weight restoration.[6]

In low-weight female athletes, the constellation of low energy availability, with or without an eating disorder, hypothalamic amenorrhea, and osteoporosis, has been termed the "female athlete triad."[7] Energy availability refers to dietary energy intake minus exercise energy expenditure. Energy availability is the amount of dietary energy remaining for other bodily functions. Some athletes resort to abnormal eating patterns, including restriction, fasting, binge eating, and purging, or may use diet pills, laxatives, diuretics, or enemas and, thus, have low energy availability. Most of these affected athletes manifest with low body fat composition, which contributes to a hypoestrogenic state, causing amenorrhea. Adolescent athletes who participate in sports in which leanness is emphasized are at higher risk of decreased bone mineralization.

Bulimia Nervosa

Diagnostic Criteria
In the *DSM-IV-TR*, BN is characterized by a regular pattern of binge eating and compensatory behaviors and an overvaluation of weight and shape (see Table 39.3). Binge eating and compensatory behaviors occur at a threshold frequency of twice

weekly for at least 3 months. A binge episode is defined as the consumption of an objectively large amount of food accompanied by a subjective feeling of being out of control during the eating episode. Often, individuals with BN alternate between binge eating and strict dieting. Binge eating typically occurs alone, involves consumption of calorie-dense foods, and is associated with abdominal discomfort and feelings of guilt, disgust, and depression. Individuals with BN engage in compensatory behaviors, including purging (self-induced vomiting, laxative, diuretic, or enema abuse) and nonpurging behaviors (excessive exercise or fasting) in efforts to counteract the effects of the binge and prevent weight gain. In the *DSM-IV-TR*, individuals are classified as purging or nonpurging type on the basis of compensatory behaviors endorsed. Proposed revisions for *DSM-5* include lowering the frequency criterion of binge/purge behavior from twice weekly to once weekly and eliminating the nonpurging subtype. Clinical features of BN are listed in Table 39.4.

Table 39.3.

Diagnostic Criteria for Bulimia Nervosa

Criterion	*DSM-IV-TR* 2000	Proposed for *DSM-5* 2013
Binge eating	Recurrent episodes of binge eating, eating in a discrete period of time (eg, within any 2-hour period), an amount of food that is definitely larger than most people would eat during a similar period of time and under similar circumstances.	No change from *DSM-IV-TR*
Compensatory behaviors	Recurrent inappropriate behaviors in order to prevent weight gain, such as self-induced vomiting; misuse of laxatives, diuretics, enemas, or other medications; fasting; or excessive exercise.	No change from *DSM-IV-TR*
Regularity	Binge eating and compensatory behaviors both occur on average at least 2 times a week for 3 months	Binge eating and compensatory behaviors both occur on average at least *once* a week for 3 months
Body image	Self-evaluation is unduly influenced by body shape and weight.	No change from *DSM-IV-TR*
No anorexia nervosa	Does not occur exclusively during episodes of anorexia nervosa.	No change from *DSM-IV-TR*
Subtype	Purging type (has regularly engaged in self-induced vomiting or the misuse of laxatives, diuretics, or enemas) or non-purging type (has used other inappropriate compensatory behaviors, such as fasting or excessive exercise, but has not regularly engaged in self-induced vomiting or the misuse of laxatives, diuretics, or enemas)	Deletion of subtype. Research has shown that individuals with nonpurging subtype closely resemble individuals with binge-eating disorder

Table 39.4.
Associated Signs and Medical Complications of Bulimia Nervosa

System	Features
Cardiovascular	Arrhythmia; mitral valve prolapse; murmur; cardiomyopathy
Musculoskeletal	Tetany; skeletal muscle myopathy
Gastrointestinal	Gastric dilation; abdominal fullness; esophagitis; gastroesophageal reflux disease or rupture; hiatal hernias; Barrett esophagus; irritable bowel syndrome; melanosis coli; atonic or cathartic colon
Oral/dental	Mouth sores; palatal scratches; dental caries; enamel erosion and gum recession; swelling of the parotid gland; submandibular adenopathy; elevated serum amylase levels
Skin	Periorbital petechiae, Russell sign (calluses over the knuckles due to induction of emesis, swelling of hands and feet, dryness, lack of hair sheen
Metabolic	Pitting edema, poor skin turgor, Chvostek signs, Trousseau sign; hypokalemia, metabolic acidosis or alkalosis secondary to purging by vomiting and/or use of diuretics and laxatives
Neurologic	Cognitive impairment; irritability

Associated Signs and Medical Complications

Patients with BN may present complaining of bloating, weakness, fatigue, dyspepsia, chest pain, and dry mouth. Physical signs may include the highly specific findings of facial swelling, sialadenosis (parotid gland hypertrophy, bilateral and nontender) or Russell sign (excoriations on dorsal aspect of hand and fingers). Oral findings may include tooth decay or discoloration, lesions, or bleeding gums. Additional signs include peripheral edema, petechiae in the skin surrounding the eyes, subconjunctival hemorrhage (resulting from increased pressure from vomiting), or angular cheilitis. Angular cheilitis may be secondary to vomiting or vitamin (often B complex) deficiencies.

Laboratory findings are not diagnostic but can be helpful in assessing medical complications. Depending on the method of purging, there can be changes in serum electrolyte concentrations. Hypokalemia, hypochloremia, and hyponatremia (associated with excess water ingestion) can be commonly seen. The serum pH can be increased or decreased from purging. There can be an elevated serum amylase. Because of electrolyte disturbances, purging may lead to weakness, tetany, and arrhythmias; diuretic overuse may cause Pseudo-Barter syndrome (hypokalemia secondary to diuretic or laxative misuse). Further complications include renal failure and electrolyte imbalances, leading to seizures. Albumin concentrations are typically normal in patients with eating disorders; if they are low, clinicians should investigate a comorbid or alternative diagnosis, such as inflammatory bowel disease.

VI

Medical complications of BN are varied, often are occult, and carry significant risk of morbidity and mortality. Gastrointestinal tract complications are often secondary to self-induced vomiting and include esophagitis, dyspepsia, gastroesophageal reflux disease, hiatal hernias, and gastric dilatation. In severe cases, self-induced vomiting may lead to Mallory-Weiss tears, aspiration pneumonia, esophageal or gastric rupture, or a pneumothorax. More commonly, delayed gastric emptying and elevated intestinal transit time lead to presenting complaints of bloating, postprandial fullness, and constipation.

It is very important to inquire about laxative abuse, as this leads to depletion of potassium bicarbonate and a resultant metabolic acidosis. Laxative and diuretic abuse or chronic dehydration may lead to renal stones. Laboratory abnormalities seen with laxative abuse include metabolic acidosis, hyperuricemia, elevated blood urea nitrogen concentration, hypocalcemia, and hypomagnesemia. Laxative abuse may lead to irritable bowel syndrome, melanosis coli, an atonic or cathartic colon, or rectal prolapse. Cessation of chronic laxative abuse may cause rapid increase in weight because of fluid retention and edema. Other times, cessation of laxative abuse leads to constipation and may be managed with increased fluid and fiber intake.

All patients with BN, especially purging subtype, should undergo electrocardiography (ECG), and abnormal results should prompt consideration of hospitalization. Self-induced vomiting and laxative and diuretic abuse may lead to electrolyte and acid base disturbances, and resultant cardiac complications may ensue. Cardiac arrhythmias and prolonged QT intervals can lead to sudden death in purging patients. T-wave changes may also be noted on ECG. Another cardiac complication noted with increased frequency in patients with BN is mitral valve prolapse.

Although no longer commercially available, ipecac abuse is associated with distinct, potentially life-threatening cardiac complications; thus, all patients must be asked about any ipecac abuse. Ipecac contains emetine, which can cause a skeletal muscle myopathy, diffuse myositis, and cardiomyopathy (which could lead to irreversible myocardial damage and cardiac failure). The development of pericardial pain, dyspnea, weakness, hypotension, or tachycardia or abnormalities detected on ECG may suggest ipecac ingestion and requires urgent medical attention.

Many endocrine abnormalities are associated with BN. Thyroid function tests may show euthyroid sick syndrome marked by low tri-iodothyronine (T_3), elevated reverse T_3, and low to normal thyroxine (T_4) and thyroid-stimulating hormone (TSH). Cortisol and growth hormone may be increased. Vasopressin depression often leads to polyuria. Patients may have irregular or absent menstruation; this may be seen in normal-weight or even overweight adolescents with BN.

Certain complaints suggest acute complications of BN. Volume depletion may lead to hypotension, dizziness, and syncope. In the case of severe abdominal pain, it is necessary to rule out gastric dilatation (perhaps requiring urgent medical intervention). Because ipecac use is associated with cardiomyopathy, any complaints of chest pain, dyspnea, hypotension, or tachycardia or abnormalities detected on ECG require urgent medical attention. In addition, hematemesis or rectal bleeding may require emergent care. Other clinical signs that suggest hospitalization may be necessary include serum potassium concentration less than 3.2 mmol/L, serum chloride concentration less than 88 mmol/L, hematemesis, cardiac arrhythmias (ie, prolonged QT), or hypothermia. Hypokalemia must be carefully corrected in a hospital setting with careful observation for cardiac instability.

Etiology of AN and BN

The etiology of eating disorders is multifactorial, dependent on sociocultural, psychological, biological, and familial factors. Both AN and BN typically have onset during adolescence, although patients frequently have a history of body image concerns and disordered eating that precede the onset of the illness.

Sociocultural factors that may increase risk of eating disorders include the Western emphasis on a thin ideal for women and a muscular ideal for men. Dieting is a behavior that increases risk for eating disorders. Further, certain populations may be at heightened risk of eating disorders. For example, sports such as ballet, gymnastics, long-distance running, ice skating, and wrestling or activities such as modeling or acting all value a slender body shape and may promote thinness and weight loss. In addition, patients with diabetes mellitus represent an at-risk group; patients with type 1 (or insulin-dependent) diabetes mellitus must adhere to strict diet plans and may underdose insulin to cause intentional weight loss. Diabetic patients with eating disorders more frequently present with ketoacidosis and vascular complications associated with poor glycemic control. Gay males may also be at increased risk. Environmental factors, including transitions from middle school to high school, the experience of a loss, and physical or sexual abuse, may also precipitate maladaptive coping responses, including eating disorders.

Psychological characteristics, such as personality or temperament, as well as comorbid psychopathology may also play a role in the development of eating disorders. Perfectionism, low self-esteem, and difficulty in regulating affect or managing emotions are personality characteristics that may be present in individuals with eating disorders. Further, a subset of patients with eating disorders, particularly those with a bulimic constellation of symptoms, may also demonstrate other impulsive behaviors, such as substance abuse, promiscuity, and self-destructive/injurious behaviors that require their own medical intervention and monitoring. Anxiety and mood disorders also often co-occur with eating disorders; although

VI

anxiety disorders most often have onset before eating disorders, mood disorders may be more likely to develop at the same time as or following the eating disorder onset.

Research in the past decade has begun to explore the genetics and heritability of eating disorders. Family and twin studies demonstrate that the risk of AN and/or BN is significantly increased in first-degree relatives of those with eating disorders, with one study indicating the relative risk of eating disorder in female relatives to be 11.3.[8,9] Further, there is growing evidence that specific symptoms, such as binge eating and self-induced vomiting, may also be heritable. Biological factors, such as obesity, may increase vulnerability to eating disorders. Neurobiological research has also demonstrated alterations in hormonal and neurohormonal systems among individuals with eating disorders. Impaired serotonergic regulation has been implicated in obesity and overeating; studies have shown patients with BN to have dysregulated serotonin function as well as lower cerebrospinal 5-HT1A levels. Ghrelin, a hormone that acts on the hypothalamus to stimulate appetite, has been shown to have an abnormal response to normal sized meals in BN patients.[10] Because patients with BN often have an abnormal satiety following normal-sized meals,[11] ghrelin may play a role in the pathogenesis in the lack of satiety that characterizes a binge episode.[10] Yet, the degree to which these neurochemical and hormonal alterations are premorbid risks rather than secondary effects of eating disorders is unclear.

Within a biopsychosocial model, the family environment may also reinforce socioculturally based thin ideal expectations. This influence may occur through modeling of healthful or unhealthful attitudes or behaviors or through direct encouragement of children or adolescents to adopt disordered eating patterns. Further, there is some evidence that a family environment characterized by enmeshment or high conflict may also increase vulnerability to eating disorders, although interpretation of this research is challenged by the fact that family dynamics may change resultant from the eating disorder.

Assessment

Given that eating disorders often involve private behaviors or secret thoughts that may not be apparent from the outside, careful assessment is critical.[12] Such an assessment involves a medical, nutritional, and psychological evaluation, and it is often pediatricians who are on the front line of screening for eating disorders in children and adolescents. Although eating disorder symptoms may be distressing to patients and often leave them feeling ashamed, lonely, or remorseful, many are ambivalent about seeking treatment and may not readily disclose their symptoms. Further, children and adolescents with eating disorders deny or minimize symptoms, either unconsciously because of a distorted perception of their behavior/ attitudes or consciously to keep clinicians from recognizing the extent of their symptoms. A strong alliance with a trusted health care professional is crucial in the success of treating the ambivalent patient. Inquiring in a direct yet caring and nonshaming manner can help many patients who are unsure how to disclose their symptoms. Data have shown that patients are more likely disclose their symptoms to a professional when directly asked.[13] With young patients, it is often important for the clinician to meet with the adolescent as well as with his or her parents to obtain a more complete perspective on the referral; the family may cite concerns about the child's diet changes, eating alone, skipping meals, and mood changes.

Obtaining a weight history (highest, lowest, current, and desired weight) can shed light on body image concerns and weight fluctuations. Evaluation will include inquiry about the amount of time spent thinking about food, calories, and weight, as patients will often report that these topics consume their thoughts and may also interfere with their ability to attend to or enjoy other activities. Detailed assessment of a 24-hour nutritional intake that will allow providers to estimate energy, macronutrient, and micronutrient intake is important to obtain. Are patients restricting or avoiding certain foods or food groups (eg, fats)? Direct assessment of pattern of eating and frequency of meals consumed provides information about whether some meals/snacks are more challenging than others and whether there may be large gaps between eating episodes. It is important to ascertain whether there are periods of time when the patient eats an unusually large amount of food in an uncontrolled way. If present, gather more details about the episodes (the length of time, feeling during episode, kinds of food eaten). Assessment should include inquiry about all compensatory behaviors, because each is associated with specific medical complications (ie, ipecac abuse and cardiomyopathy), and many patients engage in more than one compensatory behavior. Ask about vomiting, emetic drugs, laxatives, enemas, "recreational" drugs, insulin underdosing, exercise, and skipping meals. Inquiring about all compensatory measures (regardless of whether patient endorses this behavior) provides an opportunity for psychoeducation about the risks associated with each behavior (ie, after asking about ipecac use, explain risk of cardiac death). Further, it can be important to ask about unusual behaviors, such as hoarding food, chewing food and spitting it out, eating in secret, and limiting fluid consumption.

The initial laboratory evaluation should include a urinalysis; complete blood cell count with sedimentation rate; general chemistries; amylase, lipase, magnesium, phosphorous, calcium, thyroid-stimulating hormone, and serum human chorionic gonadotropin concentration for females. If there are concerns about celiac disease, then an immunoglobulin (Ig) A and serum anti-tissue transglutaminase

VI

determination are helpful. A baseline ECG is recommended. Amenorrhea can be further evaluated with determinations of follicle-stimulating hormone, luteinizing hormone, prolactin, and estradiol.[14]

Differential Diagnosis

Assessment of eating disorders should include carefully ruling out underlying medical causes of changes in weight or eating behavior. Although medical disorders may co-occur with eating disorders, if the eating disorder symptoms are better accounted for by the medical condition, an eating disorder diagnosis may not be appropriate. One should consider gastrointestinal disorders (such as celiac disease, inflammatory bowel disease, achalasia, or ulcers) and endocrine disorders (such as diabetes mellitus, Addison disease, or pituitary or thyroid dysfunction) as well as pregnancy. The clinician should consider malignancies (eg, lymphoma, central nervous system tumor) or neurologic disorders (eg, Kluver-Bucy syndrome) that may impair appetite regulation. The differential diagnosis should also include depression, substance abuse, and the illicit use of diet pills. Further, conversion disorders, schizophrenia, and mood disorders are among the psychiatric disorders that may manifest weight loss and binge/purge behavior.

Psychiatric Comorbidity

Screening for co-occurring psychiatric disorders is important. Among individuals with eating disorders, lifetime prevalence estimates of affective disorders range from 50% to 80%, and those of anxiety disorders, including obsessive compulsive disorder, generalized anxiety disorder, and social phobia, are also high, ranging from 30% to 65%.[15] Substance use disorders co-occur, particularly among individuals with bulimic symptoms, and alcohol use disorder is the strongest predictor of premature death in individuals with AN.[16] Further, screening for amphetamine misuse and other use of over-the-counter and prescribed drugs used for weight loss is indicated. Although the most commonly recognized abused substance in patients with BN is alcohol, many patients with eating disorders also use caffeine and tobacco to control appetite.[17,18] A toxicology screening is useful in assessment and ongoing monitoring for substance abuse. Personality disorders also frequently co-occur with eating disorders; avoidant or obsessive compulsive personality disorder may occur among those with AN, and borderline personality disorder has been associated with BN. Personality styles, irrespective of eating disorder diagnosis, including perfectionism, interpersonal avoidance/constriction/restraint, and affective/behavioral dysregulation, may also be important to assess, because they can be useful in informing treatment approach. For all patients with eating disorders, assessment of suicidal ideation, intent, and behavior is imperative.

Treatment

Eating disorders are complex psychiatric illnesses that require multimodal treatments. In addition to medical management, a comprehensive team comprises psychiatric/psychological care and nutrition management.[19] Depending on the severity of illness, care may be delivered with variable intensity, ranging from outpatient management to higher levels of care, including intensive outpatient (evening treatment programs), partial hospitalization, residential care, and inpatient treatment. The American Psychiatric Association provides guidelines regarding levels of care.[20]

Psychiatric Treatment

Psychotherapy

Psychotherapy is an integral component of care for the child or adolescent with an eating disorder. Individual and/or family therapy or parent training can be used to support the medical and nutritional recommendations of the team, which can be challenging for the patient or family to enact. Therapy also helps the child or adolescent identify and address underlying or associated issues which may include separation-individuation, identity development, comorbidities (such as anxiety or depression), and perfectionism, for example. Although psychotherapy is a mainstay of treatment for eating disorders, few randomized-controlled treatment studies for eating disorders in youth exist.

A notable exception to this lack of research is the body of studies supporting the use of family-based treatment for adolescent eating disorders.[21] Family-based treatment, also known as the Maudsley method because of its initial development at the Maudsley Hospital in London, is an outpatient treatment in which parents are recognized as key resources who are integral participants in the recovery process. The treatment takes an agnostic approach to the etiology of eating disorders and empowers parents to initially take more control over the child's eating to restore health; as eating disorder symptoms come under better control, the parents step back. Thus, treatment proceeds through 3 phases determined by the patient's progress, beginning with weight restoration/nutritional rehabilitation, which is managed by the parents, moving to careful return of food/eating control to the adolescent, and ending with focus on issues associated with healthy adolescent development. A number of studies have demonstrated the benefits of using family-based treatment for adolescents with AN[22] and more recently for adolescents with BN[23]; preliminary work also suggests family-based treatment may be useful in treating children, adolescents, and young adults with a wider range of eating disorders.[21]

VI

Individual psychotherapy is helpful for teenagers with eating disorders. A therapist often provides understanding, coaching, praise, and support to generate positive behavioral outcome. When individual psychotherapy is recommended for the adolescent, meetings with the patient's family must be part of the treatment as well. The goals of individual therapy will include improving nutritional health, modifying unhealthy eating attitudes and behaviors, improving self-esteem and quality of life, and treating co-existing conditions, such as depression and anxiety disorders.

Psychopharmacology

Limited data are available on the efficacy of psychiatric medications in adolescents with eating disorders. To date, there has been only one randomized-controlled clinical trial for adolescents with AN,[24] and there have been no such studies for adolescents with BN. In a small study of adolescents with AN, Biederman and colleagues[24] found that the tricyclic antidepressant amitriptyline was not effective in reducing symptoms of AN of low mood when compared with placebo or psychotherapy treatment as usual. Instead, among low-weight patients, the mainstay of treatment is weight restoration; psychiatric medications have generally not been shown to improve eating disorder outcomes, and the efficacy of these medications is likely diminished as a result of malnutrition. Hence, nutritional interventions are primary. However, psychiatric medications are often used to treat comorbid conditions, such as depression and anxiety, and are frequently prescribed, even for underweight patients. More recently, there is some evidence that atypical neuroleptics, such as olanzapine, may improve distorted body image and may assist with weight gain, although clinicians should be aware that many patients with AN will be resistant to taking a medication associated with weight gain[25]; in addition, atypical neuroleptics have been associated with long-term complications, including diabetes mellitus and dyslipidemia.

Better evidence exists for the use of psychopharmacologic interventions in adult BN. Serotonergic medications, such as selective serotonin reuptake inhibitors (SSRIs) and serotonin-norepinephrine reuptake inhibitors (SNRIs), and tricyclic antidepressants have been shown to decrease binge/purge behaviors.[26] Fluoxetine is the best-studied SSRI and the only medication approved by the Food and Drug Administration for the treatment of BN in adults. Topiramate and other antiepileptic medications have also been shown to decrease binge behaviors in those who do not tolerate serotonergic medications; however, topiramate is associated with weight loss and cognitive slowing and should be used cautiously.

Nutrition Management

The nutritional management for AN begins with the focus on weight restoration; in BN, although weight restoration may be important as well, the treatment focus is on interrupting and arresting the binge/purge cycle by establishing a regular pattern of eating.

Determining Ideal Body Weight

Nutritional management of an eating disorder begins with establishment of an initial goal weight. The goal weight is commonly the ideal weight, which is calculated using the following formula:

$$\text{Height (m}^2) \times \text{the 50}^{th} \text{ percentile body-mass index (BMI) for age and gender}$$

BMI information is available on the Centers for Disease Control and Prevention Web site for girls (http://www.cdc.gov/growthcharts/data/set1clinical/cj41l024.pdf) and for boys (http://www.cdc.gov/growthcharts/data/set1clinical/cj41l023.pdf).

Utilizing the 50th percentile BMI for age and gender as the ideal or expected BMI has the advantage of being age specific and accounts for changes in body composition that occur during puberty and adolescence.[27] However, careful consideration of the individual patient's BMI chart (and both height and weight charts) prior to the onset of the eating disorder may be informative in guiding determination of initial goal weight. For example, for the adolescent who had always tracked at the 25th percentile BMI curve, it is possible that returning to the 25th percentile would be an appropriate and justifiable goal.

Calculating Nutrition Requirements

Estimating caloric needs for eating disorders varies on the basis of physical state (eg, percent of ideal body weight), patient's recent energy intake, and risk of refeeding syndrome. Nutrition requirements will change throughout treatment and must be reevaluated frequently on the basis of rate of weight gain, laboratory levels, goal weight, and stage of treatment (inpatient versus outpatient). Overall, many factors such as age, weight, activity level, and overall state of illness can affect calorie needs for weight gain.[28] Indirect calorimetry is the most accurate method to determine energy needs; however, cost and availability make its use difficult.[29] The constant change of metabolic rate during weight restoration in underweight patients would result in requiring indirect calorimetry more frequently than is feasible to maintain accuracy.

The patient should be followed carefully by a team for continued monitoring and reevaluation during both inpatient and outpatient treatment. If the patient has severe laboratory abnormalities or is very low weight, an inpatient setting for refeeding is the safest option. Initial caloric prescription for AN can be determined using a dietary recall and can begin at estimated intake or 250 kcal above estimated intake. It should be noted that patients with AN frequently overestimate intake in a dietary recall.[30] If unable to determine actual energy intake, beginning at 1000 to 1250 kcal prior to starting the plan is generally safe.[30]

For inpatients with AN, it is recommended that 250 kcal be added to the intake prescription every 24 hours because of changes in metabolic rate and postprandial energy expenditure. Resting energy expenditure continues to increase in patients with AN throughout the weight restoration process. An increased thermic effect of food and difficulty with absorption may contribute to greater energy needs. A weight gain of 0.5 lb daily or 2 to 3 lb per week is appropriate.[29] The patient's rate of weight gain should be followed, and energy intake should be adjusted accordingly. In an inpatient setting, females often peak around 3000 to 3500 kcal/day, and males often peak around 4000 kcal/day. However, some programs recommend increasing up to 5000 kcal/day, because weight gain may not correlate with the total excess of calories consumed above basal needs.

For patients with AN being treated on an outpatient basis, energy intake is advanced at a slower pace. An increase of 500 kcal weekly is usually the maximum of what can be tolerated for energy intake advancement.[31] A gain of 1 to 2 lb weekly is appropriate. Once children and adolescents achieve a healthy weight, an increased energy prescription is needed to support future growth and development.[29]

It may be difficult to determine energy intake in patients with BN, given variability with binge/purge behaviors. Generally, 50% of kcal consumed in a binge/purge cycle should be added to total calorie count.[30] To determine energy intake for normal or overweight patients with BN, the resting energy expenditure equation (REE) covers basal needs and assumes sedentary activity levels and should prevent excessive weight gain in children.

REE:

Males 3-10 years of age: $(22.7 \times \text{wt (kg)}) + 495$

Females 3-10 years of age: $(22.5 \times \text{wt (kg)}) + 499$

Males 10-18 years of age: $(17.5 \times \text{wt (kg)}) + 651$

Females 10-18 years of age $(12.2 \times \text{wt (kg)}) + 746$

Weight loss calorie goals should be avoided regardless of overweight/obesity until an eating pattern is stabilized, because caloric restriction may trigger bingeing.[32] Patients with BN or those with a history of BN may be hypometabolic, requiring less energy intake than typically estimated for a patient of similar weight and height.

Notably, patients with BN are most often treated on an outpatient basis; higher level of care may be recommended at times for interrupting the binge/purge cycle or managing medical complications of BN.

Meal Planning

Snacks and/or supplements are helpful to increase energy and protein intake while keeping meals manageable in size. Increasing calorie-dense foods as well as providing fluids with calories may be helpful to avoid excessive fullness after eating. In addition, low-lactose foods or providing lactase supplements may decrease abdominal discomfort from nutritionally mediated lactase deficiency. Frequently, behavioral interventions are necessary to facilitate patients meeting energy intake and weight goals.[33] An eating protocol that provides clear criteria for expected energy intake, weight gain, activity, and behavior and that outlines expectations for the patients, family members, and treatment providers is a valuable tool to help patients to meet goals. The exchange list created by the American Diabetes Association in collaboration with the Academy of Nutrition and Dietetics is a helpful tool to plan meals. The exchange system groups foods into starch, protein, fruit, vegetable, milk, and fat categories and within each category indicates specific portion sizes, which provide similar nutrition content (eg, 1 serving of starch can be fulfilled by 1 slice of bread or 1/3 cup of pasta). Meals are planned by prescribing a number of exchanges from each food group. This decreases focus on calories and fat and increases emphasis on the inclusion of a variety of foods and food groups.[29] In some cases, allowing patients to make food choices can be empowering and help them to feel in control; yet for other patients, this level of control may feel overwhelming. Patients with AN may find food choices difficult despite the method of meal planning or the protocols, and there are no longitudinal outcome data to support one method of meal planning over another.[30] For normal-weight patients with BN, encouraging 3 meals and snacks daily promotes normal eating and helps the patient break the cycle of restriction and binge/purge behaviors.[34]

Nutrition Support

Oral feedings are the preferred method of restoring nutrition. The decision to start nutrition support should consider both the patient's immediate physical health and psychological health. The indications for tube feedings include refusing any oral intake, rapid weight loss despite improved oral intake or hypermetabolism, and inability to meet nutritional needs orally.[32] If enteral nutrition via tube feedings is necessary, starting at 25% of the estimated goal and increasing to initial goal over 3 to 5 days is recommended.[35] Some patients may need to have both tube feedings as well as oral nutrition to achieve nutrition and weight gain goals. Bolus feedings or nocturnal feedings are useful to provide uneaten calories or supplement intake. However, continuous feedings are less likely to result in dumping syndrome or purging. If tube feedings are initiated, typically an isotonic, fiber-containing, enteral feeding will be sufficient. Formulas containing high glucose should be avoided. If

VI

absorption or digestion is impaired, an elemental or peptide-based formula may be indicated. Parenteral nutrition should be used rarely and with caution, because it leads to the continued loss of hunger cues and increases risk of refeeding syndrome.[32,35]

Refeeding Syndrome

When starved or severely malnourished patients begin nutrition repletion, they are at risk of refeeding syndrome. As the metabolism shifts, it may result in fluid and electrolyte disorders that could cause neurologic, pulmonary, cardiac, neuromuscular, and hematologic complications.[35] Medical stabilization and safety are the initial concerns, and this stabilization period can last up to 3 weeks. Therefore, substantial weight gain cannot always be expected in this time, especially if medical complications from refeeding arise.

To prevent refeeding syndrome, advancement of energy by 250 kcal/day in addition to supplementing vitamins and minerals is essential to safely bring the patient from a catabolic to an anabolic state.[29] Frequent physical examinations as well as determinations of serum phosphorous, magnesium, and electrolyte concentrations are needed. In addition, there should be careful monitoring of the patient's vital signs, daily weights, fluid intake, and output.[29]

During the increase of energy intake, metabolic disturbances may occur, including hypophosphatemia, hypokalemia, and hypomagnesemia. Hypophosphatemia may result from the intracellular shift of serum phosphorus needed for the generation of adenosine triphosphate (ATP) in the cellular anabolic processes. Low serum concentrations of phosphorus are associated with cardiac and neuromuscular dysfunction as well as blood cell dysfunction. Hypokalemia and hypomagnesemia may increase risk of cardiac arrhythmias and gastrointestinal and neuromuscular complications. During refeeding, extracellular expansion is common, causing peripheral edema; in extreme cases, congestive heart failure may occur.[36] In the inpatient setting and occasionally in the outpatient setting, supplementary phosphorous may be given to prevent the refeeding syndrome.

Macronutrients, Fiber, and Fluids

No optimal macronutrient intake regimen has been found to be more beneficial for patients with eating disorders; however, a standard recommendation of 25% to 30% fat, 15% to 20% protein, and 50% to 55% carbohydrate may be helpful to provide a balance of macronutrients.[29,30] In patients at risk of developing refeeding syndrome, a slightly higher intake of fat and protein calories may be somewhat protective, as carbohydrate metabolism drives refeeding syndrome. Initially, when prescribing a meal plan or tube feedings, 150 to 200 g/day of carbohydrate should not be exceeded and the protein goal should be approximately 1.2 to 1.5 g/kg of ideal body weight to preserve lean body mass while feeding hypocalorically. Patient access to simple sugars and sodium should be limited to avoid the risk of refeeding syndrome. The patient's previous intake of fiber should guide how much fiber is prescribed. Excessive fiber may result in discomfort or gastrointestinal distress, and not enough fiber may contribute to constipation. Fluids should start at approximately 20 mL/kg or 1 mL/kcal and be adjusted as needed to prevent dehydration or fluid retention.[37] In both AN and BN, the initial diet should be low in salt, lactose, and fat to minimize malabsorption and edema.[36]

Micronutrients

Vitamin deficiencies are not frequently seen in patients with AN and BN. However, it is common practice to supplement the patient with a multivitamin and minerals during treatment.[30] Because AN often begins during adolescence, the critical period for bone mineral accretion, supplementation with calcium and vitamin D are recommended.[34] The current recommendation for adolescent females is 1300 mg/day of calcium and 600 IU/day of vitamin D.[38]

Longitudinal Outcome

The course and outcome of eating disorders is variable; adolescents with a shorter duration of illness have a more favorable outcome compared with adults or those with a longer duration of illness, underscoring the importance of early detection and intervention.

A recent meta-analysis of 36 quantitative studies of individuals with eating disorders found significantly elevated mortality rates,[39] and AN is associated with the highest risk of mortality among all psychiatric disorders.[40] Among adults with AN, longitudinal studies suggest the rate of mortality is 0.56% per year, which is more than 12 times higher than that for young women in the general population.[16,40] Further, the rate suicide is also elevated, with one study demonstrating a 57-fold increase in death by suicide among adult women with AN.[16] Yet, the longitudinal course and prognosis is better for adolescents. One recent analysis of multiple outcome studies for adolescents and adults with AN found that 57% recovered, 26% more had improved substantially, 17% went on to have chronic course of AN, and 2% had died.[41]

Patients with BN generally have a more favorable course. Longitudinal research suggests that approximately 50% of adult women with BN achieve full recovery from their eating disorder at 5 to 12 years of follow-up, although approximately one third of these will go on to relapse.[42] In contrast to the high mortality rates in patients with AN, mortality does not appear to be significantly increased in those with BN.[16,43] One review of 88 studies demonstrated a crude mortality rate of 0.3% during longitudinal follow-up, although the authors cautioned that this may have

VI

been an underestimate because of variable lengths of follow-up (6 months to 10 years) and low ascertainment across follow-up.[44]

Conclusions

Eating disorders are prevalent problems among adolescents, and to a lesser extent, among children. These illnesses carry the risk of severe medical and psychosocial consequences and poor long-term outcome. As such, early detection and intervention involving a multidisciplinary team is required.

References

1. American Psychiatric Association. *Diagnostic and Statistical Manual of Mental Disorders, Fourth Edition, Text Revision*. Washington, DC: American Psychiatric Publishing; 2000

2. Swanson SA, Crow SJ, Le Grange D, Swendsen J, Merikangas KR. Prevalence and correlates of eating disorders in adolescents. *Arch Gen Psychiatry*. 2011;68(7):714-723

3. Rome ES, Ammerman S, Rosen DS, et al. Children and adolescents with eating disorders: the state of the art. *Pediatrics*. 2003;111(1):e98-e107

4. Misra M, Aggarwal A, Miller KK, et al. Effects of anorexia nervosa on clinical, hematologic, biochemical, and bone density parameters in community-dwelling adolescents girls. *Pediatrics*. 2004;114(6):1574-1583

5. Grinspoon S, Thomas E, Pitts S, et al. Prevalence and predictive factors for regional osteopenia in women with anorexia nervosa. *Ann Intern Med*. 2000;133(10):790-794

6. Misra M, Katzman DK, Miller KK, et al. Physiologic estrogen replacement increases bone density in adolescent girls with anorexia nervosa. *J Bone Miner Res*. In press

7. Nattiv A, Loucks AB, Manore MM, Sanborn CF, Sundgot-Borgen J, Warren MP. American College of Sports Medicine position stand. The female athlete triad. *Med Sci Sports Exerc*. 2007;39(10):1867-1882

8. Strober M, Freeman R, Lampert C, Diamond J, Kaye W. Controlled family study of anorexia nervosa and bulimia nervosa: evidence of shared liability and transmission of partial syndromes. *Am J Psychiatry*. 2000;157(3):393-401

9. Strober M, Bulik C. Genetic epidemiology of eating disorders. In: Fairburn C, Brownell K, eds. *Eating Disorders and Obesity: A Comprehensive Handbook*. 2nd ed. New York, NY: Guilford Press; 2002:238-242

10. Monteleone P, Martiadis V, Rigamonti AE, et al. Investigation of peptide YY and ghrelin responses to a test meal in bulimia nervosa. *Biol Psychiatry*. 2005;57(8):926–931

11. Walsh BT, Kissileff HR, Cassidy SM, Dantzic S. Eating behavior of women with bulimia. *Arch Gen Psychiatry*. 1989;46(1):54-58

12. Herzog DB, Eddy KT, Beresin EV. Anorexia nervosa and bulimia nervosa. In: Dulcan MK, Wiener JM, eds. *Essentials of Child and Adolescent Psychiatry*. Washington, DC: American Psychiatric Publishing; 2006:527-560

13. Becker AE, Thomas JJ, Franko DL, Herzog DB. Disclosure patterns of eating and weight concerns to clinicians, educational professionals, family, and peers. *Int J Eat Disord.* 2005;38(1):18-23

14. Goldstein MA, Dechant EJ, Beresin EV. Eating disorders. *Pediatr Rev.* 2011;32(12):508-521

15. Herzog DB, Eddy KT. Psychiatric comorbidity in eating disorders. In: Wonderlich S, Mitchell JE, de Zwaan M, Steiger H, eds. *Annual Review of Eating Disorders.* Oxford, United Kingdom: Radcliffe Publishing Ltd; 2007:35-50

16. Keel PK, Dorer DJ, Eddy KT, Franko D, Charatan DL, Herzog DB. Predictors of mortality in eating disorders. *Arch Gen Psychiatry.* 2003;60(2):179-183

17. Burgalassi A, Ramacciotti CE, Binachi M, et al. Caffeine consumption among eating disorder patients: epidemiology, motivations, and potential of abuse. *Eat Weight Disord.* 2009;14(4):e212-e218

18. Krug I, Treasure J, Anderluh M, et al. Present and lifetime comorbidity of tobacco, alcohol and drug use in eating disorders: a European multicenter study. *Drug Alcohol Depend.* 2008;97(1-2):169-179

19. Academy for Eating Disorders. *Eating Disorders: Critical Points for Early Recognition and Medical Risk Management in the Care of Individuals with Eating Disorders.* Deerfield, IL: Academy for Eating Disorders; 2011. Available at: http://www.aedweb.org/AM/Template.cfm?Section=Medical_Care_Standards&Template=/CM/ContentDisplay.cfm&ContentID=2413. Accessed January 2, 2013

20. American Psychiatric Association. Practice guidelines for the treatment of patients with eating disorders, Third Edition. *Am J Psychiatry.* 2006:163(7 Suppl):4-54

21. Loeb KL, Le Grange D. Family-based treatment for adolescent eating disorders: current status, new applications, and future directions. *Int J Child Adolesc Health.* 2009;2(2):243-254

22. Lock J, Agras WS, Bryson S, Kraemer HC. A comparison of short- and long-term family therapy for adolescent anorexia nervosa. *J Am Acad Child Adolesc Psychiatry.* 2005;44(7):632-639

23. Le Grange D, Crosby RD, Rathouz PJ, Leventhal BL. A randomized controlled comparison of family-based treatment and supportive psychotherapy for adolescent bulimia nervosa. *Arch Gen Psychiatry.* 2007;64(9):1049-1056

24. Biederman J, Herzog DB, Rivinus TM, et al. Amitriptyline in the treatment of anorexia nervosa: a double-blind, placebo-controlled study. *J Clin Psychopharmacol.* 1985;5(1):10-16

25. Bissada H, Tasca GA, Barber AM, Bradwejn J. Olanzapine in the treatment of low body weight and obsessive thinking in women with anorexia nervosa: a randomized, double-blind, placebo-controlled trial. *Am J Psychiatry.* 2008;165(10):1281-1288

26. Broft A, Berner LA, Walsh BT. Pharmacotherapy for bulimia nervosa. In: Grilo CM, Mitchell JE. *The Treatment of Eating Disorders.* New York, NY: Guilford Press; 2010:388-401

27. Phillips S, Edlbeck A, Kirby M, Goday P. Ideal body weight in children. *Nutr Clin Pract.* 2007;22(2):240-245

VI

28. Mehler P, Andersen A. *Eating Disorders: A Guide to Medical Care and Complications.* 2nd ed. Baltimore, MD: Johns Hopkins University Press; 2008

29. Reiter CS, Graves L. Nutrition therapy for eating disorders. *Nutr Clin Pract.* 2010;25(2):122-136

30. Schebendach JE. Nutrition in eating disorders. In: Mahan LK, Escott-Stump S, eds. *Krause's Food and Nutrition Therapy.* 12th ed. St Louis, MO: Saunders/Elsevier; 2008:563-586

31. Herrin M. *Nutrition Counseling in the Treatment of Eating Disorders.* New York, NY: Brunner-Routledge; 2003

32. Fitzgerald C, Hjelmgren B. Eating disorders. In: Corkins MR, ed. *Pediatric Nutrition Support Core Curriculum.* Silver Spring, MD: American Society for Parental and Enteral Nutrition (A.S.P.E.N); 2010:204-212

33. Rosen DS; American Academy of Pediatrics, Committee on Adolescence. Clinical report: identification and management of eating disorders in children and adolescents. *Pediatrics.* 2010;126(6):1240-1253

34. Henry BW, Ozier AD; American Dietetic Association. Position of the American Dietetic Association: nutrition intervention in the treatment of anorexia nervosa, bulimia nervosa, and other eating disorders. *J Am Diet Assoc.* 2011;111(8):1236-1241

35. Kraft M, Btaiche I, Sacks G. Review of the refeeding syndrome. *Nutr Clin Pract.* 2005;20(6):625-633

36. Coughlin JW, Guarda A. Behavioral disorders affecting food intake: eating disorders and other psychiatric conditions. In: Shils ME, Shike M, Ross AC, Caballero B, Cousins RJ, eds. *Modern Nutrition in Health and Disease.* 10th ed. Philadelphia, PA: Lippincott Williams & Wilkins; 2006:1353-1361

37. Setnick J. *The Eating Disorders Clinical Pocket Guide: Quick Reference for Healthcare Providers.* Dallas, Texas: Understanding Nutrition, PC; 2005

38. Institute of Medicine, Committee to Review Dietary Reference Intakes for Vitamin D and Calcium. *Dietary Reference Intakes for Vitamin D and Calcium.* Ross AC, Taylor CL, Yaktine AL, Del Valle HB, eds. Washington, DC: National Academies Press; 2011

39. Arcelus J, Mitchell AJ, Wales J, Nielsen S. Mortality rates in patients with anorexia nervosa and other eating disorders. *Arch Gen Psychiatry.* 2011;68(7):724-731

40. Sullivan PF. Mortality in anorexia nervosa. *Am J Psychiatry.* 1995;152(7):1073-1074

41. Steinhausen HC. Outcome of eating disorders. *Child Adolesc Psychiatr Clin North Am.* 2009;18(1):225-242

42. Herzog DB, Dorer DJ, Keel PK, et al. Recovery and relapse in anorexia and bulimia nervosa: a 7.5 year follow-up study. *J Am Acad Child Adol Psychiatry.* 1999;38(7):829-837

43. Nielsen S, Moller-Madsen S, Isager T, Jorgensen J, Pagsberg K, Theander S. Standardized mortality in eating disorders – a quantitative summary of previously published and new evidence. *J Psychosomat Res.* 1998;44(3-4):413-434

44. Keel PK, Mitchell JE. Outcome in bulimia nervosa. *Am J Psychiatry.* 1997;154(3):313-321

Chapter 40

HIV Infection

Introduction

Acute and chronic infection with human immunodeficiency virus (HIV) is a worldwide problem of increasing magnitude. The World Health Organization estimates that 31.4 to 35.3 million adults and children were living with HIV in 2009, the majority of whom were in developing countries.[1] In 2009, HIV/acquired immunodeficiency syndrome (AIDS) was the cause of death worldwide in up to 260 000 children from birth through 14 years of age.[1] The number of individuals infected with HIV has been steadily declining, and the number of children dying of AIDS has also declined in the last 15 years. This trend reflects the expansion of services to prevent transmission of HIV to infants and to the wider use of antiretroviral therapy (ART) and improved prophylactic regimens worldwide. In resource-rich nations, HIV has become a chronic illness as highly active antiretroviral therapy (HAART) has become the mainstay of treatment. With the increasing number of children surviving with HIV/AIDS, the need for appropriate supportive care is paramount. Clinicians who care for children with HIV/AIDS should be aware of potential nutritional and metabolic problems and their consequences. In the past, wasting syndrome was the primary nutritional concern for HIV-infected individuals. Now, approaching 15 years since the advent of HAART, the focus on cardiometabolic and nutritional issues is expanding. Knowledge and implementation of effective nutritional therapies are important to improve medical outcomes and quality of life. With appropriate combinations of antiretroviral therapy and nutritional support, many HIV-infected children are now able to lead relatively normal lives.

Nutrition and the Immune System

In many disease states of childhood, there are well-defined associations between malnutrition, growth, and immune function.[2] Although HIV can negatively affect nutritional status, there is a reciprocal effect, as malnutrition can intensify the immunologic effects of HIV, thus leading to a destructive and negatively reinforcing relationship of malnutrition, immune dysfunction, and advancing HIV disease.[2,3] Similarly, obesity, with attendant metabolic abnormalities and type 2 diabetes mellitus—problems that currently face many children with HIV infection—can produce immune dysfunction. In both conditions, there are abnormalities in B- and T-lymphocyte immunity with increased inflammatory cytokine production, decreased response to antigen/mitogen stimulation, reduced macrophage and

VI

dendritic cell function, and natural killer cell impairment.[2,4] Table 40.1 lists the differences and similarities between the effects of protein-energy malnutrition (PEM), obesity, and HIV on the immune system.

Table 40.1.
Comparison of Body Composition, Energy Expenditure, and Immunologic Function in Protein-Energy Malnutrition (PEM), Sepsis, Obesity, and HIV Infection

Condition	Body Composition	Energy Expenditure	Immune Function
PEM (starvation)	Decreased fat leading to decreased lean body mass	Decreased	Decreased white blood cell count, cell-mediated immunity, and T-lymphocyte function; decreased immune-globulin (Ig) A and IgE; increased or decreased IgG
Sepsis	Decreased lean body mass leading to decreased fat	Increased	Activated (effective) Increased pro-inflammatory cytokines
Obesity	Increased fat mass often with truncal adiposity	Increased (based on relative increased lean)	Decreased CD4+ T-lymphocyte, CD8+ T-lymphocyte, B-lymphocyte, natural killer cell number and activity; increased oxidative burst (macrophage); increased proinflammatory cytokines
HIV	Decreased lean body mass leading to decreased fat	Unchanged to increased according to severity of infection	Increased IgG; decreased CD4+ T-lymphocyte count and function; Increased proinflammatory cytokines

Clinically, nutritional abnormalities, including failure to thrive (FTT), malnutrition, obesity, and cardiometabolic problems, are potential adverse outcomes in pediatric HIV[5] in the HAART era and can contribute to declines in health and increases in mortality. Patients who have nutritional and metabolic disturbances that result in weight loss and wasting may show a chronic inflammatory state secondary to increased viral replication or microbial translocation from the gastrointestinal tract. Furthermore, obesity and its consequences also comprise a known inflammatory disorder that compromises immune function. Inflammation and other immune responses alter nutritional status through sequestration of minerals (eg, iron and zinc), impaired absorption, increased nutrient loss, or altered nutrient utilization.[6]

Achieving and maintaining optimal nutrition can improve an individual's immune function, reduce the incidence of complications associated with HIV infection, attenuate the progression of HIV infection, improve quality of life, and ultimately, reduce mortality associated with HIV.[7]

Nutrition in Pediatric HIV for Children Naive or Resisant to Antiretroviral Therapy

Although there are different nutritional concerns in the HAART era with effective viral suppression, discussion of nutritional problems of children not receiving ART or who have become resistant to therapy with falling CD4+ T-lymphocyte counts and increasing viral loads is relevant both in resource poor nations as well as in the United States, where ART is more accessible.

An array of factors influence HIV treatment adherence, including adverse effects of medications, low self-esteem, depression, stigma experiences, cognitive impairment, substance abuse, and food insecurity and hunger.[8-11] Because of the adverse effects of HAART and lifestyle changes necessary to adhere to treatment regimens, some people choose not to take therapy or, despite a good virologic response, do not tolerate therapy.[12] Lipodystrophy is an adverse effect that could impair adherence to an otherwise successful HAART regimen in body image-conscious preadolescent and adolescent patients.[13] Adult studies have shown that lipodystrophy results in erosion of self-image and self-esteem, depression, and nonadherence with treatment regimens.[14]

Nonadherence results in immunologic and clinical deterioration and viral mutations that lead to drug resistance. Drug resistance can develop in both multidrug-experienced children and ART-naïve children who received initial regimens containing 1 or 2 drugs that incompletely suppressed viral replication.[15] Many people with HIV/AIDS already had advanced disease before HAART was introduced, and even in those who respond to treatment, viral resistance may develop, thus reducing the effectiveness of the drugs[12] and placing them at great risk of treatment failure, disease progression, nutritional problems, and potential exhaustion of treatment options.

Malnutrition and Wasting

Malnutrition and its consequences are generally more common in the child who is diagnosed with AIDS. Malnutrition in children with HIV/AIDS may be caused by several mechanisms working independently or synergistically. These causes are summarized in Table 40.2. Insufficient intake of nutrients is one factor that may lead to undernutrition. A variety of potential factors may lead to abnormal intake, as outlined in Table 40.2. For example, inflammation and ulcers of the upper gastrointestinal tract can lead to anorexia because of odynophagia, dysphagia, or abdominal pain that is associated with eating. In one series in the pre-HAART era, 70% of upper gastrointestinal tract endoscopies in HIV-infected children revealed histologic lesions.[16] These lesions can be attributable to peptic injury or infectious pathogens, such as *Candida albicans*, cytomegalovirus, or herpes simplex virus, all of which may cause inflammation and pain with swallowing or after eating.

VI

Furthermore, oral ulcers that are attributable to viral pathogens or "idiopathic" oral ulcers[17] may cause pain with eating and reduce oral intake. These opportunistic upper intestinal conditions are unusual in children who have a CD4+ T-lymphocyte count greater than 15%.[18]

Table 40.2.
Potential Causes of Malnutrition in HIV-Infected Children

Decreased Nutrient Intake
Primary anorexia Peptic disease Opportunistic infections of upper GI tract (*Candida*, CMV, HSV)[a] Idiopathic aphthous ulcers Dysgeusia (zinc deficiency) Pancreatic/hepatobiliary disease Encephalopathy
Gastrointestinal Malabsorption

Mucosal disease
    Infectious[a]
    Inflammatory
    Disaccharidase deficiency
    Protein-losing enteropathy
    Fat malabsorption
Hepatobiliary
    Sclerosing cholangitis
    Chronic pancreatitis
    Coinfection with HBV/HCV

Increased Nutritional Requirements or Tissue Catabolism
Protein wasting Increased metabolism   **Secondary to:** Fever, infections, sepsis[a] Neoplasms (Kaposi sarcoma, lymphoma)[a] Medications Proinflammatory factors
Psychosocial factors
Poverty Illness in biological family members Limited access to health care Substance abuse

GI indicates gastrointestinal; CMV, cytomegalovirus; HSV, herpes simplex virus; HBV, hepatitis B virus; HCV, hepatitis C virus.

[a] These causes are more common in children with CD4+ T-lymphocyte counts of <15%.

Malabsorption can lead to malnutrition, and a dysfunctional gastrointestinal tract can produce clinical symptoms that contribute to both morbidity and mortality in children with HIV-1 infection. The etiology of malabsorption is multifactorial but includes gastrointestinal tract mucosal abnormalities leading to macronutrient and micronutrient malabsorption. These mucosal changes can be attributable to local HIV infection of the gut or secondary enteric infections. Villous atrophy and gastrointestinal tract dysfunction are coincident with high levels of HIV-1 viral load in the gut.[19] There is evidence that certain gastrointestinal tract epithelial cells bind and selectively transfer HIV from the cells' apical to basolateral surface, where viral translocation across the epithelium encounters lamina propria macrophages and T lymphocytes.[20,21] Altered epithelial permeability may permit microbial translocation and generalized immune activation, leading to localized cytokine production and further replication of HIV.[22] High systemic levels of lipopolysaccharides as a result of bacterial translocation are associated with marked systemic immune activation that increases metabolic rate and sustains HIV infection. ART decreases levels of lipopolysaccharides and promotes CD4+ T-lymphocyte reconstitution and may subsequently decrease the systemic immune activation, although not completely.[23] As a result of either local HIV infection with associated bacterial translocation (that induces proinflammatory changes in the gastrointestinal mucosa and systemically) or of the injury caused by a secondary infection, mucosal function can be compromised with resulting malabsorption. Because of the difficulty in treating many of these infections, the diarrhea may be unremitting and predispose to severe malnutrition that may lead to eventual mortality, especially in developing nations.

A number of other causes of malnutrition should be also considered. Gastrointestinal tract bleeding attributable to mucosal ulcerations leads to loss of nutrients with the loss of blood. Opportunistic infections affect the hepatobiliary system and pancreas in addition to the gastrointestinal tract and may lead to malabsorption. The site and severity of infection vary according to the infecting organism (Table 40.3). Furthermore, HIV encephalopathy, which was present in up to 16% of children with HIV infection in the pre-HAART era,[24] albeit with lower prevalence rates with successful viral suppression,[25] may result in the physical inability to consume enough calories to sustain growth. Oral administration of feedings under this condition may also be dangerous because of the high risk of aspiration in neurologically compromised children. Finally, many medications that HIV-infected children are required to take may result in gastric irritation, vomiting, nausea, and diarrhea. These medications are listed in Table 40.4.

VI

Table 40.3.
Infectious Gastrointestinal Manifestations of HIV/AIDS

Site	Manifestations or Infecting Organisms
Oral	*Candida albicans* Herpes simplex virus Human papillomavirus Oral hairy leukoplakia Kaposi sarcoma Lymphoma
Esophagus	*Candida albicans* Cytomegalovirus Herpes simplex virus *Cryptosporidia* species Kaposi sarcoma Lymphoma
Stomach	Cytomegalovirus *Cryptosporidia* species Kaposi sarcoma *Helicobacter pylori*
Small intestine	Giardiasis *Cryptosporidia* Cytomegalovirus *Salmonella* species Enteroaggregative *Escherichia coli* *Blastocystis hominis* *Isospora belli* Rotavirus, calicivirus, astrovirus, coronavirus, picornavirus Adenovirus *Shigella* species *Mycobacterium* species Lymphoma
Colon	Cytomegalovirus *Salmonella* species *Shigella* species *Campylobacter* species *Entamoeba* species Lymphoma *Clostridium difficile* Adenovirus
Anus/rectum	Kaposi sarcoma Lymphoma Squamous cell carcinoma Papovavirus

Site	Manifestations or Infecting Organisms
Hepatobiliary	*Mycobacterium* species Cytomegalovirus *Cryptococcus, histoplasmosis* Hepatitis B, C, or D Cryptosporidiosis Kaposi sarcoma Microsporidia
Pancreas	Cytomegalovirus *Mycobacterium* species Cryptosporidiosis

Growth and Body Composition

A variety of disturbed growth patterns, most noted in the pre-HAART era, have been described for HIV-infected children,[26-31] ranging from symmetric delays in weight gain and linear growth to severe wasting with normal height. Prior to HAART, the natural history of somatic growth in HIV-infected infants was characterized by alterations in growth and body composition similar to those produced by both acute and chronic malnutrition.[26] The differences in growth patterns were likely attributable to the variable manifestations of the disease in HIV-infected children, associated with factors such as viral load and infections, as mentioned previously. In resource-rich countries in the pre-HAART era, HIV-infected children showed declines in both weight and length as early as the first 1 to 3 months of life. Sequential follow-up showed that growth of HIV-infected children remained below that of age- and gender-matched uninfected children. However, with the administration to the mother of ART[31] during the second and/or third trimester of pregnancy, transmission rates have fallen to less than 2%.[32,33] The extent to which prenatal exposure to ART and HIV affect growth will be discussed in later sections.

Several pediatric studies in the pre-HAART era have shown progressive declines in lean body mass over time in children with HIV/AIDS, whereas measures of fat stores remain constant yet low.[28,29] There is conflicting literature on whether there is more of a pattern of cachexia (preferential wasting of muscle over fat) or normal weight loss with initial loss of fat over lean body mass[34,35] in adults with HIV/AIDS. Cytokines may be responsible for some of the growth, metabolic, and immunologic effects associated with HIV infection,[36] and there are positive changes in cytokine patterns after HAART therapy.[37]

VI

Table 40.4.

HIV-Related Medications and Common Gastrointestinal and Metabolic Adverse Effects

Medication	Action	Adverse Effects
Abacavir	NRTI	Nausea, vomiting, diarrhea, abdominal pain, pancreatitis, abnormal liver function
Acyclovir	Antiviral	Nausea, abdominal pain, diarrhea, abnormal liver function
Atazanavir	PI	Nausea, diarrhea, abdominal pain, hyperbilirubinemia
Atripla (Tenofovir, Emtricitabine. Efavirenz)	Combination	Nausea, vomiting, diarrhea, abdominal pain, hepatitis, bone loss, pancreatitis, lactic acidosis
Azithromycin	Antibacterial	Nausea, vomiting, melena, jaundice
Ciprofloxacin	Antibacterial	Ileus, jaundice, bleeding, diarrhea, anorexia, oral ulcers, hepatitis, pancreatitis, vomiting, abdominal pain
Clarithromycin	Antibacterial	Nausea, diarrhea, abdominal pain, abnormal taste
Combivir (zidovudine-lamivudine)	Combination	Nausea, vomiting, abdominal pain, abnormal liver function, pancreatitis, lactic acidosis
Darunavir	PI	Nausea, vomiting, diarrhea, abdominal pain, pancreatitis, hepatitis, constipation
Didanosine (ddI)	NRTI	Nausea, vomiting, abdominal pain, pancreatitis, abnormal liver function
Efavirenz	NNRTI	Nausea, vomiting, abnormal liver function, hyperlipidemia
Emtricitabine	NRTI	Lactic acidosis, hepatomegaly, diarrhea, nausea
Epzicom (Zidovudine, Abacavir)	Combination	Nausea, vomiting, abdominal pain, abnormal liver function, lactic acidosis, pancreatitis
Erythromycin	Antibacterial	Nausea, vomiting, abdominal pain
Etravirine	NNRTI	Nausea, vomiting, diarrhea, abdominal pain, hepatitis
Fos-Amprenavir	PI	Nausea, diarrhea, vomiting, abdominal pain
Enfuvirtide	FI	Nausea, diarrhea, abdominal pain, hepatitis, pancreatitis, dry mouth, anorexia
Ganciclovir	Antiviral	Nausea, vomiting, diarrhea, anorexia, abnormal liver function
Indinavir	PI	Nausea, vomiting, abdominal pain, diarrhea, changes in taste, jaundice, abnormal liver function
Ketoconazole	Antifungal	Hepatotoxicity
Lamivudine	NRTI	Nausea, diarrhea, decreased appetite, vomiting, abdominal pain, pancreatitis, abnormal liver function

Medication	Action	Adverse Effects
Lopinavir/ ritonavir	PI	Diarrhea, nausea, vomiting, abdominal pain, lipodystrophy, hyperlipidemia
Maraviroc	EI	Nausea, constipation, diarrhea, flatulence, abdominal pain, hepatitis, dysgeusia, stomatitis,
Nelfinavir	PI	Nausea, diarrhea, fatigue, abnormal liver function, exacerbation of chronic liver disease
Nevirapine	NNRTI	Stomatitis, nausea, abdominal pain, raised gamma-glutamyl transpeptidase level, hepatotoxicity
Pentamidine	Antiparasitic	Abdominal pain, bleeding, hepatitis, pancreatitis, nausea, vomiting
Raltegravir	II	Gastritis, hepatitis, nausea, vomiting, abdominal pain, diarrhea, hyperbilirubinemia
Rifampin	Antibacterial	Abdominal pain, nausea, vomiting, diarrhea, jaundice
Rilpivirine	NNRTI	Lipodystrophy
Ritonavir	PI	Nausea, vomiting, diarrhea, abdominal pain, anorexia, pancreatitis, abnormal liver function
Saquinavir	PI	Mouth ulcers, nausea, abdominal pain, diarrhea, pancreatitis, abnormal liver function, exacerbation of chronic liver disease
Stavudine	NRTI	Nausea, vomiting, abdominal pain, diarrhea, pancreatitis, abnormal liver function, hepatic failure, lipodystrophy, hyperlipidemia, insulin resistance
Sulfonamides	Antibacterial	Hepatitis, pancreatitis, stomatitis, nausea, vomiting, abdominal pain
Tenofovir	NRTI	Nausea, vomiting, diarrhea, abdominal pain, hepatitis, bone loss, pancreatitis, flatulence
Tipranavir	PI	Hyperlipidemia, nausea, vomiting, diarrhea, abdominal pain, pancreatitis, hepatitis
Trizivir (abacavir-lamivudine-zidovudine)	Combination	Nausea, vomiting, abdominal pain, pancreatitis, abnormal liver function
Truvada (Emtricitabine, Tenofovir)	Combination	Lactic acidosis, nausea, vomiting, diarrhea, abdominal pain, hepatitis, bone loss, pancreatitis
Zidovudine (ZDV)	NRTI	Nausea, vomiting, abdominal pain, abnormal liver function

HBV indicates hepatitis B virus; FI, fusion inhibitor; II, integrase inhibitor; EE, entry inhibitor.

VI

Energy Balance

Asymptomatic chronic viral infections may have some effect on energy utilization and can predispose children to secondary infections, which in turn, can further alter energy utilization patterns. These infections can increase or shunt effective use of energy substrates from normal, healthy growth patterns to abnormal ones, as in other chronic illnesses, including cystic fibrosis, inflammatory bowel disease, congenital heart disease and childhood cancer.[38] The chronic viral activity of HIV is likely no different. Small studies of energy expenditure have shown no differences in resting energy expenditure (REE)[39-41] or total energy expenditure (TEE)[41,42] between HIV-infected children with growth failure and those with normal rates of growth. However, adults with HIV-1 infection show REE increases with severity of illness,[43] especially with secondary infection and more advanced HIV disease,[44,45] yet TEE is similar, suggesting reduced physical activity. As HIV-infected children are treated with HAART, previously noted increases in protein catabolism decrease to more normal rates, suggesting that chronic viral activity leads to increased protein catabolism and can be brought to more normal levels with successful viral suppression.[46]

Primary anorexia, described in patients with cancer and other chronic conditions, may also contribute to inadequate oral intake. It is postulated that increased proinflammatory cytokine production (eg, tumor necrosis factor [TNF], interferon-gamma, and interleukins 1 and 6) may be associated with anorexia.[47,48] In animal models, administration of exogenous TNF has produced anorexia and cachexia.[49] TNF also causes delayed gastric emptying that can increase anorexia.[50]

A few small studies have shown differences in total energy intake between HIV-infected and uninfected children, suggesting substandard intakes may relate to growth differences.[40,51] However, a large prospective study has shown that stable, HIV-infected children in an ambulatory setting whose growth was below a control group, received well over the Recommended Dietary Allowance in total calories and protein, similar to the noninfected control children.[51] Another small study showed differences in energy intake between HIV-infected and noninfected children, suggesting substandard intakes may relate to growth differences.[41] However, in this study, a higher caloric intake was associated with improvement in weight and fat mass in infected children. One large prospective study of dietary intake in HIV-infected children that spanned both the pre-HAART and HAART eras showed caloric intakes decreased (possibly because of improved gastrointestinal tract absorption and lower energy utilization with HAART), although there was a shift toward increased carbohydrates in the diet in the HAART era.[52] Intake of critical immune-modulating micronutrients, such as iron, vitamin C, and vitamin A, has been shown to be low in the earlier stages of HIV in adolescents.[53] It is generally recommended that stable HIV-infected individuals increase their energy intake by about 10% to account for the metabolic needs associated with chronic viral infection.[54] Table 40.5 reviews the phases of HIV and how these phases relate to energy balance.

Table 40.5.

Clinical Condition and Energy Balance in Pediatric HIV Infection

Potential Determinants of Energy Intake and Energy Expenditure in HIV	Resting Energy Expenditure (REE)	Energy Intake	Physical Activity	Total Energy Expenditure (TEE)
Asymptomatic phases	HIV infection is associated with increased REE[180,181] REE per kg of fat-free mass (FFM) is increased even in asymptomatic HIV-infected patients who are experiencing viral suppression while receiving HAART[12] REE is not increased in infected children with growth failure and lower amount of FFM[40]	Maintained When clinically stable, a person may indeed eat well and be more active[182] Thermic effect of food—the energy consumed during digestion, absorption, and storage of food—comprises ~10% of TEE	Activity may stimulate appetite, adequate intake may permit activity, or it may be a consequence of another factor, such as clinical well-being Voluntary physical activity fluctuates daily but generally comprises ~30% of TEE in sedentary adults	Decreased or normal TEE
Opportunistic infections (OIs), acute stress	Markedly elevated[183,184] Elevated with increased level of the inflammatory marker C-reactive protein[183] A hypometabolic pattern (associated with VO_2 and VCO_2) predominates during the acute phase of stress turning out into a hypermetabolic pattern during convalescence[185] Malabsorption and cachexia may be associated with a decrease in REE	Markedly reduced[186] Influenced by an interplay of appetite, REE, and activity level[182] Decreased caloric intake, rather than increased REE, significantly correlates with rate of weight loss[184]	Negative effect[182] Fatigue and lethargy limits activity; energy expenditure from physical activity also decreases in response to restricted dietary intake	Lower in the presence of OI The negative effect of OIs on activity-related energy expenditure exceeds the positive effect on REE, and TEE is, thus, lower in the presence of OI[182] This decrease in TEE may help conserve lean body mass by counterbalancing increased REE[187]

VI

Table 40.5. (continued)

Clinical Condition and Energy Balance in Pediatric HIV Infection

Potential Determinants of Energy Intake and Energy Expenditure in HIV	Resting Energy Expenditure (REE)	Energy Intake	Physical Activity	Total Energy Expenditure (TEE)
HIV replication, chronic inflammation	HIV replication or possibly aspects of the host immune response appear to increase the basal metabolic demands in HIV-infected adults. HAART might decrease REE by decreasing viral load; however, specific antiretroviral drugs increase REE[187] Elevated REE with increased serum levels of catabolic cytokines (IL-β and TNF-α)[188] The long duration of exposure to these cytokines in HIV infection and the potential for very high levels of production suggest that the cumulative effects of even small excesses in cytokine production over time can be clinically significant	Reduced appetite may be related to decreased CD4+ T-lymphocyte count[182] Increased REE, if uncompensated by increased energy intake, may aggravate loss of both weight and lean body mass	Negative effect[182] The level of HIV replication may impair dietary intake	Possible increases in REE caused by an ongoing acute phase response may be counterbalanced by reduced physical activity that results in normal TEE in HIV infection

Altered body composition	Patients with HIV-associated lipodystrophy have distinct metabolic abnormalities in lipid turnover[189]—elevated lipolysis and adipocyte reesterification—indicating an increase in futile cycling within the adipocyte and potential increased REE[187] Lipoatrophy syndrome is associated with increased REE[190] -The metabolic rate of skeletal muscle is increased in patients with HIV lipoatrophy[191] -Increased REE may be a form of adaptive thermogenesis caused by an inability to store triglyceride fuel normally[191] Lipodystrophy—mixed results: -Some studies revealed that HIV-infected patients with lipodystrophy had greater REE per kg of FFM than those without lipodystrophy[191-194] -Others found no difference[195] -1 study suggested that REE per kg of FFM is actually lower in HIV-infected patients with lipodystrophy[196]	Lipodystrophy has been associated with increased total energy and fat intake[194] When there is profound loss of fat, such as that seen in the generalized lipodystrophies, leptin concentrations are low and a voracious appetite is typical.	The effects of physical activity: decreased waist circumference and waist-to-hip ratio and increased lean body mass, and cardiometabolic fitness[169]
Interventions	No intervention has proven to be effective for normalizing REE	Increased caloric intake compensates for increased REE and accelerated protein turnover[180]	

VI

Gastrointestinal and Hepatobiliary Complications

The evaluation of diarrhea in patients with AIDS yields a specific cause in 50% to 85% of patients, with most being effectively treated.[55] The nonspecific AIDS enteropathy[56] may be attributable, in part, to undiagnosed infections or to HIV itself (secondary to inflammatory changes induced by HIV in mucosal lympho-cytes).[57] Several investigators have reported impaired carbohydrate, fat, and protein absorption in children with HIV/AIDS[58,59]; the extent of malabsorption is not always correlated with the degree of malnutrition.[58]

Pancreatic and biliary tract disease can also cause vomiting and abdominal pain in HIV-infected children, leading to poor oral intake or malabsorption. Pancreatic disease has been linked to medications (eg, pentamidine, 2′,3′ dideoxyinosine, sulfa medications, some protease inhibitors; Table 40.4) and opportunistic infections (eg, cytomegalovirus, *Cryptosporidium* species, and mycobacterial disease).[60,61] Biliary tract disease, including sclerosing cholangitis and papillary stenosis, has been linked to *Cryptosporidium*, cytomegalovirus, and *Microsporidia* infections.[62,63] Opportunistic infections affect the hepatobiliary system and pancreas in addition to the gastrointestinal tract and may lead to malabsorption. The site and severity of infection vary according to the infecting organism (Table 40.3).

Nutrition in Pediatric HIV With Effective Viral Suppression and Immune Reconstitution

Guidelines for treatment of HIV-infected children are evolving as new data from clinical trials become available. Currently, the treatment of choice for HIV-infected children is at least 3 drugs, which include at least 2 classes of antiretroviral drugs.[64] The term HAART refers to a combination of antiretroviral agents, generally including a protease inhibitor. This combination is highly effective against HIV replication. The risk of disease progression is inversely correlated with the age of the child, with the youngest children at greatest risk of rapid disease progression. Therefore, current recommendations for when to start therapy differ by age of the child.

In the United States, HIV-infected children generally achieve normal weight-for-age z-scores within a year of HAART initiation and experience improvement in height-for-age z-scores by 2 years.[65,66] More rapid growth reconstitution has been observed in younger children.[67] Studies of HIV-infected children in the United States/Europe have shown height gain to normal values following HAART, with the highest restoration potential in children younger than 3 years[65,68] or 3 to 5 years in a sub-Saharan Africa population.[67] Whereas HAART may improve growth by decreasing metabolic expenditure and improving nutrient absorption, adverse effects of HAART could adversely affect growth.[69]

Malnutrition in the HAART Era

HAART has had a marked effect on AIDS incidence and morbidity in children.[70,71] Nevertheless, symptomatic HIV-1 infection, including serious bacterial infections, still remains an important problem despite HAART accessibility and usage.[72] Increased cases of pneumonia in children without severe immunodeficiency at illness onset have been reported.[73] Other reports show an ongoing risk of opportunistic infections in patients who are immune reconstituted during HAART, despite a normal CD4+ T-lymphocyte count.[65,74] A functional immunologic defect, rather than a numeric reduction in CD4+ T-lymphocyte count, has been postulated to be responsible for the high risk of severe bacterial infections, including pneumonia, at least in a subset of individuals.[73]

The immune reconstitution inflammatory syndrome (IRIS) is one of the most important reasons for new or recurrent opportunistic conditions, despite achieving virologic suppression and immunologic restoration/preservation within the first months of antiretroviral treatment. This does not represent ART failure and does not generally require discontinuation of antiretroviral treatment.[64] Further, children who have injury to their lungs, brain, or other organs during prolonged and profound pretreatment immunosuppression may continue to have recurrent infections or symptoms, because the damage may not be reversed by immunologic improvement.[75]

In adults, however, the prevalence of weight loss and wasting has not changed as expected after HAART became available.[76,77] Both weight loss and wasting were found to occur in those treated successfully with HAART, those for whom HAART failed, and those who were HAART naïve.[78] The etiology of HIV-associated wasting in the HAART era continues to be multifactorial, and causes may include low socioeconomic status, poor access to care, family cultural practices, psychological factors, and medical complications of and therapies for HIV infection. Decreased nutrient intake (associated with low socioeconomic or medical factors) and altered nutrient metabolism and gastrointestinal tract dysfunction remain common in adults with HIV infection.[78]

Psychosocial Factors

Psychosocial factors are important contributors to suboptimal growth of HIV-infected children. An unstable home environment and inadequate emotional and social support may affect growth in both HIV-infected[79] and uninfected children.[80,81] Children with HIV infection are at risk of living with parents who are ill, who have limited access to social services and support, who may not be able to use food appropriately, and who may have ongoing problems with drug and substance abuse[82] and/or psychiatric illness.[83] Maternal crack and cocaine use during pregnancy can be a predictor of growth and nutritional problems for the child.[26,27] This

VI

finding is not unique for HIV, as it has been reported in other uninfected cohorts with parents who use drugs.[84] Children born to drug-using women are often small, suggesting that drugs have an effect prenatally, but the postnatal home environment is likely to influence growth as well. Studies have also determined that home care providers can both positively or negatively influence functional status of HIV-infected children.[79]

Food insufficiency is a pervasive problem in the United States, and it is most prevalent among children and younger adults.[85] Food security or sufficiency and nutrition are interlinked with HIV.[86] There is a strong association between poverty, in particular food insufficiency and hunger, with HIV treatment adherence, among socially disadvantaged people living with HIV/AIDS in the United States.[11] However, food insecurity has also been linked to high rates of obesity.[87]

Appetite Suppressant Effect of Attention-Deficit/Hyperactivity Disorder Medications

Although youths perinatally infected with HIV do not appear to be at greater risk of mental health problems than peers from similar community and home environments,[88] attention-deficit/hyperactivity disorder (ADHD) is the most commonly reported neuropsychiatric disorder in infected children.[88,89] Psychopharmacologic treatments for ADHD include stimulants and nonstimulants, atomoxetine, or methylphenidate.

Although these medications are generally well tolerated, decreased appetite[90,91] and growth attenuation[92] have been reported as one of their leading adverse effects in children. Stimulants exert a subtle, adverse influence on weight gain,[93-95] whereas nonstimulants are associated with significantly increased risks for growth delays in both height and weight beyond those attributable to HIV alone.[95] For children with comorbid HIV and ADHD, the use of stimulants to treat ADHD may exacerbate the risk of growth failure related to HIV and should be used with caution.[95]

Obesity and Cardiometabolic Disease

Obesity is an emerging health problem among adolescents[53] and adults living with HIV/AIDS.[96-99] With the institution of HAART, HIV-infected children can improve their immunologic and disease status, and their eating patterns often become similar to those in healthy children.[52] Poverty and food insecurity are among other factors that can contribute to childhood obesity that influence both HIV-infected and noninfected populations equally.[87] Immigrant families are particularly vulnerable.[100] As the prevalence of obesity increases among patients with HIV/AIDS, the cumulative risk for cardiovascular disease also increases.[101-105]

Lipodystrophy – Fat Redistribution

Coincident with the introduction of HAART, a clinical syndrome of body fat redistribution and metabolic changes was first described initially in adults[106] but is now commonly reported among children.[107-110] HIV-infected patients receiving HAART regimens have developed a syndrome of peripheral insulin resistance, hyperlipidemia, and lipodystrophy (truncal obesity, dorsocervical fat pad, and extremity and facial wasting).[106] Clinical and biochemical abnormalities associated with the lipodystrophy syndrome are shown in Table 40.6. Risk factors associated with developing the fat redistribution syndrome in adults include female gender, increasing age, family history of premature cardiovascular disease, higher pretherapy body weight, and behavioral patterns such as tobacco and alcohol use.[104] Complications associated with the fat redistribution syndrome include higher rates of diabetes mellitus and premature cardiovascular disease.[111] Medical compliance with drug therapy may be poorer because of the cosmetic adverse effects of therapy.

Table 40.6.
Clinical and Biochemical Abnormalities of the Lipodystrophy Syndrome

Clinical Features	Laboratory Features

Increased abdominal (visceral) fat
  Increased waist-to-hip ratio (more reliable in adults)
Buffalo hump
Fat atrophy
  Wasting of extremities
  Wasting of buttocks
  Loss or thinning of facial fat, prominence of
  nasolabial fold
No change to increased weight
Fatigue and weakness
	Hyperlipidemia
	  Increased triglycerides
	  Increased total cholesterol
	  Increased LDL-C
	  Decreased HDL-C
	Insulin resistance
	  Normal to increased serum glucose
	  Increased insulin
	  Increased C peptide

LDL-C indicates low-density lipoprotein cholesterol; HDL-C, high-density lipoprotein cholesterol.

Lipodystrophy is described in children as well.[13,110] Early studies in children showed that protease inhibitor therapy improved weight, weight-for-height, and mid-arm muscle circumference of HIV-infected children, independent of the concurrent decrease in HIV viral load and improved CD4+ T-lymphocyte counts.[112] The immediate treatment effects were most apparent with an improvement in weight and mid-arm muscle circumference, and there was a trend toward increased height and lean body mass. A recent study in Kenya revealed that early initiation of HAART was associated with more rapid restoration of growth.[67] In addition to the positive improvement in growth and lean body mass, however, HAART is also associated with abnormalities in fat distribution in children, although some studies report similar lean mass in HIV-infected and uninfected children.[108,113] Arpadi et al observed similar total fat, trunk fat, and percent total fat between HIV-infected and uninfected children but lower leg and higher arm fat in HIV-infected children.[114] In another study, there was decreased limb/trunk fat ratios in HIV-infected children receiving HAART when compared with healthy controls.[108] These findings suggest that both peripheral lipoatrophy, as well as central obesity, occur in these children. Further studies have shown that a majority of children develop fat redistribution within 3 years of initiating a protease inhibitor-containing regimen and that these changes progress over time.[109] Other studies have identified metabolic abnormalities induced by other specific classes of drugs. Stavudine use has been associated with lipoatrophy,[115,116] potentially by altering mitochondrial number and function.[117]

Cardiometabolic Risk

Atherosclerotic cardiovascular disease (CVD) is a leading comorbidity and cause of mortality among HIV-infected adults.[118] Several studies show that HIV-infected children, compared with healthy peers, have higher rates of CVD risk factors, including dyslipidemia, insulin resistance, obesity, and central adiposity.[101,114,119,120] HIV infection also results in prolonged chronic inflammation, thereby increasing CVD risk. In adults with HAART-related fat redistribution, several studies have suggested an increase in the risk of myocardial infarction relating to the level of viral control (increased inflammation) or to ARV exposures (including protease inhibitors and certain nucleoside reverse-transcriptase inhibitors [NRTIs]).[121-123] Exogenous obesity, common among perinatally HIV-infected youth, can also contribute to CVD risk.[124,125] Children with HIV, compared with adults with HIV, may be at even greater risk of developing premature cardiovascular disease as the lifetime exposures to factors associated with CVD risk are longer in children.

Dyslipidemia

Prior to the introduction of ART, elevated triglyceride and low-density lipoprotein (LDL) concentrations were reported and associated with HIV infection. These changes point to the effect of chronic immune activation alone on lipid metabolism. One mechanism that has been suggested includes the effect of proinflammatory cytokines (as a response to the chronic viral infection) on lipid pathways (such as lipoprotein lipase activity). After the initiation of protease inhibitor (PI) therapy, several investigators in the United States and other countries[126,127] reported a 20% to 50% rise in serum lipid concentrations of HIV-infected children. Lipid concentrations before, compared with post-PI therapy, increased but stabilized in one study.[128] However, in another study, cholesterol concentrations increased 6 months after initiation of PI-based therapy and continued to increase through the second year.[129] Other factors associated with hyperlipidemia include successful viral suppression, better CD4+ T-lymphocyte counts, and demographic factors.[130] The impact of PIs on lipid concentrations, independent of HIV, is effectively described in HIV-seronegative volunteers who developed dyslipidemia following PI treatment. Other antiretroviral agents are also associated with dyslipidemia.[131]

Insulin Resistance and Type 2 Diabetes Mellitus

Abnormal glucose homeostasis was documented in HIV-infected adults with lipodystrophy well before it was reported in children. However, insulin resistance is of particular concern in both HIV-infected children and adolescents who naturally experience a relative insulin resistance in puberty. Some studies report no difference in fasting insulin and glucose levels in children treated with PIs compared with children treated with other drugs.[132] However insulin levels become elevated across both groups after initiating HAART. Bitnun[133] surveyed several pediatric HIV cohorts and found insulin resistance with full metabolic syndrome increasingly prevalent. These symptoms slowly increased in severity with increasing age. Verkauskiene et al[134] found significantly higher fasting insulin levels in HIV-infected children with some aspect of lipodystrophy than those without.

The etiology of insulin resistance is multifactorial and has been linked with both PI and nucleoside/nonnucleoside reverse transcriptase inhibitor (NRTI/NNRTI) use singly and in combination. Exact mechanisms have not been well defined. A study by Beregszaszi et al demonstrated that insulin resistance occurs at the level of the adipose tissue and that children with lipodystrophy have more pronounced insulin resistance than those without, suggesting that metabolic changes occur as a result of the central adiposity.[135] A possible mechanism by which HAART causes insulin resistance is by direct inhibition of the transport function of the GLUT4 glucose transporter, which is responsible for insulin-stimulated glucose uptake into muscle and fat.[136] Other potential causes of insulin resistance include mitochondrial DNA (mtDNA) mutations or depletions associated with NRTI or NNRTI therapy. Although there are limited data in adults,[117,137,138] there are striking similarities between rare mitochondrial disorders, such as multiple symmetrical lipomatosis, a condition that is phenotypically very similar to HAART-associated lipodystrophy.[139] These mtDNA mutations in multiple symmetrical lipomatosis lead to impaired function of cytochrome c oxidase and a subsequent decrease in fat turnover.

Inflammatory cytokines have been linked to insulin resistance and diminished adiponectin, which affects insulin signaling and glucose homeostasis. Adipose tissue is a major determinant of insulin sensitivity, and changes associated with lipodystrophy can alter the secretion of adiponectin. Kim et al reported that patients with PI-induced lipodystrophy had increased levels of circulating inflammatory cytokines.[140] Among 18 children with lipohypertrophy, increased fasting insulin/glucose ratios were associated with decreased adiponectin even after adjustment for pubertal stage, age, and percent body fat and serum lipid concentrations.[134] A separate study of children on PI-based treatment observed reduced insulin sensitivity and impaired β-cell response.[119] Although there are fewer studies in children compared with

VI

adults, the elevated risk of diabetes mellitus in HIV-infected children on HAART is becoming increasingly clear.

Vascular Inflammation

Vascular endothelial dysfunction, a process that is associated with atherosclerosis, may occur as a result of chronic inflammation and injury in the endothelium and, in HIV infection specifically, may result from oxidative stress attributable to HAART or direct cytopathic effect of the virus.[141] In addition, dyslipidemia, insulin resistance, and chronic inflammation attributable to ongoing immune activation in HIV-infected individuals also contribute to endothelial damage. Levels of proinflammatory cytokines are higher in HIV-infected children compared with contemporary controls.[142] These vascular inflammatory biomarkers are positively correlated with higher viral load, lipids, and waist circumference.[142] These associations are similar to what is found in HIV-infected adults.[143] Furthermore, Wolf et al found that not only were levels of vascular cell adhesion molecule-1 (VCAM-1), intercellular adhesion molecule-1 (ICAM-1), and von Willebrand factor higher in untreated patients with HIV infection but also that they decreased significantly after treatment with a regimen containing either one PI or one NNRTI.[144] The extent to which these vascular inflammatory biomarkers are associated with structural evidence of atherosclerosis is unclear.

Evidence of Structural and Functional Atherosclerotic Lesions

Atherosclerotic cardiovascular risk can also be defined by several methods, including carotid intima-media thickness (cIMT) and brachial artery reactivity (or flow-mediated vasodilation). Some studies showed vascular stiffness (through flow-mediated dilation studies) and cIMT were greater in HIV-infected children than in controls,[145-147] with differences independent of known CVD risk factors and ART,[147] but others showed an association with ART, especially PIs.[145,146,148] Longitudinal follow-up in one study revealed cIMT was similar in HIV-infected children and controls.[149] Interestingly, some pre-HAART studies in children showed increased coronary artery calcifications,[150] suggesting the contribution of baseline immune activation to CVD risk.

Disorders of Bone Mineralization

Bone health must be considered when addressing the nutritional needs of HIV-infected children. Chronic inflammatory conditions like HIV infection predispose children to changes in bone metabolism, putting them at risk of low bone mineral density as they grow into adulthood. Evaluating bone density in childhood and adolescence in vulnerable populations such as HIV-infected children is important, because this time in development is critical for optimal bone mineralization for adulthood. Several studies have shown that bone mineral density of HIV-infected children are lower than national standards and compared with contemporary and socioeconomically matched cohorts.[151-154] Risk factors associated with lower bone mineral density include longer duration of HIV disease, low body mass index (BMI), history of weight loss, and previous use of steroids. Tenofovir and other antiretroviral therapies have also emerged as specific concerns for loss of bone mineral density in HIV-infected children.[155-158] Thus, baseline bone assessments are recommended (typically evaluated with dual x-ray absorptiometry), with periodic follow-up. Calcium and vitamin D intake should be optimized with supplements if necessary.

Nutritional Assessment and Interventions

Assessment

A complete baseline nutrition assessment should be performed on all patients regardless of symptoms as part of the multidisciplinary care plan, with regular follow-up care, as appropriate, to achieve care plan goals. For optimal care, it is recommended that a registered dietitian perform the nutrition evaluation and follow-up.[159]

This assessment should include a review of the medical and dietary history, nutrient analysis of usual intake, anthropometric measurements (ie, weight, height, BMI, head circumference [younger than 3 years], arm muscle circumferences, skin folds [4-sites]), and measurement of baseline biochemical values (eg, complete blood cell count, albumin, transthyretin, iron, zinc, lipid profile, and absorptive tests as indicated). When inadequate weight gain or weight loss is identified, aggressive diagnostic evaluation should be pursued to detect opportunistic infections or other inflammatory lesions of the gastrointestinal tract. With clinical symptoms, an evaluation of gastrointestinal tract absorption is indicated. Treatment of underlying infections will likely improve the response to nutritional and medical management. Determining the degree and extent of gastrointestinal tract malabsorption will help guide dietary recommendations. All HIV-infected children and adolescents should be monitored at regular intervals for metabolic problems. With clinically evident fat redistribution syndrome, a fasting serum glucose and insulin concentration should be obtained, and a homeostatic model assessment-insulin resistance (HOMA-IR) score (as a marker of insulin resistance) can be calculated as fasting insulin (U/mL) $\times$ fasting glucose (mmol/L)/22.5.[160] If abnormal, an oral glucose tolerance test, hemoglobin A_1C, and C-peptide levels should be measured. If these studies are abnormal, dietary and exercise advice and an oral hypoglycemic agent should be considered.

VI

Interventions

The approach to nutrition and nutritional interventions for HIV-infected children and adolescents are summarized in Table 40.7. Multiple strategies to improve nutritional outcomes exist, including ART, treatment of coinfections, nutritional counseling, pharmacologic agents to stimulate appetite or anabolism, and nutritional supplements. For the delay and prevention of the metabolic syndrome, emphasis should be placed on modifiable lifestyle factors.[161] Frequent nutritional assessment is necessary to determine the response to the nutritional intervention.

Table 40.7.
Nutrition Interventions for HIV-infected Children

Healthy Living With HIV
• Combination of antiretroviral drug therapy, adequate dietary intake, and frequent exercise
• Nutrition education and counseling
• Promote healthy eating habits
• Promote normal growth and development
• Self-monitoring dietary intake and weight changes
• Fad diets, including megavitamins and amino acid supplementation, should be discouraged
• Psychosocial assessment and appropriate referrals
Poor Growth, Unintentional Weight Loss, and Lean Tissue Wasting
• Careful monitoring of dietary intake and change in weight and body composition
• Assess food and nutrition security issues and provide appropriate counseling and referrals
• Increase calories and protein
• Infants: may benefit from increased caloric density of a formula by adding cereal or modular nutrient supplements (eg, glucose polymers, protein powders, medium chain triglycerides if needed and vegetable oils) or by concentrating the caloric density of the formula
• Appetite stimulants may be useful in selected patients (megestrol acetate should not be used in children who have documented insulin resistance, because this therapy may exacerbate it)
• Oral nutritional supplements are preferable
• Tube feeding: if normal food intake and optimal use of oral nutrition supplements cannot achieve sufficient energy supply
• Appropriate diagnostic studies to treat an underlying gastrointestinal disorder that results in inadequate intake should be performed prior to initiating supplemental enteral feedings
• Parenteral nutrition: should be used only in patients who are not able to feed enterally
• Multivitamin/mineral supplementation at DRI levels
Micronutrient deficiency
• Multivitamin/mineral supplementation at DRI levels
• Monitor intake of key nutrients(iron, zinc, calcium, and vitamins A and D)
• Drug-nutrient interactions should be considered
Management of symptoms that may affect nutritional status
• Dietary composition adjusted according to the degree of gastrointestinal tract dysfunction
• Nausea, vomiting: small, frequent meals; nutrient-dense beverages between meals
• Anorexia: increase nutrient density of foods; small, frequent meals; appetite stimulants
• Taste change: use stronger seasonings, avoid excessively sweet foods, offer salty foods

Diarrhea or malabsorption
- Small, frequent feedings
- Dietary composition adjusted according to the degree of gastrointestinal tract dysfunction
- Identify and manage lactose intolerance
- Semi elemental or elemental formula

Overweight/obesity and increased cardiovascular risk
- Metabolic complications of HAART should be carefully evaluated and monitored
- Promote weight loss if overweight or obese through modifications in diet and activity level
- Heart-healthy diet: reduced intake of saturated-fat, trans-fatty acids, and dietary cholesterol
- Increased fiber intake and limit simple carbohydrates
- Regular exercise: physical activity counseling or physical activity program participation
- Increase consumption of omega-3 fatty acids rich foods, such as fish (especially fatty fish such as salmon); plant sources, such as flaxseed and flaxseed oil; canola oil; soybean oil; and nuts

Loss of bone mineral density, osteopenia
- Adequate calcium and vitamin D intake
- Lactose-free dairy products for lactose-intolerant individuals
- Supplement calcium and vitamin D intakes to DRI levels for age if suboptimal intake
- Regular weight-bearing exercise
- Decrease high-phosphorous carbonated beverages intake

DRI indicates Dietary Reference Intake.

Adapted from recommendations from the Academy of Nutrition and Dietetics, American Society for Parenteral and Enteral Nutrition, European Society of Parenteral and Enteral Nutrition, and American Heart Association.[159,162,197,198]

The diet plan for infants and children with HIV/AIDS should be individualized on the basis of symptoms and ability to meet nutrient requirements. Adequacy can be assessed with food records and by frequent monitoring of growth patterns and nutrition assessment parameters. Dietary interventions for macronutrients and micronutrients according to disease stage and clinical condition are summarized in Table 40.8.

A nutrition support team should be involved to ensure optimal nutrition monitoring and care. A core team of physician, nurse-specialist, nutritionist, and social worker collaborating with other health care providers offers the best opportunity to achieve optimal nutritional health for individual patients.

Nutritional Interventions for Cardiometabolic Disease

The long-term concerns of the metabolic changes that occur with HAART are the potential cardiac implications of hyperlipidemia, insulin resistance, and obesity. Long-term evaluations in children are needed to determine the effects of HIV and its treatments on similar outcomes. There are currently no guidelines for therapeutic intervention in HIV-infected children with lipid abnormalities and insulin resistance. However, interventions should follow those recommended for non-HIV-infected children.[162-164] Therapeutic strategies to diminish the clinical and

Table 40.8.

Macronutrient and Micronutrient Needs in Pediatric HIV Infection

Nutrient	HIV Infection Factors— Clinical Situations	Recommendation/Nutrition Intervention
Energy	When secondary infections are absent and growth is adequate	Standard methods of assessing energy needs: calorie levels based on the estimated energy requirements (EER) and activity levels from the Institute of Medicine Dietary Reference Intakes (DRI) Macronutrients Report, 2002
	During illness	Stress factors Energy requirements can increase by up to 20% to 30% during infections and recovery[54]; factors that affect energy requirements include stage of disease, opportunistic infections and comorbidities, inflammation, fever, malabsorption, diarrhea, and vomiting
	Recovery phase	Catch-up growth Use equations for estimating catch-up growth requirements for both calories and protein
	Advanced disease	Up to 50% to 100% additional energy to recover and regain weight; this is best achieved through enteral or parenteral (if enteral has failed) feeding
	Overweight or obesity	Weight management: Counseling on changing eating habits and patterns Regular exercise: physical activity counseling or physical activity program participation
Protein	During periods of well-being	Acceptable macronutrient distribution ranges (AMDRs)[a] can be used to ensure sufficient intakes of essential nutrients[199]
	Period of catch-up growth	Use equation for estimating catch-up growth requirements
Fat	During periods of well-being	Provide anticipatory guidance regarding the importance of a low-fat, low-saturated fat, low-cholesterol diet for all otherwise healthy HIV-infected patients older than 2 years and their families AMDR[199]. 1-3 years: 30%-40% of total calories 4-18 years: 25%-35% of total calories
	Fat malabsorption occurs in some cases of GI enteropathy attributable to HIV or secondary infections Chronic fat malabsorption	In these cases, dietary modification of fat may be required. Supplemental medium-chain triglyceride (MCTs) and enteral formulas containing MCTs can be used to supplement caloric intake Supplementation of fat-soluble vitamins is indicated.

	Dyslipidemia	Counseling on changing eating habits and patterns per American Heart Association/American Academy of Pediatrics
Carbo-hydrate	During periods of well-being	AMDR[199]: 45%-65% of total calories Added sugars should comprise no more than 10% of total calories consumed
Fiber		A reasonable intake is 0.5 g/kg/day to a maximum of 35 g daily
Fluid	The fluid needs of individuals with HIV-infection are similar to those of their peers in their age group, although special clinical circumstances (cardiac disease, renal disease, gastrointestinal symptoms) may alter fluid requirements.	Weight: 0-10 kg: 100 mL/kg 10-20 kg: 1000 mL + 50 mL/kg over 10 kg >20 kg: 1500 mL + 20 mL/kg over 20 kg
Vitamins and minerals	Micronutrient deficiencies, as a result of acute or chronic inflammation, persist in the HAART era	Micronutrient intakes at recommended levels (DRI) need to be assured in HIV-infected children Varied diets, fortified foods, and micronutrient supplements when adequate intakes cannot be guaranteed through regular foods.
	Overall intake less than optimal	Multivitamin/mineral supplementation
Calcium and vitamin D	HIV-infected children are at increased risk for low bone mineral density Low bone mineral density	Optimize intake of calcium and vitamin D Multivitamin use has been associated with better bone mineral density[153] Supplement calcium and vitamin D if inadequate diet Calcium/vitamin D supplementation
Iron	HIV-infected children can become anemic because of a variety of nonnutritional conditions (medications, chronic illness)	Anemia should be evaluated to determine the role of nutrition intervention in treatment, such as dietary iron and supplementation of folate cr vitamin B-12

[a] AMDR is the range of intake for a particular energy source that is associated with reduced risk of chronic disease while providing intakes of essential nutrients.

VI

biochemical features of the fat redistribution syndrome in adults include oral hypoglycemic agents such as metformin[165] and troglitazone (although liver toxicity limits its use).[166] These agents have not been used extensively in children, and large-scale studies evaluating their use are not yet available. Medications to lower serum cholesterol also need to be studied in children; however, caution should be exercised in prescribing lipid-lowering medications, as there may be potential interactions between these medications and the antiretroviral medications.[167] It is clear, however, that interventions such as exercise and diet control can be useful[168,169] and, at this time, should be the primary focus in children with metabolic changes.

Nutrition in HIV-Exposed, Uninfected Children

Preventive strategies implemented during pregnancy have dramatically reduced the risk of mother-to-child transmission (MTCT) of HIV in the United States and other resource-rich countries.[1,70,170] Current preventive MTCT recommendations include ART for all HIV-infected pregnant women regardless of CD4+ T-lymphocyte count or HIV level. ARTs suppress HIV replication in the mother and provide direct prophylaxis to the infant in utero and postpartum. All recommended ART regimens to prevent MTCT include zidovudine (ZDV), an NRTI.

Despite the clear successes of the perinatal HIV prevention programs in reducing transmission rates, concern remains regarding possible adverse consequences of prenatal exposure, given that many ARTs readily cross the placenta and inhibit DNA polymerase-gamma, potentially interfering with fetal mtDNA synthesis and resulting in short- and long-term mitochondrial depletion and/or dysfunction.[171-174] The evidence regarding mitochondrial toxicity in HIV-exposed and ART-exposed children remains equivocal; some studies report no associations between mitochondrial dysfunction with perinatal ARV exposure in uninfected infants.[175,176]

Prospective comparative evaluations have shown that there are no major differences in growth among uninfected children who are born to HIV-infected women and children in the general population throughout the first years of life.[176-178] Ross et al found no difference in growth between 88 exposed children and 174 healthy controls in the United Kingdom from birth to 3 years of age.[179] The Pediatric AIDS Clinical Trials Group (PACTG) Protocol 219/076 compared growth of uninfected children receiving zidovudine or placebo, and they did not observe differences between the groups.[176] A large prospective European study investigating growth pattern of HIV-infected and uninfected children in the first 10 years of life in comparison with general British standards reported no substantial differences between the uninfected children and a reference group.[178] The European Collaborative Study[177] confirmed a lack of association between zidovudine monotherapy exposure and growth in uninfected children up to 18 months of age. However, these studies did not compare the HIV-exposed group to a socioeconomically similar group of children.

Infants and children who are exposed to HIV and ART in utero should continue to be followed for growth and nutritional abnormalities because of the aforementioned nutritional effects of these medications and the virus for children with HIV infection. These children have been exposed to factors that can alter growth in one of the most vulnerable periods of development. These children also have the greatest potential to be lost within the medical system because of the social stigma attached to HIV exposure as well as the early loss of parents and family members to HIV itself. Care should be taken to continue to track these children for growth and metabolic abnormalities as they growth through childhood and adolescence.

Conclusion

The cause of nutritional problems in children with HIV infection is complex and likely multifactorial. Although the incidence of malnutrition HIV-infected children in resource-rich countries has decreased with ART, a significant number of children continue to have problems with malnutrition and gastrointestinal tract dysfunction in the HAART era. However, greater numbers of children with HIV infection, who now have better viral suppression because of effective HIV therapies, are suffering from increasing rates of obesity, lipodystrophy, hyperlipidemia, and prediabetic and diabetic conditions and are at risk of sequelae associated with these problems. Optimal nutritional support includes complete nutritional assessment and follow-up of every child and adolescent with HIV/AIDS as well as close surveillance of children who were exposed to HIV in utero. The long-term metabolic and cardiovascular complications of HAART will shape the nutritional issues in HIV-infected children in the future.

References

1. Joint United Nations Programme on HIV/AIDS. *Global Report: Report on the Global AIDS Epidemic 2010*. Geneva, Switzerland: UNAIDS; 2010. Available at: http://www.unaids. org/en/media/unaids/contentassets/documents/unaidspublication/2010/20101123_ globalreport_en.pdf. Accessed January 3, 2013

2. Chandra RK, Kumari S. Nutrition and immunity: an overview. *J Nutr*. 1994;124(8 Suppl):1433S-1435S

3. Prendergast A, Tudor-Williams G, Jeena P, Burchett S, Goulder P. International perspectives, progress, and future challenges of paediatric HIV infection. *Lancet*. 2007;370(9581):68-80

VI

4. Cunningham-Rundles S, McNeeley DF, Moon A. Mechanisms of nutrient modulation of the immune response. *J Allergy Clin Immunol.* 2005;115(6):1119-1128

5. Majaliwa ES, Munubhi E, Ramaiya K, et al. Survey on acute and chronic complications in children and adolescents with type 1 diabetes at Muhimbili National Hospital in Dar es Salaam, Tanzania. *Diabetes Care.* 2007;30(9):2187-2192

6. Semba RD. Vitamin A and immunity to viral, bacterial and protozoan infections. *Proc Nutr Soc.* 1999;58(3):719-727

7. Mahlungulu S, Grobler LA, Visser ME, Volmink J. Nutritional interventions for reducing morbidity and mortality in people with HIV. *Cochrane Database Syst Rev.* 2007;(3):CD004536

8. Golin CE, Liu H, Hays RD, et al. A prospective study of predictors of adherence to combination antiretroviral medication. *J Gen Intern Med.* 2002;17(10):756-765

9. Arnsten JH, Demas PA, Grant RW, et al. Impact of active drug use on antiretroviral therapy adherence and viral suppression in HIV-infected drug users. *J Gen Intern Med.* 2002;17(5):377-381

10. Applebaum AJ, Reilly LC, Gonzalez JS, Richardson MA, Leveroni CL, Safren SA. The impact of neuropsychological functioning on adherence to HAART in HIV-infected substance abuse patients. *AIDS Patient Care STDS.* 2009;23(6):455-462

11. Kalichman SC, Grebler T. Stress and poverty predictors of treatment adherence among people with low-literacy living with HIV/AIDS. *Psychosom Med.* 2010;72(8):810-816

12. Batterham M, Brown D. Nutritional management of HIV/AIDS in the era of highly active antiretroviral therapy: a review. *Aust J Nutr Diet.* 2001;58(4):211-223

13. Desai N, Mullen P, Mathur M. Lipodystrophy in pediatric HIV. *Indian J Pediatr.* 2008;75:351-4.

14. Power R, Tate HL, McGill SM, Taylor C. A qualitative study of the psychosocial implications of lipodystrophy syndrome on HIV positive individuals. *Sex Transm Infect.* 2003;79(2):137-141

15. Delaugerre C, Chaix ML, Blanche S, et al. Perinatal acquisition of drug-resistant HIV-1 infection: mechanisms and long-term outcome. *Retrovirology.* 2009;6:85

16. Miller TL, McQuinn LB, Orav EJ. Endoscopy of the upper gastrointestinal tract as a diagnostic tool for children with human immunodeficiency virus infection. *J Pediatr.* 1997;130(5):766-773

17. Kotler DP, Reka S, Orenstein JM, Fox CH. Chronic idiopathic esophageal ulceration in the acquired immunodeficiency syndrome. Characterization and treatment with corticosteroids. *J Clin Gastroenterol.* 1992;15(4):284-290

18. National Institutes of Health, Health Resources and Services Administration, Working Group on Antiretroviral Therapy and Medical Management of HIV-Infected Children. *Guidelines for the Use of Antiretroviral Agents in Pediatric HIV Infection.* Rockville, MD: AIDSInfo; 2005. Available at: http://aidsinfo.nih.gov/contentfiles/PediatricGuidelines03242005016.pdf. Accessed January 3, 2013

19. Smith PD, Meng G, Salazar-Gonzalez JF, Shaw GM. Macrophage HIV-1 infection and the gastrointestinal tract reservoir. *J Leukoc Biol.* 2003;74(5):642-649

20. Meng G, Sellers MT, Mosteller-Barnum M, Rogers TS, Shaw GM, Smith PD. Lamina propria lymphocytes, not macrophages, express CCR5 and CXCR4 and are the likely target cell for human immunodeficiency virus type 1 in the intestinal mucosa. *J Infect Dis*. 2000;182(3):785-791

21. McDonald D, Wu L, Bohks SM, KewalRamani VN, Unutmaz D, Hope TJ. Recruitment of HIV and its receptors to dendritic cell-T cell junctions. *Science*. 2003;300(5623):1295-1297

22. Brenchley JM, Price DA, Schacker TW, et al. Microbial translocation is a cause of systemic immune activation in chronic HIV infection. *Nat Med*. 2006;12(12):1365-1371

23. Douek D. HIV disease progression: immune activation, microbes, and a leaky gut. *Top HIV Med*. 2007;15(4):114-117

24. Tardieu M, Le Chenadec J, Persoz A, Meyer L, Blanche S, Mayaux MJ. HIV-1-related encephalopathy in infants compared with children and adults. French Pediatric HIV Infection Study and the SEROCO Group. *Neurology*. 2000;54(5):1089-1095

25. Chiriboga CA, Fleishman S, Champion S, Gaye-Robinson L, Abrams EJ. Incidence and prevalence of HIV encephalopathy in children with HIV infection receiving highly active anti-retroviral therapy (HAART). *J Pediatr*. 2005;146(3):402-407

26. Moye J Jr, Rich KC, Kalish LA, et al. Natural history of somatic growth in infants born to women infected by human immunodeficiency virus. Women and Infants Transmission Study Group. *J Pediatr*. 1996;128(1):58-69

27. Miller TL, Easley KA, Zhang W, et al. Maternal and infant factors associated with failure to thrive in children with vertically transmitted human immunodeficiency virus-1 infection: the prospective, P2C2 human immunodeficiency virus multicenter study. *Pediatrics*. 2001;108(6):1287-1296

28. Miller TL, Evans SJ, Orav EJ, Morris V, McIntosh K, Winter HS. Growth and body composition in children infected with the human immunodeficiency virus-1. *Am J Clin Nutr*. 1993;57(4):588-592

29. Arpadi SM, Horlick MN, Wang J, Cuff P, Bamji M, Kotler DP. Body composition in prepubertal children with human immunodeficiency virus type 1 infection. *Arch Pediatr Adolesc Med*. 1998;152(7):688-693

30. Saavedra JM, Henderson RA, Perman JA, Hutton N, Livingston RA, Yolken RH. Longitudinal assessment of growth in children born to mothers with human immunodeficiency virus infection. *Arch Pediatr Adolesc Med*. 1995;149(5):497-502

31. McKinney RE Jr, Robertson JW. Effect of human immunodeficiency virus infection on the growth of young children. Duke Pediatric AIDS Clinical Trials Unit. *J Pediatr*. 1993;123(4):579-582

32. Dorenbaum A. Report of results of PACTG 316: an international phase III trial of standard antiretroviral (ARV) prophylaxis plus nevirapine (NVP) for prevention of perinatal HIV transmission [abstr]. Presented at: 8th Conference on Retroviruses and Opportunistic Infections; February 4-8, 2001; Chicago, IL

33. European Mode of Delivery Collaboration. Elective caesarean-section versus vaginal delivery in prevention of vertical HIV-1 transmission: a randomised clinical trial. *Lancet*. 1999;353(9158):1035-1039

VI

34. Mulligan K, Tai VW, Schambelan M. Cross-sectional and longitudinal evaluation of body composition in men with HIV infection. *J Acquir Immune Defic Syndr Hum Retrovirol.* 1997;15(1):43-48

35. Kotler DP, Wang J, Pierson RN. Body composition studies in patients with the acquired immunodeficiency syndrome. *Am J Clin Nutr.* 1985;42(6):1255-1265

36. de Martino M, Galli L, Chiarelli F, et al. Interleukin-6 release by cultured peripheral blood mononuclear cells inversely correlates with height velocity, bone age, insulin-like growth factor-I, and insulin-like growth factor binding protein-3 serum levels in children with perinatal HIV-1 infection. *Clin Immunol.* 2000;94(3):212-218

37. Resino S, Galan I, Perez A, et al. HIV-infected children with moderate/severe immune-suppression: changes in the immune system after highly active antiretroviral therapy. *Clin Exp Immunol.* 2004;137(3):570-577

38. Garza C. Effect of infection on energy requirements of infants and children. *Public Health Nutr.* 2005;8(7A):1187-1190

39. Alfaro MP, Siegel RM, Baker RC, Heubi JE. Resting energy expenditure and body composition in pediatric HIV infection. *Pediatr AIDS HIV Infect.* 1995;6(5):276-280

40. Arpadi SM, Cuff PA, Kotler DP, et al. Growth velocity, fat-free mass and energy intake are inversely related to viral load in HIV-infected children. *J Nutr.* 2000;130:2498-2502

41. Miller TL, Evans SE, Vasquez I, Orav EJ. Dietary intake is an important predictor of nutritional status in HIV-infected children [abstr]. *Pediatr Res.* 1997;41:85A

42. Johann-Liang R, O'Neill L, Cervia J, et al. Energy balance, viral burden, insulin-like growth factor-1, interleukin-6 and growth impairment in children infected with human immunodeficiency virus. *AIDS.* 2000;14(6):683-690

43. Melchior JC, Raguin G, Boulier A, et al. Resting energy expenditure in human immunodeficiency virus-infected patients: comparison between patients with and without secondary infections. *Am J Clin Nutr.* 1993;57(5):614-619

44. Grunfeld C, Pang M, Shimizu L, Shigenaga JK, Jensen P, Feingold KR. Resting energy expenditure, caloric intake, and short-term weight change in human immunodeficiency virus infection and the acquired immunodeficiency syndrome. *Am J Clin Nutr.* 1992;55(2):455-460

45. Hommes MJ, Romijn JA, Godfried MH, et al. Increased resting energy expenditure in human immunodeficiency virus-infected men. *Metabolism.* 1990;39(11):1186-1190

46. Hardin DS, Ellis KJ, Rice J, Doyle ME. Protease inhibitor therapy improves protein catabolism in prepubertal children with HIV infection. *J Pediatr Endocrinol Metab.* 2004;17(3):321-325

47. Morley JE, Thomas DR, Wilson MM. Cachexia: pathophysiology and clinical relevance. *Am J Clin Nutr.* 2006;83(4):735-743

48. Baronzio G, Zambelli A, Comi D, et al. Proinflammatory and regulatory cytokine levels in AIDS cachexia. *In Vivo.* 1999;13(6):499-502

49. Beutler B, Milsark IW, Cerami AC. Passive immunization against cachectin/tumor necrosis factor protects mice from lethal effect of endotoxin. *Science.* 1985;229(4716):869-871

50. Langhans W. Bacterial products and the control of ingestive behavior: clinical implications. *Nutrition*. 1996;12(5):303-315

51. Henderson RA, Talusan K, Hutton N, Yolken RH, Caballero B. Resting energy expenditure and body composition in children with HIV infection. *J Acquir Immune Defic Syndr Hum Retrovirol*. 1998;19(2):150-157

52. Sharma TS, Kinnamon DD, Duggan C, et al. Changes in macronutrient intake among HIV-infected children between 1995 and 2004. *Am J Clin Nutr*. 2008;88(2):384-391

53. Kruzich LA, Marquis GS, Carriquiry AL, Wilson CM, Stephensen CB. US youths in the early stages of HIV disease have low intakes of some micronutrients important for optimal immune function. *J Am Diet Assoc*. 2004;104(7):1095-1101

54. World Health Organization. Guidelines for an Integrated Approach to Nutritional Care of HIV-Infected Children (6 months-14 years). Geneva, Switzerland: World Health Organization; 2009. Available at: http://www.who.int/nutrition/publications/hivaids/9789241597524/en/index.html. Accessed January 3, 2012

55. Weber R, Ledergerber B, Zbinden R, et al. Enteric infections and diarrhea in human immunodeficiency virus-infected persons: prospective community-based cohort study. Swiss HIV Cohort Study. *Arch Intern Med*. 1999;159(13):1473-1480

56. Ullrich R, Zeitz M, Heise W, L'Age M, Hoffken G, Riecken EO. Small intestinal structure and function in patients infected with human immunodeficiency virus (HIV): evidence for HIV-induced enteropathy. *Ann Intern Med*. 1989;111(1):15-21

57. Kotler DP. HIV infection and the gastrointestinal tract. *AIDS*. 2005;19(2):107-117

58. Miller TL, Orav EJ, Martin SR, Cooper ER, McIntosh K, Winter HS. Malnutrition and carbohydrate malabsorption in children with vertically transmitted human immunodeficiency virus 1 infection. *Gastroenterology*. 1991;100(5 Pt 1):1296-1302

59. Yolken RH, Hart W, Oung I, Shiff C, Greenson J, Perman JA. Gastrointestinal dysfunction and disaccharide intolerance in children infected with human immunodeficiency virus. *J Pediatr*. 1991;118(3):359-363

60. Miller TL, Winter HS, Luginbuhl LM, Orav EJ, McIntosh K. Pancreatitis in pediatric human immunodeficiency virus infection. *J Pediatr*. 1992;120(2 Pt 1):223-227

61. Butler KM, Venzon D, Henry N, et al. Pancreatitis in human immunodeficiency virus-infected children receiving dideoxyinosine. *Pediatrics*. 1993;91(4):747-751

62. Bouche H, Housset C, Dumont JL, et al. AIDS-related cholangitis: diagnostic features and course in 15 patients. *J Hepatol*. 1993;17(1):34-39

63. Pol S, Romana CA, Richard S, et al. Microsporidia infection in patients with the human immunodeficiency virus and unexplained cholangitis. *N Engl J Med*. 1993;328(2):95-99

64. Panel on Antiretroviral Therapy and Medical Management of HIV Infected Children. Guidelines for the Use of Antiretroviral Agents in Pediatric HIV Infection. Rockville, MD: AIDSInfo; 2010. Available at: http://aidsinfo.nih.gov/ContentFiles/PediatricGuidelines.pdf. Accessed January 3, 2013

65. Nachman SA, Lindsey JC, Moye J, et al. Growth of human immunodeficiency virus-infected children receiving highly active antiretroviral therapy. *Pediatr Infect Dis J*. 2005;24(4):352-357

VI

66. Verweel G, van Rossum AM, Hartwig NG, Wolfs TF, Scherpbier HJ, de Groot R. Treatment with highly active antiretroviral therapy in human immunodeficiency virus type 1-infected children is associated with a sustained effect on growth. *Pediatrics*. 2002;109(2):e25

67. McGrath CJ, Chung MH, Richardson BA, Benki-Nugent S, Warui D, John-Stewart GC. Younger age at HAART initiation is associated with more rapid growth reconstitution. *AIDS*. 2011;25(3):345-355

68. Steiner F, Kind C, Aebi C, et al. Growth in human immunodeficiency virus type 1-infected children treated with protease inhibitors. *Eur J Pediatr*. 2001;160(10):611-616

69. Chantry CJ, Byrd RS, Englund JA, Baker CJ, McKinney RE Jr. Growth, survival and viral load in symptomatic childhood human immunodeficiency virus infection. *Pediatr Infect Dis J*. 2003;22(12):1033-1039

70. Centers for Disease Control and Prevention. Epidemiology of HIV/AIDS—United States, 1981-2005. *MMWR Morb Mortal Wkly Rep*. 2006;55(21):589-592

71. Resino S, Resino R, Maria Bellon J, et al. Clinical outcomes improve with highly active antiretroviral therapy in vertically HIV type-1-infected children. *Clin Infect Dis*. 2006;43(2):243-252

72. Ylitalo N, Brogly S, Hughes MD, et al. Risk factors for opportunistic illnesses in children with human immunodeficiency virus in the era of highly active antiretroviral therapy. *Arch Pediatr Adolesc Med*. 2006;160(8):778-787

73. Chiappini E, Galli L, Tovo PA, et al. Changing patterns of clinical events in perinatally HIV-1-infected children during the era of HAART. *AIDS*. 2007;21(12):1607-1615

74. Atzori C, Clerici M, Trabattoni D, et al. Assessment of immune reconstitution to Pneumocystis carinii in HIV-1 patients under different highly active antiretroviral therapy regimens. *J Antimicrob Chemother*. 2003;52(2):276-281

75. Graham SM. Non-tuberculosis opportunistic infections and other lung diseases in HIV-infected infants and children. *Int J Tuberc Lung Dis*. 2005;9(6):592-602

76. Tang AM, Jacobson DL, Spiegelman D, Knox TA, Wanke C. Increasing risk of 5% or greater unintentional weight loss in a cohort of HIV-infected patients, 1995 to 2003. *J Acquir Immune Defic Syndr*. 2005;40(1):70-76

77. Mangili A, Murman DH, Zampini AM, Wanke CA. Nutrition and HIV infection: review of weight loss and wasting in the era of highly active antiretroviral therapy from the nutrition for healthy living cohort. *Clin Infect Dis*. 2006;42(6):836-842

78. Mangili A, Gerrior J, Tang AM, et al. Risk of cardiovascular disease in a cohort of HIV-infected adults: a study using carotid intima-media thickness and coronary artery calcium score. *Clin Infect Dis*. 2006;43(11):1482-1489

79. Missmer SA, Spiegelman D, Gorbach SL, Miller TL. Predictors of change in the functional status of children with human immunodeficiency virus infection. *Pediatrics*. 2000;106(2):e24

80. Money J. The syndrome of abuse dwarfism (psychosocial dwarfism or reversible hyposomatotropism). *Am J Dis Child*. 1977;131(5):508-513

81. Boulton TJ, Smith R, Single T. Psychosocial growth failure: a positive response to growth hormone and placebo. *Acta Paediatr*. 1992;81(4):322-325

82. Children whose mothers are infected with HIV. *Commun Dis Rep CDR Wkly*. 1995;5(24):111

83. Steele RG, Nelson TD, Cole BP. Psychosocial functioning of children with AIDS and HIV infection: review of the literature from a socioecological framework. *J Dev Behav Pediatr*. 2007;28(1):58-69

84. Lifschitz MH, Wilson GS, Smith EO, Desmond MM. Fetal and postnatal growth of children born to narcotic-dependent women. *J Pediatr*. 1983;102:686-691

85. Alaimo K, Briefel RR, Frongillo EA Jr, Olson CM. Food insufficiency exists in the United States: results from the third National Health and Nutrition Examination Survey (NHANES III). *Am J Public Health*. 1998;88(3):419-426

86. Joint United Nations Programme on HIV/AIDS. UNAIDS Policy Brief: HIV, Food Security and Nutrition. Geneva, Switzerland: UNAIDS; 2008. Available at: http://data.unaids.org/pub/Manual/2008/JC1515_policy_brief_nutrition_en.pdf. Accessed January 3, 2013

87. Chilton M, Chyatte M, Breaux J. The negative effects of poverty & food insecurity on child development. *Indian J Med Res*. 2007;126(4):262-272

88. Gadow KD, Chernoff M, Williams PL, et al. Co-occuring psychiatric symptoms in children perinatally infected with HIV and peer comparison sample. *J Dev Behav Pediatr*. 2010;31(2):116-128

89. Mellins CA, Brackis-Cott E, Dolezal C, Abrams EJ. Psychiatric disorders in youth with perinatally acquired human immunodeficiency virus infection. *Pediatr Infect Dis J*. 2006;25(5):432-437

90. Didoni A, Sequi M, Panei P, Bonati M. One-year prospective follow-up of pharmacological treatment in children with attention-deficit/hyperactivity disorder. *Eur J Clin Pharmacol*. 2011;67(10):1061-1067

91. Wigal T, Greenhill L, Chuang S, et al. Safety and tolerability of methylphenidate in preschool children with ADHD. *J Am Acad Child Adolesc Psychiatry*. 2006;45(11):1294-1303

92. Pliszka S; AACAP Work Group on Quality Issues. Practice parameter for the assessment and treatment of children and adolescents with attention-deficit/hyperactivity disorder. *J Am Acad Child Adolesc Psychiatry*. 2007;46(7):894-921

93. Poulton A. Growth and sexual maturation in children and adolescents with attention deficit hyperactivity disorder. *Curr Opin Pediatr*. 2006;18(4):427-434

94. Swanson J, Greenhill L, Wigal T, et al. Stimulant-related reductions of growth rates in the PATS. *J Am Acad Child Adolesc Psychiatry*. 2006;45(11):1304-1313

95. Sirois PA, Montepiedra G, Kapetanovic S, et al. Impact of medications prescribed for treatment of attention-deficit hyperactivity disorder on physical growth in children and adolescents with HIV. *J Dev Behav Pediatr*. 2009;30(5):403-412

96. Jacobson DL, Tang AM, Spiegelman D, et al. Incidence of metabolic syndrome in a cohort of HIV-infected adults and prevalence relative to the US population (National Health and Nutrition Examination Survey). *J Acquir Immune Defic Syndr*. 2006;43(4):458-466

97. Bauer LO. Psychiatric and neurophysiological predictors of obesity in HIV/AIDS. *Psychophysiology*. 2008;45(6):1055-1063

VI

98. Amorosa V, Synnestvedt M, Gross R, et al. A tale of 2 epidemics: the intersection between obesity and HIV infection in Philadelphia. *J Acquir Immune Defic Syndr.* 2005;39(5):557-561

99. Hodgson LM, Ghattas H, Pritchitt H, Schwenk A, Payne L, Macallan DC. Wasting and obesity in HIV outpatients. *AIDS.* 2001;15(17):2341-2342

100. Morrison SD, Haldeman L, Sudha S, Gruber KJ, Bailey R. Cultural adaptation resources for nutrition and health in new immigrants in Central North Carolina. *J Immigr Minor Health.* 2007;9(3):205-212

101. Miller TL, Grant YT, Almeida DN, Sharma T, Lipshultz SE. Cardiometabolic disease in human immunodeficiency virus-infected children. *J Cardiometab Syndr.* 2008;3(2):98-105

102. Cole JW, Pinto AN, Hebel JR, et al. Acquired immunodeficiency syndrome and the risk of stroke. *Stroke.* 2004;35(1):51-56

103. Gorczyca I, Stanek M, Podlasin B, Furmanek M, Pniewski J. Recurrent cerebral infarcts as the first manifestation of infection with the HIV virus. *Folia Neuropathol.* 2005;43(1):45-49

104. Triant VA, Lee H, Hadigan C, Grinspoon SK. Increased acute myocardial infarction rates and cardiovascular risk factors among patients with human immunodeficiency virus disease. *J Clin Endocrinol Metab.* 2007;92(7):2506-2512

105. Friis-Moller N, Reiss P, Sabin CA, et al. Class of antiretroviral drugs and the risk of myocardial infarction. *N Engl J Med.* 2007;356(17):1723-1735

106. Carr A, Samaras K, Chisholm DJ, Cooper DA. Pathogenesis of HIV-1-protease inhibitor-associated peripheral lipodystrophy, hyperlipidaemia, and insulin resistance. *Lancet.* 1998;351(9119):1881-1883

107. Chantry CJ, Cervia JS, Hughes MD, et al. Predictors of growth and body composition in HIV-infected children beginning or changing antiretroviral therapy. *HIV Med.* 2010;11(9):573-583

108. Brambilla P, Bricalli D, Sala N, et al. Highly active antiretroviral-treated HIV-infected children show fat distribution changes even in absence of lipodystrophy. *AIDS.* 2001;15(18):2415-2422

109. Vigano A, Mora S, Testolin C, et al. Increased lipodystrophy is associated with increased exposure to highly active antiretroviral therapy in HIV-infected children. *J Acquir Immune Defic Syndr.* 2003;32(5):482-489

110. Miller TL. Nutritional aspects of HIV-infected children receiving highly active antiretroviral therapy. *AIDS.* 2003;17(Suppl 1):S130-S140

111. Friis-Moller N, Sabin CA, Weber R, et al. Combination antiretroviral therapy and the risk of myocardial infarction. *N Engl J Med.* 2003;349(21):1993-2003

112. Miller TL, Mawn BE, Orav EJ, et al. The effect of protease inhibitor therapy on growth and body composition in human immunodeficiency virus type 1-infected children. *Pediatrics.* 2001;107(5):e77

113. Aldrovandi GM, Lindsey JC, Jacobson DL, et al. Morphologic and metabolic abnormalities in vertically HIV-infected children and youth. *AIDS.* 2009;23(6):661-672

114. Arpadi SM, Bethel J, Horlick M, et al. Longitudinal changes in regional fat content in HIV-infected children and adolescents. *AIDS*. 2009;23(12):1501-1509

115. Arpadi SM, Cuff PA, Horlick M, Wang J, Kotler DP. Lipodystrophy in HIV-infected children is associated with high viral load and low CD4+ -lymphocyte count and CD4+ -lymphocyte percentage at baseline and use of protease inhibitors and stavudine. *J Acquir Immune Defic Syndr*. 2001;27(1):30-34

116. European Paediatric Lipodystrophy Group. Antiretroviral therapy, fat redistribution and hyperlipidaemia in HIV-infected children in Europe. *AIDS*. 2004;18(10):1443-1451

117. Gerschenson M, Shiramizu B, LiButti DE, Shikuma CM. Mitochondrial DNA levels of peripheral blood mononuclear cells and subcutaneous adipose tissue from thigh, fat and abdomen of HIV-1 seropositive and negative individuals. *Antivir Ther*. 2005;10(Suppl 2):M83-M89

118. Grinspoon SK, Grunfeld C, Kotler DP, et al. State of the science conference: Initiative to decrease cardiovascular risk and increase quality of care for patients living with HIV/AIDS: executive summary. *Circulation*. 2008;118(2):198-210

119. Bitnun A, Sochett E, Dick PT, et al. Insulin sensitivity and beta-cell function in protease inhibitor-treated and -naive human immunodeficiency virus-infected children. *J Clin Endocrinol Metab*. 2005;90(1):168-174

120. Miller TL, Orav EJ, Lipshultz SE, et al. Risk factors for cardiovascular disease in children infected with human immunodeficiency virus-1. *J Pediatr*. 2008;153(4):491-497

121. Palella FJ Jr, Phair JP. Cardiovascular disease in HIV infection. *Curr Opin HIV AIDS*. 2011;6(4):266-271

122. Friis-Moller N, Weber R, Reiss P, et al. Cardiovascular disease risk factors in HIV patients--association with antiretroviral therapy. Results from the DAD study. *AIDS*. 2003;17(8):1179-1193

123. Mary-Krause M, Cotte L, Simon A, Partisani M, Costagliola D. Increased risk of myocardial infarction with duration of protease inhibitor therapy in HIV-infected men. *AIDS*. 2003;17(17):2479-2486

124. Reiss AB. Effects of inflammation on cholesterol metabolism: impact on systemic lupus erythematosus. *Curr Rheumatol Rep*. 2009;11(4):255-260

125. DeFronzo RA. Insulin resistance, lipotoxicity, type 2 diabetes and atherosclerosis: the missing links. The Claude Bernard Lecture 2009. *Diabetologia*. 2010;53(7):1270-1287

126. Mueller BU, Sleasman J, Nelson RP Jr, et al. A phase I/II study of the protease inhibitor indinavir in children with HIV infection. *Pediatrics*. 1998;102(1 Pt 1):101-109

127. Nadal D, Steiner F, Cheseaux JJ, et al. Long-term responses to treatment including ritonavir or nelfinavir in HIV-1-infected children. Pediatric AIDS Group of Switzerland. *Infection*. 2000;28(5):287-296

128. Cheseaux JJ, Jotterand V, Aebi C, et al. Hyperlipidemia in HIV-infected children treated with protease inhibitors: relevance for cardiovascular diseases. *J Acquir Immune Defic Syndr*. 2002;30(3):288-293

129. Carter RJ, Wiener J, Abrams EJ, et al. Dyslipidemia among perinatally HIV-infected children enrolled in the PACTS-HOPE cohort, 1999-2004: a longitudinal analysis. *J Acquir Immune Defic Syndr*. 2006;41(4):453-460

VI

130. Sharma TS, Orav EJ, Duggan C, et al. Visceral adiposity and cardiac risk profiles in human immunodeficiency virus-1 infected children [abstr]. *Pediatr Res.* 2006;

131. Rhoads MP, Lanigan J, Smith CJ, Lyall EG. Effect of specific antiretroviral therapy (ART) drugs on lipid changes and the need for lipid management in children with HIV. *J Acquir Immune Defic Syndr.* 2011;57(5):404-412

132. Lainka E, Oezbek S, Falck M, Ndagijimana J, Niehues T. Marked dyslipidemia in human immunodeficiency virus-infected children on protease inhibitor-containing antiretroviral therapy. *Pediatrics.* 2002;110(5):e56

133. Bitnun A, Sochett E, Babyn P, et al. Serum lipids, glucose homeostasis and abdominal adipose tissue distribution in protease inhibitor-treated and naive HIV-infected children. *AIDS.* 2003;17(9):1319-1327

134. Verkauskiene R, Dollfus C, Levine M, et al. Serum adiponectin and leptin concentrations in HIV-infected children with fat redistribution syndrome. *Pediatr Res.* 2006;60(2):225-230

135. Beregszaszi M, Jaquet D, Levine M, et al. Severe insulin resistance contrasting with mild anthropometric changes in the adipose tissue of HIV-infected children with lipohypertrophy. *Int J Obes Relat Metab Disord.* 2003;27(1):25-30

136. Murata H, Hruz PW, Mueckler M. The mechanism of insulin resistance caused by HIV protease inhibitor therapy. *J Biol Chem.* 2000;275(27):20251-20254

137. Shikuma CM, Day LJ, Gerschenson M. Insulin resistance in the HIV-infected population: the potential role of mitochondrial dysfunction. *Curr Drug Targets Infect Disord.* 2005;5:255-262

138. Grinspoon S. Physiologic effects of GHRH in patients with HIV lipodystrophy: a model of acquired visceral adiposity. *Nat Clin Pract Endocrinol Metab.* 2006;2:355

139. Brinkman K, Smeitink JA, Romijn JA, Reiss P. Mitochondrial toxicity induced by nucleoside-analogue reverse-transcriptase inhibitors is a key factor in the pathogenesis of antiretroviral-therapy-related lipodystrophy. *Lancet.* 1999;354:1112-1115

140. Kim RJ, Wilson CG, Wabitsch M, Lazar MA, Steppan CM. HIV protease inhibitor-specific alterations in human adipocyte differentiation and metabolism. *Obesity (Silver Spring).* 2006;14(6):994-1002

141. Hurwitz BE, Klimas NG, Llabre MM, et al. HIV, metabolic syndrome X, inflammation, oxidative stress, and coronary heart disease risk : role of protease inhibitor exposure. *Cardiovasc Toxicol.* 2004;4(3):303-316

142. Miller TL, Somarriba G, Orav EJ, et al. Biomarkers of vascular dysfunction in children infected with human immunodeficiency virus-1. *J Acquir Immune Defic Syndr.* 2010;55(2):182-188

143. Baker JV, Duprez D. Biomarkers and HIV-associated cardiovascular disease. *Curr Opin HIV AIDS.* 2010;5(6):511-516

144. Wolf K, Tsakiris DA, Weber R, Erb P, Battegay M. Antiretroviral therapy reduces markers of endothelial and coagulation activation in patients infected with human immunodeficiency virus type 1. *J Infect Dis.* 2002;185(4):456-462

145. McComsey GA, O'Riordan M, Hazen SL, et al. Increased carotid intima media thickness and cardiac biomarkers in HIV infected children. *AIDS.* 2007;21(8):921-927

146. Charakida M, Donald AE, Green H, et al. Early structural and functional changes of the vasculature in HIV-infected children: impact of disease and antiretroviral therapy. *Circulation*. 2005;112(1):103-109

147. Bonnet D, Aggoun Y, Szezepanski I, Bellal N, Blanche S. Arterial stiffness and endothelial dysfunction in HIV-infected children. *AIDS*. 2004;18(7):1037-1041

148. Charakida M, Loukogeorgakis SP, Okorie MI, et al. Increased arterial stiffness in HIV-infected children: risk factors and antiretroviral therapy. *Antivir Ther*. 2009;14(8):1075-1079

149. Ross AC, O'Riordan MA, Storer N, Dogra V, McComsey GA. Heightened inflammation is linked to carotid intima-media thickness and endothelial activation in HIV-infected children. *Atherosclerosis*. 2010;211(2):492-498

150. Perez-Atayde AR, Kearney DI, Bricker JT, et al. Cardiac, aortic, and pulmonary arteriopathy in HIV-infected children: the Prospective P2C2 HIV Multicenter Study. *Pediatr Dev Pathol*. 2004;7(1):61-70

151. Mora S, Zamproni I, Beccio S, Bianchi R, Giacomet V, Vigano A. Longitudinal changes of bone mineral density and metabolism in antiretroviral-treated human immunodeficiency virus-infected children. *J Clin Endocrinol Metab*. 2004;89(1):24-28

152. Mora S, Sala N, Bricalli D, Zuin G, Chiumello G, Vigano A. Bone mineral loss through increased bone turnover in HIV-infected children treated with highly active antiretroviral therapy. *AIDS*. 2001;15(14):1823-1829

153. Jacobson DL, Spiegelman D, Duggan C, et al. Predictors of bone mineral density in human immunodeficiency virus-1 infected children. *J Pediatr Gastroenterol Nutr*. 2005;41(3):339-346

154. Arpadi SM, Horlick M, Thornton J, Cuff PA, Wang J, Kotler DP. Bone mineral content is lower in prepubertal HIV-infected children. *J Acquir Immune Defic Syndr*. 2002;29(5):450-454

155. Zuccotti G, Vigano A, Gabiano C, et al. Antiretroviral therapy and bone mineral measurements in HIV-infected youths. *Bone*. 2010;46(6):1633-1638

156. Hazra R, Gafni RI, Maldarelli F, et al. Tenofovir disoproxil fumarate and an optimized background regimen of antiretroviral agents as salvage therapy for pediatric HIV infection. *Pediatrics*. 2005;116(6):e846-e854

157. Gafni RI, Hazra R, Reynolds JC, et al. Tenofovir disoproxil fumarate and an optimized background regimen of antiretroviral agents as salvage therapy: impact on bone mineral density in HIV-infected children. *Pediatrics*. 2006;118:e711-e718

158. Vigano A, Zuccotti GV, Puzzovio M, et al. Tenofovir disoproxil fumarate and bone mineral density: a 60-month longitudinal study in a cohort of HIV-infected youths. *Antivir Ther*. 2010;15:1053-1058

159. Fields-Gardner C, Campa A. Position of the American Dietetic Association: Nutrition Intervention and Human Immunodeficiency Virus Infection. *J Am Diet Assoc*. 2010;110:1105-1119

160. Matthews DR, Hosker JP, Rudenski AS, Naylor BA, Treacher DF, Turner RC. Homeostasis model assessment: insulin resistance and beta-cell function from fasting plasma glucose and insulin concentrations in man. *Diabetologia*. 1985;28(7):412-419

VI

161. Kastorini CM, Milionis HJ, Esposito K, Giugliano D, Goudevenos JA, Panagiotakos DB. The effect of Mediterranean diet on metabolic syndrome and its components: a meta-analysis of 50 studies and 534,906 individuals. *J Am Coll Cardiol*. 2011;57(11):1299-1313

162. Krauss RM, Eckel RH, Howard B, et al. AHA Dietary Guidelines: revision 2000: a statement for healthcare professionals from the Nutrition Committee of the American Heart Association. *Stroke*. 2000;31(11):2751-2766

163. Cardiovascular risk reduction in high-risk pediatric populations. *Pediatrics*. 2007;119(3):618-621

164. McCrindle BW, Urbina EM, Dennison BA, et al. Summary of the American Heart Association's scientific statement on drug therapy of high-risk lipid abnormalities in children and adolescents. *Arterioscler Thromb Vasc Biol*. 2007;27(5):982-985

165. Hadigan C, Corcoran C, Basgoz N, Davis B, Sax P, Grinspoon S. Metformin in the treatment of HIV lipodystrophy syndrome: A randomized controlled trial. *JAMA*. 2000;284(4):472-477

166. Walli R, Michl GM, Muhlbayer D, Brinkmann L, Goebel FD. Effects of troglitazone on insulin sensitivity in HIV-infected patients with protease inhibitor-associated diabetes mellitus. *Res Exp Med (Berl)*. 2000;199(5):253-262

167. Ratz Bravo AE, Tchambaz L, Krahenbuhl-Melcher A, Hess L, Schlienger RG, Krahenbuhl S. Prevalence of potentially severe drug-drug interactions in ambulatory patients with dyslipidaemia receiving HMG-CoA reductase inhibitor therapy. *Drug Saf*. 2005;28(3):263-275

168. Malita FM, Karelis AD, Toma E, Rabasa-Lhoret R. Effects of different types of exercise on body composition and fat distribution in HIV-infected patients: a brief review. *Can J Appl Physiol*. 2005;30(2):233-245

169. Miller TL, Somarriba G, Kinnamon DD, Weinberg GA, Friedman LB, Scott GB. The effect of a structured exercise program on nutrition and fitness outcomes in human immunodeficiency virus-infected children. *AIDS Res Hum Retroviruses*. 2010;26(3):313-319

170. Suksomboon N, Poolsup N, Ket-Aim S. Systematic review of the efficacy of antiretroviral therapies for reducing the risk of mother-to-child transmission of HIV infection. *J Clin Pharm Ther*. 2007;32(3):293-311

171. Blanche S, Tardieu M, Rustin P, et al. Persistent mitochondrial dysfunction and perinatal exposure to antiretroviral nucleoside analogues. *Lancet*. 1999;354(9184):1084-1089

172. Barret B, Tardieu M, Rustin P, et al. Persistent mitochondrial dysfunction in HIV-1-exposed but uninfected infants: clinical screening in a large prospective cohort. *AIDS*. 2003;17(12):1769-1785

173. Brogly SB, Ylitalo N, Mofenson LM, et al. In utero nucleoside reverse transcriptase inhibitor exposure and signs of possible mitochondrial dysfunction in HIV-uninfected children. *AIDS*. 2007;21(8):929-938

174. Poirier MC, Divi RL, Al-Harthi L, et al. Long-term mitochondrial toxicity in HIV-uninfected infants born to HIV-infected mothers. *J Acquir Immune Defic Syndr*. 2003;33(2):175-183

175. Thorne C, Newell ML. Safety of agents used to prevent mother-to-child transmission of HIV: is there any cause for concern? *Drug Saf*. 2007;30(3):203-213

176. Culnane M, Fowler M, Lee SS, et al. Lack of long-term effects of in utero exposure to zidovudine among uninfected children born to HIV-infected women. Pediatric AIDS Clinical Trials Group Protocol 219/076 Teams. *JAMA*. 1999;281(2):151-157

177. Study EC. Exposure to antiretroviral therapy in utero or early life: the health of uninfected children born to HIV-infected women. *J Acquir Immune Defic Syndr*. 2003;32(4):380-387

178. Newell ML, Borja MC, Peckham C. Height, weight, and growth in children born to mothers with HIV-1 infection in Europe. *Pediatrics*. 2003;111(1):e52-e60

179. Ross A, Raab GM, Mok J, Gilkison S, Hamilton B, Johnstone FD. Maternal HIV infection, drug use, and growth of uninfected children in their first 3 years. *Arch Dis Child*. 1995;73(6):490-495

180. Crenn P, Rakotoanbinina B, Raynaud JJ, Thuillier F, Messing B, Melchior JC. Hyperphagia contributes to the normal body composition and protein-energy balance in HIV-infected asymptomatic men. *J Nutr*. 2004;134(9):2301-2306

181. Hommes MJ, Romijn JA, Endert E, Sauerwein HP. Resting energy expenditure and substrate oxidation in human immunodeficiency virus (HIV)-infected asymptomatic men: HIV affects host metabolism in the early asymptomatic stage. *Am J Clin Nutr*. 1991;54(2):311-315

182. Sheehan LA, Macallan DC. Determinants of energy intake and energy expenditure in HIV and AIDS. *Nutrition*. 2000;16(2):101-106

183. Garcia-Lorda P, Serrano P, Jimenez-Exposito MJ, et al. Cytokine-driven inflammatory response is associated with the hypermetabolism of AIDS patients with opportunistic infections. *JPEN J Parenter Enteral Nutr*. 2000;24(6):317-322

184. Schwenk A, Hoffer-Belitz E, Jung B, et al. Resting energy expenditure, weight loss, and altered body composition in HIV infection. *Nutrition*. 1996;12(9):595-601

185. Briassoulis G, Venkataraman S, Thompson A. Cytokines and metabolic patterns in pediatric patients with critical illness. *Clin Dev Immunol*. 2010;2010:354047

186. Macallan DC, Noble C, Baldwin C, et al. Energy expenditure and wasting in human immunodeficiency virus infection. *N Engl J Med*. 1995;333(2):83-88

187. Chang E, Sekhar R, Patel S, Balasubramanyam A. Dysregulated energy expenditure in HIV-infected patients: a mechanistic review. *Clin Infect Dis*. 2007;44(11):1509-1517

188. Roubenoff R, Grinspoon S, Skolnik PR, et al. Role of cytokines and testosterone in regulating lean body mass and resting energy expenditure in HIV-infected men. *Am J Physiol Endocrinol Metab*. 2002;283(1):e138-e145

189. Sekhar RV, Jahoor F, White AC, et al. Metabolic basis of HIV-lipodystrophy syndrome. *Am J Physiol Endocrinol Metab*. 2002;283(2):e332-337

190. Leow MK, Addy CL, Mantzoros CS. Clinical review 159: Human immunodeficiency virus/highly active antiretroviral therapy-associated metabolic syndrome: clinical presentation, pathophysiology, and therapeutic strategies. *J Clin Endocrinol Metab*. 2003;88(5):1961-1976

191. Kosmiski LA, Ringham BM, Grunwald GK, Bessesen DH. Dual-energy X-ray absorptiometry modeling to explain the increased resting energy expenditure associated with the HIV lipoatrophy syndrome. *Am J Clin Nutr*. 2009;90(6):1525-1531

VI

192. Kosmiski L, Kuritzkes D, Hamilton J, et al. Fat distribution is altered in HIV-infected men without clinical evidence of the HIV lipodystrophy syndrome. *HIV Med*. 2003;4(3):235-240

193. Kosmiski LA, Kuritzkes DR, Lichtenstein KA, et al. Fat distribution and metabolic changes are strongly correlated and energy expenditure is increased in the HIV lipodystrophy syndrome. *AIDS*. 2001;15(15):1993-2000

194. Sutinen J, Yki-Jarvinen H. Increased resting energy expenditure, fat oxidation, and food intake in patients with highly active antiretroviral therapy-associated lipodystrophy. *Am J Physiol Endocrinol Metab*. 2007;292(3):e687-e692

195. Batterham MJ. Investigating heterogeneity in studies of resting energy expenditure in persons with HIV/AIDS: a meta-analysis. *Am J Clin Nutr*. 2005;81(3):702-713

196. Van der Valk M, Reiss P, van Leth FC, et al. Highly active antiretroviral therapy-induced lipodystrophy has minor effects on human immunodeficiency virus-induced changes in lipolysis, but normalizes resting energy expenditure. *J Clin Endocrinol Metab*. 2002;87(11):5066-5071

197. Ockenga J, Grimble R, Jonkers-Schuitema C, et al. ESPEN Guidelines on Enteral Nutrition: Wasting in HIV and other chronic infectious diseases. *Clin Nutr*. 2006;25(2):319-329

198. Sabery N, Duggan C. A.S.P.E.N. clinical guidelines: nutrition support of children with human immunodeficiency virus infection. *JPEN J Parenter Enteral Nutr*. 2009;33(6):588-606

199. Institute of Medicine, Food and Nutrition Board. *Dietary Reference Intakes for Energy, Carbohydrate, Fiber, Fat, Fatty Acids, Cholesterol, Protein, and Amino Acids*. Washington, DC: National Academies Press; 2005

Chapter 41

Nutrition for Children With Sickle Cell Disease and Thalassemia

Introduction

Disorders of abnormal hemoglobin (Hb) synthesis are among the most common genetic disorders worldwide. More than 700 structural hemoglobin variants and more than 200 mutations in the alpha or globin chain subunits have been identified. Approximately 5.2% of the worldwide population are carriers for a hemoglobinopathy trait, and the global incidence of a significant hemoglobinopathy is 2.6 in 1000 live births.[1,2]

Thalassemia (Thal) is a term describing a heterogeneous group of disorders of deficient production of the alpha or beta globin chain of hemoglobin, which lead to clinical conditions characterized by varying degrees of ineffective hematopoiesis with chronic anemia, intermittent hemolysis, and iron overload. Thal has a high prevalence in Mediterranean and Asian populations, with carrier rates as high as 60% in some regions of southeast Asia, and has been increasing in incidence in the United States with recent immigration patterns. Thalassemias are classified according to which globin chain is deficient. There are 4 alpha thalassemia syndromes: silent carrier, trait, hemoglobin H, or hydrops fetalis, determined by the number (1 to 4) of genes mutated. The clinical syndromes of beta thalassemias, in contrast, are not directly correlated to the number of genes mutated. Thalassemia major is a clinical term indicating patients who are transfusion dependent, regardless of genotype. Thalassemia intermedia refers to patients with clinical symptoms that do not yet require regular transfusions. The focus of this chapter will be on nutritional complications in patients with Thal major but may also be relevant to patients with Thal intermedia.

Sickle cell disease is a general term for the group of hemoglobinopathies in which the abnormal hemoglobin variant, sickle hemoglobin, is produced and leads to a clinical condition marked by anemia and a collection of acute and chronic clinical events of vaso-occlusion caused by abnormal sickle shaped red blood cells, which are less deformable than normal erythrocytes. The hallmark is a chronic hemolytic anemia with acute and chronic tissue injury. Sickle cell anemia, the homozygous hemoglobin S state, is the most common variant type of sickle cell disease and affects more than 50 000 African American people. It is estimated that 1 in 8 African American people carries at least one Hb S gene, and the prevalence of Hb SS disease in African American newborn infants is

VI

approximately 1 in 375. Two less common types of sickle cell disease exist in the United States. Hemoglobin SC disease occurs in approximately 1 of 835 African American live births, and sickle beta-thalassemia occurs in approximately 1 in 1700 African American live births. Thus, sickle cell disease, with an autosomal-recessive inheritance pattern, is the most common medically significant genetic condition in African American children but also occurs in Americans with Mediterranean, East Indian, Middle Eastern, Caribbean, and South and Central American ancestry. The discussion that follows uses hemoglobin SS disease (SCD) as the example; it is the most common genotype and presents the greatest nutritional care challenge.

Macronutrient Intake, Requirements, and Energy Expenditure

Growth retardation, delayed pubertal development, and poor nutritional status are frequently seen both in Thal and SCD. The exact etiology of this pattern of poor growth and abnormal body composition has not been completely established, but it is generally recognized to be multifactorial, and nutritional factors likely play a major role in both clinical disorders.

In Thal, growth failure has been reported with an incidence ranging from 25% to 75% depending on the Thal syndrome and severity of disease. Linear growth, expressed as height z-score, tends to decrease with age and is commonly associated with pubertal deficits. Contributing factors to growth failure in Thal include chronic anemia, chelation toxicity, and iron-associated endocrinopathies, such as hypogonadism, hypothyroidism, and growth hormone deficiency. However, recent reports conducted mostly outside the United States suggest that nutritional inadequacy also plays a major role in growth failure and pubertal development. Several small studies have demonstrated that nutritional supplementation in toddlers with Thal improves markers of immune function and growth.[3,4] One randomized controlled trial reported that children with Thal had similar dietary intake when compared with age- and gender-matched controls, despite marked growth and body fat deficits. After increasing energy intake by 30% to 50% over an 8-week period, they observed significant improvements in weight, fat stores, and albumin and insulin-like growth factor 1 (IGF-1) levels compared with a nonsupplemented Thal group. The improvement in IGF-1 following nutritional therapy supports the notion that a component of the growth failure in Thal is related to global nutritional deficiency.

One explanation for the reduced growth rates in Thal despite seemingly adequate energy intake could be increased energy expenditure. This is quite possible, given the existence of hyperactive bone marrow and increased cardiac output attributable to chronic anemia. In one study, energy expenditure in chronically transfused adults was measured to be 12% higher than expected prior to transfusion (at the nadir of Hb concentration) and decreased to near normal levels after transfusion.[5]

Poor nutritional intake may also contribute to growth deficiencies in some patients. Few studies have explored overall dietary intake in large samples of contemporary patients with Thal. The Thalassemia Clinical Research Network recently conducted a cross-sectional analysis of dietary intake in 221 adult and pediatric patients with a variety of Thal syndromes. The results suggest that patients with Thal generally have adequate and sometimes excess intakes of macronutrients (fat and protein). However, nearly one third of the patients with Thal consumed inadequate amounts of vitamins A, D, E, and K; folate; calcium; and magnesium when compared with the Dietary Reference Intakes (DRIs) from the Institute of Medicine.[6] Dietary inadequacy also increased with increasing age group, particularly for vitamins A, C, E, and B_6; folate; thiamin; calcium; magnesium; and zinc.[6]

Dietary intake of many nutrients may also be inadequate in children with SCD. A recent large cohort study of 97 children and adolescents with SCD evaluated dietary intake longitudinally over 4 annual visits using 24-hour recall data.[7] Children receiving chronic transfusions and hydroxyurea were excluded from this study. Although the median estimated energy intake was equal to the estimated energy requirements for children with a low-active physical activity level, overall growth was suboptimal (mean height z-score -0.5 ± 1.0, weight z-score -0.8 ± 1.2), and intake of many specific micronutrients was found to be low. Specifically, intake of vitamins D and E, folate, calcium, and fiber was inadequate, with 63% to 85% of the children falling below the estimated average requirement. Additionally, similar to what is observed in Thal, there was a general decline in adequacy of dietary intake as children got older, with decreased intakes of protein; vitamins A, B_{12}, and C; riboflavin; magnesium; and phosphorus.

Growth retardation, delayed pubertal development, and poor nutritional status are also seen in children with SCD compared with healthy control children and with national reference data.[8] This is indicated by decreased body weight, height/length, arm circumference, skin fold thicknesses, and bone age. Direct measures of body composition by several research methods have shown both lower total body fat and fat-free masses.[9] Acute illness episodes in infants and young children with SCD further aggravates growth retardation and nutritional status.[10]

VI

Patients with SCD have increased energy and micronutrient requirements as a result of chronic hemolysis, increased erythropoiesis, and increased protein turnover.[11-16]

Several studies have documented increased resting energy expenditure in children and adults with SCD in the United States and other countries.[17-19] The increase is generally 10% to 20% above the predicted energy expenditure of healthy control children. Unfortunately, children with SCD do not necessarily increase energy intake to compensate for increased energy needs.[15,20] The increased resting energy expenditure has been correlated with low Hb concentrations.[21]

Although the common SCD acute vaso-occlusive event does not appear to increase resting energy expenditure,[22] these events are associated with decreased energy intakes.[10,21] Some of the new treatments for SCD, such as oral glutamine supplementation and hydroxyurea therapy, may also decrease resting energy expenditure.[23,24]

Another factor contributing to inadequate nutrient intake in children with SCD may be the emphasis placed on maintaining adequate hydration and encouraging fluid intake to help prevent dehydration precipitated vaso-occlusive events. Children with SCD also have increased fluid needs resulting from hyposthenuria, the inability of the kidneys to appropriately concentrate urine.[25] Care must be taken to avoid the increased use of fluids that contain only water and carbohydrates and few other nutrients. This may lead to inadequate intake of other dietary nutrients. Anorexia and/or nausea secondary to fever, pain, and use of analgesic medications may also contribute to poor overall intake. In addition, suboptimal intakes during periods of illness at home or in the hospital may contribute to the pattern of decreased dietary intake and poor growth, particularly in patients with severe SCD disease.

Specific Micronutrient Deficiencies

In addition to the potential increased requirement for total kilocalories, there are a number of specific essential micronutrients for which patients with SCD and Thal may be at risk of deficiency (Table 41.1).

Table 41.1.
Nutrients of Concern for Inadequacy in Sickle Cell Disease and Thalassemia

Nutrient	Sickle Cell Disease	Thalassemia	Clinical Signs Observed
Macronutrients: Kilocalories	Poor dietary quality/ nutrient density	Poor dietary quality/ nutrient density	Growth failure
	Amino acids[a]		Increased oxidative stress
Micronutrients: Fat-soluble vitamins	Vitamin A		Increased vasoocclusive crises and fever
	Vitamin D	Vitamin D	Reduced bone mineral density
	Vitamin E	Vitamin E	Increased oxidative damage
Water-soluble vitamins	Vitamin C	Vitamin C	Increased oxidative damage, decreased chelator efficacy (Thal)
	Folate and vitamin B_{12}	Folate	Ineffective erythropoiesis; increased homocysteine (SCD)
	Vitamin B_6		Increased reticulocyte count
Minerals	Zinc	Zinc	Increased vasoocclusive crises and infection (SCD), poor growth, reduced bone density (Thal)
	Calcium	Calcium	Reduced bone mineral density

[a] Although total protein intake appears adequate, SCD patients may have increased requirements for certain amino acids (glutamine, arginine).

Water-Soluble Vitamins

The most common water-soluble vitamin deficiency is folate. Folate is an essential nutrient required for normal erythropoietic activity and, therefore, may be deficient in both of these disorders, with increased needs for red cell production caused by hemolysis in SCD and chronic anemia in Thal. It has been shown that folate is readily catabolized by ferritin[26]; thus, in patients with Thal with hyperactive erythropoiesis confounded by iron overload, folate requirements are increased, and deficiencies are commonly reported.[27] Several studies have also demonstrated folate deficiency in children with SCD, along with low concentrations of vitamins B_6 and B_{12}. In one study, children with SCD remained folate deficient despite supplementation with 1 mg/day of folate, supporting the hypothesis that folate requirements are significantly increased.[28] This is of particular interest in SCD, because folate and vitamin B_{12} deficiency have been correlated with increased homocysteine concentrations.[29,30]

VI

Increased plasma homocysteine concentrations may be associated with increased risk of stroke in children with SCD.[31] Supplementation with folate, vitamin B_6, and vitamin B_{12} has been shown to decrease plasma homocysteine concentrations,[28,32] suggesting a possible role for supplementation of these vitamins. However, no studies have demonstrated that folate, vitamin B_6, and vitamin B_{12} supplementation reduces the incidence of stroke in SCD. In one study in which growth and nutritional status were assessed, vitamin B_6 status correlated positively with weight and body mass index[33] and correlated negatively with the reticulocyte count. These observations may simply reflect the overall poor nutritional status of patients with severe SCD.

Vitamin C, another essential water-soluble vitamin, serves an important antioxidant function within the cell membrane and may act to decrease osmotic fragility in SCD. Vitamin C supplementation in children with SCD has been demonstrated to reduce the percentage of irreversibly sickled cells, thus effectively increasing Hb concentration and percent fetal Hb.[34,35] It has been known for decades that vitamin C is important both in nonheme iron absorption as well as in the mobilization of iron from tissues.[36] In Thal, vitamin C deficiency has been associated with ineffective chelation.[37,38] As a result of these observations, patients are often recommended to take vitamin C supplements along with their prescribed chelator medication.

Fat-Soluble Vitamins

As a group, fat-soluble vitamins appear to be of particular concern for deficiency in patients with hemoglobinopathies. Vitamin D deficiency has received much attention in the scientific literature recently with the Institute of Medicine revised dietary guidelines for vitamin D intake[39] (see Chapter 21.I: Fat-Soluble Vitamins). Patients with Thal are at particular risk of vitamin D deficiency. In a recent study, only 18% of a sample of 361 patients with Thal residing in North America had "sufficient" concentrations of 25-hydroxyvitamin D (25-OH-D [defined as >30 ng/mL or 75 nmol/L]).[40] Other international reports have found similar levels.[41-44] As reviewed in Chapter 21.I, vitamin D has many unique hormonal functions; its active form, calcitriol (1,25-dihydroxyvitamin D_3), has been shown to affect bone and has been associated with improved cardiovascular health, immune function, and cancer prevention. Individuals with Thal may be at greater risk of vitamin D deficiency and, therefore, have a greater need for supplementation. Wood et al found a weak although significant correlation between 25-OH-D concentrations and left ventricular ejection fraction in patients with Thal ($r^2 = 0.35$).[45] In this small study, all 4 subjects with dysfunctional ejection fractions (<57%) also had low concentrations of vitamin D. More recently, Dimitriadou et al reported that parathyroid hormone concentration was higher in patients with beta thalassemia major with increased myocardial iron compared with those with normal parathyroid hormone concentrations ($P = .017$).[46] Thal patients with reduced concentrations of vitamin D have a reported 10-fold greater risk of low bone mass after controlling for age, weight z-score, and hypogonadism.[47]

Children with SCD are also at risk of vitamin D deficiency, in part because of their dark skin color. However, children with SCD have decreased serum vitamin D concentrations and decreased vitamin D and calcium intakes, even compared with healthy age-matched African American controls.[48,49] In one study of 65 children with SCD, 93% of the subjects had low serum 25-OH-D concentrations, defined as 25-OH-D <30 ng/mL (75 nmol/L). After adjustments were made for seasonal effects and age, the risk of a low serum 25-OH-D in patients with SCD was 5 times greater than in healthy African American controls. These low vitamin D concentrations may also play a role in suboptimal bone development.[50] However, no direct correlation has been demonstrated with bone density and vitamin D concentrations in children with SCD. In one small nonrandomized pilot study of 14 adults with SCD who had low bone mass and low serum vitamin D concentrations, supplementation with vitamin D and calcium over a 12-month period was able to restore concentrations to the normal range and increase bone mineral density by 3.6% to 6.5%.[51]

Given the high prevalence of low serum 25-OH-D concentrations and the potential for comorbidities in both Thal and SCD patients, vitamin D status should be monitored by measuring serum 25-OH-D concentrations every 6 months. Those who reside in Northern latitudes, are dark skinned, who customarily shroud themselves, or who have limited exposure to sunlight and have limited dietary intake of vitamin D are particularly at risk. Given that vitamin D is a fat-soluble vitamin and stored in fat tissue, it can be provided in large, infrequent doses to improve compliance. For subjects who come regularly to clinic for transfusion therapy and who have low vitamin D concentrations (<20 ng/mL [50 nmol/L]), a 50 000 IU vitamin D oral dose at time of transfusion has been used successfully to improve vitamin D status.[52]

Vitamins A and E, essential nutrients with antioxidant effects, are also frequently reported to be deficient in children and adolescents with SCD.[53-59] This is particularly important in SCD, which is a disorder marked by increased oxidative stress resulting from chronic hemolysis. In one study of young children with SCD, vitamin A status was found to be suboptimal in two thirds of the studied children and was associated with poor growth and lower hematocrit, increased episodes of pain and fever, and a 10-fold increased frequency of hospitalizations.[60] Vitamin E has been shown to help stabilize the red cell membrane, and vitamin E deficiency enhances red cell susceptibility to peroxidative damage.[61] It should be noted that several studies have suggested that chronic transfusions, although reducing the amount of hemolysis in these children, may actually increase oxidative stress and

VI

decrease antioxidant activity as result of iron overload.[62,63] This has led other scientists to explore the effects of vitamin E supplementation on iron overload-induced oxidative stress. Supplementation with 400 to 600 IU of vitamin E for 3 months in patients with either Thal intermedia or E-beta Thal has been found to reduce oxidative stress in both red and white cells[64,65] as well as reduce platelet reactivity.[66]

Zinc

Zinc is an essential trace mineral required for cell division, differentiation, and gene expression. It is critical to the function of more than 300 enzymes and, as such, it is important to a myriad of bodily functions, including development and maintenance of the immune system, bone health, vitamin A metabolism, and actions of insulin, testosterone, thyroid, and growth hormones. Zinc is a particularly important mineral for chronically transfused patients with Thal, because it is similar in size and charge to iron and has the potential to be chelated along with iron in patients treated for iron overload.

Zinc deficiency has been documented in both transfused and nontransfused patients with Thal.[67,68] A 2003 report from Iran found that 80% of adolescent patients with beta Thal exhibited poor zinc status defined by depressed plasma zinc.[69] Depletion of circulating zinc may be attributable, in part, to the presence of proximal renal tubular damage[70] with hyperzincuria, as urinary zinc is elevated fourfold in patients with Thal compared with controls.[71] Increases in urinary zinc may also be related to the presence of diabetes, a comorbidity associated with increased zinc losses.[72] Chelators used to treat iron overload may also place these patients at risk of zinc deficiency.[73] Zinc supplementation (22–90 mg/day) in young, regularly transfused but nonchelated patients with Thal has been shown to improve growth velocity.[74]

Abnormalities of zinc metabolism may also play a role in the pathology of osteoporosis in patients with Thal. Bone mineral density (BMD) z-scores are lower in males and females with severe zinc deficiency compared with Thal with normal serum zinc.[69,75] Within the last few years, others have explored the relationship between zinc deficiency and diabetes in patients with Thal. Dehshal et al found that 37% of subjects with Thal had depressed serum zinc concentrations, which were associated with lower fasting and 1-hour post-oral glucose tolerance test serum insulin concentrations.[76] Their data support the hypothesis that zinc deficiency might lead to an exacerbation of the inability of the pancreas to secrete sufficient amounts of insulin in response to glucose stimulation in patients with transfusion dependent Thal.

Zinc is also the mineral most studied in SCD, and zinc deficiency has been recognized in children with SCD for several decades.[77] Early reports showed zinc deficiency in up to 70% of adult SCD patients in one center, and a recent study demonstrated that up to 24% of children with SCD may be at risk of marginal zinc status. The exact etiology for this is not entirely clear, but there is evidence that patients with SCD have increased urinary zinc losses, and it is likely that they have increased needs resulting from chronic hemolysis and increased protein turnover.[78] A 10-mg zinc supplement taken for 1 year has been shown to improve linear growth and weight gain in prepubertal children with SCD, even in those with normal plasma zinc levels prior to supplementation.[79] This result suggests that some children with SCD in the United States with normal serum zinc concentrations may still experience a zinc-limiting growth failure. A benefit to zinc supplementation has also been demonstrated with regard to sexual maturation and decreased infections and hospitalizations.[80,81]

Amino Acids

Recent investigations have shown the amino acids L-arginine and glutamine to be deficient in patients with SCD. Glutamine is the most abundant amino acid in the body and is used preferentially in tissues containing rapidly dividing cells. When the needs for glutamine exceed the availability of plasma glutamine, glutamine may be released from body stored via increased skeletal muscle catabolism, leading to skeletal wasting and an increased metabolic rate, contributing to poor growth. Supplementation with glutamine has been shown to decrease resting energy expenditure.[23] Glutamine plays an important antioxidant role as an essential precursor in nicotinamide adenine dinucleotide phosphate biosynthesis, and red blood cell glutamine depletion has been associated with increased hemolysis and pulmonary hypertension.[82] Similarly, L-arginine deficiency has been demonstrated in patients with SCD and can contribute to oxidative stress as it is a required substrate for nitric oxide synthesis.[83] Arginine deficiency is thought to be attributable to release of arginase from red blood cells during vaso-occlusive events. A recent large cohort study demonstrated a correlation between increased arginase activity with pulmonary hypertension and increased mortality in patients with SCD.[84] One study of oral arginine supplementation demonstrated the ability to increase exhaled nitric oxide activity and, in theory, decrease pulmonary hypertension; however, the investigators were not able to show an improvement in pulmonary function.[85] However, in a previous study of 10 adolescent and adult SCD patients with pulmonary hypertension, oral arginine supplementation was shown to decrease pulmonary hypertension, as measured by echocardiography in 9 of the 10 patients.[86] Although the primary mechanism for deficiency of these amino acids is not thought to be related to poor nutritional intake, these data suggest there may be a role for supplementation beyond normal dietary intake. This is an area of continued debate and investigation.

VI

Nutritional Status in Subpopulations of SCD and Thal

Recently, Claster et al reported the circulating concentrations of a variety of essential nutrients in a convenience sample of 24 chronically transfused patients with Thal (1.9 to 25.8 y, ferritin 2089 ± 1920 ng/mL) and 43 chronically transfused patients with SCD (1.5 to 31.4 y, ferritin 3874 ± 4451 ng/mL).[63] They found surprisingly low concentrations of both water-soluble and fat-soluble vitamins in both groups. For some nutrients, more than half of the patients sampled had low serum concentrations—these included vitamins A, C, and D and selenium in both groups. Only a few nutrients were not low—serum copper, vitamin B_{12}, and gamma tocopherol, the supplemental form of vitamin E, in the Thal group. The same held true for the SCD group, with the exception that copper was abnormally elevated in this group, which is not surprising, given that copper is a marker of inflammation and SCD is a disorder marked by chronic inflammation, unlike Thal. It should be noted that vitamin B_{12} concentration was normal in the SCD cohort in this study, in contrast to previous studies. This may be because previous studies have primarily reported on nontransfused SCD patients. Circulating concentrations of many nutrients tended to decrease with increasing age; thus, younger subjects in this study tended to have higher circulating nutrient concentrations compared with older subjects. This is consistent with previous studies that have documented inadequacy of intake directly related to increasing age. Although the level of nutritional deficiency seen in this study has been shown in other studies to be associated with poor health outcomes, the small sample size and cross-sectional study design precluded a cause-and-effect conclusion.[63]

From these data, it is clear that patients with both Thal and SCD have the potential for increased requirements of some nutrients, indicating that dietary intake is inadequate. Some of the etiologies for these presumed nutritional deficiencies are presented in Table 41.2.

Table 41.2.
Etiology of Nutritional Deficiencies in Sickle Cell Disease and Thalassemia

Sickle Cell Disease	Thalassemia
• Hyposthenuria • Increased renal excretion of essential nutrients • Multiple hospitalizations resulting in poor dietary intake • Narcotic usage resulting in constipation • Overhydration leading to poor dietary intake • Increased red cell turnover leading to elevated energy expenditure • Increased inflammation leading to increased antioxidant consumption	• Increased mineral losses attributable to nonspecific chelation • Increased nontransferrin-bound iron leading to increased oxidative stress and antioxidant consumption • Ineffective erythropoietic activity and increased cardiac output leading to elevated energy expenditure

Unique Nutritional Situations

Pica and Sickle Cell Disease

Pica, the consumption and/or craving of nonfood substances, has been identified in all cultures and geographic regions but is particularly common in young children, pregnant women, nursing mothers, and individuals with mental disabilities.[87] Interestingly, pica also has a particularly high prevalence in patients with SCD.[88,89] A 2001 study from Detroit suggested that 32% of all nonpregnant SCD pediatric subjects studied reported some form of pica behavior. The most commonly consumed items were paper, fabric, dirt (geophagia), foam, and powder. There are many theories behind its cause, including compulsive neuroses, regression to oral development stage, sensory pleasure, and underlying nutritional deficiencies.[90] The most commonly linked nutritional deficiencies include the trace elements iron and zinc.[91-93] Although frequently benign, the pediatrician should be aware of these often hidden pica behaviors, given the potential for more serious medical complications, including dental injury, constipation, intestinal obstruction, lead poisoning, malabsorption of essential nutrients, and poor growth.[94]

Iron Overload in Thal: The Dogma and the Dilemma

Given the relationship between iron overload and organ dysfunction in Thal, counseling patients to consume a diet low in iron has been part of the standards of care for decades. Typically, a diet that is low in iron-rich foods, such as red and organ meats and fortified breakfast cereals, is recommended for all patients. However, there is debate regarding the effectiveness of reducing dietary iron consumption for the transfused subject. The amount of iron obtained from just one unit of packed red blood cells (200 mg) far outweighs the amount of iron obtained from a 3 oz steak (5 mg). Typical daily iron accumulation from transfusion-related iron is approximately 20 mg/day (2 transfusion units every 3 weeks), compared with iron accumulation from an iron-rich diet of approximately 4 mg (assuming 30% absorption). A low-iron diet may decrease the quality of life in some transfusion-dependent patients and/or create a false sense of security—that is, if they decrease their dietary iron intake, they may need to be less diligent with regard to chelator adherence.

For the patient with Thal who is not dependent on transfusions, reducing iron in the diet is an important part of nutritional counseling, because these patients have a tendency to overabsorb iron from the intestinal track. Black tea has been shown in one study from 1979 (n = 6 subjects) to reduce the absorption of dietary iron from plant-based foods up to 95%.[95]

VI

Nutrition and Bone Health

Bone health is another important nutritional consideration for both children with Thal and SCD. Dactylitis, seen during childhood in SCD, is a consequence of necrosis of the epiphysis and bone marrow within the fingers, resulting in permanent shortening of the carpels and metacarpals. People with SCD are also at increased risk of necrosis of the femoral head. Bone mineral content deficits are also present in children with SCD, even when adjusting for age, height, pubertal status, and lean body mass.[96] Studies would suggest this to be more common in boys, and the decreased bone mineral content is associated with delayed growth and maturation. The cortical bone compartment has been found to be most affected in studies utilizing dual energy x-ray absorptiometry and peripheral quantitative computed tomography. Multiple factors most likely contribute to this poor bone health, including decreased vitamin D and calcium intake.[97] Bone marrow hyperplasia in response to increased RBC turnover expands the marrow medullary space in long bones, thinning the cortical bone compartment. Cortical thinning likely results in increased bone fragility and increased lifelong risk of fracture. Elevations in protein and energy metabolism are also associated with increased bone turnover in SCD.[98] Increased protein turnover and decreased lean body mass may be significant when considering the concept of the bone-muscle unit. Forces produced by muscle contractions influence the restructuring of bone, and changes in muscle mass affect bone mass, size, and strength and may be relevant to SCD.

Nutritional Guidelines for SCD and Thal

Given these recent findings of inadequate nutrition in children with hemoglobinopathies, careful nutrition and growth assessment should be a routine component of care. However, there are neither nutrition intervention trials nor nutrition consensus statements to suggest a standard of care. Guidelines published by the American Academy of Pediatrics for health supervision in children with SCD in 2002[99] made no mention of routine nutritional evaluation or supplementation. A statement from the National Heart, Lung and Blood Institute (NHLBI) released in 2004[100] indicated the importance of nutritional counseling but makes no specific recommendations for monitoring. The only routine nutritional supplement recommended by the NHLBI is folate. Similarly, guidelines on the clinical management of Thal published in 2008 by the Thalassemia International Federation,[101] while recognizing the risk of multiple nutrient deficiencies, did not recommend supplementation of any individual micronutrient other than folate. Rather, it stressed a diverse, high-vegetable and low-simple carbohydrate diet to maximize ingestion of these nutrients and delay the onset of impaired glucose tolerance. However, most experts agree that there should be close monitoring of the nutritional status of patients with Thal, with inclusion of a dietitian or nutritionist in the comprehensive care team. The Northern California Comprehensive Thalassemia Center has published a set of nutritional monitoring recommendations that may provide a useful guide for clinicians (Table 41.3).[102]

Table 41.3.
Suggested Nutritional Monitoring Guidelines for Sickle Cell Disease and Thalassemia[a]

Growth/Development	Sample Type	Frequency	Adequacy
Height and weight		Monthly	^
Calculate growth velocity		Annually	
Puberty: Tanner staging		Every 6 months	
Nutritional Laboratory			
Albumin		Annually	3.5–5.0 g/dL
Folate	Serum	Annually	>3 ng/mL
Vitamin D, 25-OH-D	Serum	Every 6 months	≥30 ng/mL
Vitamin C/ascorbate	Plasma	Annually	>0.4 mg/dL
Vitamin E/alpha- and gamma-tocopherol	Serum	Annually	Age and gender dependent
Zinc	Serum (TE, F)	Annually	≥70 µg/dL
Other			
Bone densitometry		Annually, starting at 10 yrs	Z-score <−2.0

^ indicates adequacy of growth is dependent on the child's genetic potential for growth determined by the mid-parental height index; TE, all trace elements need to be collected into trace element free vacutainers; F, it is important that these are collected in the fasting state.

Adapted from: Children's Hospital & Research Center. *Standards of Care Guidelines for Thalassemia*. Oakland, CA: Children's Hospital & Research Center; 2008.

[a] For transfused patients, best to draw laboratory values prior to transfusion (eg, morning of).

May be possible to use red blood cell folate in the nontransfused patient, as it is typically a better indicator of tissue stores than serum folate.

In both groups of patients, routine, longitudinal growth and nutritional status assessment is essential to care. These data should inform a diagnosis of growth failure or malnutrition and provide the basis for planning the nutrition intervention strategy. Given the common occurrence of linear growth failure, the biological parents' heights should be obtained, recorded on the patient's growth chart, and used to assess the pattern of linear growth. It is important to remember that short stature is not a part of the genetic expression of either hemoglobinopathy, and with

VI

optimal nutritional intake, most children will be able to grow to their genetic potential for height. The care team should take this into account and not accept poor height growth as an unavoidable part of SCD or Thal. An accurate longitudinal growth (length, height, weight, head circumference) and body composition (fat stores measurements) record is essential to monitoring nutritional status and evaluating the results of nutrition intervention efforts. For children older than 10 years, the progression through pubertal development should be evaluated and documented in the physical examination every 6 months. With the exception of vitamin D, concentrations of circulating nutrients should be assessed on an annual basis and corrections made when deficiencies are observed. Given the seasonal variability in vitamin D concentrations, and the extremely high prevalence of deficiency in both SCD and Thal, it is suggested that 25-OH-D be assessed every 6 months until a patient is considered sufficient.

Conclusions

Depressed circulating concentrations of key fat- and water-soluble vitamins, as well as important essential minerals, have frequently been observed in patients with both Thal and SCD. There is increasing evidence that these patients have increased needs for certain nutrients either because of poor nutrient absorption or elevated losses or increased nutrient turnover. The etiology of frequently reported comorbidities in Thal and SCD can no longer simply be ascribed to the disease process itself or the toxic effects of transfusion-related iron overload. It is suggested that pediatric patients be monitored frequently and that nutritional deficiencies be corrected when observed to improve the overall health and quality of life in patients with hemoglobinopathies.

References

1. Weatherall DJ, Clegg JB. Inherited hemoglobin disorders: an increasing global health problem. *Bull World Health Organ*. 2001;79(8):704-712
2. Modell B, Darlison M. Global epidemiology of haemoglobin disorders and derived service indicators. *Bull World Health Organ*. 2008;86(6):480-487
3. Tienboon P. 2003.Effect of nutrition support on immunity in paediatric patients with beta-thalassaemia major. *Asia Pacific J Clin Nutr*. 12:61-65
4. Fuchs GJ, Tienboon P, Linpisarn S, et al. Nutritional factors and thalassemia major. *Arch Dis Child*. 1996;74(3):224-227
5. Vaisman N, Akivis A, Sthoeger D, et al. Resting energy expenditure in patients with thalassemia major. *Am J Clin Nutr*. 1995;61(3):582–584
6. Fung EB, Xu Y, Trachtenberg F, et al; Thalassemia Clinical Research Network. Inadequate dietary intake in patients with thalassemia. *J Acad Nutr Diet*. 2012;112(7):980-990

7. Kawchak DA, Schall JI, Zemel BS, Ohene-Frempong K, Stallings VA. Adequacy of dietary intake declines with age in children with sickle cell disease. *J Am Diet Assoc.* 2007;107(5):843-848

8. Barden EM, Kawchak DA, Ohene-Frempong K, Stallings VA, Zemel BS. Body composition in children with sickle cell disease. *Am J Clin Nutr.* 2002;76(1):218-225

9. VanderJagt DJ, Harmatz P, Scott-Emuakpor AB, Vichinsky E, Glew RH. Bioelectrical impedance analysis of the body composition of children and adolescents with sickle cell disease. *J Pediatr.* 2002;140(6):681-687

10. Malinauskas BM, Gropper SS, Kawchak DA, Zemel BS, Ohene-Frempong K, Stallings VA. Impact of acute illness on nutritional status of infants and young children with sickle cell disease. *J Am Diet Assoc.* 2000;100(3):330-334

11. Modebe O, Ifenu SA. Growth retardation in homozygous sickle cell disease: role of calorie intake and possible gender-related differences. *Am J Hematol.* 1993;44(3):149-154

12. Gray NT, Bartlett JM, Kolasa KM, Marcuard SP, Holbrook CT, Horner RD. Nutritional status and dietary intake of children with sickle cell anemia. *Am J Pediatr Hematol Oncol.* 1992;14(1):57-61

13. Salman EK, Haymond MW, Bayne E, et al. Protein and energy metabolism in prepubertal children with sickle cell anemia. *Pediatr Res.* 1996;40(1):34-40

14. Singhal A, Thomas P, Cook R, Wierenga K, Serjeant G. Delayed adolescent growth in homozygous sickle cell disease. *Arch Dis Child.* 1994;71(5):404-408

15. Singhal A, Davies P, Wierenga KJ, Ghomas P, Serjeant G. Is there an energy deficiency in homozygous sickle cell disease? *Am J Clin Nutr.* 1997;66(2):386-390

16. Buchowski MS, Townsend KM, Williams R, Chen KY. Patterns and energy expenditure of free-living physical activity in adolescents with sickle cell anemia. *J Pediatr.* 2002;140(1):86-92

17. Borel MJ, Muchowski MS, Turner EA, Peeler BB, Goldstein RE, Flakoll PJ. Alterations in basal nutrient metabolism increase resting energy expenditure in sickle cell disease. *Am J Physiol.* 1998;274(2 Pt 1):e347-e3645

18. Badaloo A, Jackson AA, Jahoor F. Whole body protein turnover and resting metabolic rate in homozygous sickle cell disease. *Clin Sci.* 1989;77(1):93-97

19. Singhal A, Davies P, Sahota A, Thomas PW, Serjeant GR. Resting metabolic rate in homozygous sickle cell disease. *Am J Clin Nutr.* 1993;57(1):32-34

20. Barden EM, Zemel BS, Kawchak DA, Goran MI, Ohene-Frempong K, Stallings VA. Total and resting energy expenditure in children with sickle cell disease. *J Pediatr.* 2000;136(1):73-79

21. Williams R, Olivi S, Mackert P, Fletcher L, Tian GL, Wang W. Comparison of energy prediction equations with measured resting energy expenditure in children with sickle cell anemia. *J Am Diet Assoc.* 2002;102(7):956-961

22. Fung EB, Malinauskis BM, Kawchak DA, et al. Energy expenditure and intake in children with sickle cell disease during acute illness. *Clin Nutr.* 2001;20:131-138

VI

23. Williams R, Olivi S, Li CS, Storm M, Cremer L, Mackert P, Wang W. Oral glutamine supplementation decreases resting energy expenditure in children and adolescents with sickle cell anemia. *J Pediatr Hematol Oncol.* 2004;26(10):619-625

24. Fung EB, Barden EM, Kawchak DA, Zemel BS, Ohene-Frempong K, Stallings VA. Effect of hydroxyurea therapy on resting energy expenditure in children with sickle cell disease. *J Pediatr Hematol Oncol.* 2001;23(9):604-608

25. Smith JA, Wethers DL. Health care maintenance. In: Embury SH, Hebbel RP, Mohandas N, Steinberg MH, eds. *Sickle Cell Disease.* New York, NY: Raven Press; 1994:739-744

26. Suh JR, Herbig AK, Stover PJ. New perspectives on folate catabolism. *Annu Rev Nutr.* 2001;21:255-282

27. Ozdem S, Kupesiz A, Yesilipek A. Plasma homocysteine levels in patients with b-thalassemia major. *Scand J Clin Lab Invest.* 2008;68(2):134-139

28. Kennedy TS, Fung EB, Kawchak DA, Zemel BS, Ohene-Frempong K, Stallings VA. Red blood cell folate and serum vitamin B_{12} status in children with sickle cell disease. *J Pediatr Hematol Oncol.* 2001;23(3):165-169

29. van der Dijs FP, Schnog JJ, Brouwer DA, et al. Elevated homocysteine levels indicate suboptimal folate status in pediatric sickle cell patients. *Am J Hematol.* 1998;59(3):192-198

30. Segal JB, Miller ER, Brereton NH, Resar LM. Concentrations of B vitamins and homocysteine in children with sickle cell anemia. *So Med J.* 2004;97(2):149-155

31. Houston PE, Rana S, Sekhsaria S, Perlin E, Kim KS, Castro OL. Homocysteine in sickle cell disease: relationship to stroke. *Am J Med.* 1997;103(3):192-196

32. van der Dijs FP, Fokkema MR, Dijck-Brouwer DA, et al. Optimization of folic acid, vitamin B12, and vitamin B6 supplements in pediatric patients with sickle cell disease. *Am J Hematol.* 2002;69(4):239-246

33. Nelson MC, Zemel BS, Kawchak DA, et al. Vitamin B_6 status of children with sickle cell disease. *J Pediatr Hematol Oncol.* 2002;24(6):463-469

34. Jaja SI, Ikotun AR, Gbenebitse S, Temiye EO. Blood pressure, hematologic and erythrocyte fragility changes in children suffering from sickle cell anemia following ascorbic acid supplementation. *J Trop Pediatr.* 2002;48(6):366-370

35. Lachant NA, Tanaka KR. Antioxidants in sickle cell disease: the in vitro effects of ascorbic acid. *Am J Med Sci.* 1986;292(1):3-10

36. Nienhuis AW. Vitamin C and iron. *N Engl J Med.* 1981;304(3):170-171

37. Wapnick AA, Lynch SR, Charlton RW, Seftel HC, Bothwell TH. The effect of ascorbic acid deficiency on desferrioxamine induced urinary iron excretion. *Br J Hematol.* 1969;17(6):563-568

38. Chapman RW, Hussain MA, Gorman A, et al. Effect of ascorbic acid deficiency on serum ferritin concentration in patients with B-thalassemia major and iron overload. *J Clin Pathol.* 1982;35(5):487-491

39. Institute of Medicine, Food and Nutrition Board. *Dietary Reference Intakes for Calcium and Vitamin D.* Washington, DC: National Academies Press; 2011

40. Vogiatzi MG, Macklin EA, Trachtenberg FL, et al. Differences in the prevalence of growth, endocrine and vitamin D abnormalities among the various thalassemia syndromes in North America. *Br J Hematol*. 2009;146(5):546-556

41. Napoli N, Carmina E, Bucchieri S, Sferrazza C, Rini GB, Di Fede G. Low serum levels of 25-hydroxy vitamin D in adults affected by thalassemia major or intermedia. *Bone*. 2006;38(6):888-892

42. Soliman A, Adel A, Wagdy M, Al Ali M, El Mulla N. Calcium homeostasis in 40 adolescents with beta-thalassemia major: a case control study of the effects of intramuscular injection of a megadose of cholecalciferol. *Pediatr Endocrinol Rev*. 2008;6(Suppl 1):149-154

43. Shamshirsaz AA, Bekheirnia MR, Kamgar M, et al. Metabolic and endocrinologic complications in beta-thalassemia major: a multicenter study in Tehran. *BMC Endocr Disord*. 2003;3(1):4

44. Tantawy AA, El Kholy M, Moustafa T, et al. Bone mineral density and calcium metabolism in adolescents with beta-thalassemia major. *Pediatr Endocrinol Rev*. 2008;6(Suppl 1):132-135

45. Wood JC, Claster S, Carson S, et al. Vitamin D deficiency, cardiac iron and cardiac function in thalassemia major. *Br J Haematol*. 2008;141(6):891-894

46. Dimitriadou M, Christoforidis A, Economou M, et al. Elevated serum parahormone levels are associated with myocardial iron load in patients with beta-thalassemia major. *Eur J Haematol*. 2010;84(1):64-71

47. Vogiatzi MG, Macklin EA, Fung EB, et al. Bone disease in thalassemia: a frequent and still unresolved problem. *J Bone Miner Res*. 2009;24(3):543-557

48. Buison AM, Kawchak DA, Schall JI, Ohene-Frempong K, Stallings VA, Zemel BS. Low vitamin D status in children with sickle cell disease. *J Pediatr*. 2004;145:622-627

49. Rovner A, Stallings VA, Kawchak DA, Schall JI, Ohene-Frempong K, Zemel BS. High risk of vitamin D deficiency in children with sickle cell disease. *J Am Diet Assoc*. 2008;108(9):1512-1516

50. Almeida A, Roberts I. Bone involvement in sickle cell disease. *Br J Hematol*. 2005;129(4):482-490

51. Adewoye AH, Chen TC, Ma Q, et al. Sickle cell bone disease: response to vitamin D and calcium. *Am J Hematol*. 2008;83(4):271-274

52. Fung EB, Aguilar C, Micaily I, Foote D, Lal A. Treatment of vitamin D deficiency in transfusion-dependent thalassemia. *Am J Hematol*. 2011;86(10):871-873

53. Marwah SS, Wheelwright D, Blann AD, et al. Vitamin E correlates inversely with non-transferrin-bound iron in sickle cell disease. *Br J Haematol*. 2001;114(4):917-919

54. Nur E, Biemond BJ, Otten HM, Brandjes DP, Schnog JJ. Oxidative stress in sickle cell disease; pathophysiology and potential implications for disease management. *Am J Hematol*. 2011;86(6):484-489

55. Ray D, Deshmukh P, Goswami K, Garg N. Antioxidant vitamin levels in sickle cell disorders. *Natl Med J India*. 2007;20(1):11-13

VI

56. Ren H, Ghebremeskel K, Okpala I, Lee A, Ibegbulam O, Crawford M. Patients with sickle cell disease have reduced blood antioxidant protection. *Int J Vitam Nutr Res*. 2008;78(3):139-147

57. Marwah SS, Blann AD, Rea C, Phillips JD, Wright J, Bareford D. Reduced vitamin E antioxidant capacity in sickle cell disease is related to transfusion status but not to sickle crisis. *Am J Hematol*. 2002;69(2):144-146

58. Hasanato R. Zinc and antioxidant vitamin deficiency in patients with severe sickle cell anemia. *Ann Saudi Med*. 2006;26(1):17-21

59. Muskiet FA, Muskiet FD, Meiborg G, Schermer JG. Supplementation of patients with homozygous sickle cell disease with zinc, alpha-tocopherol, vitamin D, soybean oil and fish oil. *Am J Clin Nutr*. 1991;54(4):736-744

60. Schall JI, Zemel BS, Kawchak DA, Ohene-Frempong K, Stallings VA. Vitamin A status and outcomes in young children with sickle cell disease. *J Pediatr*. 2004;145(1):99-106

61. Chiu D, Vichinsky E, Yee M, Kleman K, Lubin B. Peroxidation, vitamin E and sickle cell anemia. *Ann NY Acad Sci*. 1982;393:323-335

62. Walter PB, Fung EB, Killilea DW, et al. Oxidative stress and inflammation in iron-overloaded patients with β-thalassaemia or sickle cell disease. *Br J Haematol*. 2006;135(2):254-263

63. Claster S, Wood JC, Noetzli L, Carson SM, Hofstra TC, Khanna R, Coates TD. Nutritional deficiencies in iron overloaded patients with hemoglobinopathies. *Am J Hematol*. 2009;84(6):344-348

64. Pfeifer WP, Degasperi GR, Almeida MT, Vercesi AE, Costa FF, Saad ST. Vitamin E supplementation reduces oxidative stress in beta thalassemia intermedia. *Acta Haematol*. 2008;10(4):225-231

65. Tesoriere L, D'Arpa D, Butera D, et al. Oral supplements of vitamin E improve measures of oxidative stress in plasma and reduce oxidative damage to LDL and erythrocytes in beta-thalassemia intermedia patients. *Free Radic Res*. 2001;34(5):529-540

66. Unchern S, Laoharuangpanya N, Phumala N, et al. The effects of vitamin E on platelet activity in beta-thalassemia patients. *Br J Haematol*. 2003;123(4):738-744

67. Kajanchumpol S, Tatu T, Sasanakul W, Chuansumrit A, Hathirat P. Zinc and copper status of thalassemia children. *Southeast Asian J Trop Med Pub Health*. 1997;28(4):877-880

68. Arcasoy A, Cavdar AO. Changes in trace minerals (serum zinc, copper and magnesium) in thalassemia. *Acta Haematologica*. 1975;53(6):341-346

69. Bekheirnia MR, Shamshirsaz AA, Kamgar M, et al. Serum zinc and its relation to bone mineral density in beta-thalassemic adolescents. *Biol Trace Elem Res*. 2004;97(3):215-224

70. Cianciulli P, Sollecito D, Sorrentino F, et al. Early detection of nephrotoxic effects in thalassemic patients receiving deferoxamine therapy. *Kidney Int*. 1994;46(2):467-470

71. Uysal Z, Akar N, Kemahli S, Dincer N, Arcasoy A. Desferrioxamine and urinary zinc excretion in b-thalassemia major. *Pediatr Hematol Oncol*. 1993;10(3):257-260

72. Al-Refaie FN, Wonke B, Wickens DC, Aydinok Y, Fielding A, Hoffbrand AV. Zinc concentration in patients with iron-overload receiving oral iron chelator 1,2-dimethyl-3-hydroxypyrid-4-one or deferoxamine. *J Clin Pathol*. 1994;47(7):657-660

73. Maclean KH, Cleveland JL, Porter JB. Cellular zinc content is a major determinant of iron chelator-induced apoptosis of thymocytes. *Blood*. 2001;98(13):3831-3839

74. Arcasoy A, Cavdar A, Cin S, et al. Effects of zinc supplementation on linear growth in beta thalassemia (a new approach). *Am J Hematol*. 1987;24(2):127-136

75. Shamshirsaz AA, Bekheirnia MR, Kamgar M, et al. Bone mineral density in Iranian adolescents and young adults with beta-thalassemia major. *Pediatr Hematol Oncol*. 2007;24(7):469-479

76. Dehshal MH, Hooghooghi AH, Kebryaeezadeh A, et al. Zinc deficiency aggravates abnormal glucose metabolism in thalassemia major patients. *Med Sci Monit*. 2007;13(5):CR235-CR239

77. Prasad AS, Schoomaker EB, Ortega J, Brewer GJ, Oberleas D, Oelshlegel FJ. Zinc deficiency in sickle cell disease. *Clin Chem*. 1975;21(4):582-587

78. Prasad AS. Zinc deficiency in patients with sickle cell disease. *Am J Clin Nutr*. 2002;75(2):181-182

79. Zemel BS, Kawchak DA, Fung EB, Ohene-Frempong K, Stallings V. Effect of zinc supplementation on growth and body composition in children with sickle cell disease. *Am J Clin Nutr*. 2002;75(2):300-307

80. Prasad AS, Abbasi AA, Rabbani P, DuMouchelle E. Effect of zinc supplementation on serum testosterone level in adult male sickle cell anemia subjects. *Am J Hematol*. 1981;10(2):119-127

81. Prasad AS, Beck F, Kaplan J, Chandrasekar PH, Ortega J, Fitzgerald JT, Swerdlow P. Effect of zinc supplementation on incidence of infections and hospital admissions in sickle cell disease. *Am J Hematol*. 1999;61(3):194-202

82. Morris CR, Suh JH, Hagar W, et al. Erythrocyte glutamine depletion, altered redox environment, and pulmonary hypertension in sickle cell disease. *Blood*. 2008;111(1):402-410

83. Morris CR, Kuypers FA, Larkin S, Vichinsky EP, Styles LA. Patterns of arginine and nitric oxide in patients with sickle cell disease with vasoocclusive crisis and acute chest syndrome. *J Pediatr Hematol Oncol*. 2000;22(6):515-520

84. Morris CR, Kato GJ, Poljakovic M, et al. Dysregulated arginine metabolism, hemolysis-associated pulmonary hypertension, and mortality in sickle cell disease. *JAMA*. 2005;294(1):81-90

85. Sullivan KJ, Kissoon N, Sandler E, et al. Effect of oral arginine supplementation on exhaled nitric oxide concentration in sickle cell anemia and acute chest syndrome. *J Pediatr Hematol Oncol*. 2010;32(7):e249-e258

86. Morris CR, Morris SM Jr, Hagar W, et al. Arginine therapy: a new treatment for pulmonary hypertension in sickle cell disease? *Am J Respir Crit Care*. 2003;168(1):63-69

87. Sayetta RB. Pica: an overview. *Am Fam Physician*. 1986;33(5):181-185

88. Lemanek KL, Brown RT, Amstrong FD, et al. Dysfunctional eating patterns and symptoms of pica in children and adolescents with sickle cell disease. *Clin Pediatr (Phila)*. 2002;41(7):493-500

89. Ivascu NS, Sarnaik S, McCrae J, et al. Characterization of pica prevalence among patients with sickle cell disease. *Arch Pediatr Adolesc Med*. 2001;155(11):1243-1247

VI

90. Danford DE. Pica and nutrition. *Ann Rev Nutr*. 1982;2:303-322

91. Rector WG Jr. Pica: its frequency: significance in patients with iron deficiency anemia due to chronic gastrointestinal blood loss. *J Gen Intern Med*. 1989;4(6):512-513

92. Chen XC, Yin TA, He JS, et al. Low levels of zinc in hair and blood, pica, anorexia and poor growth in Chinese preschool children. *Am J Clin Nutr*. 1985;42(4):694-700

93. Lofts RH, Schroeder SR, Maier RH. Effects of serum zinc supplementation on pica behavior of persons with mental retardation. *Am J Ment Retard*. 1990;95(1):103-109

94. Robinson BA, Tolan W, Golding-Beecher O. Childhood pica: some aspects of the clinical profile in Manchester, Jamaica. *West Indian Med J*. 1990;39(1):20-26

95. de Alarcon PA, Donovan ME, Forbes GB, Landaw SA, Stockman JA III. Iron absorption in the thalassemia syndromes and its inhibition by tea. *N Engl J Med*. 1979;300(1):5-8

96. Buison AM, Kawchak DA, Schall JI, et al. Bone area and bone mineral content deficits in children with sickle cell disease. *Pediatrics*. 2005;116(4):943-949

97. Lal A, Fung EB, Pakbaz Z, Hackney-Stephens E, Vichinsky EP. Bone mineral density in children with sickle cell anemia. *Pediatr Blood Cancer*. 2006;47(7):901-906

98. Buchowski MS, de la Fuente FA, Flakoll PJ, Chen KY, Turner EA. Increased bone turnover is associated with protein and energy metabolism in adolescents with sickle cell anemia. *Am J Physiol Endocrinol*. 2001;280(3):e518-e527

99. American Academy of Pediatrics, Committee on Genetics. Health supervision for children with sickle cell disease. *Pediatrics*. 2002;109(3):526-535. Reaffirmed January 2006

100. National Heart, Lung, and Blood Institute. *The Management of Sickle Cell Disease*. Washington, DC: National Institutes of Health, National Heart, Lung, and Blood Institute; 2004. NIH Publication No. 04-2117

101. Cappellini MD, Cohen A, Eleftheriou A, Piga A, Porter J, Taher A, eds. *Guidelines for the Clinical Management of Thalassemia*. 2nd ed rev. Nicosia, Cyprus: Thalassemia International Federation; 2008

102. Northern California Comprehensive Thalassemia Center. Nutrition. In: *Standard-of-Care Clinical Practice Guidelines (2012)*. Oakland, CA: Northern California Comprehensive Thalassemia Center; 2012. Available at: http://hemonc.cho.org/thalassemia/treatment-guidelines-16.aspx. Accessed January 14, 2013

Chapter 42

Nutritional Management of Children With Kidney Disease

Introduction

Individuals with normal renal function have great latitude in the quantity (and quality) of the nutrients they can ingest. Unfortunately, individuals with kidney disease have less latitude in their nutritional choices because of decreased renal excretion and/or increased renal tubular losses. Infants and children with renal disease may have decreased appetites and insufficient energy intakes, which further limit nutrition and growth.[1] Nutritional prescriptions can be complex, and it is often necessary to restrict the intake of some nutrients (see Table 42.1) while at the same time supplementing other nutrients to maintain homeostasis and support growth. Reasonable starting points for diet prescriptions are noted in Table 42.2.

Table 42.1.
Food Sources of Selected Nutrients

Sodium	Fast food, microwavable products, and snack foods, such as chips, contribute significant sodium to the diet. Appealing to parents to make lifestyle changes for the entire family may be effective and necessary. Foods that should be limited when sodium restriction is recommended include the following: • Convenience products (frozen, packaged, or canned), including pizza, macaroni and cheese, meat stew, spaghetti, and burritos. **Use** frozen entrees with the lowest sodium content. • Cured, salted, canned, or smoked meats, including ham, corned beef, jerky, salt pork, luncheon meats, bacon, sausage, hot dogs/frankfurters, sausage, canned tuna or salmon, and sardines. **Use** fresh meats or those frozen without added sauces. • Processed cheese, cheese spreads, or buttermilk. **Use** low-sodium cheese, ricotta/mozzarella cheese, and cream cheese. • Regular canned or frozen soups and bouillon cubes, and instant soup or dried noodle cups. **Use** low-sodium soups or homemade soups without salt or bouillon cubes, and fresh-cooked pasta and grains. • Salted crackers and snack foods, such as potato chips. **Use** unsalted chips, unsalted pretzels, and unsalted popcorn or crackers. • Regular canned vegetables, vegetable juices, or those frozen with salt. **Use** fresh or frozen vegetables without added salt; if canned, use "no salt added" vegetables and sauces.

VI

Table 42.1. *(continued)*
Food Sources of Selected Nutrients

Potassium	Juices, fruits, vegetables, and nuts contribute the most significant sources of potassium to the diet. If restricted, a multivitamin supplement may be necessary to provide micronutrient needs. Herbal products may provide significant potassium and should be avoided in children. Examples of high-potassium foods: orange juice, carrot juice, avocados, bananas, cantaloupes, dried fruits (raisins, apricots, banana, etc), oranges, potatoes, sweet potatoes, tomatoes, chocolate, lentils, dried beans (cooked), and nuts. Examples of **low**-potassium foods: cranberry juice and apple juice, apples, grapes, peaches, pears, pineapple, strawberries, watermelon, green beans, lettuce, zucchini, bread, dried pasta (cooked), and tortillas.
Phosphorus	Milk and milk products, plus meat, chicken, fish, eggs, and nuts provide the most significant sources of phosphorus in the diet. Ironically, dairy products generally are the most popular protein source for children. Limiting dairy products and utilizing phosphate binders with meals is the treatment goal. Calcium supplementation may be required, because limiting phosphorus in the diet automatically limits calcium as well.

Table 42.2.
Reasonable Starting Points for Diet Prescription in Kidney Disease

Overview						
Evaluating patient and family lifestyle eating patterns may reveal areas that can be improved without limiting all sources of the nutrient in question. Ongoing nutritional follow-up is important to monitor nutrient intake and assess adequacy.						
Obtain a detailed diet history to determine current food and beverage intake. All diet changes are based on evaluation of this current intake. Focus on decreasing the amount of frequently-consumed high sources of elevated nutrients.						
Resist the temptation to restrict nutrients until there is a need demonstrated.						
The word "low" in front of a nutrient ("low sodium,""low potassium") is not a diet order. Be specific (suggestions below). "Renal" is not a diet order.						
Selective micronutrient restrictions may result in the patient refusing to consume adequate amounts of macronutrients (calories, protein, and fat). Follow-up is important to ensure adequacy of intake to meet growth needs.						
Limit as few nutrients as possible to optimize intake.						

Nutrient	Possible Diet Order	Description	Recommended Starting Points			Comments
			Weight	Outpatient	Inpatient With Severe Edema	
Sodium	3–4 g sodium (formerly No Added Salt)	Food is cooked with some salt; high sources such as pizza, hot dogs, and chips are limited or avoided	<20 kg	Begin with 2 g/day	1 g/day	A sodium restriction will automatically decrease fat intake in most children
	2 g sodium	Food is prepared with no salt; high sources are eliminated.	>20 kg	Begin with 3 g/day	2 g/day	
	1 g sodium	Food is prepared with no salt; low-sodium products are used exclusively				

Table 42.2. (continued)
Reasonable Starting Points for Diet Prescription in Kidney Disease

Nutrient	Possible Diet Order	Description	Recommended Starting Points			Comments
			Weight	Outpatient	Inpatient With Severe Edema	
Potassium	Limit food sources with high potassium content	Frequently consumed high-potassium foods (see Table 42.1) are decreased or eliminated		Limit only high sources of potassium if child is currently eating/drinking		Often, initially limiting frequently consumed foods like potatoes, bananas, and orange juice is sufficient to control serum potassium levels. Correct acidosis, bleeding, and other potential causes of elevated potassium.
Phosphorus	800 mg/day	High sources are limited to 8 ounces of milk/day or the phosphorus equivalent of cheese, yogurt, ice cream, beans, nuts		Start with 800 mg/day, smaller children will consume less because of smaller portion sizes		Infants require higher serum phosphorus levels for adequate bone mineralization. Start phosphorus binders with meals as necessary. A phosphorus limitation will automatically limit protein and potassium intake. Calcium intake may be insufficient (unless calcium binders are given).
	600 mg/day	Milk, milk products, beans, nuts, chocolate are eliminated				
Protein	Regular diet	Highest sources include meat, poultry, fish, egg, dairy products		Start with a diet history to determine need, if any, to restrict protein.		Children with rising blood urea nitrogen (BUN) levels rarely consume more than the DRI due to poor appetite and phosphorus restriction. Ensure adequate calorie intake for protein-sparing; otherwise BUN may be elevated because of protein catabolism. Protein needs are elevated in dialysis; see Table 42.5.

This chapter discusses nutritional considerations in a variety of renal conditions that affect infants, children, and adolescents. Whenever possible, evidence-based recommendations for nutritional support will be provided, and controlled studies will be cited. Unfortunately, critical studies in children are often lacking; therefore, studies performed in adults are referenced.

The Food and Nutrition Board of the Institute of Medicine has presented standards in the form of dietary reference intakes (DRIs). Previously, this information was presented as Recommended Dietary Allowances (RDAs). For the nutrients to be discussed, there is often little difference between the 2 values. Within this paper, the term RDA is used when describing experimental results performed using RDAs as standards, and the term DRI is used when noting current standards.

Urinary Tract Infections, Vesicoureteral Reflux, and Urinary Incontinence

Urinary tract infections (UTIs [often associated with vesicoureteral reflux]) are commonly seen in pediatric patients. There are no data demonstrating a clear role for special nutritional management of children with recurrent UTIs, whether or not there is associated reflux. Recurrent UTIs are associated with constipation, which often responds to dietary manipulation as part of a treatment program. In pediatrics, only one controlled study examining the effect of diet on UTIs has been performed. In this study of 84 girls, ages 3 through 14 years, the authors demonstrated a decline in recurrent UTIs after daily ingestion of 7.5 g of cranberry concentrate.[2] The experimental group of 28 girls was compared with girls in 2 control groups receiving either *Lactobacillus* products or their usual diet. In a recent meta-analysis of several studies, there is some evidence that cranberry juice, administered in varying amounts and concentrations, decreased the incidence of symptomatic UTIs over a 12-month period in adult women but not in children or individuals requiring chronic catheterization.[3] It is uncertain whether cranberry juice is effective in other susceptible groups.

Primary nocturnal enuresis is a common pediatric condition. Although it has been suggested that the introduction of a low-allergen diet can successfully cure enuresis, only 2 controlled studies are available, the number of treated patients is small, and the studies have not been replicated.[4] It is generally agreed that limiting fluid intakes in the evening or after dinner is ineffective and unwarranted. There are also no nutritional issues associated with urinary incontinence, although there is anecdotal evidence that elimination diets have been of benefit for children with nocturnal enuresis.[5]

VI

Hypertension

Epidemiologic data are abundant on the association between childhood obesity and high blood pressure.[6] Body weights track from childhood through adulthood, and there is strong evidence that obesity or increased body mass index (BMI) is related to hypertension.[7-10] Dietary modification aimed at weight stabilization (or slow weight loss in the older adolescent) to normalize BMI is appropriate.[11] The reported increase in the incidence of childhood obesity and the development of the metabolic syndrome and its implications for the development of hypertension have been noted.[12-15] It is clear that for individuals of any age, weight loss is difficult both to achieve and to maintain. In the past, attention was focused on having the individual lose most or all of their excess weight, but it has become evident that moderate weight reduction (weight loss in the range of 5%-10% of initial body weight) is also effective at lowering blood pressure.[16] The DASH (Dietary Approach to Stop Hypertension) eating plan, a low-fat, low-sodium, high-potassium diet, has been shown to be associated with modest weight loss and a significant decrease in blood pressure.[17-19]

Sodium restriction is recommended, although the safety and efficacy of long-term sodium restriction in children and adolescents has not been established.[4,20-23] In adults, lowering sodium intake has an additive effect on the decrease in blood pressure seen with the DASH diet.[24] In a meta-analysis of trials conducted in children, sodium reduction lowered mean systolic blood pressure (SBP)/diastolic blood pressure (DBP) by 1.2/1.3 mm Hg.[25] In addition, high-sodium foods are often calorie dense and should be limited. The National Health and Nutrition Examination Survey (NHANES) III noted that the average sodium intakes for children between 3 and 18 years of age ranged between 2.8 and 4.6 g/day. The Institute of Medicine, through its Food and Nutrition Board, has suggested that a much lower quantity of sodium is adequate for otherwise healthy infants and children[26] (Table 42.3). Unfortunately, it is often difficult to achieve these levels of sodium intake, but they are certainly a safe and an appropriate goal. Depending on the child's usual sodium intake, restricting sodium intake to 2 to 3 g/day may be a reasonable starting point.

Table 42.3.
Dietary Reference Intakes (DRIs): Recommended Intakes for Individuals, Macronutrients[26]

Age	Protein (g/d)	Protein g/ kg/d	Sodium g/d	Phosphorous mg/d	Calcium mg/d	Potassium g/d
Infants						
0–6 mo	9.1	1.5	0.12	100	210	0.4
7–12 mo	**11**	**1.5**	0.37	275	270	0.7
Children						
1–3 y	**13**	**1.1**	1	**460**	500	3
4–8 y	**19**	**0.95**	1.2	**500**	800	3.8
Males						
9–13 y	**34**	**0.95**	1.5	**1250**	1300	4.5
14–18 y	**52**	**0.85**	1.5	**1250**	1300	4.7
Females						
9–13 y	**34**	**0.95**	1.5	1250	1300	4.5
14–18 y	**46**	**0.85**	1.5	1250	1300	4.7

[a] Unbolded values are adequate intake (AI) the recommended average daily intake level based on observed or experimentally determined approximations or estimates of nutrient intake by a group (or groups) of apparently healthy people that are assumed to be adequate—used when an DRI cannot be determined.

[b] Values in **bold** typeface are listed as the DRI – adequate for 97.5% of the population.

Epidemiologic and clinical data have suggested that increased dietary calcium and potassium may be effective in helping to lower blood pressures,[27-32] but data on the effectiveness of potassium or calcium supplements are scant.[33] The lack of dose-response trials hinders recommendations on desirable levels of potassium intake as a means to lower blood pressure. Encouraging a diet high in fruits and vegetables is appropriate as a means of increasing dietary potassium intake and is safe in individuals with normal renal function. However, in people with significant renal impairment, potassium intake needs to be carefully monitored and/or modified.[34]

Manipulations of dietary magnesium or fiber may prove to be beneficial, but data in children are lacking.[35,36] Studies in adults and infants suggest that diets or infant formulas supplementing long-chain polyunsaturated fatty acids are associated with lower blood pressures,[37] but again, data in children are unavailable.

Kidney Stone Disorders
Most renal stones are formed of calcium and oxalate; less commonly, cystine or uric acid are the main constituents. Although there are a variety of conditions that predispose children to renal stones, there are certain common therapeutic interventions. In all cases, a high fluid intake is the primary recommendation. Children

VI

should be encouraged to drink at least 1.5 to 2 times their calculated maintenance fluid requirements (opinion-based recommendation). If necessary, children should be encouraged to get up in the middle of the night to urinate and then drink additional fluid before going back to bed. The fluids the child chooses to drink may have an effect on the child's total caloric intake, and the family should be instructed to provide at least 50% of the intake as water. A simple method to assess the adequacy of fluid intake is to tell the child/family that the urine should be clear and not yellow in color (opinion-based recommendation).

Renal sodium reabsorption is linked to the reabsorption of a variety of other chemicals, including calcium and the amino acid cystine (the source of kidney stones in the inherited condition, cystinuria). Salt-restricted diets should be advised, because high sodium intakes lead to increased sodium excretion and, hence, increased calcium and cystine excretion. Conversely, low-sodium diets lead to decreased calcium and cystine excretion. When a low-sodium diet is insufficient to lower calcium or cystine excretion, a distal tubule diuretic is often added.

In adults, protein restriction has been associated with decreased renal stone formation. Because of the importance of protein intake to growth, low-protein diets cannot be recommended, but there is little harm in limiting protein intake to the DRI for age (Table 42.2).

There is no role for dietary calcium restriction, and calcium should be provided at the level of the DRI (Table 42.3). Epidemiologic data in adults suggest that high-calcium diets may be effective in decreasing the risk of recurrent calcium stones.[38-41]

Hyperoxaluria can be divided into primary (hereditary) and secondary forms. There is no evidence that limiting dietary oxalate is of value in patients with the metabolic defects associated with primary hyperoxaluria. For children with secondary hyperoxaluria or with hypercalciuria and mild hyperoxaluria, avoidance of high-oxalate foods (see Table 42.4) is prudent.[42,43] Vitamin C should be limited to 100 mg/day or less, because ascorbate is converted to oxalate in alkaline urine.

Table 42.4.
Foods With High Oxalate Content[43]

Spinach
Rhubarb
Beets
Nuts
Chocolate
Tea
Wheat bran
Strawberries

A small percentage of children with recurrent renal stones pass stones composed predominantly of uric acid. There is no evidence that restricting the intake of foods with a high purine content alters the rate of stone formation.[44,45] The goal is to achieve but not exceed the DRI for protein (Table 42.3).

Renal Tubular Defects

Renal tubules serve to reabsorb water and chemicals lost to the body as a consequence of glomerular filtration. Within the proximal tubule, these defects may be isolated to a single compound (eg, proximal renal tubular acidosis, hypophosphatemia) or present as multiple proximal renal tubular defects, a condition known as Fanconi syndrome. Disorders within the Loop of Henle or the distal convoluted tubule are associated with the loss of electrolytes and water and/or inability to acidify urine. Each of these abnormalities results in the development of abnormal serum electrolytes and necessitates the administration of supplements.

Infants and children with proximal renal tubular acidosis (pRTA) present with short stature, failure to thrive, and hypokalemic, hypochloremic metabolic acidosis. Appropriate treatment includes the oral administration of large amounts of bicarbonate (often 10-20 mEq/kg/day) as well as supplemental potassium.

The proximal tubule is the main site for the renal reabsorption of phosphorus. A proximal tubular defect in phosphorus reabsorption leads to hypophosphatemic rickets, a condition characterized by short stature and a variety of other associated findings.[46,47] Treatment consists of phosphorus supplementation; doses of 30 to 90 mg/kg/day may be necessary, administered 3 or 4 times during the day. Unfortunately, this dose of phosphorus may cause diarrhea, and supplementation must begin with lower doses, increasing the daily intake as tolerated. Although serum calcium concentrations are often normal prior to therapy, the administration of phosphorus leads to hypocalcemia and secondary hyperparathyroidism, necessitating the concurrent administration of one of the activated forms of vitamin D. Because proximal tubule abnormalities are associated with the loss of large quantities of metabolites, replenishment must be administered multiple times per day, and in some cases, it is necessary to use continuous overnight supplementation to achieve treatment goals.

Children with distal tubular defects may have distal renal tubular acidosis (dRTA); a condition characterized by an inability to excrete an acid urine. Children with dRTA require alkali in the range of 1 to 5 mEq/kg/day, a significantly lower dose than that required by children with pRTA. Individuals with dRTA, are also at risk of developing renal calculi and nephrocalcinosis as a result of hypercalciuria and their inability to excrete acid urine. Other disorders of the Loop of Henle or distal tubule (most commonly Bartter or Gitelman syndromes) are associated with renal

VI

potassium and magnesium wasting. In these conditions, oral potassium and magnesium replacements are indicated in doses dependent on measured serum concentrations. Because these conditions are often associated with urinary sodium loss, it may be necessary add sodium chloride supplements to the diet, particularly in infants and younger children.

Nephrotic Syndrome

Nephrotic syndrome is defined clinically by the presence of proteinuria, hypoalbuminemia, edema, and hypercholesterolemia. Edema results from the abnormal salt (and water) retention seen in this condition. The mainstay of dietary therapy for children with nephrotic syndrome is sodium restriction. Although no studies have defined the optimal level to which sodium should be restricted in these children, reasonable estimates are noted in Table 42.2. This level of sodium restriction requires that the entire family adjust their eating habits, at the least by taking the salt shaker off the table, limiting processed foods, and eliminating salted snack foods. The majority of pediatric patients respond to corticosteroids and can be weaned off of steroids within 3 to 6 months. Unfortunately, most will relapse and require the reinstitution of steroid therapy. A minority of children will require the use of additional/other medications to limit proteinuria and keep them edema free. Because most forms of nephrotic syndrome recur, it should be explained to the family that it would be best for them to adopt healthy dietary habits and limit their salt intake indefinitely. Given the association between steroid use, weight gain, and hypertension, all patients would benefit from nutritional counseling as well as increased physical activity.

At times, children with severe edema may have to be hospitalized for aggressive fluid removal. One common error is the provision of intravenous "maintenance" or "partial maintenance" fluids. In the absence of intravascular volume depletion, there is no need to provide intravenous fluids, and unnecessary salt and water administration should be avoided. Although it is possible to aggressively limit oral sodium intake in hospitalized patients, very low-sodium diets are generally unpalatable, will be successful only for a limited time during the inpatient period, and are unlikely to be followed outside the hospital setting.

Serum albumin concentrations cannot be restored to normal by nutritional supplementation, and there are both animal and adult human data that demonstrate that serum albumin concentrations actually improve using low-protein diets.[48] However, no data address this in pediatric patients, and again, low protein intakes must be weighed against the concern for the development of malnutrition and poor growth in pediatric patients. Suggested protein intakes are, therefore, set no lower than the DRI for age (Table 42.3).

Infants with congenital nephrotic syndrome typically have very high levels of proteinuria and commonly develop clinical evidence of protein depletion. Nutritional care in this group of infants is complex, often requiring both enteral feeding and repeated albumin infusions to prevent severe hypoproteinemia and edema.[49] The complexity of care in this patient group makes referral to specialized pediatric centers inevitable.

Hypercholesterolemia is common in these patients, both as component of the nephrotic syndrome and steroid administration. Although prolonged hyperlipidemia is a recognized cardiovascular risk factor, it does not appear that the transient hypercholesterolemia seen in children who recovered from the nephrotic syndrome has any negative effect on cardiovascular mortality later in life.[50] Unfortunately, there are few data supporting the use of low-fat diets to lower cholesterol levels[51] and only minimal pediatric data in this condition on the use of cholesterol-lowering agents.[52] However, because in a given patient, the outcome of the nephrotic syndrome may be unknown and steroid usage as well as high-fat diets encourage weight gain, attention to dietary lipid content is prudent. Fortunately, limiting dietary sodium also limits the consumption of high-fat foods popular with children (hot dogs, pizza, and cheese). The ubiquitous presence of high-sodium, high-fat foods makes dietary recommendations complex, and families often benefit from dietary counseling by a registered dietitian. The medical and dietary approach to children with persistent nephrotic syndrome and resultant hyperlipidemia remains a dilemma. Although there is evidence that medication does lower cholesterol and low-density lipoprotein concentrations, there is currently no consensus as to the best approach to the treatment of hyperlipidemia in the young child with nephrotic syndrome.

Glomerulonephritis

Clinically, glomerulonephritis is characterized by the presence of both hematuria and proteinuria. Renal function may be reduced, and patients often develop hypervolemia and/or hypertension. If the nephrotic syndrome is also present, hyperlipidemia is likely. The nutritional management of these patients depends on how well renal function is maintained. In the setting of hypervolemia and hypertension, sodium restriction is required. There are significant differences between acute and chronic renal insufficiency, because in the former, there is little time for the development of the renal compensatory adjustments that are often seen in the

VI

chronic state. The care of children with glomerulonephritis is, therefore, dependent on whether the condition is acute or chronic as well as on the presence of associated finings, such as hypertension or the nephrotic syndrome.

Acute Renal Failure

Acute renal failure (ARF) is defined as an abrupt decline in the glomerular filtration rate (GFR) and is most often caused either by underperfusion of the kidneys (eg, during hypovolemic shock) or is the result of intrinsic renal disease. Intrinsic renal diseases are usually forms of acute glomerulonephritis or the hemolytic uremic syndrome. Acute renal failure may either be associated with low levels of urinary water output (oliguria/anuria) or with normal or even increased urine volumes (nonoliguric renal failure). In general, patients with acute renal failure cannot adjust urine output effectively, and the physician will be called on to manage fluid intakes to prevent either volume overload or depletion. Irrespective of the volume of urine output, individuals with acute renal failure are unable to control the excretion of metabolic wastes, such as urea, sodium, potassium, phosphorus, and acid. Specific dietary requirements will depend on the clinical circumstances but general recommendations are possible. When hypertension and volume overload are a concern, sodium (and often fluid volume) should be limited. Individuals with oligoanuria who are not clinically volume overloaded should receive daily fluid intakes equivalent to their urine output plus estimated insensible water loss. Potassium and phosphate intakes are often restricted, with allowable intakes based on the clinical setting.

There is no evidence to suggest that ARF, per se, leads to an increase in energy requirements. Even when ARF is associated with other conditions (eg, sepsis, multiple organ failure), recent studies using indirect calorimetry have shown that standard formulas used to compute energy requirements are inaccurate and overestimate actual energy requirements.[53,54] In the absences of direct measurements, caloric requirements should be provided at the level of the DRI for chronologic age (Table 42.5).

Table 42.5.
Recommended Energy and Protein Intakes in Children by Age[26,67,70]

Age	Predialysis		Hemodialysis		Peritoneal Dialysis	
	Energy[a]	Protein[b]	Energy[a]	Protein[b,c]	Energy[a,d]	Protein[b,e]
0-6 mo	100-110	2.2	100-110	2.6	100-110	3
6-12 mo	95-105	1.5	95-105	2	95-105	2.4
1-3 y	90	1.1	90	1.6	90	2.0
4-10 y	70	0.95	70	1.6	70	1.8-2.0
11-14 y (boys)	55	0.95	55	1.4	55	1.8
11-14 y (girls)	47	0.95	47	1.4	47	1.8
15-18 y (boys)	45	0.85	45	1.3	45	1.5
15-18 y (girls)	40	0.85	40	1.2	40	1.5

[a] kcal/kg/day.

[b] g/kg/day.

[c] Protein intakes increased by approximately 0.4 g/kg/day to account for hemodialysis losses.

[d] Note: up to 10% of the total caloric intake (10 kcal/kg/day) can be absorbed as dextrose via the dialysate. Obesity may become a concern for some children and adolescents on peritoneal dialysis.

[e] Protein requirements on peritoneal dialysis reflect the significant loss of proteins through the dialysis fluid.

Although there are good reasons to limit excess protein intake in ARF, a minimum protein intake of 1 g/kg/day is important to minimize protein catabolism. Amino acids that are not used for protein anabolism are degraded; their nitrogen contributes to excess urea production. Whenever possible, enteral nutrition should be used, but depending on the child's age and ability to tolerate enteral nutrition or to ingest solid foods, parenteral nutrition may be necessary. Except in the case of specialized commercial formulas, which limit electrolyte intake during enteral feeding, phosphorus intake and acid production are linearly related to protein intake. The best method available to maximize the efficiency of protein utilization is to provide adequate nonprotein calories. In the absence of dialysis therapy, an approximate goal is for the serum urea nitrogen concentration to increase at a rate of approximately between 10 to 20 mg/dL/day.

Nutritional goals in individuals with ARF include: maintaining appropriate hydration and electrolyte balance, providing adequate energy intake, optimizing nitrogen balance, and providing appropriate vitamin and mineral supplementation.[55] With the widespread availability of pediatric dialysis, including forms of continual renal replacement (collectively called CRRT), it is now possible to provide adequate nutritional intake for the majority of infants and children with

VI

ARF. Currently, dialysis therapies are instituted at an early stage to allow the provision of adequate nutrition.

Chronic Renal Failure

Current terminology divides chronic kidney disease (CKD) into 5 categories (Table 42.6). When renal function declines to a GFR of <60 mL/min/1.73 m² (stage 3), changes in blood chemistries become apparent and growth failure becomes more likely. The National Kidney Foundation Kidney Disease Outcomes Quality Initiative recently published consensus nutrition guidelines for the care of children with chronic kidney disease. These data are presented here in broad outlines, but the recommendations themselves are comprehensive and should be read by all involved in the care of children with CKD.[56]

Table 42.6.

National Kidney Foundation Kidney Disease Outcomes Quality Initiative Classification of the Stages of Chronic Kidney Disease (CKD)[79]

Stage	GFR (mL/min/1.73 m²)	Description	Action Plan
1	≥90	Kidney damage with normal or increased GFR	Treat primary and comorbid conditions Slow CKD progression, CVD risk reduction
2	60-89	Kidney damage with mild reduction of GFR	Estimate rate of progression of CKD
3	30-59	Moderate reduction of GFR	Evaluate and treat complications
4	15-29	Severe reduction of GFR	Prepare for kidney replacement therapy
5	<5	Kidney failure	Kidney replacement therapy

GFR indicates glomerular filtration rate; CVD, cardiovascular disease.

Spontaneous food (energy) intake is low in children with CKD.[1,55,57] Energy intake should be provided at approximately 100% to 120% of the DRI for age.[57]

There is no evidence that restricting protein intake to less than the DRI is effective at delaying progression of renal insufficiency[58,59] and some evidence that, at least in infants, low protein intakes may actually inhibit growth.[58] Because high protein intakes should also be avoided in CKD, the most appropriate recommendations are for protein intakes to be set at the DRI for age.[59-61] This is a modest restriction, because, when allowed unrestricted diets, children with CKD eat an average 120% to 150% of the DRI for protein.[1,62,63] With the progression of CKD to more severe stages, it is suggested that protein intake be limited to, at most, 110% to 120% of the DRI by stage 4 CKD.[56]

It is becoming increasingly clear that the maintenance of normal serum bicarbonate concentrations is vital in individuals with CKD. Acidosis appears to have deleterious effects on multiple aspects of metabolism, including protein degradation[64] and bone and statural growth[56] as well as a possible role in hastening the decline of GFR.[65] Current pediatric guidelines suggest that serum bicarbonate concentrations be maintained at 22 mmol/L or greater.[56] Because protein intake is related to acid formation, high protein intakes should be avoided. When necessary, acidosis can be treated with sodium bicarbonate or sodium citrate solutions.

The kidney has a remarkable ability to excrete potassium, but as renal function declines, it is reasonable to limit intake of foods with high potassium content. Hyperkalemia presenting in individuals with moderate CKD generally indicates an acute potassium overload (eg, dietary indiscretion, intravenous administration), a significant catabolic event, or dehydration. Analogous to the setting of acute renal failure, children with significant chronic renal disease may need more stringent potassium restriction.

Given the complex interplay between calcium, phosphate, vitamin D, parathyroid hormone, and the more recently discovered phosphate-controlling hormone, fibroblast growth factor 23 (FGF23), the control of serum calcium and phosphate concentrations is complex. Calcium absorption is decreased because of decreased oral intake and decreased vitamin D hydroxylation. Phosphorus excretion is dependent on renal function and urinary excretion decreases with progressive CKD, so phosphate intake should be limited to the DRI.

When serum phosphate concentrations are elevated, restriction to 80% of the DRI is suggested. In practice, these patients often receive oral calcium compounds that serve as phosphate binders as well as activated vitamin D analogues to increase enteral calcium absorption.

Poor control of serum calcium and phosphorus concentrations is associated with hyperparathyroidism, the development of metabolic bone disease, and an increased risk of cardiac calcification.[66] With the development of new activated vitamin D compounds as well as additional medications to prevent the absorption of dietary phosphate (sevelamer and lanthanum carbonate); the recent availability of a calcimimetic (cinacalcet), which decreases serum parathyroid hormone, calcium, and phosphate concentrations; and an increasing understanding of the role of FGF23, it is understandable that pediatric guidelines for the control of the metabolic bone disease associated with CKD remain in flux and subject to future modification.

VI

In the absence of hypertension or volume overload, it is reasonable to limit sodium intake to 2 to 3 g/day. When volume overload is present, sodium intake should be further limited, and diuretics may have to be administered. Because individuals drink to isotonicity, there is rarely a reason to specifically limit water intake.

One subset of children with chronic renal failure requires special mention—infants and toddlers with nonoliguric chronic renal failure, usually as a result of congenital hydronephrosis or renal dysplasia. These children may not be able to conserve sodium or bicarbonate despite advanced degrees of renal failure and often require sodium chloride and alkali supplementation. Signs of sodium depletion are often subtle and include listlessness, failure to gain weight despite adequate caloric intake, hyperkalemia, and hypercalcemia. It is reasonable to initiate supplementation with approximately 2 to 3 mEq/kg/day of sodium chloride. Substantially greater amounts of sodium may be necessary to ensure optimal growth. Sodium bicarbonate cannot substitute for sodium chloride to restore intravascular volume, and severe acidosis may not be apparent until the infants receive sufficient sodium chloride. Supplementation should be continued until the serum sodium concentration is greater than 140 mEq/L or the infant develops either hypertension or volume overload.[67]

Vitamins and Trace Minerals

With the exception of vitamin D, there is no evidence to indicate that the metabolism of fat-soluble vitamins is abnormal in CKD, and supplementation is not necessary. Vitamin A supplements should be specifically avoided, as vitamin A can accumulate in children with CKD resulting in vitamin A toxicity.[68] Vitamin E supplements are not necessary as a standard nutritional supplement.

Vitamin D has a special role in the care of these children. It is now clear that a high percentage of the normal pediatric population have suboptimal concentrations of 25-hydroxyvitamin D (25-OH-D).[69] Because 25-OH-D is converted to the active metabolite, 1,25-dihydroxyvitamin D (1,25-OH$_2$-D) primarily within the renal cortex, the combination of decreased renal mass plus low serum 25-OH-D concentrations is an early impediment to adequate to calcium absorption. Current guidelines suggest the yearly measurement of 25-OH-D concentrations with supplementation to achieve a serum 25-OH-D concentration of 20 ng/mL.[56]

Current recommendations state that well-balanced diets may not require vitamin supplementation.[70] Appropriate nutritional follow-up is required to be certain that limitations in dietary intake do not excessively restrict micronutrient intakes. Because of these concerns, supplements of the water-soluble vitamins are often provided to patients with CKD and end-stage renal disease. Excessive amounts of vitamin C can lead to increased serum oxalate concentrations. Particular attention should be paid to folate, because folate depletion can limit the effectiveness of administered erythropoietin. Hyperhomocysteinemia has been shown to be an independent predictor of heart disease. Although supplementation with vitamin B_6, folate, and vitamin B_{12} improves homocysteine concentrations in patients with normal renal function and those having undergone transplantation, there is no consensus on their efficacy in other individuals with CKD.[71]

Carnitine, a transporter of fatty acids, may be deficient in CKD, and carnitine supplementation has been suggested as a treatment for both hyperlipidemia and anemia.[72,73] Studies involving carnitine supplementation are difficult to interpret, at least in part because of the variety of dosages, time courses, and delivery methods used. There is little pediatric evidence available to support carnitine supplementation in pediatric patients and consequently routine supplementation is not recommended.[56,74,75]

There is little information available on the need for trace mineral supplementation for infants and children with CKD but it would appear that for most individuals, supplements are not required. In individual clinical situations, it may be prudent to assess serum concentrations as an approximation of body stores and supplement as necessary.

Children on Dialysis

There are 2 common forms of maintenance dialysis for children with end-stage renal disease—peritoneal dialysis and hemodialysis. The National Kidney Foundation Kidney Disease Outcomes Quality Initiative workgroup separated its recommendations for these 2 dialysis types when data existed to justify that separation.[70]

There is no evidence that dialysis, per se, is a catabolic experience requiring additional protein or caloric supplements over and above the nitrogen lost during the dialysis procedure itself, but protein requirements are increased to account for the loss of protein and amino acids during the dialysis procedure (Table 42.5). Supplemental vitamins were not routinely recommended for children whose diet achieved the recommended levels for the individual vitamins. Supplemental nutritional support (oral and/or enteral) is suggested for children who cannot consistently consume the DRIs for protein and energy or who are not growing despite good biochemical control and seemingly adequate intake.[70]

Renal Transplantation

Current immunosuppressive regimens for children after a renal transplant most often include the use of corticosteroids and calcineurin inhibitors. In part as a result of this therapy, a high percentage of children are hypertensive after transplantation.

In the initial post-transplant period, the focus of medical nutrition therapy should be on limitation of sodium (2-3 g/day), weight control, and adequate fluid intake, especially for smaller children who receive adult-size kidneys. Long-term goals include achieving or maintaining age-and gender-appropriate BMI, regular physical activity, and eating a variety of foods, including fruits and vegetables, with moderate consumption of high-fat and high-sodium foods. Adequate fluid intake remains a long-term goal. Children should have their lipid levels monitored after transplantation.[76-78]

References

1. Foreman JW, Abitbol CL, Trachtman H, et al. Nutritional intake in children with renal insufficiency: a report of the growth failure in children with renal diseases study. *J Am Coll Nutr*. 1996;15(6):579-585

2. Ferrara P, Romaniello L, Vitelli O, Gatto A, Serva M, Cataldi L. Cranberry juice for the prevention of recurrent urinary tract infections: a randomized controlled trial in children. *Scand J Urol Nephrol*. 2009;43(5):369-372

3. Jepson RG, Craig JC. A systematic review of the evidence for cranberries and blueberries in UTI prevention. *Molec Nutr Food Res*. 2007;51(6):738-745

4. Glazener CM, Evans JH, Cheuk DK. Complementary and miscellaneous interventions for nocturnal enuresis in children. *Cochrane Database Syst Rev*. 2005;(2):CD005230

5. Hjalmas K, Arnold T, Bower W, et al. Nocturnal enuresis: an international evidence based management strategy. *J Urol*. 2004;171(6 Pt 2):2545-2561

6. Sorof JM, Lai D, Turner J, Poffenbarger T, Portman RJ. Overweight, ethnicity, and the prevalence of hypertension in school-aged children. *Pediatrics*. 2004;113(3 Pt 1):475-482

7. Freedman DS, Dietz WH, Srinivasan SR, Berenson GS. The relation of overweight to cardiovascular risk factors among children and adolescents: the Bogalusa Heart Study. *Pediatrics*. 1999;103(6 Pt 1):1175-1182

8. Rosner B, Prineas R, Daniels SR, Loggie J. Blood pressure differences between blacks and whites in relation to body size among US children and adolescents. *Am J Epidemiol*. 2000;151(10):1007-1019

9. DiPietro A, Kees-Folts D, DesHarnais S, Camacho F, Wassner S. Primary hypertension at a single center: treatment, time to control, and extended follow-up. *Pediatr Nephrol*. 2009;24(12):2421-2428

10. Robinson RF, Batisky DL, Hayes JR, Nahata MC, Mahan JD. Body mass index in primary and secondary pediatric hypertension. *Pediatr Nephrol*. 2004;19(12):1379-1384

11. Rocchini AP, Katch V, Anderson J, et al. Blood pressure in obese adolescents: effect of weight loss. *Pediatrics*. 1988;82(1):16-23

12. Daniels SR, Arnett DK, Eckel RH, et al. Overweight in children and adolescents: pathophysiology, consequences, prevention, and treatment. *Circulation*. 2005;111(15):1999-2012

13. Rosenberg B, Moran A, Sinaiko A. Insulin resistance (metabolic) syndrome in children. *Panminerva Med*. 2005;47(4):229-244

14. Falkner B. Children and adolescents with obesity-associated high blood pressure. *J Am Soc Hypertens*. 2008;2(4):267-274

15. Vivian EM. Type 2 diabetes in children and adolescents—the next epidemic? *Curr Med Res Opin*. 2006;22(2):297-306.

16. Mertens IL, Van Gaal LF. Overweight, obesity, and blood pressure: the effects of modest weight reduction. *Obes Res*. 2000;8(3):270-278

17. Couch SC, Saelens BE, Levin L, Dart K, Falciglia G, Daniels SR. The Efficacy of a Clinic-Based Behavioral Nutrition Intervention Emphasizing a DASH-Type Diet for Adolescents with Elevated Blood Pressure. *J Pediatr*. 2008;152(4):494-501

18. Appel LJ, Moore TJ, Obarzanek E, et al. A clinical trial of the effects of dietary patterns on blood pressure. *N Engl J Med*. 1997;336(16):1117-1124

19. Harsha DW LP, Obarzanck E, Karanja NM, Moore TJ, Calballero B. Dietary Approaches to Stop Hypertension: a summary of study results. *J Am Diet Assoc*. 1999;99(Suppl 8):S35-S39

20. Falkner B, Michel S. Blood pressure response to sodium in children and adolescents. *Am J Clin Nutr*. 1997;65(Suppl 2):618S–621S

21. Geleijnse JM, Grobbee DE, Hofman A. Sodium and potassium intake and blood pressure change in childhood. *Br Med J*. 1990;300(6729):899-902

22. Mo R, Omvik P, Lund-Johansen P, Myking O. The Bergen blood pressure study: sodium intake and ambulatory blood pressure in offspring of hypertensive and normotensive families. *Blood Press*. 1993;2(4):278-283

23. Staessen J, Lijnen P, Thijs L, Fagard R. Salt and blood pressure in community-based intervention trials. *Am J Clin Nutr*. 1997;65(Suppl 2):661S–670S

24. Vollmer WM, Sacks FM, Ard J, et al. Effects of diet and sodium intake on blood pressure: subgroup analysis of the DASH-sodium trial. *Ann Intern Med*. 2001;135(12):1019-1028

25. He FJ, MacGregor GA. Importance of salt in determining blood pressure in children: meta-analysis of controlled trials. *Hypertension*. 2006;48(5):861-869

26. Institute of Medicine, Food and Nutrition Board. *Dietary Reference Intakes for Energy, Carbohydrate, Fiber, Fat, Fatty Acids, Cholesterol, Protein, and Amino Acids (Macronutrients)*. Washington, DC: The National Academies Press; 2002

27. Allender P, Cutler J, Follmann D, Cappuccio F, Pryer J, Elliott P. Dietary calcium and blood pressure: a meta-analysis of randomized clinical trials. *Ann Intern Med*. 1996;124(9):825-831

28. Falkner B, Sherif K, Michel S, Kushner H. Dietary nutrients and blood pressure in urban minority adolescents at risk for hypertension. *Arch Pediatr Adolesc Med*. 2000;154(9):918-922

29. Karanja N, Morris C, Rufolo P, Snyder G, Illingworth D, McCarron D. Impact of increasing calcium in the diet on nutrient consumption, plasma lipids, and lipoproteins in humans. *Am J Clin Nutr*. 1994;59(4):900-907

30. Kristal-Boneh E, Green MS. Dietary calcium and blood pressure-a critical review of the literature. *Public Health Rev*. 1990;18(4):267-300

31. Resnick L. The role of dietary calcium in hypertension: a hierarchical overview. *Am J Hypertens*. 1999;12(1 Pt 1):99-112

VI

32. Sorof J, Forman A, Cole N, Jemerin J, Morris R. Potassium intake and cardiovascular reactivity in children with risk factors for essential hypertension. *J Pediatr*. 1997;31(1 Pt 1):87-94

33. Mu J, Liu Z, Liu F, Xu X, Liang Y, Zhu D. Family-based randomized trial to detect effects on blood pressure of a salt substitute containing potassium and calcium in hypertensive adolescents. *Am J Hypertens*. 2009;22(9):943-947

34. Appel LJ; American Society of Hypertension Writing Group. ASH position paper: dietary approaches to lower blood pressure. 2010;4(2):79-89

35. Mizushima S, Cappuccio FP, Nichols R, Elliott P. Dietary magnesium intake and blood pressure: a qualitative overview of the observational studies. *J Hum Hypertens*. 1998;12(7):447-453

36. Whelton SP, Hyre AD, Pedersen B, Yi Y, Whelton PK, He J. Effect of dietary fiber intake on blood pressure: a meta-analysis of randomized, controlled clinical trials. *J Hypertens*. 2005;23(3):475-481

37. Ulbak J, Lauritzen L, Hansen H, Michaelsen K. Diet and blood pressure in 2.5-y-old Danish children. *Am J Clin Nutr*. 204;79(6):1095-1102

38. Burtis WJ, Gay L, Insogna KL, Ellison A, Broadus AE. Dietary hypercalciuria in patients with calcium oxalate kidney stones. *Am J Clin Nutr*. 1994;60(3):424-429

39. Cirillo M CC, Laurenzi M, Mellone M, Mazzacca G, De Santo NG. Salt intake, urinary sodium and hypercalciuria. *Miner Electrolyte Metab*. 1997;23(3-6):265-268

40. Hess B, Jost C, Zipperle L, Takkinen R, Jaeger P. High-calcium intake abolishes hyperoxaluria and reduces urinary crystallization during a 20-fold normal oxalate load in humans. *Nephrol Dial Transplant*. 1998;13(9):2241-2247

41. Osorio AV, Alon US. The relationship between urinary calcium, sodium, and potassium excretion and the role of potassium in treating idiopathic hypercalciuria. *Pediatrics*. 1997;100(4):675-681

42. Laminski NA MA, Kruger M, Sonnekus MI, Margolius LP. Hyperoxaluria in patients with recurrent calcium oxalate calculi: dietary and other risk factors. *Br J Urol*. 1991;68(5):454-458

43. Massey LK, Sutton RA. Modification of dietary oxalate and calcium reduces urinary oxalate in hyperoxaluric patients with kidney stones. *J Am Diet Assoc*. 1993;93(11):1305-1307

44. Cattini Perrone H, Bruder Stapleon F, Toporovski J, Schor N. Hematuria due to hyperuricosuria in children: 36-month follow-up. *Clin Nephrol*. 1997;48(5):288-291

45. La Manna A, Polito C, Marte A, Iovene A, Di Toro R. Hyperuricosuria in children: clinical presentation and natural history. *Pediatrics*. 2001;107(1):86-90

46. Reid IR, Hardy DC, Murphy WA, Teitelbaum SL, Bergfeld MA, Whyte MP. X-linked hypophosphatemia: a clinical, biochemical, and histopathologic assessment of morbidity in adults. *Medicine*. 1989;68(6):3363-52

47. Tieder M, Modai D, Samuel R, Arie R, Halabe A, Bab I, et al. Hereditary hypophosphatemic rickets with hypercalciuria. *N Engl J Med*. 1985;312(10):611-617

48. Kaysen GA, Gambertoglio J, Jiminez I, Jones H, Hutchinson F. Effect of dietary protein intake on albumin homeostasis in nephrotic patients. *Kidney Int*. 1986;29(2):572-577

49. Papez KE, Smoyer WE. Recent advances in congenital nephrotic syndrome. *Curr Opin Pediatr.* 2004;16(2):165-170

50. Lechner B, Bockenhauer D, Iragorri S, Kennedy T, Siegel N. The risk of cardiovascular disease in adults who have had childhood nephrotic syndrome. *Pediatr Nephrol.* 2004;19(7):744-748

51. D'Amico G, Gentile MG, Manna G, et al. Effect of vegetarian soy diet on hyperlipidaemia in nephrotic syndrome. *Lancet.* 1992;339(8802):1131-1134

52. Prescott WA Jr, Streetman DA, Streetman DS. The potential role of HM-CoA reductase inhibitors in pediatric nephrotic syndrome. *Ann Pharmacother.* 2004;38(12):2105-2114

53. Briassoulis G, Venkataraman S, Thompson AE. Energy expenditure in critically ill children [see comment]. *Crit Care Med.* 2000;28(4):1166-1172

54. Vazquez Martinez JL, Martinez-Romillo PD, Diez Sebastian J, Ruza Tarrio F. Predicted versus measured energy expenditure by continuous, online indirect calorimetry in ventilated, critically ill children during the early postinjury period [see comment]. *Pediatr Crit Care Med.* 2004;5(1):19-27

55. Ahithol CL, Warady BA, Massie MD, et al. Linear growth and anthropometric and nutritional measurements in children with mild to moderate renal insufficiency: a report of the growth failure in children with renal diseases study. *J Pediatr.* 1990;116(2):S46-S47

56. National Kidney Foundation, Kidney Disease Outcomes Quality Initiative. KDOQI Clinical Practice Guideline for Nutrition in Children with CKD: 2008 Update. Executive Summary. *Am J Kidney Dis.* 2009;53(3):S11-S104

57. Wingen AM, Mehls O. Nutrition in children with preterminal chronic renal failure. myth or important therapeutic aid. *Pediatr Nephrol.* 2002;17(2):111-120

58. Uuay R, Hogg R, Brewer E, Reisch J, Cunningham C, Holliday M. Dietary protein and growth in infants with chronic renal insufficiency: a report from the Southwest Pediatric Nephrology Study Group and the University of California, San Francisco. *Pediatr Nephrol.* 1994;8(1):45-50

59. Wingen AM, Fabian-Bach C, Schaefer F, Mehls O. Randomised multicentre study of a low-protein diet on the progression of renal failure in children. *Lancet.* 1997;349(9059):1117-1123

60. Hellerstein S, Holliday MA, Grupe WE, et al. Nutritional management of children with chronic renal failure. *Pediatr Nephrol.* 1987;1(2):195-211

61. Sedman A, Friedman A, Boineau F, Strife CF, Fine R. Nutritional management of the child with mild to moderate chronic renal failure. *J Pediatr.* 1996;129(2):S13-S18

62. Ratsch IM, Catassi C, Verrina E, et al. Energy and nutrient intake of patients with mild to moderate chronic renal failure compared with healthy children: an Italian multicentre study. *Eur J Pediatr.* 1992;151(9):701-705

63. Wingen AM, Fabian-Bach C, Mehls O. Evaluation of protein intake by dietary diaries and urea-N excretion in children with chronic renal failure. *Clin Nephrol.* 1993;40(2):208-215

64. Bailey JL, Wang X, England BK, Price SR, Ding X, Mitch WE. The acidosis of chronic renal failure activates muscle proteolysis in rats by augmenting transcription of genes encoding proteins of the ATP-dependent ubiquitin-proteasome pathway. *J Clin Invest.* 1996;97(6):1447-1453

VI

65. Mahajan A, Simoni J, Sheather SJ, Broglio KR, Rajab MH, Wesson DE. Daily oral sodium bicarbonate preserves glomerular filtration rate by slowing its decline in early hypertensive nephropathy. *Kidney Int*. 2010;78(3):303-309

66. Oh J, Wunsch R, Turzer M, Bahner M, Raggi P, Querfeld U, et al. Advanced Coronary and Carotid Arteriopathy in Young Adults With Childhood-Onset Chronic Renal Failure. *Circulation*. 2002;106(1):100-105

67. Wassner SJ, Baum M. Chronic renal failure: physiology and management. In: Barratt TM, Avner ED, Harmen WE, eds. *Pediatric Nephrology*. 4th ed. Baltimore, MD: Lippincott, Williams &Wilkins; 1999:115-118

68. Yatzidis H, Digenis P, Fountas P. Hypervitaminosis A accompanying advanced chronic renal failure. *Br Med J*. 1975;110(5979):352-353

69. Rovner A, O'Brien K. Hypovitaminosis D among healthy children in the United States. *Arch Pediatr Adolesc Med*. 2008;162(6):513-519

70. National Kidney Foundation, K/DOQI. Clinical practice guidelines for nutrition in chronic renal failure. *Am J Kidney Dis*. 2000;35(6 Suppl 2):S1-S140

71. Shemin D, Bostom AG, Selhub J. Treatment of hyperhomocysteinemia in end-stage renal disease. *Am J Kidney Dis*. 2001;38(4 Suppl 1):S91-S94

72. Calvani M, Benatti P, Mancinelli A, et al. Carnitine replacement in end-stage renal disease and hemodialysis. *Ann NY Acad Sci*. 2004;1033(1):52-66

73. Hurot J, Cucherat M, Haugh M, Fouque D. Effects of L-carnitine supplementation in maintenance hemodialysis patients: a systemic review. *J Am Soc Nephrol*. 2002;14(3):708-714

74. Lilien MR, Duran M, Quak JM, Frankhuisen JJ, Schroder CH. Oral L-carnitine does not decrease erythropoietin requirement in pediatric dialysis. *Pediatr Nephrol*. 2000;15(1-2):17-20

75. Schroder CH, European Pediatric Peritoneal Dialysis Working Group. The management of anemia in pediatric peritoneal dialysis patients. Guidelines by an ad hoc European committee. *Pediatr Nephrol*. 2003;18(8):805-809

76. Baker S, Barlow S, Cochran W, et al. Overweight children and adolescents: a clinical report of the North American Society for Pediatric Gastroenterology, Hepatology and Nutrition. *J Pediatr Gastroenterol Nutr*. 2005;40(5):533-543

77. Broyer M, Tete MJ, Laudat MH, Goldstein S. Plasma lipids in kidney transplanted children and adolescents: influence of pubertal development, dietary intake and steroid therapy. *Eur J Clin Invest*. 1981;11(5):397-402

78. Locsey L, Asztalos L, Kincses Z, Berczi C, Paragh G. The importance of obesity and hyperlipidaemia in patients with renal transplants. *Int Urol Nephrol*. 1998;30(6):767-775

79. Hogg R, Furth S, Lemley K, et al. National Kidney Foundation's Kidney Disease Outcomes Quality Initiative Clinical Practice Guidelines for Chronic Kidney Disease in Children and Adolescents: Evaluation, Classification and Stratification. *Pediatrics*. 2003;111(6 Pt 1):1416-1421

Chapter 43

Nutritional Management of Children With Cancer

Introduction

The maintenance of nutritional adequacy is vital for the child or adolescent undergoing cancer treatment. The inability to maintain a normal nutritional state can lead to poor tolerance of treatment, increased risk of infectious complications, and a potential diminished overall outcome. Although appropriate nutritional support is vital, there are various factors that need to be taken into consideration in the management of children with cancer. An integrative approach that builds on the "omic" technologies (ie, genomics, transcriptomics, proteomics, and metabolomics) will provide new insights into appropriate nutritional intervention strategies that recognize the interactions that occur among the nutrients that are provided with the patient's genetic background, environment, and cultural preferences.

The goal for nutrition support in children with cancer is to promote normal growth and development, minimize morbidity and mortality, and maximize quality of life. Frequently, the cancer site, extent of disease, and complications of therapy are important variables in the risk of malnutrition in pediatric patients with malignancies.[1-4] In addition to poor growth and development, malnutrition may be associated with decreased immune function (including anergy to intradermal antigens), decreased tolerance for chemotherapy, and increased rates of infection. Malnourished children with cancer have a higher risk of chemotherapy toxicity, have a higher incidence of infectious complications, and tolerate chemotherapy poorly when compared with children with normal nutritional status.[5-9]

The mechanism by which malnutrition leads to less favorable outcomes in children with cancer is currently unclear.[10-16] Nevertheless, poor nutrition negatively affects a child's physical and emotional well-being and his or her quality of life.[15,16] The pathogenesis of malnutrition in children with cancer is multifactorial and includes the effects of the tumor, the host-response to the malignancy, the effects of therapy, and psychological factors.

Nutritional Status at Diagnosis

Because childhood cancer often presents with an acute onset (eg, acute leukemia), a relatively normal nutritional status is typical at the time of diagnosis. However, children with solid tumors, especially those causing intestinal obstruction or presenting with widespread metastatic disease, may have varying degrees of malnutrition.[8] Malnutrition in pediatric oncology patients is commonly observed with advanced disease, those who relapse or who are unresponsive to treatment, and those undergoing intensive therapy.[2,5] The incidence of malnutrition has been reported to range from 6% in children with newly diagnosed leukemia to as high as 50% in patients with stage IV neuroblastoma.[6,8] Overweight or obesity is also commonplace in those with recently diagnosed cancers.[17]

Host-Related Effects

Metabolic shifts, known as cancer cachexia, have been demonstrated both in animal models and humans.[18] Cachexia is a complicated process and varies by the site of the tumor. It is marked by early satiety, weight loss, and abnormal utilization of energy from protein, fat, and carbohydrate.[18-20] Changes in substrate metabolism include an increase in protein turnover and a loss of the normal compensatory mechanisms seen in starvation, which may result in skeletal muscle depletion.[19-23] Additionally, accelerated lipolysis results in depletion of fat stores and increased free fatty acid turnover with the net effect of wasting of body fat and hyperlipidemia.[18,19] Changes in carbohydrate metabolism result in an energy-losing cycle. Studies of adult patients with large tumor burdens have shown that tumors consume glucose by anaerobic glycolysis, producing lactic acid. Lactic acidosis, during infusions of glucose, has also been reported in children with cancer.[2,5,19] The data regarding changes in a patient's metabolic rate caused by a malignancy tend to be inconsistent; mixed results have been reported in adult and small pediatric studies.[5,19,24]

The most common characteristic of cancer-associated malnutrition is anorexia. Anorexia occurs as a result of both the malignancy and the cancer therapy.[20,23] Adverse effects of chemotherapy, such as nausea, vomiting, diarrhea, mucositis, food aversion, and an altered sense of taste and smell, are major causes of anorexia in children undergoing cancer treatment. Furthermore, infection, chemotherapy-induced ulcers, delayed gastric emptying, pain, and psychological factors can play a significant role in the development of anorexia. A clear relationship exists between specific cancer treatments and the degree of anorexia, malnutrition, and growth retardation.[8,25,26]

Therapy-Related Complications

Multimodal treatments (chemotherapy, radiation, surgery, biologic and immunologic therapies) may contribute either directly or indirectly to an altered nutritional status in children with cancer. Most chemotherapeutic agents adversely affect dietary intake. In a study of 100 newly diagnosed pediatric oncology patients, 44 were found to be consuming less than 80% of their estimated caloric requirements compared with none of the controls.[2,27] Oral mucositis is one of the frequent adverse effects of intensive cancer treatment.[8,28] Many chemotherapy agents cause dysphagia, nausea, and vomiting; altered food intake; impaired digestion and absorption; and increased nutrient losses. Antineoplastic drugs can cause diarrhea, constipation, ileus, and morphologic changes in the intestine, resulting in an alteration of digestive enzyme.[8,29] Factors such as constipation related to use of vincristine or narcotics and lactose malabsorption with diarrhea as a result of upper small bowel inflammation can result in significant abdominal discomfort and loss of appetite. Toxicity of chemotherapy treatment is related to the type of agent, the dose, and combination of chemotherapeutic medications. Although new approaches in supportive care established by the Children's Oncology Group (COG) have decreased the nausea, vomiting, and mucositis associated with some of the treatment protocols, these adverse effects continue to present challenges in care of children with cancer.[30]

Radiation therapy alone or in combination with chemotherapy can severely affect one's nutritional status. The adverse effect may be influenced by dose, fractionation, location, and the field size.[8,31] Radiotherapy to the head and neck can result in anorexia, altered taste sensation, and mucositis. Radiation to the chest can cause dysphagia or swallowing difficulties. Therapy to the abdomen or pelvis can result in acute nausea and vomiting with poor food intake or late effects on intestinal mucosa leading to radiation enteritis.[8,31]

Infection is a common occurrence in children with cancer. Among the factors that contribute to an increased risk of infection are myelosuppression and changes in humoral and cellular immunity, which may result, in part, from poor nutrition.[32] A child with an infection who is myelosuppressed may experience a poor appetite with suboptimal nutritional intake. Antibiotic agents as well as antifungal agents can cause gastrointestinal and urinary losses of nutrients, malabsorption, and anorexia with associated weight loss.

Psychological Factors

The adverse effects of anticancer therapy often create many psychosocial challenges.[33] Loss of appetite, eating discomfort associated with nausea or vomiting, separation from home environment at meal time, disruption of normal life, alteration in body image, and frequent medical procedures may all have a significant effect on a child or adolescent's oral intake. A team approach that includes psychosocial, medical, nursing, and nutrition professionals may reduce some of the psychosocial effects of the malignancy and attendant therapy and thereby improve nutritional intake. Knowledge of treatment protocols and the expected adverse effects will assist in developing early intervention strategies to prevent significant nutritional deterioration.

VI

Nutritional Screening

The nutritional status of all children with cancer should be evaluated at the time of diagnosis and throughout therapy.[34,35] The purpose of a nutrition evaluation is to identify the child at risk of malnutrition and to establish baseline nutrition information for future follow-up examinations.

The following criteria are used to identify children at risk of malnutrition[34-37]:

- Total weight loss of >5% of the preillness body weight over the past month or >2% for infants
- Weight for age <5th or >85th percentile
- Stature for age <10th percentile
- Weight for stature <10th or >90th percentile
- Weight <90% of ideal body weight for stature

Note: triceps skinfold thickness <10th percentile and mid-upper arm circumference <5th percentile (arm anthropometry) appear to be more sensitive measures of malnutrition than weight for height in children with large solid tumors[36]

- Recent unexplained weight gain[34]
- Body mass index (BMI) for age <5th or >85th percentile
- Oral intake <80% of estimated needs
- No oral intake or poor intake ≥3 days[34]
- Children receiving high-dose chemotherapy or combination therapy for aggressive cancers

Nutritional Assessment

The goals for nutrition assessment are to identify and define nutrition problems, to establish individual nutrition needs and care plans, and to assess the appropriate route of nutrition. Follow-up is essential in monitoring the effectiveness of nutrition support therapy. The nutritional assessment of a child diagnosed with cancer should include:

- Medical and surgical history, including: medical tests and procedures performed as well as history of gastrointestinal tract disorders and symptoms, such as malabsorption, maldigestion, vomiting, diarrhea, and constipation
- Medication history, to include review of chemotherapy, antibiotic agents, and antifungal agents and their potential effects on nutritional status
- Physical examination to include general appearance and activity level (see below)
- Anthropometric assessment (see below)

- Biochemical and hematologic assessment (see below)
- Diet history to include:
  - Type and amount of foods or formula consumed
  - Feeding and eating patterns
  - Feeding problems and skills
  - Food allergies, aversions, sensitivities, and intolerances
  - Food preferences
  - Food intake in relation to treatment schedule
  - Supplements, herbs, and/or complementary therapies

Anthropometric Assessment

Appropriate growth of the child is the best indicator of adequate nutrition. The National Center for Health Statistics (NCHS) and WHO growth charts allow the determination of the percentile of stature (length, if ≤3 years) for age, weight for age, weight for stature (length, if ≤3 years) and head circumference for age (≤3 years [see Chapter 25: Assessment of Nutritional Status, and Appendix A: Growth Charts]). These measurements are relatively sensitive indicators of growth and are routinely used in the evaluation of the child with cancer at the time of diagnosis and throughout therapy.[7,8,36,37] The percentage of weight loss from the child's usual body weight and percentage of ideal body weight for height can be used to determine nutritional status in children with cancer.[8,37] A significant deviation from the 50th percentile weight for height is indicative of under- and overnutrition. Longitudinal data on each child's growth pattern is most helpful for detecting deviations from a child's normal growth pattern. Flattening of the weight/growth curve may be an early indicator of decreased energy and protein intake. Triceps skinfold thickness provides an index of body fat stores, and mid-upper arm muscle circumference reflects general muscle mass.[34]

Rapid weight gain throughout therapy should also be recognized, and early intervention should be implemented to prevent excessive weight gain during and after treatment. BMI (weight/height^2) is an indirect measure of lean body mass and fat stores.[37] In adolescents, BMI for age correlates with total body fatness and can be used as a screening tool to determine over- and undernutrition.[36]

Biochemical and Hematologic Assessment
(See Also Chapter 25: Assessment of Nutritional Status)

Biochemical and hematologic determinations, in combination with anthropometric data, are helpful in the evaluation of the patient's nutritional status. Serum albumin and prealbumin (transthyretin) are obtained to determine visceral protein status.

These values are altered by inadequate protein intake, impaired absorption, inadequate synthesis, chronic losses, hydration status, inflammation, and abnormal liver and renal function.[7,8,35,37] Their specificity is limited, because they are also acute-phase reactant proteins. An abnormal serum albumin concentration may often reflect the acute metabolic response to fever and infection or chronic catabolic stress from infection rather than the depletion of lean body mass. Some medications (corticosteroids, insulin) can also alter their values.[34]

The concentration of prealbumin (transthyretin), with its shorter half-life of 1.9 days versus 14 to 20 days for serum albumin, is often used to determine the effectiveness of nutrition interventions.[35] Other serum biochemical indices, such as sodium, potassium, chloride, bicarbonate, glucose, creatinine, blood urea nitrogen, calcium, phosphorous, magnesium, triglycerides, hemoglobin, hematocrit, and lymphocyte count, should be monitored closely, because dietary intake as well as chemotherapy and antibiotic medications can alter their values.

Clinical Evaluation

The clinical evaluation of the child with cancer should include monitoring for signs of muscle or fat depletion, wasting, edema, and mouth sores and must be a routine part of the comprehensive nutritional assessment. Periodic monitoring is critical for early detection of malnutrition and risks for nutrition-related complications.

Estimating Nutrient Requirements

Actual nutrient requirements of children with cancer vary with individual needs, disease activity, and treatment modalities. It is necessary to establish intake goals for calories, protein, vitamins, minerals, and fluids, especially for children receiving parenteral and enteral nutrition support. Measuring metabolic requirements by indirect calorimetry is preferred to using standardized tables, and equations estimating caloric requirements may be inaccurate.[35,38] Children receiving intensive therapy are generally less active and require less energy than their healthy counterparts. However, they may need additional calories during infections or other stresses. World Health Organization (WHO) equations estimate basal metabolic rate (BMR) with a broad range of additional calories for growth and stress. If standardized BMR values are used, correction factors should not be used.[35] Protein requirements for children with cancer are not known. Children with significant metabolic stress (eg, major surgery, infection) or increased losses may have a higher protein requirement. In injured children, daily protein requirement is typically approximately doubled, varying by age as follows: 0 to 2 years, 2 to 3 g/kg; 2 to 13 years, 1.5 to 2 g/kg; and 13 to 18 years, 1.5 g/kg.[35,39] Nitrogen balance studies can provide more accurate protein requirements for children with cancer, if appropriate or as needed.[34]

There is little information regarding vitamin and mineral requirements of children with cancer. Recommendations for vitamins and minerals are based on the Dietary Reference Intakes (DRIs) for age and gender. If the oral intake is suboptimal, or if there are increased losses of certain nutrients through malabsorption, vomiting, or diarrhea, a single or multivitamin-mineral supplement is recommended. Additional iron supplementation is not recommended for children receiving frequent blood products. It is generally accepted that children receiving methotrexate should not receive additional folic acid as a supplement.

There is mounting evidence that vitamin D may stimulate cell differentiation, promote apoptosis in transformed cells, and enhance immunocompetence.[40] Ensuring vitamin D adequacy while promoting sun-protection strategies, requires an evaluation of dietary and supplemental vitamin D in these patients.[41] For children and adolescents 1 to 18 years of age, the Recommended Dietary Allowance (RDA) is based on maintaining a serum 25-hydroxyvitamin D (25-OH-D) concentration of 50 nmol/L or 20 ng/mL. According to the Institute of Medicine, a daily intake of 400 IU of vitamin D for infants younger than 1 year and 600 IU of vitamin D for children 1 to 18 years of age is appropriate to prevent deficiency, rickets, and possibly aberrations in multiple cellular processes.[42] However, the amount necessary to support optimal health in children with cancer remains to be resolved. It is becoming increasingly apparent that excessive intake of vitamin D from dietary supplements can have adverse consequences.[40]

Mineral wasting and deficiencies associated with the adverse effects of chemotherapy are commonly seen in children. The nutrients most frequently affected include magnesium, calcium, phosphorus, potassium, and zinc.[7] Intravenous or oral electrolyte supplementation is also often needed. In these cases, monitoring of serum electrolyte concentrations is essential. The provision of adequate fluid is important throughout therapy. Fluid requirements are highly individualized; however, the following guidelines may be used as estimates of maintenance fluid requirements[37]:

<10 kg:	100 mL/kg/day
>10 kg–20 kg:	1000 mL/day plus 50 mL/kg for each kg >10 kg/day
>20 kg–30 kg:	1500 mL/day plus 20 mL/kg for each kg >20 kg/day
>30 kg:	1500 mL/m^2/day or 35 mL/kg/day

Nutritional Interventions

Nutrition interventions include oral feeding, enteral tube feeding, and parenteral nutrition. Although the oral route is the preferred method of providing nutrition, one of the challenges for children on intensive treatment protocols is their inability to eat an adequate amount of food in the face of nausea, vomiting, aversion to smells and tastes, mucositis, and stomatitis. Children should be encouraged to try calorie-dense foods. They should not be forced, threatened, or punished for not being able to eat enough food. Initial nutritional counseling regarding the effects of cancer and its treatment on nutrition is an important part of the comprehensive care of children with cancer. Information regarding appropriate food choices to meet daily nutrient requirements with or without supplements may be adequate for some children on maintenance therapy. Guidelines for management of nutritional complications attributable to therapy should be provided during initial or ongoing counseling. Reevaluations are needed periodically with changes in patient status.[35] Food safety and appropriate food handling should be a part of overall nutrition education for the caregiver.

Special diets, such as the neutropenic or low-bacteria diet, are sometimes used to minimize the introduction of pathogenic organisms into the gastrointestinal tract; however, recent studies do not support the effectiveness of such restrictions.[43-46] Appetite stimulants, such as megestrol acetate (Magace), and dronabinol (Marinol) have been used to treat weight loss in some patients experiencing cachexia, anorexia, and nausea. The benefits of these agents remain to be established, and the potential adverse effects of these drugs should be considered.

Tube Feeding

When oral intake remains inadequate, tube feedings may provide an effective and safe method of nutrition support. Although nasogastric tube feeding has been accepted for nutrition support of children with other illnesses,[47] this is generally not been the preferred long-term approach for children with cancer because of the discomfort of nasogastric tube placement, the psychological effects of alterations in body image, and poor compliance. An additional concern with nasogastric tube feeding is possible trauma to the fragile mucosal surfaces of a patient with a low platelet and white blood cell count, resulting in bacterial translocation into the blood stream. However, data support the safety and feasibility of nasogastric tube feedings for the nutritional support of children with cancer, and nasogastric tube feedings have been used successfully, mostly for short-term nutrition support.[48]

Gastrostomy tube feedings have been used for nutritional support in pediatric oncology patients with some concern for site infections, leakage of gastric contents on to the skin, and poor healing at the site.[49-51] In general, enteral tube feedings have a number of distinct advantages over parenteral nutrition.[52-54] These advantages include:

- Decreased risk of infection;
- Maintenance of structural and functional gastrointestinal tract integrity;
- Decreased potential for bacterial translocation;
- Greater ease and safety of administration;

- Decreased hepatobiliary complications; and

- Lower cost.

Tube feeding should be the first choice for nutritional support of children with an inadequate oral intake.[55] The following criteria should be considered when tube feeding is recommended:

- Patient and family consent;

- A functional gastrointestinal tract;

- The inability of the child to maintain normal nutrition by the oral route;

- The patient's status regarding nausea, vomiting, and diarrhea;

- An adequate platelet count (>20 000); and

- A normal mucosal surface in the upper gastrointestinal tract.

A team approach, including a dietitian, child life specialist, social worker, psychiatrist, oncologist, and nurses helps facilitate the successful initiation and continuation of tube feedings in a child with cancer.[48] Antiemetic and prokinetic medications are often useful adjuncts to enhance the chances for successful enteral feeding.

The optimal access route for enteral nutrition is based on anticipated duration of the tube feeding, the neurologic status of patient, and risk of aspiration. In general, nasoenteric tubes are considered for short-term use (<6 weeks), although successful long-term use of nasogastric tube feeding has been reported.[48] Other routes of enteral tube feeding include nasoduodenal, nasojejunal, gastrostomy, and jejunostomy tubes.[55] The use of a silicone or polyurethane tube with the smallest diameter (6-8 F) is recommended for nasoenteric tubes.

Enteral formulas (see Chapter 24: Enteral Nutrition) are selected on the basis of age and gastrointestinal tract function. Nutrient-dense infant formulas (≥20 kcal/oz) are appropriate choices for infants requiring oral or enteral tube feedings on the basis of their reduced fluid tolerance. Lactose-free infant formulas may be required because of chemotherapy-induced lactose intolerance. Increasing the formula concentration may increase renal solute load or cause gastrointestinal tract intolerance with abdominal distention, vomiting, or diarrhea. Thus, the concentration of a formula should be increased slowly with close monitoring of potential adverse effects. A concentrated formula may be achieved by adding "modular" supplements to standard infant formulas. Age-appropriate standard formulas may be used for patients with normal gut function. Formulas with lower osmolality are recommended for tube feedings. Children with significant compromise of the gastrointestinal tract mucosal surface may benefit from protein hydrolysate or elemental formulas.

VI

Tube feeding may be administered continuously using a feeding pump for a reliable, constant infusion rate. Continuous, rather than bolus, feeding may be better tolerated when there is delayed gastric emptying. For many children, intermittent bolus feeding is well tolerated and is more physiologic and mimics normal feeding. Nocturnal continuous feedings with daytime oral and/or bolus feedings work well to meet nutritional goals. Small bowel feedings should be considered for children with neurologic impairment who have a higher risk of aspiration and those with frequent vomiting. Continuous tube feedings may be initiated with full-strength isotonic formula at 1 to 2 mL/kg body weight per hour per day. They may be advanced by 1 to 2 mL/kg/hour per day, as tolerated, until the volume goal is achieved.[37,56]

Parenteral Nutrition

Parenteral nutrition (see Chapter 23: Parenteral Nutrition) is indicated when the child's nutrition status cannot be maintained by the enteral route.[35,57] This may occur with tumors producing gastrointestinal obstruction, severe mucositis, uncontrolled nausea and vomiting, or inability to absorb nutrients. Children receiving hematopoietic stem cell transplants with severe mucositis and enteritis, those diagnosed with typhlitis, and postsurgical patients with ascites may also be candidates for parenteral nutrition. The parenteral route may also be required to supplement enteral tube feedings. The use and risks of parenteral nutrition in children with cancer have been reviewed extensively.[55,58,59] The risk of catheter-related infections and gastrointestinal tract and metabolic complications should be considered when parenteral nutrition is selected for nutrition support of a child with normal gastrointestinal tract function. An aggressive approach with enteral tube feedings has greatly reduced the need for total parenteral nutrition, thereby reducing potential adverse effects and cost.[48]

Conclusion

Although role of diet and lifestyle in cancer prevention has received considerable attention in adults, an inadequate number of studies have examined this relationship in childhood cancers.[50] Very limited evidence suggests maternal dietary patterns during pregnancy may modify risk of germ cell tumor development in children.[60,61] Healthy lifestyle habits, including eating a healthy diet, staying physically active, and maintaining a normal weight during the maintenance phase of treatment and after treatment may help to keep a child with cancer healthy and reduce the late effects of therapy. It would be prudent to emphasize a diet consisting of a wide variety of foods, including plant food sources, whole grains, fruits, and vegetables, as illustrated in the US Department of Agriculture's "ChooseMyPlate. gov"[62] (see Appendix F: MyPlate) and suggested by the World Cancer Research

Fund/American Institute for Cancer Research.[63] Physical activity may be important for reducing depression and obesity in children during and after cancer treatment. Regular exercise may also improve muscle strength, functional mobility, and overall cardiovascular health in children with cancer.[64]

There has been an increased focus on supportive care of children with cancer. This includes efforts to develop uniform guidelines for nutritional management of children with cancer through the Children's Oncology Group[65] as well as clinical trials to investigate the role of certain nutrients, such as glutamine, arginine, omega-3 fatty acids, antioxidants, and herbal products in childhood cancer. Although much remains to be learned about appropriate personalized strategies, appropriate nutrition support is a mainstay of treatment for children with cancer.

References

1. Novy MA, Saavedra JM. Nutrition therapy for pediatric cancer patient. *Top Clin Nutr.* 1997;12:16-25

2. Bechard LJ, Adiv OE, Jaksic T, Duggan C. Nutritional supportive care. In: Pizzo P, Poplack DG, eds. *Principles and Practice of Pediatric Oncology.* Philadelphia, PA: Lippincott Williams; 2002:1285-1300

3. Reilly JJ, Weir J, McColl JH, Bison BE. Prevalence of protein-energy malnutrition at diagnosis in children with lymphoblastic leukemia. *J Pediatr Gastroenterol Nutr.* 1999;29(2):194-197

4. Elhasid R, Laor A, Lischinskys S, Postovsky S, Arush M. Nutritional status of children with solid tumors. *Cancer.* 1999;86(1):119-125

5. Mauer A, Burgess J, Donoldson S, Richard K, Stallings V, Vaneys J, Winick M. Special nutritional needs of children with malignancies: a review. *JPEN J Parenter Enteral Nutr.* 1990;14(3):315-324

6. Sala A, Pencharz P, Barr RD. Children, cancer and nutrition: a dynamic triangle. *Cancer.* 2004;100(4):677-687

7. Ladas EJ, Sacks N, Meacham L, et al. A multidisciplinary review of nutrition consideration in the pediatric oncology population: a perspective from Children's Oncology Group. *Nutr Clin Pract.* 2005;20(4):377-393

8. Barale KV, Charuhas PM. Oncology and hematopoietic cell transplant. In: Samour PQ, King K, eds. *Handbook of Pediatric Nutrition.* Sudbury, MA: Jones & Bartlett Publishers; 2005:459-481

9. Lobato-Mendizabal E, Lopez-Martinez B, Ruiz-Arguelles GJ. A critical review of the prognostic value of the nutritional status at diagnosis in the outcome of therapy of children with acute lymphoblastic leukemia. *Rev Invest Clin.* 2003;55(1):31-35

10. Lange BJ, Gerbing RB, Feusner J, et al. Mortality in overweight and underweight children with acute myeloid leukemia. *JAMA.* 2005;293(2):203-211

11. Murry DJ, Riva L, Poplack DG. Impact of nutrition on pharmacokinetics of anti-neoplastic agents. *Int J Cancer Suppl.* 1998;11:48-51

VI

12. Viana MB, Murao M, Ramos G, et al. Malnutrition as a prognostic factor in lymphoblastic leukemia: a multivariate analysis. *Arch Dis Child*. 1994;71(4):304-310

13. Taj MM, Pearson AD, Mumford DB, Price L. Effect of nutritional status on the incidence of infection in childhood cancer. *J Pediatric Hematol Oncol*. 1993;10(3):283-287

14. Barr RD, Bibson B. Nutritional status and cancer in childhood. *J Pediatr Hematol Oncol*. 2000;22(6):491-494

15. Pedrosa F, Bonilla M, Liu A, et al. Effect of malnutrition at the time of diagnosis on the survival of children treated for cancer in El Salvador and Northern Brazil. *J Pediatr Hematol Oncol*. 2000;22(6):502-505

16. Van Eys J. Benefits of nutritional intervention on nutritional status, quality of life and survival. *Int J Cancer Suppl*. 1998;11:66-68

17. Rogers PC, Meacham LR, Oeffinger KC, Henry DW, Lang BJ. Obesity in pediatric oncology. *Pediatr Blood Cancer*. 2005;45(7):881-891

18. Picton S. Aspects of altered metabolism in children with cancer. *Int J Cancer Suppl*. 1998;11:62-68

19. Langer CJ, Hoffman JP, Ottery FD. Clinical significance of weight loss in cancer patients: rationale for use of anabolic agents in the treatment of cancer-related cachexia. *Nutrition*. 2001;17(1 Suppl):S1-S20

20. Strasser F, Bruera ED. Update on anorexia and cachaexia. *Hematol Oncol Clin North Am*. 2002;160(3):589-617

21. Kurzer M, Meguid MM. Cancer and protein metabolism. *Surg Clin North Am*. 1986;66(5):969-1001

22. Pencharz P. Aggressive oral, enteral or parenteral nutrition: prescriptive decisions in children with cancer. *Int J Cancer Suppl*. 1998;11:73-75

23. Kern KA, Norton JA. Cancer cachexia. *JPEN J Parenter Enteral Nutr*. 1988;12(3):286-298

24. Truong MT, Erasmus JJ, Munden RF, et al. Focal FDG uptake in mediastinal brown fat mimicking malignancy: a potential pitfall resolved on PET/CT. *AJR Am J Roentgenol*. 2004;183(4):1127-1132

25. Katz JA, Chambers B, Everhart C, et al. Linear growth in children with acute lymphoblastic leukemia treated without cranial irradiation. *J Pediatr*. 1991;118(4 Pt 1):575-578

26. Katz JA, Pollock BH, Jacaruso D, Morad A. Final attained height in patients successfully treated for childhood acute lymphoblastic leukemia. *J Pediatr*. 1993;123(4):546-552

27. Smith DE, Stevens MC, Booth IW. Malnutrition at diagnosis of malignancy in childhood: common but mostly missed. *Eur J Pediatr*. 1991;150(5):318-322

28. Bryant R. Managing side effects of childhood cancer treatment. *J Pediatr Nurs*. 2003;18(2):113-125

29. Wohlschlaeger A. Prevention and treatment of mucositis: a guide for nurses. *J Pediatr Oncol Nurs*. 2004;21(5):281-287

30. Betcher DL, Bond D, Graner K, Lorenzen A. Chemotherapy induced nausea and vomiting. In: Altman AJ, ed. *Supportive Care of Children with Cancer*. Baltimore, MD: The John Hopkins University Press; 2004:181-199

31. Pieters RS, Marcus K, Marcus RB. Side effects of radiation therapy. In: Altman AJ, ed. *Supportive Care of Children with Cancer*. Baltimore, MD: The Johns Hopkins University Press; 2004:156-180

32. Altman AJ, Wolff LJ. The prevention of infection. In: Altman AJ, ed. *Supportive Care of Children with Cancer*. Baltimore, MD: The Johns Hopkins University Press; 2004:1-12

33. Lesko LM. Psychosocial issues in the diagnosis and management of cancer cachexia and anorexia. *Nutrition*. 1989;5(2):114-116

34. Mosby TT, Barr RD, Pencharz PB. Nutritional assessment of children with cancer. *J Pediatr Oncol Nurs*. 2009;26(4):186-197

35. Mehta NM, Compher C, A.S.P.E.N. Board of Directors. A.S.P.E.N. Clinical Guidelines: nutrition support of the critically ill child. *JPEN J Parenter Enteral Nutr*. 2009;33(3):260-276

36. Hendricks KM, Duggan C, eds. *Manual of Pediatric Nutrition*. Hamilton, Ontario: BC Decker; 2008

37. Sacks N, Ringwald-Smith K, Hale G. Nutrition support. In: Altman AJ, ed. *Supportive Care of Children with Cancer*. Baltimore, MD: The Johns Hopkins University Press; 2004:243-261

38. Mehta NM, Bechard LJ, Leavitt K, Duggan C. Cumulative energy imbalance in the pediatric intensive care unit: role of targeted indirect calorimetry. *JPEN J Parenter Enteral Nutr*. 2009;33(3):336-344

39. Institute of Medicine, Food and Nutrition Board. *Dietary Reference Intakes for Energy, Carbohydrate, Fiber, Fat, Fatty Acids, Cholesterol, Protein, and Amino Acids*. Washington, DC: National Academies Press; 2005

40. Davis CD, Milner JA. Nutrigenomics, vitamin D and cancer prevention. *J Nutrigenet Nutrigenomics*. 2011;4(1):1-11

41. Balk SJ. Ultraviolet radiation: a hazard to children and adolescents. *Pediatrics*. 2011;127(3):e791-e817

42. Institute of Medicine, Food and Nutrition Board. *Dietary Reference Intakes for Calcium and Vitamin D*. Washington, DC: National Academies Press; 2011

43. Ladas E. *The Neutropenic Diet: An Examination of Evidence*. Chicago, IL: Oncology Nutrition Dietetic Practice Group; 2002

44. Moody K, Charlson ME, Finlay J. The neutropenic diet: what is the evidence? *J Pediatr Hematol Oncol*. 2002;24(9):717-721

45. Gardner A, Mattiuzzi G, Faderl S, et al. Randomized comparison of cooked and noncooked diets in patients undergoing remission induction therapy for acute myeloid leukemia. *J Clin Oncol*. 2008;26(35):5684-5688

46. DeMille D. Have you reviewed your neutropenic diet lately? *Oncology Nutrition Connection*. 2011;19(1)

47. Heland DK, Cook DJ, Guyatt GH. Enteral nutrition in the critically ill patient: a critical review of evidence. *Intensive Care Med*. 1993;19(8):435-442

48. DeSwarte-Wallace J, Firouzbakhsh S, Finklestein J. Using research to change practice: enteral feedings for pediatric oncology patients. *J Pediatr Oncol Nurs*. 2001;18(5):217-223

VI

49. Mathew P, Bowman L, Williams R, et al. Complications and effectiveness of gastrostomy feeding pediatric cancer patients. *J Pediatr Hematol Oncol*. 1996;18(1):81-85

50. Aquino VM, Smyrl CB, Hagy R, et al. Enteral nutritional support of bone marrow transplant recipients: a prospective, randomized clinical trial comparing total parenteral nutrition with an enteral feeding program. *Cancer Res*. 1987;47(1):3309-3316

51. Skolin I, Hernell O, Larsson MV, Wahlgren C, Wahlin YB. Percutaneous endoscopic gastrostomy in children with malignant disease. *J Pediatr Oncol Nurs*. 2002;19(5):145-163

52. Ford C, Whitlock JA, Pietsch JB. Glutamine-supplemented tube feedings versus total parenteral nutrition in children receiving intensive chemotherapy. *J Pediatr Oncol Nurs*. 1997;14(2):68-72

53. Han-Markey T. Nutrition consideration in pediatric oncology. *Semin Oncol Nurs*. 2000;16(2):146-151

54. Geitch E, Winterton J, Ma L, Berg R. The gut as a portal of entry for bacteremia. *Ann Surg*. 1987;205:681-690

55. Bankhand R, Boullata J, Brantly S, et al; A.S.P.E.N. Board of Directors. A.S.P.E.N. enteral nutrition practice recommendations. *J Parenter Enteral Nutr*. 2009;33:122-167

56. Sheard NF, Clark N. Nutritional management of pediatric oncology patients. In: Baker SS, Baker RD, Davis A, eds. *Pediatric Enteral Nutrition*. London, United Kingdom: Chapman and Hall; 1994:378-398

57. Mirtallo J, Canada T, Johnson D, et al. A.S.P.E.N. special report. *JPEN J Parenter Enteral Nutr*. 2004;28(6 Suppl):S40-S70

58. Charuhas PM, Gautier ST. Parenteral nutrition in pediatric oncology. In: Baker SS, Baker RD, Davis A, eds. *Pediatric Parenteral Nutrition*. London, United Kingdom: Chapman and Hall; 1997:331-353

59. Mirtallo J, Canada T, Johnson D, et al. Safe practices for parental nutrition. *JPEN J Parenter Enteral Nutr*. 2004;28(6 Suppl):S39-S70

60. Musselman JR, Jurek AM, Johnson KJ, et al. Maternal dietary patterns during early pregnancy and the odds of childhood germ cell tumors: a Children's Oncology Group study. *Am J Epidemiol*. 2011;173(3):282-291

61. Johnson KJ, Poynter JN, Ross JA, Robison LL, Shu XO. Pediatric germ cell tumors and maternal vitamin supplementation: a Children's Oncology Group study. *Cancer Epidemiol Biomarkers Prev*. 2009;18(10):2661-2664

62. US Department of Agriculture. Available at: www.ChooseMyPlate.gov/. Accessed January 15, 2013

63. World Cancer Research Fund/American Institute for Cancer Research. *Food, Nutrition, Physical Activity, and Cancer Prevention: A Global Perspective*. Washington, DC: American Institute for Cancer Research; 2007

64. Stolley MR, Restrepo J, Sharp LK. Diet and physical activity in childhood cancer survivors: a review of the literature. *Ann Behav Med*. 2010;39(3):232-249

65. Ladas EJ, Sacks N, Brophy P, Rogers PC. Standards of nutritional care in pediatric oncology: results from a nationwide survey on the standards of practice in pediatric oncology. A Children's Oncology Group study. *Pediatr Blood Cancer*. 2006;46(3):339-344

Chapter 44

The Nutritional Aspects of Inflammatory Bowel Disease in Pediatric Patients

Introduction

Inflammatory bowel disease (IBD), most typically classified as either Crohn disease or ulcerative colitis, develops during childhood or adolescence in 25% of patients.[1] Although the incidence and prevalence of IBD varies by ethnicity and geography, recent reports suggest that the incidence, currently estimated to be approximately 7 to 20/100 000 children, is increasing globally.[2-4] Additionally, despite previous dogma, IBD is not restricted to northern regions or to European ancestry but rather has a more global and pan-ethnic distribution.[4] These data also suggest that access to care and proper diagnosis of disease may be skewing epidemiologic assessment of IBD. Furthermore, even as our molecular and genetic understanding of disease onset, progression, and response to environmental triggers expands, it is unlikely that incidence will decrease.[5]

Crohn disease and ulcerative colitis are manifest by diarrhea (often with blood), abdominal pain, fever, and anemia. Extraintestinal manifestations, such as arthritis, uveitis, liver disease, and dermatologic disorders, may accompany gastrointestinal tract-related symptoms. Crohn disease has been characterized as a disease affecting any region of the gastrointestinal tract and extending into deeper tissues, thereby causing some phenotypic hallmarks of the disease, such as strictures and fistulae. In contrast, ulcerative colitis is limited to the colon and is mostly a disease of the superficial mucosa.[6]

Because Crohn disease is more likely to affect nutrient and vitamin absorption given its distribution that involves the small intestine, it is not surprising that many children affected with IBD (Crohn, in particular) suffer from malnutrition and growth failure/delay. Furthermore, because more children are being diagnosed in areas where access to nutritional resources may be sparse, the issue of malnutrition in IBD will be confounded by other environmental factors. This chapter will highlight the problems, approaches, and challenges to managing nutrition in patients with IBD.

Growth Failure

Prevalence

Growth failure is common in children with IBD. The percentage of children with Crohn disease whose growth is negatively affected varies with the definition of

VI

growth impairment, the time at which growth impairment is diagnosed during the course of the disease, and the characteristics of the population under study (eg, children vs adolescents, tertiary referral center vs primary care practice). Impairment of linear growth or weight loss and/or failure to gain weight appropriately for age is common in these children and often occurs before the recognition of Crohn disease.[7] Thus, the reported incidence of growth failure in these children is wide and ranges from approximately 10% to 90%. Weight loss or a failure to gain weight appropriately for age may precede the decrease in height velocity, with males affected more than females.[8]

Early-onset Crohn disease, in particular, is associated with long-term impairment of linear growth. In contrast, linear growth is less often impaired at the time of diagnosis of ulcerative colitis and, in follow-up, growth impairment is much less frequently observed.[9] In patients with early-onset IBD (defined by presentation before 5 years of age), a single institution study suggested that 59% of early onset IBD patients were able to maintain or increase their height percentile over time; however, when patients with ulcerative colitis (UC) were excluded, 62% of patients with Crohn disease did not meet their adult target height.[9]

Pathophysiology

Several interrelated factors may contribute to growth impairment in children with Crohn disease. Chronic undernutrition has long been implicated as a remediable cause of growth retardation. However, a simple nutritional hypothesis fails to explain all observations related to growth patterns among children with IBD. The direct growth-inhibiting effects of proinflammatory cytokines released in the setting of acute and chronic inflammation are now well described.[10,11] Thus, enhancement of linear growth may be best achieved through both provision of adequate nutrition and control of intestinal inflammation with medications least likely to affect growth.

Role of Cytokines and Endocrine Mediators

Insulin-like growth factor-1 (IGF-1), produced by the liver in response to growth hormone (GH) stimulation, normally mediates GH effects on the growth plate of bones. The association between impaired linear growth in Crohn disease and low IGF-1 levels is well recognized. Several interrelated factors may decrease IGF-1 levels, including malnutrition, direct cytokine effects, and suppression by chronic daily corticosteroid therapy.[12]

Elevated levels of cytokines, such as tumor necrosis factor-alpha (TNF-alpha), previously called cachectin, explain, in part, the anorexia that often accompanies Crohn disease, even in the absence of symptoms. Although anti-TNF alpha antibodies reduce disease activity, a direct association between TNF-alpha and growth failure remains elusive. Animal studies also support a role for interleukin-6 (IL-6) in growth inhibition in chronic inflammatory states. Transgenic mice that overexpress IL-6 have reduced growth rates because of reduced levels of IGF-1 production.[13,14]

Aside from providing necessary nutrients, nutritional interventions can potentially improve the inflammation in IBD by modulating pro- and anti-inflammatory cytokine profiles. For instance, short-chain fatty acids influence cytokine and chemokine gene expression by intestinal epithelial cells. Transforming growth factor-beta (TGF-beta) found in human and cow milk modulates intestinal epithelial cell growth and development and has anti-inflammatory effects. An open, uncontrolled trial using a TGF-beta-2–containing polymeric formula as the sole source of nutrition in children with Crohn disease reported remission in 79% of cases, associated with down-regulation of intestinal mRNA expression of IL-1, interferon gamma (IFN-gamma), and IL-8, whereas TGF-beta-1 levels increased.[10,11,15] It remains to be seen whether the addition of anti-inflammatory cytokines to treatment protocols will prove beneficial in randomized controlled trials.

Monitoring of Nutritional Status
(See Also Chapter 25: Nutritional Assessment)

Screening and assessing children with IBD for undernutrition- (or overnutrition) is an essential component of medical care. Screening includes, at a minimum, body weight for age and height for age, with calculation of the body mass index (BMI). These data should be plotted and followed longitudinally on appropriate growth charts (available from the Centers for Disease Control and other resources, including http://www.cdc.gov/growthcharts/).

Assessment of nutritional status also includes history, physical examination, and laboratory testing. Essential is a review of recent weight changes (especially weight loss that has occurred in the setting of concomitant abdominal pain, diarrhea, and fatigue) and changes in appetite. Preillness heights need to be plotted on reference growth charts to fully appreciate the effect of chronic intestinal inflammation. A thorough dietary history should be obtained with assistance from a clinical nutritionist or a registered dietitian who can perform a 24-hour dietary intake history and/or analyze a 3- to 5-day dietary diary. Documentation of the use of medications, including corticosteroids and other immunosuppressive medications, and nutritional supplements, including vitamins and minerals, is also important. Symptoms associated with the underlying illness that might affect nutrient requirements, such as difficulty swallowing, nausea, vomiting, or diarrhea, should be documented. A review of social factors should include the home environment,

VI

economic factors, issues of food security, and access to appropriate medications. Physical examination includes anthropometric assessment of body habitus, including weight, height, BMI, head circumference in children younger than 3 years, and triceps skinfold thickness and mid-upper arm circumference to estimate body fat and muscle mass (see Chapter 25). All measurements should be recorded on appropriate standardized charts. Sexual maturation should be documented by Tanner staging. Physical signs of generalized undernutrition (eg, protein calorie malnutrition) or specific nutrient deficiencies, including skin rash, hair changes, oral lesions, hepatomegaly, clubbing of the nail beds, and edema, should be documented. Laboratory determination of serum albumin may be helpful, but interpretation is complicated by gastrointestinal losses and concurrent medication use (particularly corticosteroids). Serum albumin is better correlated with inflammation of the intestinal tract than with nutritional status in patients with IBD. Serum prealbumin (transthyretin) has a much shorter half-life (2 days) than does albumin (18–20 days) and has been used to assess the efficacy of nutrition support. Other serum proteins proposed for assessing nutritional status include serum transferrin and retinol binding protein, but these have little advantage over albumin and prealbumin.

Research techniques that assess nutritional status have not yet been widely applied to patients with IBD. Such techniques include bioelectric impedance analysis and total body electrical conductance to determine total body water and fat mass and isotopic labeling of various molecules to determine energy expenditure and metabolic turnover rates. Application of dual photon x-ray absorptiometry scanning for patients with IBD has yielded important information regarding bone mineral deficiencies among children and adolescents with IBD.[16-18]

Specific nutrient deficiencies are found in children with IBD, more commonly in Crohn disease than in ulcerative colitis, and should be considered in the nutritional assessment (see below). However, micronutrient deficiencies are likely reflective of disease activity rather than specific nutritional deficiencies.

Selected Nutrient Requirements and Nutrient Deficiencies

Daily nutrient requirements may be increased above the dietary reference intakes because of the metabolic cost of chronic disease, including inflammation, malabsorption, and diarrhea. During disease exacerbation, energy consumption in children with Crohn disease may be 20% less than the recommended dietary allowance of 2000 kcal per day. Children with Crohn disease generally have greater nutrient needs for their age, gender, and weight than do children with ulcerative colitis. The diet of pediatric patients with IBD should be well balanced, based on the US Department of Agriculture's ChooseMyPlate campaign[19] and Dietary

Reference Intakes. Dietary restrictions are avoided unless intestinal obstruction or specific abnormalities of digestion exist. Dietary supplementation of selected nutrients (eg, vitamin D, folate, and elemental iron) may be warranted.[20]

Energy

Resting energy expenditure (REE [kcal/day]) in well-nourished children with Crohn disease is not different from values obtained in healthy children when expressed per kilogram of fat free mass.[21,22] The apparent increase in REE in children with Crohn disease is a result of their lower fat-free mass. REE in well-nourished children who underwent ileocolectomy for Crohn disease decreased only about 5% after accounting for the energy expended by the resected gut. Although REE was reported to be lower in undernourished children with Crohn disease than in healthy children, when expressed in terms of lean body mass, REE was not different between the 2 groups.[23] In a subset of these undernourished children with Crohn disease, REE was 35% higher compared with malnourished female patients with anorexia nervosa, implying that adaptation of REE in children with active Crohn disease in response to weight loss is offset by the metabolic consequences of mucosal inflammation. These changes in REE are reversible with aggressive enteral refeeding. Although high-fat diets may be used more efficiently for body fat deposition in adults with Crohn disease, low-fat diets are equally as effective as high-fat diets in restoring body fat mass in undernourished children with Crohn disease.[24] Approximately 97% of dietary fat is absorbed, regardless of the quality or quantity consumed. Short-term refeeding studies in undernourished children with Crohn disease demonstrate rapid weight gain (average, 8.7 kg per 6 weeks) with dietary energy intakes that approximated 170% of REE.[24] Long-term refeeding studies in undernourished children with Crohn disease show catch-up growth, with average height and weight gains of 7 to 9 cm/year and 7 kg/year, respectively, with daily dietary energy intakes approximating 133% of recommended values for ideal body weight or 60 to 75 kcal/kg actual body weight.[25,26] Thus, energy needs may be increased above recommended dietary intakes by as little as 5% and as much as 35% in children with Crohn disease, depending on their nutritional status and the degree of inflammatory disease activity.

Protein

Whole-body protein turnover, which is increased in children with acute and chronic disease activity, can be reduced with either corticosteroid therapy or an elemental diet. Although the efficiency of dietary nitrogen absorption is high with extensively hydrolyzed formulas, refeeding studies using elemental formulas suggest that the efficiency of nitrogen utilization in children with Crohn disease depends on dietary proteins rich in aromatic and sulfur amino acids, particularly tyrosine and cystine.[27]

VI

A glutamine-enriched diet offers no advantage over a low-glutamine diet in children with Crohn disease.[28] However, the results of this study may have been flawed, insofar as glutamine supplementation occurred at the expense of a reduction in other potentially conditionally essential amino acids (glycine and proline), thereby lowering the protein quality of the diet. Short-term refeeding studies in undernourished children with Crohn disease demonstrate that lean body mass comprises 80% of body weight gain when daily dietary protein intakes approximate 3 g/kg and the protein-energy ratio of the peptide-based formulas averages 1:6.25.[24] Dietary protein deficiency is uncommon in Western diets; nevertheless, the metabolic costs of inflammation and growth on protein nutriture in children with Crohn disease remain to be defined, and no specific recommendations for quantitative and qualitative protein and/or amino acid needs can be made at this time.

Vitamins, Trace Minerals, Antioxidants

Deficiencies for virtually every vitamin, mineral, and trace element have been reported in children with Crohn disease. During disease exacerbation, dietary intakes of iron, zinc, copper, folic acid, and vitamin C may decrease on average 20% to 50% below their recommended dietary allowance.[29] Altered serum or plasma concentrations often are used to define the deficiency state; however, these values may reflect inflammation and not reflect body tissue stores or functional deficits.[30] With severe, extensive inflammation or after resection of the terminal ileum, parenteral vitamin B_{12} supplementation may be necessary. Most patients need oral or occasional parenteral iron supplementation to replace chronic and ongoing losses attributable to bleeding and malabsorption.

Vitamin D

Bone mineralization is an important consideration in the care of the growing child with IBD. The World Health Organization defines osteopenia as the loss of bone mineral and matrix z-scores >1 standard deviation (SD) and osteoporosis as matrix z-scores >2 SDs below the mean for male and female populations. High rates of osteopenia and osteoporosis are reported in pediatric patients with IBD.[31-34] Vertebral compression fracture has been reported as a presenting manifestation of the disease, and the rate of bone fracture is increased in children after corticosteroid treatment.

Gender and pubertal staging are important considerations in understanding reported rates of osteopenia and osteoporosis. In most studies, a greater proportion of adolescent boys exhibit osteoporosis. However, when osteoporosis occurs in girls with Crohn disease, it tends to persist. Because bone density is heavily influenced by growth and puberty, correction for height for age, bone age, or BMI reduces the apparent prevalence of osteoporosis. An independent risk factor may be genetic predisposition. Patient groupings can be further subdivided by disease classification

(Crohn disease vs ulcerative colitis), treatment with corticosteroids, or previous surgery. Patients with Crohn disease have far greater impairment of bone density than do patients with ulcerative colitis. Bone mineral density has consistently been reported to be low at diagnosis in pediatric patients with Crohn disease, after 2 years of treatment, and in adults with longstanding disease.[35-37]

Corticosteroids reduce calcium absorption, down-regulate calcitriol synthesis, decrease gene expression of calcium-binding protein, inhibit osteoblast proliferation, and stimulate osteoclastic bone resorption. Corticosteroid use at >7.5 mg/day, 5 g lifetime cumulative dose, or >12 months of lifetime exposure are risk factors for a low bone mineral density z-score.[38,39] Patients with newly diagnosed Crohn disease often exhibit hypercalciuria, indicating negative calcium balance, because of the effects of systemic inflammation. Serum from pediatric patients with Crohn disease inhibits osteoblastic activity in bone cell culture that is attributed to the effects of IL-6, TNF-alpha, and cytokines.[40] A genetic component certainly plays a role in the response of bone to proinflammatory cytokines (ie, noncarriage of the 240-base pair allele of the IL-1ra gene) in patients with Crohn disease. A large study of 130 IBD patients 8 to 22 years of age indicated the following as risk factors for vitamin D deficiency: dark skin complexion, winter season, early stages of disease, more severe disease, upper gastrointestinal tract involvement, and lack of vitamin D supplementation.[41]

Treatment of Bone Disease

Effective therapy of the underlying disease is the most powerful treatment for osteoporosis. Provision of adequate calcium and vitamin D is also essential. New guidelines have increased recommended intakes of calcium in growing adolescents to 1300 mg daily and increased the vitamin D recommendation to 600 IU/day.[42] Ensuring adequate calcium intake is important in patients with lactose intolerance, dietary restrictions, decreased intake, and malabsorption. Patients may be monitored by bone density assessment correlated to height for age, bone age, or BMI. Results of serum osteocalcin, a measure of bone turnover, are highly variable in adolescents.

Patients with IBD are at greater risk of physical inactivity, an independent risk factor for osteoporosis. Immobilization and bed rest compound other risk factors in patients with acute illness. Maintaining activity, encouraging full participation in sports, and minimizing bed rest are important factors. Smoking exacerbates Crohn disease and should be particularly discouraged in adolescents.[43]

The use of calcitonin has not been widely studied in children. A recent double-blind, placebo-controlled trial testing the efficacy and safety of intranasal calcitonin on bone mineral density in pediatric patients with IBD did not show any sustained efficacy.[44] Bisphosphonates inhibit osteoclasis and have been used to prevent osteoporosis and prevent the risk of fracture in adults. A Cochrane meta-analysis of 13 trials involving 842 patients showed that the use of bisphosphonate is effective in preventing and treating bone loss treated with corticosteroids.[45] Bisphosphonate use has been studied in children with osteogenesis imperfecta and other diseases.[46,47] Increasing bone strength is a separate consideration from increasing bone density. No published data support use of bisphosphonates in children with IBD. The early implementation of nutritional or immunosuppressive therapies as an alternative to chronic corticosteroid treatment may reduce the prevalence of osteoporosis in children with IBD. Recent reports of improved bone formation and bone mineral content with infliximab suggest that treatment of the underlying inflammatory state may be sufficient to improve bone health in these patients.[48,49] A recent report suggests that human growth hormone treatment may improve bone mineral content in these patients.[50]

Zinc

Zinc functions as a cofactor in more than 300 metalloenzymes. It is important in RNA and DNA synthesis, lymphocyte proliferation, cytokine production, free radical activity, and wound healing. Zinc deficiency contributes to growth retardation, anorexia, impaired cell-mediated immunity, hypogonadism, and acrodermatitis, all of which have been documented in patients with IBD. Serum zinc concentrations do not accurately reflect total body zinc depletion, because more than 95% of the zinc is intracellular, and serum concentrations depend on albumin binding availability.

Reduced serum zinc concentrations are reported in patients with Crohn disease and ulcerative colitis, and reduced zinc content is demonstrated in mucosal biopsy specimens from patients with IBD. Reduced serum zinc concentrations in Crohn disease correlate with disease activity but not with disease location or nutritional status.

In vitro epithelial cell line restitution is enhanced by supraphysiologic supplementation of zinc. Twelve patients with Crohn disease in remission received pharmacologic doses of zinc (25 mg of elemental zinc, 3 times/day for 8 weeks), which reversed increased small bowel permeability in 10 of 12 patients.[51] Zinc supplementation, as an antioxidant, in combination with selenium and vitamin E, is increasingly used in patients with IBD, with no controlled studies to confirm their value.

Folate

Folate may protect against colon cancer in patients with IBD because of its essential role in the synthesis, methylation, and repair of DNA. Epidemiologic evidence in support of an association between folate status and colon cancer was first observed in patients with ulcerative colitis.[52] Folate deficiency is poorly understood in children with IBD, with many studies showing lower serum folate concentrations compared with healthy subjects. However, recent studies suggest that folate concentrations in pediatric IBD patients may be higher than control subjects despite lower folate intakes of nearly 20% and that folate deficiency is much less common than previously thought.[53]

Nevertheless, the folic acid requirement of children with Crohn disease has not been determined. Adult patients with Crohn disease who receive total parenteral nutrition (TPN) providing 400 µg of folic acid/day have low concentrations of red blood cell folate. Red blood cell folate concentrations increased with a daily infusion of 800 µg of folic acid. Such studies lend some credence to the clinical practice of folate supplementation in subjects with Crohn disease; however, the recommended dose of folic acid (800 µg–1 mg orally daily) is empiric. Folate supplementation is also common practice for those receiving medications that may interfere with folate metabolism, such as sulfasalazine and methotrexate.

The prevalence of thromboembolic complications is increased in patients with Crohn disease because of the procoagulant effects associated with inflammation. Hyperhomocystinemia, a risk factor for venous and arterial thrombosis, is common in IBD. Hyperhomocystinemia results from genetic or environmental factors, the latter including dietary deficiencies of folate, cobalamin, and pyridoxine. Despite these relationships, hyperhomocystinemia does not appear to contribute to the development of venous or arterial thrombosis in adults with IBD, regardless of nutritional vitamin status.[54]

Antioxidants

Oxidant stress is considered important in the pathogenesis of IBD. Dietary antioxidants, such as alpha-tocopherol, ascorbic acid, and selenium, and other biologic antioxidants, such as glutathione peroxidase and glutathione, are presumed to protect cells from free radical injury. Antioxidant vitamin and mineral supplements may be of potential therapeutic value in IBD. Low serum retinol and alpha-tocopherol concentrations are found in 6% of children with IBD, although the mean serum values in children with Crohn disease, ulcerative colitis, and healthy control subjects are similar.[55] Surprisingly, alpha-tocopherol levels were similar in these patients, independent of their nutritional status and the use of multivitamin supplements. Alpha-tocopherol, beta-carotene, and gamma-tocopherol concentrations are comparable in children with Crohn disease and healthy children.[56] Others report that whole-blood concentrations of alpha-tocopherol, glutathione, and glutathione peroxidase are higher in children with Crohn disease.[57]

Evidence-based recommendations for vitamin and mineral supplementation in children with IBD are still lacking.

Nutritional Therapy for IBD

Dietary Therapy

Many parents seeking alternative therapies will try specialized and often nutritionally inadequate diets. Children and adolescents with IBD have tried gluten-free diets, diets rich in fish oils (see below), diets high or low in specific carbohydrates (eg, carbohydrate-specific diet), vegan diets, or other fad diets and supplements. However, the use of any specialized restrictive diet remains to be substantiated. As is observed in the general population, some pediatric patients with upper small bowel Crohn disease develop lactose intolerance and benefit from milk substitutes, lactase supplementation, or varying degrees of milk product limitation to alleviate symptoms associated with lactose malabsorption.

Elemental Versus Polymeric Diets

In adults, multiple meta-analyses have concluded that enteral nutrition (liquid food taken orally or by tube in the intestinal tract) as primary therapy for Crohn disease is statistically inferior to corticosteroid use in inducing clinical remission.[58] In children with Crohn disease, however, a meta-analysis indicated that no significant difference exists between corticosteroids and enteral nutrition to induce remission and suggests that enteral nutrition may indeed be a safer way to promote remission in a shorter time.[58] Treatment failures are attributable to intolerance of the defined formula diets or the tube feeding, leading to high dropout rates. In another analysis limited to randomized clinical trials involving only pediatric patients (5 trials comprising 127 patients), exclusive enteral nutrition was as effective as corticosteroid use in inducing clinical remission (13).[59] No subanalysis by type of defined formula was performed. The authors concluded that improved growth and development, without the adverse effects of steroids, made enteral nutrition a better first choice for first-line therapy in children with active Crohn disease. However, from a practical point of view, issues of compliance as well as a less favorable response rate in patients with extensive colitis (whether Crohn or ulcerative colitis) render nutritional therapy less attractive for these subgroups. Enteral nutrition is most commonly used to induce remission in children with active Crohn disease involving the small bowel (with or without proximal colonic disease) who have either growth failure or intolerable steroid-induced adverse effects.

Both elemental and polymeric diets are associated with improved disease activity scores, histologic healing, and down-regulation of proinflammatory cytokines.[15,60,61] A recent meta-analysis considered results from 9 trials including fewer than 300 patients treated with elemental and nonelemental diets.[62] No differences were observed between the groups, although the study was limited in that several types of defined formula diets were included in the nonelemental group. A double-blind, randomized trial comparing the effect of a polymeric and an elemental diet in patients with active Crohn disease was performed using 2 identical preparations except for the nitrogen source (ie, amino acid vs intact protein).[63] Remission rates were better for elemental versus polymeric formula (80% vs 55%, respectively, $P =$ .01), although the total number of patients studied was small (n = 21). Elemental diets may support mucosal healing because of their high content of glutamine. However, a recent double-blind randomized controlled trial of a glutamine-enriched polymeric diet failed to substantiate this hypothesis.[28]

An alternate explanation for the potential advantage of specific formulas for patients with Crohn disease may be the fat, rather than protein, content.[64] In an attempt to address this issue, a recent randomized and controlled double-blind trial in adults compared 2 whole-protein formulas with long-chain triglycerides supplying either 5% or 30% of total energy.[65] Remission rates in both arms of the study were low, reaching only 26% and 33% for the low and higher triglyceride formulas, respectively. Once again, a high proportion of the patients in this adult trial (21 of 54) were unable to tolerate the diet, accounting for the high failure rates. Finally, 2 studies examined the type, rather than the amount, of fat in the defined formula diet. The first showed that the use of medium-chain triglycerides did not affect the ability of an elemental diet to induce remission, achieved in approximately two thirds of patients.[24] In the second study, a polymeric diet containing 35 g of lipids per 1000 kcal high in oleic acid (79%) and low in linoleic acid (6.5%) was compared with an identical diet except for lower oleic acid (45%) and higher linoleic acid (28%) content.[25] Overall, the high–oleic acid formula induced remission in 20%, compared with 52% for a high-linoleic acid diet ($P =$ .05), suggesting that the quality of fat may be important in the therapeutic response to these diets. Both formulas were inferior to the use of corticosteroids, however (79%; $P =$ .001).[66]

With all of these results taken together, firm evidence is lacking to support the use of amino acid-, peptide-, or whole-protein–based formulas for the primary treatment of active Crohn disease. Evidence is also lacking to support the contention that formulas with anti-inflammatory cytokines, prebiotics, and probiotics are effective in the treatment of children with IBD.

Total Parenteral Nutrition as Primary Therapy
When considering studies of total parenteral nutrition (TPN) in patients with IBD, 2 points are significant. First, few studies have been conducted in children. Second, enteral nutrition is the preferred method of nutritional support for patients with IBD because of fewer complications and lower cost. Nevertheless, the use of TPN

VI

in IBD can be considered as primary or adjunct therapy when the enteral route cannot be used or the enteral route is ineffective to maintain nutritional support. TPN also is indicated in selected patients before and after surgery, including individuals who are severely undernourished or those whose disease is complicated by fistula(s), short bowel syndrome, toxic megacolon, intestinal obstruction, or perforation.

Preoperative parenteral nutrition has been shown to be efficacious in reducing postoperative complications when therapy is administered for at least 5 days. TPN given before surgery only benefits patients with IBD who are severely undernourished.[67,68] A subsequent analysis of the literature on perioperative TPN reports that preoperative TPN decreases complications by approximately 10%.[69] In contrast, when TPN is initiated only during the postoperative period, complications are about 10% higher than those observed in untreated control subjects.[66]

Bowel rest and TPN reduce intestinal inflammation and decrease disease activity in selected patients with Crohn disease. Several retrospective analyses performed since 1990 have examined the effectiveness of TPN as primary medical therapy.[70,71] The majority of patients with severe but uncomplicated Crohn colitis respond to TPN and aggressive medical therapy. However, TPN has not demonstrated any additional benefit over corticosteroids in patients with ulcerative colitis.[71]

Several studies have examined the effects of TPN on the closure of intestinal fistula(s) in patients with Crohn disease.[72] Pooled data reveal an initial closure rate of only a 44% of fistulas, and of these only 37% remain closed for an extended period of time. Short bowel syndrome may be a morbid outcome in patients with Crohn disease and repeated operations. These patients often require home TPN.

Home TPN and home enteral nutritional therapy use across the United States has been evaluated.[73] Patients with Crohn disease made up the third largest group (after neoplasms and miscellaneous), comprising 11% to 12% of patients receiving home TPN. The prevalence of the use of home TPN and home enteral nutritional therapy in the United States is as much as 10 times higher than that in other Western countries. Both therapies are relatively safe.

Fish Oil

Attention has recently been directed at the immunomodulatory role of polyunsaturated fatty acids. Increased intakes of the omega-6 fatty acid, linoleic acid, increases arachidonic acid content in the serum and cell membranes. The resulting increase in the synthesis of leukotriene B_4 and thromboxane A2 stimulates a proinflammatory response. In Japan, the incidence of Crohn disease is reported to correlate with omega-6 fatty acid intake.[74]

In contrast, the omega-3 fatty acid eicosapentaenoic acid (EPA) competes with arachidonic acid. This shifts synthesis to leukotriene B_5, a far less potent proinflammatory product, while inhibiting the synthesis of inflammatory cytokines, such as TNF-alpha, and increasing the scavenging of free radicals. Fish oil, a rich source of omega-3 fatty acids, has been investigated as therapy in patients with IBD. In adults with mild to moderate ulcerative colitis, 4 studies employing doses of 2.7 g to 4.2 g daily of omega-3 fatty acids demonstrated a modest clinical improvement and reduction of concurrent steroid requirements.[75,76] Other studies showed no benefit from fish oil treatment for maintaining ulcerative colitis in remission. A randomized controlled study of a regimen of 5 g of fish oil daily for 2 years showed no reduction in relapse rates in adults with Crohn disease.[77]

Glutamine

Glutamine supplementation maintains mucosal thickness and villus height, reduces endotoxemia, and enhances mucosal barrier function in animal models of colitis. A glutamine-enriched TPN solution prevented increased intestinal permeability to lactulose and mannitol in patients with active IBD receiving postoperative TPN.[78] However, another study in humans did not show any advantage of a glutamine-enriched polymeric diet compared with a standard diet in active Crohn disease in children.[28]

Short-Chain Fatty Acids

Colonic bacteria metabolize unabsorbed carbohydrate, protein, and fiber to form short-chain fatty acids (SCFAs), hydrogen, and carbon dioxide. The SCFAs, primarily acetate, propionate, and butyrate (ratio of 60:20:20, respectively), are weak electrolytes but constitute the predominant luminal anions in colonic fluid. Recognition that luminal SCFA concentrations are decreased in severe ulcerative colitis led to an interest in the potential role of these substances as therapy in IBD. Butyrate is a preferred metabolic substrate for colonocytes and is a trophic factor in the colon.

Initial observations with either mixtures of SCFA or butyrate alone, given as enemas, produced apparent clinical benefit.[79,80] However, prospective, randomized, placebo-controlled studies have not shown a clear therapeutic effect of SCFAs on colitis.[81,82] Thus, the role of SCFAs in maintaining mucosal integrity requires additional investigation.

Glucagon-Like Peptide-2

Glucagon-like peptide 2 (GLP-2) is a 33-amino acid member of the pituitary adenylate cyclase activating peptide glucagon hormone superfamily, with receptors located on enteric neurons, enteroendocrine cells, and subepithelial myoblasts in the gut. Recently, a synthetic analogue of GLP-2 (Teduglutide) has shown promise in phase II and III trials in adult patients with short gut syndrome and IBD.[83] Teduglutide exerts its luminal effects by enhancing crypt cell proliferation,

VI

increasing villus height and crypt depth, and decreasing intestinal permeability to macromolecules. In a study of 71 adult patients with IBD, dose-dependent response and remission rates were observed in the Teduglutide group.[84] Although studies are lacking in children with IBD, preliminary investigations into the role of GLP-2 in infants with short bowel syndrome secondary to necrotizing enterocolitis are currently ongoing.

Psychosocial Impact of Nutritional Interventions in the Care of Children With IBD

IBD represents a major, lifelong health threat that challenges the psychological resources of both the affected child and his or her family. Acute, active disease may necessitate hospital admission, causing major disruptions in children's academic, social, and family life. Most children with IBD experience considerable worry, distress, and concern about their disease and its effects on school absences, academic achievement, and participation in family and social activities away from home.

Well-conducted studies regarding the effects of nutrition support on psychosocial functioning in children with IBD are lacking. Treatment interventions can have both direct and indirect effects on psychosocial functioning. Although enteral nutrition does not entail the adverse effects of steroid treatment, it does have drawbacks. Enteral nutrition support requires high patient motivation and often involves tube feeding. Social factors, including support from family and friends, as well as peer pressure at school, are recognized as important influences on tolerance of enteral nutrition.[85]

During treatment, patients endure prolonged periods of oral food deprivation and can experience frustration because of disruption of social and family activities during meals. Enteral nutrition can be difficult for children who eat their meals at school, particularly if they are already embarrassed about the disease. Use of tube feedings and special liquid diets can also exacerbate feelings of being different and, thus, further contribute to a sense of alienation.[86] An additional consideration is that use of the feeding tube and pump apparatus makes the disease more visible, both to patients and to those around them. This can accentuate feelings of self-consciousness and heighten embarrassment in social situations. In addition, patients initially experience the insertion of a nasogastric tube as intrusive. The psychological meanings that patients attribute to treatment procedures, as well as emotional reactions such as anxiety, fear, and depression, may well be more influential than physical status in determining adherence to treatment and the success of nutritional therapies.[87]

Summary

Impairment of linear growth is common in children with Crohn disease, both before recognizing the presence of the disease and thereafter. Growth impairment is much less prevalent in pediatric patients with ulcerative colitis. Chronic undernutrition, nutrient losses, medications, and proinflammatory mediators are increasingly recognized as contributing factors to the observed growth failure in children and adolescents with Crohn disease or ulcerative colitis. Children with Crohn disease generally have greater nutrient needs based on gender, age, and weight than do those with ulcerative colitis.

Important clinical practices can enhance the growth and nutritional status of children and adolescents with IBD. These include[a]:

1. Screen and assess pediatric patients with IBD for malnutrition and growth failure. At a minimum, this includes:
   • Height, weight, and BMI followed serially and plotted on standardized reference growth charts; and
   • Biochemical tests of nutrient and micronutrient status and, in patients at high risk of bone disease, medical imaging of selected bones for mineral content and density.
2. Provide a diet based on the Dietary Reference Intakes and the 2010 Dietary Guidelines for Americans for all pediatric patients with IBD. Dietary supplementation of selected nutrients may be warranted on the basis of a nutritional assessment of the individual patient.
3. Provide adequate calcium and vitamin D intake for all children with IBD. Patients at greatest risk of osteopenia and osteoporosis may be monitored by bone mineral density assessment. Maintaining full physical activity and minimizing bed rest are important to reduce the risk of bone disease.
4. Elemental and polymeric enteral diets may be equally effective in inducing remission for active Crohn disease; enteral nutrition is considered before parenteral nutrition, because it is safer and less costly.
5. TPN is considered for nutrition support in children with IBD when the enteral route cannot be used or is ineffective in nutrition support. TPN is effective as primary therapy in pediatric patients with Crohn disease whose nutrient needs cannot be supported by enteral nutrition or who are resistant to corticosteroid therapy. Preoperative TPN may reduce postoperative complications in malnourished patients who are not candidates for enteral nutrition support.

VI

[a] Modified and reprinted with permission from Kleinman et al.[88]

6. Data are too limited to allow definitive recommendations regarding the use of glutamine, fish oil, SCFAs, GLP-2, or specific dietary restrictions as primary therapy to control inflammation in children with IBD.

7. Psychosocial dysfunction is common in children with active IBD. Total enteral and parenteral nutrition may also have negative effects on social and psychological functioning. For such children, ongoing support by a mental health professional who is experienced in helping children develop coping strategies to deal with the effects of chronic illness and the treatments used for IBD is a critical component of the child's therapy.

References

1. Kelsen J, Baldassano RN. Inflammatory bowel disease: the difference between children and adults. *Inflamm Bowel Dis*. 2008;14(Suppl 2):S9–S11

2. Lindberg E, Lindquist B, Holmquist L, Hildebrand H. Inflammatory bowel disease in children and adolescents in Sweden, 1984-1995. *J Pediatr Gastroenterol Nutr*. 2000;30(3):259-264

3. Lehtinen P, Ashorn M, Iltanen S, et al. Incidence Trends of Pediatric Inflammatory Bowel Disease in Finland, 1987-2003, a Nationwide Study. *Inflamm Bowel Dis*. 2010;17(8):1778-1783

4. Benhimol EI, Fortinsky KJ, Gozdyra P, et al. Epidemiology of pediatric inflammatory bowel disease: a systemic review of international trends. *Inflamm Bowel Dis*. 2011;17(1):423-439

5. Kugathasan S, Baldassano RN, Bradfield JP, et al. Loci on 20q13 and 21q22 are associated with pediatric-onset inflammatory bowel disease. *Nat Genet*. 2008;40(10):1211–1215

6. Van Limbergen J, Russell RK, Drummond HE, et al. Definition of phenotypic characteristics of childhood-onset inflammatory bowel disease. *Gastroenterology*. 2008;135(4):1114–1122

7. Kanof ME, Lake AM, Bayless TM. Decreased height velocity in children and adolescents before the diagnosis of Crohn's disease. *Gastroenterology*. 1988;95(6):1523–1527

8. Gupta N, Bostrom AG, Kirschner BS, et al. Gender differences in presentation and course of disease in pediatric patients with Crohn disease. *Pediatrics*. 2007;120(6):e1418-e1425

9. Ceballos C. Growth and early onset inflammatory bowel disease. *Gastroenterol Nurs*. 2008;31(2):101-104

10. Yamamoto T, Nakahigashi M, Umegae S, Kitagawa T, Matsumoto K. Impact of elemental diet on mucosal inflammation in patients with active Crohn's disease: cytokine production and endoscopic and histological findings. *Inflamm Bowel Dis*. 2005;11(6):580-588

11. Wedrychowicz A, Kowalska Duplaga K, et al. Serum concentrations of VEGF and TGF-β1 during exclusive enteral nutrition in IBD. *J Pediatr Gastroenterol Nutr*. 2011;53(2):150-155

12. Gupta N, Lustig RH, Kohn MA, McCracken M, Vittinghoff E. Sex differences in statural growth impairment in Crohn. *Inflamm Bowel Dis*. 2011;17(11):2318-2325

13. Schiechl G, Bauer B, Fuss I, et al. Tumor development in murine ulcerative colitis depends on MyD88 signaling of colonic F4/80+CD11b(high)Gr1(low) macrophages. *J Clin Invest*. 2011;121(5):1692-1708

14. Hokken-Koelega AC, Stijnen T, de Muinck Keizer-Schrama SM, Blum WF, Drop SL. Levels of growth hormone, insulin-like growth factor-I (IGF-I) and -II, IGF-binding protein-1 and -3, and cortisol in prednisone-treated children with growth retardation after renal transplantation. *J Clin Endocrinol Metab*. 1993;77(4):932–938

15. Fell JM, Paintin M, Arnaud-Battandier F, et al. Mucosal healing and a fall in mucosal pro-inflammatory cytokine mRNA induced by a specific oral polymeric diet in paediatric Crohn's disease. *Aliment Pharmacol Ther*. 2000;14(3):281-289

16. Boot AM, Bouquet J, Krenning EP, de Muinck Keizer-Schrama SM. Bone mineral density and nutritional status in children with chronic inflammatory bowel disease. *Gut*. 1998;42(2):188-194

17. Sentongo TA, Semaeo EJ, Stettler N, Piccoli DA, Stallings VA, Zemel BS. Vitamin D status in children, adolescents, and young adults with Crohn disease. *Am J Clin Nutr*. 2002;76(5):1077-1081

18. Semeao EJ, Jawad AF, Zemel BS, Neiswender KM, Piccoli DA, Stallings VA. Bone mineral density in children and young adults with Crohn's disease. *Inflamm Bowel Dis*. 1999;5(3):161-166

19. US Department of Agriculture. ChooseMyPlate. Available at: http://www.choosemyplate.gov/. Accessed January 17, 2013

20. Pappa HM, Langereis EJ, Grand RJ, Gordon CM. Prevalence and risk factors for hypovitaminosis D in young patients with inflammatory bowel disease. *J Pediatr Gastroenterol Nutr*. 2011;53(4):361-364

21. Wiskin AE, Wootton SA, Culliford DJ, Afzal NA, Jackson A, Beattie RM. Impact of disease activity on resting energy expenditure in children with inflammatory bowel disease. *Clin Nutr*. 2009;28(6):652-656

22. Hill RJ, Cleghorn GJ, Withers GD, Lewindon PJ, Ee LC, Connor F, Davies PS. Resting energy expenditure in children with inflammatory bowel disease. *J Pediatr Gastroenterol Nutr*. 2007;45(3):342-346

23. Azcue M, Rashid M, Griffiths A, et al. Energy expenditure and body composition in children with Crohn's disease: effect of enteral nutrition and treatment with prednisolone. *Gut*. 1997;41(2):203-208

24. Khoshoo V, Reifen R, Neuman MG, Griffiths A, Pencharz PB. Effect of low- and high-fat, peptide-based diets on body composition and disease activity in adolescents with active Crohn's disease. *JPEN J Parenter Enteral Nutr*. 1996;20:401-405

25. Belli DC, Seidman E, Bouthillier L, et al. Chronic intermittent elemental diet improves growth failure in children with Crohn's disease. *Gastroenterology*. 1988;94(3):603-610

26. Polk DB, Hattner JA, Kerner JA Jr. Improved growth and disease activity after intermittent administration of a defined formula diet in children with Crohn's disease. *JPEN J Parenter Enteral Nutr*. 1992;16(6):499–504

27. Vaisman N, Griffiths A, Pencharz PB. Comparison of nitrogen utilization of two elemental diets in patients with Crohn's disease. *J Pediatr Gastroenterol Nutr*. 1988;7(1):84–88

VI

28. Akobeng AK, Miller V, Stanton J, Elbadri AM, Thomas AG. Double-blind randomized controlled trial of glutamine-enriched polymeric diet in the treatment of active Crohn's disease. *J Pediatr Gastroenterol Nutr*. 2000;30(1):78–84

29. Thomas AG, Taylor F, Miller V. Dietary intake and nutritional treatment in childhood Crohn's disease. *J Pediatr Gastroenterol Nutr*. 1993;17(1):75–81

30. Ainley C, Cason J, Slavin BM, Wolstencroft RA, Thompson RP. The influence of zinc status and malnutrition on immunological function in Crohn's disease. *Gastroenterology*. 1991;100(6):1616–1625

31. Hill RJ, Brookes DS, Davies PS. Bones in pediatric Crohn. *Inflamm Bowel Dis*. 2011;17(5):1223-1228

32. Ghishan FK, Kiela PR. Advances in the understanding of mineral and bone metabolism in inflammatory bowel diseases. *Am J Physiol Gastrointest Liver Physiol*. 2011;300(2):G191-G201

33. Gokhale R, Favus MJ, Karrison T, Sutton MM, Rich B, Kirschner BS. Bone mineral density assessment in children with inflammatory bowel disease. *Gastroenterology*. 1998;114(5):902-911

34. Issenman RM, Atkinson SA, Radoja C, Fraher L. Longitudinal assessment of growth, mineral metabolism, and bone mass in pediatric Crohn's disease. *J Pediatr Gastroenterol Nutr* 1993;17(4):401-406

35. Andreassen H, Hylander E, Rix M. Gender, age, and body weight are the major predictive factors for bone mineral density in Crohn's disease: a case—control cross-sectional study of 113 patients. *Am J Gastroenterol*. 1999;94(3):824–828

36. Herzog D, Bishop N, Glorieux F, Seidman EG. Interpretation of bone mineral density values in pediatric Crohn's disease. *Inflamm Bowel Dis*. 1998;4(4):261–267

37. Warner JT, Cowan FJ, Dunstan FD, et al. Measured and predicted bone mineral content in healthy boys and girls aged 6–18 years: adjustment for body size and puberty. *Acta Paediatr*. 1998;87(3):244–249

38. Lopes L H, Sdepanian V L, Szejnfeld V L, de Morais M B, Fagundes Neto U. Risk factors for low bone mineral density in children and adolescents with inflammatory bowel disease. *Dig Dis Sci*. 2008;53(10):2746-2753

39. Semeao EJ, Jawad AF, Stouffer NO, Zemel BS, Piccoli DA, Stallings VA. Risk factors for low bone mineral density in children and young adults with Crohn's disease. *J Pediatr*. 1999;135(5):593–600

40. Hyams JS, Wyzga N, Kreutzer DL, Justinich CJ, Gronowicz GA. Alterations in bone metabolism in children with inflammatory bowel disease: an in vitro study. *J Pediatr Gastroenterol Nutr*. 1997;24(3):289–295

41. Pappa HM, Gordon CM, Saslowsky TM, Zholudev A, Horr B, Shih MC, Grand RJ. Vitamin D status in children and young adults with inflammatory bowel disease. *Pediatrics*. 2006;118(5):1950-1961

42. Institute of Medicine, Food and Nutrition Board. Dietary Reference Intakes for Calcium and Vitamin D. Washington, DC: National Academies Press; 2010

43. Rubin DT, Hanauer SB. Smoking and inflammatory bowel disease. *Eur J Gastroenterol Hepatol*. 2000;12(8):855–862

44. Pappa HM, Saslowsky TM, Filip-Dhima R, et al. Efficacy and harms of nasal calcitonin in improving bone density in young patients with inflammatory bowel disease: a randomized, placebo-controlled, double-blind trial. *Am J Gastroenterol.* 2011;106(8):1527-1543

45. Homik J, Cranney A, Shea B, et al. Bisphosphonates for steroid induced osteoporosis. *Cochrane Database Syst Rev.* 2000;(2):CD001347

46. Glorieux FH, Bishop NJ, Plotkin H, Chabot G, Lanoue G, Travers R. Cyclic administration of pamidronate in children with severe osteogenesis imperfecta. *N Engl J Med.* 1998;339(14):947-952

47. Bianchi ML, Cimaz R, Bardare M, et al. Efficacy and safety of alendronate for the treatment of osteoporosis in diffuse connective tissue diseases in children: a prospective multicenter study. *Arthritis Rheum.* 2000;43(9):1960-1966

48. Visvanathan S, van der Heijde D, Deodhar A, et al. Effects of infliximab on markers of inflammation and bone turnover and associations with bone mineral density in patients with ankylosing spondylitis. *Ann Rheum Dis.* 2009;68(2):175-182

49. Abreu MT, Geller JL, Vasiliauskas EA, et al. Treatment with infliximab is associated with increased markers of bone formation in patients with Crohn. *J Clin Gastroenterol.* 2006;40(1):55-63

50. Heyman MB, Garnett EA, Wojcicki J, et al. Growth hormone treatment for growth failure in pediatric patients with Crohn's disease. *J Pediatr.* 2008;153(5):651-658

51. Strobel CT, Byrne WJ, Ament ME. Home parenteral nutrition in children with Crohn. *Gastroenterology.* 1979;77(2):272-279

52. Lashner BA, Provencher KS, Seidner DL, et al. The effect of folic acid supplementation on the risk for cancer or dysplasia in ulcerative colitis. *Gastroenterology.* 1997;112(1):29-32

53. Heyman MB, Garnett EA, Shaikh N, et al. Folate concentrations in pediatric patients with newly diagnosed inflammatory bowel disease. *Am J Clin Nutr.* 2009;89(2):545-550

54. Oldenburg B, Fijnheer R, van der Griend R, et al. Homocysteine in inflammatory bowel disease: a risk factor for thromboembolic complications? *Am J Gastroenterol.* 2000;95(10):2825–2830

55. Bousvaros A, Zurakowski D, Duggan C, et al. Vitamins A and E serum levels in children and young adults with inflammatory bowel disease: effect of disease activity. *J Pediatr Gastroenterol Nutr.* 1998;26(2):129–135

56. Levy E, Rizwan Y, Thibault L, et al. Altered lipid profile, lipoprotein composition, and oxidant and antioxidant status in pediatric Crohn disease. *Am J Clin Nutr.* 2000;71(3):807–815

57. Hoffenberg EJ, Deutsch J, Smith S, Sokol RJ. Circulating antioxidant concentrations in children with inflammatory bowel disease. *Am J Clin Nutr.* 1997;65(5):1482–1488

58. Dziechciarz P, Horvath A, Shamir R, Szajewska H. Meta-analysis: enteral nutrition in active Crohn's disease in children. *Aliment Pharmacol Ther.* 2007;26(6):795-806

59. Heuschkel RB, Menache CC, Megerian JT, et al. Enteral nutrition and corticosteroids in the treatment of acute Crohn's disease in children. *J Pediatr Gastroenterol Nutr.* 2000;31(1):8-15

VI

60. Teahon K, Smethurst P, MacPherson A, Levi J, Menzies IS, Bjarnason I. Intestinal permeability in Crohn's disease and its relation to disease activity and relapse following treatment with elemental diet. *Eur J Gastroenterol Hepatol*. 1993;5(2):79-84

61. Leiper K, Woolner J, Mullan MM, et al. A randomised controlled trial of high versus low long chain triglyceride whole protein feed in active Crohn's disease. *Gut*. 2001;49(6):790-794

62. Zachos M, Tondeur M, Griffiths AM. Enteral nutritional therapy for inducing remission of Crohn's disease. *Cochrane Database Syst Rev*. 2001;(3)CD000542

63. Verma S, Brown S, Kirkwood B, et al. Polymeric versus elemental diet as primary treatment in active Crohn's disease: a randomized, double-blind trial. *Am J Gastroenterol*. 2000;95(3):735–759

64. Sakurai T, Matsui T, Yao T, et al. Short-term efficacy of enteral nutrition in the treatment of active Crohn's disease: a randomized, controlled trial comparing nutrient formulas. *JPEN J Parenter Enteral Nutr*. 2002;26(2):98-103

65. Leiper K, Woolner J, Mullan MM, et al. A randomised controlled trial of high versus low long chain triglyceride whole protein feed in active Crohn's disease. *Gut*. 2001;49(6):790–794

66. Gassull MA, Fernandez-Banares F, Cabre E, et al. Fat composition may be a clue to explain the primary therapeutic effect of enteral nutrition in Crohn's disease: results of a double blind randomized multicentre European trial. *Gut*. 2002;51(2):164-168

67. Han PD, Burke A, Baldassano RN, Rombeau JL, Lichtenstein GR. Nutrition and inflammatory bowel disease. *Gastroenterol Clin North Am*. 1999;28(2):423-443

68. Gouma DJ, von Meyenfeldt MF, Rouflart M, et al. Preoperative total parenteral nutrition (TPN) in severe Crohn's disease. *Surgery* 1988;103(6):648-652

69. Klein S, Kinney J, Jeejeebhoy K, et al. Nutrition support in clinical practice: review of published data and recommendations for future research directions. Summary of a conference sponsored by the National Institutes of Health, American Society for Parenteral and Enteral Nutrition, and American Society for Clinical Nutrition. *Am J Clin Nutr*. 1997;66(3):683-706

70. Sitzmann JV, Converse RL Jr, Bayless TM. Favorable response to parenteral nutrition and medical therapy in Crohn's colitis. A report of 38 patients comparing severe Crohn's and ulcerative colitis. *Gastroenterology*. 1990;99(6):1647–1652

71. Seo M, Okada M, Yao T, et al. The role of total parenteral nutrition in the management of patients with acute attacks of inflammatory bowel disease. *J Clin Gastroenterol*. 1999;29(3):270–275

72. Evans JP, Steinhart AH, Cohen Z, McLeod RS. Home total parenteral nutrition: an alternative to early surgery for complicated inflammatory bowel disease. *J Gastrointest Surg*. 2003;7(4):562-566

73. Howard L, Ament M, Fleming CR, Shike M, Steiger E. Current use and clinical outcome of home parenteral and enteral nutrition therapies in the United States. *Gastroenterology*. 1995;109(2):355–365

74. Shoda R, Matsueda K, Yamato S, Umeda N. Epidemiologic analysis of Crohn disease in Japan: increased dietary intake of n-6 polyunsaturated fatty acids and animal protein relates to the increased incidence of Crohn disease in Japan. *Am J Clin Nutr*. 1996;63(30 Suppl 8):741-745

75. Macdonald A. Omega-3 fatty acids as adjunctive therapy in Crohns disease. *Gastroenterol Nurs*. 2006;29(4):295-301

76. Belluzzi A, Brignola C, Campieri M, Pera A, Boschi S, Miglioli M. Effect of an enteric-coated fish-oil preparation on relapses in Crohn's disease. *N Engl J Med*. 1996;334(24):1557–1560

77. Lorenz-Meyer H, Bauer P, Nicolay C, et al. Omega-3 fatty acids and low carbohydrate diet for maintenance of remission in Crohn's disease. A randomized controlled multicenter trial. Study Group Members (German Crohn's Disease Study Group). *Scand J Gastroenterol*. 1996;31(8):778–785

78. Ockenga J, Borchert K, Stber E, Lochs H, Manns MP, Bischoff SC. Glutamine-enriched total parenteral nutrition in patients with inflammatory bowel disease. *Eur J Clin Nutr*. 2005;59(11):1302-1309

79. Hallert C, Bjrck I, Nyman M, Pousette A, Grnn C, Svensson H. Increasing fecal butyrate in ulcerative colitis patients by diet: controlled pilot study. *Inflamm Bowel Dis*. 2003;9(2):116-121

80. Steinhart AH, Brzezinski A, Baker JP. Treatment of refractory ulcerative proctosigmoiditis with butyrate enemas. *Am J Gastroenterol*. 1994;89(2):179–183

81. Guillemot F, Colombel JF, Neut C, et al. Treatment of diversion colitis by short-chain fatty acids. Prospective and double-blind study. *Dis Colon Rectum*. 1991;34(10):861–864

82. Breuer RI, Soergel KH, Lashner BA, et al. Short chain fatty acid rectal irrigation for left-sided ulcerative colitis: a randomised, placebo controlled trial. *Gut*. 1997;40(4):485-491

83. Jeppesen PB, Gilroy R, Pertkiewicz M, Allard JP, Messing B, O'Keefe SJ. Randomised placebo-controlled trial of teduglutide in reducing parenteral nutrition and/or intravenous fluid requirements in patients with short bowel syndrome. *Gut*. 2011;60(7):902-914

84. Yazbeck R. Teduglutide, a glucagon-like peptide-2 analog for the treatment of gastrointestinal diseases, including short bowel syndrome. *Curr Opin Mol Ther*. 2010;12(6):798-809

85. Seidman E. Nutritional therapy for Crohn's disease: lessons from the Ste-Justine Hospital experience. *Inflamm Bowel Dis*. 1997;3(1):S43–S45

86. Allison SP. Some psychological and physiological aspects of enteral nutrition. *Gut*. 1986;27(Suppl 1):18-24

87. Gray WN, Denson LA, Baldassano RN, Hommel KA. Treatment Adherence in Adolescents With Inflammatory Bowel Disease: The Collective Impact of Barriers to Adherence and Anxiety/Depressive Symptoms. *J Pediatr Psychol*. 2012;37(3):282-291

88. Kleinman RE, Baldassano RN, Caplan A, et al. Nutrition support for pediatric patients with inflammatory bowel disease: a clinical report of the North American Society for Pediatric Gastroenterology, Hepatology and Nutrition. *J Pediatr Gastroenterol Nutr*. 2004;39(1):15-27

VI

Chapter 45

Liver Disease

Introduction

The liver is the "powerhouse" for metabolic activity in the body. It is the major site for (1) the synthesis of serum proteins, such as albumin and coagulation factors; (2) urea synthesis for normal nitrogen metabolism and ammonia clearance; (3) glucose production for maintaining normoglycemia; and (4) lipid metabolism by producing lipoproteins and converting fatty acids to ketone bodies. These metabolic functions require a considerable amount of energy. The liver consumes approximately 20% of resting energy requirements while constituting only 2% of body weight.[1] Patients who have significant liver disease demonstrate impaired hepatic metabolic function as well as extrahepatic alterations in glucose (insulin resistance and impaired glucose tolerance), lipid (increased lipolytic rates), and protein (decreased protein synthesis and increased amino acid oxidation rates) metabolism.

Nutritional support of an infant or child with liver disease is dependent on the type of liver disease. Acute liver disease, such as that caused by viral hepatitis, may require no special nutritional therapy unless encephalopathy ensues. With acute liver disease, anorexia, vomiting, and diarrhea may result in acute weight loss. Malnutrition, however, is uncommon. Nutritional support of the child with chronic liver disease is influenced by the presence or absence of cholestasis. With cholestasis, fat-soluble vitamins and medium-chain triglycerides are usually required to optimize growth. Children who are anicteric but who have cirrhosis present a different challenge, because hypermetabolism, enteropathy, and increased protein oxidation may occur. Various inborn errors of metabolism that cause liver disease (ie, galactosemia, tyrosinemia, hereditary fructose intolerance, Wilson disease) have specific nutritional requirements and dietary restrictions. The success of pediatric liver transplantation has made the recognition of the importance of nutritional support in the pretransplant period imperative to optimize the success of the transplant.

Protein-energy malnutrition occurs commonly in patients with advanced liver disease and may be caused by several factors. Decreased nutrient intake occurs because of anorexia and nausea. The presence of tense ascites, especially in an infant, makes food intake much more difficult as a result of the intra-abdominal pressure on the stomach. Diminished food intake may result from depression caused by hospitalization or the unpalatable nature of many restricted diets. Malabsorption of fat and fat-soluble vitamins frequently complicates childhood chronic cholestatic liver disease. Fat and fat-soluble vitamins require a critical concentration of intraluminal bile acids for micellar solubilization. Cholestasis, with diminished bile

VI

flow, results in reduced biliary secretion of bile acids and consequent fat and fat-soluble vitamin malabsorption. Supplementation with the fat soluble vitamins A, D, E, and K is required to avoid potential deficiencies of these vitamins. Cirrhosis and portal hypertension may lead to enteropathy and malabsorption secondary to increased mesenteric venous system pressure and villous atrophy from malnutrition. Some liver diseases (Alagille syndrome, progressive familial intrahepatic cholestasis type 1 [PFIC], primary sclerosing cholangitis, hepatic fibrosis) may be associated with extrahepatic organ dysfunction, such as pancreatic insufficiency (eg, cystic fibrosis), inflammatory bowel disease, or other syndromes (eg, Joubert, Johanson-Blizzard), that will aggravate the malabsorption.

Nutritional Assessment of the Child With Liver Disease

It is imperative that any child with chronic liver disease undergo a thorough nutritional assessment to determine the degree of malnutrition, if present, and to tailor the nutritional intervention. The severity of malnutrition may not correlate with the degree of vitamin or trace mineral deficiency or the degree of hepatic dysfunction. A number of obstacles complicate the ability to accurately assess the nutritional status of a child with liver disease.

Body weight may be deceptive, because organomegaly from an enlarged liver or spleen, edema, or ascites can mask weight loss and actually increase the weight. Height (or length in infants and young children) is a better indicator of malnutrition in these children and can be a reliable tool to determine chronic malnutrition. A decrease in height/length for age percentile may be indicative of prolonged malnutrition.

In addition to weight and height/length measurements, triceps skinfold and arm circumference measurements provide a sensitive indicator of nutritional status in children with chronic liver disease. Lower extremities are more prone to peripheral edema and fluid retention than upper extremities; thus, upper extremity measurements are a better indicator of body fat stores and muscle mass. Reduced fat fold thickness and mid-upper arm circumference have been observed in children prior to measured effects in weight or height/length. In children, early reduction in fat and muscle stores reflects the preferential utilization of fat stores to conserve protein stores for energy in the malnourished state. To optimize the accuracy of anthropometric measurements, it is best to utilize a single observer using a standard technique with serial measurements.

Measurement of plasma proteins, including albumin, transferrin, prealbumin, and retinol-binding protein, which are synthesized by the liver, has been used to determine visceral protein nutriture. However, diminished serum concentrations of these proteins may not accurately reflect the body's visceral protein status. The serum concentrations of these proteins more closely correlate with the severity of liver injury rather than the degree of malnutrition as assessed by anthropometric measurements. Hypoalbuminemia in chronic liver disease patients often results from third spacing of fluid and protein in ascites or the extravascular compartment. Further, increased catabolism of albumin without a compensatory increase in albumin synthesis because of inadequate reserves and malabsorption of amino acids and peptides often makes albumin an inaccurate measure of nutritional status. Poor oral intake may further contribute to the hypoalbuminemia.

Nitrogen balance studies are difficult to evaluate in children with chronic liver disease. Impairment of hepatic urea synthesis leads to underestimation of urinary nitrogen losses. Further, ammonia accumulates in the intra- and extracellular compartments instead of being excreted by the kidneys. The creatinine-height index is a good indicator of lean body mass if renal function is unimpaired. When using the creatinine-height index, dietary protein intake, trauma, and infection must be considered, because they all can alter creatinine excretion.

Immune status is sometimes used as an indirect measure of nutritional status. However, because liver disease and, in particular, hypersplenism can result in lymphopenia, abnormal skin test results for delayed hypersensitivity, or decreased concentrations of complement irrespective of nutritional status, these immunologic markers are of limited usefulness in children with liver disease.

Another problem with using biochemical measurements to determine nutritional status in children with liver disease is that many of the drugs used to treat children with liver disease may alter blood concentrations of vitamins. For example, cholestyramine and colestipol, bile acid binding resins, may deplete enteral bile acids and interfere with fat-soluble vitamin absorption from the intestines. Diphenylhydantoin and phenobarbital increase the hepatic metabolism of vitamin D and, thus, decrease cholecalciferol concentrations in plasma.

A well-prepared 24-hour diet diary can be invaluable in assessing the usual caloric intake and should always account for use of dietary supplements or any dietary restrictions that have been imposed. Problems such as nausea, vomiting, diarrhea, or anorexia should be recorded, because these may contribute to poor intake. A careful and thorough physical examination can determine the degree of muscle wasting, depletion of subcutaneous fat, and any evidence of vitamin or mineral deficiencies.

VI

Malabsorption in Chronic Liver Disease

Fat

Steatorrhea (fat malabsorption) is frequently observed in patients with cirrhosis and/or chronic cholestasis, although the degree of biliary obstruction correlates poorly with the amount of fat excreted in the stools. Even in the absence of biliary obstruction, intraluminal bile salt concentrations are thought to be below the critical micellar concentration such that intraluminal products of lipolysis cannot form micellar solutions.[2] Typically, the prothrombin time or international normalized ratio (INR) is prolonged. A trial of parenteral vitamin K administration daily will often correct the prothrombin time or INR and suggests poor fat-soluble vitamin absorption. Anorexia, failure to thrive, ascites, prolongation of the prothrombin time or INR (unresponsive to vitamin K supplementation), and steatorrhea progress in conjunction with worsening of the underlying liver disease and cirrhosis.

Treatment with a low-fat diet supplemented with medium-chain triglyceride (MCT [C8-C12 fatty acids])-containing formulas (Pregestimil [Mead Johnson, approx. 60% MCT], Alimentum [Ross, approx 50% MCT], or Portagen [Mead Johnson, approx 87% MCT]) or MCT oil helps to decrease the degree of steatorrhea and may help to improve the nutritional status of the infant. Elemental formulas are not necessary in these infants. MCT-enhanced diets can also improve energy intake in older children with cholestasis. MCTs do not require intraluminal bile salts for micellar formation to be absorbed in the intestinal lumen. MCTs are relatively water soluble and directly absorbed into the portal circulation. However, when decompensation ensues, although steatorrhea may be diminished with MCT dietary supplementation, failure to thrive may progress.

Essential Fatty Acids

The malabsorption of fat, especially long-chain triglycerides (LCTs), and inadequate intake can lead to essential fatty acid (EFA) deficiency. EFAs are fatty acids that cannot be synthesized by desaturation or elongation of shorter fatty acids. Linoleic acid and linolenic acid are the 2 EFAs in humans. Deficiency of EFAs may result in growth impairment, a dry scaly rash, thrombocytopenia, and impaired immune function.[3] LCTs are poorly absorbed if cholestasis is present. Infants have a small linoleic acid store.[4] Cholestasis in infants places them at an increased EFA deficiency risk. Pregestimil and Alimentum provide only 7% to 14% of calories as linoleic acid. To prevent EFA deficiency, at least 3% to 4% of calories should be linoleic acid. If cholestasis is severe enough to allow 30% to 40% of dietary fat to be malabsorbed, then EFA deficiency may ensue.[5] Portagen, containing 87% MCTs and <3% EFAs, is not recommended for long-term use in children with cholestatic liver disease, because EFA deficiency may occur if supplementation is not provided.[6] Corn oil or safflower oil containing linoleic acid can be added to foods, or a lipid emulsion (Microlipid, Novartis) can be added to formula to provide additional linoleic acid.

Fat-Soluble Vitamins (See Also Chapter 21.1: Fat-Soluble Vitamins)

Bile acids in the intestinal lumen are not only important for fat absorption from the lumen but also for fat-soluble vitamin absorption. Vitamins A, D, E, and K are all dependent on intraluminal bile acid concentration. When the intraluminal bile acid concentration falls below a critical micellar concentration (1.5-2.0 mM), malabsorption of fat-soluble vitamins ensues. Cholestyramine and colestipol, bile acid binding resins, may deplete enteral bile acids and interfere with fat-soluble vitamin absorption from the intestines. Vitamin A and vitamin E require hydrolysis by an intestinal esterase that is bile acid dependent before intestinal absorption. In infants, cholestasis leads to rapid depletion of body stores of fat-soluble vitamins with both biochemical and clinical features of deficiency evident unless adequate supplementation is utilized. Evaluation for fat-soluble vitamin deficiency, supplementation, and follow-up monitoring are all necessary for infants and children with cholestasis.

To alleviate the malabsorption of fat-soluble vitamins in chronic liver disease, a double daily dose of an aqueous preparation of vitamins A, D, E, and K may be prescribed to start. Periodic determination of serum vitamin A, 25-hydroxyvitamin D (25-OH-D), and vitamin E concentrations may be necessary to optimize nutritional support and may result in supplementation of individual fat-soluble vitamins. As a surrogate for vitamin K, prothrombin time and/or INR may be serially followed.

Hypocalcemia attributable to dietary calcium deficiency or malabsorption can lead to rickets and osteopenia on bone radiographs. Large doses of vitamin D supplements (5–20 000 IU/day) may be required to correct this condition. Each fat-soluble vitamin will be discussed individually, because evaluation, supplementation, and monitoring differ.

Vitamin A

Vitamin A refers to retinol and its derivatives having similar biologic activities. The principle vitamin A compounds include retinol, retinal (retinaldehyde), retinoic acid and retinyl esters that differ in the terminal group at the end of the side chain. Dietary vitamin A predominantly is derived from animal sources (liver, fish liver oils, dairy products, kidney, eggs) and carotenoids (provitamin A, beta carotene) in darkly colored vegetables, oily fruits, and red palm oil. The Adequate Intake for vitamin A for infants is 400 to 500 μg/day. The Recommended Dietary Allowance of vitamin A for children 1 to 3 years of age is 300 μg/day, for 4 to 8 years of age is 400 μg/day, and for older children and adults is 600 to 1000 μg/day.

As a fat-soluble vitamin, vitamin A absorption can be adversely affected by cholestasis. Vitamin A nutritional status can be determined by assessing vitamin A concentration in liver tissue, corneal examination, conjunctival impression cytology, and dark-field adaptation tests (see Table 45.1).[7] Conjunctival impression cytology uses cellulose acetate filter paper that is applied to the eye and specimens are examined under a microscope and then graded based on goblet cells and epithelial cells. From a practical standpoint, determinations of serum retinol and/or retinol-binding protein are routinely used to screen for vitamin A nutritional status in children with chronic liver disease. Vitamin A deficiency is reported in 35% to 69% of children with cholestatic liver disease. However, serum concentrations of retinol and/or retinol-binding protein may not accurately reflect vitamin A sufficiency or deficiency states, particularly in cholestatic liver disease, because vitamin A is stored in the liver. The best noninvasive test of vitamin A status is the relative dose response. The relative dose response is based on the observation that if hepatic vitamin A stores are normal, plasma retinol concentration does not change significantly following a small oral loading dose of exogenous vitamin A (1500 IU; 450 μg). However, when hepatic vitamin A stores are low, the plasma retinol concentration markedly increases in response to a relatively small oral loading dose of exogenous vitamin A, reaching a peak several hours following administration. The standard relative dose response assesses plasma retinol concentration 5 hours after an oral loading dose of vitamin A. However, in children with chronic cholestasis, poor absorption of oral vitamin A may interfere with interpretation of vitamin A stores. To bypass the possibility of poor absorption, intravenous or intramuscular doses of vitamin A have been used to better assess vitamin A hepatic stores. Also, oral vitamin A in combination with oral d-alpha-tocopheryl polyethylene glycol-1000 succinate (TPGS [25 IU/kg]), a water-soluble form of vitamin E, which aids in absorption of lipid-soluble compounds, may also be used in a modified relative dose response to improve vitamin A oral absorption in cholestasis. A modified relative dose response of >20% increase at 10 hours is considered a positive test result indicative of low hepatic vitamin A stores.

Table 45.1.
Indices of Vitamin A Status

	Normal Range
Fasting serum retinol concentration	>20 μg/dL (>0.693 μmol/L)
Fasting serum retinol binding protein	>1 mg/dL
Retinol/retinol binding protein ratio	>0.8 mol/mol
Modified relative dose response (+TPGS)	<10% at 10 hours

TPGS indicates d-alpha-tocopheryl polyethylene glycol 1000 succinate.

Table 45.2.
Vitamin Supplementation in Children With Cholestasis

Vitamin	Recommended Dose	Preparation	Dose Provided
Vitamin A	Oral supplementation of vitamin A ranges from 5000–25 000 IU/day of water-miscible vitamin A	Vitamin A capsules AquADEKs drops (Axcan Pharma) Vitamin A parenteral (Aquasol A Parenteral, Mayne Pharma)	10 000 U/capsule or 25 000 U/capsule, generic 5751 IU/mL vitamin A 50 000 U/mL-15 mg retinol
Vitamin D	600–2000 IU/day 0.02 μg/kg	Oral vitamin D supplementation (Drisdol, Sanofi-Aventis) 1,25-OH vitamin D (Calcijex-Abbott, calcitriol injection)	Ergocalciferol 50 000 IU/capsule, 8000 U/mL 1 μg/mL
Vitamin E	In Infants, 50–100 IU/day In older children with vitamin E deficiency, 15–25 IU/kg/day	A-tocopherol, Aqua-E (Yasoo Health) Liqui-E (TPGS-d-alpha-tocopheryl polyethylene glycol 1000 succinate, Twinlabs)	20 IU/mL 400 IU/15 mL
Vitamin K	Daily or twice weekly dose of 2.5–10 mg, dependent upon response to therapy Subcutaneous or intravenous vitamin K administration (1–5 mg, dependent on size)	Mephyton, Anton Pharma (vitamin K₁) AquaMephyton, Merck and Co (vitamin K₁)	5-mg tablets 2 mg/mL or 10 mg/mL

Detecting vitamin A deficiency is important, because vitamin A deficiency may lead to xeropthalmia, keratomalacia, irreversible damage to the cornea of the eye, night blindness, and pigmentary retinopathy. Although these ocular findings are rare in cholestatic children, the potential for eye damage and visual disturbance is real.

Oral supplementation of vitamin A in children with liver disease ranges from 5000 to 25 000 IU/day of water-miscible vitamin A. Oral water-miscible vitamin A is not readily available for use in infants. Vitamin A capsules (8000 U/capsule, 10 000 U/capsule, 15 000 U/capsule, or 25 000 U/capsule, generic) are available. AquADEKs Pediatric Liquid (Axcan Pharma) contains 5751 IU/mL of vitamin A (www.axcan.com); vitamin A parenteral (Aquasol A Parenteral, Mayne Pharma, 50 000 U/mL-15 mg retinol) may be used for vitamin A replacement therapy intramuscularly.

Vitamin A toxicity has been well recognized and can cause hepatotoxicity. Monitoring during vitamin A supplementation is obligatory. Vitamin A toxicity may cause fatigue; malaise; anorexia; vomiting; increased intracranial pressure; painful bone lesions, including osteopenia and higher risk of fractures; hypercalcemia; and a massive desquamation dermatitis.[8] Vitamin A hepatotoxicity is associated with elevated retinyl esters and can be assayed.[9] Recent studies suggest that relatively little excess vitamin A can lead to toxicity, so close monitoring of vitamin A status and of any supplementation is warranted.[10]

Vitamin D

Vitamin D (calciferol) includes vitamin D_2 (ergocalciferol) and vitamin D_3 (cholecalciferol). Vitamin D_2 is found in very few foods naturally but is found in plants and fungi and added to supplement cow milk. Vitamin D may also be photosynthesized in the skin of vertebrates by the action of ultraviolet B radiation. Vitamin D is biologically inert and requires hydroxylation to form its biologically active hormone 1,25-dihydroxyvitamin-D (1,25-OH$_2$-D). Hydroxylation at the 1 position occurs in the kidney, and 25-hydroxylation occurs in the liver. The major biologic function of vitamin D in humans is to maintain serum calcium and phosphorus concentrations within the normal range by enhancing the efficiency of the small intestine to absorb these minerals from the diet. The adequate intake for vitamin D (calciferol) is 10 µg/day (400 IU) for infants and 15 µg/day (600 IU) for children and adults.

Vitamin D deficiency is demonstrated by its effect on calcium metabolism, resulting in hypocalcemia, hypophosphatemia, tetany, osteomalacia, and rickets. Children with chronic liver disease may develop hepatic osteodystrophy manifested by rickets, bone demineralization (osteopenia), or pathologic fractures.[11] These findings are in part the result of fat malabsorption attributable to diminished bile outflow, leading to steatorrhea and associated calcium and vitamin D malabsorption. Hypocalcemia and vitamin D insufficiency results in secondary hyperparathyroidism and increased bone resorption. Despite vitamin D repletion by supplementation to normal values, some patients continue to have poor bone mass, implying that vitamin D status alone does not account for hepatic osteodystrophy.[12] Magnesium deficiency has been proposed to play a role in the development of this bone disease.[13] Liver transplantation has demonstrated remarkable improvement in bone mineral density of these children.[14]

Clinically, bone mineral content is often assessed by dual-energy x-ray absorptiometry. Biochemical tests of vitamin D status include serum vitamin D (vitamin D_2 and D_3), 25-hydroxyvitamin D_2 (25-OH-D_2) and 25-OH-D_3, 1,25-OH$_2$-D, and vitamin-D binding protein. Serum concentrations of calcium, phosphorous, magnesium, alkaline phosphatase, and parathyroid hormone can be useful in assessing for osteomalacia, osteopenia, and rickets. Dietary calcium and phosphorus content must also be assessed. The most common indicator of vitamin D status in children with chronic cholestasis is the plasma concentration of 25-OH-D. A serum 25-OH-D concentration below 14 to 15 ng/mL is suggestive of vitamin D deficiency. Periodic assessment of serum 25-OH-D concentration, adequate sunlight exposure, and adequate dietary intake of calcium and phosphorous is recommended for cholestatic children. Vitamin D deficiency can be treated with oral vitamin D supplementation (Drisdol [ergocalciferol, 50 000 IU/capsule, 8000 U/mL Sanofi-Aventis]), usually at a dose range of 600 to 2000 IU/day. It is often possible to normalize plasma 25-OH-D concentrations in children with chronic cholestasis by providing 2-4 µg/kg/day. Serum 25-OH-D concentrations must be closely monitored along with calcium and phosphorus concentrations during supplementation.

Parenteral vitamin D preparations should be used only if patients fail to respond to oral therapy with assurance of compliance because of increased costs and risks for toxicity. Availability of various parenteral vitamin D preparations has been problematic. 1,25-OH$_2$-D (Calcijex-Abbott, calcitriol injection 1 µg/mL) at a dose of 0.02 µg/kg may be judiciously used with monitoring for vitamin D intoxication by including urine calcium-to-creatinine ratio, serum calcium and phosphorus, and serum 25-OH-D concentrations. Vitamin D toxicity may include hypercalcemia causing central nervous system depression, ectopic calcifications, hypercalciuria resulting in nephrocalcinosis, and nephrolithiasis. Bisphosphonate use for children with chronic liver disease has been limited to its use in treating hypercalcemia in children awaiting liver transplant.[15]

Vitamin E

Vitamin E refers to a group of 8 compounds including the tocopherols and the tocotrienols. The 4 major forms of vitamin E (alpha, beta, gamma, and delta) differ by the position and number of methyl group substitutions and their bioactivity. Alpha-tocopherol is the predominant form found in food and has the highest biologic activity. Gammatocopherol is found in high concentrations in soy oil. Foods high in vitamin E include grains, plants, and vegetable oils. The Recommended Dietary Intake for adequate vitamin E is 4 mg/day in infants 0 to 6 months of age, 5 mg/day in infants 7 to 12 months of age, 6 mg/day in children 1 to 3 years of age, 7 mg/day in children 4 to 8 years of age, 11 mg/day in children 9 to 13 years of age, and 15 mg/day in adults. Oral vitamin E requires solubilization by bile acids to mixed micelles and esterase hydrolysis by pancreatic or intestinal esterases that are bile acid dependent before absorption by the intestinal enterocyte. In blood, vitamin E is transported in low-density and high-density lipoprotein.

In infants and children with cholestasis, impaired secretion of bile acids results in malabsorption of vitamin E.[16] Vitamin E is the most hydrophobic of the fat-soluble

VI

vitamins and has the greatest need for bile acids intraluminally for absorption. Vitamin E absorption, as determined by an oral vitamin E tolerance test, is profoundly diminished in cholestatic children who are vitamin E deficient and can be improved by coadministration of bile acids.[15] Vitamin E is necessary to maintain the structure and function of the nervous system and muscular system. Peripheral neuropathy, ataxia, ophthalmoplegia, and muscle weakness characterize vitamin E deficiency in children with cholestasis.[17] Reversal of these findings may be accomplished before permanent injury occurs if supplementation and normalization of serum vitamin E concentrations is accomplished before 3 years of age.[18] The best predictor of vitamin E status in cholestatic children is the ratio of serum vitamin E to total serum lipids (the sum of the serum cholesterol, triglycerides, and phospholipids), because vitamin E partitions into the plasma lipoproteins that may be increased in cholestasis.[19] The serum vitamin E level may be increased into the normal range as a result of its partitioning into the plasma lipoproteins. The ratio of serum vitamin E to lipid compensates for this phenomenon. Biochemical vitamin E deficiency in older children and adults is <0.8 mg total tocopherol/g total lipid and for infants younger than 1 year is <0.6 mg/g. The target vitamin E-to-lipid ratio for correction of vitamin E deficiency is 0.8 to 1.0 mg/g. Although measurement of vitamin E in adipose tissue assesses vitamin E stores, it is impractical, because it requires adipose biopsies and is not readily available. Other functional assays of vitamin E status include red blood cell (RBC) hydrogen peroxide hemolysis and the RBC malondialdehyde release test.[20,21] Vitamin E deficiency is suggested if >10% of RBCs hemolyze on hydrogen peroxide exposure. Unfortunately, hydrogen peroxide hemolysis of RBCs or measurement of malondialdehyde (a lipid peroxidation product) may be affected by selenium or polyunsaturated fatty acids, so these tests are not specific for vitamin E deficiency. Breath ethane and pentane measurements have been used to assess antioxidant deficiency as a measure of vitamin E sufficiency.[22] Ethane and pentane are volatile gasses released during peroxidation of fatty acids. Although noninvasive, the cost, special equipment necessary for collection and detection of the gasses, and its low specificity for vitamin E deficiency because selenium deficiency also interferes make this test impractical.

To prevent vitamin E deficiency in cholestatic infants and children, vitamin E supplementation is indicated. In infants, 50 to 100 IU/day of vitamin E (alpha-tocopherol [Aqua-E, Yasoo Health], 20 IU/mL; Liqui-E, TPGS-d-alpha-tocopheryl poly-ethylene glycol 1000 succinate, 400 IU/15 mL, Twinlabs) may be prescribed. In older children with vitamin E deficiency, 15 to 25 IU/kg/day of vitamin E therapy is begun. Vitamin E dosing should not interfere with medications that might hamper its intestinal absorption (ie, cholestyramine) and may benefit from morning administration, when bile flow may be maximal after an overnight fast.

Monitoring by vitamin E-to-lipid ratio and neurologic examination will help determine the need to increase vitamin E dosing if normalization does not occur within several weeks of therapy. Vitamin E toxicity is rare and may present as bleeding in children taking anticoagulants or sepsis in neonates.

Vitamin K

Vitamin K is a member of the naphthoquinone family and has 3 forms.[23] Phylloquinone (vitamin K_1) is found in leafy vegetables, soybean oil, fruits, seeds, and cow milk. Menaquinone (vitamin K_2) is produced by intestinal bacteria. Menadione (vitamin K_3) is a synthesized form of vitamin K and has better water solubility. Because of the lack of data to estimate an average requirement, a recommended adequate intake is based on representative dietary intake data from healthy individuals. The adequate intake for vitamin K is 2.0 µg/day for infants 0 to 6 months of age, 2.5 µg/day for infants 7 to 12 months of age, 30 µg/day for children 1 to 3 years of age, 55 µg/day for children 4 to 8 years of age, 60 µg/day for children 9 to 13 years of age, and 75 µg/day for children 14 to 18 years of age. The Adequate Intake for men and women is 120 and 90 µg/day, respectively. No adverse effect has been reported for individuals consuming higher amounts of vitamin K.

Absorption of vitamin K_1 requires bile and pancreatic secretions that are impaired by cholestasis. Intestinal absorption of vitamin K_1 is an active process, while vitamin K_2 absorption is by passive diffusion. Absorbed vitamin K is incorporated into chylomicrons and is transported to the blood via the lymph. Little vitamin K is stored in the liver.

Vitamin K functions as a coenzyme during the synthesis of the biologically active form of a number of proteins involved in blood coagulation and bone metabolism. The vitamin K-dependent coagulation proteins include factors II, VII, IX, and X; protein C; and protein S.[24] Another family of vitamin K-dependent proteins includes the gla proteins. Osteocalcin is one of these proteins involved in bone mineralization.[25] Vitamin K deficiency in infancy can cause a coagulopathy resulting in intracranial bleeding.[26] In cholestatic children, malabsorption of vitamin K accompanied by antibiotic suppression of intestinal flora vitamin K production predisposes to vitamin K deficiency.[27]

Vitamin K status is frequently measured by using the prothrombin time, which is dependent on vitamin K-dependent clotting factors. If the prothrombin time is prolonged in comparison with the partial thromboplastin time, then vitamin K deficiency is likely. Liver disease may prolong the prothrombin time because of impaired synthesis of clotting factors active in the intrinsic coagulation pathway. Vitamin K concentrations may also be directly measured by high-performance liquid chromatography. Vitamin K status can also be sensitively

VI

ascertained by the plasma protein-induced in vitamin K absence (PIVKA)-II assay (enzyme-linked immunosorbent assay). Plasma PIVKA-II values greater than 3 ng/mL are indicative of vitamin K deficiency, although this test also has not proved to be clinically useful, because abnormal concentrations may also be found in healthy patients. Plasma-conjugated bilirubin, total bile acids, and severity of liver disease all have positively correlated with plasma PIVKA-II concentrations. Measurement of vitamin K-dependent clotting factors are costly, are not easily obtainable, and offer no advantage over monitoring prothrombin time for assessing vitamin K deficiency.

Vitamin K deficiency in children with cholestasis should be avoided. Supplementation with oral vitamin K should be provided (Mephyton, Aton Pharma Inc [vitamin K1], 5 mg tablets) in a daily or twice-weekly dose of 2.5 to 10 mg, dependent on response to therapy. Failure to respond to oral vitamin K supplementation may require subcutaneous or intravenous vitamin K administration (AquaMephyton, Merck and Co, [vitamin K_1], 2 mg/mL or 10 mg/mL). If administered intravenously, it should be administered slowly, not to exceed 1 mg/minute, to avoid anaphylaxis. To attempt correction of coagulopathy, vitamin K may be given subcutaneously or intravenously 3 days consecutively. Failure to respond to this regimen suggests significant hepatic dysfunction.

Water-Soluble Vitamins (See Also Chapter 21.II: Water-Soluble Vitamins)

Although in theory, decreased intake and malabsorption secondary to enteropathy are risk factors for deficiencies of water-soluble vitamins in children with chronic liver diseases, the incidence of deficiencies of these vitamins in these conditions has not been reported. Deficiencies of water-soluble vitamins in children with chronic liver disease are likely to be uncommon, because infant and enteral formulas used to feed children with chronic liver disease are supplemented with these vitamins.

Trace Elements (See Also Chapter 20: Trace Elements)

Zinc

Although children with chronic liver disease are often considered at risk of trace element deficiencies, no systematic studies of these deficiencies have been reported. Zinc is an important trace metal that is essential for normal cellular growth and differentiation, immune function, wound healing, and protein synthesis. Zinc deficiency is associated with acrodermatitis, diarrhea, and poor growth. Zinc metabolism is altered in children and adults with chronic liver disease. Infants and children with biliary atresia have been observed to have lower plasma zinc concentrations compared with controls.[28] Plasma zinc concentrations do not correlate with age, episodes of cholangitis, or repeated surgical procedures. Inappropriate urinary zinc excretion has been documented in children with chronic liver disease and hypozincemia and may be the pathogenesis for the observed deficiency in chronic liver disease.[29] Other potential causes of zinc deficiency in patients with chronic liver disease include decreased intestinal absorption, decreased dietary intake, and reduced portal-venous extraction secondary to portosystemic shunting. After liver transplantation, abnormal zinc homeostasis can rapidly improve and biochemical zinc deficiency reverses.[30] Serum zinc concentrations may not reflect total body zinc status. Identification of zinc deficiency may be difficult, although occasionally a low concentration of alkaline phosphatase, a zinc-dependent enzyme, can indicate zinc deficiency state. If clinical signs of zinc deficiency are suspected (acrodermatitis, diarrhea, and poor growth), an empiric trial of zinc supplementation is warranted. The standard dose of zinc for supplementation is 1 to 2 mg/kg/day of elemental zinc.

Copper

Copper is an essential trace element and functions as a cofactor for several important enzymes, such as lysyl oxidase, elastase, monoamine oxidase, cytochrome oxidase, ceruloplasmin, and superoxide dismutase. Deficiency of copper may be expressed by impaired activity of these enzymes. Signs of copper deficiency include neutropenia, microcytic anemia nonresponsive to iron supplementation, bone abnormalities, skin disorders, and depigmentation of hair and skin. The immune system is affected, resulting in diminished phagocytic activity of neutrophils and impaired cellular immunity. The anemia is the result of low concentrations of ceruloplasmin or ferroxidase.

Wilson disease is an autosomal-recessive disorder of copper metabolism that results in toxic effects of copper. In patients with Wilson disease, excess copper is stored in the body, especially in the liver and brain. Clinically, patients develop cirrhosis, eye lesions (Kayser-Fleisher rings), kidney abnormalities, and neurologic disease. Despite high concentrations of copper in the liver, serum concentrations of copper and ceruloplasmin are often low. Treatment includes chelation therapy with d-penicillamine or triethylenetetramine (trientine) and oral zinc therapy to reduce intestinal copper absorption. For advanced cases, liver transplantation can be life saving.

Copper is excreted into the intestinal tract via the biliary route. Thus, copper deficiency is unlikely to occur in children with cholestasis. However, in contrast, when cholestatic children receive parenteral nutrition, copper is often excluded from the trace mineral supplementation to avoid excessive accumulation of systemic copper.

Chromium

Chromium functions as a cofactor for insulin. Chromium deficiency is associated with poor growth and impaired glucose, lipid, and protein metabolism. Although peripheral insulin resistance and glucose intolerance occur in liver disease and

VI

chromium deficiency in adults, studies of the utility of chromium supplementation in adults or children with chronic liver disease are nonexistent. Chromium deficiency in infants is probably rare and only associated with protein-calorie malnutrition or prolonged parenteral nutrition without supplementation. Other than occasional development of glucose intolerance and hyperglycemia, the only indicator of chromium deficiency is the demonstration of a beneficial effect to chromium supplementation.

Manganese

Manganese is a cofactor for enzymes such as arginase, glutamate-ammonia ligase, manganese superoxide dismutase, and pyruvate carboxylase. Deficiency of manganese has not been reported in infants and children. Toxic effects of manganese accumulation in the basal ganglia are reported in adults with cirrhosis and liver disease may cause lack of coordination and balance, mental confusion, and muscle cramps and may contribute to hepatic encephalopathy. Extrapyramidal effects may resemble Parkinson disease. Because manganese is excreted in bile, children with cholestatic liver disease may develop elevated plasma concentrations.[31] Further, children with liver disease who receive parenteral nutrition, as with copper, should have manganese eliminated or reduced in trace mineral supplementation in the parenteral nutrition solutions.

Selenium

Selenium deficiency has been demonstrated in children receiving long-term parenteral nutrition without supplementation. Selenium deficiency results in macrocytosis and loss of hair and skin pigmentation.[32] Selenium is a required part of several proteins, such as selenium-dependent glutathione peroxidase, selenoprotein P, and deiodinase. Serum selenium concentration may be decreased in adults with liver disease. No studies address the distribution of selenium into bioactive forms, such as glutathione peroxidase and selenoprotein P, in patients with liver disease.

Ascites Management

Ascites development usually signifies advanced liver disease with portal hypertension. Significant hypoalbuminemia results from protein leakage into the peritoneal space and diminished albumin synthesis resulting from the liver disease. Most children with ascites have developed the condition slowly over time and are well compensated. Respiratory distress from the fluid compressing the diaphragms or concern for infected ascitic fluid (usually accompanied by fever) should prompt a paracentesis for both diagnostic and therapeutic indications. The fluid may be cultured for organisms, and a complete blood cell count and differential should be performed. Large fluid withdrawal should be avoided to prevent rapid fluid shifts from the intravascular space to the peritoneal cavity, which could result in shock, preventable with careful observation and intravascular volume replacement (preferably albumin).

Treatment of ascites begins with strict observance of sodium and fluid restriction. All sources of sodium, whether dietary or in intravenous fluids, medications, etc, must be counted. Unfortunately, food palatability is related to sodium content. A diet that is sodium free or severely sodium restricted may be highly unpalatable for a child. Assessment of urinary sodium excretion is frequently utilized to determine the adequacy of sodium restriction. Approximately 140 mEq of sodium will translate into about 1 L of water loss. Adequate calories, carbohydrates, proteins, and vitamins remain an important goal of therapy.

Fluid restriction is also an important part of the dietary treatment of ascites. A step-wise, gentle approach to fluid restriction is warranted.[33,34] If, in response to therapy, the child is losing weight, maintaining serum sodium concentrations, and showing evidence of appropriate urinary sodium excretion, then allowing the child to regulate his or her fluid intake may be acceptable. However, inappropriate fluid retention (weight gain, increasing abdominal girth), hyponatremia, or poor urinary sodium excretion should lead to fluid restriction to two thirds to three quarters of maintenance fluid therapy. Failing improvement, diuretics are then added. Spironolactone (3-6 mg/kg/day, divided twice daily) is often used as first-line diuretic therapy for ascites in children and will take approximately 5 days to begin demonstrating a noticeable effect. If additional diuretic therapy is required, addition of furosemide (1-2 mg/kg/day, divided twice daily) may be used. Diuretic dosages should be tailored to the individual child with the goal of utilizing the smallest effective dose. The goal of sodium and fluid restriction and diuretics should not be complete elimination of the ascites. Further, close monitoring of serum electrolytes, intake and output balance, and vital signs is mandatory and may require consequent nutrient supplementation or adjustments. Attention to avoiding renal compromise resulting from the restrictions is paramount.[35]

Liver Failure

Children with fulminant liver failure may develop hepatic encephalopathy (hepatic coma). Ammonia, the result of protein metabolism, is considered to be a contributing factor in the development and progression of encephalopathy. Thus, protein restriction is recommended for children with hepatic encephalopathy, and for children in deep coma, a completely protein-free diet may be warranted. However, to regenerate new liver tissue, some protein is advisable (1 g/kg/day) in children

VI

who can tolerate even small amounts so that anabolism, and not catabolism, of protein stores occurs.

Branched-chain amino acid (BCAA)-enriched formulas for enteral and parenteral use have been postulated to aid in the therapy of patients in acute or chronic liver failure in adults.[36] These formulas are expensive, and their role for children with liver failure has not been defined. Altering the type of dietary protein may benefit certain patients with chronic hepatic encephalopathy. Most but not all studies that compared vegetable with animal dietary protein found that vegetable protein diets were better tolerated than animal protein diets. Vegetable diets reduce urea production rate by increasing dietary fiber intake and increasing incorporation and elimination of nitrogen in fecal bacteria. Most patients with cirrhosis can tolerate an increasing amount of standard protein without worsening encephalopathy. Formulas with high concentrations of BCAAs (leucine, isoleucine, valine) and small amounts of aromatic amino acids (phenylalanine, tyrosine) have been proposed for use in patients with hepatic encephalopathy on the basis of the observation that the ratio of plasma BCAAs to aromatic amino acids is reduced in patients who have cirrhosis. BCAA–enriched liquid formulas, which contain approximately 35% of total amino acids as BCAAs, may be useful in a small percentage of patients with cirrhosis who are truly intolerant of increasing dietary protein. As much as 80 g of protein given as BCAA-enriched solutions has been tolerated in patients who could not tolerate 40 g of standard dietary protein. The large expense of BCAA-enriched solutions discourages their use in most settings.

The clinical efficacy of parenteral BCAA-enriched central parenteral nutrition solutions in patients with acute hepatic encephalopathy has been evaluated in clinical trials.[37] Patients who received BCAA-enriched solutions demonstrated a statistically significant improvement in mental recovery from high-grade encephalopathy during short-term (7–14 days) nutritional therapy. Considerable heterogeneity in mortality rates among studies precluded meaningful aggregation of mortality data. Although the pooled analysis of trials suggests a beneficial effect of BCAA-enriched formulas as a primary therapy in patients with acute hepatic encephalopathy, the studies have several shortcomings that limit enthusiasm for this relatively expensive therapy. The control groups usually received suboptimal, and possibly harmful, nutritional support consisting of high-dextrose solutions without amino acids. Only one study compared BCAA-enriched parenteral nutrition with a standard amino acid parenteral nutrition solution. None of the studies reported on complications associated with nutritional therapy, and none evaluated whether short-term benefits of nutritional therapy led to a long-term reduction in complications.

Protein-energy malnutrition is prevalent in children with chronic cholestasis and liver disease. Significant increases in growth and nitrogen balance are observed in children with cholestatic liver disease supplemented with BCAAs, suggesting that BCAA requirements are increased in chronic cholestasis.[38] Measurements utilizing indicator amino acid oxidation demonstrate that the mean requirement of total BCAAs in children with mild to moderate liver disease is greater than the mean requirement for the total BCAAs established in healthy children.[39]

The clinical features of hepatic encephalopathy, although well defined in adults, are not as evident in children. The Pediatric Acute Liver Failure Study Group classifies hepatic encephalopathy from stage 0 through IV. In stage 0, clinical signs or symptoms are absent, and reflexes, electroencephalogram, and neurologic signs are normal. In stages I and II, children are often inconsolable, crying, and inattentive to task and have normal or hyperreflexic reflexes. In stage III, the child may become somnolent, stuporous, and combative with hyperreflexic reflexes. In stage IV, the child is comatose, arouses with painful stimuli (stage IVa), or has no response (stage IVb) and has absent reflexes. The child may have decerebrate or decorticate posturing and abnormal, very slow delta activity on electroencephalogram. False neurotransmitters, fatty acids, mercaptans, and other toxins likely play a role in the development of encephalopathy.[40] Potential precipitating factors (sepsis, hemorrhage, medications) must be identified and proactively managed. Protein restriction may be necessary, and absorption and production of ammonia within the intestines should be prevented using lactulose or nonabsorbable antibiotics.

Lactulose, a nonabsorbable carbohydrate composed of galactose and fructose, can be metabolized by intraluminal bacteria to form organic acids.[41] The result is the acidification of the colonic pH, allowing for the conversion of NH_3 to NH_4^+ that can be trapped in the colon and then evacuated via the stools. Lactulose also causes increased numbers of stools that aids in ammonia elimination via the intestine. Patients in deep coma can have lactulose instilled directly into the colon via an enema to avoid the possibility of aspiration.

Antibiotics have also been used to diminish ammonia production intraluminally in the intestines. Neomycin and gentamicin have frequently been used in this capacity. Unfortunately, both of these antibiotics are not completely nonabsorbable. If absorbed in sufficient quantities with chronic use, ototoxicity and nephrotoxicity have been reported. Rifaximin, a minimally absorbed oral antimicrobial agent, is concentrated in the gastrointestinal tract and has broad-spectrum activity against gram-positive and gram-negative aerobic and anaerobic enteric bacteria.[42] It has a low risk of inducing bacterial resistance and has been used frequently for prevention of recurrent hepatic encephalopathy.

VI

Parenteral Nutrition-Associated Liver Disease

Parenteral nutrition-associated liver disease results from prolonged use of total parenteral nutrition (TPN) and is especially prevalent among neonates with recurrent sepsis, surgical procedures, or prematurity and leads to TPN-associated cholestasis (See Chapter 23: Parenteral Nutrition). The incidence of this problem appears to be declining as more aggressive use of enteral nutrition has been used. Prevention has involved early initiation and steady progression of enteral feedings and prevention of sepsis. Specific nutrient regimens have been attempted to diminish the risk of TPN-associated cholestasis, including use of amino acid preparations that promote a plasma amino acid pattern resembling breastfed infants, limiting potentially toxic amino acids such as methionine, adding antioxidant nutrients (eg, glutathione, vitamin E), and limiting fat and/or carbohydrate loads in at-risk infants. Further investigations are ongoing to determine efficacy of all of these treatments. Infants and older children sustaining severe liver toxicity that leads to cirrhosis and irreversible liver injury may require liver with or without small intestinal transplant as a life-saving measure.

References

1. Goldman L, Ausiello D, Bennett JC, Cecil RL, eds. *Cecil Textbook of Medicine*. 22nd ed. St Louis, MO: WB Saunders Co; 2004
2. Badley BW, Murphy GM, Bouchier IA, Sherlock S. Diminished micellar phase lipid in patients with chronic nonalcoholic liver disease and steatorrhea. *Gastroenterology*. 1970;58(6):781-789
3. Wene JD, Connor WE, DenBesten L. The development of essential fatty acid deficiency in healthy men fed fat free diets intravenously and orally. *J Clin Invest*. 1975;56(1):127-134
4. Clandinin MT, Chappell JE, Heim T, Swyer PR, Chance GW. Fatty acid utilization in perinatal de novo synthesis of tissues. *Early Hum Dev*. 1981;5(4):355-366
5. Pettei MJ, Daftary S, Levine JJ. Essential fatty acid deficiency associated with the use of a medium-chain triglyceride infant formula in pediatric hepatobiliary disease. *Am J Clin Nutr*. 1991;53(5):1217-1221
6. Kaufman SS, Scrivner DJ, Murray ND, Vanderhoof JA, Hart MH, Antonson DL. Influence of portagen and pregestimil on essential fatty acid status in infantile liver disease. *Pediatrics*. 1992;89(1):151-154
7. Feranchak AP, Gralla J, King R, et al. Comparison of indices of vitamin A status in children with chronic liver disease. *Hepatology*. 2005;42(4):782-792
8. Lippe B, Hensen L, Mendoza G, et al. Chronic vitamin A intoxication. *Am J Dis Child*. 1981;135(7):634-636
9. Smith FR, Goodman DS. Vitamin A transport in human vitamin A toxicity. *New Engl J Med*. 1976;294(15):805-808
10. Penniston KL, Tanumihardjo SA. The acute and chronic toxic effects of vitamin A. *Am J Clin Nutr*. 2006;83(2):191-201

11. Heubi JE, Hollis BW, Specker B, et al. Bone disease in chronic childhood cholestasis. 1. Vitamin D adsorption and metabolism. *Hepatology*. 1989;9(2):258-264

12. Bucuvalas JC, Heubi JE, Specker BL, Gregg DJ, Yergey AL, Vieira NE. Calcium absorption in bone disease associated with liver cholestasis during childhood. *Hepatology*. 1990;12(5):1200-1205

13. Heubi JE, Higgins JV, Argao EA, Sierra RI, Specker BL. The role of magnesium in the pathogenesis of bone disease in childhood cholestatic liver disease: a preliminary report. *J Pediatr Gastroenterol Nutr*. 1997;25(3):301-306

14. Argao EA, Balistreri WF, Hollis BW, Ryckman FC, Heubi JE. Effect of orthotopic liver transplantation on bone mineral content and serum vitamin D metabolites in infants and children with chronic cholestasis. *Hepatology*. 1994;20(3):598-603

15. Attard TM, Dhawan A, Kaufman SS, et al. Use of disodium pamidronate in children with hypercalcemia awaiting liver transplantation. *Pediatr Transplant*. 1998;2(2):157-159

16. Sokol RJ, Heubi JE, Iannaccone S, Bove KE, Balistreri WF. Mechanisms causing vitamin E deficiency during chronic childhood cholestasis. *Gastroenterology*. 1983;85(5):1172-1182

17. Guggenheim MA, Jackson V, Lilly J, et al. Vitamin E deficiency and neurologic disease in children with cholestasis: a prospective study. *J Pediatr*. 1983;102(4):577-579

18. Sokol RJ, Guggenheim MA, Iannaccone ST, et al. Improved neurologic function flowing correction of vitamin E deficiency in children with chronic cholestasis. *N Engl J Med*. 1985;313(25):1585-1586

19. Sokol RJ, Heubi JE, Iannaccone ST, et al. Vitamin E deficiency with normal serum vitamin E concentration in children with chronic cholestasis. *N Engl J Med*. 1984;310(19):1209-1212

20. Gordon HH, Nitowsky HM, Cornblath M. Studies of tocopherol deficiency in infants and children. I. Hemolysis of erythrocytes in hydrogen peroxide. *Am J Dis Child*. 1955;90(6):669-681

21. Cynamon HA, Isenberg JN, Nguyen CH. Erythrocyte malondialdehyde release in vitro: a functional measure of vitamin E status. *Clin Chim Acta*. 1985;151(2):169-176

22. Refat M, Moore TJ, Kazui M, et al. Utility of breathe ethane as a noninvasive biomarker of vitamin E status in children. *Pediatr Res*. 1991;30(5):396-403

23. Olson RE. The function and metabolism of vitamin K. *Ann Rev Nutr*. 1984;4:281-337

24. Shah DV, Suttie JW. The vitamin k dependent, in vitro production of prothrombin. *Biochem Biophys Res Commun*. 1974;60(4):1397-1402

25. Price PA, Parthemore JG, Deftos LJ. New biochemical marker for bone metabolism: measurement by radioimmunoassay of bone GLA-protein in the plasma of normal subjects and patients with bone disease. *J Clin Invest*. 1980;66(5):878-883

26. Bancroft J, Cohen MB. Intracranial hemorrhage due to vitamin K deficiency in breast fed infants with cholestasis. *J Pediatr Gastroenterol Nutr*. 1993;16(1):78-80

27. Yanofsky RA, Jackson VG, Lilly JR, et al. The multiple coagulopathies of biliary atresia. *Am J Hematol*. 1984;16(2):171-180

28. Goksu N, Ozsoylu S. Hepatic and serum levels of zinc, copper and magnesium in childhood cirrhosis. *J Pediatr Gastroenterol Nutr*. 1986;5(3):459-462

VI

29. Hambidge KM, Krebs NF, Lilly JR, Zerbe GO. Plasma and urine zinc in infants and children with EHBA. *J Pediatr Gastroenterol Nutr.* 1987;6(6):872-877

30. Narkewicz MR, Krebs N, Karrer F, Orban-Eller K, Sokol RJ. Correction of hypozincemia following liver transplantation in children is associated with reduced urinary zinc loss. *Hepatology.* 1999;29(3):830-833

31. Bayliss EA, Hambidge KM, Sokol RJ, Stewart B, Lilly JR. Hepatic concentrations of zinc, copper and managanese in infants with extrahepatic biliary atresia. *J Trace Elem Med Biol.* 1995;9(1):40-43

32. Vinton NE, Dahlstrom KA, Strobel CT, Ament ME. Macrocytosis and pseudoalbinism: manifestations of selenium deficiency. *J Pediatr.* 1987;111(5):711-717

33. Runyon BA. Treatment of patients with cirrhosis and ascites. *Semin Liv Dis.* 1997;17(3):249-260

34. Garcia-Tsao G. Current management of the complications of cirrhosis and portal hypertension: variceal hemorrhage, ascites, and spontaneous bacterial peritonitis. *Gastroenterology.* 2001;120(3):726-748

35. Sort P, Navasa M, Arroyo V, et al. Effect of intravenous albumin on renal impairment and mortality in patients with cirrhosis and spontaneous bacterial peritonitis. *N Engl J Med.* 1999;341(6):403-409

36. Cerra FB, Cheung NK, Fisher JE, et al. Disease-specific amino acid infusion (F080) in hepatic encephalopathy: a prospective, randomized, double-blind, controlled trial. *J Parenter Enteral Nutr.* 1985;9(3):288-295

37. Marchesini G, Marzocchi R, Noia M, et al. Branched-chain amino acid supplementation in patients with liver diseases. *J Nutr.* 2005;135(6 Suppl):1596S-1601S

38. Chin SE, Shepherd RW, Thomas BJ, et al. Nutritional support in children with end-stage liver disease: a randomized crossover trial of a branched-chain amino acid supplement. *Am J Clin Nutr.* 1992;56(1):158-163

39. Mager DR, Wykes LJ, Roberts EA, et al. Branched-chain amino acid needs in children with mild-to-moderate chronic cholestatic liver disease. *J Nutr.* 2006;136(1):133-139

40. Jalan R, Hayes PC. Hepatic encephalopathy and ascites. *Lancet.* 1997;350(9087):1309-1315

41. Debray D, Yousef N, Durand P. New management options for end-stage chronic liver disease and acute liver failure: potential for pediatric patients. *Paediatr Drugs.* 2006;8(1):1-13

42. Bass NM, Mullen KD, Sanyal A, et al. Rifaximin treatment in hepatic encephalopathy. *N Engl J Med.* 2010;362(12):1071-1081

Chapter 46

Cardiac Disease

Introduction

Impaired nutrition and growth is prevalent in children with congenital heart disease (CHD). Growth failure in heart disease has a multifactorial etiology and follows a pattern identical to acute and chronic protein-calorie undernutrition with wasting of body mass acutely and stunting of linear growth chronically. Cyanosis or hypoxemia, congestive heart failure (CHF), and pulmonary hypertension (pulmonary-to-systemic pressure ratio >0.4) are the sentinel features of CHD implicated in growth failure. Growth failure attributable to a congenital heart malformation may begin before birth in a newborn infant with intrauterine growth retardation. Infants with most forms of cardiac malformations (transposition of the great arteries [TGA] being a notable exception) have a lower-than-normal birth weight.[1] Approximately 6% of infants with symptomatic heart disease may present with intrauterine growth retardation.[2] In addition, extracardiac malformations or recognizable syndromes (eg, trisomy 21, trisomy 18, Turner syndrome, VACTERL association [vertebral defects, and atresia, cardiac defects, tracheo-esophageal fistula, renal anomalies, and limb abnormalities], CHARGE syndrome [coloboma, heart defect, atresia choanae, retarded growth and development, genital abnormality, and ear abnormality]) with noncardiac reasons for impaired growth are also more common in children with heart disease.[3]

Acute undernutrition, defined as reduced weight relative to the median weight predicted by length (wasting) and chronic undernutrition, based on reduced length relative to the median length predicted for age (stunting), are more prevalent among hospitalized patients with CHD. Acute undernutrition, or wasting, may affect up to one third of patients, and chronic undernutrition, or stunting, may be found in about two thirds of patients. As many as 60% of patients with left-to-right shunts and up to 70% of patients with either cyanosis or congestive heart failure meet criteria for undernutrition.[4] The most severe undernutrition may occur in severe CHF associated with ventricular septal defect (VSD), patent ductus arteriosus (PDA), TGA, or coarctation of the aorta. Infants with these defects may present as appropriate for gestational age at birth but incur early weight deficits or wasting, followed by linear growth deficits or stunting. In cyanotic (hypoxemic) lesions, such as tetralogy of Fallot or TGA, symmetric failure to thrive is observed with weight and length gain depressed concurrently. In acyanotic lesions, such as atrial septal defect (ASD), VSD, or PDA, slow weight gain predominates over linear growth retardation, especially with CHF and/or large left-to-right shunts. The incidence of growth failure is highest in patients with VSD, perhaps because of the greater prevalence of pulmonary hypertension and CHF in children with large left-to-right shunts.[5] A recent retrospective study of 123 children with CHD showed the worst growth retardation in patients with a large VSD (CHF) and tetralogy of Fallot (cyanotic heart disease). Delay in skeletal maturation as assessed by bone age is related to severity of hypoxemia in cyanotic heart disease but also is seen in CHF.[5] Conversely, asymptomatic acyanotic lesions (aortic stenosis, coarctation, pulmonary stenosis) without congestive heart failure or pulmonary hypertension may not be associated with undernutrition. Surgical repair allows normalization of most height deficits.[6]

The following text describes the components of undernutrition in CHD, the nutritional impact of the hemodynamic features of CHD, and the effects of nutrients on cardiac function, providing a basis for optimal nutritional management and monitoring.

Undernutrition in CHD

Undernutrition occurs when metabolic demands for protein or energy (expenditure) combined with nutrient losses (regurgitation or malabsorption) exceed energy and protein nutrient intake. Investigators have attempted to study each of these components of nutrient balance. In addition to deficits in these macronutrients affecting growth and body composition, clinically important deficiency in certain micronutrients may also occur.

Energy Expenditure

A number of studies have confirmed that total daily energy expenditure (TDEE), including components of physical activity, such as cardiorespiratory work associated with movement and dietary thermogenesis—the energy required to assimilate and metabolize nutrients—is increased significantly in children with CHD, with relatively insignificant increases in resting energy expenditure (REE) relative to lean body mass. TDEE comprises REE, physical activity, and dietary-induced thermogenesis. Metabolizable, or absorbed, energy intake must exceed TDEE to permit normal growth. Although REE in children with CHD seems to be similar to age-matched reference children, infants with CHD from 3 to 5 months of age have approximately 40% increased TDEE when compared with healthy control infants (94.2 + 6.9 kcal/kg/day vs 67.1 + 7.3 kcal/kg/day, respectively).[7-11]

Nutrient Losses

Some patients with CHD have abnormalities of gastrointestinal tract function or renal losses that may affect nutrition. Urinary losses of energy as glucosuria and proteinuria may be significant in certain patients with renal disease or glucose intolerance. Approximately 8% of infants with CHD have associated major gastrointestinal tract malformations, such as tracheoesophageal fistula and esophageal atresia, malrotation, or diaphragmatic hernia that generally will limit intake and cause losses of nutrients.[12] Fecal losses of energy in subclinical steatorrhea or of protein in protein losing enteropathy may be more significant and prevalent than expected, affecting up to 50% of patients with a variety of congenital heart lesions. In one study, protein-losing enteropathy was found in 8 of 21 infants with severe CHD[13] and is a major complication common to patients who undergo the Fontan procedure or have severe right-sided CHF. Steatorrhea, indicative of disturbed digestion or absorption, was found in 5 of 21 infants with CHD (1 of 8 patients with CHF and 4 of 12 cyanotic patients).[13] In these patients, mucosal small-bowel biopsies were normal. Mean resting oxygen consumption was higher in infants with CHF than in those with cyanotic heart disease.[13]

No significant malabsorption of energy or fat in stools was observed in the study of children receiving diuretics by Vaisman et al.[14] However, total body water and extracellular water excess were measured and correlated directly with fat losses and inversely with energy intake, suggesting a relationship to the degree of CHF and diuretic efficacy. Therefore, infants with increased total body water (ie, not effectively diuresed) had more malabsorption than did euvolemic diuresed patients.

Yahav et al studied malabsorption relative to energy requirements in 14 infants with CHD 2 to 36 months of age (mean age, 10.4 months).[15] Ten infants with CHF and 4 with cyanosis were studied in 3 periods of 3 to 7 days each, comparing baseline oral intake, supplemented oral intake, and nasogastric feedings of a high-caloric density formula. Nasogastric feedings of a high-caloric density formula (1.5 kcal/mL or 45 kcal/oz) were administered to 11 patients. Consistent weight gain averaging 13 g/day was observed only in patients receiving >170 kcal/kg/day, with only 50% of the children gaining weight on 149 kcal/kg/day. Increased cardiac and respiratory rates were observed in patients after feeding and were attributed to dietary thermogenesis but did not appear to be clinically significant. Minor intestinal losses of fat were observed in 3 patients and protein losing enteropathy in no patients and were not considered to be significant limiting factors in weight gain.[15]

Energy Intake

Several studies have examined energy/nutrient intake requirements of infants and young children with CHD (Table 46.1). Approximately 140 to 150 kcal/kg/day is required to effect linear growth and increase subcutaneous fat and muscle in infants with CHD and CHF. In one study of 19 infants randomly assigned to 3 groups, only the group receiving continuous 24-hour nasogastric feedings over a 5-month study period was able to achieve intakes >140 kcal/kg/day (mean, 147 kcal/kg/day).[16] Only this group of patients was able to demonstrate improved nutritional status manifested as increased weight, length, and anthropometric measures of fat and muscle stores. The groups that received either 12-hour supplemental nocturnal

VI

infusions or oral feedings alone failed to achieve such intakes and growth responses. The 12-hour oral plus infusion group received only 122 kcal/kg, well below the threshold for growth. Fatigue during oral feedings was considered a limiting factor in both of these groups. In addition, in the 12-hour infusion group, daytime oral intake (52 kcal/kg) actually dropped to approximately 50% of the prestudy mean caloric intake (98 kcal/kg). The investigators concluded that only 24-hour continuous enteral feeding by nasogastric tube of a 1-kcal/mL formula was able to provide >140 kcal/kg/day and improve nutritional status.[16]

Table 46.1.
Energy Requirements for Normal Growth in Infants With CHD

Study	Age Range	Mode	% IBW	kcal/kg/day	kcal/kg IBW
Bougle 1986[45]	2 wk–6 mo	NG	-	137	-
Vanderhoof 1982[46]	1 wk–9 mo	NG	-	120–150	-
Schwarz 1990[16]	1–10 mo	NG	82	147	120
Yahav 1985[15]	2–36 mo	NG/PO	76	149–169	113–128
Barton 1994[7]	0–3 mo	NG/PO	80	143	114
Summary:	0–36 mo	NG	80	145	115

IBW indicates ideal body weight or weight/height for age; NG, nasogastric; PO, oral.

Two studies have concluded that children with CHD who fail to grow consume insufficient calories because they reliably respond to nutritional supplementation, supporting the proposition that failure to gain weight can be simply a matter of inadequate intake, not intrinsic genetic or cardiac factors. These studies found that the type of cardiac defect did not necessarily predict or limit the response to dietary counseling and oral supplementation.[17,18]

Delayed gastric emptying[19] and gastroesophageal reflux[20] in children with CHD as well as oral aversion may be significant features that reduce voluntary intake and compromise nutrition. There may be early satiety induced by gastroparesis and gut hypomotility related to edema or hypoxia as well as by distention from hepatomegaly associated with CHF.

Hemodynamic Factors

Congestive Heart Failure

Growth failure in children with CHF is common. The pathogenesis of growth failure in CHF is not always clear and is likely multifactorial. CHF causes increased energy requirements because of increased myocardial and respiratory work and increased catecholamines as well as reduced net nutrient intake as a result of intestinal malabsorption, anorexia, or fatigability during feedings. In adults with

CHF, total energy expenditure appears to be lower than that of controls. High-protein–calorie feedings do not reverse the growth impairment, suggesting that the wasting has a metabolic basis rather than resulting from negative protein and energy balance.[21] In addition, malnutrition in adults with CHF is associated with increased right atrial pressure and tricuspid regurgitation.[22] Elevated right atrial pressures may cause intestinal protein losses and fat malabsorption and/or anorexia because of splanchnic and mesenteric venous and lymphatic congestion. In adults, REE is increased and may be caused by the increased work of breathing or elevated sympathetic innervation.[23] Cytokines, such as tumor necrosis factor, are elevated in adults with heart failure and may contribute to the cachexia seen in this condition.[24]

Oxygen consumption and basal metabolic rate are increased in infants with CHF when compared with healthy children or children with cyanotic CHD.[13,25,26] TDEE measured by the doubly (isotope) labeled water technique was increased approximately 35% in infants 2 to 8 months old with CHD with and without congestive heart failure compared with control infants in a meta-analysis of 7 small controlled studies. However, the feature of congestive heart failure did not significantly increase TDEE.[27] Traditionally, growth failure has been most common in infants with CHF attributable to pulmonary overcirculation from large left-to-right shunts, such as a VSD or atrioventricular septal defect. This has been most evident in children with a VSD and large left-to-right shunt and pulmonary hypertension.[18] Fortunately, the increasing success of complete repairs of such defects in infancy has greatly lessened this problem.

There are many possible reasons for growth failure in children with CHF. There may be insufficient caloric intake because of inability to consume adequate calories for growth, intestinal malabsorption attributable to passive congestion and/or low cardiac output, or increased metabolic demands secondary to increased work of breathing. Insufficient caloric intake could be caused by a variety of factors, including excessive fatigue with oral feeding, excessive vomiting, or iatrogenic fluid restriction and diuresis because of the severity of heart failure.[16,28] Decreased gastric capacity caused by pressure on the stomach from an enlarged, congested liver or from ascites may also interfere with the amount of nutrients a patient can ingest.[29] Children with CHF also may have abnormal intestinal function. They can have excessive intestinal protein losses secondary to elevated venous and lymphatic pressure.[13] Because of the obvious negative consequences of chronic fluid (and, thus, caloric) restriction in children, fluid restriction is now only temporarily used in patients who are either awaiting some type of intervention (eg, surgery or heart transplantation) or recovering from some type of acute process (eg, surgery, acute decompensation, pleural effusions, etc).

VI

Cyanotic Heart Disease

The role of hypoxemia as a primary cause of growth retardation in children is unclear. Cyanotic CHD (eg, tetralogy of Fallot, tricuspid atresia) with chronic hypoxemia is frequently associated with undernutrition and linear growth retardation, especially if prolonged and if complicated by CHF (TGA or single ventricle). Isolated hypoxemia or desaturation does not necessarily result in tissue hypoxia, because tissue aerobic metabolism may not be impaired until arterial oxygen partial pressure falls below 30 mm Hg, a threshold also affected by such factors as oxygen-carrying capacity determined by erythroid mass or hemoglobin and tissue perfusion. Therefore, the added complication of CHF with decreased cardiac output probably contributes to chronic tissue hypoxia limiting growth. In addition to oxygen desaturation and CHF, anemia has been identified as an important factor predicting undernutrition in CHD.[30]

Some studies have demonstrated significant differences in growth between cyanotic and acyanotic children, whereas others have failed to do so.[5] Cyanotic children without pulmonary hypertension or CHF can demonstrate a normal nutritional state with stunting of growth being more common than poor weight gain.[31] Children with cyanotic CHD have also been shown to have excessive stool protein loss.[13] Cyanotic patients with pulmonary hypertension had the worst growth, with hypoxemia or cyanosis (right-to-left shunting) and pulmonary hypertension having additive effects.[31] However, after surgical repair of cyanotic CHD, resting and total energy expenditures in these children are no different than controls.[32]

Circulatory Shunts

Cardiac lesions with nutritional implications may also be categorized by shunt direction and magnitude: left-to-right shunts are associated with CHF, and right-to-left shunts are associated with hypoxemia or cyanosis. As previously described, cyanotic patients with pulmonary hypertension appear to have the worst growth, with hypoxemia or cyanosis (right-to-left shunting) and pulmonary hypertension having additive effects.[18,31] Infants with a clinically significant VSD have similar resting energy expenditure but significantly higher TDEE than do healthy control infants, suggesting that they are unable to meet additional energy demands from physical activity or dietary thermogenesis, accounting for their growth retardation.[33]

Pulmonary Hypertension

Increased resting oxygen consumption in CHD has been demonstrated, especially in patients with CHF or pulmonary hypertension, and attributed to increased metabolic oxygen demands caused by increased catecholamine secretion and other factors. Pulmonary hypertension is a complication frequently implicated in growth failure, correlated with stunting in VSD, an acyanotic lesion.[34] Children with both cyanotic heart disease and pulmonary hypertension demonstrated both moderate to severe wasting and linear growth retardation.[31]

Management

Surgery

Significant protein-calorie undernutrition may delay surgical correction and impair postoperative recovery and growth. Growth failure has been added to the heart transplant criteria for the United Network for Organ Sharing, such that children with growth failure complicating CHD are listed at a higher status than children without growth failure.[35] Children demonstrate improvement in growth following corrective or palliative repair of a congenital heart lesion, and available data support the use of early surgical correction of major cardiac malformations to optimize growth.[9,32]

Within 1 week of surgery in infants with heart disease, energy expenditures decrease sharply to reach levels significantly below preoperative levels. By approximately 2.5 years following surgery, weight, body composition, resting energy expenditure, TDEE, or energy expended during physical activity are similar to those of healthy children without CHD.[32] Studies have demonstrated a reversal of decreased growth velocity in infants who have undergone repair of VSD, tetralogy of Fallot, and TGA in the first year of life.[36] There are conflicting data regarding somatic growth in patients who have undergone the Fontan procedure. Some studies have demonstrated improvement in growth parameters,[37] whereas others have shown persistent growth failure.[38] These differences may relate to many factors, including different malformations, timing for surgery, etc. Catch-up linear growth is more likely with corrective than palliative surgery and with early repair. Residual, although reduced, CHF or shunt may still prevent normal nutritional recovery.[36,39]

Chylothorax may complicate up to 6.5% of corrective surgeries. Biewer et al reported that most cases (71%) will resolve on a medium-chain triglyceride (MCT)-based diet administered for at least 10 days, after which customary feedings can be resumed gradually without recurrence.[40]

Nutritional Assessment

A complete nutritional history includes feeding pattern and schedule, including frequency, duration, and volume of feedings. The volume of each feeding may actually be inversely related to the duration of feeding as the child fatigues. Diaphoresis with feedings reflects autonomic stimulation effects. Gastrointestinal tract function should be assessed to identify reflux and vomiting losses, irritability attributable to esophagitis or cramping, diarrhea or constipation, and early satiety, which may respond to acid-control and motility medications or may be signs of associated anomalies. The physical examination must include accurate nude weight,

VI

length or height, and head circumference plotted on a growth curve. Consider changes in rate of growth or growth velocity as well as the relation of actual body weight to the ideal body weight predicted by height or length for age. Appropriate charts should be used for children with preterm birth, Down syndrome, Turner syndrome, or Trisomy 18. Assessment of subcutaneous fat and muscle mass may be helpful, if measured by a skilled dietitian with calipers, although dehydration or edema may affect validity. Signs of CHF, pulmonary hypertension, clubbing, cyanosis, and hepatomegaly connote increased risk of nutritional failure.

Laboratory evaluation initially should include hemoglobin, oxygen saturation, albumin, and prealbumin. Protein-losing enteropathy as a cause of hypoalbuminemia can be confirmed by fecal alpha-1-antitrypsin assay and is encountered in conditions of systemic venous hypertension, which occur with right-sided CHF, constrictive pericardial disease, or restrictive cardiac disease or after Fontan operation. A low alkaline phosphatase or cholesterol concentration may signify zinc deficiency, which may affect taste and linear growth.

Nutritional Support

The goals of nutritional intervention are to (1) achieve nutritional balance by providing sufficient energy to stop catabolism of lean body mass and sufficient protein to match nitrogen losses; (2) provide additional nutrients to restore deficits and allow growth, thus normalizing weight for height and promoting linear growth; (3) provide enteral feedings to replace parenteral nutrition, as tolerated by the gastrointestinal tract; and (4) develop and maintain oral feeding competence to enable voluntary independent feeding.

Nutrient Prescription

The optimal nutritional support should provide sufficient energy and protein not only to prevent breakdown or catabolism of protein and maintain body composition and weight but also to restore deficits and permit growth toward genetic potential. Electrolyte losses with diuretics and deficiencies in micronutrients, such as the trace minerals iron and zinc or vitamins, may be limiting factors. As a general principle, for any given level of nitrogen (or protein) provided in the diet, increasing the energy (calories) will improve nitrogen balance and protein synthesis or accretion. Similarly, for a given level of energy intake, increasing the protein intake will improve the nitrogen balance or protein accretion. If energy provided by carbohydrate and fat in the diet is below the patient's requirements, protein will be catabolized as an energy source and not used in synthesis of lean body mass. Even if sufficient calories are provided to stop gluconeogenesis and restore body glycogen and fat stores, enough protein must be provided as a nitrogen source to allow accretion of lean body protein mass and effective growth. A marginal or negative electrolyte balance, such as low net sodium or potassium intake in the setting of fluid restriction and diuretic use, required for some patients in CHF, may impair growth independent of energy and protein sufficiency. Zinc deficiency has been implicated in cases of failure to thrive, with improved growth demonstrated after supplementation.[41,42]

Energy Requirement

Additional energy above the Recommended Dietary Allowance for age is required to permit normal growth rates, with even greater amounts required to restore nutritional deficits in "catch-up" or accelerated growth. A portion of this incremental energy requirement may be explained by simply calculating needs based on the patient's ideal or median body weight predicted from body length or even head circumference. This calculation assumes that metabolic needs for energy and protein are determined by the relatively preserved brain and visceral and lean body mass with a minimal contribution from the adipose or fat mass that is depleted with undernutrition. In undernutrition, the ratio of metabolically active lean body mass to total weight is increased. For example, 150 kcal/kg of actual body weight in the typical lean child with CHD, who may be 80% of the expected or "ideal" weight for length, corresponds to 120 kcal/kg for a healthy robust infant of the same length but at ideal body weight because of increased fat mass. Therefore, energy requirements may be more reliably based on the child's "ideal" body weight for length or height (Table 46.1). (An alternative calculation of a reference weight [kg] for predicting energy requirements is the 50th percentile body mass index [BMI] for age multiplied by the patient's length in meters squared.)

Increased cardiac and respiratory work in the child with CHF, shunt, or cyanosis undoubtedly adds to the energy requirement. Increased catecholamines in CHF will increase energy expenditure, as will the demands of increased respiratory rate and hematopoiesis in cyanotic heart disease. The myocardium itself is a significant consumer of energy with demands increased with pulmonary hypertension, hypertrophy, shunting, and CHF. Barton et al[7] estimated the energy requirement for growth of an infant with CHD. The energy cost of normal tissue deposition is 21 kJ/g (5 kcal/g).[43] This energy cost is 30% less than the 31 kJ/g (7.4 kcal/g) estimated in infants with CHD receiving high-energy feedings.[44] This difference is consistent with a greater fat content (more energy per weight) of the tissue replenished in infants with CHD and is supported by measuring increased skinfold thickness during high-energy feeding.[44] Assuming 75% of the energy cost of growth is stored in this new tissue and the remainder is used during synthesis (part of TDEE), an intake of 600 kJ/kg/day (143 kcal/kg/day) is required to allow average weight gain during the first 3 months of life.[7] Table 46.1 summarizes the findings of a number of studies of energy required to achieve growth in patients with CHD, comparing requirements calculated for actual body weight and ideal body weight

VI

for height and age. The parenteral requirements for energy will be approximately 70% to 80% of these enteral estimates.

One must also consider the metabolic load imposed by feeding. Cardiac output is determined by tissue metabolic demand. As additional nutrients are provided, cardiac output must increase to oxygenate these tissues, and ventilatory demands on the lungs increase to eliminate the carbon dioxide generated by metabolic activity. This phenomenon of increased energy demands of nutrition support known as dietary thermogenesis, the thermic effect of food or specific dynamic action, varies for different nutrients, being minimal for fat metabolism and quite significant, up to 5% of calories, for carbohydrate. Carbohydrates are used for fat synthesis when carbohydrates or equivalent glucose amounts are administered at a rate exceeding 8 mg/kg/minute. This endothermic process requires energy and oxygen and liberates carbon dioxide, which must be expired. For this reason, the energy provided should be distributed between fat and carbohydrate, with fat providing at least 30% of the total caloric intake. At least 6% of fat should be long-chain triglycerides (linoleic acid, as in corn, soy, safflower oils) and some linolenic acid to provide essential fatty acids. The value and safety of additional omega-3 fatty acids beyond essential fatty acid requirements is the subject of ongoing research.

Overfeeding or overly rapid increments in nutrition support can precipitate or worsen CHF. A refeeding syndrome has been described in which overzealous nutritional support has caused complications, not only with cardiac failure, but also with conduction disturbances and dysrhythmias related to electrolyte and mineral shifts with anabolism. Provision of glucose leads to an insulin-mediated influx of potassium, and intermediary metabolism demands for phosphorus (phosphorylated intermediate metabolites and production of adenosine triphosphate) lead to an intracellular shift, causing profound hypokalemia, hypophosphatemia, hypomagnesemia, and hypocalcemia. Prolongation of QT_c interval may be observed. Sudden death suspected to be related to lethal arrhythmias, such as torsade de pointes, has been attributed to the rapid refeeding of patients accommodated to the undernourished state.

In preterm and full-term neonates with CHD, there is a higher incidence of necrotizing enterocolitis. This fact dictates gradual advancement of feeding in the newborn period and monitoring tolerance in terms of abdominal distention, accumulating gastric residual volume, and hematochezia. For those on parenteral nutrition, trophic feedings of approximately 10 mL/kg, preferably expressed human milk, for enteral and enterohepatic stimulation is beneficial.

Protein Intake
There is little discussion in the literature about nitrogen balance or protein intake in children with CHD. In general, if sufficient nonprotein energy is provided to

prevent gluconeogenesis from catabolism of dietary amino acids, provision of more protein (up to specific limits) leads to greater incorporation of protein and its nitrogen in lean body mass. Protein generally constitutes 5% to 12% of total calories, reflected in the composition of human milk and infant formulas that model human milk. Fomon and Ziegler suggested a formula caloric composition of 9% protein, 60% carbohydrate, and 31% fat provided in a density of 1 kcal/mL for infants with CHD.[47] The ratio of energy to protein in infant formulas is 30 to 50 kcal/g of protein (corresponding to nonprotein calorie-to-nitrogen ratios of 287:140). Thus, a child receiving 140 kcal/kg/day of energy would receive 2.9 to 4.25 g/kg of protein, if derived from standard or concentrated formula, with protein constituting 8% to 12% of total calories. To avoid excessive hepatic protein metabolic and renal solute load, assuming a limit of 3.5 g/kg/day of protein, the additional energy required above 120 kcal/kg based on ideal body weight for length should be provided by either glucose polymers (polycose or starch) or by fat (microlipid or oils) added to the formula, unless using a standard infant formula or human milk (see Table 46.2). These formulas are low enough in protein content that their high calorie-to-protein ratio allows concentration of the formula to achieve a higher calorie intake without exceeding the threshold for protein toler-ance. Once the child approaches 1 year of age, an intact protein-based 1-kcal/mL formula (eg, Pediasure, Kids Essential, Nutren Jr), a protein-hydrolysate (eg, Peptamen Jr), or an amino acid-based (eg, Neocate Jr, Elecare, Nutramigen AA Vivonex Pediatric) formula should be substituted for infant formula.

Table 46.2.
Protein Load in Relation to Energy Provided in Selected Formulas

Formula	Protein g/dL (% kcal)	kcal/mL	kcal/g Protein	kcal/kg @ 3.5 g/kg Protein	Protein g/kg @ 140 kcal/kg/day
Human Milk	0.9 (5)	0.69	77	268	1.83
Enfamil/Similac Pediasure/	1.4 (8)	0.67	48	167	2.9
KidEssential/Nutren Jr	3 (12)	1	33	116	4.25
Portagen	2.4 (14)	0.67	28	98	5
Nutramigen/Pregestimil	1.9 (11)	0.67	35	123	4
Peptamen Jr/Peptide	3 (12)	1	33	116	4.25
Neocate/Elecare	2 (12)	0.67	35	121	4
Vivonex Ped	2.4 (12)	0.8	33	117	4.2

VI

Protein-losing enteropathy is diagnosed by identification of hypoalbuminemia, lack of proteinuria, and positive fecal alpha-1-antitrypsin assay. Typically, protein-losing enteropathy is encountered in patients with Fontan anatomy or constrictive pericarditis. Additional protein is probably necessary, and the fat provided should be predominantly MCTs, which are transported via portal circulation, to reduce mesenteric lymphatic flow and pressures contributing to the protein loss. A similar rationale leads to the use of MCTs in patients with chylothorax or chylous ascites. Formulas with predominant MCTs as the fat source are Portagen, a lactose-free protein hydrolysate formula with 85% of its fat as MCT oil; Vivonex Pediatric (68% MCTs); Peptamen Junior (60% MCTs); Pregestimil (55% MCTs); and Alimentum (50% MCTs). The older child may be given Liposorb (85% MCTs), similar in content to Portagen. Human milk will be unable to supply these protein needs without supplementation and is very high in long-chain triglycerides, which are absorbed via the lymphatic system. Essential fatty acid deficiency can occur with MCT dominant feeding and should be monitored. Providing 2% to 4% of the total calories as essential fatty acids should prevent deficiency.

Electrolytes, Minerals, and Micronutrients
Disturbances in electrolyte and mineral homeostasis accompany diuretic therapy or refeeding. Hypokalemia or hypocalcemia may cause changes in myocardial conduction and contractility. Diuretic therapy is irrational if sodium intake is not controlled. Concentrated formulas provide an increased electrolyte and mineral load without accompanying free water, challenging renal regulation, especially in the patient on diuretic therapy for congestive heart failure. This is another argument for limiting the calorie concentration of formulas to 24 kcal/oz and providing additional caloric requirements by fat emulsion or glucose polymer additives. Potassium and chloride depletion commonly occur and may require supplementation. Calcium, magnesium, and zinc may also be depleted. Calciuria may be diminished by using chlorothiazide instead of furosemide. Calcium absorption from the gut is limited in magnesium deficiency (magnesium-dependent adenosine triphosphatase). Potassium may be spared by addition of spironolactone in selected cases.

Zinc depletion may manifest as a low-alkaline phosphatase activity and cholesterol concentration (zinc-dependent enzymatic products). Iron needs are increased in cyanotic heart disease to maintain the increased erythroid mass demanded by hypoxemia. Anemia contributes to tissue hypoxia in patients with ventricular pressure overload, volume overload, CHF, or hypoxemia/cyanosis. In aortic valve stenosis, anemia may contribute to subendocardial ischemia, causing angina or arrhythmia. In patients with a large VSD, anemia causes decreased blood viscosity and pulmonary vascular resistance, which allows increased left-to-right shunting and increased CHF and pulmonary blood flow.[48] Selenium and carnitine deficiency may occur in unsupplemented parenteral nutrition and may manifest as cardiomyopathy.

Thiamine (vitamin B_1) deficiency may present as the syndrome of wet beriberi with varying severity of CHF attributable to impaired myocardial function and impaired autonomic regulation of circulation. Clinical manifestations include edema, fatigue, dyspnea, and tachycardia with signs of CHF. Shoshin is a severe form of beriberi that may affect infants with pulmonary edema and CHF. Thiamine depletion may occur in settings of high carbohydrate intake without thiamine, as in a nursing mother on an inadequate diet or consuming alcohol and in settings of prolonged parenteral nutrition or glucose administration without a multivitamin supplement. Thiamine requirements are increased with the stress of surgery and critical illness, and losses of thiamine increase with loop diuretics such as furosemide, putting patients with CHD at risk of deficiency. Shamir et al identified thiamine deficiency in 4 of 22 children with CHD before surgery, 3 of whom had adequate thiamine intake, and 6 of 22 had thiamine deficiency after surgery. However, no relationship to the level of undernutrition, thiamine intake, or furosemide use could be proved.[49] Vitamin K-containing foods, such as green leafy vegetables, may interfere with coumadin effectiveness.

Fluids

Many patients, especially those with CHF, are restricted in fluid intake with or without diuretic treatment. Providing adequate calories in the setting of fluid restriction is challenging and requires a concentrated formula, often requiring continuous administration via nasogastric or transpyloric tube. The use of fat emulsions, such as Microlipid 4.5 kcal/mL, provides an energy-dense supplement to boost formula caloric density without increasing volume or osmolarity as well as avoiding the protein and electrolyte load incurred by concentrating formula.

Feeding Strategies

Oral or enteral feedings are preferred, and there need be no restriction in volume of formula in infants with CHF or cyanosis if they feed voluntarily. However, many patients with CHD have oral voluntary intake insufficient to supply nutrient requirements to maintain growth. The increased cardiopulmonary demands of eating or associated problems, such as gastrointestinal tract dysmotility, prematurity, and airway or pulmonary disease, may prevent adequate intake. Volume may also be restricted, especially in patients with lesions associated with CHF or pulmonary hypertension, requiring diuretic therapy, fluid, and sodium restriction. Reparative or palliative surgery may be safer if performed after achieving a target weight. Formula concentration is frequently increased to provide more energy and protein in a restricted volume. If volume is the limiting factor, a more concentrated formula will be necessary to provide up to 3.5 g/kg/day of protein, above which additional calories may be added with carbohydrates (polycose powder or liquid) or fats (Microlipid emulsion). MCTs are not miscible in formula and may contribute to diarrhea and

VI

cramping but are valuable as the principal fat source in patients with chylothorax, because most MCTs do not enter the mesenteric lymphatics. Concentrating a formula leads to increased protein and solute load, osmolarity, or tonicity and decreased free water. A recent study of postoperative infants showed that advancement to a high-concentration formula within 2 days rather than 5 days to a lower concentration safely improved energy intake and weight gain and decreased length of stay.[50]

Supplemental enteral nutrition is frequently instituted to achieve nutritional goals via nasogastric or gastrostomy tube. One study concluded that only 24-hour continuous enteral feeding by nasogastric tube of a concentrated or augmented formula is able to provide the minimum of 140 kcal/kg/day necessary to improve nutritional status.[16] Consequences of coercive oral feeding efforts or nasopharyngeal tube placement and feeding include a high incidence of oral aversion, which may prove quite refractory long after the cardiac issues have improved. Patients who are considered likely to require chronic nasogastric tube feedings for longer than 6 months should be considered early for gastrostomy tube placement. Given the possibility that gastrostomy feeding may alter gastroduodenal motility and increase gastroesophageal reflux; evidence of airway penetration; impaired airway protective reflexes, such as absent gag or cough; or lower respiratory tract disease may mandate protective antireflux surgery (Nissen fundoplication). If airway protective reflexes are intact, eg, no vocal cord dysfunction or recurrent laryngeal nerve palsy, and there is no evidence of respiratory compromise, such as reactive airway disease, laryngospasm/stridor, or aspiration pneumonia, then percutaneous gastrostomy without antireflux surgery is a safe and effective option.[51] The anatomy of the upper gastrointestinal tract should be evaluated by contrast studies to exclude associated anomalies of tracheoesophageal fistula; vascular ring; gross airway penetration, directly or with reflux; and intestinal rotational anomalies. For patients with aspiration risks who are not considered safe candidates for antireflux fundoplication surgery, transpyloric feeding with a nasojejunal or percutaneous gastrojejunal tube or direct-feeding jejunostomy are alternatives. Although transpyloric duodenal or jejunal feeding may prevent formula entry into the stomach, gastroduodenal motility may be inhibited, and duodenogastric reflux of bile or gastroesophageal reflux of acid and/or bile may still occur.

The breastfed infant may require manual or pump expression of milk if there is fatigue or problems suckling either because of inability to latch on, excessive respiratory effort, and/or tachypnea competing with sucking and swallowing. Tube feeding either fortified human milk or a high-caloric density formula continuously to augment a marginal nursing intake will be required for sufficient calories.

Parenteral nutrition is reserved for patients who cannot be fed effectively or safely by the enteral routes described previously. Examples would be patients with associated gastrointestinal tract disease, such as necrotizing enterocolitis, or those at risk of aspiration because of tachypnea or gastroesophageal reflux. Because cardiac output is determined by the demands of peripheral tissue metabolism, advancement of feedings, whether parenteral or enteral, in the patient accommodated to chronic malnutrition, should be gradual and monitored for refeeding complications. Peripheral capillary vasodilation in response to tissue anabolism can lead to high-output cardiac failure; excessive volume administration can provoke CHF and anasarca. Glucose uptake and metabolism will cause intracellular influx of potassium, magnesium, calcium, and most dramatically, phosphate. Dysrhythmias, particularly atrial arrhythmias related to changes in venous return, and ventricular arrhythmias related to conduction disturbances may be associated with electrolyte fluxes (hypokalemia, hypocalcemia, hypophosphatemia) and can manifest in changes in the corrected QT interval on electrocardiogram. Other cardiac complications of nutritional support include volume overload, increased viscosity and pulmonary artery pressures with high lipid infusions (exceeding 0.15 g/kg/hour or 3.5 g/kg/day), increased tissue metabolic demand for cardiac output, arrhythmias, and endocarditis/sepsis related to the central venous catheter.

Monitoring Outcome

Precise weights and lengths (or standing heights for patients older than 3 years) should be obtained at each encounter and plotted on the appropriate growth curve (eg, Down syndrome-specific curve, length-for-age chart for infants 0-36 months of age, height chart for children 2-18 years of age). The same dietitian should obtain measurements of mid-upper arm circumference and triceps skinfold thickness to help assess muscle and fat stores, understanding that fluid status and edema may affect the measures. Review of diet is important. The current formula and methods for mixing and adding supplements should be reviewed to eliminate errors in formulation. The family should be instructed to bring a 3- or 5-day diet record to the clinic visit for evaluation by the dietitian for nutrient analysis. Attention should be paid to total caloric intake, proportion of fat and carbohydrate intake, protein intake, and adequacy of micronutrients, including iron, zinc, and vitamins. Fluid volume intake, urinary frequency, and hydration status in the context of diuretic therapy should be assessed. More sophisticated measures of body composition, including bone mineral status, may be obtained in certain groups or research settings, if the technology such as dual energy x-ray absorptiometry or bioelectrical impedance analysis is available. Indirect calorimetry can assess resting energy expenditure and respiratory quotient to assess energy requirements and avoid overfeeding in patients in the intensive care unit. In the absence of direct measures of lean body mass or energy requirements, the surrogate parameter of weight expected for length for age or ideal body weight for length, can be helpful in estimating energy and protein requirements for the very lean or obese child (see Table 46.1). However, serial measurement of changes in weight, length, and anthropometry are the best indicators of nutrient adequacy.

VI

References

1. Levy RJ, Rosenthal A, Castaneda AR, Nadas AS. Growth after surgical repair of simple D-transposition of the great arteries. *Ann Thorac Surg*. 1978;25(3):225-230

2. Levy RJ, Rosenthal A, Fyler DC, Nadas AS. Birthweight of infants with congenital heart disease. *Am J Dis Child*. 1978;132(3):249-254

3. Rosenthal GL, Wilson PD, Permutt T, Boughman JA, Ferencz C. Birth weight and cardiovascular malformations: a population-based study. The Baltimore-Washington Infant Study. *Am J Epidemiol*. 1991;133(12):1273-1281

4. Cameron JW, Rosenthal A, Olson AD. Malnutrition in hospitalized children with congenital heart disease. *Arch Pediatr Adolesc Med*. 1995;149(10):1098-1102

5. Leitch CA. Growth, nutrition and energy expenditure in pediatric heart failure. *Progr Pediatr Cardiol*. 2000;11(3):195-202

6. Schuurmans FM, Pulles-Heintzberger CF, Gerver WJ, Kester AD, Forget PP. Long-term growth of children with congenital heart disease: a retrospective study. *Acta Paediatr*. 1998;87(12):1250-1255

7. Barton JS, Hindmarsh PC, Scrimgeour CM, Rennie MJ, Preece MA. Energy expenditure in congenital heart disease. *Arch Dis Child*. 1994;70(1):5-9

8. Leitch CA, Karn CA, Peppard RJ, et al. Increased energy expenditure in infants with cyanotic congenital heart disease. *J Pediatr*. 1998;133(6):755-760

9. Mitchell IM, Davies PS, Day JM, Pollock JC, Jamieson MP. Energy expenditure in children with congenital heart disease, before and after cardiac surgery. *J Thorac Cardiovasc Surg*. 1994;107(2):374-380

10. Huse DM, Feldt RH, Nelson RA, Novak LP. Infants with congenital heart disease. Food intake, body weight, and energy metabolism. *Am J Dis Child*. 1975;129(1):65-69

11. Menon G, Poskitt EM. Why does congenital heart disease cause failure to thrive? *Arch Dis Child*. 1985;60(12):1134-1139

12. Rosenthal A. Congenital cardiac anomalies and gastrointestinal malformations. In: Pierpont M, Moller J, eds. *Genetics of Cardiovascular Disease*. Boston, MA: Martinus Nijhoff; 1986:113-126

13. Sondheimer JM, Hamilton JR. Intestinal function in infants with severe congenital heart disease. *J Pediatr*. 1978;92(4):572-578

14. Vaisman N, Leigh T, Voet H, Westerterp K, Abraham M, Duchan R. Malabsorption in infants with congenital heart disease under diuretic treatment. *Pediatr Res*. 1994;36(4):545-549

15. Yahav J, Avigad S, Frand M, et al. Assessment of intestinal and cardiorespiratory function in children with congenital heart disease on high-caloric formulas. *J Pediatr Gastroenterol Nutr*. 1985;4(5):778-785

16. Schwarz SM, Gewitz MH, See CC, et al. Enteral nutrition in infants with congenital heart disease and growth failure. *Pediatrics*. 1990;86(3):368-373

17. Unger R, DeKleermaeker M, Gidding SS, Christoffel KK. Calories count. Improved weight gain with dietary intervention in congenital heart disease. *Am J Dis Child*. 1992;146(9):1078-1084

18. Salzer HR, Haschke F, Wimmer M, Heil M, Schilling R. Growth and nutritional intake of infants with congenital heart disease. *Pediatr Cardiol*. 1989;10(1):17-23

19. Cavell B. Gastric emptying in infants with congenital heart disease. *Acta Paediatr Scand*. 1981;70(5):517-520

20. Forchielli ML, McColl R, Walker WA, Lo C. Children with congenital heart disease: a nutrition challenge. *Nutr Rev*. 1994;52:348-353

21. Sole MJ, Jeejeebhoy KN. Conditioned nutritional requirements and the pathogenesis and treatment of myocardial failure. *Curr Opin Clin Nutr Metab Care*. 2000;3:417-424

22. Carr JG, Stevenson LW, Walden JA, Heber D. Prevalence and hemodynamic correlates of malnutrition in severe congestive heart failure secondary to ischemic or idiopathic dilated cardiomyopathy. *Am J Cardiol*. 1989;63(11):709-713

23. Freeman LM, Roubenoff R. The nutrition implications of cardiac cachexia. *Nutr Rev*. 1994;52(10):340-347

24. Feldman AM, Combes A, Wagner D, et al. The role of tumor necrosis factor in the pathophysiology of heart failure. *J Am Coll Cardiol*. 2000;35(3):537-544

25. Krauss AN, Auld PA. Metabolic rate of neonates with congenital heart disease. *Arch Dis Child*. 1975;50(7):539-541

26. Stocker FP, Wilkoff W, Miettinen OS, Nadas AS. Oxygen consumption in infants with heart disease. Relationship to severity of congestive failure, relative weight, and caloric intake. *J Pediatr*. 1972;80(1):43-51

27. Van der Kuip M, Hoos MB, Forget PP, Westerterp KR, Gemke RJ, de Meer K. Energy expenditure in infants with congenital heart disease, including meta-analysis. *Acta Paediatr*. 2003;92(8):921-927

28. Weintraub RG, Menahem S. Growth and congenital heart disease. *J Paediatr Child Health*. 1993;29(2):95-98

29. Gervasio MR, Buchanan CN. Malnutrition in the pediatric cardiology patient. *CCQ*. 1985;8(3):49-56

30. Okoromah CAN, Ekure EN, Lesi FEA, Okunowo WO, Tijani BO, Okeiyi JC. Prevalence, profile and predictors of malnutrition in children with congenital heart defects: a case-control observational study. *Arch Dis Child*. 2011;96(4):354-360

31. Varan B, Tokel K, Yilmaz G. Malnutrition and growth failure in cyanotic and acyanotic congenital heart disease with and without pulmonary hypertension. *Arch Dis Child*. 1999;81(1):49-52

32. Leitch CA, Karn CA, Ensing GJ, Denne SC. Energy expenditure after surgical repair in children with cyanotic congenital heart disease. *J Pediatr*. 2000;137(3):381-385

33. Ackerman IL, Karn CA, Denne SC, Ensing GJ, Leitch CA. Total but not resting energy expenditure is increased in infants with ventricular septal defects. *Pediatrics*. 1998;102(5):1172-1177

34. Levy RJ, Rosenthal A, Miettinen OS, Nadas AS. Determinants of growth in patients with ventricular septal defect. *Circulation*. 1978;57(4):793-797

35. Renlund DG, Taylor DO, Kfoury AG, Shaddy RS. New UNOS rules: historical background and implications for transplantation management. United Network for Organ Sharing. *J Heart Lung Transplant*. 1999;18(11):1065-1070

VI

36. Sholler GF, Celermajer JM. Cardiac surgery in the first year of life: the effect on weight gains of infants with congenital heart disease. *Aust Paediatr J.* 1986;22(4):305-308

37. Stenbog EV, Hjortdal VE, Ravn HB, Skjaerbaek C, Sorensen KE, Hansen OK. Improvement in growth, and levels of insulin-like growth factor-I in the serum, after cavopulmonary connections. *Cardiol Young.* 2000;10(5):440-446

38. Cohen MI, Bush DM, Ferry RJ Jr, et al. Somatic growth failure after the Fontan operation. *Cardiol Young.* 2000;10(5):447-457

39. Baum D, Beck RQ, Haskell WL. Growth and tissue abnormalities in young people with cyanotic congenital heart disease receiving systemic-pulmonary artery shunts. *Am J Cardiol.* 1983;52(3):349-352

40. Biewer ES, Zurn C, Arnold R, Glockler M, Schulte-Monting J, Schlensak C, Dittrich S. Chylothorax after surgery on congenital heart disease in newborns and infants—risk factors and efficacy of MCT-diet. *J Cardiothoracic Surg.* 2010;5:127-134

41. Brown KH, Peerson JM, Allen LH. Effect of zinc supplementation on children's growth: a meta-analysis of intervention trials. *Bibl Nutr Dieta.* 1998;(54):76-83

42. Walravens PA, Hambidge KM, Koepfer DM. Zinc supplementation in infants with a nutritional pattern of failure to thrive: a double-blind controlled study. *Pediatrics.* 1989;83(4):522-528

43. Payne PR, Waterlow JC. Relative energy requirements for maintenance, growth, and physical activity. *Lancet.* 1971;2(7717):210-211

44. Jackson M, Poskitt EM. The effects of high-energy feeding on energy balance and growth in infants with congenital heart disease and failure to thrive. *Br J Nutr.* 1991;65(2):131-143

45. Bougle D, Iselin M, Kahyat A, Duhamel JF. Nutritional treatment of congenital heart disease. *Arch Dis Child.* 1986;61(8):799-801

46. Vanderhoof JA, Hofshire PJ, Baluff MA, et al. Continuous enteral feedings. An important adjunct to the management of complex congenital heart disease. *Am J Dis Child.* 1982;136(9):825-827

47. Fomon SJ, Ziegler EE. Nutritional management of infants with congenital heart disease. *Am Heart J.* 1972;83(5):581-588

48. Lister G, Hellenbrand WE, Kleinman CS, Talner NS. Physiologic effects of increasing hemoglobin concentration in left-to-right shunting in infants with ventricular septal defects. *N Engl J Med.* 1982;306(9):502-506

49. Shamir R, Dagan O, Abramovitch D, Abramovitch T, Vidne BA, Dinari G. Thiamine deficiency in children with congenital heart disease before and after corrective surgery. *JPEN J Parenter Enteral Nutr.* 2000;24(3):154-158

50. Pillo-Blocka F, Adatia I, Sharieff W, McCrindle BW, Zlotkin S. Rapid advancement to more concentrated formula in infants after surgery for congenital heart disease reduces duration of hospital stay: a randomized clinical trial. *J Pediatr.* 2004;145(6):761-766

51. Ciotti G, Holzer R, Pozzi M, Dalzell M. Nutritional support via percutaneous endoscopic gastrostomy in children with cardiac disease experiencing difficulties with feeding. *Cardiol Young.* 2002;12(6):537-541

Chapter 47

Nutrition in Children With Short Bowel Syndrome

Background

Short bowel syndrome (SBS) is a complex disorder that is characterized as a malabsorptive state in the setting of a reduced length of small bowel. The complexity of this disorder stems from the nutritional, metabolic, and infectious complications that often occur as a consequence of altered anatomy and physiology. In pediatrics, SBS typically results from congenital anomalies, such as intestinal atresia, gastroschisis, midgut volvulus, and acquired causes, the most common of which is necrotizing enterocolitis (NEC [see Table 47.1]). Although the actual incidence and prevalence of SBS in the United States are not precisely known, advances in neonatal intensive care and surgical techniques will likely increase the frequency with which pediatricians will encounter such patients.

Table 47.1.
Etiology of Short Bowel Syndrome in Infants and Children

Intestinal atresia
Necrotizing enterocolitis
Gastroschisis
Midgut volvulus
Total intestinal aganglionosis
Congenital short bowel
Ischemic injury
Tumor
Radiation enteritis

There is a wide spectrum of functionality associated with SBS, but a number of patients will develop intestinal failure, defined as an inability of the small intestine to maintain adequate fluid, nutrient, and electrolyte absorption to support normal growth and development. Such patients are dependent on parenteral nutrition. Although parenteral nutrition can serve as a lifesaving treatment for patients who otherwise would not survive, its use does not come without risk. Catheter-related sepsis and parenteral nutrition-associated liver disease (PNALD) are the main contributors to the morbidity and mortality associated with chronic use of parenteral nutrition.

A number of factors have been identified that are thought to influence the prognosis of SBS (see Table 47.2).[1-3] Loss of bowel length is the most significant, because this results in reduced surface area for absorption, decreased exposure of

VI

nutrients to brush-border digestive enzymes, and decreased exposure to pancreatic and biliary secretions. It has been estimated that 10 to 30 cm of small bowel with a preserved ileocecal valve or 30 to 50 cm of small bowel without an ileocecal valve is required for successful weaning from parenteral nutrition.[4] However, because residual length is only one of several factors involved in the prognosis of these patients, there are considerable exceptions to these estimations. Recognizing the importance of these various factors can help guide the management of these patients and ultimately facilitate the process of weaning from parenteral nutrition.

Table 47.2.
Factors Affecting Prognosis of SBS

Length of residual bowel
Presence or absence of ileocecal valve
Type of enteral feeds used
Early introduction of enteral feeds
Adaptive potential of residual bowel
Frequency of infections
Health of other organs (ie, stomach, pancreas, liver, colon)

The optimal outcome for patients with SBS is to become independent from parenteral nutrition or attain what is referred to as enteral autonomy. Although there is still much to learn in this field emerging experience and data have been emerging to help us better understand how to achieve such an outcome through a physiologic mechanism known as intestinal adaptation. The act of promoting intestinal adaptation through nutritional, medical, and surgical therapies has been increasingly recognized and is now more commonly referred to as intestinal rehabilitation. Although previous estimates of survival rates have ranged from 73% to 89%, recent reports of multidisciplinary programs specializing in the field of intestinal rehabilitation have demonstrated even better outcomes.[1,5-11]

Intestinal Adaptation

Intestinal adaptation is a complex process that ensues following bowel resection. Throughout this process, the bowel undergoes both structural and functional changes in an attempt to compensate for the loss of absorptive surface area (see Table 47.3). Structurally, the villi lengthen and the bowel lengthens and dilates, both of which serve to increase the intestinal absorptive surface area.[12-15] Functionally, the bowel undergoes changes in nutrient transport, enzyme activity, and intestinal transit. Because of the innate ability of the maturing intestine to grow, infants may have an advantage for achieving better intestinal adaptation compared with older children or adults.[16-18] Small bowel length is estimated to be approximately 125 cm at 20 weeks' gestation, 200 cm at 30 weeks' gestation, and 275 cm at term.[17] An accelerated increase in bowel length during the last trimester of gestation could provide a theoretical advantage for bowel lengthening for the newborn infant.[16-18] Linear growth proceeds at a relatively rapid rate during the first year of life and continues for the next several years, although at a slower velocity. Therefore, children who undergo bowel resection earlier in life like the newborn infant are thought to have an advantage in terms of intestinal growth.

Table 47.3.
Changes Associated With Intestinal Adaptation

Increased villus height
Increased crypt depth
Increased bowel length
Increased bowel circumference
Increased bowel wall thickness
Increased enterocyte proliferation

A number of factors have been identified that influence the adaptive process, namely enteral nutrition, hormones, and growth factors. Enteral nutrients are thought to be an important stimulant for mucosal hyperplasia.[19] Complex nutrients, such as disaccharides and intact proteins, are thought to have more of a stimulatory effect compared with monosaccharides and protein hydrolysates.[20,21] However, the use of intact nutrients must be carefully weighed against the possible malabsorptive consequences. Other luminal factors, such as glutamine, fiber, and short-chain fatty acids, have been shown to be involved, but their clinical significance has yet to be clearly determined.[19] The role of hormones and growth factors have been investigated, and currently, glucagon-like peptide 2 (GLP-2) is considered one of the more important hormones involved in intestinal adaptation (see "Medical Therapies").

Intestinal Physiology

The distinct functions of the proximal versus distal small intestine have a significant effect on the management of patients with SBS. Because different segments of the small intestine may be compromised, each patient has a unique anatomy and physiology. Treatment for these patients is based on their underlying disease, which segments have been resected, and which segments are retained. To determine the optimal nutritional therapy for each patient, it is important to appreciate the various functions of each area of small intestine and the consequences of its resection.

VI

The duodenum is rarely affected in patients with SBS, perhaps because of its separate vascular supply. It is primarily responsible for the ongoing digestion of chyme (the semifluid mass of food released from the stomach) and is the preferred site of iron and folate absorption. When chyme is expelled from the stomach, the hormones secretin and cholecystokinin are released. Secretin stimulates pancreatic secretion of bicarbonate-rich fluid and of mucus-rich alkaline secretions from Brunner glands. The net effect is to neutralize the acidic chyme, establishing a pH favorable to the action of digestive enzymes. Cholecystokinin (CCK) is secreted in response to the presence of fat and protein. CCK stimulates biliary and pancreatic secretions, which promote further digestion of chyme.

The jejunum has long villi, a large absorptive surface area, and a high concentration of enzymes and transport carrier proteins. It is the primary absorptive site for most nutrients. Loss of jejunum is associated with decreased absorption attributable to loss of surface area, impaired digestion resulting from loss of brush-border enzymes, and decreased secretin and CCK with resultant compromise in pancreatic and biliary secretions. Following resection of the jejunum, however, through the process of intestinal adaptation over time, these functions of the jejunum may be acquired by the remaining bowel.

The ileum is characterized by shorter villi, more lymphoid tissue, and less absorptive capacity compared with the jejunum. Unlike the jejunum, however, 2 unique functions of the ileum cannot be acquired by other sites in the intestine following resection. The first is absorption of bile acids and vitamin B_{12}. Resections involving the ileum, therefore, can result in steatorrhea, cholelithiasis, and vitamin B_{12} deficiency. The second is the production of hormones that regulate intestinal motility. Normally, motility is more rapid in the proximal small bowel and slows in the distal ileum. Consequently, resection of the ileum may have more of an adverse effect on transit time compared with a proximal resection.

The ileocecal valve (ICV) controls the amount and rate of passage of ileal contents into the colon. Absence of the ICV shortens transit time and can lead to increased losses of fluid and nutrients. The ICV also serves to prevent reflux of colonic bacterial back into the small intestine. Reflux of colonic bacteria into the small intestine can cause mucosal inflammation, which can then lead to malabsorption.

Nutritional Assessment

The primary goals in the treatment of SBS patients are (1) to provide adequate nutrition to achieve normal growth and development; (2) to promote intestinal adaptation; and (3) to avoid complications associated with intestinal resection and use of parenteral nutrition. The first steps in assessing a child with SBS are to identify the underlying disease leading to a short gut, assess the residual anatomy, and anticipate the individual physiology of the patient on the basis of this information. Patients with intestinal atresias may not have developed a normal length of bowel in utero and, despite undergoing relatively limited resections, may be left with a significantly compromised length of bowel. Patients with gastroschisis are often compromised by a dilated, dysfunctional bowel and motility disorders, despite having a residual length that should otherwise be adequate for adaptation. NEC occurs in preterm infants and most commonly affects the terminal ileum and proximal colon. For such infants, the ICV is more likely to be resected and can contribute to more rapid transit and the development of small bowel bacterial overgrowth. The ischemic and inflammatory reactions associated with the pathogenesis of NEC can also contribute to the development of strictures.

Once the underlying diagnosis and anticipated physiology is determined, the focus becomes the assessment of the patient's nutritional status. Accurate measurements of weight, height, and head circumference obtained on a serial basis are essential. However, fluid shifts, changes in stool and ostomy output, and the presence of ascites may affect the accuracy of weight measurements. In such cases, assessment of mid-upper arm circumference and triceps skinfold thickness may provide a better representation of nutritional status.

Nutritional Management

Parenteral Nutrition

In the early postoperative stage, parenteral nutrition is used to stabilize fluid and electrolyte status. Once a postoperative ileus resolves, one can be faced with large fluid volume and electrolyte losses, along with hypergastrinemia and a need for acid suppression. Therefore, achieving adequate fluid and electrolyte balance can often pose a significant challenge. Because these losses can vary on a day to day basis, it is advantageous to use a standard parenteral nutrition solution that meets basic fluid, electrolyte, and macro- and micronutrient requirements appropriate for metabolic needs. Excessive fluid losses from ostomy output and stool losses can then be replaced based on the volume and electrolyte content of these secretions. It is preferable to measure the volume of these secretions and replace them using a separate fluid and electrolyte solution. Adjustment of parenteral nutrition should be based on daily weights; strict measurements of urine, stool, ostomy output, serum electrolytes, and triglycerides; and a liver panel (inclusive of aspartate transaminase, alanine transaminase, alkaline phosphatase, gamma glutamyl transpeptidase, total bilirubin, direct bilirubin, and albumin [see Chapter 23: Parenteral Nutrition]).

VI

Enteral Nutrition

A slow introduction of enteral feeding should be started as soon as possible after surgery. The role of early enteral feedings is important, because the process of intestinal adaptation begins as soon as 12 to 24 hours after surgical resection. Enteral nutrients stimulate the adaptive process by providing direct contact with the epithelial cells, thereby inducing villous hyperplasia and by stimulating the secretion of trophic gastrointestinal tract hormones. The use of enteral feedings is also important in the prevention of PNALD (see "Complications").

Mothers of newborn infants with SBS should be encouraged to continue with their production of human milk, because it offers several beneficial effects. In addition to the immunologic and anti-infective properties, human milk also contains growth factors, nucleotides, glutamine, and other amino acids thought to be important in the process of intestinal adaptation. Human milk from mothers of preterm infants may require fortification to increase the caloric density as well as protein concentration.

Table 47.4.

Suggested Guidelines for Advancing Enteral Feeds

Advancement of feeds are determined by:

Measure	Advance Rate by 0.5-1 mL/kg/h	No Change	Reduce Rate or Hold Feeds × 8 h, Then Restart at ¾ Previous Rate
Ostomy output (g)	<2g/kg/hr	2-3 g/kg/hr	>3 g/kg/h
Stool output (g)	<10 g/kg/day or <10 stools/day	10-20 g/kg/day or 10-12 stools/day	>20 g/kg/day or >12 stools/day
Gastric residuals (mL)	<4 times previous hour's infusion		>4 times previous hour's infusion
Signs of malabsorption			
Stool-reducing substances	<1%	1%	>1%
Dehydration	Absent		Present
Weight loss	Absent		Present

Adapted from Hendriks KM, et al. *Manual of Pediatric Nutrition Third Edition*, 2000:537-538.

When human milk is unavailable, the optimal enteral formula has not been clearly established. Some studies suggest that complex nutrients stimulate the intestinal adaptive process more effectively.[22,23] However, because of potentially compromised digestive capabilities and limited absorptive surface area, the use of an intact formula can lead to malabsorption, resulting in fluid, electrolyte, and metabolic imbalance. Because glucose, glucose polymers, medium-chain triglycerides (MCTs), and hydrolyzed proteins require less digestion, they are usually more easily tolerated. Therefore, it has become customary to use either a protein hydrolysate or amino acid-based formula (see Chapter 3: Formula Feeding of Term Infants [Web Links to Manufacturers for Product Composition and Other Information]). Observations of a higher incidence of gastrointestinal allergies in SBS and the association with successful weaning from total parenteral nutrition have also supported the use of amino acid-based formulas.[3,24]

Although fats tend to be poorly absorbed in patients with SBS, they are an important source of calories and are necessary for the prevention of essential fatty acid deficiency. MCTs are more water soluble than long-chain triglycerides and are more readily absorbed, particularly in the settings of bile acid malabsorption, liver disease, or pancreatic insufficiency. However, MCTs have slightly lower caloric density and a higher osmotic load, which can aggravate diarrhea. Long-chain triglycerides have a greater trophic effect on the small intestine and are, therefore, thought to be beneficial in stimulating intestinal adaptation. Ultimately, a combination of MCTs to maximize absorption and long-chain triglycerides to stimulate adaptation is recommended.

Carbohydrates may be difficult to tolerate, because they are rapidly metabolized to small molecules that can produce an increased osmotic load in the small intestine, resulting in high-volume stool or ostomy output. An elevation in stool reducing substances and/or a low stool pH may be indicative of carbohydrate malabsorption.

The use of soluble dietary fiber, such as pectin or guar gum, has potentially beneficial effects on colonic adaptation. Fiber can slow transit and is also fermented by bacteria in the colon to produce short-chain fatty acids. In adults, the provision of fiber and the resultant short-chain fatty acids can provide as much as 500 to 1000 calories per day. In addition, butyrate (a short-chain fatty acid) has been shown to enhance sodium and water absorption via up-regulation of sodium-hydrogen exchanges. This up-regulation, however, may be delayed initially, causing stool output to worsen before it improves.[25,26]

How to Feed

Once the appropriate source of enteral nutrition has been established, the next step is to determine the appropriate method of feeding. Continuous enteral feedings via a nasogastric or gastrostomy tube is generally preferred. Continuous enteral feeding allows for constant saturation of transport carrier proteins, thereby maximally utilizing the absorptive surface area available. Controlling the rate of feeds in this fashion may also help to reduce emesis and allow for more consistent advancement. Enteral feedings are slowly advanced, by increasing either concentration or volume, depending on their tolerance. With this regimented approach to feeding, it is also important to introduce some oral feedings, even at nonnutritive volumes, so as to

VI

stimulate the normal development of oromotor skills. Missing this window of developmental opportunity often results in significant oral aversion later in life. As an infant is advancing his or her enteral feeds, one hour's worth of volume may be given by mouth, during which time tube feedings should be held (Fig 47.1).

Fig 47.1.
Suggested Guidelines for Starting Enteral Feeds

Assess for presence of bowel sounds
Ensure no contraindications:
Marked abdominal distention
Bilious emesis
Absent bowel sounds
Decreased ostomy or stool output
Hematochezia, melena
Lactic acidosis
Cardiac and/or respiratory insufficiency
Radiographic evidence of obstruction, ileus, pneumatosis

If no contraindication, may start feeds

If yes, keep NPO on TPN/IVF

NG/G-tube/NJ/J-tube
Start at 0.5-1 mL/kg/h continuously x 24 h

Oral feeds
Start with 1 hour's worth of continuous rate
May offer QD-TID
Hold continuous tube feeds during PO feeding

NPO indicates nil per os; IVF, intravenous fluids; NG/G, nasogastric/gastrostomy; NJ/J, nasojejunal/jejunostomy; QD-TID, every day to 3 times/day.

The rate at which enteral feedings are advanced is determined by a number of factors including stool or ostomy output, and signs of malabsorption (Table 47.2). Carbohydrate malabsorption can be assessed by stool pH and reducing substances and can be an important and easily measurable factor to help in determining readiness for advancement. If feeding intolerance occurs after an increase in rate or concentration, a decrease to the previously tolerated rate or concentration should be made. Once tolerance is again established, another attempt at advancement may be made. Frequent setbacks are not uncommon. The development of diarrhea is inevitable in most patients and does not necessarily serve as a rate-limiting factor to advancing enteral feedings. As long as there is adequate weight gain, positive electrolyte and fluid balance, and lack of significant carbohydrate malabsorption as reflected by stool pH and reducing substances, advancement should continue. Once a patient achieves his or her target for enteral feedings, a gradual transition to oral/bolus feedings should be pursued. This is generally accomplished by compressing a set volume of feeds over a shorter period of time. For example, if the patient is tolerating a rate of 40 mL/hour, one could compress the feedings to be given as 48 mL/hour for 2.5 hours with 30 minutes off, then 60 mL/hour for 2 hours with 1 hour off, etc.

Medical Therapies

A number of therapeutic interventions aimed at accelerating bowel adaptation have been investigated, with somewhat disappointing results. More recently however, teduglutide, a GLP-2 analogue, has been found to have more promising effects in adults.[27] GLP-2 is a hormone secreted in response to ingestion of nutrients, has inhibitory effects on motility, decreases gastric acid secretion, and stimulates expansion of the intestinal mucosa, and its secretion has been found to be impaired in patients without a terminal ileum or colon. Recent randomized placebo-controlled trials administering GLP-2 to adult patients with SBS have showed promising results in decreasing dependency on total parenteral nutrition, which merits further investigation in pediatric patients.[28]

Bowel-Lengthening Procedures

As mentioned previously, one of the developments associated with intestinal adaptation is an increase in intestinal circumference or dilation of the bowel. Although this results in an increased absorptive surface area, such dilation can lead to compromised motility and stasis of intestinal contents, which often predisposes to the development of bacterial overgrowth. To optimize the absorptive surface area and address these adverse effects, surgical techniques to reconfigure the bowel have been pursued. For a longitudinal lengthening procedure, a dilated segment of

VI

intestine is divided along its longitudinal axis into 2 tubes, and the ends are then anastomosed in an isoperistaltic fashion (Fig 47.2). Unfortunately, this procedure is technically challenging, because it requires meticulous dissection of the mesenteric blood supply, is often complicated by the development of anatomic strictures, and ultimately has not been demonstrated to be of any significant benefit in weaning patients with SBS from total parenteral nutrition.[29]

Fig 47.2.
Longitudinal Intestinal Lengthening Procedure

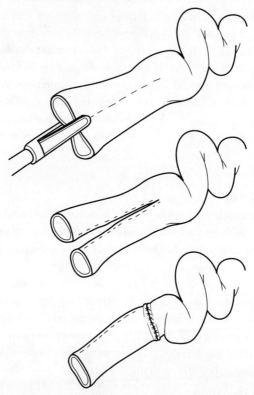

The serial transverse enteroplasty (STEP) was introduced in 2003 as a novel surgical technique for patients with SBS.[30] In contrast to the longitudinal lengthening procedure, the STEP procedure involves applying a surgical stapler perpendicular to the bowel axis from alternating sides. This creates a more normal caliber, longer lumen through which enteral contents can pass (Fig 47.3). Advantages to this technique include preservation of the vascular supply and avoiding the creation of new anastomotic sties. A study of long-term nutritional and clinical outcomes with this procedure demonstrated both improved enteral tolerance and catch-up growth.[31]

Fig 47.3.
Serial Transverse Enteroplasty Procedure

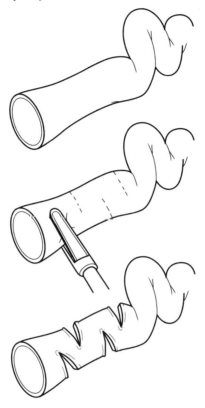

Complications

As mentioned earlier, the use of parenteral nutrition offers a life-saving therapy for patients with SBS but does not come without risk. The 2 most significant complications associated with the long-term use of parenteral nutrition include catheter-related complications and the development of PNALD. Central venous catheter complications include catheter breakage, central venous thrombosis, loss of access, and most commonly, catheter-related sepsis. The risk of infection, particularly with gram-negative organisms, may be increased in patients with SBS because of the presence of ostomies and increased stool output. The propensity for bacteria to form a biofilm of bacterial colonies adherent to the wall of the catheters can contribute to repeated line infections. Preventive measures include diligent sterile technique when manipulating catheters as well as the use of lock therapy. With lock therapy, either ethanol or an antibiotic, such as vancomycin, is instilled into the

VI

central venous catheter and left to dwell for varying durations of time in an attempt to prevent and/or breakdown the film and kill the bacteria. A recent systematic review supported the use of ethanol instillation into central venous catheters to significantly decrease the rate of catheter-related bloodstream infections in patients receiving total parenteral nutrition.[32] However, there has also been a report of increased risk of thrombosis with the use of ethanol; therefore, such therapy has not yet become established as a standard of care.[33]

PNALD occurs in 40% to 60% of infants receiving long-term total parenteral nutrition.[34,35] Histologic changes associated with PNALD include cholestasis, steatosis, steatohepatitis, fibrosis, and cirrhosis. PNALD is strongly associated with mortality. In a study of 78 children with SBS, the survival rate among those with cholestasis was approximately 20% versus 80% for those without cholestasis.[7] Multiple risk factors for the development of PNALD have been identified, including preterm birth, disrupted enterohepatic circulation of bile acids, intestinal stasis with bacterial overgrowth, catheter-related sepsis, excess glucose intake leading to steatosis, and high parenteral protein, fat, and/or energy intake.[2,3,36-38] Multiple hypotheses regarding the pathogenesis have been proposed, including altered gut hormones, bacterial overgrowth-related cholangitis, intestinal stasis-associated hepatotoxic bile acids, and deficiencies of or toxic components in the total parenteral nutrition itself.[38-40] To date, however, the etiology of PNALD is thought to be multifactorial.

Treatment strategies for the prevention of PNALD include early enteral feeding, reducing the frequency and/or duration of parenteral nutrition infusions (cycling), and avoiding sepsis. Administration of ursodeoxycholic acid may help bile flow and reduce gallbladder stasis. Recent data suggest that the reduction of omega-6 fatty acids and/or the use of omega-3 fatty acids may prevent and reverse PNALD, but further investigation is warranted.[41]

Aside from complications associated with the use of long-term parenteral nutrition, patients with SBS are at risk of developing complications inherent to their altered anatomy and physiology (Table 47.5). These include micronutrient deficiency, gastric acid hypersecretion, cholelithiasis, nephrolithiasis, bacterial overgrowth, and D-lactic acidosis.

Table 47.5.
Complications Associated With SBS

Central venous catheter related
   Loss of venous access
   Thrombosis of veins
   Line infections/sepsis

Parenteral nutrition-associated liver disease
   Cholestasis
   Steatosis
   Steatohepatitis
   Fibrosis
   Cirrhosis
   Liver failure
   Cholelithiasis
   Cholecystitis

Metabolic complications
   Fluid and electrolyte imbalance
   Micronutrient deficiency/toxicity

Metabolic bone disease
   Osteopenia
   Osteoporosis

Renal complications
   Nephrolithiasis
   Hyperoxaluria

Bacterial overgrowth
D-lactic acidosis

Gastric acid hypersecretion
   Peptic injury
   Maldigestion
   Malabsorption

Periodic surveillance of micronutrient status is recommended as part of the nutritional assessment (Table 47.6). For patients at risk of fat malabsorption attributable to ileal resection and/or associated liver or pancreatic disease, routine monitoring of fat-soluble vitamins is recommended. In addition, as a consequence of fat malabsorption, long-chain fatty acids can combine with calcium and magnesium, resulting in a deficiency of these minerals. Zinc and copper deficiencies are common in patients with SBS, particularly those with an ostomy.

Table 47.6.
Micronutrient Monitoring

Micronutrient	Mechanism for Deficiency
Fat soluble vitamins A<D<E<K	Fat malabsorption, cholestasis

Water soluble vitamins
    B_{12}
    Folate
	Gastric or ileal resection
	Proximal small bowel malabsorption

Minerals and trace elements
    Calcium
    Magnesium
    Zinc
    Iron
 	
    Copper
 	
    Selenium
	Fat malabsorption
	Fat malabsorption
	Diarrhea, ostomy losses
	Proximal small bowel malabsorption, omission from total parenteral nutrition
	Diarrhea, ostomy losses, inadequate repletion in total parenteral nutrition
	Inadequate repletion in total parenteral nutrition

Gastric acid hypersecretion results from loss of CCK and secretin secretion/feedback, both of which regulate gastrin secretion. Without this negative feedback control, gastrin concentrations are elevated, resulting in increased acid production. This can result in caustic injury to the proximal small bowel, adversely affecting its absorptive capacity. Also, because pancreatic enzymes and bile salts function optimally at a pH of 7 to 8, such hyperacidity can impair carbohydrate and protein digestion, micelle formation, and lipolysis of fat resulting in malabsorption. The suppression of acid with either H_2 blockers or proton pump inhibitors can help to improve absorption.

Compromised enterohepatic circulation of bile or bile acid malabsorption related to ileal resection may allow for cholesterol to precipitate more readily in bile because of a low concentration of bile salts. Independent of ileal resection, the chronic use of parenteral nutrition, in and of itself, has been associated with the development of biliary sludge and cholelithiasis as well.

As mentioned previously, long-chain fatty acids are able to combine with calcium and magnesium, leading to deficiency of these minerals. When this occurs, calcium becomes less available to bind to oxalate that is normally excreted in the stool in the form of calcium-oxalate. Oxalate is then reabsorbed through the colon, the permeability of which is increased when bile salts are not adequately taken up in the ileum and are, thus, present in the colon. These factors increase enteric oxalate absorption that in turn increases the risk of developing oxalate renal stones. This is a complication that can affect patients with SBS long after they have achieved intestinal adaptation. Often, such patients will need to maintain a low-oxalate diet to prevent recurrent nephrolithiasis.

Bacterial overgrowth is a common complication associated with SBS. Adverse effects include deconjugation of bile acids with resultant steatorrhea, competitive metabolism and use of enteral nutrients, synthesis of toxic metabolites including D-lactic acid, and possible translocation resulting in sepsis. Factors that can predispose to the development of bacterial overgrowth include dysmotility, stasis of intestinal contents in a dilated lumen, and absence of an ileal cecal valve allowing reflux of colonic contents into the small intestine. The organisms associated with bacterial overgrowth are usually anaerobes or gram-negative bacteria. Such bacteria can deconjugate bile salts, cause steatorrhea, and lead to mucosal inflammation, which then compromises intestinal absorption. Bacterial overgrowth should be suspected in patients who lose weight or plateau or require increasingly higher calories.

An added complication of bacterial overgrowth is the development of D-lactic acidosis. D-lactic acidosis is a rare finding in humans and results when nonabsorbed carbohydrates are metabolized by colonic bacteria. This should be suspected when there is an acidosis with an unexplained anion gap. The bacteria produce the D-isomer of lactic acid, which is unable to be metabolized by the human form of lactate dehydrogenase and can cross the blood-brain barrier. The absorption of large amounts of D-lactate can lead to a metabolic acidosis and a set of symptoms that include headache, drowsiness, confusion, behavioral disturbance, ataxia, nystagmus, and blurred vision. Treatment is with antibiotics, and prevention includes using nonabsorbable antibiotics, such as rifaximin.

Summary

SBS is a complex condition because of the nutritional, metabolic, and infectious complications that can occur from having an altered anatomy and physiology. The primary goals in the treatment of SBS are to provide adequate nutrition to achieve normal growth and development, promote intestinal adaptation, and avoid complications associated with intestinal resection and use of parenteral nutrition. These goals are best achieved by the advancement of enteral feedings, weaning from parenteral nutrition, and monitoring closely for the development of potential complications.

VI

References

1. Sondheimer JM, Cadnapaphornchai M, Sontag M, Zerbe GO. Predicting the duration of dependence on parenteral nutrition after neonatal intestinal resection. *J Pediatr.* 1998;132(1):80-84
2. Kaufman SS, Loseke CA, Lupo JV, et al. Influence of bacterial overgrowth and intestinal inflammation on duration of parenteral nutrition in children with short bowel syndrome. *J Pediatr.* 1997;131(3):356-361

3. Andorsky DJ, Lund DP, Lillehei CW, et al. Nutritional and other postoperative management of neonates with short bowel syndrome correlates with clinical outcomes. *J Pediatr*. 2001;139(1):27-33

4. Kurkchubasche AG, Rowe MI, Smith SD. Adaptation in short-bowel syndrome: Reassessing old limits. *J Pediatr Surg*. 1993;28(8):1069-1071

5. Goulet O, Baglin-Gobet S, Talbotec C, et al. Outcome and long-term growth after extensive small bowel resection in the neonatal period: A survey of 87 children. *Eur J Pediatr Surg*. 2005;15(2):95-101

6. Goulet O, Ruemmele F, Lacaille F, Colomb V. Irreversible intestinal failure. *J Pediatr Gastroenterol Nutr*. 2004;38(3):250-269

7. Quiros-Tejeira RE, Ament ME, Reyen L, et al. Long-term parenteral nutritional support and intestinal adaptation in children with short bowel syndrome: a 25-year experience. *J Pediatr*. 2004;145(2):157-163

8. Cowles RA, Ventura KA, Martinez M, et al. Reversal of intestinal failure-associated liver disease in infants and children on parenteral nutrition: Experience with 93 patients at a referral center for intestinal rehabilitation. *J Pediatr Surg*. 2010;45(1):84-87

9. Javid PJ, Malone FR, Reyes J, Healey PJ, Horslen SP. The experience of a regional pediatric intestinal failure program: Successful outcomes from intestinal rehabilitation. *Am J Surg*. 2010;199(5):676-679

10. Modi BP, Langer M, Ching YA, et al. Improved survival in a multidisciplinary short bowel syndrome program. *J Pediatr Surg*. 2008;43(1):20-24

11. Nucci A, Burns RC, Armah T, et al. Interdisciplinary management of pediatric intestinal failure: A 10-year review of rehabilitation and transplantation. *J Gastrointest Surg*. 2008;12(3):429-435

12. Dowling RH, Booth CC. Structural and functional changes following small intestinal resection in the rat. *Clin Sci*. 1967;32(1):139-149

13. Hanson WR, Osborne JW, Sharp JG. Compensation by the residual intestine after intestinal resection in the rat. II. influence of postoperative time interval. *Gastroenterology*. 1977;72(4 Pt 1):701-705

14. Sacks AI, Warwick GJ, Barnard JA. Early proliferative events following intestinal resection in the rat. *J Pediatr Gastroenterol Nutr*. 1995;21(2):158-164

15. Williamson RC. Intestinal adaptation (first of two parts). structural, functional and cytokinetic changes. *N Engl J Med*. 1978;298(25):1393-1402

16. Siebert JR. Small-intestine length in infants and children. *Am J Dis Child*. 1980;134(6):593-595

17. Weaver LT, Austin S, Cole TJ. Small intestinal length: a factor essential for gut adaptation. *Gut*. 1991;32(11):1321-1323

18. Touloukian RJ, Smith GJ. Normal intestinal length in preterm infants. *J Pediatr Surg*. 1983;18(6):720-723

19. DiBaise JK, Young RJ, Vanderhoof JA. Intestinal rehabilitation and the short bowel syndrome: part 1. *Am J Gastroenterol*. 2004;99(7):1386-1395

20. Weser E, Babbitt J, Hoban M, Vandeventer A. Intestinal adaptation. different growth responses to disaccharides compared with monosaccharides in rat small bowel. *Gastroenterology*. 1986;91(6):1521-1527

21. Vanderhoof JA, Grandjean CJ, Burkley KT, Antonson DL. Effect of casein versus casein hydrolysate on mucosal adaptation following massive bowel resection in infant rats. *J Pediatr Gastroenterol Nutr*. 1984;3(2):262-267

22. Weser E, Babbitt J, Hoban M, Vandeventer A. Intestinal adaptation. different growth responses to disaccharides compared with monosaccharides in rat small bowel. *Gastroenterology*. 1986;91(6):1521-1527

23. Clarke RM. "Luminal nutrition" versus "functional work-load" as controllers of mucosal morphology and epithelial replacement in the rat small intestine. *Digestion*. 1977;15(5):411-424

24. Bines J, Francis D, Hill D. Reducing parenteral requirement in children with short bowel syndrome: Impact of an amino acid-based complete infant formula. *J Pediatr Gastroenterol Nutr*. 1998;26(2):123-128

25. Malarese LE, O'Keefe SI, Kandil HM, Bond G, Costa G, Abu-Elmagd K. Short bowel syndrome: Clinical guidelines for nutrition management. *Nutr Clin Pract*. 2005;20(5):493-502

26. Musch MW, Bookstein C, Xie Y, Sellin JH, Chang EB. SCFA increase intestinal na absorption by induction of NHE3 in rat colon and human intestinal C2/bbe cells. *Am J Physiol Gastrointest Liver Physiol*. 2001;280(4):G687-G693

27. Drucker DJ, Erlich P, Asa SL, Brubaker PL. Induction of intestinal epithelial proliferation by glucagon-like peptide 2. *Proc Natl Acad Sci U S A*. 1996;93(15):7911-7916

28. Jeppesen PB, Gilroy R, Pertkiewicz M, Allard JP, Messing B, O'Keefe SJ. Randomised placebo-controlled trial of teduglutide in reducing parenteral nutrition and/or intravenous fluid requirements in patients with short bowel syndrome. *Gut*. 2011

29. Thompson JS, Pinch LW, Young R, Vanderhoof JA. Long-term outcome of intestinal lengthening. *Transplant Proc*. 2000;32(6):1242-1243

30. Kim HB, Fauza D, Garza J, Oh JT, Nurko S, Jaksic T. Serial transverse enteroplasty (STEP): A novel bowel lengthening procedure. *J Pediatr Surg*. 2003;38(3):425-429

31. Ching YA, Fitzgibbons S, Valim C, et al. Long-term nutritional and clinical outcomes after serial transverse enteroplasty at a single institution. *J Pediatr Surg*. 2009;44(5):939-943

32. Oliveira C, Nasr A, Brindle M, Wales PW. Ethanol Locks to Prevent Catheter-Related Bloodstream Infections in Parenteral Nutrition: A Meta-Analysis. *Pediatrics*. 2012;129(2):318-329

33. Wong T, Clifford V, McCallum Z, Shalley H, Peterkin M, Paxton G, Bines JE. Central venous catheter thrombosis associated with 70% ethanol locks in pediatric intestinal failure patients on home parenteral nutrition: a case series. *J Parenter Enteral Nutr*. 2011; Epub ahead of print

34. Buchman A. Total parenteral nutrition-associated liver disease. *JPEN J Parenter Enteral Nutr*. 2002;26(5 Suppl):S43-S48

35. Btaiche IF, Khalidi N. Parenteral nutrition-associated liver complications in children. *Pharmacotherapy*. 2002;22(2):188-211

VI

36. Beath SV, Davies P, Papadopoulou A, et al. Parenteral nutrition-related cholestasis in postsurgical neonates: multivariate analysis of risk factors. *J Pediatr Surg.* 1996;31(4):604-606

37. Colomb V, Jobert-Giraud A, Lacaille F, Goulet O, Fournet JC, Ricour C. Role of lipid emulsions in cholestasis associated with long-term parenteral nutrition in children. *JPEN J Parenter Enteral Nutr.* 2000;24(6):345-350

38. Greenberg GR, Wolman SL, Christofides ND, Bloom SR, Jeejeebhoy KN. Effect of total parenteral nutrition on gut hormone release in humans. *Gastroenterology.* 1981;80(5 Pt 1):988-993

39. Cooper A, Ross AJ III, O'Neill JA Jr, Bishop HC, Templeton JM Jr, Ziegler MM. Resolution of intractable cholestasis associated with total parenteral nutrition following biliary irrigation. *J Pediatr Surg.* 1985;20(6):772-774

40. Kubota A, Yonekura T, Hoki M, et al. Total parenteral nutrition-associated intrahepatic cholestasis in infants: 25 years' experience. *J Pediatr Surg.* 2000;35(7):1049-1051

41. Gura KM, Lee S, Valim C, et al. Safety and efficacy of a fish-oil-based fat emulsion in the treatment of parenteral nutrition-associated liver disease. *Pediatrics.* 2008;121(3):e678-e686

Chapter 48

Nutrition in Cystic Fibrosis

Introduction

Cystic fibrosis (CF) is a life-shortening, autosomal-recessive disorder that affects the sweat glands and digestive, respiratory, and reproductive systems. It is caused by mutations in the cystic fibrosis transmembrane conductance regulator (CFTR) gene, a 250 kb gene found on the long arm of chromosome 7 that encodes a chloride transport protein.[1,2] More than 1800 mutations of the CFTR gene have been reported (http://www.genet.sickkids.on.ca/cftr/app), and more are still being found; however, most occur infrequently, and approximately 10% are common enough to be well characterized (http://www.cftr2.org). Among these gene mutations, some are disease causing, some are sequence variations that do not cause CF, some are associated with single or milder organ system involvement than typically seen in CF (sometimes called "CFTR-associated disorders" or "CFTR-related metabolic syndrome"), and some have variable or unknown consequences.[3-6] The most common is the first mutation discovered, F508del, which is a 3 base pair deletion at codon 508 that leads to loss of a phenylalanine residue that, in turn, causes a protein-folding defect and a failure in processing through the cytoplasm to the epithelial surface of affected cells.[1] Approximately half of patients with CF are homozygous for F508del, and nearly 40% more have at least 1 such mutation; however, in the latter circumstance, it is the second mutation that determines genotype-phenotype implications.[4,7]

The most dramatic onset of CF is in newborn infants with intestinal obstruction caused by blockage of the terminal ileum with dehydrated meconium. This is known as meconium ileus and occurs in approximately 20% patients with CF.[8] Subsequently, among CF-affected individuals with meconium ileus, 85% to 90% will develop pancreatic exocrine insufficiency, which may be present at diagnosis or develop over the first year of life.[9] The strongest relation between the genotype and the phenotype is observed in the exocrine pancreas.[2,4,7] The majority of patients with CF have evidence of pancreatic insufficiency (PI), and most patients with the PI phenotype present with signs and symptoms of malabsorption and/or failure to thrive at an early age. A subset of patients have evidence of pancreatic dysfunction but retain sufficient residual pancreatic function to permit considerable digestion without the need for exogenous pancreatic enzyme supplements with meals. The term pancreatic sufficiency (PS) is used to describe patients with this phenotype

VI

who tend to have a milder form of CF disease.[2] Analyses of large patient cohorts have revealed that different mutations in the CFTR gene confer either the PI or the PS phenotypes.[2,4]

The lungs of infants with CF are structurally and functionally normal at birth,[10] but there is often evidence of airway obstruction and structural changes within the first few months of life.[11,12] The lungs of patients with CF are highly susceptible to infection, especially with the gram-negative bacterium *Pseudomonas aeruginosa*.[13] Intermittent, then chronic, pulmonary infection occurs over the course of months to years, leading to bronchiectasis and, ultimately, respiratory failure. Infection increases caloric requirements because of the increased work of breathing and ultimately causes premature death in 90% of affected individuals.[14]

Diagnosis

Individuals with suspected CF are identified for diagnostic evaluation after newborn screening or recognition of a positive family history or following the development of the characteristic signs and symptoms, such as steatorrhea or chronic cough. Diagnosis then may be made through various approaches, depending on age and phenotype, but ultimately, the sweat chloride test is the key to diagnosis and should be used according to published diagnostic criteria.[5]

Diagnosis Through Newborn Screening

Most cases of CF in children are now diagnosed through newborn screening, because the diagnosis is often delayed in traditional pediatric practice, despite early signs/symptoms. Newborn screening programs are organized, population-based public health services applying preventive medicine in defined regions to reduce morbidity and mortality from certain genetic disorders.[15] Newborn screening is performed by presymptomatic detection of risk using dried blood specimens from newborn infants analyzed in central laboratories that are linked to clinical follow-up programs for diagnosis (ie, a sweat chloride test) and rapid institution of specialized therapies. Newborn screening involves a system of care that includes education, screening, follow-up, diagnosis, management, evaluation, and quality assurance (http://mchb.hrsa.gov/screening).

The use of newborn screening for CF is based on initial detection of elevated immunoreactive trypsinogen (IRT) levels, which provides an opportunity for presymptomatic detection on a routine basis, before irreversible pathologic abnormality develops.[10] After the IRT test was developed in 1979 by Crossley et al,[16] it was first investigated systematically in Australia,[17] where its validity was established with a strategy that involved an initial IRT test during the first few days of life and then a repeat IRT at approximately 2 weeks of age to demonstrate persistent hypertrypsinogenemia; this became known as the IRT/IRT algorithm. However, it was obvious that false-negative test results could occur.

When it was recognized that the IRT test alone is not adequate to screen for CF,[18] investigators in Wisconsin took advantage of the discovery of the CFTR gene and its principal CF-causing mutation, F508del, to develop a 2-tiered strategy of newborn screening.[19] More specifically, because of concerns regarding suboptimal screening sensitivity of the initial high IRT cutoff and observations that the second specimens of some patients with CF showed precipitous decreases in IRT,[18] the IRT/DNA-F508del method was developed[19] to incorporate a lower IRT cutoff and a strategy that quickly applied the discovery of the F508del allele.[1] It was found that in the newborn infant, DNA analysis can be performed on small samples, including dried blood samples from Guthrie cards.[19] Moreover, the sensitivity could be improved to 97% or greater and the diagnosis could be expedited, because the IRT/DNA method can be accomplished with the initial dried blood specimen within a week of birth.[19] Subsequently, this strategy was transformed into an IRT/DNA-CFTR multimutation test involving DNA analysis for 23 to 40 CFTR mutations.[20]

After benefits, particularly nutritional advantages,[21-23] were demonstrated that outweighed the risks, the Centers for Disease Control and Prevention (CDC) recommended universal screening for CF.[24] Currently, approximately 90% of newborn infants in the United States are screened by the IRT/DNA-CFTR strategy.[25] The number of mutations in use by different states, however, varies widely,[26] because national guidelines have only recently been published,[27] and very few data have been published on what CFTR alleles are needed for specific populations.[28] The national guideline of the Clinical and Laboratory Standards Institute[29] is based on recommendations by the American College of Medical Genetics (ACMG)[25] and states the following: "The ACMG 23-mutation panel provides a high degree of sensitivity in many newborn populations and… contains only known disease-causing mutations. Therefore, it is recommended that the ACMG-23 mutations be used in IRT/DNA screening methods as the core and preferred CFTR panel. This multi-mutation panel provides advantages over simply analyzing for the F508del mutation. In addition, this panel includes the common mutations found in the United States and, when applied to NBS, appears to be satisfactory for typical newborn populations. If special circumstances such as a significant population of minorities susceptible to CF exist in a regional CF NBS program, it is recommended that other mutations beyond the ACMG-23 list be added to the CFTR panel based on compelling data."

When the CF newborn screening result is positive, follow-up evaluation is performed using the sweat chloride test. The sweat test involves collection of sweat after pilocarpine iontophoresis to stimulate sweating followed by chemical determination of the chloride concentration.[30] An elevated result provides physiological evidence of the CFTR defect. Standards for sweat chloride testing have been published,[30] although performing sweat chloride tests in newborn infants presents unique challenges. The procedure must be carried out meticulously to avoid errors, which frequently contribute to misleading values.

Overview of Therapy

Without therapeutic interventions, CF is usually fatal within the first decade of life. Current treatment is multifaceted and requires close monitoring by an expert multidisciplinary care team. This care should include regular evaluation, counseling, and intervention by expert physicians, nurses, dietitians, respiratory and/or physical therapists, and social workers. Genetic counselors, psychologists, and exercise physiologists are also important resources. A key goal is to support nutrition to promote normal growth and development. In addition, high priority should be given to effective disease education so that the family can understand and be equipped to manage this complex chronic disorder.

Guidelines for nutritional management for patients with CF have been established by the US Cystic Fibrosis Foundation since 1992[31] and were revised in 2002[32] and 2008[33] to incorporate more evidence-based recommendations. Guidelines for lung disease therapy are also available.[34-36] Most recently, guidelines for the care of infants whose CF was diagnosed early through newborn screening were published in 2009[37]; key components of early care are summarized in Table 48.1. The core objectives of CF treatment after early diagnosis through newborn screening are to prevent malnutrition, control respiratory infections, and promote mucus clearance.[37]

Table 48.1.
Important Aspects of Early Care for Newly Diagnosed Infants and Young Children With CF

Pancreatic enzyme replacement therapy (for pancreatic insufficiency)
High-calorie and high-fat diet (after human milk)
Fat-soluble vitamin supplementation (vitamins A, D, E, and K)
Salt supplements (essential to prevent fatalities)
Infection control (prevent all risky exposures)
Respiratory cultures (by vigorous oropharyngeal technique)
Antibiotic therapy as needed (goal: eradicate pseudomonas)
Airway clearance teaching and recommendations
CF education with genetic counseling (CFTR genotype)
Lifestyle counseling (promote normal/quality life)

Adapted from Borowitz et al.[37]

Nutritional Care

Goals

The goal of nutritional care in children with CF is to achieve normal growth and optimize nutritional status. Major interventions include: (1) pancreatic enzyme replacement therapy (PERT) to reduce malabsorption caused by PI; (2) a high-energy, nutrient-dense diet to compensate for fecal nutrient losses, increased energy requirement, and decreased dietary intake associated with gastrointestinal and respiratory tract complications (reduced intake is commonly reported in patients with CF who have gastroesophageal reflux disease [GERD], distal intestinal obstruction syndrome [see "Evaluation of Comorbid Medical Conditions"], and pulmonary exacerbations); and (3) vitamin/mineral supplementation to prevent micronutrient deficiencies.

Nutritional Requirements

Energy and Macronutrients

Patients with CF are at high risk of energy deficiency as a result of their increased requirement and decreased consumption. The consequence of energy deficiency leads to impaired growth in children with CF. Weight retardation and linear growth failure are common observations documented in the CF literature.[38-40] Malnutrition is particularly prevalent during times of rapid growth (ie, infancy and adolescence) as well as in patients prior to diagnosis of CF.[39,40]

Energy requirements for individual patients with CF can be estimated on the basis of predicted basal metabolic rate,[41] the degree of malabsorption, and the severity of pulmonary disease, as illustrated in Table 48.2.[32] According to this method,[32] energy requirements increase by 5% to 10% in CF children with mild CF to 20% to 50% in those with moderate-to-severe CF.

VI

Table 48.2.

Method for Estimating Energy Requirement for Patients with CF

Step I: Estimate basal metabolic rate (BMR) by using the WHO equations[41]		
	Males	**Females**
0-3 y	60.9 × wt − 54	61.0 × wt − 51
3-10 y	22.7 × wt + 495	22.5 × wt + 499
10-18 y	17.5 × wt + 651	12.2 × wt + 476
18-30 y	15.3 × wt + 679	14.7 × wt + 496
>30 y	11.6 × wt + 879	8.7 × wt + 829

Step II: Estimate energy expenditure (EE) using the following equation:
EE = BMR x (activity coefficient + disease coefficient)
    activity coefficient = 1.3 (confine to bed)
        1.5 (sedentary)
        1.7 (active)
    disease coefficient = 0 (normal lung function, ie, FEV_1 >80%)
        0.2 (moderate lung disease, ie, FEV_1 40%-79%)
        0.3 (severe lung disease, ie, FEV_1 <40%)

Step III: Estimate total energy requirement (ER), taking into account pancreatic functional status
  a. For PS patients, ie, coefficient of fat absorption (CFA) ≥93%
    ER = EE
  b. For PI patients with a CFA <93%
    ER = EE x (0.93 ÷ CFA)
  c. For PI patients whose CFA has not been determined, use 0.85 as an approximate for CFA
    ER = EE x (0.93 ÷ 0.85)

Adapted from Borowitz et al.[32]

WHO indicates World Health Organization; FEV, forced expiratory volume in 1 second.

To obtain adequate energy intake and compensate for fat malabsorption, patients with CF typically require a greater fat intake, 35% to 40% of calories,[32] than what is normally recommended for the general population (20%-35%).[42] Because fat is the most energy-dense macronutrient, fat restriction is not recommended as a mean to alleviate symptoms of malabsorption. Instead, a high-fat diet combined with adequate PERT (see "Pancreatic Enzyme Replacement Therapy" below) should be prescribed. Although not a common practice, medium-chain triglycerides (MCTs) may be used as a source of fat, because they require less lipase activity and bile salts for digestion and can be directly absorbed into the portal circulation.

With regard to macronutrients, protein poses less of a problem than does fat in the CF population. Low concentrations of serum proteins (eg, albumin, prealbumin, and retinol-binding protein), are commonly found in infants at the time of diagnosis of CF. One third to one half of infants with CF diagnosed through newborn screening programs were reported to be hypoalbuminemic.[8,43,44] Normalization of serum albumin concentration often occurs following comprehensive nutrition therapy.[45] The major risk of protein deficiency in patients with CF occurs during the first year of life, when the average requirement is at least 3 times as great as that in adulthood.[46] Infants with CF who are predominantly breastfed should be monitored closely, because human milk contains relatively low concentrations of protein, and these infants are especially prone to protein deficiency.

Essential Fatty Acids

Essential fatty acid deficiency (EFAD) has been known for decades to occur in patients with CF.[8,47-52] In patients who are adequately treated, clinical evidence of EFAD is rare, although biochemical abnormalities of essential fatty acids remain common.[50-52] The major fatty acid abnormalities found in patients with CF are low serum concentrations of linoleic (18:2, omega-6) and docosahexaenoic (22:6, omega-3) acids, normal or mildly decreased concentrations of arachidonic acid (20:4, omega-6), and elevated concentrations of palmitoleic, oleic (18:1, omega-9) and eicosatrienoic (20:3, omega-9) acids. In EFAD, oleic acid is converted to eicosatrienoic acid, which is commonly referred to as the "pathologic triene," because its increase in EFAD coupled with the usual decrease in arachidonic acid leads to a high triene-to-tetraene ratio.[45,51,52] A net energy deficit secondary to PI and increased energy requirements is the most common cause of EFAD in patients with CF. However, a primary metabolic defect in fatty acid metabolism has also been postulated.[51,53]

It has been demonstrated conclusively that linoleic acid deficiency associated with impaired growth[52,54,55] is manifested by abnormal serum fatty acid profiles early in infancy,[45] potentially affecting approximately 90% of patients with CF with PI.[9] Most importantly, recent studies demonstrated that achieving normal growth in the first 2 years of life depends not only on sufficient energy intake but also normal essential fatty acid status.[55]

Despite the above evidence, essential fatty acid supplementation for patients with CF remains controversial for 2 reasons. First, not all patients respond to oral supplementation, and normalizing plasma linoleic acid concentration is particularly difficult in patients with CF with meconium ileus.[8,48] Second, omega-6 fatty acids, including linoleic acid and its metabolite arachidonic acid, have been proposed to play a role in CF inflammation.[56-60] In the 2009 Cystic Fibrosis Foundation infant care guidelines,[37] clinical trials to "answer questions related to essential fatty acid supplementation in infants" are recommended as a research priority to resolve this long overdue controversy.

VI

Fat-Soluble Vitamins

Deficiencies of fat-soluble vitamins in untreated CF are highly prevalent.[8,43,59-65] Studies of infants with CF diagnosed through newborn screening revealed that 20% to 40% had low serum retinol, 35% had low serum 25-hydroxyvitamin D (25-OH-D), and 40% to 70% had low serum alpha-tocopherol[8,43,64] concentrations.

Vitamin A deficiency was the first micronutrient deficit demonstrated in patients with CF. Vitamin D insufficiency is increasingly reported in both children and adults with CF[65-68] and is directly linked to poor bone mineralization.[66] Vitamin E deficiency can lead to hemolytic anemia.[62] In addition, early, prolonged vitamin E deficiency has been shown to be associated with cognitive dysfunction later in life.[69]

Vitamin K deficiency has not been routinely demonstrated in patients with CF; those with severe cholestatic liver disease, short-bowel syndrome, and lung disease requiring frequent antibiotic use are at greater risks of vitamin K deficiency.[63,70,71] Low concentrations of vitamin K are also seen in patients with CF not taking appropriate vitamin supplementation. Vitamin K status can be evaluated by prothrombin time or the more sensitive PIVKA (proteins induced in vitamin K absence) measurement.

In patients with CF, vitamin supplementation is necessary to prevent deficiencies. A standard, age-appropriate multivitamin supplement should be given to all patients with CF. Additional supplementation with fat-soluble vitamins is needed; recommended doses[32,37] are summarized in Table 48.3. If blood concentrations of vitamins A, D, and E are low despite supplementation, it is important to evaluate patient adherence to and timing of recommended vitamin intakes. Fat-soluble vitamins are absorbed most effectively when taken with fat-containing meals and pancreatic enzymes.

Table 48.3.
Fat-Soluble Vitamin Supplementation for Children With CF

Age	Vitamin A (IU)	Vitamin E (IU)	Vitamin D (IU)	Vitamin K (mg)[a]
0-12 mo	1500	40-50	400	0.3-0.5
1-3 y	5000	80-150	600-800[b]	0.3-0.5
4-8 y	5000–10 000	100-200	600-800[b]	0.3-0.5
>8 y	10 000	200-400	600-800[b]	0.3-0.5

Adapted from Borowitz et al[32] and Borowitz et al.[37]

[a] Currently, commercially available products do not have ideal doses for supplementation. Prothrombin time or, ideally, PIVKA-II levels should be checked in patients with liver disease, and vitamin K dose should be titrated as indicated.

[b] New recommendation from Institute of Medicine, Food and Nutrition Board. *Dietary Reference Intakes for Calcium and Vitamin D.* Washington, DC: The National Academies Press; 2011.

Minerals and Electrolytes

For patients with CF, sodium is of great concern, because they lose large amounts of sodium in their sweat; salt depletion can be catastrophic, leading to severe hyponatremic dehydration and shock.[72] In addition, there has been concern that marginal or low body sodium may limit the growth of children with CF.[73] Young infants with CF are particularly at risk of hyponatremia, hypochloremic dehydration with metabolic alkalosis, irritability, and lethargy. Therefore, electrolyte status should be evaluated if there is any suspicion of electrolyte depletion, such as exposure to high environmental temperatures, overbundling, or excessive sweating. Serum sodium concentrations do not accurately reflect total body sodium; urinary sodium in relation to creatinine is a better indicator of sodium status in infants.

Because of increased risk of hyponatremia, infants with CF should receive salt supplementation. Current guidelines recommend a daily dose of 1/8 teaspoon of table salt, which contains 12.5 mEq of sodium, for infants younger than 6 months.[37] For infants 6 to 12 months of age, ¼ teaspoon per day, but not to exceed 4 mEq/kg/day, was recommended.[37] In older children and adolescents with CF, routine sodium supplementation may not be necessary,[32] because the average American diet contains an overabundance of sodium.[42] However, sodium supplements are required in conditions that may cause prolonged sweat loss.

Low calcium intake and suboptimal bone density accrual are of concerns even in the general pediatric population.[74] Children with CF have a higher risk of bone demineralization because of malabsorption of nutrients needed for bone health (eg, calcium, vitamins D and K), reduced physical activity, increased periods of bed rest in association with pulmonary exacerbations, pulmonary inflammation with increased inflammatory cytokines, and use of medications, such as glucocorticoid therapy.[67] The relative contributions of these factors to the development of bone disease in patients with CF remain to be elucidated. Few data are available regarding calcium supplementation in improving bone health in the CF population. A recent double-blind, cross-over, randomized trial with 15 children with CF 7 to 13 years of age demonstrated that supplementation with calcium (1000 mg), vitamin D_3 (2000 IU), or both for 6 months did not change serum calcium and 25-OH-D concentrations and bone mineral gain, compared with the control group (400 IU of vitamin D_3).[75]

Studies with stable isotopes have reported increased fecal zinc losses and decreased zinc absorption in infants and children with CF.[76,77] Zinc deficiency affects growth and vitamin A status but is difficult to diagnose, because serum zinc concentration is not an adequate measure of zinc status. Therefore, current Cystic Fibrosis Foundation guidelines recommend a trial of zinc supplementation, 1 mg/

VI

kg/day of elemental zinc for 6 months, for children with CF experiencing poor growth despite adequate caloric intake and pancreatic enzyme supplementation.[32,37]

Anemia in patients with CF has been reported with varying prevalence as high as 33%, with iron deficiency proposed to be the main cause.[78] Chronic lung inflammation may also alter iron metabolism. Patients with CF with advanced pulmonary disease have been shown to have low serum ferritin concentrations.[78,79] In the general pediatric population, the importance of diagnosis and prevention of iron deficiency has been emphasized recently, stemming from new evidence showing the adverse, long-term, and irreversible effect on neurodevelopment and behavior caused by iron deficiency.[80] In children with CF, chronic lung inflammation poses additional risk of iron deficiency and anemia. In the setting of chronic inflammation, serum transferrin receptor concentrations are a more sensitive indicator of iron status than serum ferritin, because the latter is an acute phase reactant.

Nutritional Assessment and Monitoring

Frequent assessment and monitoring of nutritional status for patients with CF are essential to ensure early detection of any deterioration and prompt initiation of intervention. Patients with CF are most vulnerable to malnutrition with delayed diagnosis, during times of rapid growth (ie, infancy and adolescence), and during pulmonary exacerbations. It should be emphasized that with comprehensive nutritional assessment and intervention, infants with CF diagnosed early through newborn screening can achieve normal growth throughout childhood.[26,27] Most importantly, optimizing growth and nutritional status is critical for children with CF, because malnutrition worsens lung disease and reduces survival.[38,81]

Assessment of nutritional status for children with CF must include anthropometric, biochemical, clinical, and dietary assessments. Current recommendations for these assessments[32,37] are summarized in Table 48.4.

Anthropometric Assessment
Anthropometric assessment, with an emphasis on physical growth, is the most important component of nutritional assessment in children with CF. Accurate and sequential measurements of head circumference (0-3 years), recumbent length (0-2 years), height (2-20 years), weight (0-20 years), weight for length (0-2 years), and body mass index (BMI [2-20 years]) should be obtained at each clinic visit using standardized techniques. These measurements should be plotted on the 2000 CDC growth charts[82] and/or the 2009 World Health Organization growth charts (0-2 years)[83] to determine sex- and age-specific percentiles.

According to recommendations from the Cystic Fibrosis Foundation, children with CF should aim at maintaining weight-for-length (age 0-2 years) and BMI percentiles (age 2 years and older) above the 50th percentile to support better lung function.[33,37] With regard to linear growth, in addition to determining height-for-age percentile, it is important to evaluate whether the child's height is reaching his or her genetic potential. This can be estimated by using parental heights to calculate a target height range or an adjusted height percentile.[32,84] A child with CF whose height is below his or her genetic potential is considered at risk and should be evaluated.[32,85]

In addition to weight and length/height percentiles, weight gain and length/height velocity are more sensitive indicators of growth and should be evaluated when growth faltering is observed.[32,37] Other anthropometric assessments, such as measurements of skinfold thickness (eg, mid-upper arm circumference, triceps skinfold thickness, etc) provide additional information on body composition (ie, lean body mass and subcutaneous fat stores). However, skinfold thickness measurements are prone to measurement errors, and reference standards are not available for all ages of children.

Biochemical Assessment

Monitoring biochemical indices of nutritional status is essential in patients with CF. Current guidelines,[32,37] summarized in Table 48.4, recommend routine measurements of serum protein (albumin), vitamin A (retinol), vitamin D (25-OH-D) and vitamin E (alpha-tocopherol) concentrations. With regard to iron, the 2002 guidelines[32] have not been updated and only recommended measurement of hemoglobin and hematocrit to detect anemia.

Assessment of essential fatty acids is not routinely performed but only as indicated (eg, in children with CF experiencing failure to thrive).[32] However, recent findings on the relationships between abnormal essential fatty acid status and growth in children with CF[52,55] warrant the consideration of routine monitoring of essential fatty acid status in infants and young children with CF (Table 48.4). Similarly, routine measurements of vitamin K, calcium, zinc, and sodium concentrations are not regarded as necessary according to current guidelines[32,37] but may be needed in individual patients, as explained in Table 48.4.

Clinical Assessment

Clinical assessment of nutritional status in children with CF focuses on evaluation of the severity of maldigestion and malabsorption caused by PI. The clinical signs and symptoms of PI include abdominal discomfort (bloating, flatus, pain), steatorrhea (frequent, malodorous, greasy stools), and the presence of meconium ileus, constipation, or distal intestinal obstruction syndrome (DIOS).

PI should be identified by assessing exocrine pancreatic functional status.[86] Objective tests include (1) duodenal measurement of pancreatic enzymes and bicarbonate; (2) 72-hour fecal fat balance study; and (3) fecal elastase-1 in spot

Table 48.4.
Nutritional Assessment and Monitoring in Children With CF^a

Age at Visit	At Diagnosis	Early Infancy (0-6 mo)					Late Infancy (7-12 mo)			Second year of life		Age 2-20 y	
	1 mo	2 mo	3 mo	4 mo	5 mo	6 mo	8 mo	10 mo	12 mo	Every 2-3 mo	24 mo	Every 3 mo	Annually
Anthropometric assessment													
Weight, length/height	x^a	x	x	x	x	x	x	x	x	x	x	x	
Head circumference (up to age 3 y)	x	x	x	x	x	x	x	x	x	x	x		
Body mass index (ages >2 y)												x	
Skinfold measures													x
Pubertal status (Tanner stages)													x^b
Biochemical assessment													
Complete blood cell count		x					x		x				
Albumin		x					x		x				
Essential fatty acids (EFAs)^c		x					x		x				

Vitamins A, D, and E		X				X			X		
Vitamin K[d], zinc,[e] and sodium[f]											
Calcium and bone status[g]											
Clinical assessment											
Pancreatic functional status	X										
Dietary assessment											
Energy and nutrient intake[h]		X	X	X	X	X	X	X	X	X	X
Feeding/eating behavior				X		X				X	

[a] Recommended in the 2002 (32) and/or 2009 (37) Cystic Fibrosis Foundation guidelines, except where indicated.

[b] Starting at age 9 years for girls and 10 years for boys until sexual maturation completes; by self-assessment (patient, or parent and patient) or physician assessment using Tanner stage system (118, 119); annual question as to menarchal status for girls.

[c] The 2002 guidelines recommended checking EFA status on in children with failure to thrive (32). On the basis of abundant literature (see text) and recent new findings (55), routine monitoring of EFA status in young infants and at age 1 year and 2 years is recommended.

[d] In patients with liver disease or if patient has hemoptysis or hematemesis (32); recommended tests include PIVKA-II (preferred) or prothrombin time.

[e] In children with poor growth despite adequate caloric intake and pancreatic enzyme replacement therapy (32, 37); no recommended test, because serum zinc concentration does not reflect zinc sufficiency; instead, a trial of zinc supplementation should be given (see text).

[f] In patients exposed to heat stress who become dehydrated; recommended tests include serum sodium and spot urine sodium (32).

[g] In patients >8 years of age if risk factors are present (see text); recommended tests include serum calcium, phosphorus, ionized parathyroid hormone, and dual-energy x-ray absorptiometry.

[h] A review of enzymes, vitamins, minerals, oral or enteral formulas, herbal or botanical products, and other complementary and alternative medicine.

stool samples. Among these, the 72-hour fecal fat balance study has been the gold standard, which yields a quantitative measure of fat absorption that is used not only to define PI but also as an estimate of energy requirement (Table 48.2). However, 72-hour fecal fat balance study is cumbersome and not well accepted by patients with CF and care providers. Measurement of fecal elastase-1 in a small random stool sample has become the preferred method to assess PI in most CF centers.[86,87] Elastase-1 is one of many enzymes secreted by the pancreas and appears directly related to pancreatic acinar function.[86] Unlike other enzymes that may be degraded by intraluminal proteases, elastase-1 has the physical property of being stable as it transits the intestinal tract. As water is withdrawn from the intestinal contents in the colon, elastase-1 concentration increases, making it easy to measure in stool. In addition, elastase-1 is stable through a wide range of pH and temperatures, making it ideal to collect at home. Fecal elastase-1 can be performed with an enzyme-linked immunosorbent assay.[86,87] Values less than 100 µg/g of stool are indicative of PI; values greater than 200 µg/g of stool are consistent with PS.[86,87]

Dietary Assessment

Assessments of energy requirements and dietary intake are important ways of determining whether the patient is in negative energy balance. Evaluation of dietary intake is best performed by dietitians specializing in the care of patients with CF. For patients with good nutritional status, the dietitian may assess dietary habits and the quality of dietary intake using a 24-hour dietary recall. However, for patients with suboptimal nutritional status, a 3- to 7-day prospective food record is the best way to obtain quantitative estimates of energy and nutrient intakes. This assessment can then be used as the basis for initiating appropriate nutritional intervention.

Patient and Parent Education

Education of patients and their caregivers is a vital and routine component of the multidisciplinary care of patients with CF.[32,37] A solid grounding in the special nutritional needs of a patient with CF should be established at diagnosis. This should include an explanation of the role of the pancreas and how enzyme replacement therapy helps to improve maldigestion. Parents should be given specific instructions on how to provide an appetizing, high-energy, nutritionally balanced diet, particularly with a liberal use of fat to provide extra calories. It is important to communicate the expectation that most children with CF are able to grow and gain weight normally. Patients and their parents require education about the importance of fat-soluble vitamins. Details on when to administer enzymes and vitamins must be reviewed on several occasions. For older children, the pediatrician should ensure that there is adequate understanding of the nature of the disease process, and concerns about adherence should be emphasized and assessed at each follow-up visit.

Specific Guidelines for Nutritional Management

Diagnosis and Treatment of Malabsorption

Diagnosis of Pancreatic Insufficiency

Exocrine pancreatic function should be assessed in the following situations: (1) at or shortly after diagnosis to provide objective evaluation of pancreatic status before enzyme therapy is initiated; and (2) to monitor patients with PS for evidence of developing fat maldigestion, particularly when frequent bulky bowel movements or unexplained weight loss occur. The preferred test for assessment of pancreatic functional status is fecal elastase-1 concentration, as described previously. Fecal elastase-1 concentration is not diagnostic by itself but aids in defining PS (>200 µg/g) or PI (<100 µg/g). This test does not quantitate the degree of malabsorption.

Pancreatic Enzyme Replacement Therapy

There is a strong association between genotype and pancreatic phenotype.[2,4,7] PERT should be started if the patient is known to have 2 CFTR mutations associated with PI or objective evidence of PI.[37] PERT should not be started in infants with a CFTR mutation known to be associated with PS, unless there are unequivocal signs or symptoms of malabsorption.[37]

In some infants with CF diagnosed through newborn screening, PI is not present at the time of diagnosis but develops later in infancy or even early childhood.[9] Therefore, it is important to repeat fecal elastase-1 measurement in infants who initially have PS, especially when gastrointestinal tract symptoms appear or poor weight gain occurs. Children with CF who have laboratory evidence of PI should be started on PERT, even in the absence of signs or symptoms of fat malabsorption.

Pancreatic enzymes are extracts of porcine origin containing amylase, proteases, and lipase. A large variety of enzyme products have been available. However, many were marketed without formal testing. In 2004, the US Food and Drug Administration (FDA) issued a notice requiring that manufacturers submit a new drug application for pancreatic enzyme products. As of 2010, there were 3 FDA-approved products. The activity of these enzymes varies considerably according to specific batches and the commercial manufacturer. Enzyme potency is based on the content of amylase, protease, and lipase in each capsule. However, many caregivers use lipase content to determine enzyme dosing to treat fat maldigestion. Commercial products are sold in capsules with varying lipase activity, ranging from 4200 to 24 000 lipase units/capsule.

The enteric coated forms of pancreatic enzymes vary considerably in their biochemical coating, biophysical dissolution properties, and size of microspheres or microtablets.[88,89] There are few carefully performed clinical studies comparing the different formulations, and few in vivo data are available that demonstrate the

VI

superiority of a single product. In fact, all currently available enzyme products fail to completely correct nutrient malabsorption in all patients with CF.[90] The reasons are multiple, are likely to vary from patient to patient, and in some cases, may be attributable to factors unrelated to failed pancreatic digestion.[91] The enteric coating of enzyme microsphere or microtablets require a pH >5.2 to 6.0 for dissolution to occur in the proximal intestine, which may be acidic in the patient with CF. Some patients with CF and PI have gastric acid hypersecretion and a deficiency of bicarbonate secretion from the pancreaticobiliary tree. This may result in a more acidic proximal intestinal environment, which may decrease dissolution or be below the ideal optimal pH for maximal pancreatic enzyme activity and may hasten the inactivation of enzymes especially lipase within the small intestine. Histamine (H_2) antagonists or proton-pump inhibitors may be used to improve the intestinal milieu, but studies have revealed mixed results.[92,93] Even if nutrient digestion is achieved, malabsorption of nutrients may occur because of thick intestinal mucus, which may affect the unstirred water layer, reducing absorption of fatty acids in the small intestinal epithelium.[94] Nevertheless, enzymes do improve nutrient digestion and absorption in patients with CF, but the caregiver must be aware of the less-than-ideal efficacy of these products in individual patients.

Dosing Guidelines

To date, no studies have been performed in infants to determine the optimal dose of PERT. Data are insufficient with regard to the association of enzyme dose to macronutrient content, coefficient of fat absorption, or growth.[33] Until reliable data are available, dosing is based on consensus recommendations established by the Cystic Fibrosis Foundation and the FDA.[32,33,95] These include: 500 to 2500 U of lipase/kg of body weight/meal; or <10 000 U of lipase/kg/day; or <4000 U of lipase/gram of dietary fat/day. These guidelines were established when it was recognized that many CF centers were giving excessive doses of enzymes, which is strongly associated with a severe intestinal complication termed fibrosing colonopathy.[95,96]

Response to PERT by individual patients will vary considerably, in part because of differences in gastric acid secretion, as will their required dosing schedule. Although dosing is best calculated using U of lipase/g of fat ingested, it is, perhaps, more practical to use a dosing schedule with weight-adjusted guidelines.[32,33,37] Weight-adjusted guidelines, with a limit of 4000 U lipase/g fat or 2500 U lipase/kg/meal beyond 1 year of age, would avoid overdosing.

Enzyme Administration

There are no convincing data concerning timing of enzyme dosing with meals, but for practical reasons, it is recommended that enzymes be taken in 2 to 3 divided doses before and during meals.[97] Theoretically, this will result in more even mixing and gastric emptying of enzymes, although this has not been clinically proven. Enzymes are not required with simple carbohydrates (eg, hard candy, popsicles, pop, Jello) but are needed for foods containing fat, protein, and starch (rice, potatoes, etc).

Adjunctive Therapy

H_2 antagonists and proton-pump inhibitors inhibit gastric acid and, in some cases, may improve enzyme activity either by: (1) by decreasing gastric acidity, resulting in less destruction of unprotected conventional powder enzymes in the stomach; or (2) by increasing pH in the upper intestine, allowing for more rapid dissolution of the enteric coating and optimal conditions for enzymes to catalyze nutrients. As mentioned, efficacy of this treatment is not clear, as results in 1 study demonstrated proton-pump inhibitors to be helpful,[92] whereas another found no benefit.[93] Caregivers of children with CF should be cautioned that there are no safety data on the long-term use of these medications in children.

Infants and Young Children (Through Two Years of Age) With Newly Diagnosed CF

Initial Visits and Coordination With Primary Care Physician

The majority of young infants with CF diagnosed through newborn screening appear to be totally healthy to the parents, and the diagnosis of CF is largely unexpected. Therefore, the psychosocial impact on the family must be carefully addressed at the initial visits.[37] Infants with newly diagnosed CF should be seen at an accredited CF center, ideally within 24 to 72 hours of diagnosis. At the first visit, adequate time for the family to receive comprehensive education and counseling is very important. Disbelief, anger, and anxiety about the new diagnosis are likely, which affects the retention of information. Basic information should be provided in the clearest of terms, and information should be conveyed in a sensitive, empathetic, and positive manner. A variety of formats should be used to provide information, including verbal, written, and audiovisual. Information should be repeated or understanding should be assessed at subsequent visits.

Introduction to other CF clinicians, namely the nurse, dietitian, respiratory therapist, and social worker, should occur with the first 2 visits.[37] This allows key components of nutrition and airway clearance to be taught and facilitates the development of relationships with team members. A genetic counselor should meet with the family within 2 months of diagnosis to discuss, in greater depth, how mutations in the CFTR gene cause CF and the implications for other family members.[37] Equally important, the positive outlook for infants with newly diagnosed CF should be reinforced and a sense of hope should be instilled.

VI

The pivotal role that both parents and primary care provider play as part of the CF team should be emphasized at the early visits.[37] Coordination with the primary care physician is essential, as families will be making numerous visits to their primary care provider and CF center during the first 2 years of life. Therefore, regular and open trilateral communications among the family, the primary care physician, and the CF center should be established. Communication between the primary care physician and the CF center is critical to ensure that parents do not get conflicting messages, because many CF care goals are different from those of standard pediatric care (eg, an emphasis on the need for the CF child to be "chubby" versus concerns about obesity in the general pediatric population).

Types of Feeding

Special attention to growth and nutrition early in life is essential, because it is a time of extraordinary growth; healthy infants double their birth weight by 4 to 6 months of age and triple it by 1 year.[82] The first 6 months of life represent a unique window of opportunity to promote optimal growth, whereas poor growth during this critical period may be irreversible.[27] The Cystic Fibrosis Foundation recommends that children reach a weight-for-length status of the 50th percentile by 2 years of age, with an emphasis on achieving this goal early in infancy.[33,37] However, optimal nutritional care to achieve this goal has not been defined.

Human Milk Versus Infant Formula

The basic principles of infant feeding for healthy term infants apply to feeding infants with CF. However, optimal feeding (ie, human milk, infant formula, or combination) to meet the increased nutritional requirement for infants with CF is unknown. The benefits of breastfeeding for healthy infants are widely recognized.[98] However, human milk may be nutritionally inadequate in caloric density, protein, essential fatty acids, and sodium to meet the increased requirements of CF infants, especially for those with meconium ileus or PI, who are at greater risks of poor growth and malnutrition.[8,9,43,99-102] On the other hand, human milk's antimicrobial constituents are likely to offer protection against respiratory infections.[103-106] The breastfeeding issue was less relevant before nationwide implementation of newborn screening, when CF was diagnosed in infants at a median age of 8 to 9 months,[107] an age when most infants would no longer be breastfed; now, the breastfeeding issue is of prime importance.

Breastfeeding was historically discouraged for infants with CF because of concerns about protein energy malnutrition, which manifests as hypoproteinemia, hyponatremia, edema, and anemia.[9,43,99-102] Despite these reports, a 1990 survey demonstrated that 77% of CF centers encouraged breastfeeding, with nearly 37% of CF centers recommending exclusive breastfeeding.[108] Similar trends were confirmed by a 2004 survey.[109] The most recent 2009 Cystic Fibrosis Foundation infant care guidelines[37] reaffirmed the 2002 recommendation[32] to suggest human milk as the initial type of feeding for infants with CF on the basis of surprisingly little evidence from only one US[109] and 2 European studies.[110,111] Of utmost importance, the Cystic Fibrosis Foundation guidelines[37] do not specify the exclusivity or the duration of breastfeeding. Therefore, whether exclusive breastfeeding promotes optimal growth and provides respiratory benefits for infants with CF remains to be elucidated. A recent study from Wisconsin revealed that exclusive breastfeeding for less than 2 months was associated with adequate growth and protected against *Pseudomonas aeruginosa* infections during the first 2 years of life.[112] On the other hand, exclusive breastfeeding longer than 2 months was associated with attenuated growth without additional reduction in respiratory infections.[112] More studies are needed to evaluate the long-term risks on growth faltering associated with prolonged exclusive breastfeeding (ie, whether attenuated growth persists or catch-up growth occurs after 2 years of age) and to investigate whether the protection from respiratory infection associated with breastfeeding leads to better pulmonary function later in life in children with CF.

Standard Formula Versus Special Formula
There is limited evidence to address whether formula-fed infants with CF and PI should consume special formula (eg, predigested formula containing protein hydrolysates and/or medium-chain triglycerides). Among 3 studies conducted in the 1980s and 1990s, 1 reported similar nutritional status between infants with CF fed hydrolyzed and standard formulas,[113] another showed better anthropometric measures in infants fed hydrolysates,[114] and the third study found improved fat and nitrogen absorption in infants fed semi-elemental formula when PERT was not given.[115] These conflicting results led the Cystic Fibrosis Foundation to conclude that there was insufficient evidence to recommend a special formula for formula-fed infants with CF.[37]

It is also unclear whether human milk and standard formula should be fortified routinely to increase caloric and nutrient densities for feeding infants with CF who are growing adequately, for the purpose of sustaining normal growth or preventing growth faltering. This is another urgent nutritional issue recommended by the CF Foundation for research.[37]

Complementary Foods
Infants with CF should be introduced to solid foods at the same age as healthy infants, (ie, 4-6 months of life), according to recommendations from the American Academy of Pediatrics. Nutrient- and calorie-dense foods, such as meat, which will enhance weight gain and provide a good source of iron and zinc,[80] are ideal as first

VI

foods for infants with CF. Human milk or formula should continue to be fed through the first year of life. Thereafter, in a thriving child, whole cow milk is recommended, because generally, efforts are made to maximize caloric intake.

As infants are introduced to table foods, it is important that families and primary care physicians understand that most children with CF need a balanced diet that is moderately high in fat to meet their nutritional requirement, which is different from the usual nutritional education given to families with healthy children for overweight and obesity prevention. For example, families should buy whole milk for the child with CF and lower-fat milk for other children. During the second year of life, children establish self-feeding skills, food preferences, and dietary habits. Dietitians caring for children with CF should inquire about feeding behaviors to promote positive interactions and to prevent negative behaviors.

Enzyme Dose and Administration

PERT should be given with human milk and formulas, including elemental and MCT-containing formulas, and all foods. An initial dose of 2000 to 5000 U of lipase for each 120-mL feeding is recommended.[37] As the infant grows and the volume of intake increases, the dose is adjusted to up to 2500 U lipase/kg/feeding, not to exceed a maximal daily dose of 10 000 U lipase/kg/day.[37] Enzyme dose in relation to caloric/fat intake and weight gain should be evaluated at each visit. The goal is to prescribe enzyme doses that are sufficient but not excessive to support optimal weight gain while minimizing the risk of fibrosing colonopathy. Nevertheless, caution to avoid fibrosing colonopathy may lead to excessive conservatism in enzyme dosing, as revealed from the Cystic Fibrosis Foundation registry data that average enzyme dose tended to be at the low end of weight-based dosing early in life.

In infants with CF, PERT should be offered before feeding, mixed with 2 to 3 mL (½ teaspoon) applesauce, and given by spoon.[37] Other strained fruit can be tried if applesauce is not taken, but parents should be encouraged to use only 1 type of food to avoid problems with potential food refusal if many different types of food are used as the vehicle for enzyme delivery.

After 1 year of age, children can be offered enteric-coated products, mixed with 1 type of food. Swallowing of capsules is encouraged as soon as parents consider the child is ready. This varies considerably from patient to patient but occurs usually around 4 to 5 years of age. If children continue to experience difficulties swallowing capsules, parents should open the capsule and sprinkle the beads in the mouth which can be ingested by drinking a liquid. Children should be discouraged from chewing the capsules, as this will destroy the protective coating of enzymes.

Energy Intake and Nutrient Supplementation

Sufficient energy intake is critical in infants with CF, and the best indicators that energy requirement is met are maintenance of normal growth or achievement of catch-up growth. In addition to energy intake, adequate intakes of essential fatty acids and micronutrients, such as zinc and sodium, are needed to promote normal growth.

All infants with CF should receive standard, age-appropriate water-soluble vitamins plus fat-soluble vitamins A, D, E, and K, as recommended by the Cystic Fibrosis Foundation guidelines (Table 48.3). Because of increased risk of hyponatremia, sodium supplementation is especially important for infants with CF,[37] particularly in those fed human milk, which contains very low amount of sodium. Older infants receiving solid foods are also likely to have low sodium intake, because infant foods contain no added salt. Infants younger than 6 months with CF should receive a daily dose of 1/8 teaspoon of table salt; this amount should be increased to ¼ teaspoon for infants 6 to 12 months of age.[37]

Children With CF (Age 2-20 Years)

Toddlers to Preschool Age (2-4 Years)

Children in this age group are developing self-feeding skills, food preferences, and dietary habits. Food intake and physical activity vary from day to day. For these reasons, close monitoring of dietary habits, energy intake, and growth are important. Routinely adding calories to table foods may help with maintaining optimal growth at this stage. The importance of serving calorie-dense foods (such as providing whole milk and avoiding low-fat foods) should be emphasized.

Studies have demonstrated that toddlers with CF have longer meal times than do their peers without CF, yet still do not meet the Cystic Fibrosis Foundation's dietary recommendations for increased energy intake.[116] As the duration of meal times increases, difficult behaviors also occur more frequently.[117] Therefore, dietary counseling should include assessment of eating behaviors. One strategy to address behavioral problems is to limit mealtimes to 15 minutes for toddlers and use snack times as mini-meals. Another strategy is to teach parents alternative ways of responding to their child who eats slowly or negotiates what he or she will eat. The importance of establishing positive mealtime interactions should be emphasized.

School Age (4-10 Years)

Children in this age group are at risk of declining growth for various reasons. They typically participate in a variety of activities, leading to limited time for meals and snacks. They also begin to be exposed to peer pressure and may begin self-managing their disease. These life changes may affect compliance with prescribed therapies, such as pancreatic enzymes and fat-soluble vitamins. In addition, acceptance and

VI

understanding by teachers and fellow students may be lacking, further compounding stress for a child with CF. Encouraging children to help in meal planning and preparation maybe helpful in improving food intake.

It is important to begin monitoring bone health at this age.[66] Bone health can be evaluated by history (traumatic bone fracture), physical examination (poor growth, back pain), and radiologic and laboratory assessment. According to current guidelines,[66] children age 8 and older with CF who are at risk of poor bone health (ie, poor growth, poor lung function, history of bone fracture, delayed puberty, or chronic use of glucocorticoids) should be screened by dual energy x-ray absorptiometry to assess their bone mass. In addition, serum calcium, phosphorus, and 25-OH-D concentration and parathyroid hormone level should be measured annually.[66]

Preadolescence and Adolescence (10-18 Years)

This stage represents another vulnerable period for developing malnutrition because of increased nutritional requirements associated with accelerated growth, puberty, and high levels of physical activity. In addition, pulmonary disease often becomes more severe in this period, increasing energy requirement. This is also the age when other complications, such as CF-related diabetes mellitus (see comorbid conditions below), begin to occur more frequently, which further increases the risk of poor growth and malnutrition.

Puberty is often delayed in adolescents with CF; it usually is related to growth failure and poor nutritional status rather than to a primary endocrine disorder. Assessment of puberty should be performed annually beginning at 9 years of age in girls and 10 years of age in boys by a standardized self-assessment or physical examination.[118,119] In addition to plotting weight and height on growth charts, evaluating height and weight velocity in association with Tanner stages[118] can be very useful in identifying delayed or attenuated pubertal growth.

Nutritional counseling should be directed toward the patient rather than the parents. Teenagers may be more receptive to efforts to improve muscular strength and body image as a justification for better nutrition than emphasis on weight gain and improved disease status.

Nutrition Intervention for Poor Growth and Malnutrition

In the era prior to newborn screening, children would often have failure to thrive as the presenting symptom of CF. Although all states and the District of Columbia are performing newborn screening for CF, there will still be cases diagnosed clinically (either patients born prior to before newborn screening was implemented or patients missed by newborn screening). Such children could be severely malnourished at diagnosis. Young infants with CF have high energy requirements and frequently have significant malabsorption, which may require several adjustments to enzyme therapy in the first year after diagnosis. If poor weight gain is observed or the patient is failing to exhibit catch-up growth, careful assessment of energy intake and malabsorption is needed. Careful assessment for underlying pulmonary exacerbation also should be conducted, because inadequate control of respiratory infections is still a common basis of growth faltering.

Dietary Intervention
Oral Supplementation
For infants experiencing inadequate weight gain, increasing caloric density of the feedings is the first step. This can be achieved by fortifying human milk or by concentrating formula. For infants who are eating solids, additional calories can be added to infant cereal with the addition of carbohydrate polymers (eg, Polycose) and/or fats (eg, vegetable oil, MCT oil, or Microlipids).

Dietary modification should begin by adding high-calorie foods to the child's regular diet without dramatically increasing the amount of food consumed. For example, margarine or butter may be added to many foods, and half and half can be used in place of milk or water when preparing canned soup. If dietary modification is ineffective, use of an energy supplement may be introduced. However, it is important to ensure that the energy supplement is not used as a substitute for normal food intake.

Enteral Feedings
For children with growth deficits that do not improve with oral supplementation, enteral feeding should be initiated.[32,37] The goals of enteral feeding should be explained to the patient and family (ie, as a supportive therapy to improve quality of life and outcome), and their acceptance and commitment to this intervention should be realistically assessed.

Enteral feeding can be delivered via nasogastric tubes, gastrostomy tubes, or jejunostomy tubes. The choice of enterostomy tube and technique for its placement should be based on the expertise of the CF center. Nasogastric tubes are appropriate for short-term nutritional support in highly motivated patients. Gastrostomy tubes are more appropriate for patients who need long-term enteral nutrition. Jejunostomy tubes may be indicated in patients with severe gastroesophageal reflux; use of predigested or elemental formula may be needed with jejunostomy feeding.

Standard enteral feeding formulas (complete protein, long-chain fat) are typically well tolerated.[32] Calorically dense formulas (1.5-2.0 kcal/mL) are usually required to provide adequate energy. Nocturnal infusion is encouraged to promote normal eating patterns during the day. Initially, 30% to 50% of estimated energy requirement may be provided overnight. Pancreatic enzymes should be given with enteral feedings; however, optimal dosing regimen is unclear with overnight feeding.

VI

Behavioral Intervention

To increase dietary intakes, caregivers of young children with CF may engage in ineffective feeding practices, such as coaxing, commanding, physical prompts, and parental feeding. Adolescents with CF may intentionally skip pancreatic enzymes to achieve a certain body image. An in-depth assessment of eating behavior, feeding patterns, and family interactions at mealtimes should be performed in patients with CF at risk of experiencing malnutrition. If negative behaviors are present, behavioral intervention should be used in conjunction with dietary intervention to improve intake. Referral for more in-depth behavioral therapy is also encouraged.

Evaluation of Comorbid Medical Conditions

SEVERE MALABSORPTION

A large number of patients with CF continue to have malabsorption despite adequate dosing with potent pancreatic enzymes.[89] Subjective symptoms, such as abdominal bloating or cramps, or bulky stools cannot reliably assess the severity of malabsorption.[86] Instead, objective assessment is advocated by a 72-hour fat collection while eating a regular diet and the prescribed dose of enzymes. If severe fat malabsorption is identified (fecal fat losses exceeding 20% of intake) and is clearly contributing to abdominal symptoms or malnutrition, the dose of enzymes could be increased up to the maximum recommended amount. Alternatively, inhibition of gastric acid secretion with an H_2 antagonist or a proton-pump inhibitor may raise intestinal pH and improve the efficacy of enzyme therapy. Several weeks after the adjustment to therapy has been made, the individual patient should be reassessed by a repeat 72-hour fecal fat collection.

GASTROESOPHAGEAL REFLUX DISEASE

GERD is quite common in infants with CF,[120] particularly in those with respiratory disease. Drugs to suppress gastric acid may be indicated if reflux is severe. A predigested formula offers no advantage and should be only considered in individuals who have had significant bowel resection following complicated meconium ileus.[113]

DISTAL INTESTINAL OBSTRUCTION SYNDROME

Distal intestinal obstruction syndrome (DIOS) is unique to CF.[121] It is characterized by cramping abdominal pain, which may be periumbilical or in the right lower quadrant. A mass is usually palpable in the ileocecal area. It should be emphasized that simple constipation is a common problem in individuals with CF. Consequently, a careful history, abdominal examination, and abdominal radiography are indicated when abdominal pain attributable to DIOS is suspected to distinguish it from constipation and other CF-associated complications, such as intussusception and appendiceal abscess.

DIOS is treated with several different approaches. If the DIOS is severe, a balanced electrolyte solution (used for cleansing the bowel prior to colonoscopy) is very effective in relieving the subacute obstruction. Complete bowel obstruction is an absolute contraindication to the use of these solutions. Volumes of 4 to 8 L, delivered at 1 L/hour, are usually required for a complete cleanout in children >10 years of age. In younger children, the electrolyte solution should be administered at a rate of 10 to 40 mL/kg/hour for 4 to 6 hours until the stools no longer have any solid material. N-acetylcysteine and, in severe cases, large-volume enemas with hyperosmolar contrast agents are also used. More recently, a polyethylene glycol solution without electrolytes has been used by some clinicians to help with the management of DIOS and/or constipation in CF. Anecdotal reports suggest that this solution, a powder mixed with any choice of beverage, at doses of approximately 17 to 34 g, once or twice per day, is effective in children with CF. Most patients who have an episode of DIOS are prone to have recurrent episodes, and it is logical for these patients to maintain a bowel regimen using polyethylene glycol, although there are no published studies.[121]

CF-RELATED DIABETES

Adolescents and adults with CF and PI are at increased risk of developing CF-related diabetes mellitus. The prevalence of CF-related diabetes mellitus is reported to be between 5% and 15% in children <18 years of age and up to 50% in adults with CF.[122-125] In many instances, patients exhibit no clear-cut signs or symptoms of diabetes. Furthermore, determination of hemoglobin A1C is not a reliable test for the diagnosis of CF-related diabetes mellitus. The diagnosis should be considered in any patient who is exhibiting weight loss or poor weight gain. In 2010, the Cystic Fibrosis Foundation recommended annual screening for CF-related diabetes mellitus by a modified oral glucose-tolerance test after the age of 10 years.[124,125] In the patient who has CF-related diabetes mellitus, high-energy meals and snacks are encouraged, but energy needs and insulin requirements must be carefully balanced. Foods high in simple sugars may be limited according to insulin needs. Multidisciplinary care and the support of an endocrinologist are essential. In individuals who have impaired glucose tolerance, close monitoring by both the CF and endocrine teams are required, because these patients are at increased risk of developing CF-related diabetes mellitus.

VI

Conclusions

The clear associations between nutritional status and clinical outcomes in CF mandate careful nutritional assessment, management, and monitoring of all patients with CF. In recent years, with new knowledge arising from newborn screening research, there has been a shift away from the idea that malnutrition is inevitable for most patients with CF toward the more optimistic view that normal nutrition and growth are possible if early diagnosis and aggressive nutritional monitoring and therapy are accomplished for each patient. This task is best accomplished by involving a multidisciplinary team that includes a dietitian in the care and management of patients with CF. In this way, the goals of normal growth and prevention of malnutrition can be attained, which will improve the prognosis and quality of life for patients with CF.

References

1. Kerem B, Rommens JM, Buchanan JA, et al. Identification of the cystic fibrosis gene: genetic analysis. *Science*. 1989;245(4922):1073-80.

2. Kerem E, Corey M, Kerem BS, et al. The relation between genotype and phenotype in cystic fibrosis - analysis of the most common mutation (delta F508). *N Engl J Med*. 1990;323(22):1517-1722

3. De Boeck K, Wilschanski M, Castellani C, et al. Cystic fibrosis: terminology and diagnostic algorithms. *Thorax*. 2006;61(7):627-635

4. Castellani C, Cuppens H, Macek M Jr, et al. Consensus on the use and interpretation of cystic fibrosis mutation analysis in clinical practice. *J Cyst Fibros*. 2008;7(3):179-196

5. Farrell PM, Rosenstein BJ, White TB, et al. Cystic Fibrosis Foundation guidelines for diagnosis of cystic fibrosis in newborns through older adults: Cystic Fibrosis Foundation consensus report. *J Pediatr*. 2008;153(2):S4-S14

6. Borowitz D, Parad RB, Sharp JK, et al. Cystic Fibrosis Foundation practice guidelines for the management of infants with cystic fibrosis transmembrane conductance regulator-related metabolic syndrome during the first two years of life and beyond. *J Pediatr*. 2009;155(6 Suppl 1):S106-S116

7. Kristidis P, Bozon D, Corey M, et al. Genetic determination of exocrine pancreatic function in cystic fibrosis. *Am J Hum Genet*. 1992;50(6):1178-1184

8. Lai HC, Kosorok MR, Laxova A, Davis LA, FitzSimmon SC, Farrell PM. Nutritional Status of Patients with Cystic Fibrosis with Meconium Ileus: A comparison with patients without meconium ileus and diagnosed early through neonatal screening. *Pediatrics*. 2000; 105(1 Pt 1):53-61

9. Bronstein MN, Sokol RJ, Abman SH, et al. Pancreatic insufficiency, growth, and nutrition in infants identified by newborn screening as having cystic fibrosis. *J Pediatr*. 1992; 120(4 Pt 1):533-540

10. Bedrossian CWM, Greenberg SC, Singer DB, Hansen J, Rosenberg H. The lung in cystic fibrosis: a quantitative study including prevalence of pathologic findings among different age groups. *Hum Pathol*. 1976;7(2):195-204

11. Linnane BM, Hall GL, Nolan G, Brennan S, Stick SM, Sly PD, et al. Lung function in infants with cystic fibrosis diagnosed by newborn screening. *Am J Respir Crit Care Med* 2008;178(12):1238-1244

12. Mott LS. Gangell CL, Murray CP, Stick SM, Sly PD, Arest CF. Bronchiectasis in an asymptomatic infant with cystic fibrosis diagnosed following newborn screening. *J Cyst Fibros*. 2009;8(4):285-287

13. Li Z, Kosorok MR, Farrell PM, et al. Longitudinal development of mucoid Pseudomonas aeruginosa infection and lung disease progression in children with cystic fibrosis. *JAMA*. 2005;293(5):581-588

14. Cystic Fibrosis Foundation. *National Cystic Fibrosis Patient Registry Annual Data Report*. Bethesda, MD: Cystic Fibrosis Foundation; 2009

15. Allen DB, Farrell PM. Newborn screening: principles and practice. *Adv Pediatr*. 1996;43:231-270

16. Crossley JR, Elliott RB, Smith PA. Dried-blood spot screening for cystic fibrosis in the newborn. *Lancet*. 1979;1(8114):472-474

17. Wilcken B, Chalmers G. Reduced morbidity in patients with cystic fibrosis detected by neonatal screening. *Lancet*. 1985;2(8468):1319-1321

18. Rock MJ, Mischler EH, Farrell PM, Bruns WT, Hassemer DJ, Laessig RH, et al. Newborn screening for cystic fibrosis is complicated by the age-related decline in immunoreactive trypsinogen levels. *Pediatrics*. 1990;85(6):1001-1007

19. Gregg RG, Simantel A, Farrell PM, et al. Newborn screening for cystic fibrosis in Wisconsin: comparison of biochemical and molecular methods. *Pediatrics*. 1997;99(6):819-824

20. Comeau AM, Parad RB, Dorkin HL, et al. Population-based newborn screening for genetic disorders when multiple mutation DNA testing is incorporated: a cystic fibrosis newborn screening model demonstrating increased sensitivity but more carrier detections. *Pediatrics*. 2004;113(6):1573-1581

21. Farrell PM, Kosorok MR, Laxova A, et al. Nutritional benefits of neonatal screening for cystic fibrosis. *N Engl J Med*. 1997;337(14):963-969

22. Farrell PM, Kosorok MR, Rock MJ, et al. Early diagnosis of cystic fibrosis through neonatal screening prevents severe malnutrition and improves long-term growth. *Pediatrics*. 2001;107(1):1-12

23. Balfour-Lynn IM. Newborn screening for cystic fibrosis: evidence of benefit. *Arch Dis Child*. 2008;93(1):7-9

24. Grosse SD, Boyle CA, Botkin JR, et al. Newborn screening for cystic fibrosis: evaluation of benefits and risks and recommendations for state newborn screening programs. *MMWR Recomm Rep*. 2004;53(RR-13):1-36

25. Fritz A, Farrell P. Estimating the annual number of false negative cystic fibrosis newborn screening tests. *Pediatr Pulmonol*. 2012;47(2):207-208

26. Earley MC, Laxova A, Farrell PM, et al. Development of a DNA-based CF newborn screening proficiency testing program. *Clin Chim Acta*. 2011;412(15-16):1376-1381

27. Farrell P, Cutting GR, Earley MC, et al. *Newborn Screening for Cystic Fibrosis: Approved Guideline*. Wayne, PA: Clinical and Laboratory Standards Institute; 2011

28. Baker MW, Groose M, Hoffman G, Rock M, Levy H, Farrell PM. Optimal DNA tier for the IRT/DNA algorithm: lessons learned from CFTR mutation results in Wisconsin's 1994-2008 cystic fibrosis newborn screening program. *J Cyst Fibros*. 2011;10(4):278-281

VI

29. Watson MS, Cutting GR, Desnick RJ, et al. Cystic fibrosis population carrier screening: 2004 revision of American College of Medical Genetics mutation panel. *Genet Med.* 2004;6(5):387-391

30. LeGrys VA, Yankaskas JR, Quittell LM, Marshall BC, Mogayzel PJ. Diagnostic sweat testing: the Cystic Fibrosis Foundation guidelines. *J Pediatr.* 2007;151(1):85-89

31. Ramsey BW, Farrell PM, Pencharz P; The Consensus Committee. Nutritional assessment and management in cystic fibrosis. *Am J Clin Nutr.* 1992;55(1):108-116

32. Borowitz D, Baker RD, Stallings V. Consensus report on nutrition for pediatric patients with cystic fibrosis. *J Pediatr Gastroenterol Nutr.* 2002;35(3):246-259

33. Stallings VA, Stark LJ, Robinson KA, Feranchak AP, Quinton H; Clinical Practice Guidelines on Growth and Nutrition Subcommittee. Evidence-based practice recommendations for nutrition-related management of children and adults with cystic fibrosis and pancreatic insufficiency: results of a systematic review. *J Am Diet Assoc.* 2008;108(5):832-839

34. Flume PA, O'Sullivan BP, Robinson KA, et al. Cystic fibrosis pulmonary guidelines: chronic medications for maintenance of lung health. *Am J Respir Crit Care Med.* 2007;176(10):957-969

35. Flume PA, Robinson KA, O'Sullivan BP, et al. Cystic fibrosis pulmonary guidelines: airway clearance therapies. *Respir Care.* 2009;54(4):522-537

36. Flume PA, Mogayzel PJ Jr, Robinson KA, Goss CH, Rosenblatt RL, Kuhn RJ, et al. Cystic fibrosis pulmonary guidelines: treatment of pulmonary exacerbations. *Am J Respir Crit Care Med.* 2009;180(9):802-808

37. Borowitz D, Robinson KA, Rosenfeld M, et al. Cystic fibrosis foundation evidence-based guidelines for management of infants with cystic fibrosis. *J Pediatr.* 2009;155(6 Suppl):S73-S93

38. Kraemer R, Rudeberg A, Hadorn B, Rossi E. Relative underweight in cystic fibrosis and its prognostic value. *Acta Paediatr Scand.* 1978;67(1):33-37

39. Lai HC, Kosorok MR, Sondel SA, et al. Growth status in children with cystic fibrosis based on National Cystic Fibrosis Patient Registry data: evaluation of various criteria to identify malnutrition. *J Pediatr.* 1998;132(3 Pt 1):478-485

40. Lai HC, Corey M, FitzSimmons SC, Kosorok MR, Farrell PM. Comparison of growth status in patients with cystic fibrosis in the United States and Canada. *Am J Clin Nutr.* 1999;69(3):531-538

41. World Health Organization. Energy and protein requirements. WHO Tech Rep Ser, No. 724, 1985;924:000.

42. US Department of Agriculture, US Department of Health and Human Services. *Dietary Guidelines for Americans, 2010.* 7th ed. Washington, DC: US Government Printing Office; 2010

43. Sokol RJ, Reardon MC, Accurso FJ, et al. Fat-soluble vitamin status during the first year of life in infants with cystic fibrosis identified by screening of newborns. *Am J Clin Nutr.* 1989;50(5):1064-1071

44. Benabdeslam H, Garcia I, Bellon G, Gilly R, Revol A. Biochemical assessment of the nutritional status of cystic fibrosis patients treated with pancreatic enzyme extracts. *Am J Clin Nutr.* 1998;67(5):912-918

45. Marcus MS, Sondel SA, Farrell PM, et al. Nutritional status of infants with cystic fibrosis associated with early diagnosis and intervention. *Am J Clin Nutr*. 1991;54(3):578-585

46. Institute of Medicine, Food and Nutrition Board. *Dietary Reference Intakes for Energy, Carbohydrate, Fiber, Fat, Fatty Acids, Cholesterol, Protein, and Amino Acids (Macronutrients)*. Washington, DC: National Academies Press; 2002

47. Farrell PM, Mischler EH, Engle MJ, Brown DJ, Lau S. Fatty acid abnormalities in cystic fibrosis. *Pediatr Res*. 1985;19(1):104-109

48. Lloyd-Still JD, Bibus DM, Powers CA, Johnson SB, Holman RT. Essential fatty acid deficiency and predisposition to lung disease in cystic fibrosis. *Acta Paediatr*. 1996;85(12):1426-1432

49. Roulet M, Frascarolo P, Rappaz I, Pilet M. Essential fatty acid deficiency in well nourished young cystic fibrosis patients. *Eur J Pediatr*. 1997;156(12):952-956

50. Strandvik B, Gronowitz E, Enlund F, Martinsson T, Wahlstrom J. Essential fatty acid deficiency in relation to genotype in patients with cystic fibrosis. *J Pediatr*. 2001;139(5):650-655

51. Strandvik B. Fatty acid metabolism in cystic fibrosis. *N Engl J Med*. 2004;350(6):605-607

52. Maqbool A, Schall JI, Garcia-Espana JF, Zemel BS, Strandvik B, Stallings VA. Serum linoleic acid status as a clinical indicator of essential fatty acid status in children with cystic fibrosis. *J Pediatr Gastroenterol Nutr*. 2008;47(5):635-644

53. Bhura-Bandali FN, Suh M, Man SF, Clandinin MT. The F508del mutation in the CFTR alters control of essential fatty acid utilization in epithelial cells. *J Nutr*. 2000;130(12):2870-2875

54. vanegmond AWA, Kosorok MR, Koscik R, Laxova A, Farrell PM. Effect of linoleic acid intake on growth of infants with cystic fibrosis. *Am J Clin Nutr*. 1996;63(5):746-752

55. Shoff SM, Ahn HY, Davis L, Lai H; Wisconsin CF Neonatal Screening Group. Temporal associations among energy intake, plasma linoleic acid, and growth improvement in response to treatment initiation after diagnosis of cystic fibrosis. *Pediatrics*. 2006;117(2):391-400

56. Freedman SD, Blanco PG, Zaman MM, et al. Association of cystic fibrosis with abnormalities in fatty acid metabolism. *N Engl J Med*. 2004;350(6):560-569

57. Beharry S, Ackerley C, Corey M, et al. Long-term docosahexaenoic acid therapy in a congenic murine model of cystic fibrosis. *Am J Physiol Gastrointest Liver Physiol*. 2007;292(3):G839-G848

58. Werner A, Bongers MEJ, Bijvelds MJ, de Jonge HR, Verkade HJ. No indications for altered essential fatty acid metabolism in two murine models for cystic fibrosis. *J Lipid Res*. 2004;45(12):2277-2286

59. Andersson C, Al-Turkmani MR, Savaille JE, et al. Cell culture models demonstrate that CFTR dysfunction leads to defective fatty acid composition and metabolism. *J Lipid Res*. 2008;49(8):1692-1700

60. Al-Turkmani MR, Andersson C, Alturkmani R, et al. A mechanism accounting for the low cellular level of linoleic acid in cystic fibrosis and its reversal by DHA. *J Lipid Res*. 2008;49(9):1946-1954

VI

61. Lancellotti L, D'Orazio C, Mastella G, Mazzi G, Lippi U. Deficiency of vitamins E and A in cystic fibrosis is independent of pancreatic function and current enzyme and vitamin supplementation. *Eur J Pediatr.* 1996;155(4):281-285

62. Wilfond BS, Farrell PM, Laxova A, Mischler E. Severe hemolytic anemia associated with vitamin E deficiency in infants with cystic fibrosis. Implications for neonatal screening. *Clin Pediatr (Phila).* 1994;33(1):2-7

63. Durie PR. Vitamin K and the management of patients with cystic fibrosis. *CMAJ.* 1994;15(7):933-936

64. Feranchak AP, Sontag MK, Wagener JS, Hammond KB, Accurso FJ, Sokol RJ. Prospective, long-term study of fat-soluble vitamin status in children with cystic fibrosis identified by newborn screen. *J Pediatr.* 1999;135(5):601-610

65. Chavasse RJ, Francis J, Balfour-Lynn I, Rosenthal M, Bush A. Serum vitamin D levels in children with cystic fibrosis. *Pediatr Pulmonol.* 2004;38(2):119-122

66. Aris RM, Merkel PA, Bachrach LK, et al. Consensus statement: guide to bone health and disease in cystic fibrosis. *J Clin Endocrinol Metab.* 2005;90(3):1888-1896

67. Chavasse RJ, Francis J, Balfour-Lynn I, Rosenthal M, Bush A. Serum vitamin D levels in children with cystic fibrosis. *Pediatr Pulmonol.* 2004;38(2):119-122

68. Stephenson A, Brotherwood M, Robert R, Atenafu E, Corey M, Tullis E. Cholecalciferol significantly increases 25-hydroxyvitamin D concentrations in adults with cystic fibrosis. *Am J Clin Nutr.* 2007;85(5):1307-1311

69. Koscik RL, Farrell PM, Kosorok MR, et al. Cognitive function of children with cystic fibrosis: deleterious effect of early malnutrition. *Pediatrics.* 2004;113(6):1549-1558

70. van Hoorn JH, Hendriks JJ, Vermeer C, Forget PP. Vitamins K supplementation in cystic fibrosis. *Arch Dis Child.* 2003;88(11):974-975

71. Conway SP, Wolfe SP, Brownlee KG, et al. Vitamin K status among children with cystic fibrosis and its relationship to bone mineral density and bone turnover. *Pediatrics.* 2005;115(5):1325-1331

72. Corneli HM, Gormley CJ, Baker RC. Hyponatremia and seizures presenting in the first two years of life. *Pediatr Emerg Care.* 1985;1(4):190-193

73. Ozcelik U, Gocmen A, Kiper N, Coskun T, Yilmaz E, Ozguc M. Sodium chloride deficiency in cystic fibrosis patients. *Eur J Pediatr.* 1994;153(11):829-831

74. Greer FR, Krebs NF; American Academy of Pediatrics, Committee on Nutrition. Optimizing bone health and calcium intakes of infants, children and adolescents. *Pediatrics.* 2006;117(2):578-585

75. Hillman LS, Cassidy JT, Popescu MF, Hewett JE, Kyger J, Robertson JD. Percent true calcium absorption, mineral metabolism, and bone mineralization in children with cystic fibrosis: effect of supplementation with vitamin D and calcium. *Pediatr Pulmonol.* 2008;43(8):772-780

76. Easley D, Krebs N, Jefferson M, Miller L, Erskine J, Accurso F. Effect of pancreatic enzymes on zinc absorption in cystic fibrosis. *J Pediatr Gastroenterol Nutr.* 1998;26(2):136-139

77. Krebs NF, Westcott JE, Arnold TD, Kluger BM, Accurso FJ, Miller LV. Abnormalities in zinc and homeostasis in young infants with cystic fibrosis. *Pediatr Res.* 2000;48(2):256-261

78. von Drygalski A, Biller J. Anemia in cystic fibrosis: incidence, mechanisms, and association with pulmonary function and vitamin deficiency. *Nutr Clin Pract.* 2008;23(5):557-563

79. Pond MN, Morton AM, Conway SP. Functional iron deficiency in adults with cystic fibrosis. *Respir Med.* 1996;90(7):409-413

80. Baker RD, Greer FR; American Academy of Pediatrics, Committee on Nutrition. Clinical report: diagnosis and prevention of iron deficiency and iron-deficiency anemia in infants and young children (0-3 years of age). *Pediatrics.* 2010;126(5):1040-1050

81. Milla CE. Association of nutritional status and pulmonary function in children with cystic fibrosis. *Curr Opin Pulmonol Med.* 2004;10(6):505-509

82. Kuczmarski RJ, Ogden CL, Grummer-Strawn LM, et al. CDC Growth Charts: United States. *Adv Data.* 2000;(314):1-27

83. World Health Organization. The WHO Child Growth Standards. Geneva, Switzerland: World Health Organization; 2009. Available at: www.who.int/childgrowth/en/. Accessed January 18, 2013

84. Zhang Z, Shoff SM, Lai HJ. Incorporating genetic potential when evaluating stature in children with cystic fibrosis. *J Cystic Fibrosis.* 2010;9(2):135-142

85. Lai HJ. Classification of nutritional status in patients with cystic fibrosis. *Curr Opin Pulmonol Med.* 2006;12(6):422-427

86. Borowitz D. Update on the evaluation of pancreatic exocrine status in cystic fibrosis. *Curr Opin Pulmonol Med.* 2005;11(6):524-527

87. Borowitz D, Baker SS, Duffy L, Baker RD, Fitzpatrick L, Gyamfi J, et al. Use of fecal elastase-1 to classify pancreatic status in patients with cystic fibrosis. *J Pediatr.* 2004;145(3):322-326

88. Carroccio A, Pardo F, Montalto G, et al. Effectiveness of enteric-coated preparations on nutritional parameters in cystic fibrosis. A long-term study. *Digestion.* 1988;41(4):201-206

89. Durie P, Kalnins D, Ellis L. Uses and abuses of enzyme therapy in cystic fibrosis. *J R Soc Med.* 1998;91(Suppl 34):2-13

90. Kalnins D, Corey M, Ellis L, Durie PR, Pencharz PB. Combining unprotected pancreatic enzymes with pH-sensitive enteric-coated microspheres does not improve nutrient digestion in patients with cystic fibrosis. *J Pediatr.* 2005;146(4):489-493

91. Borowitz D, Durie PR, Clarke LL, et al. Gastrointestinal outcomes and confounders in cystic fibrosis. *J Pediatr Gastroenterol Nutr.* 2005;41(3):273-285

92. Heijerman HG, Lamers CB, Bakker W. Omeprazole enhances the efficacy of pancreatin (pancrease) in cystic fibrosis. *Ann Intern Med.* 1991;114(3):200-201

93. Francisco MP, Wagner MH, Sherman JM, Theriaque D, Bowser E, Novak DA. Ranitidine and omeprazole as adjuvant therapy to pancrelipase to improve fat absorption in patients with cystic fibrosis. *J Pediatr Gastroenterol Nutr.* 2002;35(1):79-83

94. Laiho KM, Gavin J, Murphy JL, Connett GJ, Wootton SA. Maldigestion and malabsorption of 13C labelled tripalmitin in gastrostomy-fed patients with cystic fibrosis. *Clin Nutr.* 2004;23(3):347-353

VI

95. Borowitz DS, Grand RJ, Durie PR. Use of pancreatic enzyme supplements for patients with cystic fibrosis in the context of fibrosing colonopathy. Consensus Committee. *J Pediatr*. 1995;127(5):681-684

96. FitzSimmons SC, Burkhart GA, Borowitz D, et al. High-dose pancreatic-enzyme supplements and fibrosing colono-pathy in children with cystic fibrosis. *N Engl J Med*. 1997;336(18):1283-1289

97. Brady MS, Rickard K, Yu PL, Eigen H. Effectiveness of enteric coated pancreatic enzymes given before meals in reducing steatorrhea in children with cystic fibrosis. *J Am Diet Assoc*. 1992;92(7):813-817

98. American Academy of Pediatrics, Section on Breastfeeding. Policy statement: breastfeeding and the use of human milk. *Pediatrics*. 2012;129(3):e827-e841

99. Fleisher DS, DiGeorge AM, Barness LA, Cornfeld D. Hypoproteinemia and edema in infants with cystic fibrosis of the pancreas. *J Pediatr*. 1964;64:341-348

100. Lee PA, Roloff DW, Howatt WF. Hypoproteinemia and anemia in infants with cystic fibrosis: a presenting symptom complex often misdiagnosed. *JAMA*. 1974;228(5):585-588

101. Nielsen OH, Larsen BF. The incidence of anemia, hypoproteinemia, and edema in infants as presenting symptoms of cystic fibrosis: a retrospective survey of the frequency of this symptom complex in 130 patients with cystic fibrosis. *J Pediatr Gastroenterol Nutr*. 1982;1(3):355-359

102. Fustik S, Jacovska T, Spirevska L, Koceva S. Protein-energy malnutrition as the first manifestation of cystic fibrosis in infancy. *Pediatr Int*. 2009;51(5):678-683

103. Wright AL, Holberg CJ, Martinez FD, Morgan WJ, Taussig LM. Breast feeding and lower respiratory tract illness in the first year of life. Group Health Medical Associates. *BMJ*. 1989;14(299):946-949

104. Heinig MJ. Host defense benefits of breastfeeding for the infant. Effect of breastfeeding duration and exclusivity. *Pediatr Clin North Am*. 2001;48(1):105-123

105. Ietta F, Romagnoli R, Liberatori S, et al. Presence of macrophage migration inhibitory factor in human milk: evidence in the aqueous phase and milk fat globules. *Pediatr Res*. 2002;51(5):619-624

106. Oddy WH, Sly PD, de Klerk NH, et al. Breast feeding and respiratory morbidity in infancy: a birth cohort study. *Arch Dis Child*. 2003;88(3):224-228

107. Accurso FJ, Sontag MK, Wagener JS. Complications associated with symptomatic diagnosis in infants with cystic fibrosis. *J Pediatr*. 2005;147(3 Suppl):S37-S41

108. Luder E, Kattan M, Tanzer-Torres G, Bonforte RJ. Current recommendations for breast-feeding in cystic fibrosis centers. *Am J Dis Child*. 1990;144(10):1153-1156

109. Parker EM, O'Sullivan BP, Shea JC, Regan MM, Freedman SD. Survey of breast-feeding practices and outcomes in the cystic fibrosis population. *Pediatr Pulmonol*. 2004;37(4):362-367

110. Holiday KE, Allen JR, Waters DL, Gruca MA, Thompson SM, Gaskin KJ. Growth of human milk-fed and formula-fed infants with cystic fibrosis. *J Pediatr*. 1991;118(1):77-79

111. Colombo C, Costantini D, Zazzeron L, Faelli N, Russo MC, Ghisleni D, et al. Benefits of breastfeeding in cystic fibrosis: a single-centre follow-up survey. *Acta Paediatr.* 2007;96(8):1228-1232

112. Jadin, S, Wu GS, Zhang Z, et al. Growth and pulmonary outcomes during the first two years of life of breastfed and formula-fed infants diagnosed through the Wisconsin routine cystic fibrosis newborn screening program. *Am J Clin Nutr.* 2011;93(5):1037-1047

113. Ellis L, Kalnins D, Corey M, Brennan J, Pencharz P, Durie P. Do infants with cystic fibrosis need a protein hydrolysate formula? A prospective, randomized comparative trial. *J Pediatr.* 1998;132(2):270-276

114. Farrell PM, Mischler EH, Sondel SA, Palta M. Predigested formula for infants with cystic fibrosis. *J Am Diet Assoc.* 1987;87(10):1353-1356

115. Canciani M, Mastella G. Absorption of a new semielemental diet in infants with cystic fibrosis. *J Pediatr Gastroenterol Nutr.* 1985;4(5):735-740

116. Powers SW, Patton SR, Byars KC, Mitchell MJ, Jelalian E, Mulvihill MM. Caloric intake and eating behavior in infants and toddlers with cystic fibrosis. *Pediatrics.* 2002;109(5):e75-e85

117. Stark LJ, Opipari-Arrigan L, Quittner AL, Bean J, Powers SW. The effects of an intensive behavior and nutrition intervention compared to standard of care on weight outcomes in CF. *Pediatr Pulmonol.* 2011;46(1):31-35

118. Tanner JM, Whitehouse RH. Clinical longitudinal standards for height, weight, height velocity, weight velocity, and stages of puberty. *Arch Dis Child.* 1976;51(3):170-179

119. Morris NM, Udry JR. Validation of a self-administered instrument to assess stage of adolescent development. *J Youth Adolesc.* 1980;9:271-280

120. Heine RG, Button BM, Olinsky A, Phelan PD, Catto-Smith AG. Gastro-oesophageal reflux in infants under 6 months with cystic fibrosis. *Arch Dis Child.* 1998;78(1):44-48

121. van der Doef HP, Kokke FTM, van der Ent CK, Houwen RH. Intestinal obstruction syndromes in cystic fibrosis: meconium ileus, distal intestinal obstruction syndrome, and constipation. *Curr Gastro Rep.* 2011;13:265-270

122. Lanng S, Thorsteinsson B, Lund-Andersen C, Nerup J, Schiotz PO, Koch C. Diabetes mellitus in Danish cystic fibrosis patients: prevalence and late diabetic complications. *Acta Paediatr.* 1994;83(1):72-77

123. Solomon MP, Wilson DC, Corey M, Kalnins D, Zielenski J, Tsui LC. Glucose intolerance in children with cystic fibrosis. *J Pediatr.* 2003;142(2):128-132

124. Laguna TA, Nathan BM, Moran A. Managing diabetes in cystic fibrosis. *Diabetes Obes Metab.* 2010;12(10):858-864

125. Moran A, Becker D, Casella SJ, et al. Epidemiology, pathophysiology, and prognostic implications of cystic fibrosis-related diabetes: a technical review. *Diabetes Care.* 2010;33(12):2677-2683

VI

Chapter 49

The Ketogenic Diet

Introduction

The ketogenic diet is a high-fat, low-carbohydrate, and minimal-protein diet designed to mimic the fasting state. It is used most commonly to treat intractable epilepsy but is also a primary therapy for some metabolic defects involving glucose transport and metabolism. The diet increases the body's reliance on fatty acids rather than on glucose for energy. This chapter briefly reviews the history, physiology, mechanism of action, indications, efficacy, and contraindications of the ketogenic diet. The emphasis is on implementing and maintaining the classic ketogenic diet while preventing and managing its complications. Alternative dietary therapies for epilepsy, including the medium-chain triglyceride (MCT) oil version of the ketogenic diet, the low-glycemic index treatment, and the modified Atkins diet, are also described.

History

The benefits of fasting for seizure control have been known for ages.[1] Although the first scientific report did not appear until 1911 in France, fasting for seizure therapy was used by Hippocrates and was also recommended in the Bible (Mark 9:14-29). In the United States, the first report of fasting as a treatment for epilepsy was presented to the American Medical Association in 1921 by endocrinologist HR Geyelin (New York Presbyterian Hospital) on the basis of his observation of patients treated by the osteopath HW Conklin (Battle Creek, Michigan), who believed that epilepsy could be caused by toxic secretions from intestinal Peyer patches. Because fasting is not a practical long-term treatment, RM Wilder (Mayo Clinic) described a high-fat, low-carbohydrate, "ketogenic" diet to mimic fasting; the first efficacy studies of this ketogenic diet by MG Peterman (1925, Mayo Clinic) and FB Talbot (1926, Massachusetts General Hospital) showed remarkable efficacy, with 50% to 60% of patients becoming seizure free.[2] Interest in the diet waned after the introduction of phenytoin in 1938, but a resurgence of interest in the diet occurred in the 1990s, in part because of the advocacy of the Charlie Foundation (http://www.charliefoundation.org) and in part because of the media attention surrounding the 1997 movie *First Do No Harm*.[1] The diet is currently administered at major medical centers around the United States as well as in at least 41 other countries.[3] A list of dietary centers following patients on the ketogenic diet can be found on the Charlie Foundation Web site (http://www.charliefoundation.org/hospitals.html).

VI

Physiologic Basis

The ketogenic diet is based on the brain's ability to obtain 30% to 60% or more of its energy during fasting from serum ketone bodies derived from beta-oxidation of fatty acids.[4-8] Some of the most relevant aspects are briefly reviewed here (Fig 49.1).

Fig 49.1.
Summary of ketogenesis. HSL indicates hormone sensitive lipase; CPT I, carnitine palmitoyltransferase I; AcAcCoA, acetoacetyl CoA; CoA, coenzyme A; mHS, mitochondrial HMG-CoA synthease; HMG, 3-hydroxy-3-methyl glutaric acid; HL, HMG-CoA lyase; AcAc, acetoacetate. Adapted from Mitchell and Fukao.[6]

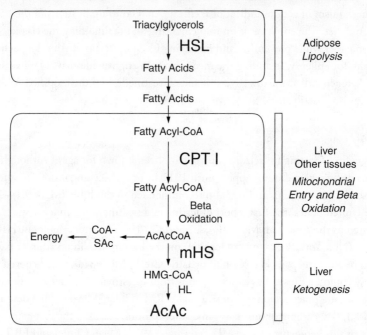

Fasting lowers serum glucose concentration, resulting in a low insulin-to-glucagon ratio. The decrease in this ratio and changes in other hormones, such as epinephrine, stimulate lipolysis in adipocytes. The free fatty acids released into the blood cannot cross the blood-brain barrier and, therefore, cannot be used directly to sustain brain metabolism. Instead, fatty acids are converted by the liver to ketone bodies that cross the blood-brain barrier and serve as a major energy source for the brain.

Fatty acids from lipolysis undergo beta-oxidation to acetyl coenzyme A (acetyl CoA) in the mitochondria of liver, cardiac muscle, and skeletal muscle cells. Acetyl CoA ordinarily condenses with oxaloacetate to enter the tricarboxylic acid cycle

(TCA cycle or Krebs cycle). However, liver oxaloacetate is low during fasting, because it is used to synthesize glucose. The liver, therefore, converts excess acetyl CoA to acetoacetate and then to beta-hydroxybutyrate, 2 ketone bodies, which are then released into the bloodstream and cross the blood-brain barrier.

In the brain, as in other tissues, beta-hydroxybutyrate and acetoacetate are converted back to acetyl CoA and enter the TCA cycle, yielding biosynthetic carbon compounds and energy (in the form of reduced nicotinamide adenine dinucleotide [NADH] and reduced flavin adenine dinucleotide [$FADH_2$]). The mitochondrial electron transport chain then oxidizes NADH and $FADH_2$ to yield adenosine triphosphate (ATP).

Beta-oxidation of fatty acids in the liver occurs in the mitochondrial matrix; therefore, free fatty acids must cross the outer and inner mitochondrial membranes. The carnitine cycle is required for this transmembrane transport of long-chain fatty acids but not for short- or medium-chain fatty acids.[9]

Mechanisms of Action

The anticonvulsant mechanism of the ketogenic diet remains unknown, although many hypotheses have been proposed. Originally, ketone bodies were thought to act directly as anticonvulsants when crossing the blood-brain barrier.[10] However, their importance in the mechanism of action of the ketogenic diet has been questioned over the years. Evidence suggests that the ketone body, acetone, may have a direct anticonvulsant effect on neurons, but further research is necessary to determine the mechanism involved.[11] Other ketone bodies, acetoacetate and beta-hydroxybutyrate, do not appear to act directly on synapses, nor do they appear to directly alter neurotransmitter function; however, they may serve a neuroprotective role against free radical damage.[12,13]

Ketone bodies may also indirectly contribute to the anticonvulsant effect by acting as metabolic substrates. Research suggests that the metabolism of ketone bodies by the TCA cycle may increase levels of glutamate and, thereby, increase levels of gamma-aminobutyric acid (GABA), a major inhibitory neurotransmitter.[14] Ketone body metabolism may also induce mitochondrial biogenesis, which may raise seizure threshold by enhancing resistance to metabolic stress.[15] Additionally, the metabolism of ketone bodies may activate ATP-sensitive potassium channels and, thus, reduce the neuronal firing rates.[16]

It is also possible that the anticonvulsant mechanism of the ketogenic diet is associated with physiologic consequences other than the production and metabolism of ketone bodies. For example, because glucose uptake increases during seizures, the decreased availability of glucose as an energy source may provide an anticonvulsant effect.[17] In addition, a glycolytic inhibitor, 2-deoxy-D-glucose, has

VI

been effective against multiple seizure models, suggesting that reducing glycolysis may provide seizure control.[18] Decreased insulin or glucose concentrations may also provide antiseizure efficacy by inhibiting the mammalian target of Rapamycin (mTOR) signaling pathway, which has been implicated in epileptogenesis.[19] Finally, elevated levels of polyunsaturated fatty acids may act to raise seizure threshold by modulating sodium, calcium, and potassium channels.[20,21]

Despite the many hypotheses that have been proposed, none have been universally accepted. The ketogenic diet likely has multiple mechanisms of action, given the complex nature of the metabolic changes involved.

Indications

Intractable Epilepsy

Historically, the ketogenic diet has been most commonly used in the treatment of intractable epilepsy. It effectively treats multiple seizure types (including generalized seizures and partial-onset seizures[22,23]) and epilepsy syndromes (including Lennox-Gastaut syndrome,[24,25] Landau Kleffner syndrome [acquired epileptic aphasia],[26] Dravet syndrome [severe myoclonic epilepsy of infancy],[24,27,28] Doose syndrome [myoclonic-astatic epilepsy of early childhood],[29,30] and West syndrome [infantile spasms],[31-33]) as well as childhood and juvenile absence epilepsy.[34] It is also effective for seizures caused by tuberous sclerosis complex[35,36] and other inherited disorders.

Traditionally, the ketogenic diet has been considered too difficult for use as a first-line agent and has been treated as a last resort. Furthermore, like other treatments, the ketogenic diet is associated with a risk of adverse events (see "Adverse Effects"). However, the majority of the 2009 expert consensus panel felt that the ketogenic diet should be strongly considered after a patient has failed 2 antiepileptic drugs.[37]

The ketogenic diet is indicated for patients of all ages. In most studies, efficacy in adolescents and adults is similar to that in children,[38-40] although some studies suggest slightly lower tolerability in older patients.[23] A ketogenic formula can also be effectively administered to formula-fed infants and gastrostomy tube-fed children (see "Calculation of the Ketogenic Diet").[41-43]

Inborn Metabolic Disorders

The ketogenic diet is the preferred treatment for 2 congenital disorders affecting glucose metabolism and transport: pyruvate dehydrogenase complex deficiency (PDHD)[44,45] and glucose transporter type 1 (GLUT1) deficiency.[46,47] Pyruvate dehydrogenase normally converts pyruvate (from glycolysis) to acetyl CoA, which normally enters the TCA cycle. GLUT1 is responsible for facilitated transport of glucose across the blood-brain barrier. In both disorders, mutations result in an inability of the brain to use glucose as its primary energy substrate. The ketogenic diet should be considered soon after diagnosis of these metabolic disorders.

Experimental Uses

Preliminary evidence suggests that the ketogenic diet may be an effective treatment for other disorders, including Alzheimer disease, Parkinson disease, amyotrophic lateral sclerosis (ALS), autism spectrum disorders, depression, headaches, narcolepsy, traumatic brain injury, hypoxic/ischemic brain injury, glycogenosis type V (McArdle disease), cardiac ischemia, certain types of cancer,[48] type 2 diabetes mellitus,[49] polycystic ovary syndrome,[50] and bipolar disorder.[51] However, the efficacy and safety have not been established for any of these indications; therefore, the use of the diet for each of these conditions should be considered strictly experimental.

Efficacy

Since the early 1920s, multiple case series and open label studies, mostly retrospective, have been published describing the efficacy of the ketogenic diet for intractable epilepsy. Most studies have not found that age, sex, seizure type, or etiology made a difference in response to the diet. The most recent meta-analysis, published in 2006, of 1084 patients from 19 studies published between 1970 and 2003 showed 84% of patients achieving >50% reduction in seizure frequency compared with baseline, with 52% of patients achieving ≥90% reduction and 24% of patients achieving complete seizure control.[52]

The first randomized controlled trial of the ketogenic diet was published in 2008.[22] One hundred and forty-five children ages 2 to 16 years with intractable epilepsy (failure to respond to at least 2 antiepileptic drugs and at least 7 seizures per week) were randomly assigned to a treatment group, in which initiation of the diet took place immediately, or to a control group, in which initiation of the diet was delayed for 3 months. After 3 months, seizure frequency had decreased to a mean of 62% of baseline in the treatment group and had increased to 137% of baseline in the control group, and 38% of children in the treatment group had >50% seizure reduction compared with 6% of children in the control group. Furthermore, 7% of those on the diet had a >90% reduction in seizure frequency compared with none in the control group. Of note, there was no significant difference in the efficacy of the treatment between generalized and focal epilepsy syndromes. These results provide substantial evidence that the ketogenic diet is an effective treatment for patients with intractable epilepsy.

This conclusion is further supported by the observation that patients who have failed trials of 2 antiepileptic drugs have a limited chance of achieving seizure control with a third antiepileptic drug. On the ketogenic diet, such patients with intractable epilepsy have approximately a one third chance of achieving seizure control and another one third chance of attaining a meaningful but incomplete reduction in seizures. Even patients who do not experience decreased seizure frequency may still benefit from the diet: many patients on the ketogenic diet have reduced seizure intensity, improved alertness, improved behavior, and reduced number or dosage of antiepileptic drugs. In a prospective study, significant improvements in developmental quotient, attention, and social functioning were observed in 34 children who continued on the ketogenic diet for 1 year.[53]

Contraindications

The ketogenic diet is absolutely contraindicated for patients with the following: fatty acid oxidation defects (including defects involving fatty acid transportation, enzymes of beta-oxidation, and ketone body production), primary carnitine deficiency or other carnitine cycle defects, pyruvate carboxylase deficiency, or porphryia.[37] Candidates for the ketogenic diet should be screened for metabolic disorders, including a comprehensive metabolic blood panel, prior to diet initiation. Although high-fat diets can exacerbate ketotic hypoglycemia, the ketogenic diet is not absolutely contraindicated in this condition but requires careful monitoring.[54]

Cotherapy with some drugs may increase the risk of certain adverse events; however, no drugs are absolutely contraindicated with the ketogenic diet. Because cotherapy may provide optimal seizure control for some patients, the risks and benefits must be weighed. Furthermore, all medications must be reviewed for carbohydrate content (see "Concurrent Medications and Occult Carbohydrates").

Patients using the ketogenic diet and carbonic anhydrase inhibitors (including acetazolamide, topiramate, and zonisamide) may be at increased risk of metabolic acidosis and renal stones.[55,56] In particular, ketogenic diet and zonisamide cotherapy, but not ketogenic diet and topiramate cotherapy, is associated with an elevated rate of nephrolithiasis compared with the ketogenic diet alone. However, with adequate hydration and appropriate prophylaxis with a buffering agent, such as potassium citrate, as well as careful monitoring of urine calcium, creatinine, citrate, pH, specific gravity, occult hematuria, and serum bicarbonate, carbonic anhydrase inhibitors and the ketogenic diet can usually be safely coadministered.

Cotherapy with valproate is also somewhat controversial. Rare adverse events associated with valproate include acute pancreatitis and hepatic failure. Long-term use of valproate can also induce carnitine deficiency. It has been suggested, therefore, that cotherapy with valproate and the ketogenic diet may induce hepatotoxicity by a carnitine-related mechanism in some patients or elevate the risk of other adverse effects, such as pancreatitis.[9,57] However, recent studies have not found that valproate elevates the risk of adverse events on the ketogenic diet.[58,59] Liver function, pancreatic amylase, and carnitine should be monitored carefully in patients cotreated with valproate and the ketogenic diet; however, valproate is not an absolute contraindication to the ketogenic diet.

Adverse Effects

Common short-term adverse effects of the ketogenic diet include dehydration, hypoglycemia, acidosis, vomiting, diarrhea, constipation, and loss of appetite.[59] These complications are generally treated symptomatically. The first 3 symptoms may be prevented with a diet protocol that includes no fasting, no fluid restriction, and prophylactic potassium citrate (see "Initiation Protocol"). Constipation is very common and can usually be managed with medication, such as polyethylene glycol (MiraLax) or through dietary manipulation, such as increasing fluid and fiber intake, adding MCT oil, or supplementing with carnitine.

Common longer-term adverse effects include growth retardation, renal stones, hypertriglyceridemia, bone mineral content loss, increased bruising, irritability, and lethargy. Some patients on the ketogenic diet may be more susceptible to infection, but it is unclear whether impaired immune function is attributable to the diet or whether patients on the diet have impaired immune function for other reasons.[60] Rare but serious adverse events have been reported with the ketogenic diet, including acute (possibly hypertriglyceridemia-induced) pancreatitis,[61] cardiomyopathy associated with prolonged QT_c interval,[62] and iron-deficiency anemia.[59] Hepatotoxicity and Fanconi renal tubular acidosis have been reported in a few patients cotreated with the ketogenic diet and valproate,[57] but this combination has been used in many other patients without adverse effects.[58]

Growth Retardation

There have been several reports demonstrating growth retardation of children on the ketogenic diet.[63-66] Changes in weight-for-age percentile appear to be greatest within the first several months on the diet, and the greatest changes in height-for-age percentile occur only after 6 months on the diet. Younger children on the diet for longer periods of time may be at greater risk of growth retardation. However, a recent study of the use of ketogenic diet-formula for infantile spasms found that the infants' weight-for-height z-score remained stable throughout their first year of treatment.[31] Also, a recent study of the long-term effects of the ketogenic diet found that growth appeared to improve after discontinuation of the diet; however, 40% of the subjects were still $<10^{th}$ percentile height for age after the diet was discontinued.[67] The risk of growth retardation, especially with long-term treatment, should be considered when weighing the risks and benefits of the ketogenic diet. Height

VI

and weight should be monitored closely (at least every 3 months). Protein and total kilocalories should be adjusted in patients with suboptimal growth.

Renal Stones

Although older studies have indicated that renal calculi occur in approximately 3% to 10% of children treated with the ketogenic diet,[68-69] the incidence may currently be lower because of recent changes to the diet initiation and maintenance protocols at some hospitals, including the elimination of fluid restriction and preinitiation fasting, as well as prophylactic use of potassium citrate or other buffering agents.[56,70] Certain medications (eg, zonisamide) may increase the risk of calculi (see "Contraindications"). Calculi may be composed of uric acid, calcium oxalate, or calcium phosphate. Patients with hematuria (gross or microscopic), crystalluria, abdominal pain, or flank pain should be evaluated for possible nephrolithiasis. Analgesia and hydration are appropriate for acute episodes, and lithotripsy, and/or medical or surgical extraction may be indicated in some cases. Further incidence may be prevented by liberalization of fluids and alkalinization of urine with potassium citrate or other buffering agents.

Lipid Profiles

Abnormal lipid profiles, including elevated triglyceride, total cholesterol, and low-density lipoprotein concentrations, as well as decreased high-density lipoprotein concentration, are frequently seen in patients on the ketogenic diet, but they appear to normalize after discontinuation of the diet.[67,70] The long-term consequences of these alterations in lipid profile are unknown.

Bone Mineral Content

As with antiepileptic drugs, long-term use of the ketogenic diet may increase risk of osteopenia, osteoporosis, and bone fractures.[59,64,72] Although all patients on the ketogenic diet are supplemented with vitamin D and calcium, this may not be sufficient in preventing bone loss. As suggested by the 2009 expert consensus panel, periodic dual energy x-ray absorptiometry (DEXA) screening for bone health should be considered for patients receiving the ketogenic diet for long-term use.[37]

The Keto Team

The ketogenic diet requires a multidisciplinary team approach. At the heart of the "keto team" are the patient and his or her family, a neurologist, a dietitian, a pediatrician, and a nurse. The inpatient pediatric house staff, a gastroenterologist, the hospital foodservice staff, a social worker, a pharmacist, and other specialists are typically involved as well. Close coordination and excellent communication are mandatory. Implementing the ketogenic diet is very time intensive for families and for clinicians.

Calculation of the Ketogenic Diet

The ketogenic diet is traditionally calculated at a 4:1 ketogenic ratio (4 g of fat for every 1 g of protein and carbohydrate), although this ratio may be modified to suit the needs of individual patients. Lower ratios may be necessary to meet some patients' protein requirements or to improve tolerability. During follow-up, the diet may be recalculated with an increased or decreased ketogenic ratio if necessary for improved seizure control or with increased calories and/or protein if necessary for growth.

The energy requirements of children with intractable epilepsy, especially those with impaired mobility, often differ substantially from other children. In preinitiation consultation, the dietitian collects and analyzes a 3-day food record, measures height and weight, and assesses activity level. After considering all of these variables, an energy recommendation for the ketogenic diet can be formulated.

The calculation of macronutrient requirements for the ketogenic diet is outlined in Table 49.1. Menus should be calculated by, or in consultation with, a registered dietitian with experience in the ketogenic diet. These calculations can be made by hand, but the process is greatly facilitated by ketogenic diet software (eg, KetoCalculator, Nutricia North America). Many families rely exclusively on menus calculated by the dietitian; some parents learn to calculate menus for their own children. Menus are calculated to the nearest g, and foods should be weighed to the nearest tenth of a g.

Table 49.1 Ketogenic Diet Macronutrient Calculations

1. Calculate calories needed per day (Example: 15 kg child × 68 kcal/kg/day = 1000 kcal per day)
2. Calculate number of dietary units needed per day[a] (For example, on a 4:1 diet, each dietary unit (4 g fat + 1 g protein or carbohydrate) = 40 kcal. (1000 kcal/day)/(40 kcal/unit) = 25 units/day)
3. Calculate the number of g of fat required per day (Fat: 25 units/day × 4 g/unit = 100 g per day)
4. Calculate the remainder of units/kcal, allotted to protein and carbohydrate (Protein and carbohydrate: 25 units/day × 1 g/unit = 25 g/day)
5. Maintain at least the minimum protein requirement (1 g/kg/day) (Protein: 1 g/kg/day × 15 kg = 15 g/day of protein)
6. Calculate remainder, allotted to carbohydrate (Carbohydrate: 25 g/day − 15 g/day protein = 10 g/day carbohydrate)
7. Divide the allotments into the number of meals per day

[a] The calories per dietary unit vary with the ratio of the ketogenic diet as follows: for a 2:1 diet, 22 kcal per dietary unit; for a 3:1 diet, 31 kcal per dietary unit; for a 4:1 diet, 40 kcal per dietary unit; and for a 5:1 diet, 49 kcal per dietary unit.

In constructing menus to satisfy the daily allotment of macronutrients, fat (from heavy cream, butter or margarine, oils, mayonnaise, and other sources) is a critical part of the equation. Heavy cream (36% fat) may be drunk, whipped, or flavored and frozen as ice cream. Consistent use of the same brand of heavy cream and careful calculations using nutritional tables[73] or standard software are mandatory. Once fat is allotted, protein sources (eg, meat, fish, poultry, eggs, and cheese) are added, taking into account the protein already present in cream. Carbohydrate-containing foods (eg, fruits and vegetables) are added last, taking into account the carbohydrates already present in cream, protein sources, and medications. Small quantities of certain "free foods" (eg, a lettuce leaf, 2 macadamia nuts, or 2 olives) may be added to increase dietary flexibility and palatability.

Ketogenic formulas are available for gastrostomy tube-fed children and formula-fed infants. They can also be used as meal replacements for patients eating by mouth. Ross Carbohydrate Free soy-based formula (RCF), which is combined with a glucose polymer (Polycose, Ross) and emulsified safflower oil (Microlipid, Novartis Nutrition) to yield the desired ketogenic ratio, is primarily used for tube feedings. There is also a milk-based formula (KetoCal, Nutricia North America), which is available in 3 versions: a powdered 4:1 ratio, a powdered 3:1 ratio, and a ready-to-consume 4:1 ratio that contains fiber. These formulas can be used for tube feedings and in patients eating by mouth.

Micronutrient Supplementation

The ketogenic diet is deficient in several vitamins (including vitamin D and B vitamins) and minerals (including magnesium, potassium, and calcium). Children on the ketogenic diet must receive supplements of these vitamins and minerals. Parents must understand that these supplements are not elective. Prior to understanding these vitamin requirements in the 1920s and 1930s, patients developed serious complications of vitamin and mineral deficiencies. Patients should receive an age-appropriate low-carbohydrate multivitamin every day, as well as a carbohydrate-free calcium supplement with vitamin D.[37] Because carnitine is important for fatty acid transport, carnitine concentrations should be routinely monitored. Valproate cotherapy may increase the risk of carnitine deficiency.[74] Patients who develop carnitine deficiency should receive carnitine supplementation.[9]

Initiation Protocol

Prior to scheduling diet initiation, parents should meet with the ketogenic dietitian. In addition to assessing the patient's anthropometric and nutritional status, the dietitian educates the family about the ketogenic diet and the initiation protocol, as well as psychosocial issues associated with the ketogenic diet. Laboratory studies (complete blood cell count, complete metabolic panel, lipid profile, pancreatic functions, electrolytes, uric acid, magnesium, phosphorus, carnitine, beta-hydroxybutyrate, and urinalysis) are performed to detect any possible contraindications and to establish baseline levels. The family should commit to maintain the diet under close supervision for at least 3 months to determine whether the diet will be effective.

Traditionally, the ketogenic diet is initiated with a 24- to 48-hour fast, followed by the introduction of ketogenic meals once the patient is in documented ketosis (large ketones on urine dipstick). In recent years, this approach has been called into question; some medical centers have introduced modified initiation protocols that do not involve fasting. Although some evidence suggests that fasting leads to a quicker onset of ketosis and seizure control,[75] other studies do not support this claim and show that nonfasting protocols may be more easily tolerated and may reduce the likelihood of some complications (including symptomatic acidosis, hypoglycemia, and electrolyte imbalances).[76-78] Thus, this approach remains controversial.

Whether fasting or not, standard practice is to initiate the ketogenic diet on an inpatient basis. However, 2 retrospective studies have shown that it is possible to successfully initiate the ketogenic diet on an outpatient basis.[78,79] Hospital admission has many benefits: it allows monitoring for adverse events, treatment of acute complications, and adjustment of medications. Furthermore, it provides an ideal opportunity for the keto team to meet with the patient and family to provide education and support.

If a classic fasting protocol is used (eg, Johns Hopkins), the patient is asked to fast after dinner the night prior to the admission. After 48 hours of fasting, ketogenic meals are introduced, first at one third of calculated calories for 24 hours, then at two thirds of calculated calories for 24 hours, then at full strength.[73] Alternatively, using 1 nonfasting protocol (Massachusetts General Hospital), full-strength ketogenic meals are given from day 1. Under another protocol (Children's Hospital of Pennsylvania), full-calorie meals are given from day 1 at a 1:1 ketogenic ratio. The ratio is then increased daily to 2:1, 3:1, and finally 4:1.[76]

During the course of the hospital admission, blood glucose concentration is generally monitored every 6 hours, or more often if hypoglycemia is detected, until the child is in ketosis and tolerating the full ketogenic diet. Once eating the diet and in ketosis, the child is monitored clinically and blood glucose measurements are performed only if there are symptoms of hypoglycemia. Unless the child is symptomatic, blood glucose concentrations as low as 25 mg/dL are not treated. Urine

VI

ketone dipsticks are typically checked every void. Serum bicarbonate is checked every 24 hours, and the prescribed potassium citrate dose is adjusted accordingly.

The traditional ketogenic diet involves restricted fluid intake on the basis of the observation that urine ketones may decrease with increased hydration. However, fluid intake generally does not affect serum beta-hydroxybutyrate, which is a more reliable indicator of ketosis than urine ketones.[80] To reduce the risk of dehydration and nephrolithiasis, many practitioners now recommend a nonfluid-restricted ketogenic diet.[69,77] Preliminary data suggest that fluid liberalization does not decrease efficacy.

During initiation, all children are supplemented with a multivitamin, calcium, and vitamin D supplement. On the basis of evidence of reduced risk of renal stones, children may also be prophylactically supplemented with potassium citrate.[56,70]

Maintenance and Follow-Up

A child on the ketogenic diet requires close supervision by his or her pediatric neurologist/epileptologist, dietitian, and pediatrician. Ketogenic diet clinic follow-up visits typically occur at 2 weeks, 1 month, 3 months, and every 3 months thereafter. More frequent visits may be necessary for infants to insure adequate nutrition and growth.[65] At these visits, height and weight are measured, and routine laboratory studies are performed, as during the preinitiation consult. The child's parents or caregivers should provide records of seizure frequency, food diaries, and records of urine dipsticks for ketones to the neurologist and the dietitian. The majority of the 2009 expert consensus panel suggested routine urine ketosis evaluation by parents several times per week.[37] Clinicians should ask about common adverse effects. The diet may be adjusted at these visits to optimize growth and seizure control.

Minor viral illnesses and more serious infections typically make it difficult to maintain ketosis and may increase metabolic acidosis. During intercurrent illnesses, breakthrough seizures can often be managed with a benzodiazepine pulse (eg, lorazepam or diazepam).

Concurrent Medications and Occult Carbohydrates

Most oral drug formulations and almost all syrups contain carbohydrates in the form of sugars, starches, or reduced carbohydrates such as glycerin. Parents and caregivers should be instructed to check with the dietitian before giving any new prescription or over-the-counter medications to children on the ketogenic diet. They should also be made aware that some toothpastes, lotions (including sun-screen), and shampoos contain carbohydrates, such as sorbitol, which can be absorbed transdermally. Hidden sources of carbohydrates should be considered if seizure exacerbations occur.

Likewise, physicians who care for children on the ketogenic diet should consult with the dietitian and with appropriate references regarding choice of medications.[81,82] A compounding pharmacy should be identified that can prepare carbohydrate-free drug formulations, and the hospital pharmacist may be contacted for inpatient hospital stays, including diet initiations. During inpatient hospital stays, physicians, pharmacists, and nursing staff should be reminded to avoid intravenous solutions containing dextrose, glucose, or other sugars. Any added carbohydrates in medication formulations must be included in diet calculations.

Adjusting the Diet for Optimal Seizure Control

The experienced pediatric neurologist and dietitian will learn to adjust the ketogenic diet like an antiepileptic drug. Breakthrough seizures may occur at times of day when ketosis is suboptimal; in these cases, the diet may be adjusted to optimize seizure control. For example, breakthrough seizures on waking in the morning might be treated with a small, high-fat snack at bedtime (eg, olives) to help sustain ketosis overnight.

Discontinuation of the Ketogenic Diet

According to the 2009 expert consensus panel, consideration to discontinue the diet should be given to children who have not experienced a reduction in seizure frequency after 3 months or who have experienced 2 years of seizure freedom; however, longer duration may be necessary for children with tuberous sclerosis complex, GLUT-1, or PDHD.[37] Occasionally, children who experience significant improvement stay on the ketogenic diet for many years.[64] Such patients should be monitored at a major pediatric epilepsy center.

Weaning by reducing the ketogenic ratio should take place gradually over several months. If seizures recur during the weaning process, the diet can be immediately reincreased to the original ratio without necessitating hospital admission. A recent retrospective study of 557 children initiated on the ketogenic diet found that 80% of children who reached seizure freedom remained seizure free after the diet had been discontinued.[83] The risk of recurrence was highest for children with abnormal electroencephalograms within 12 months of discontinuation, structural brain abnormalities on magnetic resonance imaging, and tuberous sclerosis complex. However, the majority of patients who experienced a recurrence of seizures after discontinuation were able to regain seizure control with the ketogenic diet or anticonvulsants.

Alternative Dietary Therapy

Although the ketogenic diet has been used for more than 90 years with good efficacy, many patients are unable to tolerate its restrictions and find it unpalatable. Therefore, several variations on the classic ketogenic diet have been introduced.

In the 1970s, Huttenlocher introduced the MCT oil version of the ketogenic diet.[84] Because MCT oil is, gram-for-gram, more ketogenic than other fats, the MCT diet allows liberalized quantities of protein and carbohydrate. Recently, a randomized controlled trial found no difference in efficacy and tolerability between the MCT oil diet and classic ketogenic diet.[85] However, the MCT oil diet tends to have increased adverse effects of bloating, nausea, and vomiting.

In 2002, the low-glycemic index treatment (LGIT) was developed at Massachusetts General Hospital as a liberalized alternative to the traditional ketogenic diet.[86] This approach permits greater total intake of carbohydrate than the traditional ketogenic diet (40–60 g/day) but limits foods to those with a glycemic index of <50 relative to glucose (ie, foods that produce a relatively low increase in blood glucose per g of carbohydrate). In 2 recent retrospective studies, the efficacy of LGIT approached that of the ketogenic diet but with fewer adverse effects. In 1 study of 15 patients, 57% of the population had ≥50% reduction from baseline seizure frequency after a mean follow-up period of 15 months.[87] In a larger series of 76 children, 66% of patients had >50% reduction from baseline seizure frequency at 12 months.[88] LGIT has also proved effective in patients with epilepsy associated with tuberous sclerosis complex and Angelman syndrome. In a retrospective study of LGIT in 15 patients with tuberous sclerosis complex, 47% experienced a >50% reduction in seizure frequency after 6 months.[89] In a prospective study of LGIT in 6 children with Angelman syndrome, 67% experienced a >90% reduction in seizure frequency after 4 months.[90]

The modified Atkins diet, developed at Johns Hopkins Hospital as another alternative to the classic ketogenic diet, was first described in 2003.[91] This approach initially restricts carbohydrates to 10 g/day in children and 15 g/day in adults during the first month of treatment and then gradually increases daily carbohydrate intake by 5 g/month to the limit of 30 g/day. Once implementation is complete, most patients receive a 1:1 to 2:1 ketogenic diet.[92] In a study of 20 children with intractable epilepsy, the 6-month efficacy of the modified Atkins diet was similar to that observed in the ketogenic diet: approximately one third of patients experienced >90% reduction in seizure frequency, one third experienced 50% to 90% reduction, and one third experienced <50% reduction.[93] The modified Atkins diet has also proved effective in adults with intractable epilepsy.[94,95]

Reductions in seizure frequency on LGIT and modified Atkins diet suggest that successful dietary therapy for epilepsy may not require ketosis at the level once thought necessary. These observations have interesting implications for the possible mechanisms of action of the ketogenic diet.

Conclusions

The ketogenic diet is the most effective available treatment for intractable epilepsy, although it carries with it a significant risk of adverse effects. An expert keto team is required to ameliorate this risk and to guide patients and families through diet initiation and maintenance. Parents should attempt the ketogenic diet only with the guidance of an experienced dietitian, neurologist, and support staff.

References

1. Bailey EE, Pfeifer HH, Thiele EA. The use of diet in the treatment of epilepsy. *Epilepsy Behav.* 2005;6(1):4-8
2. Wheless JW. History and origin of the ketogenic diet. In: Stafstrom CE, Rho JM, eds. *Epilepsy and the Ketogenic Diet.* Totowa, NJ: Humana Press; 2004:31-50
3. Kossoff EH, McGrogan JR. Worldwide use of the ketogenic diet. *Epilepsia.* 2005;46(2):280-289
4. Cullingford TE. Molecular regulation of ketogenesis. In: Stafstrom CE, Rho JM, eds. *Epilepsy and the Ketogenic Diet.* Totowa, NJ: Humana Press; 2004:201-215
5. Nordli DR, DeVivo DC. Effects of the ketogenic diet on cerebral energy metabolism. In: Stafstrom CE, Rho JM, eds. *Epilepsy and the Ketogenic Diet.* Totowa, NJ: Humana Press; 2004:179-184
6. Mitchell GA, Fukao T. Inborn errors of ketone body metabolism. In: Scriver CR, Beaudet AL, Sly WS, Valle D, eds. *The Metabolic and Molecular Bases of Inherited Disease.* New York, NY: The McGraw-Hill Companies Inc; 2001:2327-2356
7. Sankar R, Sotero de Menezes M. Metabolic and endocrine aspects of the ketogenic diet. *Epilepsy Res.* 1999;37(3):191-201
8. Table: Williamson DH. Ketone body metabolism during development. *Fed Proc.* 1985;44:2342-2346
9. De Vivo DC, Bohin TP, Coulter DL, et al. L-carnitine supplementation in childhood epilepsy: current perspectives. *Epilepsia.* 1998;39(11):1216-1225
10. Wilder RM. The effects of ketonemia on the course of epilepsy. *Mayo Clin Bull.* 1921;2:307-308
11. Likhodii S, Nylen K, Burnham WM. Acetone as an anticonvulsant. *Epilepsia.* 2008;49(Suppl 8):83-86
12. Thio LL, Wong M, Yamada KA. Ketone bodies do not directly alter excitatory or inhibitory hippocampal synaptic transmission. *Neurology.* 2000;54(2):325-331
13. Kim DY, Davis LM, Sullivan PG, et al. Ketone bodies are protective against oxidative stress in neocortical neurons. *J Neurochem.* 2007;101(5):1316-1326

VI

14. Yudkoff M, Daikhin Y, Melø TM, Nissim I, Sonnewald U, Nissim I. The ketogenic diet and brain metabolism of amino acids: relationship to the anticonvulsant effect. *Annu Rev Nutr.* 2007;27:415-430

15. Bough KJ, Wetherington J, Hassel B, et al. Mitochondrial biogenesis in the anticonvulsant mechanism of the ketogenic diet. *Ann Neurol.* 2006;60(2):223-235

16. Yellen G. Ketone bodies, glycolysis, and KATP channels in the mechanism of the ketogenic diet. *Epilepsia.* 2008;49(Suppl 8):80-82

17. Greene AE, Todorova MT, Seyfried TN. Perspectives on the metabolic management of epilepsy through dietary reduction of glucose and elevation of ketone bodies. *J Neurochem.* 2003;86(3):529-537

18. Stafstrom CE, Ockuly, JC, Murphree L, Valley MT, Roopra A, Sutula TP. Anticonvulsant and antiepileptic actions of 2-deoxy-Dglucose in epilepsy models. *Ann Neurol.* 2009;65(4):435-477

19. McDaniel SS, Rensing NR, Thio LL, Yamada KA, Wong M. The ketogenic diet inhibits the mammalian target of rapamycin (mTOR) pathway. *Epilepsia.* 2011;52(3):e7-e11

20. Xu XP, Erichsen D, Börjesson SI, Dahlin M, Amark P, Elinder F. Polyunsaturated fatty acids and cerebrospinal fluid from children on the ketogenic diet open a voltage-gated K channel: a putative mechanism of antiseizure activity. *Epilepsy Res.* 2008;80(1):57-66

21. Taha AY, Ryan MA, Cunnane SC. Despite transient ketosis, the classic high-fat ketogenic diet induces marked changes in fatty acid metabolism in rats. *Metabolism.* 2005;54(9):1127-1132

22. Neal EG, Chaffe H, Schwartz RH, et al. The ketogenic diet for the treatment of childhood epilepsy: a randomised controlled trial. *Lancet Neurol.* 2008;7(6):500-506

23. Maydell BV, Wyllie E, Akhtar N, et al. Efficacy of the ketogenic diet in focal versus generalized seizures. *Pediatr Neurol.* 2001;25(3):208-212

24. Dressler A, Stöcklin B, Reithofer E, et al. Long-term outcome and tolerability of the ketogenic diet in drug-resistant childhood epilepsy—The Austrian experience. *Seizure.* 2010;19(7):404-408

25. Trevathan E. Infantile spasms and Lennox-Gastaut syndrome. *J Child Neurol.* 2002;17(Suppl2):2S9-2S22

26. Bergqvist AG, Chee CM, Lutchka LM, Brooks-Kayal AR. Treatment of Acquired Epileptic Aphasia With the Ketogenic Diet. *J Child Neurol.* 1999;14(11):696-701

27. Korff C, Laux L, Kelley K, Goldstein J, Koh S, Nordli D. Dravet syndrome (severe myoclonic epilepsy in infancy): a retrospective study of 16 patients. *J Child Neurol.* 2007;22(2):185-194

28. Caraballo RH, Cersosimo RO, Sakr D, Cresta A, Escobal N, Fejerman N. Ketogenic diet in patients with Dravet syndrome. *Epilepsia.* 2005;46(9):1539-1544

29. Kilaru S, Bergqvist AG. Current treatment of myoclonic astatic epilepsy: clinical experience at the Children's Hospital of Philadelphia. *Epilepsia.* 2007;48(9):1703-1707

30. Caraballo RH, Cerosimo RO, Sakr D, Cresta A, Escobal N, Fejerman N. Ketogenic diet in patients with myoclonic-astatic epilepsy. *Epileptic Disord.* 2006;8(2):151-155

31. Numis AL, Yellen MB, Chu-Shore CJ, Pfeifer HH, Thiele EA. The relationship of ketosis and growth to the efficacy of the ketogenic diet in infantile spasms. *Epilepsy Res.* 2011;96(1-2):172-175

32. Hong AM, Turner Z, Hamdy RF, Kossoff EH. Infantile spasms treated with the ketogenic diet: prospective single-center experience in 104 consecutive infants. *Epilepsia.* 2010;51(8):1403-1407

33. Kossoff EH, Hedderick EF, Turner Z, Freeman JM. A case-control evaluation of the ketogenic diet versus ACTH for new-onset infantile spasms. *Epilepsia.* 2008;49(9):1504-1509

34. Groomes LB, Pyzik PL, Turner Z, Dorward JL, Goode VH, Kossoff EH. Do patients with absence epilepsy respond to ketogenic diets? *J Child Neurol.* 2011;26(2):160-165

35. Coppola G, Klepper J, Ammendola E, et al. The effects of the ketogenic diet in refractory partial seizures with reference to tuberous sclerosis. *Eur J Pediatr Neurol.* 2006;10(3):148-151

36. Kossoff EG, Thiele EA, Pfeifer HH, McGrogan JR, Freeman JM. Tuberous sclerosis complex and the ketogenic diet. *Epilepsia.* 2005;46(10):1684-1686

37. Kossoff EH, Zupec-Kania BA, Amark PE, et al. Optimal clinical management of children receiving the ketogenic diet: Recommendations of the International Ketogenic Diet Study Group. *Epilepsia.* 2009;50(2):304-317

38. Sperling MR, Nei M. The ketogenic diet in adults. In: Stafstrom CE, Rho JM, eds. *Epilepsy and the Ketogenic Diet.* Totowa, NJ: Humana Press; 2004:103-109

39. Mady MA, Kossoff EH, McGregor AL, Wheless JW, Pyzik PL, Freeman JM. The ketogenic diet: adolescents can do it, too. *Epilepsia.* 2003;44(6):847-851

40. Sirven J, Whedon B, Caplan D, et al. The ketogenic diet for intractable epilepsy in adults: preliminary results. *Epilepsia.* 1999;40(12):1721-1726

41. Hosain SA, La Vega-Talbott M, Solomon GE. Ketogenic diet in pediatric epilepsy patients with gastrostomy feeding. *Pediatr Neurol.* 2005;32(2):81-83

42. Kossoff EH, McGrogan JR, Freeman JM. Benefits of an all-liquid ketogenic diet. *Epilepsia.* 2004;45(9):1163

43. Nordli DR Jr., Kuroda MM, Carroll J, et al. Experience with the ketogenic diet in infants. *Pediatrics.* 2001;108(1):129-133

44. Weber TA, Antognetti MR, Stacpoole PW. Caveats when considering ketogenic diets for the treatment of pyruvate dehydrogenase complex deficiency. *J Pediatr.* 2001;138(3):390-395

45. Wexler ID, Hemalatha SG, McConnell J, et al. Outcome of pyruvate dehydrogenase deficiency treated with ketogenic diets. Studies in patients with identical mutations. *Neurology.* 1997;49(6):1655-1661

46. Leen WG, Klepper J, Verbeek MM, et al. Glucose transporter-1 deficiency syndrome: the expanding clinical and genetic spectrum of a treatable disorder. *Brain.* 2010;133(Pt 3):655-670

47. Klepper J. Glucose transporter deficiency syndrome (GLUT1DS) and the ketogenic diet. *Epilepsia.* 2008;49(Suppl 8):46-49

VI

48. Barañano KW, Hartman AL. The ketogenic diet: uses in epilepsy and other neurologic illnesses. *Curr Treat Options Neurol.* 2008;10(6):410-419

49. Yancy WS Jr, Foy M, Chalecki AM, Vernon MC, Westman EC. A low-carbohydrate, ketogenic diet to treat type 2 diabetes. *Nutr Metab (Lond).* 2005;2:34

50. Mavropoulos JC, Yancy WS, Hepburn J, Westman EC. The effects of a low-carbohydrate, ketogenic diet on the polycystic ovary syndrome: a pilot study. *Nutr and Metab (Lond).* 2005;2:35

51. Yaroslavsky Y, Stahl Z, Belmaker RH. Ketogenic diet in bipolar illness. *Bipolar Disord.* 2002;4(1):75

52. Henderson CB, Filloux FM, Alder SC, et al. Efficacy of the ketogenic diet as a treatment option for epilepsy: meta-analysis. *J Child Neurol.* 2006;21(3):193-198

53. Pulsifer MB, Gordon JM, Brandt J, Vining EPG, Freeman JM. Effects of ketogenic diet on development and behavior: preliminary report of a prospective study. *Dev Med Child Neurol.* 2001;43(5):301-306

54. DeVivo DC, Pagliara AS, Prensky AL. Ketotic hypoglycemia and the ketogenic diet. *Neurology.* 1973; 23(6):640-649

55. Takeoka M, Riviello JJ Jr, Pfeifer H, Thiele EA. Concomitant treatment with topiramate and ketogenic diet in pediatric epilepsy. *Epilepsia.* 2002;43(9):1072-1075

56. Paul E, Conant KD, Dunne IE, et al. Urolithiasis on the ketogenic diet with concurrent topiramate or zonisamide therapy. *Epilepsy Res.* 2010;90(1-2):151-156

57. Ballaban-Gil K, Callahan C, O'Dell C, Pappo M, Moshé S, Shinnar S. Complications of the ketogenic diet. *Epilepsia.* 1998(7);39:744-748

58. Lyczkowski DA, Pfeifer HH, Ghosh S, Thiele EA. Safety and tolerability of the ketogenic diet in pediatric epilepsy: effects of valproate combination therapy. *Epilepsia.* 2005;46(9):1533-1538

59. Kang HC, Cheung DE, Kim DW, Kim HD. Early- and late-onset complications of the ketogenic diet for intractable epilepsy. *Epilepsia.* 2004;45(9):1116-1123

60. Woody RC, Steele RW, Knapple WL, Pilkington NS. Impaired neutrophil function in children with seizures treated with the ketogenic diet. *J Pediatr.* 1989;115(3):427-430

61. Stewart WA, Gordon K, Camfield P. Acute pancreatitis causing death in a child on the ketogenic diet. *J Child Neurol.* 2001;16(9):682

62. Best TH, Franz DN, Gilbert DL, Nelson DP, Epstein MR. Cardiac complications in patients on the ketogenic diet. *Neurology.* 2000;4(12):2328-2330

63. Neal EG, Chaffe HM, Edwards N, Lawson MS, Schwartz RH, Cross JH. Growth of children on classical and medium-chain triglyceride ketogenic diets. *Pediatrics.* 2008;122(2):e334-e340

64. Groesbeck DK, Bluml RM, Kossoff EH. Long-term use of the ketogenic diet in the treatment of epilepsy. *Dev Med Child Neurol.* 2006;48(12):978-981

65. Vining EP, Pyzik P, McGrogan J, et al. Growth of children on the ketogenic diet. *Dev Med Child Neurol.* 2002;44(12):796-802

66. Williams S, Basualdo-Hammond C, Curtis R, Schuller R. Growth retardation in children with epilepsy on the ketogenic diet: a retrospective chart review. *J Am Diet Assoc.* 2002;102(3):405-407

67. Patel A, Pyzik PL, Turner Z, Rubenstein JE, Kossoff EH. Long-term outcomes of children treated with the ketogenic diet in the past. *Epilepsia.* 2010;51(7):1277-1282

68. Furth SL, Casey JC, Pyzik PL, et al. Risk factors for urolithiasis in children on the ketogenic diet. *Pediatr Nephrol.* 2000;15(1-2):125-128

69. Kielb S, Koo HP, Bloom DA, Gaerber GJ. Nephrolithiasis associated with the ketogenic diet. *J Urol.* 2000; 164(2):464-466

70. McNally MA, Pyzik PL, Rubenstein JE, Hamdy RF, Kossoff EH. Empiric use of potassium citrate reduces kidney-stone incidence with the ketogenic diet. *Pediatrics.* 2009;124(2):e300-e304

71. Nizamuddin J, Turner Z, Rubenstein JE, Pyzik PL, Kossoff EH. Management and risk factors for dyslipidemia with the ketogenic diet. *J Child Neurol.* 2008;23(7):758-761

72. Bergqvist AC, Schall JI, Stallings VA, Zemel BS. Progressive bone mineral content loss in children with intractable epilepsy treated with the ketogenic diet. *Am J Clin Nutr.* 2008;88(6):1678-1684

73. Freeman JM, Kossoff EH, Freeman JB, Kelly MT. *The Ketogenic Diet: A Treatment for Children and Others with Epilepsy.* 4th ed. New York, NY: Demos Medical Publishing; 2007

74. Coppola G, Epifanio G, Auricchio G, Federico RR, Resicato G, Pascotto A. Plasma free carnitine in epilepsy children, adolescents and young adults treated with old and new antiepileptic drugs with or without ketogenic diet. *Brain Dev.* 2006;28(6):358-365

75. Kossoff EH, Laux LC, Blackford R. When do seizures usually improve with the ketogenic diet? *Epilepsia.* 2008;49(2):329-333

76. Bergqvist AG, Schall JI, Gallagher PR, Cnaan A, Stallings VA. Fasting versus gradual initiation of the ketogenic diet: a prospective, randomized clinical trial of efficacy. *Epilepsia.* 2005;46(11):1810-1819

77. Kim DW, Kang HC, Park JC, Kim HD. Benefits of the nonfasting ketogenic diet compared with the initial fasting ketogenic diet. *Pediatrics.* 2004;114(6):1627-1630

78. Wirrell EC, Darwish HZ, Williams-Dyjur C, Blackman M, Lange V. Is a fast necessary when initiating the ketogenic diet? *J Child Neurol.* 2002;17(3):179-182

79. Vaisleib II, Buchhalter JR, Zupanc ML. Ketogenic diet; outpatient initiation, without fluid, or caloric restrictions. *Pediatr Neurol.* 2004;31(3):198-202

80. Gilbert DL, Pyzik PL, Freeman JM. The ketogenic diet: seizure control correlates better with serum beta-hydroxybutyrate than with urine ketones. *J Child Neurol.* 2000;15(12):787-790

81. Karvelas G, Lebel D, Carmant L. The carbohydrate and caloric content of drugs [Appendix]. In: Stafstrom CE, Rho JM, eds. *Epilepsy and the Ketogenic Diet.* Totowa, NJ: Humana Press; 2004:311-344

82. McGhee B, Katyal N. Avoid unnecessary drug-related carbohydrates for patients consuming the ketogenic diet. *J Am Diet Assoc.* 2001;101(1):87-101

83. Martinez CC, Pyzik PL, Kossoff EH. Discontinuing the ketogenic diet in seizure-free children: recurrence and risk factors. *Epilepsia.* 2007;48(1):187-190

84. Huttenlocher PR, Wilbourn AJ, Signore JM. Medium-chain triglycerides as a therapy for intractable childhood epilepsy. *Neurology.* 1971;21(11):1097-1103

VI

85. Neal EG, Chaffe H, Schwartz RH, et al. A randomized trial of classical and medium-chain triglyceride ketogenic diets in the treatment of childhood epilepsy. *Epilepsia*. 2009;50(5):1109-1117

86. Pfeifer HH, Thiele EA. Low glycemic index treatment: a liberalized ketogenic diet for treatment of intractable epilepsy. *Neurology*. 2005;65:1810-1812

87. Coppola G, D'Aniello A, Messana T, et al. Low glycemic index diet in children and young adults with refractory epilepsy: first Italian experience. *Seizure*. 2011;20(7):526-528

88. Muzykewicz DA, Lyczkowski DA, Memon N, Conant KD, Pfeifer HH, Thiele EA. Efficacy, safety, and tolerability of the low glycemic index treatment in pediatric epilepsy. *Epilepsia*. 2009;50(5):1118-1126

89. Larson AM, Pfeifer HH, Thiele EA. Low glycemic index treatment for epilepsy in tuberous sclerosis complex. 2012;99(1-2):180-182

90. Thibert RL, Pfeifer HH, Larson AM, et al. Low glycemic index treatment for seizures in Angelman syndrome. 2012;53(9):1498-1502

91. Kossoff EH, Krauss GL, McGrogan JR, Freeman JM. Efficacy of the Atkins diet as therapy for intractable epilepsy. *Neurology*. 2003;61(12):1789-1791

92. Kossoff EH, Dorward JL. The modified Atkins diet. *Epilepsia*. 2008;49(Suppl 8):37-41

93. Kossoff EH, McGrogan JR, Bluml RM, Pillas DJ, Rubenstein JE, Vining EP. A modified Atkins diet is effective for the treatment of pediatric epilepsy. *Epilepsia*. 2006;47(2):421-424

94. Kossoff EH, Rowley H, Sinha SR, Vining EP. A prospective study of the modified Atkins diet for intractable epilepsy in adults. *Epilepsia*. 2008;49(2):316-319

95. Carrette E, Vonck K, de Herdt V, et al. A pilot trial with modified Atkins' diet in adult patients with refractory epilepsy. *Clin Neurol Neurosurg*. 2008;110(8):797-803

Chapter 50

Nutrition and Oral Health

Introduction

The oral health of children living in resource-rich countries has improved over the last 2 decades in a remarkable way, but there are many children who continue to suffer the ill effects of dental decay.[1] Dental caries is a preventable disease that still affects approximately 42% of children 2 to 11 years old.[2] The prevalence of early childhood caries (ECC) has increased significantly in children 2 to 5 years of age.[2] By kindergarten age, 40% of children have experienced ECC.[3] It has been reported that ECC is 5 times more common than asthma.[4] However, segments of the population continue to experience a disproportionate amount of caries and have a difficult time obtaining care. Children who experience ECC tend to remain at high risk of caries in the primary as well as the permanent dentition.[5] Children have a 32 times greater chance of having caries by 3 years of age if they come from a low socioeconomic background, eat sugary foods, and have a mother with a low education level.[6]

Dental Caries—an Infectious Disease

The group of cariogenic bacteria that is well established to have the strongest association with caries is *Streptococcus mutans*, which metabolizes sucrose to lactic acid. These bacteria are detectable in children's mouths on the oral mucosa prior to the eruption of the primary teeth.[7,8] The predominant source of these bacteria seems to be the mother's own saliva. Studies have demonstrated fidelity of maternal transfer of *S mutans* as high as 71% and as low as 41%.[9,10] Dental caries is an infectious disease, because children colonized with acid-producing bacteria have a greater risk of developing caries. These findings give support for prenatal counseling to establish a healthy oral cavity to reduce the mother's overall concentrations of *S mutans*.

As carbohydrate intake increases, *S mutans* colonizes in plaque and metabolizes carbohydrates, creating an acidic environment. This provides for a drop in the plaque pH, and demineralization of the enamel can occur. Saliva, a pH buffering agent, also contains calcium and phosphate and promotes remineralization of enamel by hydroxyapatite formation. In the presence of fluoride, the hydroxyapatite in the outer layer of enamel is transformed into fluoridated hydroxyapatite and fluorapatite, which are less soluble than hydroxyapatite in an acidic environment. If demineralization exceeds remineralization over time, cavitation of the enamel

VI

surface will occur, leading to frank caries. As the carious lesion continues to grow in size, eventually the pulp/nerve of the tooth will become involved, leading to pain, infection, early tooth loss, and potential crowding problems. Severe dental infections can lead to hospitalizations and emergency surgeries for removal of infected teeth.

Dietary Influences

ECC, in many cases, is thought to be the result of the inappropriate use of a bottle or sippy cup while sleeping or its unsupervised use during the day with a liquid other than water. Early childhood caries usually affects the maxillary anterior teeth first, followed by the primary molars. The lower anterior teeth are usually not involved because of the protective nature of the tongue. A study by Kaste and Gift[11] demonstrated that approximately 95% of children 6 months to 5 years of age have used a bottle at some time, with nearly 20% of these children using a bottle in bed with contents other than water. More than 8% of children 2 to 5 years of age still used a bottle. Most infant formulas have been shown to be acidogenic and promote the development of caries.[12]

There have also been reports of ECC associated with at-will breastfeeding. The role at-will breastfeeding plays in contributing to ECC has been controversial.[13] Although there have been some studies that have implicated this practice with caries, this may be misleading if the remainder of the child's diet is overlooked. On the basis of an in vitro study by Erickson et al[14] (Table 50.1), human milk was demonstrated to be a poor buffering agent when acid from other carbohydrate sources were added. With the addition of sucrose to human milk, the rate of in vitro caries formation was faster than for sucrose alone. It was concluded from this study that human milk alone was not cariogenic. However, if a child is given a sugar-rich food in combination with on-demand breastfeeding, the combination is highly cariogenic. Once the first tooth erupts, the American Academy of Pediatric Dentistry (AAPD) recommends that breastfeeding should be limited to normal meal times and not at will while sleeping.[15] Because of the decrease in salivary flow during sleep, there is a decrease in the clearance of sugars from formula, human milk, juices, etc, by saliva in the mouth. This, in-turn, allows these substrates to have an increased cariogenic effect.

Table 50.1.
Relative Decay Potential of Beverages[12,14]

Source	Relative Decay Potential
Standards	
Water	0.00
10% sucrose solution	1.00
Human milk	
Human milk alone	0.01
Human milk with 10% sucrose	1.30
Formula[a]	
Soy-based, lactose free	0.68-1.11
Standard cow milk	0.51-0.62
Extensively hydrolyzed	0.01
Other beverages	
Yo-J[b] (yogurt-based drink)	0.32
Apple juice	0.80
Orange juice	0.85
Grape juice	0.74
Fruit drinks (10% juices)	0.93
Soft drinks ("soda" or "pop")	1.05

[a]The Committee on Nutrition recommends the use of iron-supplemented (not low-iron supplemented) formulas for infants being fed formula.

[b] Kemps LLC, St Paul, MN.

VI

In the United States, by 1 year of age, almost 90% of infants have been introduced to fruit juice. Some juice products contain more sugar than some soft drinks.[16] Juice should be limited to 4 to 6 oz per day in children younger than 5 years[17,18] (see Chapter 6). Sucrose, glucose, and fructose found in fruit juices are probably the main sugars associated with ECC. A study by Neff[19] suggests that fructose and glucose are as cariogenic as sucrose in their abilities to cause a decrease in the oral pH. In addition, starchy foods, such as breads or biscuits, have been shown to cause a variable pH decrease. As the levels of starch increased, the acid production found in plaque also increased.[20]

The frequency of eating and drinking also plays a role in the decay process for children. Children who are constantly snacking and drinking sugar-containing substances are at higher risk of developing caries than are children who eat 3 meals and few snacks per day. The more frequent the dietary intake, the greater the risk of caries. The amount of calories that can be attributed to sugars has increased by 16% between 1982 and 1996. Today, 155 pounds of sugar are eaten by the average person annually, which is equivalent to 39 teaspoons per day.[16] Consumption of soft drinks has been on the rise, with 56% to 85% of school-aged children consuming at least 1 serving of soda each day and some children consuming even greater amounts.[21] Between 1989 and 1995, the consumption of carbonated beverages increased by 41% in children 12 to 17 years of age. The increased intake of soda, which has no nutritional value, is associated with a decreased consumption of milk and a decreased intake of important nutrients, such as vitamin A, calcium, magnesium, and B vitamins.[16] Between 1965 and 1996, the intake of dairy products decreased by as much as 30% while the intake of soft drinks doubled.[22] Marshall and coauthors documented that the modern consumption of soda pop, powdered beverages, and 100% fruit juice was associated with increased caries risk.[23] The consumption of sports and energy drinks by children and adolescents has also increased. Most sports and energy drinks have a pH in the acidic range that causes erosion of enamel (pH 3-4). Citric acid incorporated in these types of beverages is highly erosive to tooth structure causing irreversible demineralization.[24]

Given the high sugar content and highly acidic nature of soft drinks, demineralization of the teeth occurs in the presence of bacteria, eventually leading to tooth decay.[21] Studies by Erickson et al (Table 50.1)[12,14] have demonstrated the decay potential of several beverages, including infant formulas. Parents must be reminded that they should not allow their child to continually drink or sip out of a bottle or sippy cup containing these sweetened drinks. Consumption of these drinks should be confined to meal or snack times only. Parents also need to be vigilant about giving their children sugar containing vitamins, dried fruit, and sticky candies without proper toothbrushing and flossing.

The teeth are most susceptible to caries during first few years after eruption because of their immaturity. In addition to the lack of maturation, there is a possibility that the teeth may have structural defects or hypoplastic areas. This can be the result of hereditary diseases, birth trauma, preterm birth, low birth weight, infections, malnutrition, metabolic disorders, and chemical toxicity.[25] Enamel defects may be common in newborn infants, ranging from 12.8% in children weighing >2500 g to more than 62% in those born preterm with very low birth weight (<1500 g).[26] In children who had been intubated at birth, left-sided defects of the maxillary anterior teeth occurred twice as frequently as right-sided defects. Defects were noted to have occurred in 85% of the 40 intubated children in this study, compared with approximately 22% of nonintubated children.[27] Chronically ill children are also at high risk of developing ECC. These children can have increased enamel hypoplastic areas as well. In addition, many of these children may be comforted with bottles containing sweetened liquids or frequently ingest medications that have high sugar content. This allows the teeth to be surrounded by a constant source of sugar, leading to rapid demineralization of the enamel. Enamel erosions have also been reported in children with gastroesophageal reflux disease.[28]

Poor nutritional intake has resulted not only in ECC but also an increase in childhood obesity. In 2007-2008, 31.7% of children 2 to 19 years of age were above the 85th percentile for BMI (classified as overweight), 16.9% were above the 95th percentile (classified as obese), and 11.9% were above the 97th percentile. This high prevalence of obesity is also seen at very young ages, as 9.5% of infants and toddlers were at or above the 95th percentile for weight for length. The newest data from 2009-2010 reveal that the prevalence of obesity in children and adolescents was 16.9%—unchanged from 2007-2008.[29] This increase in weight can partially be attributed to foods that are packaged for convenience, making them easy targets for snacking. Many of them contain sucrose and other refined carbohydrates that are highly cariogenic, leading not only to weight gain but also caries formation.[30] In counseling these patients, it is important that bad dietary habits be dealt with as early as possible to limit the possible lifetime implications.

The Costs Are Enormous

The prevalence of caries in children 3 to 5 years old participating in the US Head Start program has been reported as high as 90% in some groups.[31] Untreated dental decay leads to pain, poor eating, infection, speech problems, crowding of the permanent teeth, and self-esteem issues. In a study by Acs,[32] 8.7% of children with ECC weighed less than 80% of their ideal weight, compared with only 1.7% of the control group. In addition, 19.1% of children with ECC were in the 10th percentile or less for weight, compared with only 7% of the control group. ECC has also been implicated in contributing to other health problems, such as otitis media.

Treatment for ECC often has to be completed in the operating room under general anesthesia because of the amount of treatment required and the situational anxiety of the child. The costs of dental treatment in a hospital setting can be very expensive. Treatment of ECC is expensive to society, and the child's overall health and well-being can be compromised.

Nutritional Effects

The teeth may reflect nutritional disturbances that occur during their formation. Tooth development begins during the second month of embryonic life, and by 8 years of age, the crowns of all permanent teeth except the third molars are formed. Enamel and dentin have no powers of biologic regeneration, and any defect in their structure is permanent.

A published longitudinal study[33] of Peruvian children confirmed previous studies in animals and indirect epidemiologic evidence in humans that suggested a cause-and-effect relationship between early malnutrition and increased dental caries. The study also reported the eruption of primary teeth was significantly delayed.

Vitamin A deficiency during tooth formation is reported to interfere with calcification and result in hypoplasia of the enamel.[34] The effect of vitamin C deficiency in humans occurs chiefly in the gingival and periodontal tissues. The gingiva is bright red with a swollen, smooth, shiny surface that may become boggy, ulcerate, and bleed.[34] When vitamin D deficiency occurs during childhood, eruption of the deciduous and permanent teeth is delayed, and the sequence of eruption is disturbed. Histologically, widening of the predentin layer, the presence of interglobular dentin, and interference with enamel formation has been reported. Some authors report hypoplasia of the enamel with a symmetrical distribution of thinning and pitting enamel defects.[34] In riboflavin deficiency, glossitis begins with soreness of the tip and lateral margins of the tongue. The tongue surface appears reddened and coarsely granular. The lips are pale, and cheilosis develops at the oral commissures.[34] Niacin deficiency leads to pellagra. In the acute stages, the oral mucosa becomes fiery red and painful, accompanied by profuse salivation. As pellagra progresses, the epithelium of the tongue sloughs[34] (see Chapter 21.II).

Fluoride: Background

Water fluoridation was named as one of the top 10 public health achievements in the 20th century by the Centers for Disease Control and Prevention. Since the introduction of water fluoridation and topical fluorides, there has been a significant reduction in caries. Studies have shown that caries in the primary teeth of children have decreased by as much as 60% with fluoridation. Fluoride has been shown to reduce dental decay by 3 specific mechanisms: (1) it reduces the solubility of enamel; (2) it reduces the bacteria's ability to produce acid; and (3) it promotes remineralization.[35,36] At one time, fluoride was thought to exert a pre-eruptive effect on teeth through the use of prenatal fluoride, but now it is generally accepted that its main benefit is topical in nature.[37] Systemically, fluoride exerts its topical effects through secretion into the saliva from the salivary glands.

Fluoridation protects more than 195 million individuals throughout the United States. As of 2008, approximately 72.4% of the US water public supply was fluoridated.[38] The benefits of fluoridation extend across all ethnic groups and income and education levels. The cost of water fluoridation is $0.50/person annually in larger communities and up to $3.00/person annually in smaller communities.[35]

Fluoride Supplements

For children living in a fluoride-deficient area, fluoride supplements may be of some benefit. Table 50.2 shows the most recent guidelines on fluoride supplementation that have been accepted by the American Academy of Pediatric Dentistry and AAP.[36,39]

Table 50.2.
Fluoride Supplementation Schedule[a,36,39]

Age	Fluoride Concentration in Local Water Supply, ppm		
	<0.3	0.3-0.6	>0.6
Birth–6 mo	0.00	0.00	0.00
6 mo–3 y	0.25	0.00	0.00
3–6 y	0.50	0.25	0.00
6 y–at least 16 y	1.00	0.50	0.00

[a] Must know fluoride values of drinking water prior to making a prescription. All values are mg of fluoride supplement/day.

When considering whether a fluoride supplement is needed, more time should be spent considering all sources of fluoride that a child may have access to on a given day. Allowing the criterion of no fluoride in the community water to dictate the need for a fluoride prescription may be premature and lead to an overall underestimation of the child's total fluoride intake on a daily basis. For example, a child may be living in a nonfluoridated community but attend school in an area where fluoride is at optimal levels. If the fluoride content of a child's water source is unknown, then it is important to have the water tested at a local laboratory for the fluoride content before prescribing a fluoride supplement. Foods and beverages that are processed in communities with optimally fluoridated water are consumed not only in the area where they are processed but also can be shipped to a neighboring community that is nonfluoridated. This added benefit of fluoride is termed the "halo" or "diffusion" effect and can benefit people in nonfluoridated communities. According to an evidence-based clinical recommendation from the American Dental Association (ADA), a child's overall risk of decay should be high before prescribing a fluoride supplement.[40]

As a result of the widespread availability of fluoride, the difference in the decay rate in communities with fluoridated water compared with those that do not have fluoridated water has lessened. According to Burt, the question was raised as to the need for fluoride supplements in the United States, given the fact that fluoride can be found in so many various sources, such as drinking water, toothpaste, gels, rinses, professionally applied fluorides, and processed foods and beverages. The argument was made that the evidence for the benefit of fluoride supplements when used from birth or soon after was weak and that supplements were a risk factor for fluorosis.[41] It is essential, as ways to reduce caries are devised, that the risks of fluorosis are minimized. Given that as a guideline, it could be concluded that the risk of using fluoride supplements outweigh the benefits, if the risk of fluorosis has been established.

Some may argue that fluoride supplements should not be eliminated. Moss stated that dietary supplements alone are unlikely to be the cause of the reported increase in fluorosis because compliance continues to be extremely poor.[42] Other authors have also noted the lack of compliance of patients with prescriptions.[43,44] In addition, few children use supplements for more than a year and a half at best.[42] Horowitz stated[43] that it would be wrong in his opinion to eliminate the availability of dietary fluoride supplementation as a caries-preventive regimen. Many children are still at high risk of dental caries and, for a variety of reasons, may not have access to fluoridated drinking water or professionally administered fluoride regimens. Horowitz went on to say that postponing the use of fluoride supplements until 2 or 3 years of age, as some propose, will reduce the supplements' potential effectiveness in caries prevention. Some studies have shown the greatest benefit for the primary and permanent teeth is when fluoride supplements are given before 2 years of age.[45] In addition, a downward revision in dosage is very different from the recommendation for the elimination of fluoride supplements altogether.[43]

Prescriptions for supplemental fluoride should be specific about when and how the supplement is to be given. Fluoride ingested on an empty stomach is 100%

bioavailable, whereas fluoride administered with milk or a meal will not be completely absorbed. The best time to administer the supplement is at bedtime or at least 1 hour before eating.[46] Another factor that may need to be considered in assessing a child's total fluoride exposure is the increasing popularity of bottled water and home water-filtration systems—the question is what effect these may have on the total fluoride content. The majority of bottled water sold on the market today does not contain adequate amounts of fluoride (0.7-1.2 parts per million [ppm]). In a 1994 study of 39 different bottled water brands, 34 of them had fluoride concentrations less than 0.3 ppm.[47] Home water-treatment systems also have the ability to reduce fluoride levels. It has been well established that reverse osmosis and distillation units remove significant amounts of fluoride. Therefore, it is conceivable that a preschool child could live in an optimally fluoridated area but not receive adequate amounts of fluoride. A common type of home water-filtration is the carbon or charcoal filter systems. Generally, they do not remove significant amounts of fluoride. Studies have also shown that water softeners caused no significant changes in fluoride concentrations.[48,49] The optimum concentration of fluoride in the drinking water ranges from 0.7 to 1.2 ppm. This range effectively reduces dental decay while minimizing the risk of dental fluorosis. In 2011, the US Department of Human and Health Services and Environmental Protection Agency recommendation for fluoride concentration in public water systems was changed from being a range to specifically 0.7 ppm.[50]

Fluoride Varnish

The topical application of fluoride varnish has been shown to prevent or reverse enamel demineralization.[51] Fluoride varnishes typically contain 5% sodium fluoride (NaF), which is equivalent to 2.26% or 22 600 ppm fluoride ion.[52] Fluoride varnish is approved by the US Food and Drug Administration (FDA) for the treatment of dentin hypersensitivity associated with the exposure of root surfaces or as a cavity varnish. However, the FDA has not approved the use of fluoride as a caries-reducing agent. There continues to be an increasing body of evidence indicating that fluoride varnish is effective in caries reduction.[52] The ADA endorses the use of fluoride varnish for caries prevention,[53] Until the FDA approves the use of fluoride varnish as a caries prevention modality, its use in this manner is considered "off-label"; not unlike many pediatric medications. The ADA in 2006 issued an evidence-based clinical recommendation for the application of fluoride varnish at 3-month intervals for patients at high caries risk.[53] The 2008 AAP policy on preventive oral health intervention recommends that pediatricians apply fluoride varnish in children who are assessed to have significant risk of dental caries and who are unable to establish a dental home.[54]

VI

Fluorosis

How much fluoride a child should receive on a daily basis varies with both age and body weight. Table 50.3 demonstrates the adequate intake of fluoride from all sources on a daily basis to be 0.05 mg/kg per day.[55] This is the amount of fluoride needed for optimal health without the risk of fluorosis. It has been calculated by gender and age group. The maximum level has been set at 0.10 mg/kg per day for infants, toddlers, and children up to 8 years of age. For older children who are not at risk of fluorosis, the upper limit has been set at 10 mg/day.[55]

Table 50.3.
Dietary Reference Intakes for Fluoride[55]

Age Group	Adequate Intake (mg/day)	Tolerable Upper Intake (mg/day)
Infants 0-6 mo	0.01	0.7
Infants 7-12 mo	0.5	0.9
Children 1-3 y	0.7	1.3
Children 4-8 y	1.0	2.2
Children 9-13 y	2.0	10
Boys 14-18 y	2.0	10
Girls 14-18 y	3.0	10
Males 19 y and older	4.0	10
Females 19 y and older	3.0	10

Over the past several years, an increase in enamel fluorosis has been noted in both optimally fluoridated and nonfluoridated areas. Fluorosis is the result of too much fluoride and affects approximately 22% of children. Of these children, 94% have only mild cases of fluorosis.[35] This condition results in a change in the appearance of the teeth when higher-than-optimal levels of fluoride are ingested before 7 years of age, during the calcification stage of tooth development. Dental fluorosis is a cosmetic effect with few known health problems. The risk of fluorosis can be greatly reduced by proper supervision of children around the use of fluoride-containing products. Clinically, fluorosis can range from minor white lines running across the teeth to a more severe form that exhibits a very chalky appearance with possible pitting and brown staining.

One factor that has contributed to the overall increase in fluorosis has been the inappropriate prescribing of fluoride supplements for children already in optimally fluoridated communities. Pendrys[56] found that inappropriate supplementation accounted for 25% of the fluorosis cases of children living in an optimally fluoridated area.

In Europe and Canada, fluoride supplement schedules are used as guidelines for only children considered to be at high risk of caries, and fluoride supplementation does not start until the child reaches 3 years of age.[41] One reason for this may be the fact that there are many alternative forms of fluoride to choose from today.

Many studies over the past few years have shown strong evidence of an association between dental fluorosis and the use of fluoride toothpaste in early childhood. A study conducted in Asheville, NC, found that using a fluoride toothpaste before 2 years of age increased a child's chances of developing fluorosis by 3 times.[57] Another study conducted in Canada showed that 72% of the fluorosis cases could be attributed to early fluoride toothpaste use during the first 2 years of life.[58] It is recommended that children should not use fluoridated toothpaste until after reaching the age of 2, and then, they should use only a small pea-sized amount. Over the past several years, many companies have marketed toothpaste with special colors and flavors to increase use by children. There is concern this type of marketing may encourage children to use more toothpaste and potentially ingest significant amounts of fluoride, thereby contributing to dental fluorosis. A study by Adair[52] demonstrated that children used significantly more children's toothpaste than adult brands and that they brushed their teeth for a longer period of time.[59] His study demonstrated that approximately 50% of the children expectorated and approximately 25% rinsed after brushing. The number of children who rinsed and expectorated was even smaller.[59] Parents should be reminded of the need to supervise their preschool children during toothbrushing to ensure that the proper amount of toothpaste is used, regardless of whether their water is optimally fluoridated or not. Parents should encourage their children to expectorate and rinse with water as soon as possible to lessen the amount swallowed. Horowitz stated that, because nearly all children use fluoride toothpaste and relatively few take fluoride supplements, fluoride toothpaste undoubtedly has had a greater overall effect on the rate of fluorosis in the United States than have fluoride supplements.[43]

Having considered the risks and benefits of fluoride, the idea of assessing the child's overall risk of developing caries becomes important. One can look at the child's previous dental history, family history, medical complications, diet, hygiene, fluoride status, and use of chronic medications in determining a child's risk of developing caries and the need for a fluoride supplement. The AAPD has also established a Caries-Risk Assessment Tool[60] (available at http://aapd.org/media/Policies_Guidelines/P_CariesRiskAssess.pdf) that will help in determining what a child's risk of developing future decay could be and help in forming an overall treatment plan for a child.

VI

Fluoride Toxicity

Although fluoride has been shown to be beneficial, it can be toxic to children if taken in high doses. The acute toxic dose of fluoride has been determined to be 5 mg/kg, for which medical intervention will be necessary. Because most toothpaste products on the market in the United States contain fluoride, it is theoretically possible for a child to ingest enough toothpaste to lead to toxicity. The probable toxic dose for a 1-year-old (10-kg) child is contained in 50 mL of a toothpaste with 1000 ppm of fluoride. For a 5-year-old (19-kg) child, it is found in 95 mL. For these reasons, parents are to be reminded that close supervision of all fluoride products is essential for their children. Children should be encouraged not to swallow or eat toothpaste. All fluoride products should be stored out of reach of young children. Symptoms include nausea, vomiting, electrolyte imbalance, arrhythmias, central nervous system excitation, and coma followed by death within a few hours.[61]

Role of the Pediatrician

Tooth decay is the most common chronic disease of childhood. Despite the clear importance of health insurance, an estimated 1.3 million children with special health care needs were uninsured during the period of 1994-1995. These children were disproportionately represented among low-income families. It was also pointed out that there are access problems for some children with special health care needs, despite having insurance.[62] Children with dental problems lose more than 51 million school hours annually, and substantial numbers of children with untreated caries are seen in emergency departments around the United States.[63,64] According to 1 study, 27% of the children that were seen had never been to the dentist. For those who were 3.5 years and younger, this was the first visit for 52% of the children.[64] Only 1 in 5 children covered by Medicaid received preventive oral care for which they were eligible.[65]

The infectious nature of dental caries, its early onset, and the potential of early interventions require an emphasis on preventive oral care in the primary pediatric setting.[65] Most caries in children today occur in approximately 25% of children. These children could greatly benefit from early referral for appropriate care. Pediatric primary health care professionals see many more children than do dentists and can provide early intervention. An early examination of children may identify children at greatest risk of dental disease. The presence of plaque on the upper front teeth of infants is predictive of future caries. In a study of children 19 months of age, the prevalence of plaque was the best predictor of future caries risk in 91% of the children.[66] Undetected caries can present dramatically if left untreated. When the decay spreads to the nerve of the tooth, infection can result, leading to a cellulitis and potentially death.

The AAPD and AAP recommend that all infants obtain an oral health risk assessment by their primary health care professional or other qualified professional by 6 months of age. This risk assessment should be obtained using the Caries-Risk Assessment Tool[60] (available at http://aapd.org/media/Policies_Guidelines/P_CariesRiskAssess.pdf). A child should see a dentist by 12 months of age.[15,67]

The number of dentists available to treat young children with significant dental disease is insufficient and declining, and it is essential for primary health care professionals to help ensure timely oral screenings. Fewer than 3% of dentists are trained as pediatric specialists, and only approximately 1 pediatric dentist exists for every 15 pediatricians in the United States.[68] There are approximately 6400 practicing pediatric dentists. The number of pediatric dental residency training program positions continues to increase. The goal of reducing children's oral health disparities also supports increased integration of dentistry with medicine and other health disciplines. Children with special health care needs have the potential for significant oral-systemic interactions, which necessitates integrated approaches. Although hospitalized children typically receive complete pediatric examinations, it is rare that their oral health and its effects on the systemic health are fully evaluated.[65] These children require additional oral health promotion efforts by pediatricians if poor oral health and significant oral health problems are to be eliminated. These children face such complex and demanding health care needs, oral health issues tend to be of secondary concern. As a result, these children often suffer avoidable dental problems that further affect the quality of their life. The more demanding a child's medical issues, the more necessary it is to ensure early and timely referral for dental care.[68]

US Surgeon General David Satcher called for a national oral health plan to eliminate disparities in oral health for all Americans. Surgeon General Satcher stated, "Everyone has a role in improving and promoting oral health. Together we can work to broaden public understanding of the importance of oral health and its relevance to general health and well-being, and to ensure that existing and future preventive, diagnostic, and treatment measures for oral diseases and disorders are made available to all Americans."[4]

VI

References

1. Nowak AJ. Rationale for the timing of the first oral evaluation. *Pediatr Dent.* 1997;19(1):8-11
2. Dye BA, Tan S, Smith V, et al. Trends in oral health status: United States, 1988-1994 and 1999-2004. *Vital Health Stat.* 2007;11(248):1-17

3. Pierce KM, Rozier RG, Vann WF Jr. Accuracy of pediatric primary care providers' screening and referral for early childhood caries. *Pediatrics*. 2002;109(5):e82

4. Oral health in America: a report of the Surgeon General. *J Calif Dent Assoc*. 2000;28(9):685-695

5. Li Y, Wang W. Predicting caries in permanent teeth from caries in primary teeth: an eight-year cohort study. *J Dent Res*. 2002;81(8):561-566

6. Nowak AJ, Warren JJ. Infant oral health and oral habits. *Pediatr Clin North Am*. 2000;47(5):1043-1066

7. Berkowitz RJ. Mutans streptococci: acquisition and transmission. *Pediatr Dent*. 2006;28(2):106–109

8. Kohler B, Bratthall D, Krasse B. Preventive measures in mothers influence the acquisition of *Streptococcus mutans* in their infants. *Arch Oral Biol*. 1983;28(3):225–231

9. Li Y, Caulfield PW. The fidelity of initial acquisition of mutans streptococci by infants from their mothers. *J Dent Res*. 1995;74(2):681-685

10. Mitchell SC, Ruby JD, Moser S, et al. Maternal transmission of mutans Streptococci in severe-early childhood caries. *Pediatr Dent*. 2009;31(3):193-201

11. Kaste LM, Gift HC. Inappropriate infant bottle feeding. Status of the Healthy People 2000 objective. *Arch Pediatr Adolesc Med*. 1995;149(7):786-791

12. Sheikh C, Erickson PR. Evaluation of plaque pH changes following oral rinse with eight infant formulas. *Pediatr Dent*. 1996;18(3):200-204

13. Valaitis R, Hesch R, Passarelli C, Sheehan D, Sinton J. A systematic review of the relationship between breastfeeding and early childhood caries. *Can J Public Health*. 2000;91(6):411-417

14. Erickson PR, Mazhari E. Investigation of the role of human breast milk in caries development. *Pediatr Dent*. 1999;21(2):86-90

15. American Academy of Pediatric Dentistry, Clinical Affairs Committee, Infant Oral Health Subcommittee, Council on Clinical Affairs. Guideline on infant oral health care, pediatric dentistry reference manual. *Pediatr Dent*. 2010-2011;33(6 Reference Manual): 1-334

16. Falco MA. The lifetime impact of sugar excess and nutrient depletion on oral health. *Gen Dent*. 2001;49(6):591-595

17. American Academy of Pediatrics, Committee on Nutrition. The use and misuse of fruit juice in pediatrics. *Pediatrics*. 2001;107(5):1210-1213

18. Marshall TA. Diet and nutrition in pediatric dentistry. *Dent Clin North Am*. 2003;47(2):279-303

19. Neff D. Acid production from different carbohydrate sources in human plaque in situ. *Caries Res*. 1967;1(1):78-87

20. Mormann JE, Muhlemann HR. Oral starch degradation and its influence on acid production in human dental plaque. *Caries Res*. 1981;15(2):166-175

21. Kaplowitz G, Forman M, Aaronson SA, eds. *The Dangers of Soda Pop*. Academy of Dental Therapeutics and Stomatology; 2004. Available at: http://www.colgateprofessional.com/ColgateProfessional/Home/US/EN/ProfessionalEd/PDFs/SodaPopCourse.pdf. Accessed January 18, 2013

22. Cavadini C, Siega-Riz AM, Popkin BM. US adolescent food intake trends from 1965 to 1996. *Arch Dis Child*. 2000;83(4):18-24

23. Marshall TA, Levy SM, Broffitt B, Warren JJ, Eichenberger-Gilmore JM, Burns TL, Stumbo PJ. Dental Caries and Beverage Consumption in Young Children. *Pediatrics*. 2003;112(3 Pt 1):e184-e191

24. American Academy of Pediatrics, Committee on Nutrition and the Council on Sports Medicine and Fitness. Sports drinks and energy drinks for children and adolescents: are they appropriate? *Pediatrics*. 2011;127(6):1182-1189

25. Seow WK. Enamel hypoplasia in the primary dentition: a review. *ASDC J Dent Child*. 1991;58:441-452

26. Seow WK, Humphrys C, Tudehope DI. Increased prevalence of developmental dental defects in low birth-weight, prematurely born children: a controlled study. *Pediatr Dent*. 1987;9(3):221-225

27. Seow WK, Brown JP, Tudehope DI, O'Callaghan M. Developmental defects in the primary dentition of low birth-weight infants: adverse effects of laryngoscopy and prolonged endotracheal intubation. *Pediatr Dent*. 1984;6(1):28-31

28. Linnett V, Seow WK. Dental erosion in children: a literature review. *Pediatr Dent*. 2001;23(1):37-43

29. Ogden CL, Carroll MD, Bit BK, et al. Prevalence of obesity trends in body mass index among US children and adolescents, 1999-2010. *JAMA*. 2012;307(5):483-490

30. Adair SM. Dietary counseling—time for a nutritionist in the office? *Pediatr Dent*. 2004;26(5):389

31. Tinanoff N, O'Sullivan DM. Early childhood caries: overview and recent findings. *Pediatr Dent*. 1997;19(1):12-16

32. Acs G, Lodolini G, Kaminsky S, Cisneros GJ. Effect of nursing caries on body weight in a pediatric population. *Pediatr Dent*. 1992;14(5):302-305

33. Alvarez JO, Caceda J, Woolley TW, et al. A longitudinal study of dental caries in the primary teeth of children who suffered from infant malnutrition. *J Dent Res*. 1993;72(12):1573-1576

34. Neville BW, Damm DD, Allen CM, Bouquot JE. *Oral and Maxillofacial Pathology*. 3rd ed. St Louis, MO: Saunders Elsevier; 2009

35. American Dental Association. Fluoridation Facts. Chicago, IL: American Dental Association; 2005. Available at: www.ada.org/sections/newsAndEvents/pdfs/fluoridation_facts.pdf. Accessed January 19, 2013

36. American Academy of Pediatric Dentistry, Council on Clinical Affairs. Guideline on fluoride therapy. *Pediatr Dent*. 2010-2011;33(6 Reference Manual):153-156

37. Hellwig E, Lennon AM. Systemic versus topical fluoride. *Caries Res*. 2004;38(3):258-262

38. Center for Disease Control and Prevention, Community Water Fluoridation. 2008 Water Fluoridation Statistics. Available at: www.cdc.gov/fluoridation/statistics/2008stats.htm. Accessed January 19, 2013

39. American Academy of Pediatrics, Committee on Nutrition. Fluoride supplementation for children: interim policy recommendations. *Pediatrics*. 1995;95(5):777

VI

40. Rozier RG, Adair S, Graham F, et al. Evidence-based clinical recommendations on the prescription of dietary fluoride supplements for caries prevention: a report of the American Dental Association Council on Scientific Affairs. *J Am Dent Assoc*. 2010;141(12):1480-1489

41. Burt BA. The case for eliminating the use of dietary fluoride supplements for young children. *J Public Health Dent*. 1999;59(4):269-274

42. Moss SJ. The case for retaining the current supplementation schedule. *J Public Health Dent*. 1999;59:259-262

43. Horowitz HS. The role of dietary fluoride supplements in caries prevention. *J Public Health Dent*. 1999;59(4):205-210

44. Adair SM. Overview of the history and current status of fluoride supplementation schedules. *J Public Health Dent*. 1999;59(4):252-258

45. Mellberg JR, Ripa LW. *Fluoride in Preventive Dentistry: Theory and Clinical Applications*. Chicago, IL: Quintessence Publishing Co; 1983

46. Shulman ER, Vallejo M. Effect of gastric contents on the bioavailability of fluoride in humans. *Pediatr Dent*. 1990;12(4):237-240

47. Tate WH, Chan JT. Fluoride concentrations in bottled and filtered waters. *Gen Dent*. 1994;42(4):362-366

48. Robinson SN, Davies EH, Williams B. Domestic water treatment appliances and the fluoride ion. *Br Dent J*. 1991;171(3-4):91-93

49. Warren JJ, Levy SM. Current and future role of fluoride in nutrition. *Dent Clin North Am*. 2003;47(2):225-243

50. US Environmental Protection Agency. EPA and HHS announce new scientific assessments and actions on fluoride [press release]. January 7, 2011. Available at: http://yosemite.epa.gov/opa/admpress.nsf/3881d73f4d4aaa0b85257359003f5348/86964af577c37ab285257811005a8417!OpenDocument. Accessed January 19, 2013

51. Castellano JB, Donly KJ. Potential remineralization of demineralized enamel after application of fluoride varnish. *Am J Dent* 2004;17(6):462-464

52. Beltran-Aguilar ED, Goldstein J. Fluoride varnishes: a review of their clinical use, cariostatic mechanisms, efficacy, and safety. *J Am Dent Assoc*. 2000;131(5):589-596

53. American Dental Association Council on Scientific Affairs. Professionally applied topical fluoride. Evidence-based clinical recommendations. *J Am Dent Assoc*. 2006;137(8):1151-1159

54. American Academy of Pediatrics, Section on Pediatric Dentistry and Oral Health. Preventive oral health intervention for pediatricians. *Pediatrics*. 2008;122(6):1387-1394

55. Institute of Medicine, Food and Nutrition Board. *Dietary Reference Intakes for Calcium, Phosphorus, Magnesium, Vitamin D, and Fluoride*. Washington, DC: National Academies Press; 1997

56. Pendrys DG. Risk of fluorosis in a fluoridated population. Implications for the dentist and hygienist. *J Am Dent Assoc*. 1995;126(12):1617-1624

57. Lalumandier JA, Rozier RG. The prevalence and risk factors of fluorosis among patients in a pediatric dental practice. *Pediatr Dent*. 1995;17(1):19-25

58. Osuji OO, Leake JL, Chipman ML, Nikiforuk G, Locker D, Levine N. Risk factors for dental fluorosis in a fluoridated community. *J Dent Res*. 1988;67(12):1488-1492

59. Adair SM, Piscitelli WP, McKnight-Hanes C. Comparison of the use of a child and an adult dentifrice by a sample of preschool children. *Pediatr Dent*. 1997;19(2):99-103

60. American Academy of Pediatric Dentistry, Council on Clinical Affairs. Caries-risk Assessment and Management for infants, children, and adolescents. *Pediatric Dentistry Reference Manual*. 2010-2011;33(6 Reference Manual):110-117

61. Whitford GM. Fluoride in dental products: safety considerations. *J Dent Res*. 1987;66(5):1056-1060

62. Newacheck PW, McManus M, Fox HB, Hung YY, Halfon N. Access to health care for children with special health care needs. *Pediatrics*. 2000;105(4 Pt 1):760-766

63. Gift HC, Reisine ST, Larach DC. The social impact of dental problems and visits. *Am J Public Health*. 1992;82(12):1663-1668

64. Sheller B, Williams BJ, Lombardi SM. Diagnosis and treatment of dental caries-related emergencies in a children's hospital. *Pediatr Dent*. 1997;19(8):470-475

65. Mouradian WE, Wehr E, Crall JJ. Disparities in children's oral health and access to dental care. *JAMA*. 2000;284(20):2625-2631

66. Alaluusua S, Malmivirta R. Early plaque accumulation—a sign for caries risk in young children. *Community Dent Oral Epidemiol*. 1994;22(5 Pt 1):273-276

67. Hale KJ; American Academy of Pediatrics, Section on Pediatric Dentistry. Oral health risk assessment timing and establishment of the dental home. *Pediatrics*. 2003;111(5 Pt 1):1113-1116

68. Edelstein BL. Public and clinical policy considerations in maximizing children's oral health. *Pediatr Clin North Am*. 2000;47(5):1177-1189

VI

Chapter 51

Community Nutrition Services

Introduction

Promoting the nutritional health of children and their families is a common goal of the nutrition services offered by a wide variety of public and private agencies, organizations, and individuals in communities across the nation. These include federal government agencies; state health and education departments; local health agencies, such as city and county health departments; community health centers; health maintenance and preferred provider organizations; hospital and ambulatory outpatient clinics; nutritionists and dietitians in public and private practice; voluntary health agencies, such as the American Diabetes Association and the American Heart Association; social service agencies; elementary and secondary schools; colleges and universities; and business and industry.

Nutrition Services Provided Through Federal, State, and Local Health and Nutrition Agencies

Each year, Congress appropriates funds for a variety of nutrition and health programs, many of which are targeted to low-income mothers and children. Such programs are administered at the national level by the US Department of Agriculture (USDA) and the US Department of Health and Human Services (DHHS). USDA services include Child Nutrition Programs (National School Lunch Program, School Breakfast Program, Summer Food Service Program, and Child and Adult Care Food Program); the Special Supplemental Nutrition Program for Women, Infants, and Children (WIC); the Supplemental Nutrition Assistance Program (SNAP; formerly known as the Food Stamp Program); and the Commodity Supplemental Food Program. Services of the DHHS include maternal and child health services block grant programs; preventive health services block grant programs; Early and Periodic Screening, Diagnostic, and Treatment (EPSDT) services under Medicaid; Indian Health Services, and programs from the Centers for Disease Control and Prevention (CDC). There are also programs such as community health centers and migrant health projects that serve at-risk populations.[1]

In addition to federal support, considerable state and local funds also support child health programs. An example of a local resource is community-based food programs that are nonprofit, nongovernmental, grass-roots, self-help community developmental programs. One such resource is Feeding America (formerly known as America's Second Harvest), which coordinates a vast network of local food pantries and meal programs across the country. Many of these food programs are tied to other services that low-income mothers and children may need.

Physicians and other primary health care professionals should be knowledgeable about local food and nutrition programs so they can assist families to become informed consumers and appropriate referrals can be made. An informed health care professional can also serve as an advocate to strengthen policy and budget decisions that guide the provision of quality, cost-effective nutrition programs focused on improving the health of the nation.

Although nutrition services were introduced into public health programs as early as the late 1920s, Title V of the Social Security Act of 1935 (Pub L No. 74-721) initiated the federal-state partnership for maternal and child health that served as the major impetus for the development of nutrition services for mothers and children.[2] A census of public health nutrition personnel in 1999-2000 showed that approximately 10 904 public health nutritionists are employed in federal, state, and local public health agencies.[3] Public health nutritionists provide a wide range of services related to core public health functions, including assessment, assurance, and policy development. Public health nutritionists provide direct clinical services (eg, screening, assessment, nutrition counseling, monitoring); population-based research; development and implementation of nutrition services and policies that focus on disease prevention and health promotion; provision of technical assistance to a range of providers and consumers; collection and analysis of health-related data, including nutrition surveillance and monitoring; investigation and control of disease, injuries, and responses to natural disasters; protection of the environment, housing, food, water, and workplaces; public information, education, and community mobilization; quality assurance; training and education; leadership, planning, policy development, and administration; targeted outreach and linkage to personal services; and other direct clinical services.[4]

Many community nutrition services include screening, education, counseling, and treatment to improve the nutritional status of an individual or a population. These services are designed to meet the preventive, therapeutic, and rehabilitative health care needs of all segments of the population. The focus of nutrition services in an agency is based on several factors, including the mission of the agency, funding, analysis of data from a community-needs assessment, resources, and politics.[5] Public agencies provide nutrition services for individuals throughout the life cycle, provided in a variety of inpatient and outpatient settings. The broadest range of nutrition services may be most evident in community-based nutrition programs, in which services are based on core public health functions. The physician and other primary health care professionals must know where these services are provided in their community. Professional and federal resources for nutrition services are listed in Table 51.1. The Maternal and Child Health (MCH) Library at

Table 51.1.
Selected Professional and Federal Resources for Nutrition Services

Selected Professional Nutrition Organizations
Academy of Nutrition and Dietetics (AND) 120 S. Riverside Plaza, Suite 2000 Chicago, IL 60606-6995 Phone: 800-877-1600; Consumer Nutrition Hot Line: 800-366-1655 www.eatright.org
School Nutrition Association (SNA) 700 S. Washington Street, Suite 300 Alexandria, VA 22314 Phone: 703-739-3900; Fax 703-739-3915 www.schoolnutrition.org
Association of State and Territorial Public Health Nutrition Directors PO Box 1001 Johnstown, PA 15907-1001 Phone: 814-255-2829 http://www.astphnd.org/
National WIC Association 2001 S Street, NW, Suite 580 Washington, DC 20009-3405 Phone: 202-232-5492; fax: 202-387-5281 http://www.nwica.org/
American Public Human Services Association (APHSA) 810 First Street, NE Suite 500 Washington, DC 20002 Phone: 202-682-0100 Fax: 202-289-6555 http://www.aphsa.org/Home/home_news.asp
Feeding America 35 E. Wacker Drive, Suite 2000 Chicago, IL 60601 Phone: 800-771-2303 www.feedingamerica.org (Web site has a search function to locate local services)
Selected Federal Resources
US Department of Agriculture Resources
US Department of Agriculture Food and Nutrition Service (FNS) 3101 Park Center Drive Alexandria, VA 22302 Phone: 703-305-2062 Information on USDA nutrition assistance programs including associated research, nutrition education initiatives, such as WIC Loving Support Breastfeeding Campaign, Team Nutrition, Eat Smart Play Hard, State Nutrition Action Plans (SNAP), and Food Stamp Nutrition Education, are found at: http://www.fns.usda.gov/fns/. Fact sheets on the USDA nutrition assistance programs are available at: http://www.fns.usda.gov/cga/FactSheets/ProgramFactSheets.htm.

VII

Table **51.1.** (*continued*)
Selected Professional and Federal Resources for Nutrition Services

US Department of Agriculture Center for Nutrition Policy and Promotion (CNPP) 3101 Park Center Drive Alexandria, VA 22302 Phone: 703-305-7600 The CNPP develops and promotes dietary guidance that links scientific research to the nutrition needs of consumers. For information on CNPP resources, the Dietary Guidelines for Americans, and MyPyramid, see http://www.cnpp.usda.gov/.
US Department of Agriculture Cooperative State Research, Education, and Extension Service (CSREES) 1400 Independence Avenue, SW, Stop 2201 Washington, DC 20250-2201 Phone: 202-720-7441 The CSREES provides linkages between federal and state components of a broad-based national agricultural higher education, research, and extension system designed to address national problems and needs related to agriculture, the environment, human health and well-being, and communities; see http://www.csrees.usda.gov/.
National Agricultural Library (NAL) US Department of Agriculture Abraham Lincoln Building 10301 Baltimore Avenue Beltsville, MD 20705-2351 Phone: 301-504-5414 (for FNIC); Fax: 301-504-6409 (for FNIC) http://www.nal.usda.gov/ The NAL sponsors the Food and Nutrition Information Center (FNIC), the Healthy Meals Resource System for schools and child care programs, the WIC Works Resource System, the Food Stamp Nutrition Connection Resource System, and the USDA/FDA Foodborne Illness Education Information Center. The FNIC/NAL also sponsors the "Nutrition.gov" Web site, which provides easy access to the best food and nutrition information from across the federal government.
US Department of Health and Human Services Resources
Centers for Disease Control and Prevention Division of Nutrition and Physical Activity 4770 Buford Highway, Mailstop K25 Atlanta, GA 30341 Phone: 770-488-6042 Information and resources on infant and child nutrition, physical activity, and the obesity epidemic are available from the CDC Web site at http://www.cdc.gov/nccdphp/dnpa.
Food and Drug Administration 5600 Fishers Lane Rockville, MD 20857 For general inquiries: 1-888-INFO-FDA (1-888-463-6332) For Office of Public Affairs: 301-827-6250 This Web site is a central source of information about FDA activities and resources and includes a section on consumer advice and publications on food safety and nutrition: www.fda.gov.

Table 51.1.
Selected Professional and Federal Resources for Nutrition Services

The National Center for Education in Maternal and Child Health (NCEMCH) Georgetown University Box 571272 Washington, DC 20057-1272 Phone: 202-784-9770; fax 202-784-9777 Funded by the Maternal and Child Health Bureau, Health Resources and Services Administration, Department of Health and Human Services, the NCEMCH Web site (www.ncemch.org) provides online access to NCEMCH initiatives, educational resources, and publications; a virtual MCH library and MCH databases; bibliographies; and knowledge paths.
US Department of Health and Human Services 200 Independence Avenue, SW Washington, DC 20201 For more information by mail, write: National Health Information Center PO Box 1133 Washington, DC 20013-1133 Phone: 301-565-4167 Toll Free: 1-800-336-4797 The HealthierUS initiative is a national effort, sponsored by the Department of Health and Human Services and the Executive Office of the President, to improve people's lives, prevent and reduce the costs of disease, and promote community health and wellness. See the Web site, which includes information on nutrition, physical activity, and healthy choices: www.HealthierUS.gov.
National Heart, Lung, and Blood Institute PO Box 30105 Bethesda, MD 20824-0105 Phone: 301-592-8573 or toll-free 866-35-WECAN *We Can!* or "Ways to Enhance Children's Activity and Nutrition" is a national education program from the National Institutes of Health designed for families and caregivers to help children 8 to 13 years of age achieve a healthy weight. This program offers communities and families resources including materials for healthcare providers, physicians, and parents. See the Web site: http://wecan.nhlbi.nih.gov.
Indian Health Service The Reyes Building 801 Thompson Avenue, Ste. 400 Rockville, MD 20852-1627 Phone: 301-443-1083 For information on how the Indian Health Service works to improve the health of patients with nutrition related diseases, and prevent these illnesses in future generations through interventions in schools, community health programs, and hospital and clinic based services, see the Web site: http://www.ihs.gov.

VII

Georgetown University maintains the MCH Organizations Database (http://
mchlibrary.info/databases/about_org.html), which lists more than 2000 government, professional, and voluntary organizations involved in MCH activities,
primarily at a national level. This is a useful resource for pediatricians and other
primary care providers. Qualified providers of nutrition services include physicians,
registered dietitians (RDs) and/or licensed dietitians, licensed nutritionists, nurses,
and other qualified professionals. The Academy of Nutrition and Dietetics (AND),
the largest organization of professional dietitians and nutritionists, has identified
qualified providers as RDs and other qualified professionals who meet licensing and
other standards prescribed at the state level.[6]

Health and Nutrition Agencies: A Nutrition Resource to Provide Services and Identify Qualified Providers

Federal, state, and local health and nutrition agencies, particularly those employing
public health nutritionists, can be helpful resources for physicians and other
primary health care professionals. Nutritionists provide extensive technical assistance to clients and their families and physicians, especially for children with special
health care needs. One example is services for children with an inborn error of
metabolism. The diet prescription includes special medical formulas and foods that
are modified to meet medical and socioeconomic needs. The formulas and foods are
expensive, and the costs are generally not reimbursed by insurance companies.
Many states have provisions for coverage for special formulas and foods.[7] Physicians
should contact the special needs program of their state health department for
information about patient eligibility for coverage for these formulas and foods and
procedures for obtaining them.

Another example in which a nutritionist and nutrition services are instrumental
in supporting feeding and growth is an early intervention program. In an early
intervention program, nutritionists work with the child's family, other team
members, and the child's primary health care professional to optimize development
from birth to 3 years of age.[8] This national early intervention program for infants
and toddlers with disabilities and their families was created by Congress in 1986
under the Education for All Handicapped Children Act (Pub L No. 94-142
[1975]), which then became the Individuals with Disabilities Education Act (Pub L
No. 101-476 [1990]), and is administered by states. To be eligible for services,
children must be younger than 3 years and have a confirmed disability or established developmental delay as defined by the state, in 1 or more of the following
areas of development: physical, cognitive, communication, social-emotional, and/or
adaptive. A complete evaluation of the child and family must be conducted, at no
cost to the family, to determine whether a child is eligible for this early intervention

program. The evaluation would include an assessment of the child's nutritional history and dietary intake; anthropometric, biochemical, and clinical variables; feeding skills and feeding problems; and food habits and food preferences. If a child and family are found eligible for services, the parents and a team will develop a written plan (individualized family service plan [IFSP]) for providing early intervention services to the child and, as necessary, to the family. The child's and family's IFSP can include nutrition, or nutrition may be listed as another service that the child receives but is not provided or paid for by the early intervention program. Depending on the child's assessed nutritional needs, a qualified nutritionist, as a member of the IFSP team, would develop and monitor appropriate goals and objectives to address any nutritional needs and also make referrals to appropriate community resources to carry out nutrition goals, if needed. For more information on disabilities in infants, toddlers, children, and youth and the Individuals with Disabilities Education Act, which is the law authorizing special education and the early intervention program, see the Web site of the National Dissemination Center for Children with Disabilities (www.nichcy.org).

Other types of nutrition services provided by many state and local health agencies include nutrition counseling, classes on specific aspects of nutrition (eg, infant feeding, breastfeeding, diet and prevention of heart disease, and weight management), radio and cable television programs on nutrition topics, publications and educational materials on a wide range of topics for the lay public, and nutrition seminars and workshops. Local nutrition education resources are available from the USDA-funded Cooperative Extension Service. This service provides up-to-date information about the science of nutrition and its practical application in planning low-cost, nutritious meals. Many nutrition publications provided by the Cooperative Extension Service and other public health agencies are available in various foreign languages and for clients with low literacy skills.[5,9] The National Institute of Food and Agriculture (formerly the Cooperative State Research, Education, and Extension Service) of the USDA operates the Expanded Food and Nutrition Education Program in all 50 states and in American Samoa, Guam, Micronesia, Northern Marianas, Puerto Rico, and the Virgin Islands. The Expanded Food and Nutrition Education Program is designed to assist limited-resource audiences in acquiring the knowledge, skills, attitudes, and behavior changes necessary to follow nutritionally sound diets and to contribute to their personal development and improvement of the total family diet and nutritional well-being (for more information, see http://www.csrees.usda.gov/nea/food/efnep/efnep.html).

The director of the nutrition department at the state health department is another excellent resource for identifying specific state, regional, or national resources and services. Similar information can be obtained from the Association of

VII

State and Territorial Public Health Nutrition Directors (Table 51.1). The state affiliate of the AND or the AND consultant directory can help identify an RD with specific clinical expertise (Table 51.1). Consumers may also call the AND consumer hotline number and speak directly to an RD who can assist them with answers to general questions ranging from food labeling to food sanitation and other topics.

In addition to federal, state, and local health agencies, agencies such as visiting nurse associations, the American Diabetes Association, the American Heart Association, health maintenance organizations, and hospital inpatient and out-patient departments frequently employ personnel with nutrition expertise. They usually provide technical consultation in nutrition to physicians and nurses and nutrition counseling to patients and other agencies in the community. An increasing number of RDs have also established private or independent practices.

Nutrition-Assistance Programs

National policy has long provided for publicly supported nutrition-assistance programs to safeguard the health of individuals whose nutrition status is compromised because of poverty or complex physiologic, social, or other stressors. The National School Lunch Act of 1946 (Pub L No. 79-396) provided for a major federal role in food service for school children. Two major types of nutrition-assistance programs are operated nationally by the USDA: the Supplemental Nutrition Assistance Program and the special nutrition programs that include the Child Nutrition Programs and WIC. The USDA Food and Nutrition Service (FNS) provides updated fact sheets on each of its nutrition-assistance programs (Table 51.1).

Supplemental Nutrition Assistance Program

SNAP—formerly known as the Food Stamp Program—is a nutrition-assistance program that enables people with low income to buy nutritious food and make healthy food choices within a limited budget.[10] It is the largest of the federal nutrition-assistance programs. States have the option to include nutrition education activities to SNAP participants and eligible individuals as part of their administrative services. Every state now conducts nutrition education activities for current and potential SNAP clients. The average monthly household benefit level in fiscal year 2008 was $227. SNAP benefits are provided on an electronic card that is used by participants at authorized retail stores to buy food. SNAP benefits redeemed at local stores not only provide nutrition benefits for the participants but also provide an economic boost to the local community. Every $5 in new SNAP benefits generates $9.20 in total community spending.

SNAP is a federal program but it is administered by state and local agencies. As an entitlement program, it is available to all who meet the eligibility standards. However, only 56% of those who are eligible actually participate in SNAP. Half of the participants are children and another 8% are older than 60 years. The FNS, which oversees SNAP, offers numerous resources and tools to help community and faith-based organizations, state and local offices, food retailers, and other health and social service providers teach their clients with low income about the nutrition benefits of food stamps and help them enroll. These materials are available free online (Document7http://www.fns.usda.gov/snap/outreach/default.htm).

To qualify for SNAP benefits, a person must apply through a local SNAP office and have income and resources under certain limits. The FNS Web site offers the "step 1" online prescreening tool (http://http://www.snap-step1.usda.gov/fns/) in English and Spanish, which privately tells users whether they may be eligible for benefits and how much they could receive. The FNS Web site also provides SNAP application and local office locators (http://www.fns.usda.gov/snap/outreach/map.htm) and state SNAP information/hotline numbers (Document7http://www.fns.usda.gov/snap/contact_info/hotlines.htm).

School Nutrition Programs

The National School Lunch Program (NSLP), the School Breakfast Program (SBP), and the Special Milk Program are administered in most states by the state education agency, which enters into agreements with officials of local schools or school districts to operate nonprofit food services. Most public and private schools in the United States participate in the NSLP. Participating schools can receive cash subsidies and USDA-donated foods regardless of the number of children eligible for free lunch program. Any public or nonprofit private school of high school grade or less is eligible. Public and licensed, nonprofit, private residential child care institutions, such as orphanages, community homes for disabled children, juvenile detention centers, and temporary shelters for runaway children, are also eligible. For more information on USDA school meals programs, visit http://www.fns.usda.gov/cnd.

Schools participating in the federal school meals programs agree to serve nutritious meals at a reduced price or free to children who are determined to be eligible on the basis of uniform national poverty guidelines, determined annually by the DHHS. A child's eligibility to receive reduced-price or free meals is based on their household size and income. Additionally, a child from a household currently certified to receive SNAP benefits or benefits under the Food Distribution Program on Indian Reservations or Temporary Assistance to Needy Families (TANF) is categorically eligible for free benefits. Foster children are also categorically eligible to receive school meals. The school meals program provides federal subsidies for

VII

program meals served to children from all income levels; however, free and reduced-price meals served to children determined to be eligible by income criteria are subsidized at a higher rate.

Federal nutrition requirements are specified in program regulations to ensure that the nutrition goals of the school meal programs are met. The nutrient standards, averaged over a week's menu cycle, are one third and one quarter of the Recommended Dietary Allowances for protein, vitamin A, vitamin C, iron, calcium, and calories for various age/grade groupings for school lunch and school breakfast, respectively. There are also limits for total fat (no more than 30% of calories) and saturated fat (less than 10% of calories).

Through the 1994 Healthy Meals for Healthy Children Act (Pub L No. 104-149), the USDA, in 1995, undertook the first major reform in the nutritional quality of school meals since the program began, with the School Meals Initiative for Healthy Children. In addition to the Recommended Dietary Allowances for key nutrients, starting in 1996, school were also required to comply with the Dietary Guidelines for Americans (DGAs), which call for less fat, saturated fat, cholesterol, and sodium and more fruits, vegetables, and grains. The Dietary Guidelines for Americans are the cornerstone of federal nutrition policy and nutrition education activities. They are jointly issued and updated every 5 years by the USDA and DHHS. The *MyPlate* food guidance system, which recently replaced the *MyPyramid* guidance system, provides food-based guidance to help implement the recommendations of the DGAs. The DGAs provide authoritative advice for people 2 years and older about how good dietary habits can promote health and reduce risks of major chronic diseases. For more information the DGAs, see http://www.dietaryguidelines .gov and for more information on *MyPlate*, see http://www.choosemyplate.gov.

To help schools implement the updated nutritional standards, the USDA launched the Team Nutrition initiative in June 1995. In addition to expanding training and technical assistance resources for schools, Team Nutrition brings together public and private networks to promote food choices for a healthy diet through 6 channels: the classroom, food service providers, the media, the entire school, families, and the community. Team Nutrition funds a limited number of competitive grants to states each year for Team Nutrition initiatives at the state and local levels. The Nutrition, Education and Training Program, authorized in 1978, funds grants to the states for nutrition activities and develop the infrastructure for the delivery of the Team Nutrition materials within the states. More information on Team Nutrition can be found at http://teamnutrition.usda.gov.

The Special Milk Program reduces the cost of each half-pint of milk served to children by providing cash reimbursement at an annually adjusted rate. A school district can choose to provide milk free to children who meet the eligibility guidelines. This program is available only to schools, child care institutions, and summer camps that do not participate in other federal meal service programs. At present, the Special Milk Program allows flavored milks and reduced-fat milks.

School Wellness Policies

Under the Child Nutrition and WIC Reauthorization Act of 2004 (Public Law No. 108-265), each local educational agency participating in a program authorized by the National School Lunch Act or the Child Nutrition Act of 1966 (Public Law No. 89-642) was required to establish a local school wellness policy by school year 2006. The purpose of implementing local wellness policies is to create healthy school nutrition environments that promote healthy eating and physical activity for students.

The legislation placed the responsibility of developing and implementing a wellness policy at the local level so that the individual needs of each local educational agency can be addressed. Preventing childhood obesity is a collective responsibility requiring family, school, community, corporate, and governmental commitments. The key is to implement changes through coordinated and collaborative efforts from all sectors. For more information, visit the USDA Web site at http://teamnutrition.usda.gov/Healthy/wellnesspolicy.html.

The American Academy of Pediatrics (AAP) has encouraged its members to become involved in assisting their local school districts in developing and implementing school wellness policies. The AAP and the AND are cooperating with the Action for Healthy Kids, a national nonprofit organization, to address the epidemic of overweight, undernourished, and sedentary youth through tangible changes in the school environment. Useful information for how pediatricians can become involved in school wellness policies is available (www.actionforhealthykids.org).

Child and Adult Care Food Program

The Child and Adult Care Food Program (CACFP) provides cash reimbursement and USDA Foods for the provision of meals and snacks to facilities providing nonresidential child care for children. Institutions eligible to participate include nonprofit childcare centers, Head Start centers, and family or group child care homes. Some for-profit child care centers serving children from families with low income may also be eligible to participate in the program.

Although federal subsidies continue to be provided for meals served to children from all income levels, program benefits are primarily directed to needy children. Children 12 years and younger are eligible to receive up to 2 meals and 1 snack each day at a child care home or center. Children who reside in homeless shelters may receive up to 3 meals each day. Migrant children 15 years and younger and people with disabilities, regardless of their age, are eligible to receive reimbursable

VII

meals. After-school care snacks and meals are available to children through 18 years of age. For more information on the Child and Adult Care Food Program, visit the Web site (http://www.fns.usda.gov/cnd/care).

Summer Food Service Program

The Summer Food Service Program (SFSP) provides nutritious meals for children 18 years and younger during school vacations at centrally located sites, such as schools or community centers in neighborhoods with low incomes, or at summer camps. Meals are served free to all eligible children and must meet the nutritional standards established by the USDA. Sponsors of the program must be public or private nonprofit schools, public agencies, or private nonprofit organizations. For more information on the Summer Food Service Program, visit the Web site (http://www.fns.usda.gov/cnd/summer).

Supplemental Food Programs

WIC

The WIC program is the premiere public health nutrition program serving low-income, nutritionally at-risk pregnant, breastfeeding, and nonbreastfeeding postpartum women, infants, and children up to 5 years of age. The WIC program is administered at the federal level by the FNS of the USDA and was created by Congress to serve as an adjunct to health care during critical times of growth and development. The benefits of the WIC program include nutritious supplemental foods, nutrition education, and referrals for health and social services, which are all provided to participants at no cost. Many studies show that the WIC program has made many contributions toward improving maternal and child health and saving children's lives.[11-14]

The WIC program is available in all 50 states, 34 Indian Tribal Organizations, American Samoa, the District of Columbia, Guam, Puerto Rico, the Virgin Islands, and the Commonwealth of the Northern Marianas Islands. As of 2011, these state agencies administered the WIC program through 2200 local agencies and 9000 clinic sites. Of the 8.7 million people who received WIC benefits each month in fiscal year 2011, approximately 4.6 million were children, 2.07 million were infants, and 2.04 million were women. Services under WIC are provided in county health departments, hospitals, mobile clinics (vans), community centers, schools, public housing sites, Indian reservations, migrant health centers and camps, and Indian Health Service facilities.

Since the piloting of the WIC program in 1972, funding has grown to approximately $6.73 billion yearly. Program funds are allocated to state agencies according to a formula that considers both administrative and food costs. The average monthly food package cost for fiscal year 2011 was $42.99.

The food packages provided for the different categories of WIC participants are designed to provide nutrients frequently lacking in the diets of the target population. The Institute of Medicine (IOM) recently reviewed the WIC food packages and provided their recommendations for revising the foods offered in the program in their final report, "WIC Food Packages: Time for a Change."[15] In response to the IOM recommendations, FNS published regulations that would implement the first comprehensive revisions to the WIC food packages since 1980. The proposed changes to the food packages largely follow recommendations made by the IOM and align with the DGAs and infant feeding practice guidelines of the AAP.

The revised food packages continue to provide the same food categories and add new food categories as well as optional substitutions for some food categories, to better meet the needs of the diverse population of WIC participants. All WIC state agencies had to implement the revised food packages by October 1, 2009. The revised food packages included:

- Addition of fruits and vegetables for women and children—participants may choose fruits and vegetables (fresh and processed) that provide ethnic variety and appeal.

- Addition of soy-based beverage and tofu as milk alternatives for women and children, although medical documentation is required for children to ensure the child's health care provider is aware that milk is being replaced with soy-based beverage or tofu.

- Addition of whole-grain foods for women and children—participants may choose whole-grain cereals, whole-wheat bread, brown rice, bulgur, oatmeal, whole-grain barley, or soft corn or whole-wheat tortillas, depending on state option.

- Reductions in some food allowances, including milk, cheese, eggs, and juice for women and children—the new food packages are consistent with dietary recommendations from the DGAs, and the reductions in some food allowances allow a more balanced food package to be provided. Women who are exclusively breastfeeding receive the most variety and largest quantity of food.

- Provision of only fat-reduced milk to women and children 2 years and older and only whole milk to children between 1 and 2 years of age. Whole milk would be available for women and children older than 2 years only with medical documentation.

- Revision of infant food packages—infants will receive food packages designed for the categories of fully breastfeeding, partially breastfeeding, or fully formula feeding. Compared with previous food packages, partially breastfed

VII

infants receive less infant formula to allow mothers to breastfeed their infants more, and there is no routine issuance of infant formula in the first month of life to support the establishment of breastfeeding. Jarred infant foods (fruits and vegetables) have been added for all infants 6 months and older, and the quantity of infant formula is reduced. Jarred infant food meat has been added for fully breastfed infants 6 months and older, and juice has been eliminated from infant food packages. Low-iron infant formula is no longer authorized.

- For the complete provisions and requirements for foods in the WIC food packages, refer to the full regulation at www.fns.usda.gov/wic. Although federal regulations specify the minimum nutritional requirements for the WIC foods, state agencies determine which foods, under the new regulation, to include on state authorized food lists.

The revised food packages promote and support the establishment of successful, long-term breastfeeding; provide WIC participants with a wide variety of foods, including fruits, and vegetables and whole grains; provide less saturated fat and cholesterol and more fiber to women and children; reinforce the nutrition messages provided to participants; and provide WIC state agencies greater flexibility in prescribing food packages to accommodate the cultural food preferences of WIC participants.

Nutrition education is an important benefit of the WIC program. Efforts are made to provide client-centered nutrition education that focuses on the individual participant's nutritional needs, cultural preferences, and education level. Breastfeeding promotion and support activities are an important component of WIC nutrition education.

The WIC Farmers' Market Nutrition Program provides additional coupons to WIC recipients that can be used to buy fresh fruits and vegetables from authorized farmers, farmers markets, or roadside stands.

For more information on the WIC program, see the WIC Web site at http://www.fns.usda.gov/wic.

Food Distribution Programs

These programs include the Commodity Supplemental Food Program, the Emergency Food Assistance Program, the Food Distribution Program on Indian Reservations, the Nutrition Services Incentive Program (formerly the Nutrition Program for the Elderly), and Schools/Child Nutrition USDA Foods Programs, which include the NSLP, Summer Food Service Program, and the Child and Adult Care Food Program.

Commodity Supplemental Food Program

The Commodity Supplemental Food Program operates in 38 states (including the District of Columbia) and on 2 Indian reservations. The program provides food packages to low-income pregnant, lactating, and postpartum women up to 1 year, to infants and children up to 6 years of age, and to elderly people 60 years or older.

Like the WIC program, the Commodity Supplemental Food Program provides food packages to supplement the diets of participants. The foods offered include infant formula and cereal, nonfat dry and low-fat ultra–high-temperature fluid milk, juice, farina, oats, ready-to-eat cereal, rice, pasta, peanut butter, dried beans or peas, canned meat, poultry, or fish, and canned fruits and vegetables. Food packages through the Commodity Supplemental Food Program do not provide a complete diet but, rather, are good sources of the nutrients typically lacking in the diets of the target population.

Unlike the WIC program, the Commodity Supplemental Food Program distributes food rather than vouchers for redemption at grocery stores. Eligible people cannot participate concurrently in both programs. In fiscal year 2010, an average of more than 518 000 people each month participated in the Commodity Supplemental Food Program, including more than 497 000 elderly people and more than 21 000 women, infants, and children. In instances in which a woman, infant, or child is unable to participate in WIC, the Commodity Supplemental Food Program serves as an additional (and important) food assistance resource within the community about which pediatric health care professionals should be informed.

State agencies set eligibility standards, store the food, and select local public and nonprofit private agencies to which they distribute the food. Local agencies determine the eligibility of applicants, distribute the foods, and provide nutrition education and referrals for health care and social services. In addition to donated food, the USDA provides funds to cover some program administrative costs. For more information on the Commodity Supplemental Food Program, see the Web site (http://www.fns.usda.gov/fdd/programs/csfp).

The Emergency Food Assistance Program

The Emergency Food Assistance Program is a federal program, administered by the USDA, that helps supplement the diets of low-income Americans, including elderly people, by providing them with emergency food and nutrition assistance at no cost. Under the Emergency Food Assistance Program, the USDA makes USDA foods available to state distributing agencies. States provide the food to

VII

local agencies that they have selected, usually food banks, which in turn distribute the food to soup kitchens and food pantries that directly serve the public. These organizations distribute the USDA foods for household consumption or use them to prepare and serve meals in a congregate setting. Recipients of food for home use must meet income eligibility criteria set by the states. States also provide the food to other types of local organizations, such as community action agencies, which distribute the foods directly to households in need. State agencies receive the food and supervise overall distribution. For more information on the Emergency Food Assistance Program, see the Web site (http://www.fns.usda.gov/fdd/programs/tefap). For additional information about disaster relief and federal disaster programs, see http://www.fns.usda.gov/FDD/programs/fd-disasters/about_disasters.htm.

Food Distribution Program on Indian Reservations

The Food Distribution Program on Indian Reservations provides USDA foods to low-income households on Indian reservations and to American Indian households residing in approved areas near reservations or in Oklahoma. Many households participate in the Food Distribution Program on Indian Reservations, as an alternative to the SNAP, because they do not have easy access to SNAP offices or authorized food stores. The program is administered at the federal level by the Food and Nutrition Service (FNS). The Food Distribution Program on Indian Reservations is administered locally by either Indian Tribal Organizations or an agency of a state government. As of 2010, there are approximately 276 tribes receiving benefits through 100 Indian Tribal Organizations and 5 state agencies. Average monthly participation for fiscal year 2010 was 84 609 individuals.

Each month, participating households receive a food package to help them maintain a nutritionally balanced diet. Participants may select from more than 70 products, including: frozen ground beef, beef roast, and chicken; canned meats, poultry, and fish; canned fruits and vegetables, canned soups, and spaghetti sauce; macaroni and cheese, pastas, cereals, rice, and other grains; cheese, egg mix, nonfat dry and evaporated milk, and low-fat ultra-high temperature fluid milk; flour, cornmeal, low-fat bakery mix, and reduced sodium crackers; low-fat refried beans, dried beans, and dehydrated potatoes; canned juices and dried fruit; peanuts and peanut butter; and light buttery spread and vegetable oil. Participants on most reservations can choose fresh produce instead of canned fruits and vegetables. For more information on the Food Distribution Program on Indian Reservations, see the Web site (http://www.fns.usda.gov/fdd/programs/fdpir).

Where to Seek Nutrition Assistance for Clients

Nutrition-assistance programs are usually administered at the local level by the following agencies:

1. Local school food authority: NSLP, School Breakfast Program, and Special Milk Program.
2. State and local health, social services, education, or agriculture agencies; public or private nonprofit health agencies; and Indian Tribal Organizations or groups recognized by the US Department of the Interior: WIC; Food Distribution Program on Indian Reservations; Summer Food Service Program; Child and Adult Care Food Program; the Emergency Food Assistance Program; Commodity Supplemental Food Program.
3. Local social services, human services, or welfare department: SNAP.
4. Community or faith-based organizations.

Other Federal Agencies Providing Nutrition Services to Improve Pediatric Health and Well-Being

CDC Nutrition and Physical Activity Program to Prevent Obesity and Other Chronic Diseases

The CDC administers the state-based Nutrition and Physical Activity Program to Prevent Obesity and Other Chronic Diseases. This program is based on a cooperative agreement between the CDC Division of Nutrition and Physical Activity and 28 state health departments. The program was established in fiscal year 1999 to prevent and control obesity and other chronic diseases by supporting states in developing and implementing nutrition and physical activity interventions, particularly through population-based strategies (eg, policy-level changes, environmental supports).

States receive funding from the program to work to prevent and control obesity and other chronic diseases through these strategies: balancing caloric intake and expenditure, increasing physical activity, increasing consumption of fruits and vegetables, decreasing television-viewing and other screen time, and increasing breastfeeding. The program also helps states work to reduce soft-drink consumption and decrease portion size. States funded by the program partner with stakeholders in government, academia, industry, and other areas to create statewide health plans—one of the most important ways to help guide state efforts. State plans promote working with a variety of partners and using all available resources to prevent and control obesity and other chronic diseases. For more information on CDC programs and campaigns, research reports, surveillance data, training modules, nutrition education, and related resources, see the Web site (http://www.cdc.gov/nccdphp/dnpa).

VII

Maternal and Child Health Services

The Title V MCH block grant program provides states with federal funds that support a wide variety of health services, including nutrition services. Title V seeks to improve the health of all mothers and children (including children with special health care needs) by assessing needs, setting priorities, and providing programs and services. Specifically, the Title V MCH program seeks to:

1. Ensure access to quality care, especially for those with low-incomes or limited availability of care;
2. Reduce infant mortality;
3. Provide and ensure access to comprehensive prenatal and postnatal care to women (especially low-income and at-risk pregnant women);
4. Increase the number of children receiving health assessments and follow-up diagnostic and treatment services;
5. Provide and ensure access to preventive and child care services as well as rehabilitative services for certain children;
6. Implement family-centered, community-based, systems of coordinated care for children with special health care needs; and
7. Provide toll-free hotlines and assistance in applying for services to pregnant women with infants and children who are eligible for Medicaid.

On the basis of a comprehensive 5-year needs assessment, state Title V MCH programs identify their priority needs and develop a program plan and state performance measures to address these needs, to the extent that they are not addressed by the program's 18 national performance measures. Each state is unique in the type of services they provide under their Title V MCH block grant. The conceptual framework for the services of the Title V MCH block grant is a pyramid, which includes 4 tiers of services (ie, direct health care services, enabling services [such as coordination with Medicaid and WIC services], population-based services, and infrastructure building services). The MCH block grant program is the only federal program that provides services at all 4 levels, including state population-based capacity and infrastructure-building services and which targets the entire population and not only the low-income population.

In 2006, the Health Resources and Services Administration's Maternal and Child Health Bureau (MCHB) included a new national performance measure that addresses the "percentage of children, ages 2 to 5 years, receiving WIC services with a body mass index at or above the 85th percentile." Another national performance measure, which had previously focused on the percentage of "mothers who breastfeed their infants at hospital discharge," was revised to reflect the percentage of "mothers who breastfeed their infants at 6 months of age."

The Title V Information System electronically captures data reported in the annual Title V MCH block grant applications and reports on 59 states, territories, and jurisdictions. State-reported financial data, program data, and information on key measures and indicators of MCH in the United States are posted on the Title V Information System Web site (https://mchdata.hrsa.gov/tvisreports/).

In addition to the formula block grants to states, Title V supports activities under the Special Projects of Regional and National Significance grants and the Community Integrated Service Systems grants. Activities supported under Special Projects of Regional and National Significance include MCH research, training, breastfeeding promotion and support, nutrition services, and a broad range of other MCH initiatives and grant projects. The Community Integrated Service Systems program seeks to improve the health of mothers and children by funding projects for the development and expansion of integrated health, education, and social services at the community level. Additional information on MCHB-funded programs is available on the MCHB Web site (http://http://mchb.hrsa.gov/).

The EPSDT program is the child health component of Medicaid. The EPSDT program is required in every state and is designed to improve the health of low-income children by financing appropriate and necessary pediatric services. State Title V agencies can play an important role in fulfilling the potential of EPSDT services. Federal rules encourage partnerships between state Medicaid and Title V agencies to ensure better access to and receipt of the full range of screening, diagnostic, and treatment services.

Bright Futures, initiated in 1990, is a longstanding, major effort of the MCHB and its partners to improve the quality of health promotion and prevention for infants, children, and adolescents and their families. Over the years, Bright Futures has evolved to encompass a vision, a philosophy, and a set of expert guidelines, tools, and other resources to implement a practical developmental approach to providing health supervision for children of all ages, from birth through adolescence.

Recognizing the need for more in-depth materials in certain areas to complement the guidelines, the MCHB launched the Building Bright Futures Project to foster the implementation of the Bright Futures health supervision guidelines by publishing practical tools and materials and by providing technical assistance and training. Using *Bright Futures: Guidelines for Health Supervision of Infants, Children, and Adolescents* as a cornerstone document, a series of implementation guides have been developed. Included in the *Bright Futures* series are the first, second, and upcoming third editions of *Bright Futures: Nutrition*[16] and the first edition of *Bright Futures: Physical Activity*.[17] Through a cooperative agreement between

VII

MCHB and the AAP, the third edition of the *Bright Futures in Practice* is available (www.brightfutures.aap.org)

Conclusion

As the key provider of child health care, the pediatrician has a major role in ensuring that nutrition services for children include assessment of nutritional status and provision of a safe food supply adequate in quality and quantity, nutrition counseling, and nutrition education for children and parents. As the primary expert on health in the community and as a concerned citizen, the pediatrician, in coordination with other members of the health care team, including the nutritionist or dietitian and nurse, can provide meaningful leadership in the formulation of sound nutrition policy and the education of legislators, administrators, and others who influence the response of the community to the nutritional needs of its children.

References

1. Eagan MC, Oglesby AC. Nutrition services in the maternal and child health program: a historical perspective. In: Sharbaugh CO, Egan MC, eds. *Call to Action: Better Nutrition for Mothers, Children, and Families.* Washington, DC: National Center for Education in Maternal and Child Health; 1991:73-92

2. US Department of Health and Human Services. *Healthy People 2010. With Understanding and Improving Health and Objectives for Improving Health.* 2nd ed. Washington, DC: US Government Printing Office; 2000

3. McCall M, Keir B. *Survey of the Public Health Nutrition Workforce 1999-2000.* Alexandria, VA: US Department of Agriculture; 2003

4. Institute of Medicine. *The Future of the Public's Health in the 21st Century.* Washington, DC: National Academies Press; 2003

5. Edelstein S. *Nutrition in Public Health: Handbook for Developing Programs and Services.* 2nd ed. Sudbury, MA: Jones and Bartlett Publishers; 2005

6. American Dietetic Association. Position of the American Dietetic Association: cost-effectiveness of medical nutrition therapy. *J Am Diet Assoc.* 1995;95(1):88-91

7. An Act Further Regulating Insurance Coverage for Certain Inherited Diseases. Massachusetts Session Law. Chapter 384 §1-11 (1993). Available at: http://archives.lib.state.ma.us/actsResolves/1993/1993acts0384.pdf. Accessed January 19, 2013

8. Bayerl CT, Ries J, Bettencourt MF, Fisher P. Nutritional issues of children in early intervention programs: primary care team approach. *Semin Pediatr Gastrointest Nutr.* 1993;4:11-15

9. Owen AY, Splett PL, Owen GM, Frankle RT. *Nutrition in the Community. The Art and Science of Delivering Services.* 4th ed. Boston, MA: McGraw-Hill; 1999

10. *Myths and Facts About Food Stamp Benefits and the Elderly*. Alexandria, VA: Food and Nutrition Service, US Department of Agriculture; 2007. Available at: http://www.fns .usda.gov/snap/outreach/pdfs/myths-elderly.pdf. Accessed January 19, 2013

11. US General Accounting Office. *Early Intervention: Federal Investments Like WIC Can Produce Savings: Report to Congressional Requesters*. Washington, DC: US General Accounting Office; 1992. Publication No. GAO/HRD-92-18

12. Mathematica Policy Research Inc. *The Savings in Medicaid Costs for Newborns and Their Mothers From Prenatal Participation in the WIC Program*. Alexandria, VA: Food and Nutrition Service, US Department of Agriculture; 1991

13. Bitler MP, Currie J. Does WIC work? The effects of WIC on pregnancy and birth outcomes. *J Policy Anal Manage*. 2005;24(1):73-91

14. Henchy W. *WIC in the States: Thirty-One Years of Building a Healthier America*. Washington, DC: Food Research and Action Center; 2005. Available at: http://www.frac .org/WIC/2004_Report/Full_Report.pdf. Accessed November 2, 2007

15. Institute of Medicine. *WIC Food Packages: Time for a Change*. Washington, DC: National Academies Press; 2006

16. Holt K, Wooldridge N, Story M, Sofka D. *Bright Futures Nutrition*. 3rd ed. Elk Grove Village, IL: American Academy of Pediatrics; 2011

17. Patrick K. *Bright Futures in Practice: Physical Activity*. Arlington, VA: National Center for Education in Maternal and Child Health; 2001

Chapter 52

Food Labeling

Introduction

In 1990, the Nutrition Labeling and Education Act (NLEA [Pub L No. 101-535]) was enacted, mandating numerous changes in food labeling. Before that time, nutrition labeling on food products was voluntary, except for those that contained added nutrients or carried nutrition claims. As Americans became more interested in nutrition, food label regulations were revised to provide nutrition information that would help consumers make food choices to meet national dietary recommendations.

The NLEA took effect in 1994, when the labels of most packaged foods were required to feature the new "Nutrition Facts" panel.[1] Labeling is voluntary for fresh fruits and vegetables and raw meat, poultry, and seafood. For these raw foods, nutrition information may be printed on the package or on pamphlets or posters displayed near the food in the supermarket. Food labeling is regulated by the US Food and Drug Administration (FDA), with the exception of meat and poultry products, which are regulated by the US Department of Agriculture (USDA).

Ingredient Labeling

Ingredient labeling is an important source of information for consumers about the composition of packaged foods. Both FDA and USDA regulations require that food products with 2 or more ingredients provide a listing of ingredients in descending order of their prominence by weight by their common, specific names.[2,3] The source of some ingredients must be stated by name to help people with specific food needs because of religious or health reasons. These include protein hydrolysates and caseinate as a milk derivative in foods that claim to be nondairy. Certified color additives must also be listed by name (eg, FD&C Blue No. 1 or FD&C Yellow No. 5).

For families with food allergies, it is essential to read the ingredient listings on food labels to determine the presence of the 8 major allergens (milk, egg, wheat, soy, peanuts, tree nuts, fish, and crustacea). Because food and beverage manufacturers are continually making ingredient changes, food-allergic people and their caregivers should read the ingredient declaration or "Contains..." statement on the food label of every product purchased, each time it is purchased and consumed (or served).

In January 2006, food allergen labeling requirements of the Food Allergen Labeling and Consumer Protection Act (FALCP [Pub L No. 108-282]) became effective on FDA-regulated food and beverage products.[4] The Act defined the 8 major food allergens and requires 1 of 2 options for ingredient labeling of food products:

VII

1. Immediately following the ingredient declaration, the label states "Contains" followed by the name of the food source from which the major food allergen is derived (eg, "Contains milk, egg, walnuts."). In the case of tree nuts, fish, or shellfish, each specific food in these classes that is an ingredient in the food must be declared (ie, salmon, cod, crab, pecan, hazelnut) rather than the group listing.
2. Within the ingredient declaration, in parentheses following the common or usual name of the allergenic ingredient, the label presents the name of the food source from which the major food allergen is derived—for example, "…whey (milk)…"

An ingredient listing, especially a long list of ingredients, may contain both options for labeling of the major food allergens.

The Nutrition Facts Panel

The food label carries a variety of nutrition information (Fig 52.1, Fig 52.2, and Fig 52.3) in the Nutrition Facts panel that indicates the amount of targeted macronutrients and micronutrients. Simplified or shortened formats may be used for products that contain insignificant amounts (amount declarable as zero in labeling; generally less than 0.5 g) of certain mandatory label nutrients. Package size constraints may also dictate different formats.

The following provides more details about the various features of the Nutrition Facts panel for foods for adults and children older than 4 years (Fig 52.1):

1. Serving size: Serving sizes are standardized for different food categories based on the average amount of food eaten at one time, using data from national food consumption surveys. Sizes do not always match serving sizes specified in My Plate. Two measurements are provided: common household and metric measures.
2. Calories: Total calories in one serving are identified. In addition, calories from fat per serving are also included on the panel.
3. Nutrients: Information about the content of nutrients most related to today's health concerns must be listed. These nutrients include fat, saturated fat, trans fat, cholesterol, sodium, total carbohydrate, fiber, sugars, protein, vitamins A and C, calcium, and iron. Other nutrients are listed voluntarily, and if foods contain insignificant amounts of a required nutrient, that nutrient may be omitted from the label. Information about other nutrients is required in 2 cases: (1) if a claim is made about the nutrients on the label, or (2) if the nutrients are added to the food, as in the case of fortified foods (eg vitamin D). Nutrient amounts can be listed in 1 of 2 ways: in the metric amount or as a percentage of the Daily Value. Percentage of Daily Value is used only for vitamins and minerals, except for sodium and potassium. Amounts can be listed both as a metric amount and percentage of Daily Value on the same label for all other ingredients (Fig 52.1).

Fig 52.1.
Nutrition Label Format, Food for Ages Greater Than 4 Years

Nutrition Facts
Serving Size 1 cup (228g)
Servings Per Container 2

Amount Per Serving
Calories 260   Calories from Fat 120

% Daily Value*

Total Fat 13g	**20%**
Saturated Fat 5g	**25%**
Trans Fat 2g	
Cholesterol 30mg	**10%**
Sodium 660mg	**28%**
Total Carbohydrate 31g	**10%**
Dietary Fiber 0g	**0%**
Sugars 5g	
Protein 5g	

Vitamin A 4%   •   Vitamin C 2%
Calcium 15%   •   Iron 4%

* Percent Daily Values are based on a 2,000 calorie diet.
Your Daily Values may be higher or lower depending on your calorie needs:

	Calories:	2,000	2,500
Total Fat	Less than	65g	80g
Sat Fat	Less than	20g	25g
Cholesterol	Less than	300mg	300mg
Sodium	Less than	2,400mg	2,400mg
Total Carbohydrate		300g	375g
Dietary Fiber		25g	30g

Calories per gram:
Fat 9   •   Carbohydrate 4   •   Protein 4

Fig 52.2.
Nutrition Label Format, Food for Children Under 2 Years

Nutrition Facts
Serving Size 1 cup (228g)
Servings Per Container 2

Amount Per Serving
Calories 260   Calories from Fat 120

% Daily Value*

Total Fat 13g	**20%**
Saturated Fat 5g	**25%**
Trans Fat 2g	
Cholesterol 30mg	**10%**
Sodium 660mg	**28%**
Total Carbohydrate 31g	**10%**
Dietary Fiber 0g	**0%**
Sugars 5g	
Protein 5g	

Vitamin A 4%   •   Vitamin C 2%
Calcium 15%   •   Iron 4%

* Percent Daily Values are based on a 2,000 calorie diet.
Your Daily Values may be higher or lower depending on your calorie needs:

	Calories:	2,000	2,500
Total Fat	Less than	65g	80g
Sat Fat	Less than	20g	25g
Cholesterol	Less than	300mg	300mg
Sodium	Less than	2,400mg	2,400mg
Total Carbohydrate		300g	375g
Dietary Fiber		25g	30g

Calories per gram:
Fat 9   •   Carbohydrate 4   •   Protein 4

Fig 52.3.
Nutrition Label Format, Food for Children Under 4 Years

Nutrition Label Format, Food for Children under 4

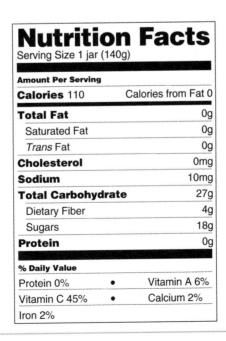

Nutrition Facts
Serving Size 1 jar (140g)

Amount Per Serving
Calories 110   Calories from Fat 0

Total Fat	0g
Saturated Fat	0g
Trans Fat	0g
Cholesterol	0mg
Sodium	10mg
Total Carbohydrate	27g
Dietary Fiber	4g
Sugars	18g
Protein	0g

% Daily Value

Protein 0%	•	Vitamin A 6%
Vitamin C 45%	•	Calcium 2%
Iron 2%		

VII

4. Daily Values: The "% Daily Value" characterizes how the amount of a nutrient in a food or beverage contributes to a moderate, varied, and balanced diet. The term Daily Value is an umbrella term for 2 sets of reference values: daily reference values (DRVs) and Recommended Daily Intakes (RDIs). The DRVs are set for total fat, saturated fat, cholesterol, total carbohydrate, dietary fiber, sodium, potassium, and protein. They are established for adults and children 4 years or older on the basis of current nutrition recommendations. DRVs for cholesterol, sodium, and potassium are set at a constant level for all caloric intakes. DRVs for total fat, saturated fat, cholesterol, total carbohydrate, sodium, potassium, dietary fiber, and protein are based on a 2000-kcal reference diet (Table 52.1). Current Dietary Reference Intakes are listed in Appendix E.

5. Label footnotes: A reference chart for a 2000- and a 2500-kcal diet also appears on the bottom of some Nutrition Facts panels (Fig 52.1). It suggests the amounts of fat, saturated fat, cholesterol, and sodium not to exceed and the amounts of carbohydrate and dietary fiber to consume. Some labels also show the number of calories supplied by 1 g of fat, carbohydrate, and protein.

Table 52.1.

Daily Values Used to Calculate % Daily Value for Nutrition Facts Panel[a]

Food Component	Daily Value for Adults and Children Older Than 4 Years
Daily Reference Values	
Total fat	65 g[b]
Saturated fat	20 g[b]
Cholesterol	300 mg
Sodium	2400 mg
Potassium	3500 mg
Total carbohydrate	300 g[b]
Dietary fiber	25 g[c]
Protein	50 g[b]

[a] Based on a 2000-kcal diet for adults and children older than 4 years.

[b] Daily value based on a 2000-kcal reference diet.

[c] Daily value based on 11.5 g/1000 kcal.

Food Labels for Infants Younger Than 2 Years and Children Between 2 and 4 Years of Age

Food labels on products designed for infants younger than 2 years and children between 2 and 4 years of age are different from food labels on adult products. Specifically, infant food labels (foods for children younger than 2 years) differ in the listing of calories from fat, saturated fat, and cholesterol, percentages of Daily Value, and serving sizes. Fat information is not detailed for infant food (except for total grams) because of the concern that adults may mistakenly apply this information to controlling the calories provided by fat for their infants (Fig 52.2).

The percentages of Daily Value for fat, cholesterol, sodium, potassium, carbohydrates, and fiber are not listed, because the reference values have not been established for infants and children younger than 4 years. Protein is listed in grams per serving and as a percentage of the Daily Value on foods for infants and children younger than 4 years. The Daily Value used to calculate other nutrient percentages are calculated based on the RDI for each population (Fig 52.2 and 52.3).

Serving sizes of foods for infants and children younger than 4 years are based on government reference amounts and are smaller than typical adult servings.

Nutrition Claims

Nutrient content claims are those that characterize the amount of a nutrient in a food, using terms such as free, low, reduced, less, more, added, good source, and high. Using these terms in connection with a specific nutrient is strictly defined (Table 52.2).

Infant food labels may carry claims for vitamins and minerals. Claims about protein, fat, and sodium or the content of certain nutritional ingredients (ie, salt and sugar) are not allowed on products intended for infants younger than 2 years.

Claims about nonnutrient ingredients (eg, preservatives), the identification of ingredients (eg, made with apples), and taste (eg, unsweetened) are allowed.

Juice Labeling

There are specific labeling requirements for juice. Since 1994, the percentage of juice must be specified on the food label if a beverage claims to contain fruit or vegetable juice.[5] Label statements must be declared using the language, "Contains [x] percent [name of fruit or vegetable] juice," "[x] percent juice," or a similar phrase (eg, Contains 50% apple juice"). If a beverage contains minor amounts of juice for flavoring, the product may use the term "flavor," "flavored," or "flavoring" with a fruit or vegetable name, as long as the product does not bear the term "juice" (other than in the ingredient declaration) and does not visually depict the fruit or vegetable from which the flavor is derived. If the beverage contains no juice, but appears to contain juice, the label must state, "Contains no [name of fruit or vegetable] juice," or similar statements. These percentage juice statements appear near the top of the information panel of the beverage label.

VII

Table 52.2.
Nutrition Claims

	Definition, per Serving
Calories	
Calorie free	<5 kcal
Low calorie	≤40 kcal
Reduced or fewer calories	At least 25% fewer calories[a]
Light or lite	One third fewer calories or 50% less fat[a]
Sugar	
Sugar free	<0.5 g
Reduced sugar or less sugar	At least 25% less sugars
No added sugar; without added sugar; no sugar added	No sugars added during processing or packaging, including ingredients that contain sugars, such as juice or dry fruit
Fat	
Fat free	<0.5 g
Low fat	≤3 g
Reduced or less fat	At least 25% less fat[a]
Light or lite	One third fewer calories or 50% less fat[a]
Saturated fat	
Saturated fat free	<0.5 g
Low saturated fat	≤1 g saturated fat and no more than 15% of calories from saturated fat
Reduced or less saturated fat	At least 25% less saturated fat[a]
Cholesterol	
Cholesterol free	<2 mg cholesterol and <2 g fat
Low cholesterol	≤20 mg cholesterol and <2 g saturated fat
Reduced or less cholesterol	At least 25% less cholesterol[a] and <2 g saturated fat
Sodium	
Sodium free	<5 mg
Very low sodium	≤35 mg
Low sodium	≤140 mg
Reduced or less sodium	At least 25% less sodium[a]
Light in sodium	50% less sodium[a]

	Definition, per Serving
Fiber	
High fiber	≥5 g[b]
Good source of fiber	2.5 to 4.9 g
More or added fiber	At least 2.5 g more or added[a]
Other Claims	
High, rich in, excellent source of [name of nutrient]	≥20% of daily value[a]
Good source of, contains, provides [name of nutrient]	10% to 19% of daily value[a]
More, enriched, fortified, added [name of nutrient]	≥10% or more of daily value more or added[a]
Lean[c]	<10 g fat, (<4.5 g saturated fat, and <95 mg cholesterol)
Extra lean[c]	<5 g fat, <2 g saturated fat, and <95 mg cholesterol
Healthy	Meets standards for "low" fat and saturated fat; contains ≤480 mg sodium; ≤60 mg cholesterol; and contains at least 10 percent daily value for vitamin A, vitamin C, calcium, iron, protein, or fiber

[a] Compared with a standard serving size of the traditional food.

[b] Must also meet the definition for low fat, or the level of fat must appear next to the high-fiber claim.

[c] On meat, poultry, seafood, and game meats.

Gluten-Free Labeling

In August 2013, the FDA published its final rule to define the term "gluten free" for voluntary use in the labeling of foods. The rule allows manufacturers to label a food "gluten-free" if the food does NOT contain any of the following[6]:

1. An ingredient that is any type of wheat, rye, or barley or crossbreeds of these grains.
2. An ingredient derived from these grains and that has not been processed to remove gluten.
3. An ingredient derived from these grains and that has been processed to remove gluten, if it results in the food containing 20 or more parts per million of gluten.
4. 20 ppm or more gluten.

VII

"Gluten-free" will remain a voluntary claim that can be used at the manufacturer's discretion and is not required information. Therefore, this claim should not appear in the ingredient statement on the Nutrition Facts label and can be included on the front of the package.

Health Claims

In addition to nutrient content claims, a food label may bear claims about the health benefits of the food or a component of the food. Products must meet strict nutrition requirements before they can carry these claims associating foods, nutrients, or substances with reduced risk of a disease or condition. Health claims are not allowed on the food labels of products intended for children younger than 2 years.

To date, the FDA, on the basis of scientific evidence, has authorized 12 health claims.[7] Although the wording on packages may differ, the following summarizes the allowed claims that link disease with food and nutrients:

1. Calcium and osteoporosis: Physical activity and a calcium-rich diet may reduce the risk of osteoporosis, a condition in which the bones become soft or brittle.
2. Fat and cancer: A diet low in total fat may reduce the risk of some cancers.
3. Saturated fat and cholesterol and heart disease: A diet low in saturated fat and cholesterol may reduce the risk of heart disease.
4. Fiber-containing grain products, fruits, and vegetables, and cancer: A low-fat diet rich in fiber-containing grain products, fruits, and vegetables may reduce the risk of some cancers.
5. Fruits, vegetables, and grain products that contain fiber and heart disease: A diet low in saturated fat and cholesterol and rich in fruits, vegetables, and grain products that contain some types of dietary fiber may reduce the risk of heart disease.
6. Sodium and high blood pressure: A low-sodium diet may reduce the risk of high blood pressure, which is a risk factor for heart attacks and strokes.
7. Fruits and vegetables and some cancers: A low-fat diet rich in fruits and vegetables (foods that are low in fat and may contain dietary fiber, vitamin A, or vitamin C) may reduce the risk of some cancers.
8. Folic acid and neural tube birth defects: Women who consume 0.4 mg of folic acid daily may reduce their risk of giving birth to a child affected with a neural tube defect.
9. Noncariogenic carbohydrate sweeteners (sugar alcohols, sucralose) and dental caries: Frequent eating of foods high in sugars and starches as between-meal snacks can promote tooth decay. The [name of sugar alcohol, or sucralose] used to sweeten this food may reduce the risk of dental caries.

10. Soluble fiber from certain foods and risk of coronary heart disease: Soluble fiber from [name of food (eg, oat bran, psyllium, or barley fiber)], as part of a diet low in saturated fat and cholesterol, may reduce the risk of heart disease.

11. Soy protein and risk of coronary heart disease: Diets low in saturated fat and cholesterol that include 25 g of soy protein a day may reduce the risk of heart disease. One serving of [name of food] provides [x] g of soy protein.

12. Plant sterol or stanol esters and risk of coronary heart disease: Diets low in saturated fat and cholesterol that include 2 servings of foods that provide a daily total of at least 1.3 g of vegetable oil sterol esters in 2 meals may reduce the risk of heart disease. A serving of [name of the food] supplies [x] g of vegetable oil sterol esters. Diets low in saturated fat and cholesterol that include 2 servings of foods that provide a daily total of at least 3.4 g of vegetable oil stanol esters in 2 meals may reduce the risk of heart disease. A serving of [name of the food] supplies [x] g of vegetable oil stanol esters.

To bear a health claim, each food must not exceed (unless exempted by FDA) specified levels of fat, saturated fat, cholesterol, and sodium.

In addition to the above health claims, the FDA Modernization Act of 1997 (FDAMA [Pub L No. 105-115]) established an additional route to establish health claims. FDAMA procedures allow a health claim to be made if it is based on a published authoritative statement, currently in effect, about the relationship between a nutrient and a disease or health-related condition to which the claim refers, issued by a scientific body of the US government with official responsibility for public health protection or research directly relating to human nutrition (eg, *Dietary Guidelines for Americans* from USDA and DHHS; DRI reports from the National Academy of Sciences).

In July 1999, the first such health claim was established related to whole-grain foods and reduced risk of heart disease and cancer. The health claim states: Diets rich in whole-grain foods and other plant foods and low in total fat, saturated fat, and cholesterol, may help reduce the risk of heart disease and certain cancers. To qualify for the claim, a food must contain 51% or more whole-grain ingredients per serving, be low in fat, and meet other general criteria for health claims.

In October 2000, a second FDAMA health claim was established related to potassium-containing foods and reduced risk of high blood pressure and stroke. The health claim states: Diets containing foods that are good sources of potassium and low in sodium may reduce the risk of high blood pressure and stroke. To qualify for the claim, a food must be a good source of potassium and low in sodium, total fat, saturated fat, and cholesterol (see "Nutrition Claims").

In December 2003, a third FDAMA health claim was established related to whole-grain foods with moderate fat content and reduced risk of heart disease. The health claim states: Diets rich in whole-grain foods and other plant foods may help reduced the risk of heart disease. To qualify for the claim, a food must contain 51% or more grain ingredients as whole grain and meet other FDA-specified criteria. These foods do not have to be low fat (<3 g per serving) but must contain <6 g of fat per serving and must meet other criteria for saturated fat, cholesterol, and sodium and have <0.5 g of trans fat per serving.

Structure/Function Claims

A food label may also include a structure/function claim that describes the role of a nutrient or dietary ingredient intended to affect normal structure or function in humans. Structure/function claims can be used on FDA-regulated conventional foods and dietary supplements and are often added to a label claim when a "health claim" cannot be made for a food or an ingredient. The FDA published final regulations defining the types of structure or function claims permitted on dietary supplement labels in February 2000.[8] Structure/function claims can be made on labels with only modest levels of evidence, and companies are not required to presubmit labels for approval; however, for a structure/function claim made for a dietary supplement, notification must be submitted to the FDA no later than 30 days after marketing. The FDA has recently urged companies to presubmit labels to avoid the need for postmarket surveillance. The FDA can take action against a structure/function claim if it can prove that the label is blatantly false or misleading. The FDA enforcement authority is through courts, however, because there is no administrative remedy established by legislation. For a comparison of structure/function claims and health claims, see Table 52.3.

Table 52.3.
Structure/Function Claims Versus Health Claims on Food Labels

Structure/Function Claim	Health Claim
Enhances the immune system	Protects against infection
For babies with colic	Prevents colic in babies
Builds stronger bones	Prevents fractures

Additional examples of structure/function claims that have been found on food label marketed for children are as follows:

- Proven to help build a strong immune system
- Now with prebiotics similar to those found in human milk
- Easy to digest
- Supports healthy growth and development
- Prebiotics to support digestive health
- Calcium for strong bones
- Nucleotides, prebiotics, and carotenoids for immune support
- For bedtime feeding
- For spit-up
- For fussiness and gas
- Docosahexaenoic acid (DHA) to help support brain and eye development
- Good bacteria specially formulated to help strengthen your baby's digestive system, which can protect against the development of allergies
- Antioxidants help maintain cell integrity
- May contribute to heart health

Package Dating

Package dating on labels provides a measure of a product's freshness. Although the FDA does not regulate most package dating, FDA food labeling law and regulations require that such information is truthful and not misleading. *Open dates* are calendar dates that are imprinted or stamped on a food label that indicate to the consumer the freshness and safety of the product. Open dates are stated alpha-numerically (eg, Oct 15) or numerically (eg, 10-15 or 1015). An open date might be featured as:

1. Pull or "sell by" date: This is the last day that the manufacturer recommends sale of the product. Usually, the date allows for additional storage and use time at home.
2. Freshness or quality assurance date: This date suggests how long the manufacturer believes the food will remain at peak quality. The label might read, "Best if used by October 2007." However, the product may be used after this date. A "freshness date" has a different meaning than the word "fresh" printed on the label, which often suggests that a food is raw or unprocessed.

3. Pack date: The date when the food was packaged or processed.
4. Expiration date: The last day the product should be eaten. State governments regulate these dates for perishable foods, such as milk and eggs. The FDA requires expiration dates on infant formula.

Front-of-Package Nutrition Rating Systems and Symbols

Over the past 30 years, there has been substantial growth in the number of front-of-package (FOP) symbols and rating systems designed to summarize nutritional profiles of food products for the consumer. In response to this, Congress in 2009 directed the Centers for Disease Control and Prevention (CDC) to undertake a study with the Institute of Medicine (IOM) to examine and provide recommendations regarding FOP nutrition rating systems and symbols.[9] In 2010, Congress directed the CDC to continue the study, for which the FDA and later the USDA Center of Nutrition Policy and Promotion provided support.[10] This has resulted in 2 reports from the IOM on FOP labeling.[9,10] The 2010 IOM report reviewed 20 representative systems that had been introduced into the marketplace[9] to make the nutrition information on packages easier to understand and, thereby, simplify the decision-making process at the point of purchase for the consumer. They had been developed by the food industry, governments, and nonprofit organizations. The first of the FOP labeling systems was developed in 1987 by the American Heart Association (AHA) with its Heart Guide symbol to signal the consumer that a food was heart friendly. In 2006, the United Kingdom Food Standards Agency recommended that food manufacturers and retailers in the United Kingdom place traffic light labels (red, amber, and green) on the front of food packages to help consumers make healthier food choices.[9] In 2008, ConAgra introduced the Start Making Choices program, an FOP nutrition rating system based on the USDA Food Pyramid, illustrating the contribution of various food groups to a healthier diet. However, despite the proliferation of FOP nutrition rating systems, there is little evidence to show that they have encouraged healthier food choices and purchase decisions.[10]

As many consumers have difficulty in evaluating product healthfulness on the Nutrition Facts panel, a well-designed and simplified FOP labeling system would more likely be used by consumers unable to understand or are less motivated to use the Nutrition Facts panel, given time constraints at the point of purchase. Therefore, the 2012 IOM report,[11] which extended the 2010 IOM report[10] on FOP labeling systems, recommended that the FDA develop, test, and implement a single, standardized FOP system to appear on all food and beverage products, consistent with 2010 *Dietary Guidelines for Americans*, that included the following 8 characteristics: (1) a simple, standard symbol that would translate the Nutrition Facts panel on each product into a quickly and easily grasped health meaning, making healthier food options unmistakable; (2) display calories in common household measure serving sizes and give 0 to 3 points based on quantities of saturated and trans fats, sodium, and added sugars; (3) appear on all grocery store products; (4) appear in a consistent location across all products; (5) practical to implement and consistent with current nutrition labeling regulations; (6) integrated with the Nutrition Facts panel so that the FOP system and the Nutrition Facts panel are mutually reinforcing; (7) provide a nonproprietary, transparent translation of nutritional information into health meaning; and (8) prominent and useful to consumers through an ongoing frequently refreshed program of promotion integrating the efforts of all concerned parties.

Implementation of this system will require further modifications and/or exemptions to current FDA regulations and development of both new regulations and food group specifications for establishing evaluative criteria.

In the meantime, a voluntary FOP labeling program, "Facts Up Front," was adopted by the Grocery Manufacturers Association and the Food Marketing Institute in 2011. It includes 4 basic icons on the principal display panel that provide information on calories, saturated fat, sodium, and total sugar content.[11] In a letter to the Grocery Manufacturers Association and the Food Marketing Institute in December 2011, the FDA viewed the "Facts Up Front" and basic icons as nutrient content claims subject to all the requirements of the Agency's regulations.[12] However, the FDA recognized that the standardized, nonselective presentation of the 4 basic icons on a company's product line would alleviate some of its concerns regarding the potential for product labeling to mislead consumers by presenting only the "good news" about nutrient content of the front of the package (selecting only the favorable nutrient information for the label). The FDA also acknowledged in its letter that, if the "Facts Up Front" program were uniformly adopted by the food industry, it may contribute to the FDA's public health goals by fostering public awareness of the nutrient content of foods in the marketplace and the ability to make healthy food choices. The FDA agreed to work with industry to evaluate the "Facts Up Front" system to ensure that it promotes public health and is useful to consumers.[12] The FDA's strategic plan for 2012-2016 includes a provision not only to explore the front-of-pack nutrition labeling opportunities but also to update the Nutrition Facts panel and serving sizes.[13]

Conclusion

Food labeling helps consumers and parents make food choices to meet dietary recommendations by providing specific information about the content of certain nutrients in the product. This information, currently contained in the nutrition facts panel on the back of the package, may be used to compare foods, to choose foods that help provide a balance of recommended nutrients, and to build meals and a total diet that is moderate, varied, and balanced. In addition, ingredient declarations are useful for consumers to make food choices based on religious, cultural, health, or food allergy concerns.

Food labels may contain both health claims and structure/function claims, but these are not without controversy. The US Government Accountability Office recently released a report encouraging the FDA to protect consumers from false or misleading label claims made by private industry.[12] There are no FDA guidelines for FOP nutrition rating systems and symbols, although the IOM has recommended that such a uniform symbol system would help consumers identify and choose products that are more consistent than others with the 2010 *Dietary Guidelines for Americans* for saturated and trans fats, sodium, and added sugars. There is currently no timetable for instituting a national FOP labeling system as recommended by the IOM, which will require cooperation of all interested parties in private industry and government as well as consumers. In the meantime, a voluntary "Facts Up Front" labeling system, which adopts some of the IOM's recommendations, has been adopted by private industry and is being monitored for its effectiveness in promoting healthy food choices by consumers.

References

1. US Food and Drug Administration. *Focus on Food Labeling: An FDA Consumer Special Report*. Washington, DC: Government Printing Office; 1993
2. 21 CFR §101.4 (2012)
3. 9 CFR §317.2c (2008); and 9 CFR §381.118 (2008)
4. Food Allergen Labeling and Consumer Protection Act. Pub L No. 108-282 (2006)
5. 21 CFR §101.30 (2011)
6. US Food and Drug Administration. Food Labeling; Gluten-Free Labeling of Foods. *Federal Register*. 2013;78(150):47154-47179
7. 21 CFR §101.72–§101.83 (2012)
8. US Food and Drug Administration. Structure/Function Claims Dietary Supplements/ Conventional Foods. Available at: http://www.fda.gov/Food/LabelingNutrition/ LabelClaims/StructureFunctionClaims/default.htm. Accessed January 19, 2013
9. Institute of Medicine. *Examination of Front-of-Packaging Nutrition Rating Systems and Symbols: Phase I Report*. Washington, DC: National Academies Press; 2010
10. Institute of Medicine. *Front-of-Packaging Nutrition Rating Systems and Symbols: Promoting Healthier Choices*. Washington, DC: The National Academies Press; 2012

11. News Release. GMA and FMI Announce 'Facts Up Front' as Theme for Front-of-Pack Labeling Program Consumer Education Campaign. Sept 22, 2011. Available at: http://www.gmaonline.org/news-events/newsroom/gma-and-fmi-announce-facts-up-front-as-theme-for-labeling-program-consumer-/. Accessed January 19, 2013

12. US Food and Drug Administration. FDA Letter of Enforcement Discretion to GMA/FMI re "Facts Up Front." December 13, 2011. Available at: http://www.fda.gov/Food/LabelingNutrition/ucm302720.htm. Accessed January 19, 2013

13. US Food and Drug Administration. FDA Foods and Veterinary Medicine Program Strategic Plan 2012 – 2016. Available at: http://www.fda.gov/downloads/AboutFDA/CentersOffices/OfficeofFoods/UCM273732.pdf. Accessed January 19, 2013

VII

Chapter 53

Food Safety: Infectious Disease

Introduction

In the United States, an estimated 48 million cases of foodborne illness occur every year, resulting in approximately 128 000 hospitalizations and 3000 deaths.[1] More than 200 infectious and noninfectious agents have been associated with foodborne and waterborne illness with a wide range of clinical manifestations; these agents include bacteria, viruses, parasites and their toxins, marine organisms and their toxins, and chemical contaminants including heavy metals.[2-6] Infants, children, pregnant women, the elderly, and immunocompromised people are particularly vulnerable to more severe forms of foodborne illnesses.[7,8]

Prevention of foodborne illness remains a continuing challenge. As more people live with immunocompromising conditions, the risks of infection and severe illness from foodborne pathogens may rise. Furthermore, identification of new pathogens and established pathogens in unexpected food vehicles will likely occur.[9] Increased importation of food and international travel increases the potential for exposure to novel or rare pathogens, and centralization of food processing in the United States and widespread distribution of commercial products increases the risk of large, national foodborne illness outbreaks if a problem occurs.[9,10]

Because primary care practitioners are often the first to be contacted by people with foodborne illness, an understanding of the possible causes, spectrum of illness, diagnostic methods, and public health importance of foodborne infections is crucial, not only for initial patient treatment, but also to ensure timely reporting to public health authorities for accurate surveillance. Understanding the diversity and nature of foodborne pathogens and associated vehicles of transmission is crucial to recognize, control, and prevent foodborne disease outbreaks. This chapter will focus on: (1) the epidemiology of infectious foodborne disease; (2) the clinical manifestations, testing, and management of foodborne illness; (3) foodborne disease surveillance; (4) control and prevention; and (5) resource materials available.

Epidemiology of Foodborne Disease

Although foodborne illness can be caused by many pathogens, several pathogens have been recognized as frequent or severe causes of foodborne disease. It is estimated that 59% of foodborne illness in the United States is caused by viruses, 39% by bacteria, and 2% by parasites.[1] Norovirus is the leading cause of foodborne illness (58%) in the United States attributable to known pathogens, followed by nontyphoidal *Salmonella* species (11%), *Clostridium perfringens* (10%), and *Campylobacter* species (9%). However, nontyphoidal *Salmonella* species are the leading cause of foodborne illness hospitalizations (35%) and deaths (28% [Table 53.1]).[1] Although less common, *Listeria monocytogenes*, *Clostridium botulinum*, and *Toxoplasma gondii* can also cause serious foodborne illness.

Table 53.1.
Pathogens Accounting for the Majority of Illnesses, Hospitalizations, and Deaths From Foodborne Illness in the United States[1]

Pathogen	Estimated Number of Illnesses	Estimated Number of Hospitalizations	Estimated Number of Deaths
Norovirus	5 461 731	14 663	149
Salmonella, nontyphoidal	1 027 561	19 336	378
Clostridium perfringens	965 958	438	26
Campylobacter species	845 024	8463	76
Staphylococcus aureus	241 148	1064	6
Escherichia coli (STEC) O157:H7	63 153	2138	20
Toxoplasma gondii	86 686	4428	327
Listeria monocytogenes	1591	1455	255

Most cases of foodborne illness are sporadic and are not part of recognized outbreaks. Investigations of foodborne disease outbreaks provide critical information about food vehicles, emerging pathogens, and food production and preparation practices associated with illness. Of the 1034 foodborne outbreaks reported to the Centers for Disease Control and Prevention (CDC) in 2008, 479 (46%) were caused by a single laboratory-confirmed etiologic agent, of which viruses accounted for 49%, bacteria accounted for 44%, chemicals and toxins accounted for 6%, and parasites accounted for 1% (Table 53.2).[11] Among outbreaks with a single, laboratory-confirmed etiology, norovirus was the most common pathogen, causing 49% of outbreaks, followed by *Salmonella*—the most common bacterial pathogen—causing 23% of outbreaks. Etiology was not determined in 34% of outbreaks.[12] New foodborne pathogens continue to emerge, including non-O157:H7 Shiga toxin-producing *Escherichia coli* (STEC), *Cyclospora* species, and multidrug-resistant *Salmonella* species.[12]

Table 53.2.

Confirmed and Suspected Causes of Single-Etiology Foodborne Outbreaks Reported to the National Outbreak Reporting System, CDC, 2008[11]

Etiology	Etiology Confirmed	Etiology Suspected	Total
Bacterial			
Salmonella	110	7	117
Clostridium perfringens	21	19	40
Escherichia coli, Shiga toxin-producing	36	—	36
Campylobacter	21	4	25
Bacillus cereus	3	12	15
Staphylococcus enterotoxin	6	8	14
Shigella	6	—	6
Clostridium botulinum	4	—	4
Other bacterial	1	2	3
Listeria	3	—	3
Vibrio parahaemolyticus	1	—	1
Vibrio other		1	1
Escherichia coli, enterotoxigenic	—	—	—
Brucella species	—	—	—
Yersinia enterocolitica	—	—	—
Total	**212**	**53**	**265**
Chemical and toxin			
Scombroid toxin/histamine	10	2	12
Ciguatoxin	11	3	14
Cleaning agents	—	3	3
Heavy metals	2	—	2
Other chemical	1	1	2
Mycotoxins	1	—	1
Paralytic shellfish poison	1	—	1
Plant/herbal toxins	1	—	1
Neurotoxic shellfish poison	—	—	—
Puffer fish tetrodotoxin	—	—	—
Other natural toxins	—	—	—
Total	**27**	**9**	**36**
Parasitic			
Cyclospora species	3	—	3
Cryptosporidium species	2	—	2
Giardia species	1	—	1
Trichinella species	—	—	—
Other parasitic	—	—	—
Total	**6**	**—**	**6**

VII

Table 53.2. *(continued)*
Confirmed and Suspected Causes of Single-Etiology Foodborne Outbreaks Reported to the National Outbreak Reporting System, CDC, 2008[11]

Etiology	Etiology Confirmed	Etiology Suspected	Total
Viral			
Norovirus	233	123	356
Hepatitis A	1	—	1
Rotavirus	—	1	1
Other viral	—	1	1
Total	234	125	359
Known etiology	479	187	666
Unknown etiology[a]	—	—	350
Multiple etiologies	11	7	18
Total	490	194	1034

[a] An etiologic agent was not confirmed or suspected based on clinical, laboratory, or epidemiologic information.

Infectious and noninfectious agents of foodborne disease can be acquired from a variety of sources, with some linked more frequently with specific foods (see also Chapter 54: Food Safety: Pesticides, Industrial Chemicals, Toxins, Antimicrobial Preservatives, Irradiation, Food Contact Substances). For instance, outbreaks of *Salmonella* serotype Enteritidis infections are commonly associated with eggs and poultry meat, and *E coli* O157:H7 outbreaks are frequently associated with ground beef, leafy greens, and unpasteurized dairy products. Listeriosis in people at high risk is frequently associated with consuming ready-to-eat meats and unpasteurized dairy products.[13] *Salmonella* and *Campylobacter* infections in infants and children have been associated with riding in a shopping cart next to raw meat or poultry products.[14-16]

A wide variety of contaminated foods have caused foodborne illness outbreaks. In 2008, the most commonly implicated food commodities in foodborne disease outbreaks were poultry, beef, and finfish.[11] However, new foods continue to be identified as causes of outbreaks, including bagged spinach, carrot juice, peanut butter, raw cookie dough, and hot peppers. Table 53.3 lists examples of recent foodborne disease outbreaks in the United States by location, food vehicle, and etiology, indicating the diversity in vehicles and pathogens. Several recent outbreaks have predominantly affected children and adolescents, including an *E coli* O:157:H7 outbreak associated with consumption of raw cookie dough and a *Salmonella* Wandsworth outbreak associated with a vegetable-coated snack.

Table 53.3.
Examples of Recent Foodborne Outbreaks in the United States by Location, Vehicle, and Cause

Pathogen	Food Vehicle	Where	Year	No. Cases	Ref.
Salmonella Montevideo	Pepper-coated salami products	Multistate	2009	272	49
Salmonella Saintpaul	Alfalfa sprouts	Multistate	2009	228	50
Salmonella Typhimurium	Peanut butter and peanut butter-containing products	Multistate	2008	714	51
Salmonella Saintpaul	Jalapeno or serrano peppers	Multistate	2008	1500	52
Clostridium perfringens	Casserole with ground turkey and beef	Wisconsin	2008	>100	53
Escherichia coli O157:H7	Ground beef	Multistate	2008	64	54
Salmonella I 4,5,12:i:-	Frozen pot pies	Multistate	2007	401	55
Listeria monocytogenes	Pasteurized milk	Massachusetts	2007	5	56
Salmonella Litchfield	Fruit salad	New Jersey	2007	30	57
Salmonella Wandsworth	Vegetable-coated snack food	Multistate	2007	69	58
Campylobacter jejuni	Unpasteurized milk and fresh cheese	Kansas	2007	67	59
Clostridium botulinum	Canned chili sauce	Multistate	2007	5	60
Salmonella Newport	Unpasteurized Mexican-style cheese	Multistate	2006	85	61
Vibrio parahaemolyticus	Raw shellfish	Multistate	2006	177	62
Clostridium botulinum	Carrot juice	Multistate, Canada	2006	6	63
E coli O157:H7	Prepackaged spinach	Multistate	2006	183	64
Salmonella Schwarzengrund	Dry dog food	Multistate	2006	79	65
Salmonella Newport	Tomatoes	Multistate	2005	25	66
Norovirus	Food handler	Michigan	2005	23	67
Vibrio parahaemolyticus	Raw oysters	Alaska	2004	62	68
Cyclospora	Uncooked snow peas	Pennsylvania	2004	96	69
Salmonella Typhimurium	Ground beef	Multistate	2004	31	70
E coli O169:H41	Coleslaw	Tennessee	2003	36	71
Cryptosporidium	Ozonated apple cider	Ohio	2003	23	72
Hepatitis A	Green onions	Pennsylvania	2003	601	73

Animal contact can also be a cause of illnesses attributable to pathogens usually transmitted through foods. Poultry including baby chicks, turtles and other reptiles, amphibians such as aquatic frogs, and animals in petting zoos have been implicated in past *Salmonella* and *E coli* O157:H7 outbreaks.[17-20] Although illness can be acquired through direct animal contact (ie, touching or petting the animal), animals can also be an indirect source of infection through cross-contamination, when food or food-preparation surfaces become contaminated with feces from an infected animal.[21] This may occur when cages or aquariums are cleaned in the kitchen (in the sink or on surfaces), when pets carrying pathogens are allowed to roam in the house, and when proper handwashing or surface cleaning is not performed before food preparation after contact with the animal, animal's environment, or pet food.

Clinical Manifestations

Table 53.4 describes 5 clinical/epidemiologic profiles into which illnesses caused by most foodborne agents can be categorized. These profiles were derived from national data on foodborne outbreaks including incubation period, duration of illness, percentage of affected people with vomiting or fever, and vomiting-to-fever ratio.[22] These syndromes include: vomiting-toxin, diarrhea-toxin, diarrheogenic *E coli* syndrome, norovirus syndrome, and *Salmonella*-like syndrome. Most foodborne illness results in gastrointestinal tract symptoms, such as vomiting, diarrhea, and abdominal cramps.[3,6] Neurologic manifestations are less common but may include paresthesias (fish, shellfish, and monosodium glutamate), hypotonia and descending paralysis (*Clostridium botulinum*), and a variety of other neurologic signs and symptoms (fish, shellfish, mushrooms). Systemic manifestations are varied and are associated with a variety of causes, including *Brucella* species, *Listeria* species, *Toxoplasma* species, *Trichinella* species, *Vibrio* species, and hepatitis A virus. Pregnant women with listeriosis can experience a mild flu-like illness, and the infection may result in miscarriage, stillbirth, preterm delivery, or severe illness in the newborn infant.[13] Other complications or sequelae of enteric illnesses include hemolytic-uremic syndrome (HUS) associated with *E coli* O157:H7 and other STEC infection, reactive arthritis associated with *Campylobacter* and *Salmonella* enteritis, and Guillain-Barré syndrome after *Campylobacter* infection.[23-27]

Laboratory Testing

Because the presenting symptoms are common to many causes, many infectious and noninfectious agents must be considered in people suspected of having foodborne illness, and establishing an etiologic diagnosis may be difficult on clinical grounds alone. Testing clinical specimens is often the only way to establish a diagnosis;

Table 53.4.
Distinct Foodborne Pathogen Syndromes[22]

Syndrome	Incubation Period (h)	Duration (h)	Vomiting (%)	Fever (%)	Vomiting/ Fever Ratio[a]	Main Causative Agents[b]
Vomiting-toxin	1.5–9.5	6.3–24	50–100	0–28	0–4.3	Chemical
						Bacillus cereus
						Staphylococcus aureus
						Clostridium perfringens
Diarrhea-toxin	10–13.0	12–24	3.6–20	2.3–10	0.40–1.3	Bacillus cereus
						Clostridium perfringens
Escherichia coli-like	48–120	104–185	3.1–37	13–25.3	0.25–1.1	E coli
Norovirus-like	34.5–38.5	33–47	54–70.2	37–63	0.70–1.7	Norovirus
Salmonella-like	18.0–88.5	63–144	8.9–51	31–81	0.20–1.0	Campylobacter
						Norovirus
						Salmonella
						Shigella

Table adapted from: Hall JA, Goulding JS, Bean NH, Tauxe RV, Hedberg CW. Epidemiologic profiling: evaluating foodborne outbreaks for which no pathogen was isolated by routine laboratory testing: United States, 1982-9. Epidemiol Infect. 2001;127(3):381-387

[a] Ratio of proportion vomiting to proportion with fever.

[b] Viral and bacterial pathogens were listed as a main causative agent of each syndrome if ≥25% of the foodborne outbreaks included in the Hall et al study fit the clinical/epidemiologic syndrome.

however, frequently, specimens are not obtained for laboratory testing. For individual cases of illness, collecting specimens for laboratory diagnosis should be considered for the following conditions: (1) in patient populations more likely to develop severe illness, including infants, children, the elderly, pregnant women, and immunocompromised hosts; (2) in patients with underlying gastrointestinal tract disease that might increase the risk of enteric infection and serious illness, such as inflammatory bowel disease, malignancy, prior gastrointestinal tract surgery, or radiation; use of gastric acid inhibitors; malabsorption syndromes; and other structural or functional conditions; (3) in the presence of specific signs and symptoms that are more consistent with bacterial infection or severe illness, including bloody diarrhea; severe abdominal pain and fever; sudden onset of nausea, vomiting or diarrhea; dehydration associated with diarrhea; neurologic involvement, including cranial nerve palsies, motor weakness, and paresthesias; and evidence of HUS; and (4) under circumstances raising public health issues, such as travel, hospitalization, occupation, child care or nursing home attendance, or when an illness outbreak is suspected. The occurrence of neurologic signs and symptoms and HUS are particularly worrisome because of the potential for life-threatening complications.

Laboratory testing of stool specimens may include at least one of the following: stool cultures for bacteria, polymerase chain reaction (PCR) assays of stool for viruses and bacteria, microscopic examination of stool for parasites and fecal leukocytes, and direct antigen detection tests of stool culture broths and blood cultures. Collaboration and communication with clinical microbiology laboratory personnel and local public health officials will help optimize laboratory testing, as detection of some organisms may not be part of the routine testing procedures for clinical laboratories and may require health care providers to make special test requests with submission of the specimen. Other tests may be available only through public health laboratories or large commercial laboratories. For example, many clinical laboratories do not routinely test patients with diarrhea for *E coli* O157:H7 and other STEC. The CDC recommends that all stool specimens submitted for routine enteric pathogen testing from patients with acute community-acquired diarrhea should be cultured for *E coli* O157:H7 and tested simultaneously for non-O157 STEC by an assay that detects Shiga toxins. Testing should be performed regardless of whether blood or white blood cells are present or absent in the stool, because not all patients with STEC infection will have bloody diarrhea or fecal leukocytes.[28] Serologic testing can be useful in the diagnosis of some foodborne diseases, such as trichinosis and toxoplasmosis. As yet, there is no commercial laboratory test approved by the US Food and Drug Administration (FDA) available for diagnosis of norovirus infection in individuals, but state public health laboratories and the CDC routinely test stools by polymerase chain reaction (PCR) assays. In 2011, the FDA allowed marketing of an enzyme immunoassay test (RIDASCREEN, r-Biopharm) to aid in preliminary identification of norovirus as a cause of an acute gastrointestinal tract illness outbreak, but the test is not sensitive enough to be used to diagnose individual patients with norovirus infection.[29] More detailed information on laboratory procedures for identification of foodborne pathogens can be obtained from clinical and microbiology specialists and local or state public health personnel.

For suspected outbreaks of foodborne disease involving gastrointestinal tract symptoms, stools should always be collected for laboratory testing when possible. Important clues for investigating and determining the etiology of an outbreak of foodborne illness include obtaining information about the incubation period, duration of illness, and clinical signs and symptoms. If a foodborne disease outbreak is suspected, appropriate clinical specimens should be submitted for laboratory testing, and the local public health authorities should be notified.

Management

Enteric infections generally are self-limited conditions that require supportive care and fluid and electrolyte therapy (see also Chapter 29: Oral Therapy for Acute Diarrhea). Patients should be monitored closely for signs and symptoms of dehydration. When possible, oral rehydration solutions should be used for fluid replacement in children with mild to moderate dehydration; severely dehydrated patients require intravenous fluids.[30] Routine use of antimicrobial agents is not indicated for the treatment of acute, community-acquired diarrheal illness in the United States, because most illnesses are caused by viruses, are self-limited, and are not shortened by antimicrobial therapy.[3] Depending on the etiology, antimicrobial therapy might be indicated for patients at higher risk of severe or invasive illness (eg, patients with immunocompromising conditions, infants, pregnant women). In some instances, it may eradicate fecal shedding of the causative organism, prevent transmission of the enteropathogen, abbreviate clinical symptoms, or prevent future complications. However, antimicrobial therapy can prolong the duration of *Salmonella* excretion into the stool and has been identified as a risk factor in *E coli* O157:H7 infection for progression to HUS.[31,32] Antibiotic treatment may also disrupt the normal gut flora and exacerbate diarrhea, particularly because some pathogens have developed resistance to certain antibiotics. Therefore, careful consideration of the illness etiology and the medical history of the patient are important prior to treatment.

Botulism is a medical and public health emergency. Health care providers should immediately report any suspected case of botulism to their state health department. Additional emergency consultation is available through CDC's 24-hour botulism service (telephone, 770-488-7100) to assist health care providers in the diagnosis and management of botulism. Administration of botulinum antitoxin early in the course of illness can prevent the progression of neurologic dysfunction. Heptavalent botulinum antitoxin, an equine-derived antitoxin, is available through CDC to treat noninfant botulism.[33] Botulism Immune Globulin (BabyBIG) is available through the California Infant Botulism Treatment and Prevention Program to treat infant botulism,[34] but physicians should first consult their state health department when infant botulism is suspected.

A primer on foodborne diseases developed by the American Medical Association, the American Nurses Association–American Nurses Foundation, CDC, FDA, and the Food Safety and Inspection Service of the US Department of Agriculture (USDA/FSIS) contains information about causes of foodborne illness, clinical considerations, patient scenarios, and patient handout material and resources.[3] Guidelines endorsed by the American Academy of Pediatrics (AAP) for the management of acute gastroenteritis in children are available.[30,35] DPDx is a website developed by CDC's Division of Parasitic Diseases to aid in the diagnosis of parasitic diseases; diagnostic assistance through telediagnosis is available. The AAP *Red Book* also provides additional clinical, diagnostic, and treatment information for specific pathogens.[36] Vaccines are not available for most foodborne illnesses, but hepatitis A vaccine is safe, effective, and recommended by the Advisory Committee on Immunization Practices (ACIP) for all children and for people at increased risk of hepatitis A, including travelers to areas with high or intermediate endemicity of hepatitis A infection. Typhoid fever vaccines are also available for travelers to areas where there is an increased risk of exposure to *Salmonella* Typhi.

Surveillance for Foodborne Diseases

The CDC collects information on enteric disease outbreaks through the National Outbreak Reporting System (NORS). This surveillance system is passive in that it relies on state health departments reporting outbreaks to CDC. The data collected help monitor foodborne disease outbreak etiologies, types of implicated food vehicles, and contributing factors (eg, factors that resulted in contamination of a food vehicle). Data from this surveillance system need to be interpreted with caution, because not all outbreaks may be detected, investigated, or reported by local or state health departments because of variations in patient care, clinical diagnostic capabilities and practice, public health reporting, and public health resources. The NORS surveillance system is important for monitoring trends in foodborne disease outbreaks, describing the various types of foodborne pathogens, determining the risk of exposure attributable to different types of foods, and summarizing factors that contributed to the outbreaks.

PulseNet USA, the national molecular subtyping network for foodborne disease surveillance, was started in 1996 to enhance foodborne disease outbreak detection and investigation.[37] More than 75 public health and food regulatory laboratories, including all state health departments, participate in PulseNet USA and routinely perform pulsed-field gel electrophoresis (PFGE) of *Campylobacter* species, *E coli* O157:H7, *Shigella* species, *Listeria* species, and *Salmonella* species using standardized methods. The resulting PFGE pattern is a molecular "fingerprint" of the bacteria. The PFGE patterns are shared electronically, allowing PulseNet-affiliated public health laboratories to rapidly compare the PFGE patterns of bacteria isolated from ill people and determine whether they are likely to be part of the same outbreak or attributable to the same exposure. Public health officials perform regular searches of the PFGE databases, looking for clusters of isolates that are indistinguishable by PFGE, which might indicate an outbreak. Clusters identified by PulseNet are referred to the CDC and state epidemiologists for investigation.

Because of the extensive food distribution system in the United States, contaminated foods may be distributed to people in many locations, with few ill people in a specific location. PulseNet has been useful in the detection of foodborne disease outbreaks, including these widely dispersed outbreaks, by quickly compiling information on genetic profiles of bacterial isolates from ill people and food specimens across the country.[10,37] However, an inherent limitation of PulseNet is that laboratory-confirmation of infection and a bacterial isolate are required for case detection, thus, emphasizing the importance that appropriate laboratory testing be performed by clinicians evaluating patients with gastrointestinal illness. Together, the real-time acquisition of PFGE patterns from PulseNet and routine reporting of enteric disease outbreaks through NORS allow for more thorough outbreak detection and control.

Surveillance for norovirus and other enteric viruses historically has been performed by the CDC on receipt of specimens from presumed norovirus outbreaks.[38] However, all state public health laboratories have established the capacity to routinely detect norovirus in specimens collected from persons involved in outbreaks, and many foodborne outbreaks of norovirus are now confirmed locally and reported to the CDC via NORS. Additionally, CalciNet, an electronic norovirus outbreak surveillance network consisting of 21 local, state, and federal public health and regulatory laboratories, was launched in 2009.[29] CalciNet-affiliated laboratories perform genotyping of norovirus using reverse-transcriptase PCR and share the resulting sequences electronically. CalciNet aims to identify links between norovirus outbreaks to help identify common food vehicles, trends, and emerging strains. However, because most clinical laboratories do not test for norovirus, widespread outbreaks of foodborne illness presenting as dispersed sporadic illnesses may remain undetected.

In 1996, the CDC's Emerging Infection Program, in collaboration with participating state departments of health, USDA/FSIS, and FDA, initiated the Foodborne Diseases Active Surveillance Network (FoodNet).[39,40] FoodNet conducts population-based, active, laboratory surveillance for 9 foodborne pathogens, including the bacterial pathogens *Salmonella* species, *Shigella* species, *Campylobacter* species, STEC, including *E coli* O157:H7, *Listeria monocytogenes*, *Yersinia* excluding *Yersinia* pestis, *Vibrio* species, and the parasitic organisms *Cryptosporidium* species and *Cyclospora* species. FoodNet encompasses a surveillance population of 46 million people (15% of the US population) and consists of more than 650 clinical laboratories that test specimens in the FoodNet sites. In addition to collecting laboratory-diagnosed cases of foodborne pathogens, investigators at FoodNet sites conduct active surveillance for HUS, a serious complication of STEC infection.

Bacterial agents including *Salmonella* species, *Campylobacter* species, and *Shigella* species are the most frequently identified causes of laboratory-confirmed illness in FoodNet.[40] Table 53.5 shows the incidence by age group, total number of cases, and death rate among people infected with specific pathogens under surveillance in 2010.

VII

Pathogens with the highest incidence in children younger than 5 years are *Salmonella* species, *Campylobacter* species, *Shigella* species, *Cryptosporidium* species, and STEC.[40] Rates of *Campylobacter, E coli* O157:H7, *Listeria, Shigella,* and *Yersinia* infection have showed sustained declines compared with the rates reported from 1996-1998, but rates have increased for *Vibrio* infections and remain unchanged for *Salmonella* infections.[40] Fig 53.1 shows trends in incidence of infection by selected FoodNet pathogens in 2010 compared with the 1996-1998 baseline. Through active surveillance and additional studies, FoodNet produces estimates of the burden and sources of foodborne diseases in the United States, which can be used to help develop and evaluate new foodborne illness prevention and control strategies. For example, after measures to control foodborne disease have been implemented, such as Hazard Analysis and Critical Control Point (HACCP) measures, FoodNet surveillance monitors for changes in bacterial and parasitic infection rates that may correspond to these efforts.

Fig 53.1.
Trends in selected pathogens in Foodborne Diseases Active Surveillance Network (FoodNet) sites. Relative rates of laboratory-confirmed infections with *Campylobacter*, Shiga toxin-producing *Escherichia coli* (STEC) O157, *Listeria*, *Salmonella*, and *Vibrio* compared with 1996—1998 baseline rates, by year.[a,40,41]

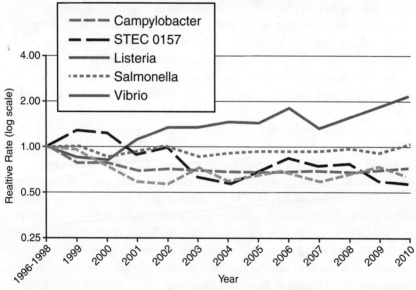

From: Centers for Disease Control and Prevention. Vital signs: incidence and trends of infection with pathogens transmitted commonly through food—Foodborne Diseases Active Surveillance Network, 10 U.S. Sites, 1996–2010. *MMWR Morb Mortal Wkly Rep.* 2011;60(22):729-772.
[a] The position of each line indicates the relative change in the incidence of that pathogen compared with 1996–1998. The absolute incidences of these infections cannot be determined from this graph. Data for 2010 are preliminary.

Table 53.5.
Incidence of Laboratory-Confirmed Infection by Age Group, Total Cases, and Deaths, FoodNet 2010[a,40]

Pathogen	Incidence Rate[b] by Age Group (y)					Total Cases		Total Deaths	
	<5	5-9	10-19	20-59	≥60	No.	Rate	No.	CFR[c]
Bacteria									
Campylobacter species	24.4	10.6	10.1	13.3	13.9	6365	13.6	8	0.1
Listeria species	0.3	0.03	0.05	0.1	1.1	125	0.3	16	12.8
Salmonella species	69.5	21.4	12.2	12.3	17.0	8256	17.6	29	0.4
Shigella species	16.4	11.7	2.2	2.5	1.1	1780	3.8	0	0.0
STEC[c] O157	3.3	2.5	1.1	0.5	0.7	442	0.9	2	0.5
STEC non-O157	5.0	1.1	1.3	0.5	0.5	451	1.0	1	0.2
Vibrio species	0.0	0.3	0.2	0.4	0.8	193	0.4	6	3.1
Yersinia species	1.9	0.4	0.2	0.2	0.4	159	0.3	1	0.6
Parasites									
Cryptosporidium species	5.1	2.7	2.5	2.60	2.5	1290	2.8	5	0.4
Cyclospora species	0.0	0.0	0.02	0.1	0.1	28	0.1	0	0.0

Adapted from: Centers for Disease Control and Prevention. Vital signs: incidence and trends of infection with pathogens transmitted commonly through food—Foodborne Diseases Active Surveillance Network, 10 US Sites, 1996–2010. *MMWR Morb Mortal Wkly Rep.* 2011;60(22):729-772

[a] Data are preliminary.

[b] Per 100 000 population for FoodNet areas.

[c] Case fatality ratio (CFR) = number of deaths/total cases.

[d] Shiga toxin-producing *Escherichia coli*.

Food Safety and Prevention of Foodborne Illness

From 1993 through 1997, the most commonly reported food preparation practices that contributed to foodborne disease were improper holding temperatures of food and poor personal hygiene of preparers of food.[41] Since these findings, both general and specific measures aimed at food production and processing industries, retail and food service providers, and consumers have been established to improve foodborne disease prevention throughout the farm-to-table continuum.

Prevention and control measures aimed at the food industry have been broadly implemented to prevent foodborne illness. Education targeted toward retail and food service operators with an emphasis on safe food handling practices during preparation, cooking, and storage of food and pathogen-control measures during food production and processing have been implemented.[42] In 1996, the USDA/

VII

FSIS introduced comprehensive pathogen-reduction and HACCP systems requirements for meat and poultry processors. HACCP regulations for seafood processing became effective in 1997. The FDA Food Code, last updated in 2009, is a model regulatory code that assists local, state, and tribal food regulatory authorities by providing them with official, scientifically rigorous guidelines for regulating the retail and food service segment of the industry (restaurants and grocery stores and institutions such as nursing homes).[43] In 2010, the FDA created the Reportable Food Registry program, which requires the food industry to report to the FDA food items that have a "reasonable probability" of causing serious adverse health consequences or death to humans or animals. In 2011, The Food Safety Modernization Act (Pub L No. 111-353) was signed into law. The Act provides the FDA with new enforcement authorities designed to achieve higher rates of compliance with prevention- and risk-based food safety standards, including for foreign food producers. It also provides new authorities in response to food contamination events, such as mandatory recall of foods, and a focus on enhanced surveillance, outbreak detection and response. Additional measures have been enacted that are specific for defined food products and have been associated with a decline in the incidence of foodborne infections.[40,44] These measures have included increased attention to good agriculture practices aimed at fresh fruit and vegetables, increased regulation of imported foods, food safety education, irradiation of meat, pasteurization of dairy products, new egg safety regulations, and the use of technology during food production to prevent or mitigate food contamination.[42,44,45] Information about these and other measures enacted to reduce foodborne disease can be found at various Web sites shown in the directory of resources (Table 53.6).

Food safety in the home is also critical for preventing foodborne illness. Cleanliness is a major factor in preventing foodborne illness. Hands should be washed with warm, soapy water for 20 seconds before preparing any foods and after handling uncooked eggs or raw meat, poultry, seafood, and their juices. The cleaning of surfaces in the kitchen is also important to preventing cross-contamination during food preparation. Microorganisms can be transmitted in the kitchen via hands, cutting boards, utensils, and countertops. Cross contamination from one food item to another is a major problem when handling raw meat, poultry, seafood, and eggs. In addition to hand washing, cutting boards, utensils, and countertops should be washed with hot, soapy water after preparing each food item. Contamination of foods with viruses is particularly easy when preparing food. Any contact of bare, contaminated hands with food subsequently eaten without heating has the potential to transmit virus and cause infection. Individuals who have recently had vomiting or diarrhea should refrain from preparing and serving food. In addition, food preparation surfaces can become contaminated with viruses; this contamination can be unapparent and may resist disinfection with common products. In the home, 1 teaspoon of unscented, liquid chlorine bleach per quart of clean water can also be used to sanitize surfaces; it should be left on the surface for about 10 minutes to be effective, then rinsed clean. Once cutting boards become excessively worn or develop hard-to-clean grooves, replace them. Hands should always be washed after using the bathroom; changing diapers; tending to a sick person; blowing one's nose, coughing, or sneezing; or handling pets or their food or cages to prevent contamination of foods or preparation surfaces.

Normal cooking of foods will kill most pathogens that cause foodborne illness. Eggs should be cooked until both yolk and white are firm; all poultry (ground, whole, parts) should be cooked until it has an internal temperature of 165°F; whole cuts of meat, such as pork, steaks, roasts, and chops, should be cooked to an internal temperature of 145°F as measured with a food thermometer placed in the thickest part of the meat and then allowed to rest for 3 minutes before carving or consuming; fish should be cooked to 145°F and until it is opaque and flakes easily with a fork; ground meat, especially hamburger meat, should be cooked to 160°F. Because bacteria grow at room temperature, hot foods should be maintained at 140°F or higher and cold foods at 40°F or lower. Perishables, prepared foods, and leftovers should be refrigerated or frozen within 2 hours of preparation with minimal handling. Foods should be defrosted in the refrigerator, under cold running water or in a microwave, and foods should be marinated in the refrigerator.

These measures are especially relevant for specific high-risk segments of the population, including infants, children, the elderly, immunocompromised people, and pregnant women.[8] These high-risk populations should avoid eating or drinking raw (unpasteurized) milk or raw milk products, raw or partially cooked eggs or raw egg products, raw or undercooked meat and poultry, raw or undercooked fish or shellfish, unpasteurized juices, and raw sprouts. Furthermore, certain deli meats, luncheon meats, and hot dogs should only be eaten once they have been reheated to steaming hot. Honey should not be fed to infants younger than 12 months because of the risk of infant botulism. Physicians and parents should be aware that powdered infant formulas, although heat-treated during processing, are not sterile, in contrast to liquid formulas that are nutritionally designed for consumption by preterm or low birth weight infants.[46] "Transition" infant formulas that are generally used for preterm or low birth weight infants after hospital discharge are available in both nonsterile powder form and commercially sterile liquid form. Because of the risk of *Cronobacter sakazakii* infection (formerly *Enterobacter sakazakii*), which can cause meningitis, sepsis, and necrotizing enterocolitis in infants,[47,48] the FDA recommends that powdered infant formulas not be used in neonatal intensive care settings unless no alternative is available.[46] Parents should be

VII

Table 53.6.
Directory of Online Resources for Prevention of Foodborne Illness

Surveillance, Reporting, and Outbreaks
Estimates of Foodborne Illness in the United States (CDC): http://www.cdc.gov/foodborneburden/
Nationally Notifiable Conditions: http://www.cdc.gov/osels/ph_surveillance/nndss/phs/infdis.htm#top
CSTE's Index of State Reportable Conditions list: http://www.cste.org/dnn/LinkClick.aspx?fileticket=KVo%2fcS9UR5Q%3d&tabid=145&mid=667
CDC's OutbreakNet/ Outbreak Response Team: http://www.cdc.gov/outbreaknet/

Diagnosis and Management of Suspected Foodborne Illness
Diagnosis and Management of Foodborne Illnesses: A Primer for Physicians and Other Health Care Professionals (CDC): http://www.cdc.gov/mmwr/PDF/rr/rr5304.pdf
Managing Acute Gastroenteritis Among Children: Oral Rehydration, Maintenance, and Nutritional Therapy (CDC): http://www.cdc.gov/mmwr/PDF/RR/RR5216.pdf
CDHS Infant Botulism Treatment and Prevention Program: http://www.infantbotulism.org/
Updated Norovirus Outbreak Management and Disease Prevention Guidelines (CDC): http://www.cdc.gov/mmwr/preview/mmwrhtml/rr6003a1.htm?s_cid=rr6003a1_w
CDC Parasites Transmitted by Food: http://www.cdc.gov/parasites/food.html
CDC DPDx (for parasites): http://www.dpd.cdc.gov/dpdx/Default.htm
FDA Bad Bug Book: http://www.fda.gov/Food/FoodSafety/FoodborneIllness/FoodborneIllnessFoodbornePathogensNaturalToxins/BadBugBook/default.htm
Recommendations for Diagnosis of Shiga Toxin-Producing *Escherichia coli* Infections by Clinical Laboratories: http://www.cdc.gov/mmwr/preview/mmwrhtml/rr5812a1.htm

Food Safety

CDC Food Safety: http://www.cdc.gov/foodsafety/

FDA Food Safety: http://www.fda.gov/Food/FoodSafety/default.htm

USDA/FSIS: http://www.fsis.usda.gov/Home/index.asp

Food Safety Modernization Act (2011): http://www.fda.gov/Food/FoodSafety/FSMA/default.htm

FDA Food Code: http://www.fda.gov/food/foodsafety/retailfoodprotection/foodcode/default.htm

FDA Reportable Registry for Industry: http://www.fda.gov/food/foodsafety/foodsafetyprograms/rfr/default.htm

Compendium of Measures to Prevent Disease Associated with Animals in Public Settings, 2009: http://www.cdc.gov/mmwr/preview/mmwrhtml/rr5805a1.htm

Food Safety Consumer Education Resources

FoodSafety.gov: http://www.foodsafety.gov/

The Basics: Clean, Separate, Cook, and Chill: http://www.foodsafety.gov/keep/basics/index.html

Safe Minimum Cooking Temperatures: http://www.foodsafety.gov/keep/charts/mintemp.htm

Be Food Safe campaign: http://www.befoodsafe.org/

Fight BAC!® Partnership for Food Safety Education campaign: http://www.fightbac.org/

CDC Food Safety and Raw Milk: http://www.cdc.gov/foodsafety/rawmilk/raw-milk-index.html

CDC Reptiles, Amphibians, and *Salmonella*: http://www.cdc.gov/Features/SalmonellaFrogTurt e/

encouraged to separate infants and children from raw meat and poultry products while shopping and to place children in the shopping cart child seats rather than the baskets.[16]

Food safety education materials aimed at consumers are available online through several organizations (Table 53.6, Food Safety Consumer Education Resources). Current consumer messaging from the Partnership for Food Safety Education's Fight BAC!® campaign (http://www.fightbac.org/) emphasizes 4 simple steps that can be done when preparing food to help prevent food poisoning—clean, separate, cook, and chill—which focus on hand washing and surface cleaning, prevention of cross contamination, cooking of food at proper temperatures, and prompt and appropriate refrigeration of food before and after cooking or preparation:

1. *CLEAN: Wash Hands and Surfaces Often*

   Bacteria can be spread throughout the kitchen and get onto hands, cutting boards, utensils, counter tops and food. To Fight BAC!® always:

   - Wash your hands with warm water and soap for at least 20 seconds before and after handling food and after using the bathroom, changing diapers, and handling pets.

   - Wash your cutting boards, dishes, utensils, and counter tops with hot soapy water after preparing each food item and before you go on to the next food.

   - Consider using paper towels to clean up kitchen surfaces. If you use cloth towels, wash them often in the hot cycle of your washing machine.

   - Rinse fruits and vegetables under running tap water, including those with skins and rinds that are not eaten.

   - Rub firm-skin fruits and vegetables under running tap water or scrub with a clean vegetable brush while rinsing with running tap water.

2. *SEPARATE: Don't Cross-Contaminate*

   Cross-contamination is how bacteria can be spread. When handling raw meat, poultry, seafood and eggs, keep these foods and their juices away from ready-to-eat foods. Always start with a clean scene—wash hands with warm water and soap. Wash cutting boards, dishes, countertops, and utensils with hot soapy water.

   - Separate raw meat, poultry, seafood, and eggs from other foods in grocery shopping cart, in grocery bags, and in the refrigerator.

   - Use one cutting board for fresh produce and a separate one for raw meat, poultry, and seafood.

   - Never place cooked food on a plate that previously held raw meat, poultry, seafood, or eggs.

3. *COOK: Cook to Proper Temperatures*
   Food is safely cooked when it reaches a high enough internal temperature to kill the harmful bacteria that cause foodborne illness. Use a food thermometer to measure the internal temperature of cooked foods. The best way to Fight BAC!® is to:

   - Use a food thermometer that measures the internal temperature of cooked meat, poultry, and egg dishes to make sure that the food is cooked to a safe internal temperature (Table 53.7).

Table 53.7.
Safe Minimum Cooking Temperatures

Food	Minimum Internal Temperature
Ground beef, ground pork, ground veal, ground lamb	160°F
Ground turkey, ground chicken	165°F
Beef, lamb, and veal steaks and roasts	145°F and allow to rest at least 3 minutes
Poultry, including chicken and turkey (ground, whole, or parts), duck, and goose	165°F
Pork chops, ribs, and roasts	145°F and allow to rest at least 3 minutes
Eggs	Until yolk and white are firm
Egg dishes	160°F
Fish	145°F
Stuffing, casseroles, and leftovers	165°F

Adapted from http://www.foodsafety.gov/keep/charts/mintemp.html (Accessed January 21, 2013) and http://www.fsis.usda.gov/is_it_done_yet/Thermometer_Placement_and_Temps/index.asp (Accessed January 21, 2013).

   - Cook all raw beef, pork, lamb and veal steaks, chops, and roasts to a minimum internal temperature of 145°F as measured with a food thermometer before removing meat from the heat source. For safety and quality, allow meat to rest for at least 3 minutes before carving or consuming.[a] All poultry should reach a safe minimum internal temperature of 165°F as measured with a food thermometer. Check the internal temperature in the innermost part of the thigh and wing and the thickest part of the breast with a food thermometer.

   - Cook ground meat, in which bacteria can be spread during grinding, to at least 160°F. Information from the CDC links eating undercooked ground

[a] Updated to reflect new USDA cooking guidelines announced May 24, 2011. Available at: http://www.fsis.usda.gov/is_it_done_yet/brochure_text/index.asp#5.

beef with a higher risk of illness. Remember, color is not a reliable indicator of doneness. Use a food thermometer to check the internal temperature of your burgers.

- Cook eggs until the yolk and white are firm, not runny. Do not use recipes in which eggs remain raw or only partially cooked.

- Cook fish to 145°F or until the flesh is opaque and separates easily with a fork.

- Make sure there are no cold spots in food (where bacteria can survive) when cooking in a microwave oven. For best results, cover, stir, and rotate food for even cooking. If there is no turntable, rotate the dish by hand once or twice during cooking.

- Bring sauces, soups and gravy to a boil when reheating. Heat other leftovers thoroughly to 165°F.

4. *CHILL: Refrigerate promptly*

Refrigerate foods quickly, because cold temperatures slow the growth of harmful bacteria. Do not overstuff the refrigerator. Cold air must circulate to help keep food safe. Keeping a constant refrigerator temperature of 40°F or below is one of the most effective ways to reduce the risk of foodborne illness. Use an appliance thermometer to be sure the temperature is consistently 40°F or below. The freezer temperature should be 0°F or below.

- Refrigerate or freeze meat, poultry, eggs, and other perishables as soon as you get home from the store.

- Never let raw meat, poultry, eggs, cooked food, or cut fresh fruits or vegetables sit at room temperature more than 2 hours before putting them in the refrigerator or freezer (1 hour when the temperature is >90°F).

- Never defrost food at room temperature. Food must be kept at a safe temperature during thawing. There are 3 safe ways to defrost food: in the refrigerator, in cold water, and in the microwave. Food thawed in cold water or in the microwave should be cooked immediately.

- Always marinate food in the refrigerator.

- Divide large amounts of leftovers into shallow containers for quicker cooling in the refrigerator.

- Use or discard refrigerated food on a regular basis. Check the Cold Storage Chart (http://www.fightbac.org/storage/documents/coldstoragechart_fnl.pdf) for optimum storage times.

References

1. Scallan E, Hoekstra R, Angulo F, et al. Foodborne illness acquired in the United States—major pathogens. *Emerg Infect Dis*. 2011;17(1):7-15

2. Bryan F. *Diseases Transmitted by Foods (A Classification and Summary)*. 2nd ed. Atlanta, GA: Centers for Disease Control and Prevention; 1982

3. Centers for Disease Control and Prevention. Diagnosis and management of foodborne illnesses: a primer for physicians and other health care professionals. *MMWR Recomm Rep*. 2004;53(RR-4):1-33

4. Yoder J, Roberts V, Craun GF, et al. Surveillance for waterborne disease and outbreaks associated with drinking water and water not intended for drinking—United States, 2005-2006. *MMWR Surveill Summ*. 2008;57(9):39-62

5. Pickering LK. Approach to the diagnosis and management of gastrointestinal tract infections. In: Long SS, Pickering LK, Prober CG, eds. *Principles and Practice of Pediatric Infectious Diseases*. 3rd ed. Churchill Livingstone Elsevier; 2008:377-383

6. Guerrant RL, Van Gilder TJ, Steiner TS, et al. Practice guidelines for the management of infectious diarrhea. *Clin Infect Dis*. 2001;32(3):331-351

7. Koehler KM, Lasky R, Fein SB, et al. Population-based incidence of infection with selected bacterial enteric pathogens in children younger than five years of age, 1996-1998. *Pediatr Infect Dis J*. 2006;25(2):129-134

8. Gerba CP, Rose JB, Haas CN. Sensitive populations: who is at the greatest risk? *Int J Food Microbiol*. 1996;30(1-2):113-123

9. Tauxe RV. Emerging foodborne pathogens. *Int J Food Microbiol*. 2002;78(1-2):31-41

10. Sobel J, Griffin P, Slutsker L, Swerdlow D, Tauxe R. Investigation of multistate foodborne disease outbreaks. *Public Health Rep*. 2002;117(1):8-19

11. Centers for Disease Control and Prevention. Surveillance for foodborne disease outbreaks—United States, 2008. *MMWR Morb Mortal Wkly Rep*. 2011;60(35):1197-1202

12. Lynch M, Painter J, Woodruff R, Braden C. Surveillance for foodborne-disease outbreaks—United States, 1998-2002. *MMWR Surveill Summ*. 2006;55(10):1-42

13. Swaminathan B, Gerner-Smidt P. The epidemiology of human listeriosis. *Microbes Infect*. 2007;9(10):1236-1243

14. Fullerton KE, Ingram LA, Jones TF, et al. Sporadic Campylobacter infection in infants: a population-based surveillance case-control study. *Pediatr Infect Dis J*. 2007;26(1):19-24

15. Jones TF, Ingram LA, Fullerton KE, et al. A case-control study of the epidemiology of sporadic Salmonella infection in Infants. *Pediatrics*. 2006;118(6):2380-2387

16. Patrick M, Mahon B, Zansky S, Hurd S, Scallan E. Riding in shopping carts and exposure to raw meat and poultry products: prevalence of, and factors associated with, this risk factor for Salmonella and Campylobacter infection in children younger than 3 years. *J Food Prot*. 2010;73(6):1097-1100

17. Centers for Disease Control and Prevention. Multistate outbreaks of Salmonella infections associated with live poultry—United States, 2007. *MMWR Morb Mortal Wkly Rep*. 2009;58(2):25-29

VII

18. Harris Julie R, Neil Karen P, Behravesh Casey B, Sotir Mark J, Angulo Frederick J. Recent multistate outbreaks of human *Salmonella* infections acquired from turtles: a continuing public health challenge. *Clin Infect Dis*. 2010;50(4):554-559

19. Centers for Disease Control and Prevention. Outbreak of Shiga toxin-producing *Escherichia coli* O157 infection associated with a day camp petting zoo—Pinellas County, Florida, May-June 2007. *MMWR Morb Mortal Wkly Rep*. 2009;58(16):426-428

20. Centers for Disease Control and Prevention. Multistate outbreak of human *Salmonella typhimurium* infections associated with aquatic frogs—United States, 2009. *MMWR Morb Mortal Wkly Rep*. 2010;58(51):1433-1436

21. Mermin J, Hoar B, Angulo F. Iguanas and *Salmonella marina* infection in children: a reflection of the increasing incidence of reptile-associated salmonellosis in the United States. *Pediatrics*. 1997;99(3):399-402

22. Hall JA, Goulding JS, Bean NH, Tauxe RV, Hedberg CW. Epidemiologic profiling: evaluating foodborne outbreaks for which no pathogen was isolated by routine laboratory testing: United States, 1982-9. *Epidemiol Infect*. 2001;127(3):381-387

23. Brooks JT, Sowers EG, Wells JG, et al. Non-O157 Shiga toxin-producing *Escherichia coli* infections in the United States, 1983-2002. *J Infect Dis*. 2005;192(8):1422-1429

24. Griffin P, Tauxe R. The epidemiology of infections caused by *Escherichia coli* O157: H7, other enterohemorrhagic *E. coli*, and the associated hemolytic uremic syndrome. *Epidemiol Rev*. 1991;13(1):60-98

25. Hannu T, Mattila L, Rautelin H, et al. Campylobacter-triggered reactive arthritis: a population-based study. *Rheumatology (Oxford)*. 2002;41(3):312-318

26. Warren CP. Arthritis associated with *Salmonella* infections. *Ann Rheum Dis*. 1970;29(5):483-487

27. Mishu B, Ilyas AA, Koski CL, et al. Serologic evidence of previous *Campylobacter jejuni* infection in patients with the Guillain-Barre syndrome. *Ann Intern Med*. 1993;118(12):947-953

28. Gould LH, Bopp C, Strockbine N, et al. Recommendations for diagnosis of shiga toxin-producing *Escherichia coli* infections by clinical laboratories. *MMWR Recomm Rep*. 2009;58(RR-12):1-14

29. Centers for Disease Control and Prevention. Updated norovirus outbreak management and disease prevention guidelines. *MMWR Recomm Rep*. 2011;60(RR-3):1-15

30. Centers for Disease Control and Prevention. Managing acute gastroenteritis among children: oral rehydration, maintenance, and nutritional therapy. *MMWR Recomm Rep*. 2003;52(RR-16):1-16

31. Wong CS, Jelacic S, Habeeb RL, Watkins SL, Tarr PI. The risk of hemolytic-uremic syndrome after antibiotic treatment of *Escherichia coli* O157:H7 infections. *N Engl J Med*. 2000;342(26):1930-1936

32. Aserkoff B, Bennett JV. Effect of antibiotic therapy in acute salmonellosis on the fecal excretion of Salmonellae. *N Engl J Med*. 1969;281(12):636-640

33. Centers for Disease Control and Prevention. Investigational heptavalent botulinum antitoxin (HBAT) to replace licensed botulinum antitoxin AB and investigational botulinum antitoxin E. *MMWR Morb Mortal Wkly Rep*. 2010;59(10):299

34. Arnon SS, Schechter R, Maslanka SE, Jewell NP, Hatheway CL. Human botulism immune globulin for the treatment of infant botulism. *N Engl J Med.* 2006;354(5):462-471

35. American Academy of Pediatrics. Statement of endorsement: managing acute gastroenteritis among children: oral rehydration, maintenance, and nutritional therapy. *Pediatrics.* 2004;114(2):507

36. Pickering LK, Baker CJ, Kimberlin DW, Long SS, eds. *Red Book: 2012 Report of the Committee on Infectious Diseases.* 29th ed. Elk Grove Village, IL: American Academy of Pediatrics; 2012

37. Gerner-Smidt P, Hise K, Kincaid J, et al. PulseNet USA: a five-year update. *Foodborne Pathog Dis.* 2006;3(1):9-19

38. Blanton LH, Adams SM, Beard RS, et al. Molecular and epidemiologic trends of caliciviruses associated with outbreaks of acute gastroenteritis in the United States, 2000–2004. *J Infect Dis.* 2006;193(3):413-421

39. Centers for Disease Control and Prevention. Foodborne disease active surveillance network, 1996. *MMWR Morb Mortal Wkly Rep.* 1997;46(12):258-261

40. Centers for Disease Control and Prevention. Vital signs: incidence and trends of infection with pathogens transmitted commonly through food—foodborne diseases active surveillance network, 10 U.S. sites, 1996—2010. *MMWR Morb Mortal Wkly Rep.* 2011;60(22):749-755

41. Bryan FL, Guzewich JJ, Todd ECD. Surveillance of foodborne disease III. Summary and presentation of data on vehicles and contributory factors; their value and limitations. *J Food Prot.* 1997;60:701-714

42. Tauxe RV. Food safety and irradiation: protecting the public from foodborne infections. *Emerg Infect Dis.* 2001;7(3 Suppl):516-521

43. US Food and Drug Administration. FDA Food Code 2009. http://www.fda.gov/Food/FoodSafety/RetailFoodProtection/FoodCode/FoodCode2009/default.htm. Accessed January 19, 2013

44. Centers for Disease Control and Prevention. Achievements in public health, 1990-1999: safer and healthier foods. *MMWR Morb Mortal Wkly Rep.* 1999;48(40):905-913

45. Billy TJ, Wachsmuth IK. Hazard analysis and critical control point systems in the United States Department of Agriculture regulatory policy. *Rev Sci Tech.* 1997;16(2):342-348

46. US Food and Drug Administration. Health professionals letter on Enterobacter sakazakii infections associated with use of powdered (dry) infant formulas in neonatal intensive care units. Available at: http://www.fda.gov/Food/FoodSafety/Product-SpecificInformation/InfantFormula/AlertsSafetyInformation/ucm111299.htm. Accessed January 19, 2013

47. Bowen AB, Braden CR. Invasive *Enterobacter sakazakii* disease in infants. *Emerg Infect Dis.* 2006;12(8):1185-1189

48. van Acker J, de Smet F, Muyldermans G, Bougatef A, Naessens A, Lauwers S. Outbreak of nNecrotizing enterocolitis associated with *Enterobacter sakazakii* in powdered milk formula. *J Clin Microbiol.* 2001;39(1):293-297

VII

49. Centers for Disease Control and Prevention. *Salmonella montevideo* infections associated with salami products made with contaminated imported black and red pepper—United States, July 2009–April 2010. *MMWR Morb Mortal Wkly Rep.* 2010;59(50):1647-1650

50. Centers for Disease Control and Prevention. Outbreak of *Salmonella* serotype *Saintpaul* infections associated with eating alfalfa sprouts—United States, 2009. *MMWR Morb Mortal Wkly Rep.* 2009;58(18):500-503

51. Cavallaro E, Date K, Medus C, et al. *Salmonella Typhimurium* infections associated with peanut products. *N Engl J Med.* 2011;365(7):601-610

52. Behravesh CB, Mody RK, Jungk J, et al. 2008 outbreak of *Salmonella Saintpaul* infections associated with raw produce. *N Engl J Med.* 2011;364(10):918-927

53. Centers for Disease Control and Prevention. *Clostridium perfringens* infection among inmates at a county jail—Wisconsin, August 2008. *MMWR Morb Mortal Wkly Rep.* 2009;58(6):138-141

54. Centers for Disease Control and Prevention. Two multistate outbreaks of Shiga toxin-producing *Escherichia coli* infections linked to beef from a single slaughter facility—United States, 2008. *MMWR Morb Mortal Wkly Rep.* 2010;59(18):557-560

55. Centers for Disease Control and Prevention. Multistate outbreak of *Salmonella* infections associated with frozen pot pies—United States, 2007. *MMWR Morb Mortal Wkly Rep.* 2008;57(47):1277-1280

56. Centers for Disease Control and Prevention. Outbreak of *Listeria monocytogenes* infections associated with pasteurized milk from a local dairy—Massachusetts, 2007. *MMWR Morb Mortal Wkly Rept.* 2008;57(40):1097-1100.

57. Centers for Disease Control and Prevention. Salmonella Litchfield outbreak associated with a hotel restaurant—Atlantic City, New Jersey, 2007. *MMWR Morb Mortal Wkly. Rep.* 2008;57(28):775-779

58. Sotir MJ, Ewald G, Kimura AC, et al. Outbreak of *Salmonella wandsworth* and *Typhimurium* infections in infants and toddlers traced to a commercial vegetable-coated snack food. *Pediatr Infect Dis J.* 2009;28(12):1041-1046

59. Centers for Disease Control and Prevention. Campylobacter jejuni infection associated with unpasteurized milk and cheese—Kansas, 2007. *MMWR Morb Mortal Wkly Rep.* 2009;57(51):1377-1379

60. Centers for Disease Control and Prevention. Botulism associated with commercially canned chili sauce—Texas and Indiana, July 2007. *MMWR Morb Mortal Wkly Rep.* 2007;56(30):767-769

61. Centers for Disease Control and Prevention. Outbreak of multidrug-resistant *Salmonella enterica* serotype *Newport* infections associated with consumption of unpasteurized Mexican-style aged cheese—Illinois, March 2006–April 2007. *MMWR Morb Mortal Wkly Rep.* 2008;57(16):432-435

62. Centers for Disease Control and Prevention. *Vibrio parahaemolyticus* infections associated with consumption of raw shellfish—three states, 2006. *MMWR Morb Mortal Wkly Rep.* 2006;55(31):854-856

63. Sheth AN, Wiersma P, Atrubin D, et al. International outbreak of severe botulism with prolonged toxemia caused by commercial carrot juice. *Clin Infect Dis.* 2008;47(10):1245-1251

64. Centers for Disease Control and Prevention. Ongoing multistate outbreak of *Escherichia coli* serotype O157:H7 infections associated with consumption of fresh spinach—United States, September 2006. *MMWR Morb Mortal Wkly Rep.* 2006;55(38):1045-1056

65. Behravesh CB, Ferraro A, Deasy M III, et al. Human *Salmonella* infections linked to contaminated dry dog and cat food, 2006-2008. *Pediatrics.* 2010;126(3):477-483

66. Greene SK, Daly ER, Talbot EA, et al. Recurrent multistate outbreak of *Salmonella newport* associated with tomatoes from contaminated fields, 2005. *Epidemiol Infect.* 2008;136(2):157-165

67. Centers for Disease Control and Prevention. Multisite outbreak of norovirus associated with a franchise restaurant—Kent County, Michigan, May 2005. *MMWR Morb Mortal Wkly Rep.* 2006;55(14):395-397

68. McLaughlin JB, DePaola A, Bopp CA, et al. Outbreak of *Vibrio parahaemolyticus* gastroenteritis associated with Alaskan oysters. *N Engl J Med.* 2005;353(14):1463-1470

69. Centers for Disease Control and Prevention. Outbreak of cyclosporiasis associated with snow peas—Pennsylvania, 2004. *MMWR Morb Mortal Wkly Rep.* 2004;53(37):876-878

70. Centers for Disease Control and Prevention. Multistate outbreak of *Salmonella* Typhimurium infections associated with eating ground beef—United States, 2004. *MMWR Morb Mortal Wkly Rep.* 2006;55(7):180-182

71. Devasia RA, Jones TF, Ward J, et al. Endemically acquired foodborne outbreak of enterotoxin-producing *Escherichia coli* serotype O169:H41. *Am J Med.* 2006;119(2):168.e7-168.e10

72. Blackburn BG, Mazurek JM, Hlavsa M, et al. Cryptosporidiosis associated with ozonated apple cider. *Emerg Infect Dis.* 2006;12(4):684-686

73. Wheeler C, Vogt TM, Armstrong GL, et al. An outbreak of hepatitis A associated with green onions. *N Engl J Med.* 2005;353(9):890-897

VII

Chapter 54

Food Safety: Pesticides, Industrial Chemicals, Toxins, Antimicrobial Preservatives, Irradiation, and Food Contact Substances

Introduction

Foods available in the United States are among the safest found in the world. Nonetheless, there are a wide variety of nonnutritive chemical substances found in the food supply that may have health and safety implications for infants and children. A rising challenge has been the monitoring of foods imported from more than 150 countries and territories. Imported foods now constitute 15% of the US food supply, including 60% of fresh fruits and vegetables and 80% of seafood.[1]

In contrast to the usually defined illnesses associated with microbial contamination of foods, the safety issues related to nonmicrobial substances in foods are less well understood and result in effects that may be subclinical and, thus, difficult to document. However, toxicity resulting from exposures over brief periods (days to weeks) does occur, as evidenced by melamine-related deaths in 2007. Melamine is a metabolite of a pesticide and is used in a variety of products, including tableware and paper. In 2007, following deaths of household pets attributable to renal failure, melamine was identified as a contaminant in vegetable proteins imported into the United States from China and used as ingredients in pet food. The addition of melamine artificially increases readings of protein content. Subsequently, melamine-contaminated infant formula was linked to urinary tract ailments in nearly 300 000 infants and the deaths of 6 infants attributed to kidney failure in China.[2]

The chronic effects of nonmicrobial substances in foods are generally more significant for the fetus and young child than for adults because of potential neurotoxic and developmental effects. Infants and children are often more sensitive than adults to environmental chemicals for a number of reasons.[3] Increased susceptibility may result from the greater intake of foods per unit of body weight. This is especially true for foods, such as milk, that are a part of the diet of most infants and young children. The immaturity of developing organ systems is another potential hazard, especially for the nervous, immune, and endocrine systems, and particularly during sensitive periods of development when relatively brief insults may result in later long-term effects. The pharmacokinetic properties of nonmicrobial substances in foods can vary greatly because of the immaturity of organs, such as the liver and kidneys, and the changes in the amounts of body fat and extracellular water. These properties can lead to differential and often higher dose exposures

VII

for children as compared with adults. For chronic effects, prevention of exposure is more significant than most treatments.

US Food Safety Regulations

The primary responsibility for food safety in the United States resides with the US Food and Drug Administration (FDA) and the US Department of Agriculture (USDA) Food Safety and Inspection Service (FSIS). The FSIS regulates meat, poultry, catfish, and processed egg products. The FDA has jurisdiction over 80% of the food supply, including seafood, dairy, and produce and all other products not regulated by the FSIS. The Environmental Protection Agency (EPA) also plays a role in food safety as it is responsible for setting limits (tolerances) on pesticide residues in food and animal feed. The CDC has responsibility for ongoing surveillance; response to; and detection, investigation, and monitoring of foodborne and waterborne illness, including emerging pathogens and antimicrobial resistance patterns. A dozen other agencies also have limited roles, including the National Marine Fisheries Service (NMFS) in the Department of Commerce, which conducts voluntary, fee-for-service inspections of seafood safety and quality, and the Department of Homeland Security, which coordinates agencies' food security activities.

Regulation protecting food and drink from being misbranded and adulterated was first passed by Congress in 1906 and significantly expanded in the Federal Food, Drug, and Cosmetic Act of 1938 (Pub L No. 75-717). A major amendment, the Food Quality and Protection Act of 1996 (Pub L No. 104-170), changed how pesticides in foods are regulated and increased attention to pesticide-related food safety issues for infants and children (see sidebar). Up until the passage of the Food Quality and Protection Act, the allowable levels of pesticide residues in food were intended to protect adult health. In response to Act requirements, by 2006, the EPA had established regulatory limits ("tolerances") on more than 9500 pesticides and pledged to reevaluate every active ingredient of pesticides every 15 years. The tolerance limits represent the maximum amount of pesticides that may legally remain in or on food and animal feed. When the tolerance is exceeded in foods, the FDA can take action to remedy the situation.

Regulations

Food Quality Protection Act of 1996

- Established single health-based standards for all pesticides in food. Benefits, in general, cannot override the health-based standard.

- Prenatal and postnatal effects are to be considered.

- In the absence of data confirming the safety to infants and children, because of their special sensitivities and exposures, an additional uncertainty factor of up to 10X can be added to the safety values.

- Aggregate risk (the sum of all exposures to the chemical) and cumulative risk (the sum of all exposures to chemicals with similar mechanisms of action) must be considered in establishing safe levels.

- Risks are to be determined for both 1 year and lifetime exposure.

- Endocrine disrupters are to be included in the evaluation of safety.

- Called for EPA review of existing pesticide registrations. Expedited review is possible for safer pesticides.

Food Safety Modernization Act of 2011

- Gave the FDA authority to order a recall of food products, whereas in the past FDA could only issue recalls of infant formula, and all other recalls were voluntarily issues by food manufacturers and distributors.

- Calls for more frequent inspections and for those inspections to be based on risk.

- Increases FDA's ability to oversee food produced in foreign countries and imported into the United States. Allows the FDA to prevent a food from entering the country if the facility has refused US inspection.

- Mandates that food facilities must have a written plan identifying possible safety issues of their products and further to outline steps that would help prevent those problems from occurring.

- Establishes science-based standards for the safe production and harvesting of fruits and vegetables.

- Allows exemptions from the produce safety standards for small farms that sell directly to consumers (eg, roadside stand or farmer's market).

In response to new challenges in food safety, the Food Safety Modernization Act was signed in 2011 (Pub L No. 111-353).[4] This Act expands FDA authority (see Sidebar) by increasing preventative actions to address the challenges of imported food and the increasing consumption of raw or minimally processed foods and to better protect a US population with increasing numbers of most vulnerable individuals, including older adults, young children, pregnant women, and immune-compromised individuals.

VII

Sources of Concern for Chemical Food Safety

Chemical substances that are potentially toxic may occur in foods. Contaminants enter the food supply in a variety of ways, including: residues of substances (eg, pesticides) deliberately applied to food during agricultural practices; contaminants from industrial practices (dioxins, metals, flame retardants, and perchlorates); contaminants that are naturally occurring toxins (eg, aflatoxin, vomitoxin); chemicals, such as colorings and flavorings and preservatives deliberately added to food during processing; and substances used in food contact materials or food processing byproducts (eg, adhesives, paper, plastics). This chapter presents an overview of this topic; for additional information, see *Pediatric Environmental Health*, published by the American Academy of Pediatrics (AAP) in 2011.[3]

Pesticides

Pesticides represent a broad classification of chemicals that are applied to kill or control insects, unwanted plants, molds, or unwanted animals (eg, rodents). Pesticides include insecticides, herbicides, fungicides, rodenticides, and fumigants. Although these products can increase both yield and quality of produce, pesticide residues are found on many foods, and chronic low-level exposure is common.

The residues an individual ingests from various foods are determined by the amount of pesticide applied to the crop; the time between application and harvesting, processing, or storage; the type of processing; the treatment of the food in the home; and the amount of the food ingested. Pesticide exposures have been linked to a wide variety of acute and chronic effects.[3]

The USDA and FDA each operate programs to assess pesticides residues on foods sold in the United States. The USDA operates the Pesticide Data Program. Results of this program provide statistically representative data on pesticides in the US food supply. Rotating panels of commodities are selected for testing, which, in 2009, included analysis of 13 244 of samples of 20 types of fruits and vegetables (81% of samples) and samples of beef, catfish, and water. In 2009, pesticide residues exceeding the established tolerance were detected in 0.3% of samples tested, and residues with no established tolerance were found in 2.7% of samples.[5] Among the various fruits and vegetables selected for testing, more than 90% of apples, grapes, strawberries, cilantro, potatoes, and oranges contained pesticide residues, but nearly all were below the tolerance level.

The FDA provides an annual summary of its pesticide-monitoring program.[6] FDA sampling strategies include focused sampling and targeted sampling of food that may be suspect for violations. In 2008, 5053 samples (28% domestically grown foods) were collected and analyzed by the FDA program. Pesticide residues were detected in 35.8% of domestic samples and in 27.7% of imported samples. Residues in violation of allowed tolerances were found in 0.9 % of the domestic samples and 4.7% of the imported samples (see Table 54.1); 13% were for levels exceeding tolerance limits and 87% were for detection of residue for pesticides lacking tolerance limits; thus, detection of the chemical represents a violative level. FDA also reports data from the Total Diet Study, which evaluates approximately 280 table-ready foods for more than 200 different components, including elements (toxic and nutrient), pesticide residues, industrial chemicals, volatile organic compounds, radionuclides, and folate, and includes an analysis of approximately 30 infant and toddler foods. Nearly all table-ready foods analyzed have nondetectable or very low pesticide levels.[7]

Table 54.1.

US Food and Drug Administration Pesticide Residue Monitoring Program, Fiscal Year 2009[6]

Food	% of Samples Above the Violative Level	
	Domestic	Imports
Grains and grain products	0	1.2
Milk/dairy products/eggs	0	0
Fish/shellfish/other aquatic products/aquaculture seafood group	0	0
Fruits	0	4.8
Vegetables	1.7	4.4
Other[a]	2.6	8.3

[a] Mostly nuts, seeds, oils, honey, candy, spices, multiple food products, and dietary supplements.

Pesticide Exposures From Foods

In a national sample of individuals ages 6 to 59 years, among 44 pesticide metabolites examined, 29 were detectable in most people; organophosphate and organochlorine insecticides were the most prevalent.[8] The food supply is the most important source of exposure for these insecticides, as organophosphates were banned for use in the home in 2000, and organochlorines (eg, p,p'-dichlorodiphenyltrichloroethane [DDT], dieldrin, and chlordane) were banned in the United States 20 to 30 years earlier.[9,10] Pyrethroids, which have replaced organophosphates for most uses, are now detectable in 75% of the national sample.[11] Food residues are the most important source of exposure to pyrethroids for children and adolescents.

VII

The FDA does not monitor pesticide usage in home gardens or enforce appropriate use in that setting. Excessive applications or too short a time between application and harvesting can result in greater residue levels than are tolerated in commercially produced foods. For detailed information on pesticides in foods, see the AAP statement on pesticide exposure in children.[9]

Effects of Pesticides in Children

Acute pesticide poisoning in US children is rarely seen, but chronic low-level exposures are common. Serious acute poisoning from pesticides most often follows unintentional ingestion.[10] Although pesticides in the food chain are not the major source for acute pesticide exposure in infants and children, such events do occur.

Of the pesticides, the insecticides are most likely to cause acute illness. Pyrethroids commonly in use have features at presentation that are similar to organophosphates and carbamates, both of which are acetylcholinesterase inhibitors, but pyrethroid symptoms dissipate with only supportive care in approximately 24 hours.[9] Organophosphates have greatest toxicity of the 3 types because of irreversible binding of the acetylcholinesterase inhibitor. Treatment varies according to which type of pesticide has been ingested, so obtaining an accurate history is key.[9] Additional details on differentiating the pesticides and their treatments are found in AAP statements from the Committee on Environmental Health.[9,10]

Recent prospective cohort studies have demonstrated adverse effects of early-life exposure to organophosphates and organochlorine pesticides on neurodevelopment and behavior. Several papers have reviewed the evidence.[12-15] Ongoing studies have enrolled pregnant women living in urban or rural areas, objectively assessed their routinely encountered chronic exposures during pregnancy, and evaluated their children into the preschool ages. These studies report significant associations of higher levels of pesticide exposures with children's poorer cognitive development and increased scores on measures assessing pervasive developmental disorder, inattention, and attention-deficit/hyperactivity disorder. In the National Health and Nutrition Examination Survey sample of US children 8 to 15 years of age, those with higher urinary concentrations of organophosphate metabolites more often had a diagnosis of attention-deficit/hyperactivity disorder.[16] Studies are underway to elucidate genetic influences of risk for pesticide effects in children and further identify mechanistic pathways of neurodevelopment and other metabolic effects in animal models. These studies are evaluating effects at levels of pesticide exposure commonly encountered in US urban and rural samples.

In general, one can assume that exposure in utero and early in infancy would be more harmful to the developing nervous system than exposure later in childhood.

Reducing Pesticide Exposure From Foods

People can reduce their pesticide exposures by purchasing organic foods.[17] A study of children placed on an organic diet for 5 consecutive days demonstrated a marked decrease in their urinary excretion of metabolites of organophosphate insecticides during the organic diet phase.[18] In 2002, the USDA defined organically-grown food as food grown and processed using no synthetic fertilizers or pesticides. Producers and handlers must be certified by a USDA-accredited certifying agent to sell, label, or represent their product as "100% organic" or "organic" (at least 95% organic).[19] An estimated two thirds of US consumers purchase organic foods sometimes, and 28% purchase it weekly[20]; organic products cost up to 40% more than conventionally grown products. Organically grown fruits and vegetables have not been shown to have higher nutritional value.[17]

Food-preparation measures can also reduce pesticide residue on food. Measures that can be recommended to parents include (http://www.epa.gov/pesticides/food/tips.htm):

- Thoroughly wash and scrub fresh fruits and vegetables with cold or warm running tap water before consumption. However, not all pesticides can be removed by washing.
- Peel fruits and vegetables when possible. Discard the outer leaves of leafy vegetables, such as lettuce and cabbage.
- Trim the fat from meats and the skin and fat from poultry and fish.
- Avoid pesticide use on home-grown fruits and vegetables.

Industrial Chemicals

Another source of contaminants is chemicals dispersed in the environment from industrial processes that have entered the food chain. These chemicals may precipitate from the atmosphere into water, onto soil or directly onto food crops and directly contaminate underground or surface waters that may, in turn, affect the water supply for irrigation or consumption. Industrial chemicals that contaminate food during processing are termed "food contact substances" and are covered in a separate section.

The most ubiquitous group of compounds resulting from industrial production is termed "persistent toxic substances," which includes a class of compounds known as persistent organic pollutants (POPs). A wide variety of persistent toxic substances are encountered in the environment, more than 50 of which are monitored in the US National Health and Nutrition Examination Survey. Many of these substances are present in measurable levels in the majority of individuals tested in the United States.[21]

VII

There were 12 original POPs—all chlorinated compounds—but additional, diverse compounds have been added to the list. POPs include polychlorinated biphenyls (PCBs), polychlorinated dibenzofurans (PCDFs), polychlorinated dibenzo-p-dioxins (PCDDs, including tetrachlorodibenzo-p-dioxin [TCDD], a particularly potent dioxin), organochlorines (eg, chlordane, heptachlor, DDT and its derivatives), polybrominated biphenyls (PBB), polybrominated diphenyl ethers (PBDEs), and a host of others (aldrin, dieldrin, endrin, hexachlorobenzene, mirex and toxaphene). The ongoing use of many of these chemicals has been extensively curtailed by international treaty. Information on these chemicals to supplement that presented below is found in the 2011 edition of *Pediatric Environmental Health* from the AAP.[3]

PCBs were originally used by the electrical industry as insulators and dielectrics; PCDFs appear as contaminants after extreme heating of PCBs. PCDDs were formed as contaminants in the production of hexachlorophene, pentachlorophenol, and several herbicides, including Agent Orange (a defoliant during the Vietnam War). PBDEs have been used primarily as flame retardants and continue to be extensively used in a variety of consumer products, such as home/office furnishings and electronics.[22]

Another commonly encountered persistent toxic substance is perchlorate. Perchlorate is used in solid rocket fuel, propellants, and explosives. It is a contaminant of drinking water and is associated with elevated thyroid-stimulating hormone concentrations when iodine concentration is low.[23] Women with lower iodine and higher perchlorate concentrations have higher concentrations of thyroid-stimulating hormone.[24]

Persistence in the Environment

These toxic chemicals persist in the environment and have accumulated in produce grown in contaminated soils. Because of their lipophilic nature, they bioaccumulate in the fat tissue of many animal-based foods, including meat, eggs, dairy products, and fish (both saltwater and freshwater varieties), with sport fish from contaminated waters generally being the most concentrated food source of such chemicals. Because of their use in many household products, PBDEs in household dust is a significant source for toddlers, who ingest more dust than adults, but food sources are of primary importance for all other ages.[25]

When ingested by humans in food, these toxicants bioaccumulate in human fat. Persistent toxic substances, often acquired over many years, are transferred to the fetus from maternal stores and appear in human milk, because they are fat soluble and are not significantly metabolized.

Effects

In addition to the child developmental and behavioral effects of organochlorine exposure discussed in the previous section, many of these compounds are thought to have endocrine-disrupting properties. In adults, higher levels of PCBs, organochlorine pesticides, and PBDEs have been associated with risk of diabetes and metabolic syndrome in National Health and Examination Survey samples.[21,26-28] Among women recruited from a predominantly Mexican-immigrant community in California, higher PBDE blood concentrations were associated with reduced fertility.[29] PBDEs have direct toxic effects on the developing nervous system and impair the thyroid hormone system, which is a critical component of early brain development.[30,31] In a study of 210 children in Mexico, after adjusting for potential confounders, higher cord blood PBDE concentrations were associated with lower assessments of development at 12, 24, and 36 months of age and IQ at 48 and 72 months of age.[32]

The carcinogenic potential of the dioxins has also been recognized by the EPA. TCDD, which causes chloracne in humans, is classified as a known human carcinogen.[33] Food, particularly fat-containing animal products (including seafoods), are the major sources of these organic pollutants.[34] The most recent assessment of dioxin and dioxin-like compounds (ie, PCDDs, PCDFs, and dioxin-like PCBs) in the US meat and poultry supply was conducted in 2007-2008 with samples from slaughterhouses.[35] Compared with a previous survey in the mid-1990s, the basic congener profiles for each animal type were fairly constant and the overall levels of these substances may have decreased, but changes in analytic methods may also play a role in report findings. In the recent survey, the USDA tested fat samples in cattle, hogs, young chickens, and young turkeys and found relatively higher levels of these compounds in cattle and turkeys compared with chickens and hogs.

No specific treatments are known, and the prevention of excessive intake is the only therapeutic approach. To reduce food-related exposures, reducing the ingestion of the fats found in animals, dairy products, and fish are the basis of the recommendations currently proposed. Because these persistent toxic substances are minimally metabolized and excreted, intakes are cumulative over years. Fish vary in their fat content by species, and the level of contamination varies with species, location, body size, and the type of feeding, especially in farmed fish.[36] Because of the variation in the contamination in fresh water fish, states in which contaminated fish may be found publish fish advisories about where such fish may exist, with recommendations on their consumption by pregnant women, lactating mothers, and young children. Recommendations to reduce the intake of dioxin-like compounds

VII

in the diet, especially for children, young women, women who may become pregnant, and lactating mothers,[37] include:

- Choose lean cuts of meat and trim all visible fat before cooking.
- Choose fish with lower fat content and lower levels of contamination and remove visible fat and skin before cooking.
- Use low-fat or fat-free dairy products routinely.
- Reduce the amount of butter or lard used in the preparation of foods.
- Cook meats and fish by broiling, grilling, or other methods that allow fat to be drained away.
- Do not save or reuse rendered fats.

Metal Compounds

Another group of compounds that may contaminate food are metals. The metals most commonly found in food are mercury and lead.

Mercury

Mercury is primarily released into the environment by natural and industrial processes, particularly the burning of fossil fuels.[3] Coal-burning power plants remain the largest single source of mercury emissions in the United States. Mercury-containing rains go into lakes, rivers, and oceans, where the mercury is biotransformed by bacteria to methylmercury. Methylmercury, a potent neuro-developmental toxicant, is bioconcentrated up the aquatic food chain. Methylmercury has also been used as a fungicide on seed grains. Consumption of mercury-treated seed grains had caused widespread mercury poisoning among people in Iraq and China.[38]

Fish consumption is the source of most human mercury exposure in the United States. Chronic effects of methylmercury ingestion have been noted in the offspring of mothers who had elevated concentrations in their bodies. The EPA has determined a reference dose (RfD) for methylmercury at 0.1 µg/kg/day (to achieve a cord blood mercury concentration <5.8 µg/L) on the basis of protecting the fetal brain from damage. Because mercury is concentrated in the fetus, a maternal blood mercury concentration of 3.5 µg/L would be expected to achieve a fetal blood mercury concentration of 5.8 µg/L.[39] Analysis of data from adult women gathered in the 1999-2004 National Health and Nutrition Examination Surveys identified 10.4% with a mercury concentration above 3.5 µg/L and 4.7% of women with mercury concentration above 5.8 µg/L. Risk of elevated mercury concentrations was highest among women living in the Northeast or who were of Asian descent or had higher income.[40] Mercury concentrations in many ocean fish and shellfish have been evaluated.[41] Predatory fish generally have the highest mercury levels. Mercury concentrations in freshwater fish vary by location, and many are also highly contaminated. States' fish consumption advisories include data on mercury as well as PCBs with guidance on which fish to limit intakes and which to avoid either because of mercury and/or PCBs and other POPs. A national listing of fish advisories is available on the EPA Web site (http://water.epa.gov/scitech/ swguidance/fishshellfish/fishadvisories/index.cfm). Updated information can be obtained from state EPA offices.

Marine and freshwater fish and shellfish are important components of a balanced, healthy diet. Fish is high in protein and low in saturated fat and contains essential vitamins and minerals and long-chain omega-3 fatty acids (see Chapter 17: Fats and Fatty Acids). Unfortunately, fish are vulnerable to contamination by toxic industrial pollutants, such as mercury, as well as lipophilic chemicals, such as PCBs, dioxins, flame retardants, and others. These pollutants accumulate in fish flesh (as in the case of methylmercury) or fatty tissue (as in the case of PCBs), exposing people who eat them. Mothers can pass on these pollutants to their offspring both in utero and via human milk, and children may also be exposed to these harmful chemicals directly through eating fish. For some populations, locally caught fish may be the only good alternative for a nutritious diet. Finding the balance between acquiring the nutritional benefits from adequate fish consumption and avoiding the toxicity from consumption of polluted fish is a challenge. The suggested potential beneficial effects on child IQ from fish intake (>2 meals/week) during pregnancy must be weighed against negative effects from mercury in the fish.[42] If fish with lower mercury concentrations are available, then it is prudent to substitute these rather than eat fish that have methylmercury advisories. Many commercial fish have low concentrations of methylmercury.

The FDA has set a regulatory limit for methylmercury in commercial fish of 1 ppm (1 µg/g). The FDA has issued an advisory to pregnant women, women of childbearing age, nursing mothers, and young children to avoid consumption of shark, king mackerel, swordfish, and tilefish. For other types of fish, including canned light tuna, the FDA has advised that consumption by children, pregnant women, and those who may become pregnant be kept below 12 ounces per week.[43] (Canned albacore and fresh tuna have approximately 3 times higher methylmercury concentration than canned light tuna.) Mercury content of many various commercial seafood varieties can be found on the FDA Web site (see Table 54.2 for a partial list).

VII

Table 54.2.
Mercury Concentration in Selected Commercial Seafood (1990-2010)[a]

Seafood	Mean Mercury Concentration (ppm)
	Highest Levels
Tilefish (Gulf of Mexico)	1.450
Shark	0.979
Swordfish	0.995
Mackerel king	0.730
	Moderate Levels
Orange roughy	0.571
Grouper (all species)	0.448
Bass Chilean	0.354
Tuna (fresh/frozen, yellowfin)	0.354
Tuna (canned, albacore)	0.350
Monkfish	0.181
	Lowest Levels
Tuna (canned, light)	0.128
Trout, freshwater	0.071
Crab	0.065
Scallops	0.003
Catfish	0.025
Pollock	0.031
Salmon (fresh/frozen)	0.022
Tilapia	0.013
Clams	0.009
Salmon (canned)	0.008
Shrimp	0.009

[a] Selected data from FDA.[41] Other contaminants, such as PCBs, may alter the safety of eating particular fish.

The federal government does not regulate the levels of mercury or other contaminants, such as PCBs or dioxins, in fish caught for sport. Because of the potential for mercury contamination, states have issued advisories recommending public limits or the avoidance of consuming certain fish caught for sport from specific bodies of water. These include freshwater species, such as trout, walleye, pike, muskie, and bass, which may have concentrations of mercury that would result in substantial exposure. States in which PCBs or dioxins in fish have been a problem, such as those around the Great Lakes, have advisories concerning the consumption of noncommercial fish, and these should be available from the state health department. PCBs are stored mainly in the fat. Trimming the fat, removing the skin, and filleting the fish can lower PCB concentrations in fish by about 50%.

In general, guidelines for selecting safer fish focus on several major points (see Sidebar). Women of childbearing age and all children should (1) avoid varieties of fish known to be highly contaminated; (2) know and follow local and federal fish consumption guidelines; (3) eat a wide variety of the least contaminated fish; and (4) limit weekly fish meals depending on which varieties are chosen. In general, leaner, smaller, and younger wild fish are least likely to be heavily polluted.

Fish Recommendations

Advice from the EPA on selecting healthier varieties of fish:

- **Do Not Eat (high mercury content):** swordfish, shark, king mackerel, and tilefish.

- **Eat up to 12 oz (2 average meals)** of fish and shellfish weekly.

  - Choose varieties that are low in mercury: most commonly canned light tuna, salmon, shrimp, pollock, catfish.

  - If choosing a fish variety with a moderate level of mercury, such as albacore "white" tuna, limit intake to 6 oz/week and select a low-mercury fish for the other fish meal.

- **Check local advisories about the safety of sport fish.** If no advice is available, eat up to 6 oz (1 average meal) per week of fish you catch from local waters, but do not consume any other fish during that week. A listing of national and state fish advisories can be found at the EPA Web site: http://water.epa.gov/scitech/swguidance/fishshellfish/fishadvisories/index.cfm.

Lead, Manganese, Cadmium

Although most lead exposure in the United States is not from food sources, there are many foods that can sometimes be identified as contributing to a child's lead burden. Some types of candy imported from other countries, primarily Mexican-style candy, and powdered snack mix have been found to be contaminated with lead. A pictorial index of more than 70 Mexican candies identified with elevated lead in the product or wrapping is available at http://www2.ocregister.com/multimedia/lead/. Contaminated Mexican candies were of the traditional style, such as lollipops coated with chili, or powdery mixtures of ingredients, such as salt,

VII

lemon flavoring, and chili powder. In 2005, the FDA set a recommended maximum lead level in candy likely to be consumed frequently by small children at 0.1 ppm, above which the FDA may consider enforcement.[44] Other foods found to have elevated lead have most commonly been supplements, ethnic remedies, and spices (see *Pediatric Environmental Health*[3] for additional details).

In June 2010, the Joint Food and Agriculture Organization of the United Nations and World Health Organization Expert Committee on Food Additives rejected its prior provisional tolerable weekly intake of lead of 25 µg/kg and recommended limiting lead intake to <0.3 µg/kg per day for a child and 1.2 µg/kg per day for an adult. These new recommendations were shown to be associated with negligible change to child IQ (0.5 IQ point loss) and limited adult blood pressure increase (1 mm Hg).[45]

Lead is taken up by growing plants, with highest concentration in the root and lowest in the fruit. Measurable amounts of lead in edible roots and shoots have been identified in urban gardens.[46]

Another metal that may have toxic effects on infants is manganese, which is an essential trace element in human metabolism.[47] Elevated blood concentrations have been associated with neurologic problems in children, such as hyperactivity and learning disabilities,[48] although these associations are controversial and remain to be validated. Soy products are enriched in aluminum and manganese.[49] For example, soy-based formulas contain 200 to 300 µg of manganese/L compared with other formulas that contain 77 to 100 µg/L[50] (see also Chapter 4: Formula Feeding of Term Infants). It should be emphasized, however, that no examples of neurotoxicity have been associated with the ingestion of soy formulas.[49] Manganese is also a natural component of water,[51] with an estimated 6% of US domestic groundwater wells exceeding the US health reference level of 300 µg/L.[48] The bioavailability of dietary manganese is very low (~1%–5%); manganese bioavailability is approximately 1.5 to 2 times greater in drinking water, compared with other dietary sources.

Cadmium is another metal with a long biological half-life (>20 years) and potential neurotoxicity. It is found in foods such as tofu, leafy vegetables, grains, and shellfish. Foods grown in cadmium-contaminated soils may also contribute to higher cadmium concentrations.

Toxins

A wide variety of toxins are found in various foods. These toxins may be endogenously produced or the product of other organisms or bacteria that inhabit the food product.

Various varieties of seafood can produce toxins. The most commonly encountered is deadly tetrodotoxin produced by puffer fish. The meat of some varieties of puffer fish is considered a delicacy in Japan, and several deaths attributable to respiratory failure after eating puffer fish prepared incorrectly occur annually. Several other varieties of mollusks, frogs, newts, and fish also produce tetrodotoxin.

Many varieties of seafood acquire toxin from the ingestion by fish of toxin-producing algae. The most significant algae are the dinoflagellates like *Gymnodinium breve*, which produces a severe neurotoxin and is the cause of the Red Tide, *Gambierdiscus,* which produces the most common fish toxin, ciguatera, and a large number of others that produce toxins affecting shellfish[52] see Table 54.3).

Table 54.3.
Toxins in Seafoods[52]

Organism Producing Toxin	Toxin	Seafood Affected	Health Effects
Gambierdiscus species	Ciguatera	Barracudas, groupers, snappers, jacks, mackerel, triggerfish	Acute symptoms of the gastrointestinal tract, central nervous system, and cardiovascular system; self-limited; usually subsides in several days
Many dinoflagellates	Saxitoxin derivatives Polyethers Brevetoxins Domoic acid	Mussels, clams, cockles, scallops Mussels, oysters, scallops Shellfish from the Florida coast Mussels	Paralytic shellfish poisoning Diarrheic shellfish poisoning Neurotoxic shellfish poisoning Amnesic shellfish poisoning
Various bacteria	Histamine, also called scombrotoxin	Tuna, mahi mahi, bluefish, sardines, mackerel, amberjack, abalone Note: may also be in Swiss cheese	Burning mouth, upper body rash, hypotension, headache, pruritus, vomiting, and diarrhea

Cooking does not remove seafood toxins, although they may become diluted. These toxins are generally found among seafood varieties in certain geographic areas, whereas the same varieties of seafood in other geographic areas lack toxins. To limit risk of exposures to seafood toxins, the following general suggestions are made:

- Do not use any seafood (fish or shellfish) that looks, smells, or tastes odd.
- Buy seafood from reputable sources.
- Buy only fresh seafood that is refrigerated or properly iced.
- Do not buy cooked seafood if displayed in the same case as raw fish.
- Do not buy frozen seafood with torn, open, or crushed package edges.
- Keep seafood refrigerated immediately after buying it.

VII

Naturally occurring toxins also can be found with a wide variety of other foods, including mushrooms, corn, beans, and apples. The frequency of illness reported to result from these toxins is low, but no specific data are available. The rarity of case reports may be related to lack of recognition of specific toxidromes.[52] Decreasing risk for children is through avoidance. Mushroom toxins are classified in 4 groups: protoplasmic poisons, neurotoxins, gastrointestinal irritants, and disulfiram toxins. They are found in a wide variety of mushrooms, which are not easily distinguished from nontoxic varieties. They are not inactivated by cooking. Pyrrolizidine alkaloids are usually associated with home remedies that are derived from legumes and other plants. Phytohemagglutinins are found primarily in red kidney beans that are raw or only partially cooked, as in slow cookers and in salads. Grayanotoxin is found in honey that comes from rhododendrons. Like most others in this group, the symptoms are usually acute. Aflatoxins are fungal in origin and may affect corn, nuts and milk.[30] Aflatoxin ingestion increases risk of liver cancer, especially in individuals testing positive for hepatitis B virus.[53]

Two fungal toxins, patulin and fumonisin, are more widespread and are specifically addressed by the FDA. Patulin can be found in apple juice and apple juice products, if production includes rotten or partially rotted apples. Preprocessing water treatments and visually removing rotted and damaged fruit by hand are effective measures to reduce patulin concentrations in apple juice. At the maximum recommended concentration for patulin in juice, 50 μg/kg, it is possible for infants and small children to exceed the allowable limit of 0.43 μg/kg of body weight. There are only chronic effects of patulin ingestion, and these occur with long-term consumption. Toxicologic studies in animals indicate premature death, fetotoxic, and embryotoxic effects and possible immunologic effects.[54] Studies in humans have not been performed, but consumption of apple juice should be limited to 4 to 6 oz/day for children 1 to 6 years old and 8 to 12 oz/day for older children (see also Chapter 7: Feeding the Child). However, intakes above the tolerable daily limit of patulin would occur less often by lowering the accepted maximum recommended concentration for patulin in juice from 50 to 25 μg/kg rather than applying a guideline on juice intake.[55]

Fumonisin is a mycotoxin. More than 10 types have been found worldwide[56] in corn and corn products, such as corn flour, corn meal, and grits. They have been found to be at very low levels in ready-to-eat breakfast cereals. They are not found in corn syrup. Low levels are found in corn chips and tortillas as well as in popcorn. The toxicity of the fumonisins in animals includes leukoencephalomalacia in horses, pulmonary edema in pigs, and liver, kidney, cardiac, and atherogenic effects in experimental animals. Rats and mice have been shown to develop liver cancers in chronic feeding experiments.[57] Fumosin has been associated with increased incidence of esophageal cancer and neural tube defects in subsistence maize farming communities.[58-60] Guidance on fumonisin levels in human foods and animal feeds has been established by the FDA.[57]

Antimicrobial Preservatives

Among the approaches used in achieving food preservation by inhibiting growth of undesirable microorganisms is the use of chemical agents exhibiting antimicrobial activity. These chemicals may be either synthetic compounds intentionally added to foods or naturally occurring, biologically derived substances—"naturally occurring antimicrobials" of plant, animal, or microbial origin.[61] The FDA maintains a listing of more than 3000 substances classified as GRAS (generally regarded as safe) which can be added to foods for coloring, flavoring, or preservation purposes.[62] GRAS preservatives include the traditional substances, such as salt, sugar, vinegar, alcohol, or smoke. Other substances may be found naturally in some foods or be naturally occurring substances (for instance, of bacterial origin) that are found in the food as it exists or are added to other foods.[63] The most common food preservatives are the organic acids or their salts or derivatives: sorbic acid and benzoic acid are the most common, but others include propionic, citric, acetic, lactic, sulfites, and others. Additionally, lipid materials, such as monoacylglycerols (from partially hydrolyzed fat), phenols, lytic enzymes such as egg white lysozyme, peroxidases and oxidases such as glucose oxidase, bacteriocins such as nisin, and hydrogen peroxide may be used. No specific toxicity to any of these substances is known. Disodium ethylene-diaminetetraacetic acid (EDTA), the natural antioxidant vitamin E, and synthetic antioxidants (butylated hydroxyanisole [BHA] and butylhydroxytoluene [BHT]) are also commonly used. The FDA considers these to be GRAS substances at levels allowed in foods in the United States. Sodium nitrates and nitrites have long been used for meat preservatives to enhance the cured meat flavor and color. The maximum amount of nitrite allowed in smoked and cured fish and meat is 200 ppm. Concern for development of methemoglobinemia in infants resulting from nitrate ingestion is generally from well water or plant nitrates (eg, naturally occurring in green beans, carrots, squash, spinach, and beets).[64]

Food Irradiation

Food irradiation is a process by which food is exposed to a controlled source of ionizing radiation to prolong shelf-life and reduce food losses, to improve microbiologic safety, and/or to reduce the use of chemical fumigants and additives. The dose of the ionizing radiation determines the effects of the process on foods. Food is generally irradiated at levels from 10 Gy to 50 kGy (1 kGy = 1000 Gy), depending

VII

on the goals of the process. Low-dose irradiation (up to 1 kGy) is used primarily to delay ripening of produce or to kill or render sterile insects and other higher organisms that may infest fresh food. Medium-dose irradiation (1-10 kGy) reduces the number of pathogens and other microbes on food and prolongs shelf life. High-dose irradiation (>10 kGy) sterilizes food.

Food irradiation is regulated by the FDA as a food additive. The USDA also has regulatory responsibilities for some types of foods irradiated for defined purposes. All petitioners for FDA approval of food irradiation must complete a process that ensures that food irradiated for a specific purpose under precise conditions will remain radiologically, toxicologically, and microbiologically safe and nutritionally adequate.[65]

Currently, all irradiated food sold in the United States must be labeled with the international sign of irradiation, the radura (Fig 54.1) and the statement "treated with radiation" or "treated by irradiation." Manufacturers may optionally add a statement with the purpose (eg, "to control spoilage"). Current rules do not require food services to identify irradiated foods they serve.

Fig 54.1.
The radura is the international symbol indicating that a food has been irradiated.

The FDA is considering rules that will allow some irradiated foods (those in which the irradiation has caused no material change in the food) to be marketed without any labeling as having been irradiated.[66] The proposed change also would not require foods that have incorporated irradiated foods as ingredients to be labeled.

Radiologic Safety

Neither the food nor the packaging materials become radioactive as a result of food irradiation.[67,68] The sources of radiation approved for use in food irradiation are limited to those producing energy too low to induce subatomic particles or cause chain reactions.

Toxicologic Safety

Radiation absorbed by food causes a host of chemical reactions proportional to the dose of radiation applied. The desired reactions involve disrupting the DNA of spoilage and disease causing microbes and pests. Undesired reactions could involve creation of toxic compounds. A number of approaches involving hundreds of studies have been employed over decades to determine whether such toxic compounds are created during irradiation and, if created, whether they are unique to the irradiation process (versus canning, freezing, drying, etc) or created in amounts large enough to cause harm. With improved analytic techniques, a class of compounds have been identified and proposed as a marker of food irradiation. These compounds, known as 2-alkylcyclobutanones, are derived from irradiation of fatty acids in food in a dose-dependent way. However, a recent study has also identified these compounds in foods not radiated.[69] Little is known about their toxicity, but there is evidence that some of these chemicals could be tumor promoters.[70,71] Nonetheless, multigenerational animal feeding studies and analytical chemical modeling studies have failed to identify any unusual toxicity associated with consumption of irradiated foods.[72-74] In fact, irradiated food often contains fewer changed molecules (also called radiolytic products) than food processed in conventional ways. For example, heat-processed foods can contain 50 to 500 times more changed products molecules than irradiated foods.[75] Further, radiation treatment can reduce postharvest losses and use of chemical fumigants, such as methyl bromide.

Microbiologic Safety

Irradiation kills microbes primarily by fragmenting DNA. The sensitivity of organisms increases with the complexity of the organism. Thus, viruses are most resistant to destruction by irradiation, and insects and parasites are most sensitive. Spores, cysts, toxins and prions are quite resistant to the effects of irradiation, because they are in highly stable resting states or are not living organisms. The conditions under which irradiation takes place (ie, temperature, humidity, and atmospheric content) can affect the dose required to achieve the food-processing goal. Regardless, the quality of the food to be irradiated must be high, without heavy microbial contamination, for irradiation to achieve food-processing goals at any level.

VII

When irradiation is used at nonsterilizing doses, the possibility of persistent pathogens is always present. Although it is true that pathogen loads can be substantially reduced using this technique, it is always possible for foods to become recontaminated. Irradiation does not obviate the need for strict application of safe food handling techniques including adequate storage, hygienic preparation and complete cooking, particularly of high-risk foods, such as foods of animal origin, precooked processed foods, or imported foods.[76]

Nutritional Value

As with any food-processing technique, irradiation can have a negative effect on some nutrients. It does not significantly damage carbohydrates or proteins, nor does it change the bioavailability or quantity of minerals or trace elements in foods. Slight loss of essential polyunsaturated fatty acids does occur with irradiation, but fats and oils that are major dietary sources of these nutrients tend to become rancid when irradiated and are not good candidates for this kind of treatment.[77]

Vitamin loss is the largest nutritional concern when foods are irradiated. Vitamin losses are most dramatic when studied in pure solutions. Whole foods exert a protective effect on vitamins, because most of the radiation dose is absorbed by macromolecules (proteins, carbohydrates and fats). Losses can be minimized by irradiating at low temperatures, at low doses, and by excluding oxygen and light.[78] When studied in pure solution, the water-soluble vitamins most sensitive to irradiation are thiamin (B_1), pyridoxine (B_6) and riboflavin (B_2). Vitamin C is converted by irradiation to dehydroascorbic acid (DHAA), which behaves like ascorbic acid in humans, thus preserving nearly normal vitamin C activity after irradiation. Vitamin B_{12}, niacin, and pantothenic and folic acids are resistant to irradiation. Of the fat-soluble vitamins, E and A are sensitive. Plant carotenes are relatively resistant, and vitamins D and K are quite resistant to irradiation.[75]

Thiamine loss can be 50% or more under some conditions in some foods. Loss is enhanced with increased irradiation doses, increased storage time after irradiation, and cooking after irradiation. Rich sources of thiamin include whole-grain cereals, legumes, nuts, pork, brown rice, milk, and other foods that have been fortified. If all sources of thiamine come from irradiated products, a deficiency condition could develop, but this is unlikely in the United States. Irradiation losses of pyridoxine (found in meat; whole grains; vegetables, such as potatoes, corn, and soybeans; and fortified cereals) are not as severe as with thiamine, and deficiency states are even less likely to develop. The biological availability of riboflavin (found in meat, milk, eggs, green vegetables, whole grains, and legumes) can be paradoxically increased after irradiation by shortening required cooking time. For example, dried legumes irradiated at high dose require less than a quarter of the cooking time of untreated

Food Safety: Pesticides, Industrial Chemicals, Toxins, Antimicrobial Preservatives, **1271**
Irradiation, and Food Contact Substances

legumes, and measured riboflavin is higher in irradiated versus nonirradiated cooked samples.[75]

Vitamin E loss can be significant. A study of effects of radiation plus heat shows that nonirradiated rolled oats lost 17% of their vitamin E after 10 minutes of cooking and 40% after 30 minutes of cooking, whereas rolled oats treated with 1 kGy lost 17% of their vitamin E after irradiation, 27.5% after cooking for 10 minutes, and 57% after cooking for 30 minutes.[75] Many of the sources of vitamin E, cereal grains, seed oils, peanuts, soybeans, milk fat, and turnip greens, are unlikely to be treated with radiation and should provide for adequate alternative sources in a balanced and varied diet. Preformed vitamin A is found primarily in milk fat (vitamin A-fortified milk) and eggs. Thus far, only eggs are approved for irradiation. Furthermore, plant carotenes found in dark green and yellow vegetables are converted by the body into vitamin A and are relatively resistant to irradiation.

Although a few vitamins are significantly affected by irradiation, in general, irradiated food is quite nutritious. As long as a diet is balanced and food choices are varied, deficiency states are unlikely to develop.

Palatability

Taste, texture, color, and smell are all components of palatable foods. Some foods, particularly foods with high fat content, could suffer unacceptable changes in these qualities when irradiated. However, modified conditions, such as excluding oxygen from the atmosphere (oxidation can make food rancid), lowering the temperature, excluding light, reducing water content, or lowering the radiation dose can minimize or eliminate these changes. Use of low-dose radiation can reduce chemical changes to food to the point where only chemical analysis could detect a change. A welcome consequence of modifying irradiation conditions to preserve palatability is that the same modifications can also minimize vitamin loss.

Conclusion

Irradiation is increasingly suggested as an important adjunct to improving food safety and availability, including reducing post-harvest losses, reducing use of chemical fumigants, and extending shelf-life without significantly changing foods, inducing radioactivity, or leaving harmful or toxic residues.[66,79,80] Current rules by the FDA for food irradiation are listed in Table 54.4. The most important health benefit of irradiation is inactivation of pathologic microorganisms. Irradiated foods can be safely used as part of a balanced and varied diet. However, it is important to remember that irradiation of food does not substitute for careful food handling from farm to fork. Widespread use of food irradiation would necessitate construction of additional irradiation facilities in the United States and other countries. The benefits of expanding this technology and the risks involved must be thoroughly debated. Pediatricians should participate in the dialogue. As with any technology, unforeseen consequences are possible; therefore, careful monitoring and continuous evaluation of this and all food processing techniques are prudent precautions. (For more information, see the AAP technical report on food irradiation.[65]

Table 54.4.
Irradiated Foods Approved by the FDA

Food	Purpose of Irradiation	Maximum Dose, kGy	Year of Rule
Wheat and wheat products	Insect disinfestations	0.5	1963
Potatoes	Sprout inhibition	0.15	1964
Spices and dried vegetable seasoning	Microbial control	10	1983
Dry and dehydrated enzyme preparations	Microbial control	10	1985
Pork	Trichinosis control	1	1985
Fresh fruits and vegetables	Insect control and delay of physiological growth	1	1986
Spices and dried vegetable seasoning	Microbial control	30	1990
Poultry meat	Inactivation of pathogens, eg, *Salmonella* species	3	1990
Raw/frozen red meat (including beef and pork products)	Inactivation of pathogens, eg, *Escherichia coli O157:H7*	4.5/7	1997; 2000
Pet food and animal feed	Sterilization	50	2000
Fresh shell eggs	Inactivation of *Salmonella* species	3	2000
Seeds for sprouting	Pathogen control	8	2000
Molluscan shellfish (fresh/frozen)	Inactivation of pathogens, eg, *Vibrio* species	5/5.5	2005
Fresh iceberg lettuce and fresh spinach	Foodborne pathogens and shelf-life extension	4	2008

Adapted with permission from Stefanova R et al.[66]

Nonnutritive Additives

Food-Contact Substances

Food-contact substances are defined by the FDA as substances used in food-contact materials, including adhesives, dyes, coatings, paper, paperboard, and polymers (plastics), that may come into contact with food as part of packaging or processing equipment but are not intended to be added directly to food.[81] They confer no nutritional value to food. The FDA maintains a list of more than 3000 approved food contact substances.[82] Approvals under this process are proprietary; thus, they are specific to the manufacturer identified and under the conditions stated in the application.

Although direct food additives undergo toxicologic testing prior to approval based on structure/activity relationships as well as anticipated human exposure levels,[83] testing of indirect food additives is based primarily on anticipated exposure levels. For cumulative exposures <0.5 parts per billion (ppb), no safety tests are recommended. At cumulative exposures between 0.5 ppb and <50 ppb (1.5 µg/person/day to <150 µg/person/day), testing to evaluate carcinogenicity using gene toxicity tests (by checking for gene mutations in bacteria or evaluating in mammalian or rodent cell lines) is required. Cumulative exposures between 50 ppb and 1 ppm (150 µg/person/day to 3 mg/person/day) require testing for gene toxicity, as described previously, and also include evaluations of subchronic oral toxicity in a rodent species and nonrodent species,[84] which includes exposure for 90 consecutive days at a minimum of 3 dose levels for each sex group.[83] For cumulative exposures at or greater than 1.0 ppm, the FDA normally requires that an application for use of the substance as a food additive (with appropriate testing) be completed. Petitioners for new indirect additive approvals may apply for an exemption from regulation if they can satisfy the agency that exposures will not exceed the regulatory threshold of 0.5 ppb or involve the use of a regulated food additive for which the dietary exposures are at or below 1% of the acceptable dietary intake.[85] Since 1996, more than 100 substances have received exemptions.[86] This regulatory approach is based on the concept that "the dose makes the poison," and adverse human health effects are unlikely for most substances when exposure levels are very small. The exposure level is calculated from laboratory generated migration data of the chemical into food simulants and estimates of the total daily intake of the substance in food for an adult.[85] Additional calculations to estimate daily intake of indirect food additives of infants, children, or adolescents are not routinely performed as part of the approval process.

Many common packaging materials were approved for use prior to the 1958 Food Additives Amendment to the Food, Drug, and Cosmetics Act (Pub L No. 85-929) and were, thus, "grandfathered in" for continued use as "prior approved" substances. Some of these substances are plasticizers like the phthalate esters (used in polyvinyl chloride [PVC] plastics, inks, dyes, and adhesives in food packaging), nonyl phenol (used in PVC, juice boxes, and lid gaskets), and bisphenol A (BPA) (these were found in some baby bottles, water bottles, and can liner enamels). Data have been accumulating to elucidate the endocrine disrupting capacity of plasticizers and the exposure levels at which toxicity might occur, including identifying

VII

varying responses to high and low levels that deviate from the traditional dose-response curves.[87] In particular, in laboratory experiments, fetal, newborn, and young animals are very sensitive to even very low doses (sometimes picomolar to nanomolar) of chemicals having estrogenic effects.[88] A variety of studies have found associations of BPA and phthalates with various endocrinologic and other effects in adults and children.[3]

An observational study in preschool children verified that BPA could be found in more than 50% of solid food and liquid food samples and suggested that 99% of exposures of preschool children originated in the diet.[89] The National Health and Nutrition Examination Survey examined children as young as 6 years of age and found that urinary BPA was detectable in 93% of individuals sampled, with concentrations highest in children.[90]

BPA and phthalate exposures can be modified by attention to use of plastics with foods and drinks. Routine use of polycarbonate containers for cold beverages for 1 week was found to increase urinary BPA concentration by 69%,[91] whereas a 3-day intervention during which individuals ate "fresh food" (those with limited packaging) and avoided use of plastic cookware reduced BPA and phthalate urinary excretion by more than 50%.[92] A study of 455 commercially available plastic products found that most (even those labeled as BPA free) had some estrogenic activity; however, release of such chemicals was higher when the products were placed under stress conditions (eg, microwaving, ultraviolet radiation, hot water).[93] It is difficult to discern types of plastics, because labeling is not required by federal law. Food-handling recommendations that could potentially reduce exposures to plastics are listed below ("Reducing Exposures").

Housewares

In the past, the FDA typically has not required review of food-contact articles used exclusively in the home or in restaurants. Many such articles have short contact times or are made of materials such as alloys and ceramics, so they are deemed to pose little likelihood of migration to food.[85] However, several chemicals sometimes found on products in the home and that can be transferred to foods have important health concerns.

The FDA began regulating lead in glazes used on dishes made in the United States in the 1980s and further strengthened regulations in the 1990s. Dishes made in the United States before these regulations took effect may contain lead. Some imported ceramics contain lead. Of particular concern have been pottery from Mexico and ceramic ware from China. As the dishes wear or become chipped or cracked, lead can leach from the dishes into foods. Hot foods or acidic foods or drinks stored in such glazed containers may more rapidly leach metals from the glaze. Even some imported dishes labeled as "lead free" have been found to contain unsafe amounts of lead. There are many safe alternatives, so using such dishes should be avoided. Lead contamination of drinking water represents another source for some children. Lead can leach into water from service pipes, solder, and fixtures. The only way to tell whether water has lead is to test it. The concentration of lead in drinking water can sometimes be reduced by flushing the system, but the time needed for this varies by locale, so local authorities should be consulted. Cold water should always be used for cooking and drinking. Most water filters remove lead.[94] See *Pediatric Environmental Health* from the AAP[3] for more information.

Since its creation in the 1970s, the use of the nonstick surfaced cooking pan has been a major contributor to substantial human exposure of polyfluoroalkyl chemicals, particularly perfluorooctanoic acid, which is found in nonstick surfaced cooking pans and microwave popcorn bags, along with many other widely used household products.[95] Small amounts of polyfluoroalkyl chemicals are emitted into the environment when new nonstick cookware is used.[96] Polyfluoroalkyl chemicals bioaccumulate, but concentrations in children are generally higher than those in adults.[97] Exposure of the fetus and child to polyfluoroalkyl chemicals raises concerns about neurotoxicity and potential mutagenicity.[3] Epidemiologic studies have found increased risk of ADHD[98] and higher blood cholesterol concentrations[99] with higher exposure. Studies associating perfluoroalkyl chemicals with fetal outcomes are mixed.[100] The Scientific Advisory Board of the EPA has recommended that perfluorooctanoic acid be considered a likely human carcinogen.[101] New cookware has higher emissions that wane with repeated use. Good ventilation practices reduce exposures.

Reducing Exposures

Chemicals can and will migrate from processing equipment, packaging materials, and storage containers into foods. A reasonable approach is to develop food preparation and storage practices that will minimize exposures. The following suggestions should help to minimize unnecessary exposure to indirect food contaminants.

- Avoid routine use of single-serving packaging. Such packaging maximizes contact between food and the packaging materials.
- When possible, buy fresh food to minimize contact with packaging materials.
- Use heat-safe glass or crockery when cooking or reheating food in the microwave. Heat increases migration of many contaminants into food, particularly foods containing fats. Do not use plastic in the microwave.
- Make sure a generous air space separates the surface of stored food from cling wraps used to seal containers. Avoid using cling wraps when microwaving foods.

VII

- Avoid placing plastics in the dishwasher.
- Look to the recycling code on the bottom of products to find the plastic type. Avoid plastics with recycling code No. 3 (phthalates), No. 6 (styrenes), and No. 7 (BPA) unless plastics labeled No. 7 are labeled as "biobased" or "greenware," meaning that they are made from corn and do not use bisphenol A. Plastic codes No. 1, 2, 4, and 5 are considered safer alternatives. For fact sheets on phthalates and BPA, see http://www.aoec.org/pehsu/facts.html.
- If using nonstick cookware products, new cookware should be used in well-ventilated environments until it "ages" sufficiently to have minimal emission when heated.[3]

Finally, pediatricians are in an ideal position to provide important input and continued encouragement to regulatory agencies to ensure that the special exposures and vulnerabilities of children to toxic exposures remain under consideration as food-related materials and processes are developed, reviewed, and revised.

Chemical Byproducts From Food Processing

Food-processing technologies include many processes, such as drying, salting, fermentation, acidification, freeze-drying, freezing, irradiation, pasteurization, canning, pulsed electric field, ohmic heating, high-hydrostatic pressure treatment, and others. All of these approaches are used to increase safety while maintaining palatability and nutrient value. All of these approaches also have the capacity to create chemical changes in the food that may be detrimental. As analytical technology has improved, so has the ability to identify more chemical byproducts in processed foods.

Acrylamide, a known neurotoxicant and possible human carcinogen and reproductive toxicant, is one such food processing chemical byproduct.[102] Once thought to be only of significance in the occupational setting, in 2002 acrylamide was found in carbohydrate-containing foods treated with high heat through frying, roasting, or baking but not boiling or steaming. It is a product of the incomplete combustion of organic matter. It is mainly found in foods made from plants, such as potatoes (French fries, potato chips), grains (crackers, cereals, corn chips), or coffee.[103] Furans are another group of chemicals identified in 2004 in a wide range of foods, particularly formed during traditional processing like canning, and have been measured in commercially available foods, such as soups, sauces, beans, pasta meals, and baby foods and also foods like crackers, potato chips, and tortilla chips.[104] The risk posed by dietary exposure to these possible human carcinogens is not yet well understood, and no regulatory actions have been implemented.

These chemical byproducts of processing create unknown risks to children. A precautionary approach would be to use a wide variety of healthy foods in children's diets, and to use fresh ingredients as much as is feasible.

References

1. US Government Accountability Office. Lisa Shames, Director. Testimony before the Subcommittee on Oversight and Investigations, Committee on Energy and Commerce, House of Representatives. GAO Food Safety. FDA Could Strengthen Oversight of Imported Food by Improving Enforcement and Seeking Additional Authorities. Washington, DC: Government Accountability Office; May 6, 2010. Publication No. GAO-10-699T. Available at: http://www.gao.gov/new.items/d10699t.pdf. Accessed January 20, 2013

2. Pediatric Environmental Health Specialty Units. Fact Sheets. Advisory About Melamine for Health Professionals. Washington, DC: Pediatric Environmental Health Specialty Units; October 2009. Available at: http://www.aoec.org/pehsu/facts.html. Accessed January 20, 2013

3. American Academy of Pediatrics, Council on Environmental Health. *Pediatric Environmental Health*. Etzel RA, Balk SJ, eds. 3rd ed. Elk Grove Village, IL: American Academy of Pediatrics; 2011

4. US Food and Drug Administration. The New FDA Food Safety Modernization Act (FSMA). Available at: http://www.fda.gov/food/foodsafety/fsma/default.htm. Accessed January 20, 2013

5. US Department of Agriculture. Pesticide Data Program. May 24, 2011. Available at: http://www.ams.usda.gov/AMSv1.0/pdp. Accessed January 20, 2013

6. US Food and Drug Administration. Residue Monitoring Reports. Available at: http://www.fda.gov/Food/FoodSafety/FoodContaminantsAdulteration/Pesticides/ResidueMonitoringReports/ucm228867.htm. Accessed January 20, 2013

7. US Food and Drug Administration. Total Diet Study Analytical Results. Available at: http://www.fda.gov/Food/FoodSafety/FoodContaminantsAdulteration/TotalDietStudy/ucm184293.htm. Accessed January 20, 2013

8. Centers for Disease Control and Prevention, National Center for Environmental Health, Division of Laboratory Sciences. *National Report on Human Exposure to Environmental Chemicals*. Atlanta, GA: Centers for Disease Control and Prevention; 2005. NCEH Pub. No. 05-0570. Available at: http://www.cdc.gov/exposurereport/. Accessed January 20, 2013

9. Roberts JR, Karr CJ; American Academy of Pediatrics, Council on Environmental Health. Technical report: pesticide exposure in children. *Pediatrics*. 2012;130(6):e1765-e1788

10. American Academy of Pediatrics, Council on Environmental Health. Policy statement: pesticide exposure in children. *Pediatrics*. 2012;130(6):e1757-e1763

11. Riederer AM, Bartell SM, Barr DB, Ryan PB. Diet and nondiet predictors of urinary 3-phenoxybenzoic acid in NHANES 1999–2002. *Environ Health Perspect*. 2008;116(8):1015–1022

12. Rosas LG, Eskenazi B. Pesticides and child neurodevelopment. *Curr Opin Pediatr*. 2008;20(2):191-197

VII

13. Eskenazi B, Rosa LG, Marks AR, et al. Pesticide toxicity and the developing brain. *Basic Clin Pharmacol Toxicol*. 2008;102(2):228-236

14. Jurewicz J, Hanke W. Prenatal and childhood exposure to pesticides and neurobehavioral development: review of epidemiological studies. *Int J Occup Med Environ Health*. 2008;21(2):121-132

15. Eubig PA, Aguiar A, Schantz SL. Lead and PCBs as risk factors for attention deficit/hyperactivity disorder. *Environ Health Perspect*. 2010:118(12):1654-1667.

16. Bouchard MF, Bellinger DC, Wright RO, Weisskopf MG. Attention-deficit/hyperactivity disorder and urinary metabolites of organophosphate pesticides. *Pediatrics*. 2010;125(6):e1270-e1277

17. Silverstein J, Foreman J; American Academy of Pediatrics, Committee on Nutrition and Council on Environmental Health. Organic foods: health and environmental advantages and disadvantages. *Pediatrics*. 2012;130(5):e1406-e1415

18. Lu C, Toepel K, Irish R, et al. Organic diets significantly lower children's dietary exposure to organophosphorus pesticides. *Environ Health Perspect*. 2006;114(2):260–263

19. US Department of Agriculture, National Organic Program. Organic Labeling and Marketing Information. Updated April 2008. Available at: http://www.ams.usda.gov/AMSv1.0/getfile?dDocName=STELDEV3004446&acct=nopgeninfo/. Accessed January 20, 2013

20. US Department of Agriculture. Emerging Issues in the US Organic Industry Economic Research Service, June 2009. Available at: http://www.ers.usda.gov/publications/eib55/eib55.pdf. Accessed January 20, 2013

21. Lee DH, Lee IK, Steffes M, Jacobs DR Jr. Extended analyses of the association between serum concentrations of persistent organic pollutants and diabetes. *Diabetes Care*. 2007;30(6):1596-1598

22. Lorber M. Exposure of Americans to polybrominated diphenyl ethers. *J Expo Sci Environ Epidemiol*. 2008;18(1):2–19

23. Cao Y, Blount BC, Valentin-Blasini L, Bernbaum JC, Phillips TM, Rogan WJ. Goitrogenic anions, thyroid-stimulating hormone, and thyroid hormone in infants. *Environ Health Perspect*. 2010;118(9):1332-1337

24. Blount BC, Valentin-Blasini L, Osterloh JD, Mauldin JP, Pirkle JL. Perchlorate exposure of the US population, 2001-2002. *J Expo Sci Environ Epidemiol*. 2007;17(4):400-407

25. Frederiksen M, Vorkamp K, Thomsen M, Knudsen LE. Human internal and external exposure to PBDEs—a review of levels and sources. *Int J Hyg Environ Health*. 2009;212(2):109–134

26. Lee DH, Lee IK, Song KE, Steffes M, Toscano W, Baker BA, Jacobs DR Jr: A strong dose-response relation between serum concentrations of persistent organic pollutants and diabetes: results from the National Health and Examination Survey. *Diabetes Care*. 2006;29(7):1638-1644

27. Lim JS, Lee DH, Jacobs DR Jr. Association of brominated flame retardants with diabetes and metabolic syndrome in the U.S. population, 2003-2004. *Diabetes Care*. 2008;31(9):1802-1807

28. Lee DH, Lee IK, Porta M, Steffes M, Jacobs DR Jr. Relationship between serum concentrations of persistent organic pollutants and the prevalence of metabolic syndrome among non-diabetic adults: results from the National Health and Nutrition Examination Survey 1999–2002. *Diabetologia*. 2007;50(9):1841–1851

29. Harley K, Marks A, Chevrier J, Bradman A, Sjödin A, Eskenazi B. PBDE concentrations in women's serum and fecundability. *Environ Health Perspect*. 2010;118(5):699–704

30. Dingemans MM, van den Berg M, Westerink RH. Neurotoxicity of brominated flame retardants: (in)direct effects of parent and hydroxylated polybrominated diphenyl ethers on the (developing) nervous system. *Environ Health Perspect*. 2011;119(7): 900–907

31. Schreiber T, Gassmann K, Götz C, et al. Polybrominated diphenyl ethers induce developmental neurotoxicity in a human in vitro model: evidence for endocrine disruption. *Environ Health Perspect*. 2010;118(4):572-578

32. Herbstman JB, Sjödin A, Kurzon M, et al. Prenatal exposure to PBDEs and neurodevelopment. *Environ Health Perspect*. 2010;118(5):712-719

33. National Library of Medicine. Toxicology Data Network. 2,3,7,8-Tetrachlorodibenzo-p-dioxin. Available at: http://toxnet.nlm.nih.gov/cgi-bin/sis/search/a?dbs I hsdb:@ term+@DOCNO+4151. Accessed January 20, 2013

34. Domingo JL, Bocio A. Levels of PCDD/PCDFs and PCBs in edible marine species and human intake: a literature review. *Environ Int*. 2007;33(3):397-405

35. US Department of Agriculture. DIOXIN 08 Survey: Dioxins and Dioxin-Like Compounds in the U.S. Domestic Meat and Poultry Supply. October 2009. Available at: http://www.fsis.usda.gov/PDF/Dioxin_Report_1009.pdf. Accessed January 20, 2013

36. Institute of Medicine. *Dioxins and Dioxin-Like Compounds in the Food Supply: Strategies to Decrease Exposure*. Washington, DC: National Academies Press; 2003. Available at: http://books.nap.edu/catalog/10763.html. Accessed January 20, 2013

37. US Food and Drug Administration. Questions and Answers about Dioxins. May 2010. Available at: http://www.fda.gov/Food/FoodSafety/FoodContaminantsAdulteration/ChemicalContaminants/DioxinsPCBs/ucm077524.htm#g12. Accessed January 20, 2013

38. Clarkson TW, Magos L, Myers GJ. Human exposure to mercury: the three modern dilemmas. *J Trace Elem Exp Med*. 2003;16(18):321-343

39. Stern AH, Smith AE. An assessment of the cord blood-maternal blood methylmercury ratio: implications for risk assessment. *Environ Health Perspect*. 2003;113(1):155-163

40. Mahaffey KR, Clickner RP, Jeffries RA. Adult women's blood mercury concentrations vary regionally in USA: association with patterns of fish consumption (NHANES 1999-2004). *Environ Health Perspect*. 2009;117(1):47-53

41. US Food and Drug Administration. Mercury Levels in Commercial Fish and Shellfish (1990-2010). Available at: http://www.fda.gov/food/foodsafety/product-specificinformation/seafood/foodbornepathogenscontaminants/methylmercury/ucm115644.htm. Accessed January 20, 2013

42. Oken E, Radesky JS, Wright RO, et al. Maternal fish intake during pregnancy, blood mercury levels, and child cognition at age 3 years in a US cohort. *Am J Epidemiol*. 2008;167(10):1171-1181

VII

43. US Environmental Protection Agency. What You Need to Know About Mercury in Fish and Shellfish. 2004 EPA and FDA Advice For: Women Who Might Become Pregnant, Women Who are Pregnant, Nursing Mothers, Young Children. Publication No. PA-823-R-04-005. Washington, DC: US Environmental Protection Agency; March 2004

44. US Food and Drug Administration. Lead in Candy Likely To Be Consumed by Small Children. Guidance for Industry. Lead in Candy Likely To Be Consumed Frequently by Small Children: Recommended Maximum Level and Enforcement Policy. November 2006. Available at: http://www.fda.gov/food/guidancecomplianceregulatoryinformation/guidancedocuments/Chemicalcontaminantsandpesticides/ucm077904.htm. Accessed January 20, 2013

45. Food and Agricultural Organization of the United Nations and World Health Organization. Joint FAO/WHO Expert Committee on Food Additives: Summary and Conclusions, 73rd meeting, June 2010. Available at: http://www.fao.org/ag/agn/agns/jecfa/JECFA73%20Summary%20Report%20Final.pdf. Accessed January 20, 2013

46. Finster ME, Gray KA, Binns HJ; for the Safer Yards Project. Lead levels of edibles grown in contaminated residential soils: a field survey. *Sci Total Env.* 2004;320(2-3):245-257

47. US Environmental Protection Agency. 2003a. Health Effects Support Document for Manganese. Washington, DC: US Environmental Protection Agency, Office of Water; 2003. Publication No. EPA-822-R-03-003. Available at: http://www.epa.gov/safewater/ccl/pdfs/reg_determine1/support_cc1_magnese_healtheffects.pdf. Accessed January 20, 2013

48. Wasserman GA, Liu X, Parvez F, et al. Water manganese exposure and children's intellectual function in Araihazar, Bangladesh. *Environ Health Perspect.* 2006;114(1): 124–129

49. Aschner JL, Aschner M. Nutritional aspects of manganese homeostatis. *Mol Aspects Med.* 2005;26(4-5):353-362

50. Davidsson L, Almgren A, Juillerat MA, Hurrell RF. Manganese absorption in humans: the effect of phytic acid and ascorbic acid in soy formula. *Am J Clin Nutr.* 1995;62(5):984-987

51. US Environmental Protection Agency. Regulatory Determinations for Priority Contaminants on the First Drinking Water Contaminant Candidate List. Available at: http://www.epa.gov/ogwdw/ccl/pdfs/reg_determine1/support_cc1_magnese_dwreport.pdf. Accessed January 20, 2013

52. US Food and Drug Administration. Foodborne Pathogenic Microorganisms and Natural Toxins Handbook (Bad Bug Book). 03/03/2011. Available at: http://www.cfsan.fda.gov/~mow/intro.htm. Accessed January 20, 2013

53. Henry SH, Bosch FX, Bowers JC. Aflatoxin, hepatitis and worldwide liver cancer risks. *Adv Exp Med Biol.* 2002;504:229-233

54. US Food and Drug Administration. Patulin in Apple Juice, Apple Juice Concentrates and Apple Juice Products. September 2001. Available at: http://www.fda.gov/Food/FoodSafety/FoodContaminantsAdulteration/NaturalToxins/ucm212520.htm. Accessed January 20, 2013

55. Baert K, De Meulenaer B, Verdonck F, et al. Variability and uncertainty assessment of patulin exposure for preschool children in Flanders. *Food Chem Toxicol.* 2007;45(9); 1745-1751

56. US Food and Drug Administration. Background Paper in Support of Fumonisin Levels in Corn and Corn Products Intended for Human Consumption. November 9, 2001. Available at: http://www.fda.gov/Food/FoodSafety/FoodContaminantsAdulteration/NaturalToxins/ucm212899.htm. Accessed January 20, 2013

57. US Food and Drug Administration. Guidance for Industry: Fumonisin Levels in Human Foods and Animal Feeds; Final Guidance. Contains Nonbinding Recommendations. November 9, 2001. Available at: http://www.fda.gov/Food/GuidanceComplianceRegulatoryInformation/GuidanceDocuments/ChemicalContaminantsandPesticides/ucm109231.htm. Accessed January 20, 2013

58. Gelderblom WC, Abel S, Smuts CM, et al. Fumonisin-induced hepatocarcinogenesis: Mechanisms related to cancer initiation and promotion. *Environ Health Perspect.* 2001;109(S2):291–300

59. Marasas WF, Riley RT, Hendricks KA, et al. Fumonisins disrupt sphingolipid metabolism, folate transport, and neural tube development in embryo culture and in vivo: a potential risk factor for human neural tube defects among populations consuming fumonisin contaminated maize. *J Nutr.* 2004;134(4):711–716

60. Sun G, Wang S, Hu X, et al. Fumonisin B1 contamination of home-grown corn in high-risk areas for esophageal and liver cancer in China. *Food Addit Contam.* 2007;24(2): 181–185

61. Council for Agricultural Science and Technology. Naturally Occurring Antimicrobials in Food. Task Force Report 132. Ames, IA: Council for Agricultural Science and Technology; 1998

62. US Food and Drug Administration. Everything Added to Food in the United States (EAFUS). Available at: http://www.fda.gov/food/foodingredientspackaging/ucm115326.htm. Accessed January 20, 2013

63. Tiwari BK, Valdramidis VP, O'Donnell CP, Muthukumarappan K, Bourke P, Cullen PJ. Application of natural antimicrobials for food preservation. *J Agric Food Chem.* 2009;57(140):5987–6000

64. Greer FR, Shannon M; American Academy of Pediatrics Committee on Nutrition and Committee on Environmental Health. Infant methemoglobinemia: the role of dietary nitrate in food and water. *Pediatrics.* 2005;116(3):784-786

65. Shea KM; American Academy of Pediatrics, Committee on Environmental Health. Irradiation of food: a technical report. *Pediatrics.* 2000;106(6):1505-1510

66. Stefanova R, Vasilev NV, Spassov SL. Irradiation of food, Current legislation framework, and detection of irradiated foods. *Food Anal Methods.* 2010;3(3):225-252

67. World Health Organization. *Safety and Nutritional Adequacy of Irradiated Food.* Geneva, Switzerland: World Health Organization; 1994

68. Urbain WM. *Food Irradiation.* Orlando, FL: Academic Press Inc; 1986:16

69. Variyar PS, Chatterjee S, Sajilata MG, Singhal RS, Sharma A. Natural existence of 2-alkylcyclobutanones. *J Agric Food Chem.* 2008;56(24):11817-11823

70. Raul F, Gosse F, Delincee H, et al. Food-borne radiolytic compounds (2-alkylcyclobutanones) may promote experimental colon carcinogenesis in laboratory animal. *Nutr Cancer.* 2002;44(2):189-191

VII

71. Rao CV. Do irradiated foods cause or promote colon cancer? *Nutr Cancer*. 2003;46(2):107-109

72. US Department of Health and Human Services, Food and Drug Administration. Irradiation in the production, processing, and handling of food. *Federal Regist*. 1986;51:13376-13399

73. World Health Organization. *Safety and Nutritional Adequacy of Irradiated Food*. Geneva, Switzerland: World Health Organization; 1994

74. World Health Organization. High-Dose Irradiation: Wholesomeness of Food Irradiated With Doses Above 10 kGy. Report of a Joint FAO/IAEA/WHO Study Group. Geneva, Switzerland: World Health Organization; 1999. WHO Technical Report Series No. 890

75. Diehl J. *Safety of Irradiated Food*. 2nd ed. New York, NY: Marcel Dekker; 1995

76. World Health Organization. WHO 5 Keys to Safer Food. Available at: http://www.who.int/foodsafety/consumer/5keys/en/index.html. Accessed January 20, 2013

77. World Health Organization. *Safety and Nutritional Adequacy of Irradiated Food*. Geneva, Switzerland: World Health Organization; 1994

78. Murano EA, ed. *Food Irradiation: A Source Book*. Ames, IA: Iowa State University Press; 1995

79. Osterholm MT, Norgan AP. The role of food irradiation in food safety. *N Engl J Med*. 2004;350(18):1898-1901

80. Thayer DW. Irradiation of food—helping to ensure food safety. *N Engl J Med*. 2004;350(18):1811-1812

81. US FDA. List of Indirect Food Additives used in Food Contact Substances. Updated September 2010. Available at: http://www.fda.gov/Food/FoodIngredientsPackaging/ucm115333.htm. Accessed January 20, 2013

82. US Food and Drug Administration. Inventory of Effective Food Contact Substance (FCS) Notifications. Available at: http://www.fda.gov/Food/FoodIngredientsPackaging/FoodContactSubstancesFCS/ucm116567.htm. Accessed January 20, 2013

83. US Food and Drug Administration. *Guidance for Industry and Other Stakeholders. Toxicological Principles for the Safety Assessment of Food Ingredients. Redbook 2000*. Revised July 2007. Available at: http://www.fda.gov/Food/GuidanceComplianceRegulatoryInformation/GuidanceDocuments/FoodIngredientsandPackaging/Redbook/default.htm. Accessed January 20, 2013

84. US Food and Drug Administration. *Guidance for Industry: Preparation of Food Contact Notifications for Food Contact Substances: Toxicology Recommendations*. Revised April 2002. Available at: http://www.fda.gov/Food/GuidanceComplianceRegulatoryInformation/GuidanceDocuments/FoodIngredientsandPackaging/ucm081825.htm#iva2. Accessed January 20, 2013

85. US Food and Drug Administration. Guidance for Industry: Submitting Requests under 21 CFR 170.39 Threshold of Regulation for Substances Used in Food-Contact Articles. Available at: http://www.fda.gov/Food/GuidanceComplianceRegulatoryInformation/GuidanceDocuments/FoodIngredientsandPackaging/ucm081833.htm. Accessed January 20, 2013

86. US Food and Drug Administration. Threshold of Regulation Exemptions. Available at: http://www.fda.gov/Food/FoodIngredientsPackaging/FoodContactSubstancesFCS/ucm093685.htm. Accessed January 20, 2013

87. Vandenberg LN, Maffini MV, Sonnenschein C, Rubin BS, Soto AM. Bisphenol-A and the great divide: A review of controversies in the field of endocrine disruption. *Endocr Rev*. 2009;30(1):75–95

88. vom Saal FS, Nagel SC, Timms BG, Welshons WV. Implications for human health of the extensive bisphenol A literature showing adverse effects at low doses. *Toxicology* 2005;212(2-3):244–252

89. Wilson NK, Chuang JC, Morgan MK, Lordo RA, Sheldon LS. An observational study of the potential exposures of preschool children to pentachlorophenol, bisphenol-A, and nonylphenol at home and daycare. *Environ Res*. 2007;103(1):9-20

90. Calafat AM, Ye X, Wong LY, Reidy JA, Needham LL. Exposure of the U.S. population to bisphenol A and 4-tertiary-octylphenol: 2003-2004. *Environ Health Perspect*. 2008;116(1):39-44

91. Carwile JL, Luu HT, Bassett LS, et al. Polycarbonate bottle use and urinary bisphenol A concentrations. *Environ Health Perspect*. 2009;117(9):1368-1372

92. Rudel RA, Gray JM, Engel CL, et al. Food packaging and bisphenol a and bis(2-ethyhexyl) phthalate exposure: findings from a dietary intervention. *Environ Health Perspect*. 2011;119(7):914-920

93. Yang CZ, Yaniger SI, Jordan VC, Klein DJ, Bittner GD. Most plastic products release estrogenic chemicals: a potential health problem that can be solved. *Environ Health Perspect*. 2011;119(7):989-996

94. Rogan WJ, Brady MT; American Academy of Pediatrics, Committee on Environmental Health and Committee on Infectious Diseases. Technical report: drinking water from private wells and risks to children. *Pediatrics*. 2009;123(6):e1123-e1137

95. Calafat A, Wong L, Kuklenyik Z, Reidy J, Needham L. Polyfluoroalkyl chemicals in the U.S. population: data from the National Health and Nutrition Examination Survey (NHANES) 2003-2004 and comparisons with NHANES 1999-2000. *Environ Health Perspect*. 2007;115(11):1596-602

96. Sinclair E, Kim S, Akinleye H, Kannan K. Quantitation of gas-phase perfluoroalkyl surfactants and fluorotelomer alcohols released from nonstick cookware and microwave popcorn bags. *Environ Sci Technol*. 2007;41(4):1180-1185

97. Toms LL, Calafat AM, Kato K, et al. Polyfluoroalkyl chemicals in pooled blood serum from infants, children, and adults in Australia. *Environ Sci Technol*. 2009;43(11):4194–4199

98. Hoffman K, Webster TF, Weisskopf MG, Weinberg J, Vieira VM. Exposure to polyfluoroalkyl chemicals and attention deficit/hyperactivity disorder in U.S. children 12-15 years of age. *Environ Health Perspect*. 2010;118(12):1762-1767

99. Nelson J, Hatch E, Webster T. Exposure to polyfluoroalkyl chemicals and cholesterol, body weight, and insulin resistance in the general U.S. population. *Environ Health Perspect*. 2010;118(8):197–202

100. Olsen GW, Butenhoff JL, Zobel LR. Perfluoroalkyl chemicals and human fetal development: an epidemiologic review with clinical and toxicological perspectives. *Reprod Toxicol*. 2009;27(3-4):212-230

VII

101. US Environmental Protection Agency. Perfluorooctanoic Acid (PFOA) and Fluorinated Telomers: Risk Assessment. Available at: http://www.epa.gov/opptintr/pfoa/pubs/pfoarisk.html. Accessed January 20, 2013

102. US Food and Drug Administration. Acrylamide Questions and Answers. Acrylamide. Available at: http://www.fda.gov/Food/FoodSafety/FoodContaminantsAdulteration/ChemicalContaminants/Acrylamide/ucm053569.htm, Accessed 07/02/2011.

103. US Food and Drug Administration. Acrylamide in Food. Available at: http://www.fda.gov/Food/FoodSafety/FoodContaminantsAdulteration/ChemicalContaminants/Acrylamide/default.htm. Accessed January 20, 2013

104. US Food and Drug Administration. Furan. Available at: http://www.fda.gov/Food/FoodSafety/FoodContaminantsAdulteration/ChemicalContaminants/Furan/default.htm. Accessed January 20, 2013

Appendix A

Appendix A - 1
Set I

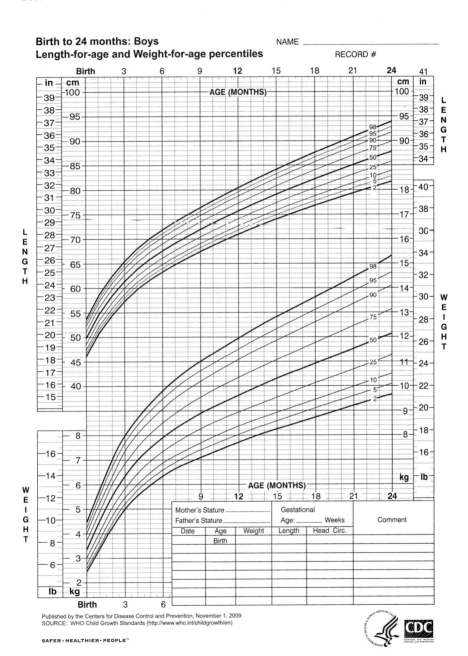

Birth to 24 months: Boys
Length-for-age and Weight-for-age percentiles

NAME _____

RECORD # _____

Published by the Centers for Disease Control and Prevention, November 1, 2009
SOURCE: WHO Child Growth Standards (http://www.who.int/childgrowth/en)

SAFER · HEALTHIER · PEOPLE™

Birth to 24 months: Boys
Head circumference-for-age and
Weight-for-length percentiles

NAME _____

RECORD # _____

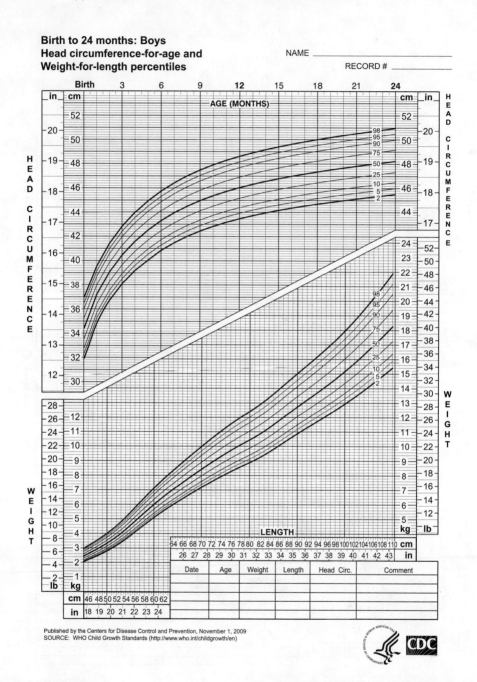

Published by the Centers for Disease Control and Prevention, November 1, 2009
SOURCE: WHO Child Growth Standards (http://www.who.int/childgrowth/en)

Birth to 24 months: Girls
Length-for-age and Weight-for-age percentiles

NAME _____

RECORD # _____

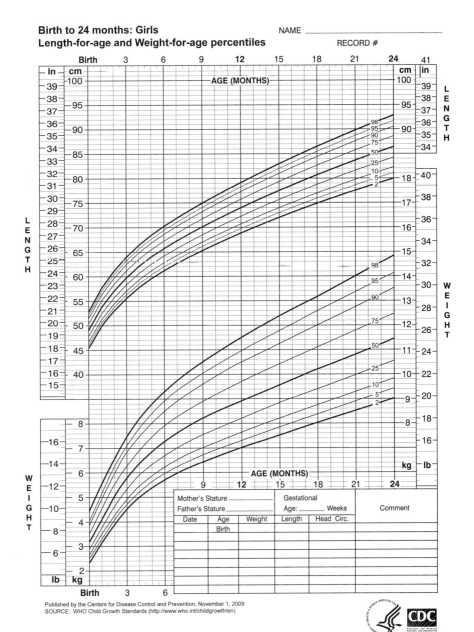

Mother's Stature _____
Father's Stature _____

Gestational
Age: _____ Weeks

Comment

Date	Age	Weight	Length	Head Circ.	
Birth					

Published by the Centers for Disease Control and Prevention, November 1, 2009
SOURCE: WHO Child Growth Standards (http://www.who.int/childgrowth/en)

CDC

APP

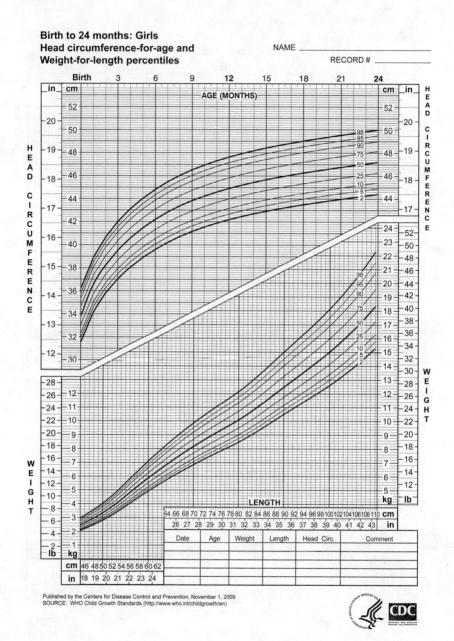

Birth to 24 months: Girls
Head circumference-for-age and
Weight-for-length percentiles

NAME _____

RECORD # _____

Published by the Centers for Disease Control and Prevention, November 1, 2009
SOURCE: WHO Child Growth Standards (http://www.who.int/childgrowth/en)

2 to 20 years: Boys
Stature-for-age and Weight-for-age percentiles 5th to 95th

NAME _____

RECORD # _____

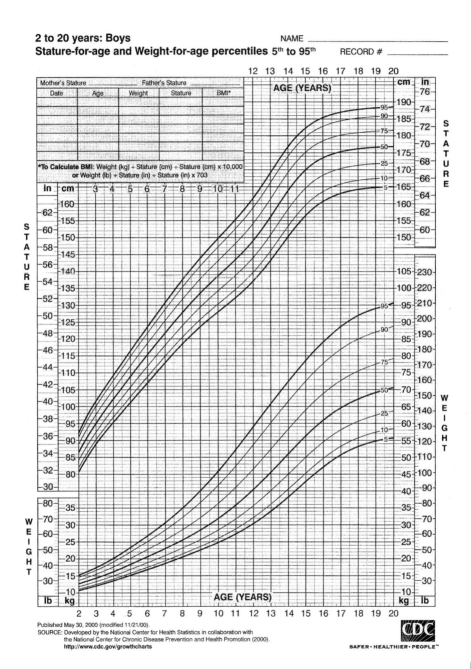

Published May 30, 2000 (modified 11/21/00).
SOURCE: Developed by the National Center for Health Statistics in collaboration with
the National Center for Chronic Disease Prevention and Health Promotion (2000).
http://www.cdc.gov/growthcharts

SAFER · HEALTHIER · PEOPLE™

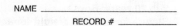

2 to 20 years: Boys
Body mass index-for-age percentiles 5th to 95th

NAME _____

RECORD # _____

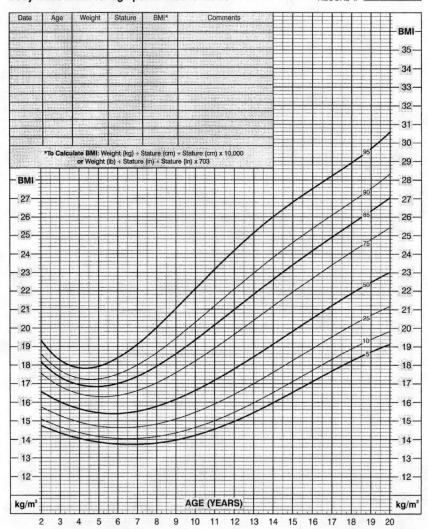

*To Calculate BMI: Weight (kg) ÷ Stature (cm) ÷ Stature (cm) x 10,000
or Weight (lb) ÷ Stature (in) ÷ Stature (in) x 703

SOURCE: Developed by the National Center for Health Statistics in collaboration with
the National Center for Chronic Disease Prevention and Health Promotion (2000).
http://www.cdc.gov/growthcharts

2 to 20 years: Girls
Stature-for-age and Weight-for-age percentiles 5th to 95th

NAME _____

RECORD # _____

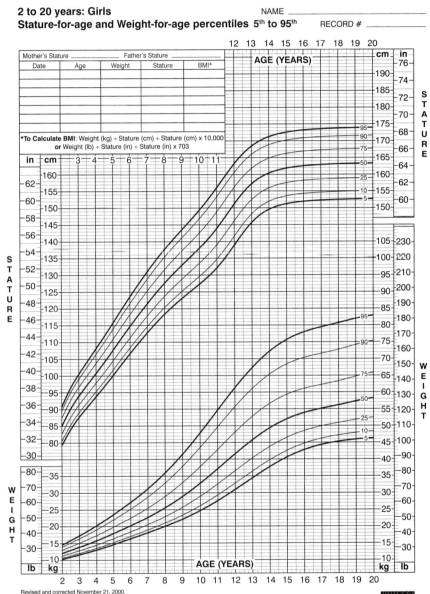

Revised and corrected November 21, 2000.
SOURCE: Developed by the National Center for Health Statistics in collaboration with
the National Center for Chronic Disease Prevention and Health Promotion (2000).
http://www.cdc.gov/growthcharts

2 to 20 years: Girls
Body mass index-for-age percentiles 5th to 95th

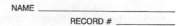

NAME _____

RECORD # _____

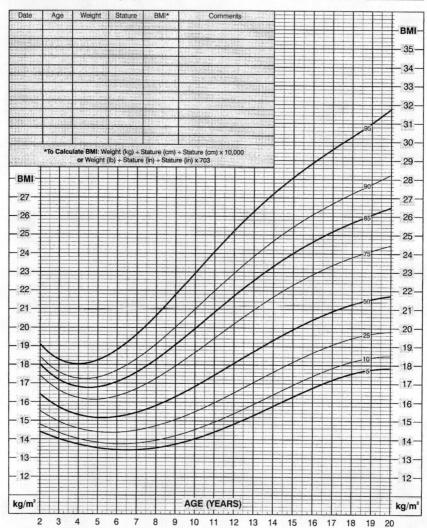

*To Calculate BMI: Weight (kg) ÷ Stature (cm) ÷ Stature (cm) x 10,000
or Weight (lb) ÷ Stature (in) ÷ Stature (in) x 703

SOURCE: Developed by the National Center for Health Statistics in collaboration with
the National Center for Chronic Disease Prevention and Health Promotion (2000).
http://www.cdc.gov/growthcharts

Weight-for-stature percentiles: Boys

NAME _____

RECORD # _____

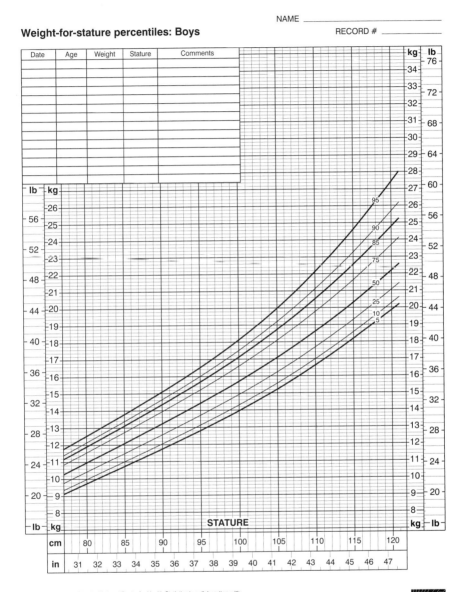

STATURE

SOURCE: Developed by the National Center for Health Statistics in collaboration with
the National Center for Chronic Disease Prevention and Health Promotion (2000).
http://www.cdc.gov/growthcharts

APP

Weight-for-stature percentiles: Girls

NAME _____

RECORD # _____

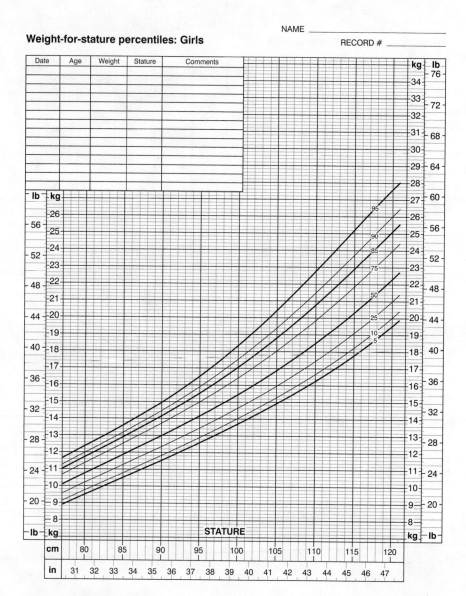

Date	Age	Weight	Stature	Comments

SOURCE: Developed by the National Center for Health Statistics in collaboration with
the National Center for Chronic Disease Prevention and Health Promotion (2000).
http://www.cdc.gov/growthcharts

Appendix A - 1
Set II

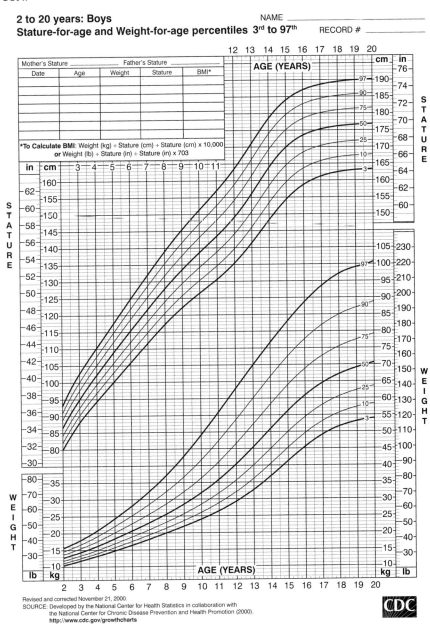

2 to 20 years: Boys
Stature-for-age and Weight-for-age percentiles 3rd to 97th

NAME _____

RECORD # _____

Revised and corrected November 21, 2000.
SOURCE: Developed by the National Center for Health Statistics in collaboration with
the National Center for Chronic Disease Prevention and Health Promotion (2000).
http://www.cdc.gov/growthcharts

2 to 20 years: Boys
Body mass index-for-age percentiles 3rd to 97th

NAME _____

RECORD # _____

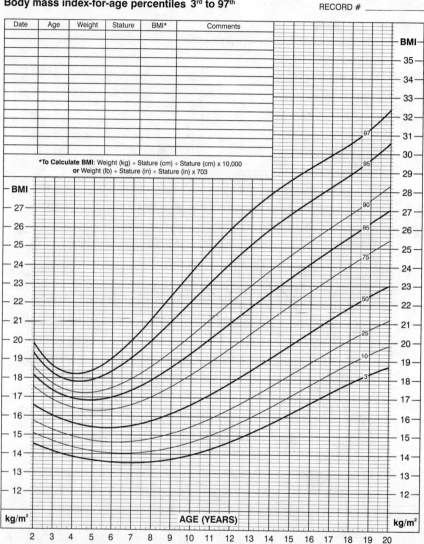

*To Calculate BMI: Weight (kg) ÷ Stature (cm) ÷ Stature (cm) x 10,000
or Weight (lb) ÷ Stature (in) ÷ Stature (in) x 703

SOURCE: Developed by the National Center for Health Statistics in collaboration with
the National Center for Chronic Disease Prevention and Health Promotion (2000).
http://www.cdc.gov/growthcharts

2 to 20 years: Girls
Stature-for-age and Weight-for-age percentiles 3rd to 97th

NAME _____

RECORD # _____

Mother's Stature _____	Father's Stature _____			
Date	Age	Weight	Stature	BMI*

*To Calculate BMI: Weight (kg) ÷ Stature (cm) ÷ Stature (cm) x 10,000
or Weight (lb) ÷ Stature (in) ÷ Stature (in) x 703

AGE (YEARS)

STATURE

WEIGHT

Revised and corrected November 21, 2000.
SOURCE: Developed by the National Center for Health Statistics in collaboration with
the National Center for Chronic Disease Prevention and Health Promotion (2000).
http://www.cdc.gov/growthcharts

2 to 20 years: Girls
Body mass index-for-age percentiles 3rd to 97th

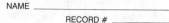

NAME _____

RECORD # _____

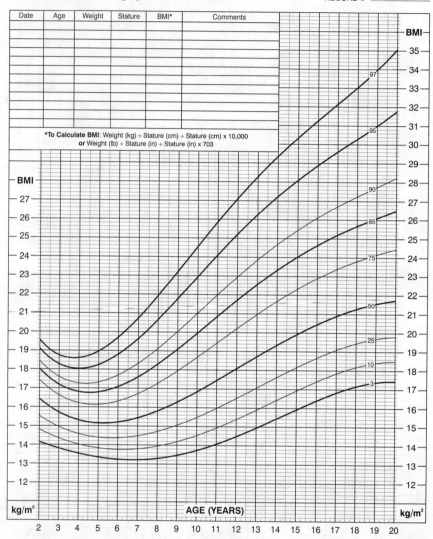

Date	Age	Weight	Stature	BMI*	Comments

*To Calculate BMI: Weight (kg) ÷ Stature (cm) ÷ Stature (cm) x 10,000
or Weight (lb) ÷ Stature (in) ÷ Stature (in) x 703

AGE (YEARS)

SOURCE: Developed by the National Center for Health Statistics in collaboration with
the National Center for Chronic Disease Prevention and Health Promotion (2000).
http://www.cdc.gov/growthcharts

Appendix A - 2

Fig. A-2.1

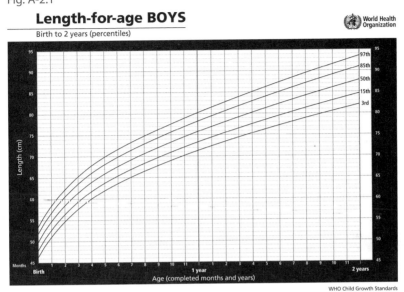

WHO Child Growth Standards

Fig. A-2.2

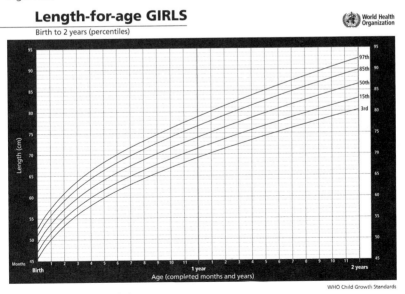

WHO Child Growth Standards

http://www.who.int/childgrowth/en/

Fig. A-2.3

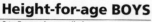

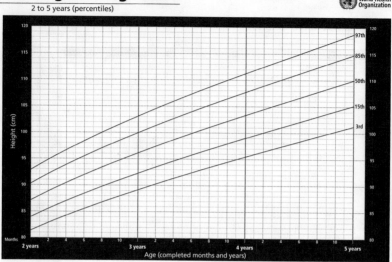

Fig. A-2.4

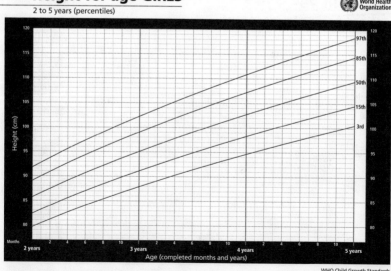

http://www.who.int/childgrowth/en/

Fig. A-2.5

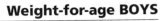

Weight-for-age BOYS

Birth to 5 years (percentiles)

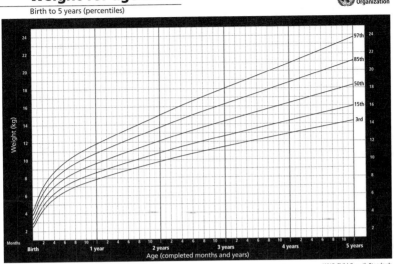

WHO Child Growth Standards

Fig. A-2.6

Weight-for-age GIRLS

Birth to 5 years (percentiles)

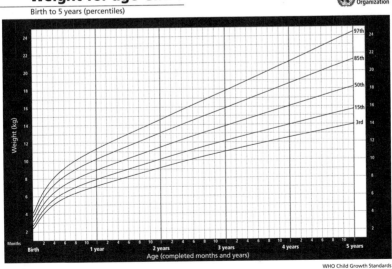

WHO Child Growth Standards

http://www.who.int/childgrowth/en/

Fig. A-2.7

Weight-for-length BOYS
Birth to 2 years (percentiles)

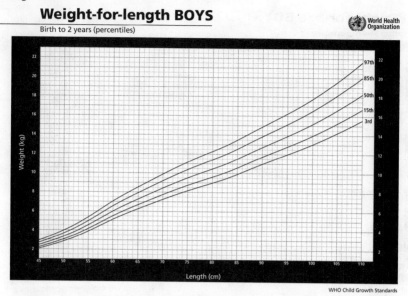

Length (cm)

WHO Child Growth Standards

Fig. A-2.8

Weight-for-length GIRLS
Birth to 2 years (percentiles)

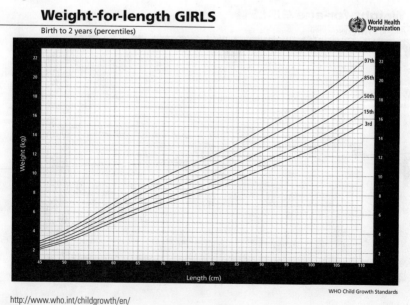

Length (cm)

http://www.who.int/childgrowth/en/

WHO Child Growth Standards

Fig. A-2.9

Weight-for-height BOYS

World Health
Organization

2 to 5 years (percentiles)

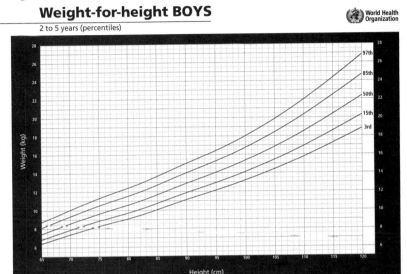

WHO Child Growth Standards

Fig. A-2.10

Weight-for-height GIRLS

World Health
Organization

2 to 5 years (percentiles)

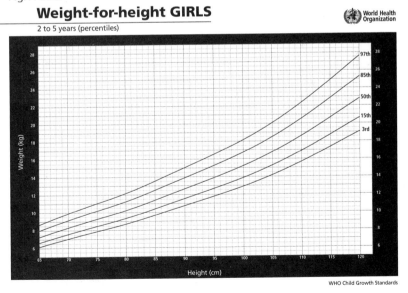

WHO Child Growth Standards

http://www.who.int/childgrowth/en/

APP

Fig. A-2.11

BMI-for-age BOYS

Birth to 5 years (percentiles)

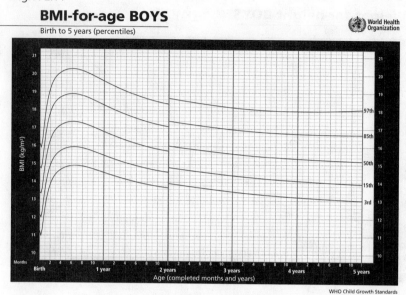

WHO Child Growth Standards

Fig. A-2.12

BMI-for-age GIRLS

Birth to 5 years (percentiles)

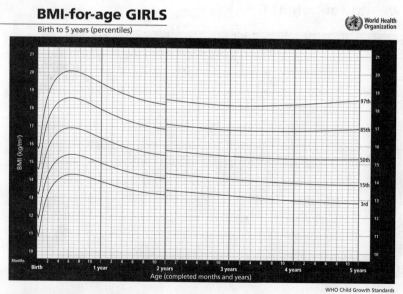

WHO Child Growth Standards

http://www.who.int/childgrowth/en/

Fig. A-2.13

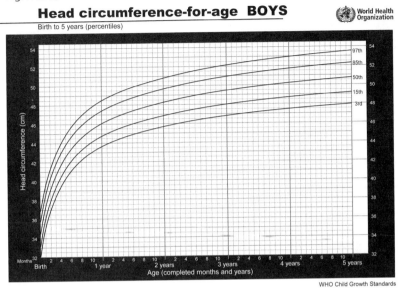

Fig. A-2.14

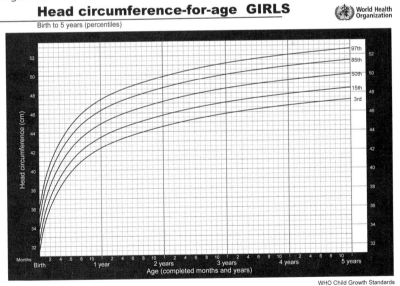

Appendix A - 3

Fig. A-3.1

Intrauterine Growth Curves   Name _____

Record # _____

FEMALES

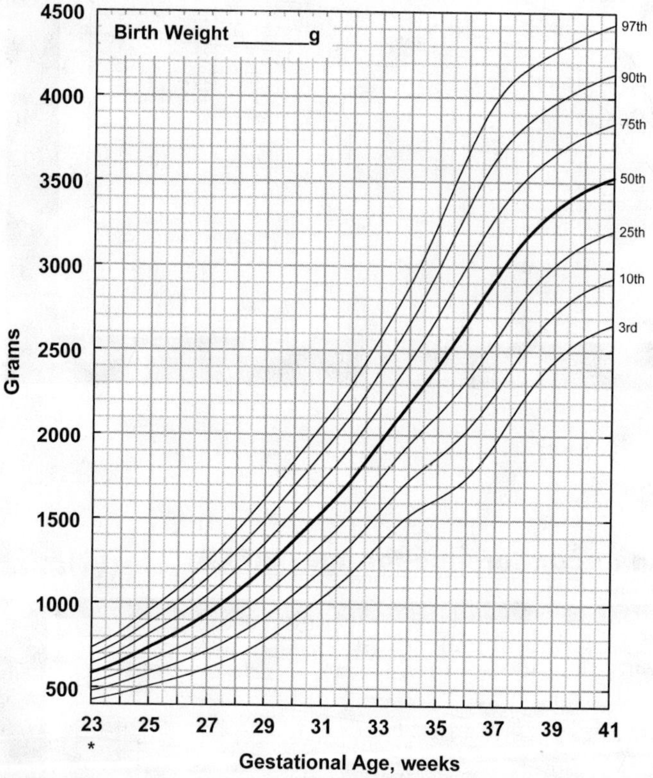

Birth Weight _____ g

Reproduced with permission from: Olsen IE, Groveman S, Lawson ML, Clark R, Zemel B. New intrauterine growth curves based on U.S. data. *Pediatrics*, Volume 125, Pages e214-e244. Copyright 2010 by the American Academy of Pediatrics. Data source: Pediatrix Medical Group

BIRTH SIZE ASSESSMENT

Date of birth: / / (wks GA)	Select one
Large-for-gestational age (LGA) >90th percentile	☐
Appropriate-for-gestational age (AGA) 10-90th percentile	☐
Small-for-gestational age (SGA) <10th percentile	☐

* 3rd and 97th percentiles on all curves for 23 weeks should be interpreted cautiously given the small sample size.

Fig. A-3.2

Page 2

Name _____

Record # _____

FEMALES

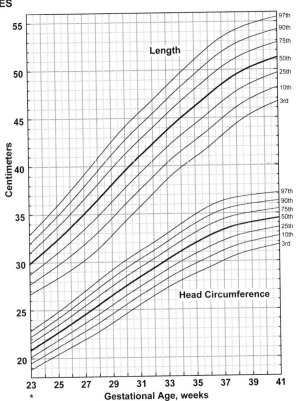

Reproduced with permission from: Olsen IE, Groveman S, Lawson ML, Clark R, Zemel B. New intrauterine growth curves based on U.S. data. *Pediatrics*, Volume 125, Pages e214-e244. Copyright 2010 by the American Academy of Pediatrics. Data source: Pediatrix Medical Group

Date																
GA (wks)																
WT (g)																
L (cm)																
HC (cm)																

* 3rd and 97th percentiles on all curves for 23 weeks should be interpreted cautiously given the small sample size.

APP

Fig. A-3.3

Intrauterine Growth Curves   Name _____

MALES   Record # _____

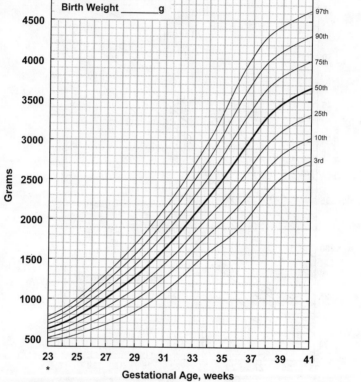

Reproduced with permission from: Olsen IE, Groveman S, Lawson ML, Clark R, Zemel B. New intrauterine growth curves based on U.S. data. *Pediatrics*, Volume 125, Pages e214-e244. Copyright 2010 by the American Academy of Pediatrics. Data source: Pediatrix Medical Group

BIRTH SIZE ASSESSMENT:

Date of birth: / / (wks GA)	Select one
Large-for-gestational age (LGA) >90th percentile	☐
Appropriate-for-gestational age (AGA) 10-90th percentile	☐
Small-for-gestational age (SGA) <10th percentile	☐

* 3rd and 97th percentiles on all curves for 23 weeks should be interpreted cautiously given the small sample size.

Fig. A-3.4

Page 2

Name _____

Record # _____

MALES

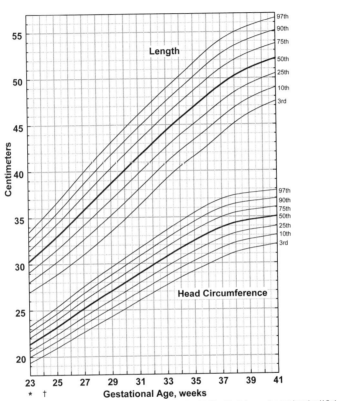

Reproduced with permission from: Olsen IE, Groveman S, Lawson ML, Clark R, Zemel B. New intrauterine growth curves based on U.S. data. *Pediatrics*, Volume 125, Pages e214-e244. Copyright 2010 by the American Academy of Pediatrics. Data source: Pediatrix Medical Group

Date																
GA (wks)																
WT (g)																
L (cm)																
HC (cm)																

* 3rd and 97th percentiles on all curves for 23 weeks should be interpreted cautiously given the small sample size.
† Male head circumference curve at 24 weeks all percentiles should be interpreted cautiously as the distribution of data is skewed left.

Appendix A - 4

Fig. A-4.1

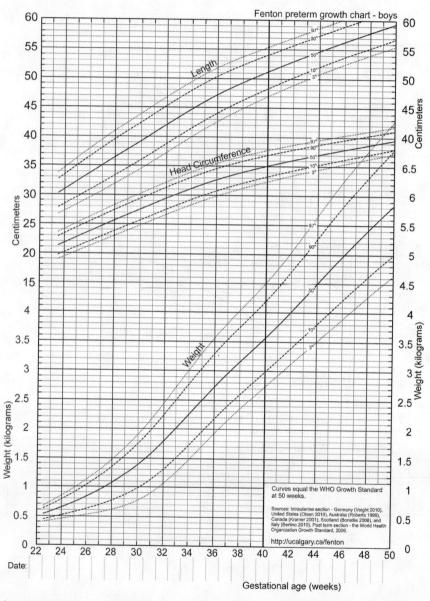

Fenton preterm growth chart - boys

Curves equal the WHO Growth Standard at 50 weeks.

Sources: Intrauterine section - Germany (Voight 2010), United States (Olsen 2010), Australia (Roberts 1999), Canada (Kramer 2001), Scotland (Bonellie 2008), and Italy (Bertino 2010). Post term section - the World Health Organization Growth Standard, 2006.

http://ucalgary.ca/fenton

Reproduced with permission from Fenton TR, Kim JH. A systematic review and meta-analysis to revise the Fenton growth chart for preterm infants. *BMC Pediatr.* 2013;13:59. doi:10.1186/1471-2431-13-59

Fig. A-4.2

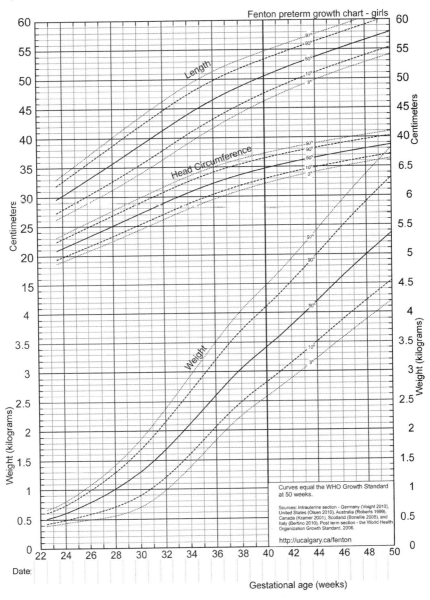

Fenton preterm growth chart - girls

Curves equal the WHO Growth Standard at 50 weeks.

Sources: Intrauterine section - Germany (Voight 2010), United States (Olsen 2010), Australia (Roberts 1999), Canada (Kramer 2001), Scotland (Bonellie 2008), and Italy (Bertino 2010). Post term section - the World Health Organization Growth Standard, 2006.

http://ucalgary.ca/fenton

Reproduced with permission from Fenton TR, Kim JH. A systematic review and meta-analysis to revise the Fenton growth chart for preterm infants. *BMC Pediatr.* 2013;13:59.
doi:10.1186/1471-2431-13-59

Appendix A - 5

Fig. A-5.1
Low Birth Weight Growth Charts

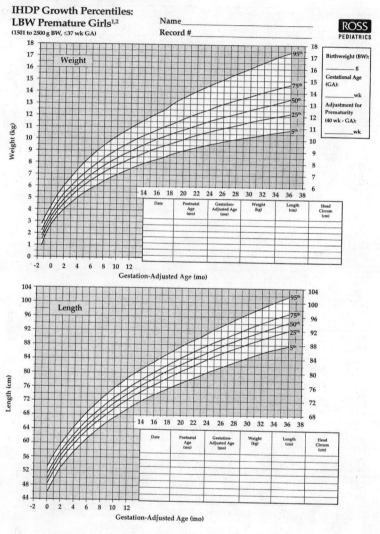

IHDP Growth Percentiles:
LBW Premature Girls[1,2]
(1501 to 2500 g BW, ≤37 wk GA)

Name_____

Record #_____

ROSS
PEDIATRICS

Birthweight (BW):

_____ g

Gestational Age
(GA):

_____ wk

Adjustment for
Prematurity
(40 wk - GA):

_____ wk

Fig. A-5.2

IHDP Growth Percentiles: LBW Premature Girls[1,2]

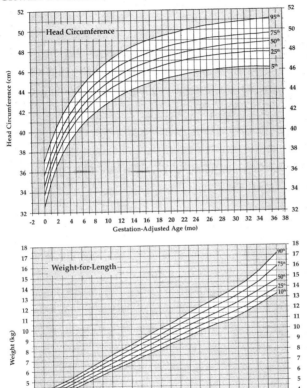

References
1. Guo SS, Roche AF, Chumlea WC, et al: Growth in weight, recumbent length, and head circumference for preterm low-birthweight infants during the first three years of life using gestation-adjusted ages. *Early Hum Dev* 1997;47:305-325.
2. Guo SS, Wholihan K, Roche AF, et al: Weight-for-length reference data for preterm, low-birth-weight infants. *Arch Pediatr Adolesc Med* 1996;150:964-970. Copyright: 1996, American Medical Association.

Acknowledgment
IHDP studies were supported by grants from the Robert Wood Johnson Foundation, Pew Charitable Trusts, and the Bureau of Maternal and Child Health, US Department of Health and Human Services. The IHDP growth percentile graphs were prepared by S.S. Guo and A.F. Roche, Wright State University, Yellow Springs, Ohio. IHDP, its sponsors and the investigators do not endorse specific products.

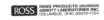

ROSS PRODUCTS DIVISION
ABBOTT LABORATORIES INC.
COLUMBUS, OHIO 43215-1724

Provided as a service of
Similac NeoSure™
Infant Formula With Iron

Fig. A-5.3

IHDP Growth Percentiles:
LBW Premature Boys[1,2]
(1501 to 2500 g BW, ≤37 wk GA)

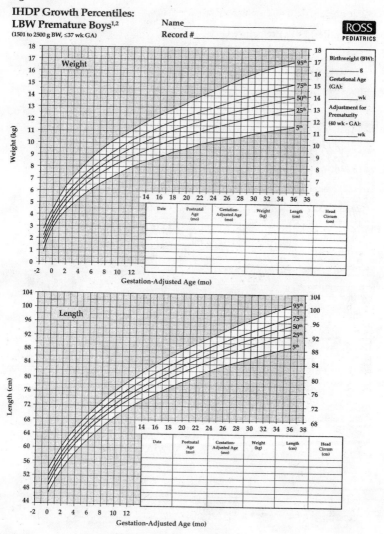

Fig. A-5.4

IHDP Growth Percentiles: LBW Premature Boys[1,2]

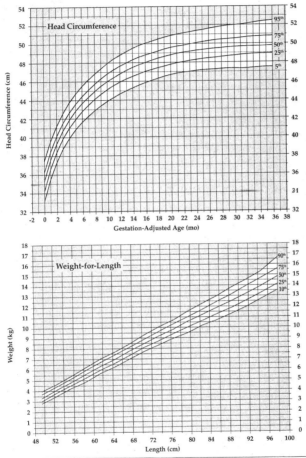

References

1. Guo SS, Roche AF, Chumlea WC, et al: Growth in weight, recumbent length, and head circumference for preterm low-birthweight infants during the first three years of life using gestation-adjusted ages. *Early Hum Dev* 1997;47:305-325.

2. Guo SS, Wholihan K, Roche AF, et al: Weight-for-length reference data for preterm, low-birth-weight infants. *Arch Pediatr Adolesc Med* 1996;150:964-970. Copyright: 1996, American Medical Association.

Acknowledgment

IHDP studies were supported by grants from the Robert Wood Johnson Foundation, Pew Charitable Trusts, and the Bureau of Maternal and Child Health, US Department of Health and Human Services. The IHDP growth percentile graphs were prepared by S.S. Guo and A.F. Roche, Wright State University, Yellow Springs, Ohio. IHDP, its sponsors and the investigators do not endorse specific products.

© 1999 Abbott
A7222/MARCH 1999
LITHO IN USA

ROSS PRODUCTS DIVISION
ABBOTT LABORATORIES INC.
COLUMBUS, OHIO 43215-1724

Provided as a service of
Similac NeoSure™
Infant Formula With Iron

APP

Fig. A-5.5

IHDP Growth Percentiles:
VLBW Premature Girls[1,2]
(≤1500 g BW, ≤37 wk GA)

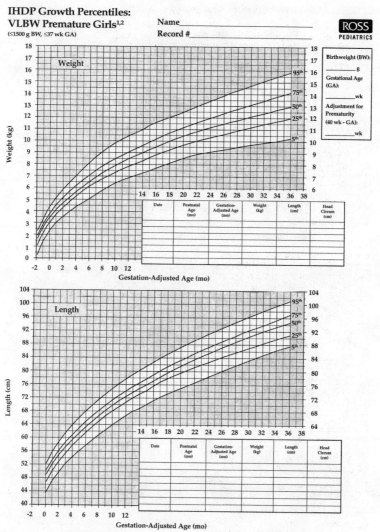

Fig. A-5.6

IHDP Growth Percentiles: VLBW Premature Girls[1,2]

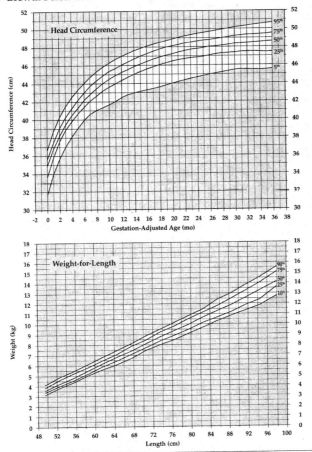

References

1. Guo SS, Roche AF, Chumlea WC, et al: Growth in weight, recumbent length, and head circumference for preterm low-birthweight infants during the first three years of life using gestation-adjusted ages. *Early Hum Dev* 1997;47:305-325.

2. Guo SS, Wholihan K, Roche AF, et al: Weight-for-length reference data for preterm, low-birth-weight infants. *Arch Pediatr Adolesc Med* 1996;150:964-970. Copyright: 1996, American Medical Association.

Acknowledgment

IHDP studies were supported by grants from the Robert Wood Johnson Foundation, Pew Charitable Trusts, and the Bureau of Maternal and Child Health, US Department of Health and Human Services. The IHDP growth percentile graphs were prepared by S.S. Guo and A.F. Roche, Wright State University, Yellow Springs, Ohio. IHDP, its sponsors and the investigators do not endorse specific products.

© 1999 Abbott
A7220/MARCH 1999
LITHO IN USA

ROSS PRODUCTS DIVISION
ABBOTT LABORATORIES INC.
COLUMBUS, OHIO 43215-1724

Provided as a service of
Similac NeoSure™
Infant Formula With Iron

Fig. A-5.7

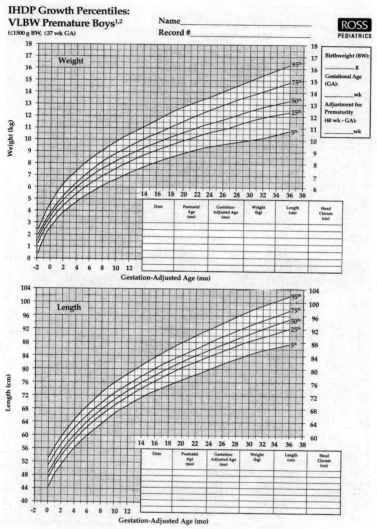

IHDP Growth Percentiles:
VLBW Premature Boys[1,2]
(≤1500 g BW, ≤37 wk GA)

Name_____

Record #_____

ROSS
PEDIATRICS

Birthweight (BW):

_____ g

Gestational Age
(GA):

_____ wk

Adjustment for
Prematurity
(40 wk - GA):

_____ wk

Fig. A-5.8

IHDP Growth Percentiles: VLBW Premature Boys[1,2]

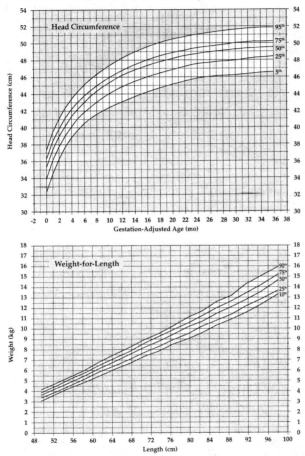

References

1. Guo SS, Roche AF, Chumlea WC, et al: Growth in weight, recumbent length, and head circumference for preterm low-birthweight infants during the first three years of life using gestation-adjusted ages. *Early Hum Dev* 1997;47:305-325.

2. Guo SS, Wholihan K, Roche AF, et al: Weight-for-length reference data for preterm, low-birth-weight infants. *Arch Pediatr Adolesc Med* 1996;150:964-970. Copyright: 1996, American Medical Association.

Acknowledgment

IHDP studies were supported by grants from the Robert Wood Johnson Foundation, Pew Charitable Trusts, and the Bureau of Maternal and Child Health, US Department of Health and Human Services. The IHDP growth percentile graphs were prepared by S.S. Guo and A.F. Roche, Wright State University, Yellow Springs, Ohio. IHDP, its sponsors and the investigators do not endorse specific products.

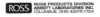 ROSS PRODUCTS DIVISION
ABBOTT LABORATORIES INC.
COLUMBUS, OHIO 43215-1724

Provided as a service of
Similac NeoSure™
Infant Formula With Iron

APP

Appendix A - 6

Fig. A-6.1

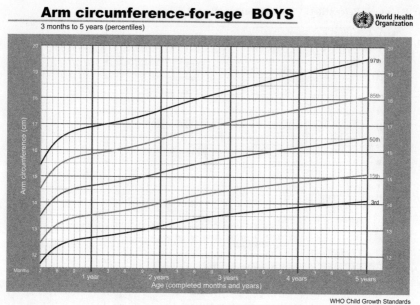

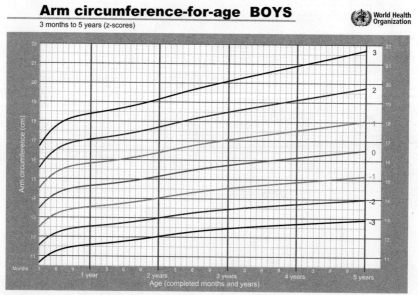

Fig. A-6.2

Arm circumference-for-age GIRLS

World Health Organization

3 months to 5 years (percentiles)

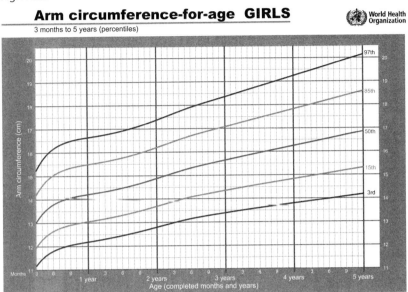

WHO Child Growth Standards

Arm circumference-for-age GIRLS

World Health Organization

3 months to 5 years (z-scores)

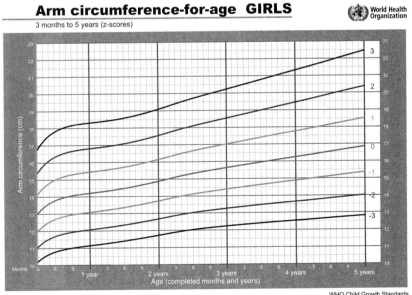

WHO Child Growth Standards

http://www.who.int/childgrowth/en/

Appendix A - 7

Fig. A-7.1

Simplified field tables

1-month weight increments (g) BOYS Birth to 12 months (percentiles)											World Health Organization
Interval	1st	3rd	5th	15th	25th	50th	75th	85th	95th	97th	99th
0 - 4 wks	182	369	460	681	805	1023	1229	1336	1509	1575	1697
4 wks - 2 mo	528	648	713	886	992	1196	1408	1524	1724	1803	1955
2 - 3 mo	307	397	446	577	658	815	980	1071	1228	1290	1410
3 - 4 mo	160	241	285	403	476	617	764	845	985	1041	1147
4 - 5 mo	70	150	194	311	383	522	666	746	883	937	1041
5 - 6 mo	-17	61	103	217	287	422	563	640	773	826	927
6 - 7 mo	-76	0	42	154	223	357	496	573	706	758	859
7 - 8 mo	-118	-43	-1	111	181	316	457	535	671	724	827
8 - 9 mo	-153	-77	-36	77	148	285	429	508	646	701	806
9 - 10 mo	-183	-108	-66	48	120	259	405	486	627	683	790
10 - 11 mo	-209	-132	-89	27	100	243	394	478	623	680	791
11 - 12 mo	-229	-150	-106	15	91	239	397	484	635	695	811
WHO Growth Velocity Standards											

Fig. A-7.2

Simplified field tables

2-month weight increments (g) BOYS Birth to 24 months (percentiles)											World Health Organization
Interval	1st	3rd	5th	15th	25th	50th	75th	85th	95th	97th	99th
0-2 mo	1144	1338	1443	1720	1890	2216	2552	2737	3054	3179	3418
1-3 mo	1040	1211	1303	1549	1701	1992	2296	2463	2753	2868	3088
2-4 mo	675	810	884	1081	1202	1438	1685	1822	2059	2154	2336
3-5 mo	455	576	642	820	930	1145	1371	1496	1715	1802	1970
4-6 mo	291	404	466	634	738	941	1156	1277	1486	1569	1731
5-7 mo	165	271	330	487	585	778	982	1096	1294	1374	1528
6-8 mo	79	182	230	300	486	673	871	982	1175	1252	1402
7-9 mo	16	117	172	323	417	601	797	907	1098	1174	1322
8-10 mo	-41	60	115	266	360	544	739	848	1039	1115	1261
9-11 mo	-92	10	67	219	315	502	700	810	1003	1079	1227
10-12 mo	-132	-28	30	187	286	478	681	795	992	1070	1221
11-13 mo	-169	-62	-2	159	260	458	666	782	984	1064	1218
12-14 mo	-202	-92	-31	133	236	437	648	766	969	1050	1206
13-15 mo	-230	-119	-58	109	212	414	626	744	947	1028	1183
14-16 mo	-250	-138	-75	93	197	401	614	731	935	1016	1170
15-17 mo	-262	-148	-84	87	193	399	615	734	939	1020	1176
16-18 mo	-272	-155	-90	84	192	401	619	739	945	1027	1183
17-19 mo	-281	-162	-97	79	188	398	617	737	944	1025	1181
18-20 mo	-291	-170	-104	73	182	393	611	731	937	1018	1173
19-21 mo	-299	-178	-111	67	176	387	605	725	929	1010	1164
20-22 mo	-307	-185	-118	61	171	382	599	719	923	1003	1156
21-23 mo	-314	-191	-123	57	167	378	596	715	919	999	1151
22-24 mo	-320	-196	-128	53	164	376	594	713	917	997	1149

WHO Growth Velocity Standards

Fig. A-7.3

Simplified field tables

6-month weight increments (g) BOYS Birth to 24 months (percentiles)											World Health Organization
Interval	1st	3rd	5th	15th	25th	50th	75th	85th	95th	97th	99th
0-6 mo	2940	3229	3387	3810	4072	4580	5114	5412	5929	6136	6534
1-7 mo	2342	2611	2759	3157	3406	3893	4411	4701	5210	5413	5809
2-8 mo	1736	1968	2096	2443	2662	3093	3555	3816	4275	4461	4821
3-9 mo	1319	1523	1636	1945	2141	2530	2949	3188	3609	3779	4112
4-10 mo	1030	1217	1321	1607	1789	2152	2546	2771	3169	3331	3647
5-11 mo	806	982	1080	1351	1524	1871	2249	2465	2849	3005	3311
6-12 mo	642	813	909	1175	1346	1688	2062	2277	2658	2813	3116
7-13 mo	515	683	778	1042	1212	1553	1927	2141	2521	2675	2978
8-14 mo	415	582	676	938	1106	1445	1816	2028	2404	2557	2856
9-15 mo	341	506	599	858	1024	1359	1725	1934	2304	2453	2746
10-16 mo	291	455	547	805	970	1301	1662	1868	2232	2379	2665
11-17 mo	258	422	515	772	937	1267	1624	1827	2184	2329	2609
12-18 mo	236	400	493	750	914	1241	1593	1793	2143	2284	2558
13-19 mo	221	386	479	735	898	1222	1569	1765	2108	2246	2513
14-20 mo	212	377	470	725	887	1207	1549	1741	2077	2212	2472
15-21 mo	206	372	465	719	880	1196	1533	1721	2050	2182	2435
16-22 mo	202	368	460	713	872	1184	1515	1700	2021	2150	2397
17-23 mo	198	363	455	706	863	1171	1496	1677	1992	2117	2358
18-24 mo	195	360	451	700	855	1158	1478	1656	1964	2086	2321
WHO Growth Velocity Standards											

Fig. A-7.4

Simplified field tables

1-month weight increments (g) GIRLS Birth to 12 months (percentiles)											World Health Organization
Interval	1st	3rd	5th	15th	25th	50th	75th	85th	95th	97th	99th
0 - 4 wks	280	388	446	602	697	879	1068	1171	1348	1418	1551
4 wks - 2 mo	410	519	578	734	829	1011	1198	1301	1476	1545	1677
2 - 3 mo	233	321	369	494	571	718	869	952	1094	1150	1256
3 - 4 mo	133	214	259	376	448	585	726	804	937	990	1090
4 - 5 mo	51	130	172	286	355	489	627	703	833	885	983
5 - 6 mo	-24	52	93	203	271	401	537	611	739	790	886
6 - 7 mo	-79	-4	37	146	214	344	480	555	684	734	832
7 - 8 mo	-119	-44	-2	109	178	311	450	526	659	711	811
8 - 9 mo	-155	-81	-40	70	139	273	412	489	623	675	776
9 - 10 mo	-184	-110	-70	41	110	245	385	464	598	652	754
10 - 11 mo	-206	-131	-89	24	95	233	378	459	598	653	759
11 - 12 mo	-222	-145	-102	15	88	232	383	467	612	670	781
WHO Growth Velocity Standards											

Fig. A-7.5

Simplified field tables

2-month weight increments (g) GIRLS Birth to 24 months (percentiles)											World Health Organization
Interval	1st	3rd	5th	15th	25th	50th	75th	85th	95th	97th	99th
0-2 mo	968	1128	1216	1455	1604	1897	2210	2386	2696	2820	3062
1-3 mo	890	1030	1107	1317	1450	1714	2000	2163	2452	2569	2799
2-4 mo	625	740	804	978	1088	1307	1545	1681	1922	2020	2213
3-5 mo	451	556	615	773	874	1074	1290	1413	1632	1720	1894
4-6 mo	295	395	450	600	695	883	1085	1200	1403	1486	1646
5-7 mo	170	267	321	468	560	742	938	1048	1243	1321	1473
6-8 mo	76	175	229	377	469	651	846	955	1147	1223	1372
7-9 mo	3	103	157	306	399	581	775	883	1072	1147	1293
8-10 mo	-59	40	95	243	336	517	708	814	999	1073	1215
9-11 mo	-104	-3	53	203	297	478	670	776	960	1033	1174
10-12 mo	-135	-31	26	179	274	458	652	759	944	1018	1159
11-13 mo	-163	-57	1	157	254	441	637	745	932	1005	1147
12-14 mo	-185	-78	-19	140	238	428	626	736	924	999	1142
13-15 mo	-204	-95	-35	127	227	420	621	732	924	999	1144
14-16 mo	-219	-108	-47	118	220	416	622	735	930	1007	1154
15-17 mo	-231	-118	-55	112	216	418	627	743	943	1021	1172
16-18 mo	-243	-128	-64	106	212	417	631	750	954	1035	1189
17-19 mo	-255	-139	-75	97	205	413	631	751	959	1041	1199
18-20 mo	-267	-151	-86	88	196	407	628	751	962	1046	1206
19-21 mo	-279	-162	-97	79	188	402	626	750	965	1050	1213
20-22 mo	-291	-174	-109	67	178	393	620	745	963	1049	1214
21-23 mo	-305	-189	-124	53	164	381	608	735	954	1040	1207
22-24 mo	-318	-202	-137	39	150	367	596	723	942	1029	1197
WHO Growth Velocity Standards											

Fig. A-7.6

Simplified field tables

6-month weight increments (g) GIRLS Birth to 24 months (percentiles)											
Interval	1st	3rd	5th	15th	25th	50th	75th	85th	95th	97th	99th
0-6 mo	2701	2924	3049	3395	3620	4079	4597	4902	5462	5697	6170
1-7 mo	2174	2381	2498	2822	3033	3462	3946	4231	4753	4971	5409
2-8 mo	1684	1877	1985	2286	2480	2878	3324	3586	4063	4262	4660
3-9 mo	1279	1461	1563	1846	2030	2403	2821	3064	3506	3689	4054
4-10 mo	964	1140	1240	1514	1692	2052	2451	2682	3099	3271	3610
5-11 mo	725	900	999	1271	1446	1799	2186	2409	2807	2969	3288
6-12 mo	549	725	824	1007	1271	1618	1996	2211	2592	2746	3047
7-13 mo	425	603	702	975	1147	1489	1857	2065	2430	2577	2862
8-14 mo	340	519	619	891	1063	1400	1760	1962	2314	2454	2726
9-15 mo	284	465	565	838	1009	1343	1697	1895	2238	2375	2638
10-16 mo	249	431	532	805	975	1309	1660	1855	2194	2329	2588
11-17 mo	230	412	513	785	956	1288	1639	1834	2173	2307	2566
12-18 mo	221	401	501	772	942	1275	1627	1823	2163	2299	2560
13-19 mo	216	394	492	762	931	1264	1617	1815	2158	2296	2560
14-20 mo	211	386	484	751	920	1253	1608	1807	2155	2294	2563
15-21 mo	204	377	474	740	908	1242	1599	1800	2151	2292	2565
16-22 mo	193	365	461	726	894	1228	1586	1788	2143	2285	2561
17-23 mo	178	348	444	708	876	1210	1569	1772	2128	2271	2549
18-24 mo	161	330	425	689	857	1191	1551	1754	2111	2254	2533
WHO Growth Velocity Standards											

World Health Organization

APP

Fig. A-7.7

Simplified field tables

2-month length increments (cm) BOYS Birth to 24 months (percentiles)											World Health Organization
Interval	1st	3rd	5th	15th	25th	50th	75th	85th	95th	97th	99th
0-2 mo	5.9	6.4	6.6	7.3	7.7	8.5	9.3	9.7	10.4	10.6	11.1
1-3 mo	4.7	5.2	5.4	6.0	6.3	7.0	7.7	8.0	8.6	8.9	9.3
2-4 mo	3.4	3.8	4.0	4.6	4.9	5.6	6.2	6.6	7.2	7.4	7.8
3-5 mo	2.3	2.7	3.0	3.5	3.9	4.5	5.1	5.5	6.1	6.3	6.7
4-6 mo	1.7	2.0	2.3	2.8	3.1	3.7	4.3	4.7	5.2	5.4	5.9
5-7 mo	1.3	1.6	1.8	2.3	2.7	3.2	3.8	4.1	4.7	4.9	5.3
6-8 mo	1.0	1.4	1.6	2.1	2.4	3.0	3.5	3.8	4.4	4.6	5.0
7-9 mo	0.9	1.3	1.5	2.0	2.3	2.8	3.4	3.7	4.2	4.4	4.8
8-10 mo	0.8	1.2	1.4	1.8	2.1	2.7	3.2	3.5	4.1	4.3	4.6
9-11 mo	0.7	1.1	1.3	1.7	2.0	2.6	3.1	3.4	3.9	4.1	4.5
10-12 mo	0.7	1.0	1.2	1.7	1.9	2.5	3.0	3.3	3.8	4.0	4.4
11-13 mo	0.6	0.9	1.1	1.6	1.8	2.4	2.9	3.2	3.7	3.9	4.3
12-14 mo	0.5	0.8	1.0	1.5	1.8	2.3	2.8	3.1	3.6	3.8	4.2
13-15 mo	0.4	0.7	0.9	1.4	1.7	2.2	2.8	3.1	3.5	3.7	4.1
14-16 mo	0.3	0.7	0.8	1.3	1.6	2.1	2.7	3.0	3.5	3.7	4.0
15-17 mo	0.3	0.6	0.8	1.2	1.5	2.1	2.6	2.9	3.4	3.6	4.0
16-18 mo	0.2	0.5	0.7	1.2	1.5	2.0	2.5	2.8	3.3	3.5	3.9
17-19 mo	0.2	0.5	0.7	1.1	1.4	1.9	2.5	2.8	3.3	3.5	3.9
18-20 mo	0.1	0.4	0.6	1.1	1.4	1.9	2.4	2.7	3.2	3.4	3.8
19-21 mo	0.0	0.4	0.5	1.0	1.3	1.8	2.4	2.7	3.2	3.4	3.8
20-22 mo	0.0	0.3	0.5	1.0	1.3	1.8	2.4	2.7	3.2	3.4	3.7
21-23 mo	0.0	0.3	0.4	0.9	1.2	1.8	2.3	2.6	3.1	3.3	3.7
22-24 mo	0.0	0.2	0.4	0.9	1.2	1.7	2.3	2.6	3.1	3.3	3.7

WHO Growth Velocity Standards

Fig. A-7.8

Simplified field tables

6-month length increments (cm) BOYS Birth to 24 months (percentiles)											World Health Organization
Interval	1st	3rd	5th	15th	25th	50th	75th	85th	95th	97th	99th
0-6 mo	13.8	14.5	14.9	15.9	16.5	17.7	18.8	19.4	20.4	20.8	21.6
1-7 mo	11.0	11.7	12.1	13.1	13.6	14.7	15.8	16.4	17.4	17.8	18.5
2-8 mo	8.8	9.5	9.8	10.7	11.3	12.3	13.3	13.9	14.8	15.2	15.9
3-9 mo	7.3	7.9	8.2	9.1	9.6	10.6	11.5	12.1	13.0	13.3	14.0
4-10 mo	6.3	6.9	7.2	8.0	8.5	9.4	10.3	10.8	11.7	12.0	12.6
5-11 mo	5.7	6.2	6.5	7.3	7.8	8.6	9.5	10.0	10.8	11.1	11.7
6-12 mo	5.3	5.8	6.1	6.8	7.3	8.1	8.0	9.4	10.2	10.5	11.0
7-13 mo	5.0	5.6	5.8	6.5	6.9	7.7	8.5	9.0	9.7	10.0	10.5
8-14 mo	4.8	5.3	5.6	6.3	6.7	7.4	8.2	8.6	9.3	9.6	10.1
9-15 mo	4.7	5.1	5.4	6.0	6.4	7.2	7.9	8.3	9.0	9.3	9.8
10-16 mo	4.5	4.9	5.2	5.8	6.2	6.9	7.6	8.0	8.7	9.0	9.4
11-17 mo	4.3	4.8	5.0	5.6	6.0	6.7	7.4	7.8	8.4	8.7	9.2
12-18 mo	4.1	4.6	4.8	5.4	5.8	6.5	7.2	7.6	8.2	8.4	8.9
13-19 mo	4.0	4.4	4.6	5.2	5.6	6.3	7.0	7.3	8.0	8.2	8.7
14-20 mo	3.8	4.3	4.5	5.1	5.4	6.1	6.8	7.1	7.8	8.0	8.5
15-21 mo	3.7	4.1	4.3	4.9	5.3	5.9	6.6	7.0	7.6	7.8	8.3
16-22 mo	3.6	4.0	4.2	4.8	5.1	5.8	6.5	6.8	7.4	7.7	8.1
17-23 mo	3.4	3.9	4.1	4.7	5.0	5.6	6.3	6.7	7.3	7.5	7.9
18-24 mo	3.3	3.7	4.0	4.5	4.9	5.5	6.2	6.5	7.1	7.3	7.8
WHO Growth Velocity Standards											

Fig. A-7.9

Simplified field tables

2-month length increments (cm) GIRLS Birth to 24 months (percentiles)											World Health Organization
Interval	1st	3rd	5th	15th	25th	50th	75th	85th	95th	97th	99th
0-2 mo	5.3	5.8	6.1	6.7	7.1	7.9	8.7	9.1	9.7	10.0	10.5
1-3 mo	4.2	4.6	4.8	5.4	5.7	6.4	7.0	7.4	8.0	8.2	8.6
2-4 mo	3.0	3.4	3.7	4.2	4.5	5.2	5.8	6.1	6.7	6.9	7.3
3-5 mo	2.2	2.6	2.8	3.4	3.7	4.3	4.9	5.2	5.8	6.0	6.4
4-6 mo	1.6	2.0	2.2	2.7	3.0	3.6	4.2	4.5	5.0	5.2	5.6
5-7 mo	1.3	1.6	1.8	2.3	2.6	3.2	3.7	4.0	4.5	4.7	5.1
6-8 mo	1.1	1.4	1.6	2.1	2.4	3.0	3.6	3.9	4.4	4.6	4.9
7-9 mo	1.0	1.3	1.5	2.0	2.3	2.9	3.4	3.7	4.2	4.4	4.8
8-10 mo	0.9	1.2	1.4	1.9	2.2	2.7	3.3	3.6	4.1	4.3	4.6
9-11 mo	0.8	1.2	1.3	1.8	2.1	2.6	3.2	3.4	3.9	4.1	4.5
10-12 mo	0.7	1.1	1.3	1.7	2.0	2.5	3.1	3.3	3.8	4.0	4.3
11-13 mo	0.7	1.0	1.2	1.6	1.9	2.4	3.0	3.2	3.7	3.9	4.2
12-14 mo	0.6	0.9	1.1	1.6	1.8	2.4	2.9	3.2	3.6	3.8	4.2
13-15 mo	0.5	0.8	1.0	1.5	1.8	2.3	2.8	3.1	3.6	3.8	4.1
14-16 mo	0.4	0.7	0.9	1.4	1.7	2.2	2.8	3.0	3.5	3.7	4.1
15-17 mo	0.3	0.7	0.9	1.3	1.6	2.2	2.7	3.0	3.5	3.7	4.0
16-18 mo	0.3	0.6	0.8	1.3	1.6	2.1	2.7	2.9	3.4	3.6	4.0
17-19 mo	0.2	0.5	0.7	1.2	1.5	2.0	2.6	2.9	3.4	3.6	3.9
18-20 mo	0.1	0.5	0.7	1.2	1.4	2.0	2.5	2.8	3.3	3.5	3.8
19-21 mo	0.1	0.4	0.6	1.1	1.4	1.9	2.5	2.8	3.2	3.4	3.8
20-22 mo	0.0	0.4	0.6	1.0	1.3	1.9	2.4	2.7	3.2	3.4	3.7
21-23 mo	0.0	0.3	0.5	1.0	1.3	1.8	2.4	2.6	3.1	3.3	3.7
22-24 mo	0.0	0.3	0.5	0.9	1.2	1.8	2.3	2.6	3.1	3.3	3.6
WHO Growth Velocity Standards											

Fig. A-7.10

Simplified field tables

6-month length increments (cm) GIRLS
Birth to 24 months (percentiles)

World Health Organization

Interval	1st	3rd	5th	15th	25th	50th	75th	85th	95th	97th	99th
0-6 mo	12.8	13.5	13.9	14.8	15.4	16.5	17.6	18.2	19.2	19.6	20.4
1-7 mo	10.5	11.1	11.5	12.3	12.9	13.9	14.9	15.5	16.4	16.8	17.5
2-8 mo	8.7	9.3	9.6	10.4	10.9	11.8	12.8	13.3	14.2	14.5	15.2
3-9 mo	7.4	8.0	8.3	9.0	9.5	10.3	11.2	11.7	12.6	12.9	13.5
4-10 mo	6.6	7.1	7.4	8.1	8.5	9.3	10.2	10.7	11.4	11.8	12.4
5-11 mo	6.0	6.5	6.8	7.5	7.9	8.7	9.5	9.9	10.7	11.0	11.6
6-12 mo	5.6	6.1	6.4	7.0	7.4	8.2	9.0	9.5	10.2	10.5	11.1
7-13 mo	5.4	5.8	6.1	6.7	7.1	7.9	8.7	9.1	9.8	10.1	10.7
8-14 mo	5.1	5.6	5.8	6.4	6.8	7.6	8.4	8.8	9.5	9.8	10.3
9-15 mo	4.9	5.3	5.6	6.2	6.6	7.3	8.1	8.5	9.2	9.5	10.0
10-16 mo	4.7	5.1	5.3	6.0	6.4	7.1	7.8	8.3	9.0	9.2	9.8
11-17 mo	4.5	4.9	5.2	5.8	6.2	6.9	7.6	8.0	8.7	9.0	9.5
12-18 mo	4.3	4.7	5.0	5.6	6.0	6.7	7.4	7.8	8.5	8.8	9.3
13-19 mo	4.1	4.6	4.8	5.4	5.8	6.5	7.2	7.6	8.3	8.6	9.1
14-20 mo	4.0	4.4	4.6	5.2	5.6	6.3	7.1	7.5	8.2	8.4	9.0
15-21 mo	3.8	4.2	4.5	5.1	5.4	6.1	6.9	7.3	8.0	8.2	8.8
16-22 mo	3.7	4.1	4.3	4.9	5.3	6.0	6.7	7.1	7.8	8.0	8.6
17-23 mo	3.5	4.0	4.2	4.8	5.1	5.8	6.5	6.9	7.6	7.9	8.4
18-24 mo	3.4	3.8	4.0	4.6	5.0	5.6	6.3	6.7	7.4	7.7	8.2

WHO Growth Velocity Standards

Fig. A-7.11

Simplified field tables

2-month head circumference increments (cm) BOYS Birth to 12 months (percentiles)											World Health Organization
Interval	1st	3rd	5th	15th	25th	50th	75th	85th	95th	97th	99th
0-2 mo	3.0	3.3	3.5	3.9	4.2	4.7	5.2	5.5	5.9	6.1	6.5
1-3 mo	2.2	2.4	2.5	2.8	3.0	3.4	3.7	3.9	4.3	4.4	4.7
2-4 mo	1.6	1.8	1.9	2.1	2.2	2.5	2.8	3.0	3.2	3.3	3.6
3-5 mo	1.3	1.4	1.5	1.7	1.8	2.1	2.3	2.5	2.7	2.8	3.0
4-6 mo	1.0	1.1	1.2	1.4	1.5	1.7	2.0	2.1	2.3	2.4	2.6
5-7 mo	0.7	0.8	0.9	1.1	1.2	1.4	1.7	1.8	2.0	2.1	2.3
6-8 mo	0.5	0.6	0.7	0.9	1.0	1.2	1.4	1.5	1.8	1.8	2.0
7-9 mo	0.3	0.4	0.5	0.7	0.8	1.0	1.2	1.3	1.5	1.6	1.8
8-10 mo	0.2	0.3	0.4	0.6	0.7	0.9	1.1	1.2	1.4	1.5	1.6
9-11 mo	0.1	0.2	0.3	0.5	0.6	0.8	1.0	1.1	1.3	1.3	1.5
10-12 mo	0.0	0.1	0.2	0.4	0.5	0.7	0.9	1.0	1.2	1.2	1.4
WHO Growth Velocity Standards											

Fig. A-7.12

Simplified field tables

6-month head circumference increments (cm) BOYS Birth to 24 months (percentiles)											World Health Organization
Interval	1st	3rd	5th	15th	25th	50th	75th	85th	95th	97th	99th
0-6 mo	6.8	7.1	7.3	7.9	8.2	8.9	9.5	9.9	10.6	10.8	11.3
1-7 mo	5.2	5.5	5.7	6.1	6.4	6.9	7.5	7.8	8.3	8.6	9.0
2-8 mo	4.0	4.3	4.4	4.8	5.1	5.5	6.0	6.2	6.7	6.9	7.2
3-9 mo	3.2	3.4	3.6	3.9	4.1	4.5	4.9	5.2	5.6	5.7	6.0
4-10 mo	2.6	2.8	2.9	3.2	3.4	3.8	4.2	4.4	4.8	4.9	5.2
5-11 mo	2.1	2.3	2.4	2.7	2.9	3.2	3.6	3.8	4.1	4.2	4.5
6-12 mo	1.7	1.9	2.0	2.3	2.4	2.7	3.1	3.2	3.6	3.7	3.9
7-13 mo	1.4	1.6	1.7	1.9	2.1	2.4	2.7	2.0	3.1	3.2	3.4
8-14 mo	1.1	1.3	1.4	1.6	1.8	2.0	2.3	2.5	2.8	2.9	3.1
9-15 mo	0.9	1.1	1.2	1.4	1.5	1.8	2.1	2.2	2.5	2.6	2.8
10-16 mo	0.8	0.9	1.0	1.2	1.3	1.6	1.8	2.0	2.2	2.3	2.5
11-17 mo	0.7	0.8	0.9	1.1	1.2	1.4	1.7	1.8	2.0	2.1	2.3
12-18 mo	0.5	0.7	0.8	0.9	1.1	1.3	1.5	1.6	1.8	1.9	2.1
13-19 mo	0.5	0.6	0.7	0.8	1.0	1.2	1.4	1.5	1.7	1.8	1.9
14-20 mo	0.4	0.5	0.6	0.8	0.9	1.1	1.3	1.4	1.6	1.7	1.8
15-21 mo	0.3	0.5	0.5	0.7	0.8	1.0	1.2	1.3	1.5	1.6	1.7
16-22 mo	0.3	0.4	0.5	0.6	0.8	0.9	1.1	1.3	1.4	1.5	1.7
17-23 mo	0.2	0.4	0.4	0.6	0.7	0.9	1.1	1.2	1.4	1.5	1.6
18-24 mo	0.2	0.3	0.4	0.6	0.7	0.9	1.0	1.2	1.3	1.4	1.5
WHO Growth Velocity Standards											

Fig. A-7.13

Simplified field tables

2-month head circumference increments (cm) GIRLS Birth to 12 months (percentiles)										World Health Organization
Interval	1st	3rd	5th	15th	25th	50th	75th	85th	95th	97th	99th
0-2 mo	2.8	3.1	3.2	3.6	3.9	4.4	4.8	5.1	5.5	5.7	6.0
1-3 mo	1.9	2.1	2.3	2.6	2.8	3.1	3.5	3.6	4.0	4.1	4.3
2-4 mo	1.4	1.6	1.7	1.9	2.1	2.3	2.6	2.8	3.1	3.2	3.4
3-5 mo	1.1	1.2	1.3	1.6	1.7	2.0	2.2	2.4	2.6	2.7	2.9
4-6 mo	0.8	1.0	1.1	1.3	1.4	1.7	1.9	2.0	2.3	2.4	2.5
5-7 mo	0.6	0.8	0.8	1.0	1.2	1.4	1.6	1.8	2.0	2.1	2.2
6-8 mo	0.4	0.6	0.6	0.8	1.0	1.2	1.4	1.5	1.7	1.8	2.0
7-9 mo	0.3	0.4	0.5	0.7	0.8	1.0	1.2	1.3	1.5	1.6	1.8
8-10 mo	0.2	0.3	0.4	0.5	0.6	0.8	1.1	1.2	1.4	1.4	1.6
9-11 mo	0.1	0.2	0.3	0.4	0.5	0.7	0.9	1.1	1.2	1.3	1.5
10-12 mo	0.0	0.1	0.2	0.4	0.5	0.7	0.9	1.0	1.1	1.2	1.4
WHO Growth Velocity Standards										

Fig. A-7.14

Simplified field tables

6-month head circumference increments (cm) GIRLS Birth to 24 months (percentiles)											World Health Organization
Interval	1st	3rd	5th	15th	25th	50th	75th	85th	95th	97th	99th
0-6 mo	6.2	6.6	6.8	7.3	7.6	8.3	8.9	9.3	10.0	10.2	10.7
1-7 mo	4.9	5.1	5.3	5.7	6.0	6.5	7.0	7.3	7.9	8.1	8.5
2-8 mo	3.8	4.1	4.2	4.6	4.8	5.2	5.7	5.9	6.4	6.5	6.9
3-9 mo	3.1	3.3	3.4	3.8	4.0	4.3	4.7	5.0	5.4	5.5	5.8
4-10 mo	2.5	2.7	2.9	3.1	3.3	3.7	4.0	4.2	4.6	4.7	5.0
5-11 mo	2.1	2.3	2.4	2.6	2.8	3.1	3.5	3.7	4.0	4.1	4.3
6-12 mo	1.7	1.9	2.0	2.2	2.4	2.7	3.0	3.2	3.5	3.6	3.8
7-13 mo	1.4	1.6	1.7	1.9	2.0	2.3	2.6	2.8	3.1	3.2	3.4
8-14 mo	1.2	1.3	1.4	1.6	1.8	2.0	2.3	2.5	2.7	2.8	3.0
9-15 mo	1.0	1.1	1.2	1.4	1.5	1.8	2.1	2.2	2.5	2.6	2.7
10-16 mo	0.8	0.9	1.0	1.2	1.4	1.6	1.9	2.0	2.2	2.3	2.5
11-17 mo	0.7	0.8	0.9	1.1	1.2	1.5	1.7	1.8	2.1	2.2	2.3
12-18 mo	0.5	0.7	0.8	1.0	1.1	1.3	1.6	1.7	1.9	2.0	2.2
13-19 mo	0.4	0.6	0.7	0.9	1.0	1.2	1.4	1.6	1.8	1.9	2.0
14-20 mo	0.4	0.5	0.6	0.8	0.9	1.1	1.4	1.5	1.7	1.8	1.9
15-21 mo	0.3	0.4	0.5	0.7	0.8	1.1	1.3	1.4	1.6	1.7	1.8
16-22 mo	0.2	0.4	0.5	0.6	0.8	1.0	1.2	1.3	1.5	1.6	1.7
17-23 mo	0.2	0.3	0.4	0.6	0.7	0.9	1.1	1.2	1.4	1.5	1.6
18-24 mo	0.1	0.3	0.4	0.5	0.6	0.8	1.1	1.2	1.3	1.4	1.5
WHO Growth Velocity Standards											

Appendix B

Appendix B.
Recommended Nutrient Levels of Infant Formulas (per 100 kcal)[a]

Nutrient	Range Minimum	Maximum
Protein, g	1.8[b]	4.5[b]
Fat, g	3.3 (30% of kcal)	6.0 (54% of kcal)
Linoleic acid (18:2ω-6) mg	300 (2.7% of kcal)	
Vitamins		
A, IU	250 (75 μg)[c]	750 (225 μg)[c]
D, IU	40 (1 μg)[d]	100 (2.5 μg)[d]
K, μg[e]	4	...
E, IU	0.7 (0.5 mg)[f] at least 0.7 IU (0.5 mg)/g linoleic acid	...
C (ascorbic acid), mg	8	...
B₁ (thiamine), μg	40	...
B₂ (riboflavin), μg	60	...
B₆ (pyridoxine), μg	35[g]	...
B₁₂, μg	0.15	...
Niacin, μg	250 (or 0.8 mg niacin equivalents)	...
Folic acid, μg	4	
Pantothenic acid, μg	300	
Biotin, μg	1.5[h]	
Choline, mg	7[h]	
Inositol, mg	4[h]	
Minerals		
Calcium, mg	60[j]	...
Phosphorus, mg	30[j]	...
Magnesium, mg	6	...
Iron, mg[i]	0.15	3.0
Iodine, μg	5	75
Zinc, mg	0.5	...
Copper, μg	60	...
Manganese, μg	5	...
Sodium, mg	20 (0.9 mEq)	60 (2.6 mEq)
Potassium, mg	80 (2.1 mEq)	200 (5.1 mEq)
Chloride, mg	55 (1.6 mEq)	150 (4.2 mEq)

[a] From the US Infant Formula Act of 1980, Amended 1986. For additional information, see 21 CFR 107, available at the following: http://www.access.gpo.gov/nara/cfr/waisidx_09/21cfr107_09.html.
[b] Biologically equivalent to or better than casein. If protein of lower quality used, minimum is increased in proportion. In no case, protein with biological value <70%.
[c] Retinol equivalents.
[d] Cholecalciferol.
[e] Any vitamin K added shall be in the form of phylloquinone.
[f] all-rac-α-tocopherol equivalents.
[g] At least 15 μg for each g protein in excess of 18 g/100 kcal.
[h] Naturally present in milk-based formulas; addition required only nonmilk-based formulas.
[i] If contains ≥1 mg/100 kcal, must be labeled as formula "with iron."
[j] Calcium-phosphorus ratio should be no less than 1.1 or more than 2.

Appendix C

Appendix C.
Increasing the Caloric Density of Infant Formula

Using Concentrated Liquid: Most concentrated liquids contain 40 kcal/fl oz and when diluted 1:1, produce a formula that contains 20 kcal/fl oz. If a more concentrated final formula is desired using these products, use the upper part of the Table. For the few concentrated liquid products that contain 38 kcal/fl oz and normally produce a formula with 19 kcal/fl oz, more concentrated formulas can be made using the lower part of the Table.

Concentrated Liquid One Can	Added Water	Approximate Yield fl oz	Approximate Final Caloric Density - kcal/fl oz
Using Concentrated Liquid That Normally Produces a Formula With 20 kcal/fl oz			
13 fl oz	13 fl oz	26 fl oz	20
13 fl oz	11 fl oz	24 fl oz	22
13 fl oz	9 fl oz	22 fl oz	24
13 fl oz	6 fl oz	19 fl oz	27
13 fl oz	4.5 fl oz	17.5 fl oz	30
Using Concentrated Liquid That Normally Produces a Formula With 19 kcal/fl oz			
13 fl oz	13 fl oz	26 fl oz	19
13 fl oz	10 fl oz	23 fl oz	21
13 fl oz	8 fl oz	21 fl oz	24
13 fl oz	5 fl oz	18 fl oz	27
13 fl oz	4 fl oz	17 fl oz	29

Using Powder:

Because of the variability of scoop sizes for different formulas from different manufacturers and the variability of household measures, no single set of recipes can be provided that is safe for all products. Some manufacturers provide recipes for their specific products on their Web sites. In the absence of such information, contact the manufacturer directly.

Increasing Caloric Density Using Other Additives:
- Medium-chain triglyceride oil provides 7.7 kcal/mL; 1 teaspoon provides 38 kcal.
- Vegetable oils provide 40 kcal per teaspoon.
- Polycose liquid contains 60 kcal/fluid ounce; Polycose powder contains 8 kcal per teaspoon.

Note that increasing caloric density using fat and/or carbohydrate should be performed with caution, because the additional energy (calories) effectively decreases the density (amount per 100 kcal) of all other nutrients.

Appendix D

Appendix D-1

Formulas for Low Birth Weight and Preterm Infants (per L)

	Similac Special Care 24[a] Liquid (Abbott Nutrition, Columbus, OH)	Enfamil Premature 24[a] Fe & (low Fe) Liquid (Mead Johnson, Evansville, IN)	GoodStart Premature 24[a] cal Liquid (Nestle, Fremont, MI)	Similac Special Care 24[a] HP Liquid (Abbott Nutrition, Columbus, OH)	Enfamil Premature High Protein 24[a] Liquid (Mead Johnson, Evansville, IN)	GoodStart Premature 24[a] High Protein Liquid, Nestle, Fremont, MI)
Energy, kcal	806	810	812	812	811	812
Protein, g	22[b]	24[b]	24.3[c]	26.8[b]	28[b]	29.2[c]
Fat, g	43.8	41	42.2	44.1	40.8	42.2
Polyunsaturated, g	8.3	10.3	9.3			9.3
Monounsaturated, g	3.5	4.5	12			13
Saturated, g	32	26.2[d]	18.5			15.7
Linoleic acid, g	5.7	8.5	8.0			8.0
MCT	50%	40%	40%	50%	40%	40%
Soy	30%	40%	29%	30%		29%
Safflower	-	-	29%			29%
Coconut	20%	20%	-	18%		
DHA	0.25%	0.32% FA	0.32% FA	0.25%	0.32%FA	0.32%
ARA	0.40%	0.64% FA	0.64% FA	0.40%	0.64%FA	0.64%
Carbohydrate, g	86.1	90	85.2	81	85	78.7
Lactose %	50%	40%	50%	50%		50%
Glucose polymers %	50%	60%	50% (malto-dextrin)	50%		50% (malto-dextrin)
Mineral						
Calcium, mg	1460	1340	1331	1461	1340	1331
Phosphorus, mg	730	670	690	812	670	690
Magnesium, mg	100	73	81	97.4	73	81
Iron, mg	3.0	14.6 (4.1)	14.6	14.6	14.6	14.6
Zinc, mg	12.2	12.2	10.6	12.2	12.2	10.6
Manganese, μg	100	51	56.8	97	51	56.8
Copper, μg	2030	1010	1217	2029	970	1217
Iodine, μg	50	200	284	49	200	284
Sodium, mEq	15	13.9	20.4	15.2	13.9	20.4
Potassium, mEq	27	21	25	26.8	21	25
Chloride, mEq	19	19.4	19.7	18.6	19.4	19.7

Similac Special Care 30 Cal Liquid (Abbott Nutrition, Columbus, OH)	Enfamil Premature 30 cal Liquid, Mead Johnson, Evansville, IN)	Neosure 22 Cal Liquid (Abbott Nutrition, Columbus, OH)	Enfacare 22 Cal Liquid (Mead Johnson, Evansville, IN)	GoodStart Nourish 22 cal Liquid (Nestle, Fremont, MI)	Similac Special Care 20 Liquid (Abbott Nutrition, Columbus, OH)	Enfamil Premature 20 Fe & (low Fe) Liquid, Mead Johnson, Evansville, IN)	Good Start, 20 cal premature Liquid, (Nestle, Fremont, MI)
1014	1010	746	740	744	676	676	676
30.4[b]	30[b]	20.8[b]	21[b]	20.8[c]	20.3[b]	20[b]	20.3[c]
67.1	52	41	39	38.7	36.7	34	35.2
		-	-	8.2			7.7
		-	-	20.6			10
		-	-	10			15.4
		5.6	7.1	6.7		8.5	6.7
50%	40%	25%		20%	50%	40%	40%
30%		45%		18%	30%	40%	29%
				60%			29%
18%		29%			18%	20%	
0.21%	32%FA	0.25%	0.32%	0.32%	0.25%	.32%FA	.32%FA
0.33%	64%FA	0.40%	0.64%	0.64%	0.40%	.64%FA	.64% FA
78.4	112	75.1	79	78.1	69.7	74	71
50%				60%	50%	40%	50%
50%				40% (malto-dextrin)	50%	60%	50% (maltodextrin)

1826	1670	781	890	893	1217	1120	1109
1014	840	461	490	484	676	560	575
122	91	67.0	59	74	81	61	67.6
18.3	18.3	13.4	13.3	13.4	12	12.2 (3.4)	12.2
15.22	15.2	8.9	9.0	8.9	10.1	10.1	8.8
122	64	74	111	52	81	43	47.3
2536	1220	893	890	893	1691	810	1015
61	250	112	111	149	41	169	237
19.0	25.7	10.7	11.3	11.3	12.6	16.7	16.2
33.5	26.3	27.0	20.2	20	22.3	16.9	20.8
23.2	24.2	15.7	16.5	15.7	15.5	17.2	16.2

Appendix D-1 *(continued)*
Formulas for Low Birth Weight and Preterm Infants (per L)

	Similac Special Care 24[a] Liquid (Abbott Nutrition, Columbus, OH)	Enfamil Premature 24[a] Fe & (low Fe) Liquid (Mead Johnson, Evansville, IN)	GoodStart Premature 24[a] cal Liquid (Nestle, Fremont, MI)	Similac Special Care 24[a] HP Liquid (Abbott Nutrition, Columbus, OH)	Enfamil Premature High Protein 24[a] Liquid (Mead Johnson, Evansville, IN)	GoodStart Premature 24[a] High Protein Liquid, Nestle, Fremont, MI)
Vitamin						
A, USP Units	10 081	10 100	8116	10 144	10 100	8116
D, USP Units	1210	1950	1461	1217	1950	1461
E, USP Units	32.3	51	48.7	32.5	51	48.7
K, μg	97	65	65	97.4	73	65
Thiamine (B$_1$), μg	2016	1620	1623	2029	1620	1623
Riboflavin (B$_2$), μg	5000	2400	2435	5032	2400	2435
Pyridoxine (B$_6$), μg	2016	1220	1623	2029	1220	1623
B$_{12}$, μg	4.4	2	2	4.5	2	2
Niacin (B$_3$), mg	40.3	32	32.5	40.6	32	32.5
Folic acid (B$_9$), μg	298	320	365	300	320	365
Pantothenic acid (B$_5$), mg	15.3	9.7	11.4	15.4	9.7	11.4
Biotin (B$_7$), μg	298	32	40.6	300	32	40.6
C (ascorbic acid), mg	298	162	243	300	162	243
Choline, mg	81	162	122	81	162	122
Inositol, mg	48.4	360	284	325	360	284

[a] 24 kcal/oz; 81 kcal/dL.

[b] Nonfat milk, whey protein concentrate.

[c] Partially hydrolyzed whey protein.

[d] Included 17.4 g MCT oils.

Similac Special Care 30 Cal Liquid (Abbott Nutrition, Columbus, OH)	Enfamil Premature 30 cal Liquid, Mead Johnson, Evansville, IN)	Neosure 22 Cal Liquid (Abbott Nutrition, Columbus, OH)	Enfacare 22 Cal Liquid (Mead Johnson, Evansville, IN)	GoodStart Nourish 22 cal Liquid (Nestle, Fremont, MI)	Similac Special Care 20 Liquid (Abbott Nutrition, Columbus, OH)	Enfamil Premature 20 Fe & (low Fe) Liquid, Mead Johnson, Evansville, IN)	Good Start, 20 cal premature Liquid, (Nestle, Fremont, MI)
12 681	12 700	2604	3330	3348	8454	850	6764
1522	2400	521	520	595	1014	1620	1217
40.6	64	26.8	30	30	27	43	40.6
122	91	81.8	59	60	81	54	54
2536	2000	1302	1480	1116	1691	1350	1353
6290	3000	1116	1480	1488	4193	2000	2029
2536	2000	744	740	744	1691	1010	1353
5.58	2.5	2.9	2.2	1.9	3.7	1.7	1.7
50.7	41	14.5	14.8	11.2	33.8	27.0	27.1
375	410	186	192	186	250	270	304
19.2	12.2	6.0	6.3	7.4	12.8	8.1	9.5
375.3	41	67	44	22	250	27	33.8
375	200	112	118	149	250	135	203
101	200	119	178	179	68	135	101
406	450	260	220	223	271	300	237

APP

Appendix D-2
Human Milk Fortifiers for Preterm Infants[a]

Nutrient	Enfamil Powder Human Milk Fortifier (4 pkt), Mead Johnson, Evansville, IN	Similac Powder Human Milk Fortifier (4 pkt), Abbott Nutrition, Columbus, OH	Prolact+ H2MF (20 mL), Prolacta Bioscience, Monrovia, CA	Similac Liquid Human Milk Fortifier (4 pkt), Abbott Nutrition, Columbus, OH	Enfamil Liquid Fortifier (4 vials), Mead Johnson, Evansville, IN
Energy (kcal)	14	14	28	27.4	30
Protein (g)	1.1	1.0	1.2	1.4	2.24
Fat (g)	1	0.36	1.8	1.1	2.32
Linoleic acid (mg)	90	0	Unknown	Unknown	230 (includes ARA 20 mg)
α-Linolenic acid (mg)	11	0	Unknown	4	28 (includes DHA 12 mg)
Carbohydrate (g)	1.1	1.8	1.8	3.2	<1.2
Minerals					
Calcium (mg)	90	117	103	140.4	116
Phosphorus (mg)	50	67	54	80	63.2
Magnesium (mg)	1	7	4.7	8.6	1.84
Iron (mg)	1.44	0.35	0.1	0.4	1.76
Zinc (mg)	0.72	1	0.7	1.2	0.96
Manganese (μg)	10	7.2	<12	8.5	10
Copper (μg)	44	170	64	208	60
Sodium (mEq)	0.48	0.65	1.6	0.94	1.18
Potassium (mEq)	0.51	1.6	1.28	2.12	1.16
Chloride (mEq)	0.25	1.1	0.8	1.5	0.79
Vitamins					
A (IU)	950	620	61.2	788	1160
D (IU)	150	120	26	140	188
E (IU)	4.6	3.2	0.4	3.9	5.6
K (μg)	4.4	8.3	<0.2	9.7	5.68
Thiamine (B$_1$) (μg)	150	233	4	275	184
Riboflavin (B$_2$) (μg)	220	417	15	492	264
Niacin (B$_3$) (mg)	3	3.57	52.4	4.18	3.68
Pantothenate (B$_5$) (mg)	0.73	1.5	74.8	1.78	0.92
Pyridoxine (B$_6$) (μg)	115	211	4.1	248	140
Biotin (B$_7$) (μg)	2.7	26	Unknown	30.2	3.36
Folate (B$_9$) (μg)	25	23	5.4	27.3	30.8
B$_{12}$ (μg)	0.18	0.64	0.05	0.33	0.64
C (ascorbate) (mg)	12	25	<0.2	30.8	15.2

[a] As of August 1, 2013.

ARA indicates arachidonic acid; DHA, docosahexaenoic acid.

Appendix E

Appendix E-1

Dietary Reference Intakes: Recommended Intakes for Individuals, Food and Nutrition Board, Institute of Medicine, The National Academies of Sciences

	Infants 0–6 mo	Infants 7–12 mo	Children 1–3 y	Children 4–8 y	Males 9–13 y	Males 14–18 y	Females 9–13 y	Females 14–18 y	Pregnancy ≤18 y	Lactation ≤18 y
Carbohydrate (g/day)	60*	95*	130	130	130	130	130	130	175	210
Total Fiber (g/day)	ND	ND	19*	25*	31*	38*	26*	26*	28*	29*
Fat (g/day)	31*	30*	ND	ND	ND	ND	ND	ND	ND	ND
n-6 Polyunsaturated Fatty Acids (g/day) (Linoleic Acid)	4.4*	4.6*	7*	10*	12*	16*	10*	11*	13*	13*
n-3 Polyunsaturated Fatty Acids (g/day) (α-Linolenic Acid)	0.5*	0.5*	0.7*	0.9*	1.2*	1.6*	1.0*	1.1*	1.4*	1.3*
Protein (g/kg/day)	1.52*	1.2*	1.05*	0.95*	0.95*	0.85*	0.95*	0.85*	1.1*	1.3*
Vitamin A (µg/d)a	400*	500*	300	400	600	900	600	700	750	1200
Vitamin C (mg/d)	40*	50*	15	25	45	75	45	65	80	115
Vitamin D (IU/d)b,c	400*	400*	600	600*	600	600*	600	600	600	600
Vitamin E (mg/d)d	4*	5*	6	7	11	15	11	15	15	19
Vitamin K (mg/d)	2.0*	2.5*	30*	55*	60*	75*	60*	75*	75*	75*

NOTE: This table (taken from the DRI reports, see www.nap.edu) presents Recommended Dietary Allowances (RDAs) in **bold type** and Adequate Intakes (AIs) are in ordinary type followed by and asterisk (*).

(*). RDAs and AIs may both be used as goals for individual intake. RDAs are set to meet the needs of almost all individuals in a group (97%–98%). For healthy breastfed infants, the AI is the mean intake. The AI for other life stage and gender groups is believed to cover needs of all individuals in the group, but lack of data or uncertainty in the data prevent being able to specify with confidence the percentage of individuals covered by this intake.

a As retinol activity equivalents (RAEs). 1 RAE = 1 µg retinol, 12 µg β-carotene, 24 µg α-carotene, or 24 µg β-cryptoxanthin in foods. The RAE for dietary provitamin A carotenoids is twofold greater than retinol equivalents (REs), whereas the RAE for preformed vitamin A is the same as RE.

b As cholecalciferol. 1 µg cholecalciferol = 40 IU vitamin D.

c In the absence of adequate exposure to sunlight.

d As α-tocopherol. α-Tocopherol includes *RRR*-α-tocopherol, the only form of α-tocopherol that occurs naturally in foods, and the *2R*-stereoisomeric forms of α-tocopherol (*RRR*-, *RSR*-, *RRS*-, and *RSS*-α-tocopherol) that occur in fortified foods and supplements. It does not include the *2S*-stereoisomeric forms of α-tocopherol (*SRR*-, *SSR*-, *SRS*-, and *SSS*-α-tocopherol), also found in fortified foods and supplements.

Appendix E-1 (continued)

Dietary Reference Intakes: Recommended Intakes for Individuals, Food and Nutrition Board, Institute of Medicine, The National Academies of Sciences

	Infants 0–6 mo	Infants 7–12 mo	Children 1–3 y	Children 4–8 y	Males 9–13 y	Males 14–18 y	Females 9–13 y	Females 14–18 y	Pregnancy ≤18 y	Lactation ≤18 y
Thiamin (mg/d)	0.2*	0.3*	0.5	0.6	0.9	1.2	0.9	1.0	1.4	1.4
Riboflavin (mg/d)	0.3*	0.4*	0.5	0.6	0.9	1.3	0.9	1.0	1.4	1.6
Niacin (mg/d)e	2*	4*	6	8	12	16	12	14	18	17
Vitamin B$_6$ (mg/d)	0.1*	0.3*	0.5	0.6	1.0	1.3	1.0	1.2	1.9	2.0
Folate (µg/d)f,h,i	65*	80*	150	200	300	400	300	400g	600h	500
Vitamin B$_{12}$ (µg/d)	0.4*	0.5*	0.9	1.2	1.8	2.4	1.8	2.4	2.6	2.8
Pantothenic acid (mg/d)	1.7*	1.8*	2*	3*	4*	5*	4*	5*	6*	7*
Biotin (µg/d)	5*	6*	8*	12*	20*	25*	20*	25*	30*	35*
Choline^g (mg/d)	125*	150*	200*	250*	375*	550*	375*	400*	450*	550*

e As niacin equivalents (NE). 1 mg of niacin = 60 mg of tryptophan; 0–6 months = preformed niacin (not NE).

f As dietary folate equivalents (DFE). 1 DFE=1 µg food folate = 0.6 µg of folic acid from fortified food or as a supplement consumed with food = 0.5 µg of a supplement taken on an empty stomach.

g Although AIs have been set for choline, there are few data to assess whether a dietary supply of choline is needed at all stages of the life cycle, and it may be that the choline requirement can be met by endogenous synthesis at some of these stages.

h In view of evidence linking folate intake with neural tube defects in the fetus, it is recommended that all women capable of becoming pregnant consume 400 µg from supplements or fortified foods in addition to intake of food folate from the diet.

i It is assumed that women will continue consuming 400 µg from supplements or fortified food until their pregnancy is confirmed and they enter prenatal care, which ordinarily occurs after the end of the periconceptional period—the critical time for formation of the neural tube.

Appendix E-1

Dietary Reference Intakes: Recommended Intakes for Individuals, Food and Nutrition Board, Institute of Medicine, The National Academies of Sciences

	Infants 0–6 mo	Infants 7–12 mo	Children 1–3 y	Children 4–8 y	Males 9–13 y	Males 14–18 y	Females 9–13 y	Females 14–18 y	Pregnancy ≤18 y	Lactation ≤18 y
Calcium (mg/d)	200*	260*	700	1000	1300	1300	1300	1300	1300	1300
Chromium (µg/d)	0.2*	5.5*	11*	15*	25*	35*	21*	24*	29*	44
Copper (µg/d)	200*	220*	340	440	700	890	700	890	1000	1300
Fluoride (mg/d)	0.01*	0.5*	0.7*	1*	2*	3*	3*	3*	3*	3*
Iodine (µg/d)	110*	130*	90	90	120	150	120	150	220	290
Iron (mg/d)	0.27*	11	7	10	8	11	8	15	27	10
Magnesium (mg/d)	30*	75*	80	130	240	410	240	360	400	360
Manganese (mg/d)	0.003*	0.6*	1.2*	1.5*	.9*	2.2*	1.6*	1.6*	2.0*	2.6*
Molybdenum (µg/d)	2*	3*	17	22	34	43	34	43	50	50
Phosphorus (mg/d)	100*	275*	460	500	1250	1250	1250	1250	1250	1250
Selenium (µg/d)	15*	20*	20	30	40	55	40	55	60	70
Zinc (mg/d)	2*	3	3	5	8	11	8	9	12	13
Potassium (g/d)	0.4*	0.7*	3.0*	3.8*	4.5*	4.7*	4.5*	4.7*	4.7*	5.1*
Sodium (g/d)	0.12*	0.37*	1.0*	1.2*	1.5*	1.5*	1.5*	1.5*	1.5*	1.5*
Chloride (g/d)	0.18*	0.57*	1.5*	1.9*	2.3*	2.3*	2.3*	2.3*	2.3*	2.3*

NOTE: This table presents Recommended Dietary Allowances (RDAs) in **bold type** and Adequate Intakes (AIs⁻ are in ordinary type followed by and asterisk (*). RDAs and AIs may both be used as goals for individual intake. RDAs are set to meet the needs of almost all individuals in a group (97–98%). For healthy breastfed infants, the AI is the mean intake. The AI for other life stage and gender groups is believed to cover needs of all individuals in the group, but lack of data or uncertainty in the data prevent being able to specify with confidence the percentage of individuals covered by this intake.

APP

Appendix E-2

Dietary Reference Intakes (DRIs): Tolerable Upper Intake Levels (UL[a]), Food and Nutrition Board, Institute of Medicine, The National Academies of Sciences

	Infants 0–6 mo	Infants 7–12 mo	Children 1–3 y	Children 4–8 y	Males/Females 9–13 y	Males/Females 14–18 y	Pregnancy ≤18y	Lactation ≤18y
Vitamin A (µg/d)[b]	600	600	600	900	1700	2800	2800	2800
Vitamin C (mg/d)	ND[f]	ND	400	650	1200	1800	1800	1800
Vitamin D (IU/d)	1000	1500	2500	3000	4000		4000	4000
Vitamin E (mg/d)[c,d]	ND	ND	200	300	600	800	800	800
Vitamin K (µg/d)	ND	ND	ND	ND	ND	ND	ND	ND
Thiamin (mg/d)	ND	ND	ND	ND	ND	ND	ND	ND
Riboflavin (mg/d)	ND	ND	ND	ND	ND	ND	ND	ND
Niacin (mg/d)[d]	ND	ND	10	15	20	30	30	30
Vitamin B$_6$ (mg/d)	ND	ND	30	40	60	80	80	80
Folate (µg/d)[d]	ND	ND	300	400	600	800	800	800
Vitamin B$_{12}$ (mg/d)	ND	ND	ND	ND	ND	ND	ND	ND
Pantothenic Acid (mg/d)	ND	ND	ND	ND	ND	ND	ND	ND
Biotin (µg/d)	ND	ND	ND	ND	ND	ND	ND	ND
Choline (mg/d)	ND	ND	1.0	1.0	2.0	3.0	3.0	3.0
Carotenoids[e]	ND	ND	ND	ND	ND	ND	ND	ND
Arsenic[b]	ND[f]	ND	ND	ND	ND	ND	ND	ND
Boron (mg/d)	ND	ND	3	6	11	17	17	17
Calcium (mg/d)	1000	1500	2500	2500	3000	3000	3000	3000
Chromium	ND	ND	ND	ND	ND	ND	ND	ND

Copper (µg/d)	ND	ND	1000	3000	5000	8000	8000	8000
Fluoride (mg/d)	0.7	0.9	1.3	2.2	10	10	10	10
Iodine (µg/d)	ND	ND	200	300	600	900	900	900
Iron (mg/d)	40	40	40	40	40	45	45	45
Magnesium (mg/d)c	ND	ND	65	110	350	350	350	350
Manganese (mg/d)	ND	ND	2	3	6	9	9	9
Molybdenum (µg/d)	ND	ND	300	600	1100	1700	1700	1700
Nickel (mg/d)	ND	ND	0.2	0.3	0.6	1.0	1.0	1.0
Phosphorus (mg/d)	ND	ND	3	3	4	4	3.5	4
Potassium	ND	ND	ND	ND	ND	ND	ND	ND
Selenium (µg/d)	45	60	90	150	280	400	400	400
Silicond	ND	ND	ND	ND	ND	ND	ND	ND
Sulfate	ND	ND	ND	ND	ND	ND	ND	ND
Vanadium (mg/d)e	ND	ND	ND	ND	ND	ND	ND	ND
Zinc (mg/d)	4	5	7	12	23	34	34	34
Sodium (g/d)	ND	ND	1.5	1.9	2.2	2.3	2.3	2.3
Chloride (g/d)	ND	ND	2.3	2.9	3.4	3.6	3.6	3.6

a UL = The maximum level of daily nutrient intake that is likely to pose no risk of adverse effects. Unless otherwise specified, the UL represents total intake from food, water, and supplements. Due to lack of suitable data, ULs could not be established for vitamin K, thiamin, riboflavin, vitamin B_{12}, pantothenic acid, biotin, or carotenoids. In the absences of ULs, extra caution may be warranted in consuming levels above recommended intakes.

b As preformed vitamin A only.

c As α-tocopherol; applies to any form of supplemental α-tocopherol.

d The ULs for vitamin E, niacin, and folate apply to synthetic forms obtained from supplements, fortified foods, or a combination of the two.

e β-Carotene supplements are advised only to serve as a provitamin A source for individuals at risk of vitamin A deficiency.

f ND = Not determinable due to lack of data of adverse effects in this age group and concern with regard to lack of ability to handle excess amounts.

APP

Appendix F

Fig. F-1
ChooseMyPlate

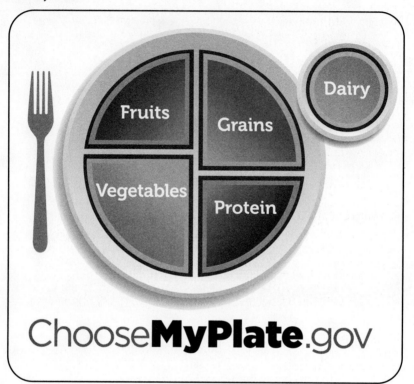

Fig. F-2

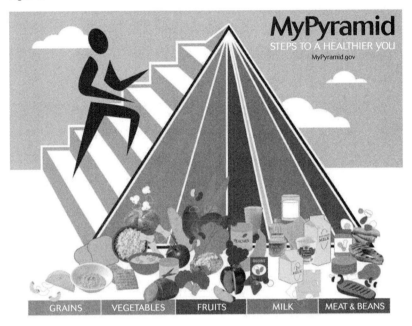

Illustration of mini-poster from the US Department of Agriculture's MyPyramid, which provides food-based guidance for professionals and the public to help implement the recommendations of the Dietary Guidelines for Americans for people 2 years and older (for Web version of poster, see http://www.mypyramid.gov/downloads/MiniPoster.pdf).

Fig. F-3.A
Simplified version.

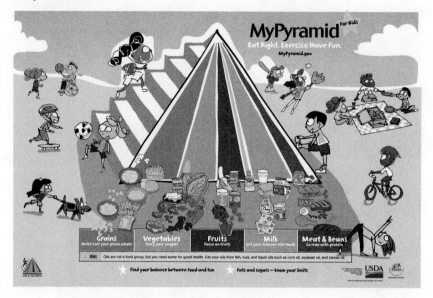

Fig. F-3.B
Advanced version.

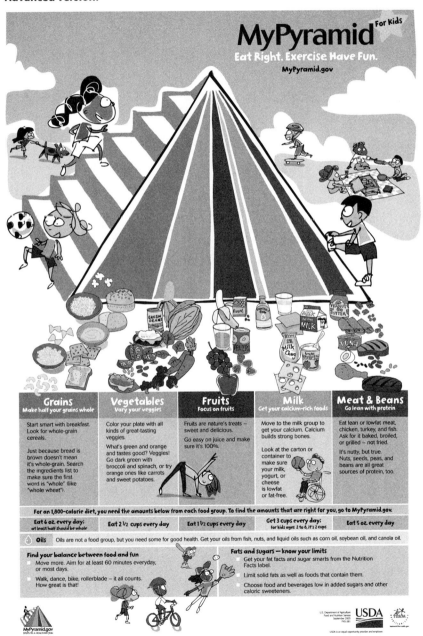

Fig. F-4

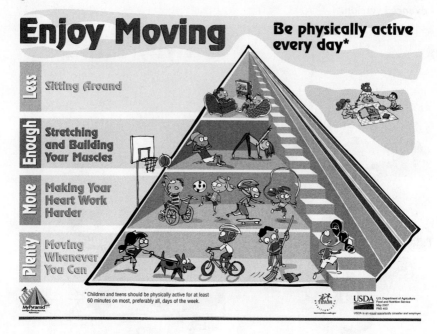

Appendix G

Food-Drug Interactions

Food-drug interactions occur when an ingested food or nutrient alters the effects of a medication. Conversely, medications can alter the effects of vitamins, minerals, and other nutrients in the body and may also interfere with food intake by affecting appetite. Medications can stimulate or suppress appetite.

Food components can enhance, delay, or decrease drug absorption. Some nutrients can alter metabolism by binding with drug ingredients to reduce their absorption, or speed their elimination. Some medications *should* be administered with food, in order to minimize gastrointestinal distress, or to maximize the drug's effect. Certain nutrients found in food and/or antacids have the ability to bind up certain medications in the stomach, decreasing the absorption of the drug from the stomach into the bloodstream. However, some nutrients can interfere with drug absorption, thereby reducing the efficacy of the drug. In these cases, it is advisable to administer these medications on an empty stomach. A food-drug interaction occurs when a medication affects food or a nutrient in food.

Some well-known food-drug interactions include MAO inhibitors with tyramine-containing foods, such as red wine and aged cheese, and warfarin with green, leafy vegetables and other foods high in vitamin K. There are many food-drug interactions reported in the literature, of varying clinical significance.

In recent years, there has been increased awareness of the potential for medications to interact with grapefruit juice. Drugs that interact with grapefruit and/or grapefruit juice undergo cytochrome p450 oxidative metabolism in the intestinal wall or liver. Grapefruit juice contains substances that have been demonstrated to affect the cytochrome p450 (CYP) system by binding to the isoenzyme as a substrate and impairing first-pass metabolism, by direct inactivation or inhibition of the enzyme. This seems to result in a selective down-regulation of CYP3A4 in the small intestine. For certain drugs which are known to be metabolized this way, less drug is metabolized prior to absorption, so more drug reaches the systemic circulation, leading to higher blood levels, and potential increases in therapeutic and/or toxic effects. If patients are accustomed to ingesting grapefruit juice while on chronic medications, it is best that they avoid significant increases or decreases in the amount of grapefruit juice they are ingesting.

In addition, drugs can affect metabolism of minerals and vitamins. Examples of this include low folate levels in patients on chronic anticonvulsant therapy, and diuretics causing electrolyedepletion. Laxatives can decrease the absorption of many vitamins and minerals.

Many factors determine the clinical significance of food-drug interactions. These include, but are not limited to the dosage of the drug, the dosage form, and patient factors. Patient factors include age, size, and health status, as well as when the food was consumed in relation to the medication. Identifying a food-drug interaction may not mean that the offending agent must be completely avoided. In some cases, adjustments can be made to allow for the medication to administered in a way that avoids or minimizes the interaction, such as with food, or on an empty stomach.

Medications may affect food intake and nutritional status by causing adverse effects such as taste disturbance, dry mouth, or stomatitis and esophagitis. Gastrointestinal effects caused by medications may result in decreased food intake by making it difficult or unappealing for patients to eat. There are also medications that can stimulate appetite, resulting in weight gain. In the case of medications like cypropheptadine and megestrol, this side effect is used for the patient's benefit.

The following tables provide some specific information about food-drug interactions, and issues related to medication administration. Please be advised that this is not a substitute for clinical judgment. Readers are advised to consult current references, because clinical information frequently changes. Although this is a comprehensive list, there could be omissions and changes. Thus, the absence of a medication does not necessarily mean that it is not associated with an interaction.

Appendix G
Drug-Nutrient Interactions

G – 1	Drugs for Which Absorption Is Increased by Food
G – 2	Drugs for Which Absorption May Be Delayed by Food
G – 3	Drugs That Should Be Administered on an Empty Stomach
G – 4	Drugs That Should Be Administered With Food
G – 5	Miscellaneous Food-Nutrient Effects
G – 6	Drug-Grapefruit Juice Interactions

Appendix G - 1
Drugs for Which Absorption Is Increased by Food

Atovaquone (administer with a high-fat meal)
Atovaquone/proguanil
Azithromycin (food increases AUC; extended-release tablets should be administered with food)
Cefpodoxime
Cefuroxime
Erythromycin
Griseofulvin (administer with a high-fat meal)
Morphine sulfate (oral solution)
Nitrofurantoin
Theophylline sustained release (food may induce sudden release of QD sustained-release preparation)

Appendix G - 2
Drugs for Which Absorption May Be Delayed by Food or Milk (drugs in this category should either be administered on an empty stomach or taken consistently with regard to food)

Medication Name	Comments
Acetaminophen	Rate may decreased by food
Amitriptyline	Increased fiber may decrease effect
Ampicillin	Food decreases rate and extent of absorption
Aripiprazole	High-fat meal delays time to peak plasma level
Cephalosporins	Food may delay absorption
Ciprofloxacin	Dairy products/minerals decrease concentration food decreases rate of absorption enteral feeds decrease plasma concentration by >30%
Digoxin	Increased fiber or pectin may decrease absorption; food may decrease peak serum concentration
Diltiazem	Food may increase absorption
Fluoxetine	Food may delay absorption by 1-2 h
Furosemide	Avoid acidic solutions; food may decrease serum levels
Glipizide	Rate of absorption, not extent, delayed by food delayed release of insulin with food
Lansoprazole	Food decreases bioavailability
Metronidazole	Peak serum concentration decreased and delayed
Omeprazole	Mixing 20-mg capsule with applesauce may decrease peak plasma concentration; unknown clinical significance
Penicillin	Food or milk may decrease absorption
Trazodone	Rate of absorption, not extent, delayed by food
Valproic acid	Rate of absorption, not extent, delayed by food
Zafirlukast	Food decreases absorption by 40%

APP

Appendix G - 3
Drugs That Should Be Administered on an Empty Stomach

Ampicillin
Amprenavir (avoid antacids and high-fat meals)
Atenolol
Captopril
Ceftibuten
Cloxacillin
Dicloxacillin
Didanosine
Diltiazem
Efavirenz
Erythromycin base: avoid citrus and carbonated drinks, may administer with food to decrease gastrointestinal distress
Indinavir
Iron: avoid milk and antacids
Isoniazid
Itraconazole oral solution
Ketoconazole: administer 2 h prior to antacids; may administer with food to decrease gastrointestinal distress
Lansoprazole
Levofloxacin oral solution
Loracarbef
Metronidazole (may administer with food if gastrointestinal distress occurs)
Mycophenolate
Nifedipine
Omeprazole
Rifampin (may administer with food to decrease gastrointestinal distress)
Tacrolimus (separate antacids by at least 2 h)
Tetracycline
Zafirlukast

Appendix G - 4
Drugs That Should Be Administered With Food

Allopurinol: after meals with fluid	Itraconazole capsules
Atovaquone	Ketorolac
Amoxicillin/clavulanate	Lithium
Aspirin	Mebendazole
Baclofen	Methylprednisolone
Bromocriptine	Naproxen
Carvedilol	Nelfinavir
Carbamazepine	Nitrofurantoin
Cefpodoxime tablets	Olsalazine
Chloroquine	Potassium
Cimetidine	Prednisone
Diclofenac	Ritonavir
Divalproex	Salsalate
Doxycycline	Saquinavir
Fludrocortisone	Sevelamer
Fenoprofen	Spironolactone
Glyburide	Sulfasalazine
Hydrocortisone	Sulindac
Hydroxychloroquine	Ticlopidine
Ibuprofen	Trazodone
Indomethacin	Valproic acid

Appendix G – 5
Miscellaneous Food-Nutrient Effects

Drug or Class	Nutrient	Comment
Albuterol	Glucose	May cause hyperglycemia
	Potassium	May cause hypokalemia
Amiloride	Potassium	May cause hyperkalemia
Amphotericin	Magnesium	Causes electrolyte wasting
	Potassium	
	Sodium	
Aspirin	Folate	May cause folate deficiency
	Vitamin C	May increase vitamin C excretion
	Iron	May cause iron deficiency anemia

Appendix G – 5 *(continued)*
Miscellaneous Food-Nutrient Effects

Captopril	Potassium	May cause small increases in serum potassium
	Zinc	May cause zinc deficiency (long-term)
Ciprofloxacin	Enteral feeds	Enteral feeds may interfere with absorption
	Caffeine	May increase caffeine concentration
Cisplatin	Magnesium	Causes magnesium depletion
Cholestyramine	Fat-soluble vitamins	May result in deficiency
Corticosteroids	Glucose	May cause hyperglycemia
Digoxin	Calcium	May cause arrhythmias due to inotropic effect
	Antacids, fiber	May decrease digoxin effects
	Licorice	Avoid natural licorice
Ethambutol	Aluminum salts	May decrease absorption of ethambutol
Furosemide	Calcium	May cause electrolyte depletion
	Magnesium	
	Potassium	
	Sodium	
Gabapentin	Glucose	May cause fluctuations in glucose and weight gain
Glipizide, glyburide	Alcohol	Disulfiram-like reaction with alcohol
Insulin	Concentrated sugar	Can increase insulin requirement
Isoniazid	Pyridoxine	Isoniazid is a B_6 antagonist
Isotretinoin	Vitamin A	May result in increased toxicity
Lithium	Sodium	Maintain constant sodium intake
	Caffeine	Caffeine may decrease lithium effects to avoid toxicity
MAOIs	Tyramine	Dietary tyramine can cause hypertensive crisis
Methotrexate	Folic acid	Folic acid may decrease effects
Metronidazole	Alcohol	Causes disulfuram-like reaction
Mineral oil	Fat-soluble vitamins	May decrease absorption of fat-soluble vitamins
NSAIDs	Potassium	May cause hyperkalemia in patients w/renal impairment or on supplements, or potassium-sparing diuretics
Omeprazole, Lansoprozole	Acid	Acid-labile drug, administer w/beads intact
Pancreatic enzymes	Calcium carbonate	May increase drug effect
	Magnesium hydroxide	
Phenobarbital	Protein	Be consistent with protein intake
	Vitamin C	Displaces drug from binding sites
	Vitamin D	Deficiency may result from malabsorption

Phenytoin	Enteral feeds	May interfere with phenytoin absorption
	Folate	High-dose folic acid may reverse drug effects
	Calcium	Phenytoin decreases absorption
	Vitamin D	May interfere with phenytoin metabolism
	Vitamin C	Displaces drug from binding sites
	Glucose	May cause hypoglycemia
Primidone	Folic acid	Megaloblastic anemia due to folate deficiency may occur
Propranolol	Protein rich foods	May result in increased propranolol effects
Spironolactone	Potassium	May cause hyperkalemia, avoid supplements
Sulfasalazine	Folic acid	May inhibit abosrption of folate
Terbutaline	Glucose, potassium	May cause hyperglycemia, hypokalemia
Theophylline	Caffeine	May cause increased theophylline toxicity
Thiazide diuretics	Magnesium	May cause electrolyte depletion
	Sodium	
	Potassium	
Trimethoprim	Folate	May cause folate depletion
Valproic acid	Carbonated beverages	Avoid carbonated beverages with syrup
	Carnitine	May cause carnitine deficiency with hyperammonemia
Warfarin	Vitamin K	May inhibit response to warfarin
	Vitamins A, C, E	May alter prothrombin time
Zidovudine	Folate, B_{12}	Deficiency may increase myelosuppression

Appendix G - 6
Drug-Grapefruit Juice Interactions

Drug	Effect of Grapefruit Juice on Drug Concentration	Clinical Significance	Onset
Amlodipine	Increases	Minor	Delayed
Atorvastatin	Increases	Moderate	Rapid
Buspirone	Increases	Moderate	Rapid
Carbamazepine	Increases	Moderate	Rapid
Cisapride	Increases	Major	Rapid
Clomipramine	Increases	Moderate	Delayed
Cyclosprine	Increases	Moderate	Delayed
Diazepam (all benzodiazepines)	Increases	Moderate	Rapid
Felodipine	Increases	Moderate	Rapid
Fentanyl	Increases	Moderate	Unknown

Appendix G - 6 *(continued)*
Drug-Grapefruit Juice Interactions

Indinavir	Decreases	No dose changes needed per manufacturer	Not applicable
Itraconazole	Decreases area under the curve by 30%	Moderate	Rapid
Lovastatin	Increases	Moderate	Rapid
Methylprednisolone	Increases	May be significant	Unknown
Midazolam	Increases	Moderate	Rapid
Nicardipine	Increases	Moderate	Unknown
Nifedipine	Increases	Moderate	Rapid
Nimodipine	Increases	Moderate	Rapid
Nisoldipine	Increases	Moderate	Rapid
Pimozide	Increases	Major	Rapid
Quinidine	Unknown	Moderate	Rapid
Saquinavir	Increases drug level	Moderate	Rapid
Sertraline	Increases	Moderate	Delayed
Simvastatin	Increases	Moderate	Rapid
Sirolimus	Increases	Moderate	Delayed
Tacrolimus	Increases	Moderate	Delayed
Triazolam	Increases	Minor	Rapid
Zolpidem	Increases	Minor	Unknown

References:

Bland SE. Drug-food interactions. *J Pharm Soc Wisc*. 1998;Nov-Dec:28-35

Elbe D. Drug commentary: grapefruit juice-drug interactions. *BC Pharmacy*. 1998;7:18-19

Global RPH: The Clinician's Ultimate Reference. Available at: www.globalrph.com. Accessed January 31, 2013

Kane G, Lipsky J. Drug-grapefruit juice interactions. *Mayo Clin Proc*. 2000;75(9):933-942

Kirk J. Significant drug-nutrient interactions. *Am Fam Phys*. 1995;51(5):1175-1182

Lexi-Comp Online. Pediatric & Neonatal Lexi-Drugs Online. Hudson, OH: Lexi-Comp Inc; January 29, 2011

Maka D, Murphy L. *Drug-Nutrient Interactions: A Review. Advanced Practice in Acute & Critical Care*. 2000; 11(4)580-588

Merck Manual of Diagnosis and Therapy. Whitehouse Station, NJ: Merck Inc; 2011

Micromedex Healthcare Series [Internet database]. Greenwood Village, CO: Thomson Reuters (Healthcare) Inc. Available at: http://www.micromedex.com/products/hcs/. Accessed January 31, 2013

Appendix H

Appendix H.
Calories and Electrolytes in Beverages

Beverages Calories and Selected Electrolytes (per fl oz)[a]				
Beverage	Energy, kcal	Sodium, mg	Potassium, mg	Phosphorous, mg
Regular Soft Drinks				
Cola or pepper cola	11–13	1–3	0–1	3
Decaffeinated cola	13	1	1	3
Lemon-lime (clear)	12	3	0	0
Orange	15	4	1	0
Grape	13	5	0	0
Root beer	13	4	0	0
Ginger ale	10	2	0	0
Tonic water	10	2	0	0
Diet Soft Drinks				
Diet cola or pepper cola	1	2	2	3
Decaffeinated diet cola or pepper cola	0	1	2	3
Diet lemon-lime	0	2	1	0
Diet root beer	0	5	3	1
Club soda, seltzer, and sparkling water	0	6	1	0
Apricot nectar, canned	18	1	36	3
Apple juice, unsweetened	14	1	31	2
Cranberry juice cocktail, bottled	17	1	4	0
Grape juice, canned, unsweetened	19	2	33	4
Grapefruit juice, canned, unsweetened	12	0	47	3
Orange juice, raw	14	0	62	5
Pear nectar, canned	19	1	4	1
Peach nectar, canned	17	2	12	2
Pineapple juice, canned, unsweetened	17	1	41	3
Tomato juice, canned, without salt added	5	3	70	5

[a] From US Department of Agriculture, Agricultural Research Service. USDA National Nutrient Database for Standard Reference, Release 23. 2010. Available at: http://www.ars.usda.gov/ba/bhnrc/ndl. Accessed January 31, 2013

APP

Appendix I

Appendix I-1
Selected Food Sources Ranked by Amount of Dietary Fiber and Calories per Standard Portion

Food	Standard Portion Size	Calories in Standard Portion	Dietary Fiber in Standard Portion (g)
Beans (navy, pinto, black, kidney, white, great northern, lima), cooked	½ cup	104–149	6.2–9.6
Bran ready-to-eat cereal (100%)	⅓ cup (about 1 oz)	81	9.1
Split peas, lentils, chickpeas, or cowpeas, cooked	½ cup	108–134	5.6–8.1
Artichoke, cooked	½ cup hearts	45	7.2
Pear	1 medium	103	5.5
Soybeans, mature, cooked	½ cup	149	5.2
Plain rye wafer crackers	2 wafers	73	5.0
Bran ready-to-eat cereals (various)	⅓–¾ cup (about 1 oz)	88–91	2.6–5.0
Asian pear	1 small	51	4.4
Green peas, cooked	½ cup	59–67	3.5–4.4
Whole-wheat English muffin	1 muffin	134	4.4
Bulgur, cooked	½ cup	76	4.1
Mixed vegetables, cooked	½ cup	59	4.0
Raspberries	½ cup	32	4.0
Sweet potato, baked in skin	1 medium	103	3.8
Blackberries	½ cup	31	3.8
Soybeans, green, cooked	½ cup	127	3.8
Prunes, stewed	½ cup	133	3.8
Shredded wheat ready-to-eat cereal	½ cup (about 1 oz)	95–100	2.7–3.8
Figs, dried	¼ cup	93	3.7
Apple, with skin	1 small	77	3.6
Pumpkin, canned	½ cup	42	3.6
Greens (spinach, collards, turnip greens), cooked	½ cup	14–32	2.5–3.5
Almonds	1 oz	163	3.5
Sauerkraut, canned	½ cup	22	3.4
Whole-wheat spaghetti, cooked	½ cup	87	3.1
Banana	1 medium	105	3.1
Orange	1 medium	62	3.1
Guava	1 fruit	37	3.0
Potato, baked, with skin	1 small	128	3.0

Appendix I-1 *(continued)*
Selected Food Sources Ranked by Amount of Dietary Fiber and Calories per Standard Portion

Oat bran muffin	1 small	178	3.0
Pearled barley, cooked	½ cup	97	3.0
Dates	¼ cup	104	2.9
Winter squash, cooked	½ cup	38	2.9
Parsnips, cooked	½ cup	55	2.8
Tomato paste	¼ cup	54	2.7
Broccoli, cooked	½ cup	26–27	2.6–2.8
Okra, cooked from frozen	½ cup	26	2.6

Source: US Department of Agriculture, Agricultural Research Service, Nutrient Data Laboratory. 2009. USDA National Nutrient Database for Standard Reference, Release 22. Available at: http://www.ars.usda.gov/research/publications/publications.htm?seq_no_115=243584. Accessed January 31, 2013

Appendix I-2
Available Over-the-Counter Fiber Preparations

Brand	Form	Fiber Sources	Fluid
Benefiber	Caplets	Wheat dextrin, microcrystalline cellulose	No
	Stick packs	Wheat dextrin	4- to 8-oz/packet
	Tablets	Wheat dextrin, cellulose	No
	Powder	Wheat dextrin	4-8 oz/tbsp
Citrucel	Caplets	Methylcellulose	8 oz/dose
	Powder	Methylcellulose	8 oz/tbsp
Fiber Choice	Tablets	Inulin, cellulose	No
FiberCon	Caplets	Calcium polycarbophil	8 oz/dose
Metamucil	Capsules	Psyllium husk	8 oz/dose
	Powder	Psyllium husk	8 oz/dose
	Wafers	Psyllium husk	8 oz/dose
	Clear and natural	Inulin	8 oz/dose
Senokot	Tablets	Hydroxy-anthracene glycosides	8 oz/dose
Ultra-Fiber	Caplets	Psyllium, oat bran, orange fiber, apple fiber, prune fiber	8 oz/dose
Fiber Gummies	Gummies	Polydextrose	No

Appendix J

Appendix J-1

Approximate Calcium Contents of 1 Serving of Some Common Foods That Are Good Sources of Calcium

Food	Serving Size	Calcium Content, mg	No. of Servings to Equal Calcium Content in 1 Cup of Low-Fat Milk
Dairy foods			
Whole milk	1 cup (244 g)	276	1.1
Low-fat (1%) milk	1 cup (244 g)	305	—
Nonfat milk	1 cup (245 g)	299	1.02
Yogurt, nonfat, fruit variety	6 oz (170 g)	258	1.2
Frozen yogurt, vanilla, soft serve	½ cup (72 g)	103	3.0
Cheese, cheddar	1 1-oz slice (28 g)	202	1.5
Cheese, pasteurized, processed, American	1 3/4-oz slice (21 g)	144	2.1
Cheese, ricotta, part skim milk	½ cup (124 g)	337	0.9
Nondairy foods			
Salmon, sockeye canned, drained, with bones	3 oz (85 g)	188	1.6
Tofu, firm, prepared with calcium sulfate and magnesium chloride	½ cup (126 g)	253	1.2
White beans, cooked, boiled	1 cup (179 g)	161	1.9
Broccoli, cooked, boiled, drained	1 cup, chopped (156 g)	62	4.9
Collards, cooked, boiled, drained	1 cup, chopped (190 g)	266	1.1
Baked beans, canned	1 cup (253 g)	126	2.4
Tomatoes, canned, stewed	1 cup (255 g)	87	3.5
Foods fortified with calcium			
Calcium-fortified orange juice	1 cup (240 mL)	500	0.6
Selected calcium-fortified cereal	¾ cup (30 g)	1000	0.3
Instant oatmeal, fortified, plain, prepared with water	½ cup (117 g)	94	3.2
English muffin, plain, enriched, with calcium propionate	1 muffin (57 g)	93	3.3
Low-fat calcium-fortified soy milk[a] (all flavors)	1 cup (240 mL)	199	1.5

From US Department of Agriculture, Agricultural Research Service. 2010. USDA National Nutrient Database for Standard Reference, Release 23. Nutrient Data Laboratory Home Page. Available at: http://www.ars.usda.gov/ba/bhnrc/ndl. Accessed January 31, 2013.

[a] Native soy milk contains 63 mg of calcium per cup (240 mL).

Appendix J-2.
Calcium Content of Foods, mg per Serving[a]

100	150	200	250
15 Brazil nuts	1 cup ice cream	1 oz cheddar or Muenster cheese	1 cup almonds
2 cups instant farina, dry	1 cup oysters	1 oz Swiss or Parmesan cheese	1 cup milk
1 cup cooked kale	1 cup cooked rhubarb	3 oz sardines with bones	1 cup low-fat chocolate milk
3 tbsp molasses	1 oz feta or mozzarella cheese	1 cup low-fat soy milk with added calcium (all flavors)	½ cup ricotta cheese
1 cup cooked navy beans	3 oz canned salmon with bones		6 medium stalks broccoli
1 cup sunflower seeds	1 cup cottage cheese, regular or low fat		½ cup tofu, with calcium sulfate
5 tbsp maple syrup	1 cup cooked dandelion greens		½ cup cooked collards
1 cup beet greens			1 cup cooked spinach
1 cup unfortified soymilk, original/vanilla			8 oz low-fat fruit yogurt

[a]Values are approximate.

From US Department of Agriculture, Agricultural Research Service. 2010. USDA National Nutrient Database for Standard Reference, Release 23. Nutrient Data Laboratory Home Page. Available at: http://www.ars.usda.gov/ba/bhnrc/ndl. Accessed January 31, 2013.

Appendix K

Appendix K:
Iron Content of Selected Foods

Food	Portion	Iron, mg
Apricots, raw	3 medium	0.41
Avocado, California	1 medium	0.83
Banana, raw	1 medium	0.31
Black-eyed peas, boiled	½ cup	1.8
Bread, white	1 slice	0.94
Bread, whole wheat	1 slice	0.68
Broccoli, boiled	½ cup	0.52
Brussels sprouts	½ cup	0.94
Butter	1 tsp	0.00
Cheddar cheese	1 oz (1 slice)	0.19
Chicken, light and dark, without skin, roasted	3.5 oz	1.20
Chocolate, semisweet	1 oz	0.89
Chocolate, sweet	1 oz	0.78
Clams, raw	3 oz	1.38
Cream of wheat, instant, cooked	¾ cup	8.98
Egg, white	1 large	0.03
Egg, whole	1 large	0.88
Egg, yolk	1 large	0.46
Frankfurter, beef	1 frank, 8/lb	0.86
Frankfurter, turkey	1 frank, 10/lb	0.66
Garbanzos, canned	½ cup	1.62
Grape juice, from frozen concentrate	8 oz	0.25
Grapes, red or green, raw	1 cup	0.54
Halibut, cooked	3 oz	0.17
Ham, 95% lean meat	1 oz	0.29
Hamburger, extra lean, broiled, medium	3 oz	2.41
Lettuce, iceberg	1 leaf	0.06
Lettuce, romaine, shredded	½ cup	0.23
Liver (beef)	3 ½ oz	4.85
Liver (pork)	3 ½ oz	23.12
Milk, 2%	8 oz	0.05
Molasses	1 tbsp	0.94
Navy beans, canned	½ cup	2.42
Oatmeal, cooked with water	¾ cup	1.57

Appendix K: *(continued)*
Iron Content of Selected Foods

Food	Portion	Iron, mg
Orange juice, from frozen concentrate	8 oz	0.99
Oysters, raw (Eastern)	6 medium	3.87
Papaya nectar, canned	8 oz	0.85
Peanut butter, smooth	1 tbsp	0.30
Potato, baked with skin	6 ½ oz	1.87
Prune juice, canned	½ cup	1.51
Prunes, dried, cooked	½ cup	1.64
Raisins, seedless	⅔ cup	1.80
Rice, brown, cooked	1 cup	0.82
Rice, white, enriched	1 cup	1.90
Soybeans, green, boiled	½ cup	2.25
Spinach, boiled	½ cup	3.21
Tomato juice, no added salt	½ cup	0.52
Tortilla, corn	1 (1 oz)	0.66
Yeast, baker's	1 oz	0.62
Yogurt, low fat (12 g protein per 8-oz serving)	8 oz	0.18

From US Department of Agriculture, Agricultural Research Service. 2010. USDA National Nutrient Database for Standard Reference, Release 23. Nutrient Data Laboratory Home Page. Available at: http://www.ars.usda.gov/ba/bhnrc/ndl. Accessed January 31, 2013.

Appendix L

Appendix L.
Zinc Content of Common Household Portions of Selected Foods

Food	Portion	Zinc, mg
Fish (flounder, tuna, salmon)	3 oz	0.33
Oysters, Eastern, wild, raw	6 medium	33.01
Crab	3 oz	3.24
Poultry 　　Dark meat 　　Light meat	 3 oz 3 oz	 2.48 1.23
Beef, tenderloin	3 oz	3.43
Pork, loin	3 oz	2.46
Bologna	3 oz	0.40
Liver (pork)	3 oz	4.90
Whole egg	1 large	0.65
Dried lentils	½ cup	4.59
Milk, whole	1 cup	0.90
Cheese (cheddar)	1 oz	0.88
Bread 　　White 　　Wheat	 1 slice 1 slice	 0.21 0.51
Rice 　　White, unenriched 　　Brown	 ½ cup ½ cup	 0.29 0.61
Cornmeal (cooked)	½ cup	0.52
Oatmeal (cooked)	½ cup	1.17
Bran flakes	1 oz	1.42
Corn flakes	1 oz	0.08

From US Department of Agriculture, Agricultural Research Service. 2010. USDA National Nutrient Database for Standard Reference, Release 23. Nutrient Data Laboratory Home Page. Available at: http://www.ars.usda.gov/ba/bhnrc/ndl. Accessed January 31, 2013

Appendix M

Appendix M:
Parenteral Nutrition Solutions

Product (Manufacturer)	Solutions Designed for Infants							
	Aminosyn PF 10% (Abbott)	TrophAmine 10% (BBraun)	Premasol 10% (Baxter)	Aminosyn 3.5% (Abbott)	Aminosyn II 3.5% (Abbott)	FreAmine III 10% (McGaw)	Travasol 10% (Clintec)
Essential Amino Acids (g/100 mL)							
Isoleucine	0.760	0.820	0.820	0.252	0.231	0.690	0.600
Leucine	1.200	1.400	1.400	0.329	0.350	0.910	0.730
Lysine	0.677	0.820	0.820	0.252	0.368	0.730	0.580
Methionine	0.180	0.340	0.340	0.140	0.060	0.530	0.400
Phenylalanine	0.427	0.48	0.480	0.154	0.104	0.560	0.560
Threonine	0.512	0.420	0.420	0.182	0.140	0.400	0.420
Tryptophan	0.180	0.200	0.200	0.056	0.070	0.150	0.180
Valine	0.673	0.780	0.780	0.280	0.175	0.660	0.580

Appendix M: *(continued)*
Parenteral Nutrition Solutions

Product (Manufacturer)	Solutions Designed for Infants						
	Aminosyn PF 10% (Abbott)	TrophAmine 10% (BBraun)	Premasol 10% (Baxter)	Aminosyn 3.5% (Abbott)	Aminosyn II 3.5% (Abbott)	FreAmine III 10% (McGaw)	Travasol 10% (Clintec)
Nonessential Amino Acids (g/100 mL)							
Alanine	0.698	0.540	0.540	0.448	0.348	0.710	2.070
Arginine	1.227	1.200	1.200	0.343	0.356	0.950	1.150
Histidine[a]	0.312	0.480	0.480	0.105	0.105	0.280	0.480
Proline	0.812	0.680	0.680	0.300	0.253	1.120	0.680
Serine	0.495	0.380	0.380	0.147	0.186	0.590	0.500
Taurine	0.070	0.025	0.025	–	–	–	–
Tyrosine	0.044	0.240	0.240	0.031	0.095	–	0.040
Glycine	0.385	0.360	0.360	0.448	0.175	1.400	1.030
Glutamic acid	0.820	0.500	0.500	–	0.258	–	–
Aspartic acid	0.527	0.320	0.320	–	0.245	–	–
Cysteine	–	<0.016	<0.016	–	–	–	–
N-ac-L-tyrosine	0.044	0.240	0.240	–	–	–	–
Nitrogen (g/100 mL)	1.52	1.55	1.55	0.55	0.54	1.53	1.65

[a] Histidine is considered an essential amino acid in infants and in renal failure.

Appendix N

Selected Enteral Products for Special Indications[a]

Product	Energy, kcal/L	Protein Source, g/L	Carbohydrate Source, g/L	Fat Source, g/L	Fiber g/L	Purpose
Benecalorie (Nestle)	330/41.3 g (1.5 oz)	Ca caseinate	7	None	0	High-oleic sunflower oil	33	High-calorie protein/fat-based liquid modular supplement, nutritionally incomplete
Beneprotein (Nestle)	25/7 g (1 scoop)	Whey protein isolates	6	None	0	None	0	Protein powder modular supplement, nutritionally incomplete
Boost Breeze (Nestle)	1060	Whey protein isolate	38	Sugar, corn syrup	230	None	0	Fat-free clear liquid oral supplement, incomplete nutrition
Boost (Nestle)	1010	Milk-protein concentrate	42	Corn syrup solids, sucrose	180	Canola, high-oleic sunflower, and corn oils	17	Nutritionally complete, lactose-free oral supplement
Boost Glucose Control (Nestle)	1060	Na and Ca caseinates (milk), L-arginine	58.2	Tapioca dextrin, fructose, corn syrup solids	84	Canola oil	14.8	Adult formula specifically formulated for use in the dietary management of diabetes mellitus
Boost High Protein (Nestle)	1010	Milk protein concentrate, Na and Ca caseinate	61	Corn syrup solids, sucrose	139	Canola, high-oleic sunflower, and corn oils	23	High-protein, nutritionally complete oral supplement
Boost Plus (Nestle)	1520	Na and Ca caseinate, milk protein concentrate	59	Corn syrup solids, sucrose	190	Canola, high-oleic sunflower, and corn oils	58	High-calorie nutritionally complete oral supplement
Boost Kids Essentials 1.0 (Nestle)	1000	Na and Ca caseinate, whey protein concentrate	30	Sucrose, maltodextrins	135	High-oleic sunflower, soybean and medium-chain triglyceride (MCT) oils	38	Complete formula for children 1–13 y
Boost Kids Essentials 1.5 (Nestle)	1498	Na and Ca caseinate, whey protein concentrate	42	Sucrose, maltodextrins	165	High-oleic sunflower soybean and MCT oils	75	High-calorie complete formula for children 1–13 y

Appendix N-1. (continued)
Selected Enteral Products for Special Indications[a]

Product		Protein source		CHO source		Fat source		Fiber	Comments
Boost Kids Essentials 1.5 w/ fiber (Nestle)	1498	Na and Ca caseinate, whey protein concentrate	42	Sucrose, maltodextrins	165	High-oleic sunflower, soybean and MCT oils	75	9	High-calorie complete formula for children 1–13 y with soluble and insoluble fiber
Carnation Breakfast Lactose Free (Nestle)	1000	Ca caseinate	35	Corn syrup solids, sucrose	132.4	Canola and corn oils, soy lecithin	36.8		Lactose-free, gluten-free, low-residue oral supplement
Carnation Breakfast Lactose Free Plus (Nestle)	1500	Ca caseinate	52.4	Corn syrup solids, sucrose	176.4	Canola and corn oils, soy lecithin	68		High-calorie, lactose-free, gluten-free, low-residue oral supplement
Carnation Breakfast Lactose Free VHC (Nestle)	2240	Ca-potassium caseinate, isolated soy protein	90	Corn syrup solids, sucrose	196.8	Canola and corn oils, soy lecithin	122.4		Very high-calorie, lactose-free, gluten-free, low-residue oral supplement
Compleat (Nestle)	1070	Chicken, Na caseinate, pea puree	48	Corn syrup, maltodextrin, fruits, vegetables	128	Canola oil, chicken	40	6.0	Blenderized tube feed formulated from traditional foods
Compleat Pediatric (Nestle)	1000	Chicken, Na caseinate, pea puree	38	Hydrolyzed cornstarch, fruits, vegetables, apple juice, corn syrup solids, fruits, vegetables, cranberry juice	130	High-oleic sunflower, soybean, MCT (18%) oils, canola oil, chicken	39	6.8	Intact protein, formulated from traditional foods including meats, vegetables, and fruit; for children 1–10 y
Crucial (Nestle)	1500	Hydrolyzed casein, L-arginine	94	Maltodextrin	134	MCT oil (50%), deodorized fish oil, soy oil, soy lecithin	68		High-calorie and protein peptide-based formula designed for critically ill patients
Diabeti-Source AC (Nestle)	1200	Soy protein, L-arginine	60	Corn syrup, fructose, tapioca dextrin, vegetables, fruits	100	Oil, Menhaden oil	59	15	Traditional food ingredients, designed for abnormal glucose tolerance and stress-induced hypoglycemia
Duocal (Nutricia)	492/100 g powder	None	0	Hydrolyzed cornstarch	72.7	Corn, coconut, MCT (35%) oils	22.3		Carbohydrate and fat calorie modular supplement, nutritionally incomplete

Product	kcal/L	Protein source	Protein (g)	Carbohydrate source	CHO (g)	Fat source	Fat (g)	Fiber (g)	Description
EleCare Jr. (1 kcal/mL) (Abbott)	1000	Free L-amino acids	31	Corn syrup solids	106.7	High-oleic safflower oil, MCT (33%) and soy oils	49.1		Nutritionally complete elemental formula for children 1 y and older who require an amino acid-based medical food
Ensure (Abbott)	1060	Milk protein concentrate, soy protein isolate	38	Corn syrup, sucrose, maltodextrin	171	Corn, canola, soy oils	25	4	Nutritionally complete oral formula
Ensure Bone Health (Abbott)	917	Ca and Na caseinates, soy protein isolate	42	Sucrose, maltodextrin	129	Corn, soy oils	25	0	Supplemental higher protein oral nutrition with extra calcium and vitamin D
Ensure Enlive (Abbott)	1010	Whey protein isolate	35	Corn maltodextrin, sucrose	217	None	0	0	High-calorie, fat-free, clear liquid oral supplement, nutritionally incomplete
Ensure High Protein (Abbott)	875	Milk protein concentrate, soy protein isolate, Ca caseinate	104	Sucrose, maltodextrin	96	High-oleic safflower oil	10	12	High-protein, low-fat, low-sugar oral formula with prebiotic fiber
Ensure Immune Health (Abbott)	1040	Milk protein concentrate, soy protein isolate	38	Sucrose, maltodextrin	175	Corn, canola, soy oils	25	12	Supplemental oral nutrition with prebiotic fiber (FOS)
Ensure Plus (Abbott)	1458	Milk protein concentrate, soy protein isolate	54	Maltodextrin, sucrose	204	Corn, soy oils	46	4	High-calorie, complete oral supplement
EO28 Splash (Nutricia)	1000	Free amino acids	25	Maltodextrin, sucrose	146	Fractionated coconut oil (MCT 35%), canola, high-oleic sunflower oils	35		Elemental, flavored, oral formula for children >1 y with severe gastrointestinal tract (GI) impairment
Glucerna 1.0 (Abbott)	1000	Na and Ca caseinate, soy protein	41.8	Corn maltodextrin, fructose	95.6	High-oleic safflower oil, canola oil, soy oil	54.4	14.4	Complete oral or tube feeding for patients with diabetes mellitus
Glucerna 1.2 (Abbott)	1200	Na caseinate, soy protein isolate, milk protein concentrate	60	Corn maltodextrin, isomaltulose, fructose, sucromalt	114.5	High-oleic safflower oil, canola oil, soy oi, marine oil	60	16.1	Higher-calorie complete oral or tube feeding for patients with diabetes mellitus or altered glucose metabolism due to illness or trauma

APP

Appendix N-1. *(continued)*
Selected Enteral Products for Special Indications[a]

Product									Comments
Glucerna 1.5 (Abbott)	1500	Na and Ca caseinate, soy protein	82.5	Corn maltodextrin, isomaltulose, fructose, sucromalt	133.1	High-oleic safflower oil, canola oil, soy oil	75	16.1	High-calorie, high-protein complete oral or tube feeding for patients with diabetes or altered glucose metabolism due to illness or trauma
Impact (Nestle)	1000	Na and Ca caseinate, L-arginine	56	Maltodextrin	130	Palm kernel, safflower oil, high-oleic sunflower oil, menhaden oil	28		Designed for critically ill patients without high energy needs
Impact with fiber (Nestle)	1000	Na and Ca caseinate, L-arginine	56	Maltodextrin	140	Palm kernel, safflower oil, high-oleic sunflower oil, menhaden oil	28	10	Designed for critically ill patients who have fiber needs but not high energy needs
Impact Glutamine (Nestle)	1300	Wheat protein hydrolysate, free amino acids, sodium caseinate	78	Maltodextrin	150	Palm kernel, safflower oil, high-oleic sunflower oil, menhaden oil	43	10	High glutamine (15 g/L), immune-enhancing enteral formula for critically ill patients
Impact 1.5 (Nestle)	1500	Na and Ca caseinate, L-arginine	84	Maltodextrin, corn syrup solids	140	Palm kernel, safflower oil, high-oleic sunflower oil, menhaden oil and MCT (55%) oil	69		High-calorie, high-protein formula designed for critically ill patients
Isosource HN (Nestle)	1200	Soy protein isolate	53	Corn syrup	160	Canola and MCT oils	39		High-nitrogen, high-calorie soy protein formula
Isosource 1.5 (Nestle)	1500	Na caseinate	68	Maltodextrin, sucrose	168	Canola, soybean, and MCT oils	65	8	High-nitrogen, high-calorie complete formula with fiber
Jevity 1 Cal (Abbott)	1060	Na and Ca caseinate, soy protein isolate	44.3	Corn maltodextrin, corn syrup solids, soy fiber	154.7	Canola, corn, and MCT oils	34.7	14.4	Isotonic, fiber-containing nutritionally complete tube feeding formula

Product		Protein source		Carbohydrate source		Fat source			Description
Jevity 1.2 Cal (Abbott)	1200	Na and Ca caseinate, soy protein isolate	55.5	Corn maltodextrin, corn syrup solids, fructo-oligosaccharides, soy fiber, oat fiber	169.4	Canola, corn, and MCT oils	39.3	18	Higher-calorie, high-protein, fiber-containing tube feeding formula
Jevity 1.5 Cal (Abbott)	1500	Na and Ca caseinate, soy protein isolate	63.8	Corn maltodextrin, corn syrup solids, fructo-oligosaccharides, soy fiber, oat fiber	215.7	Canola, corn, and MCT oils	49.8	22	High-calorie, high-protein, fiber containing tube feeding formula
MCT oil (Nestle)	116 kcal/tbsp 8.3 kcal/g	None	0	None	0	Coconut oil	14 g/tbsp		Modular fat supplement or substitute for patients with long-chain fatty acid malabsorption – directly absorbed into portal vein, nutritionally incomplete
Microlipid (Nestle)	68 kcal/tbsp	None	0	None	0	Safflower oil	7.5 g/tbsp		Modular fat emulsion (50%) for special use in oral or tube feeding formulas, nutritionally incomplete
Neocate Jr. (Nutricia)	1000	Free amino acids	33	Corn syrup solids	104	Fractionated coconut oil (MCT), canola and high-oleic safflower oils	50		Nutritionally complete elemental formula for children 1–10 y with severe GI tract impairment
Neocate Jr. with Prebiotics (Nutricia)	1000	Free amino acids	33	Corn syrup solids, fructo-oligosaccharides, inulin	104	Fractionated coconut oil (MCT), canola and high-oleic safflower oils	50	4	Nutritionally complete elemental formula with prebiotic fiber for children 1–10 y with severe GI tract impairment
Nepro (Abbott)	1800	Ca, Mg, and Na caseinate, milk protein isolate	81	Corn syrup solids, sucrose, corn maltodextrin, fructo-oligosaccharides	161	High-oleic safflower oil and canola oil	96		Very high-calorie, complete oral or tube feeding designed for patients on dialysis
NovaSource Pulmonary (Nestle)	1500	Na and Ca caseinates	75	Corn syrup, sugar	150	Canola and MCT (20%) oils	68	8	High-calorie and –nitrogen formula, designed for pulmonary patients

Appendix N-1. (continued)
Selected Enteral Products for Special Indications[a]

Product		Protein source		Carbohydrate source		Fat source			Description
NovaSource Renal (Nestle)	2000	Na and Ca caseinate, L-arginine	74	Corn syrup, fructose	200	High-oleic sunflower, corn, and MCT (14%) oils	100		Very high-calorie, -vitamin and -mineral profile specifically formulated for dialysis patients, TetraBrik Pak
Nutren 1.0 (Nestle)	1000	Ca and K caseinate	40	Maltodextrin, corn syrup solids	127	Canola, MCT (25%), corn oils, soy lecithin	38		Complete liquid nutrition for patients with normal calorie and protein needs
Nutren 1.0 With fiber (Nestle)	1000	Ca and K caseinate	40	Maltodextrin, corn syrup solids	127	Canola, MCT (25%), corn oils, soy lecithin	38	14	Complete liquid nutrition with fiber
Nutren 1.5 (Nestle)	1500	Ca and K caseinate	60	Maltodextrin, sucrose	169	MCT (50%), canola, corn oils, soy lecithin	68		Complete high-calorie liquid nutrition for high calorie needs or limited volume tolerance, 50% MCT oil
Nutren 2.0 (Nestle)	2000	Ca and K caseinate	80	Corn syrup solids, maltodextrin, sucrose	196	MCT (75%), canola oil, soy lecithin, corn oil	104		Very high-calorie, severe fluid restriction, 75% MCT oil
Nutren Glytrol (Nestle)	1000	Ca and K caseinate	45	Maltodextrin, modified corn starch, pea fiber, gum arabic, oligofructose	100	Canola, high-oleic safflower oil, MCT, soy lecithin	47.6	15.2	Complete nutrition for patients with hyperglycemia
Nutren Jr (Nestle)	1000	Casein, whey (50%)	30	Maltodextrin, sucrose	110	MCT (25%), canola, and soybean oils, soy lecithin	49.6		Balanced formula designed to meet needs of children 1–10 y; oral or enteral
Nutren Jr With fiber (Nestle)	1000	Casein, whey (50%)	30	Maltodextrin, sucrose, pea fiber, oligofructose	110	MCT (25%), canola, and soybean oils, soy lecithin	49.6	6	Balanced formula with prebiotic fiber designed to meet needs of children 1–10 y; oral or enteral
Nutren Pulmonary (Nestle)	1500	Ca and K caseinate	68	Maltodextrin	100	Canola, MCT (40%), corn oils, soy lecithin	94.8		High fat content, designed to reduce CO_2 production for use in pulmonary patients

Product	kcal/L	Protein source	Protein (g)	Carbohydrate source	CHO (g)	Fat source	Fat (g)	Fiber	Description
Nutren Replete (Nestle)	1000	Ca and K caseinate	62	Maltodextrin	113	Canola, MCT, soy lecithin	34		Very high-protein complete formula to support healing from surgery, burns, and pressure ulcers
NutriHep (Nestle)	1500	L-amino acids, whey protein (50% branched-chain amino acids)	40	Maltodextrin, modified corn starch	290	MCT (70%), canola, soy lecithin, and corn oils	21.2		High branched-chain amino acids, low aromatic and ammonogenic amino acids for patients with liver disease
Optimental (Abbott)	1000	Whey protein hydrolysate, partially hydrolyzed Na caseinate, free arginine	51.3	Corn maltodextrin, sucrose, fructo-oligosaccharides	138.7	Marine oil, MCT structured lipid, cano a and soybean o ls	28.4	5	Complete elemental oral or tube feeding formula designed for patients with malabsorptive conditions
Osmolite 1 Cal (Abbott)	1060	Na and Ca caseinates, soy protein isolate	44.3	Corn maltodextrin, corn syrup solids	143.9	Canola, corn, and MCT oils, soy lecithin	34.7		Isotonic, nutritionally complete, high-nitrogen, formula for oral or tube feeding
Osmolite 1.2 Cal (Abbott)	1200	Na and Ca caseinates	55.5	Corn maltodextrin	157.5	High-oleic safflower, canola, and MCT oils, soy lecithin	39.3		Higher-calorie, high-nitrogen, low-residue complete oral or tube feeding
Osmolite 1.5 Cal (Abbott)	1500	Na and Ca caseinates, soy protein isolate	62.7	Corn maltodextrin	203.6	High-oleic safflower, canola, and MCT oils, soy lecithin	49.1		High-calorie, high-protein, low-residue complete nutrition for oral or tube feeding use
Oxepa (Abbott)	1500	Na and Ca caseinates	62.7	Sucrose, corn maltodextrin	105.3	Canola, MCT, marine, and borage oils, soy lecithin	93.8		High-calorie, complete tube feeding formula for critically ill patients with acute lung injury, acute respiratory distress syndrome, and systemic inflammatory response syndrome
Pediasure (Abbott)	1013	Milk protein concentrate, whey protein concentrate, soy protein isolate	30	Sucrose, corn maltodextrin, fructo-oligosaccharides	139	High-oleic safflower, soy, MCT, and *Crypthecodinium cohnii* oils	38	4	Complete oral or tube feeding formula designed for patients 1-13 years

Appendix N-1. *(continued)*

Selected Enteral Products for Special Indicationsª

Product (Manufacturer)		Protein source		Carbohydrate source		Fat source			Description
Pediasure and Pediasure Enteral, with fiber (Abbott)	1013	Milk protein concentrate, soy protein isolate	30	Sucrose, corn maltodextrin, soy fiber, fructo-oligosaccharides	139	High-oleic safflower, soy, MCT, and C cohnii oils	38	13	Complete oral or tube feeding formula with fiber designed for patients 1–13 y
Pediasure 1.5 Cal (Abbott)	1476	Milk protein concentrate	59	Corn maltodextrin	160	High-oleic safflower, soy, MCT, and C cohnii oils	67.5		High-calorie complete oral or tube feeding formula designed for patients 1–13 y
Pediasure 1.5 Cal with Fiber (Abbott)	1476	Milk protein concentrate	59	Corn maltodextrin, fructo-oligosaccharides, oat fiber, soy fiber	164.6	High-oleic safflower, soy, MCT, and C. Cohnii oils	67.5	12.7	High-calorie complete oral or tube feeding formula with fiber designed for patients 1–13 y
Pediasure Peptide (formerly Vital Jr) (Abbott)	1000	Whey protein hydrolysate, hydrolyzed Na caseinate	30	Corn maltodextrin, sucrose, fructo-oligosaccharides	133.8	Structured lipid (interesterified canola/MCT), MCT, canola oil	40.5	3	Peptide-based complete oral or tube feeding formula for patients 1–13 y with malabsorption
Pepdite Jr. (Nutricia)	1000	Hydrolyzed protein (pork, soy), free amino acids	31	Corn syrup solids	106	Fractionated coconut oil (MCT-35%), canola, high-oleic safflower oils	50		Nutritionally complete semi-elemental formula for children 1–10 y with GI tract impairment
Peptamen (Nestle)	1000	Enzymatically hydrolyzed whey	40	Maltodextrin, corn starch	127	MCT (70%), soybean oil, soy lecithin	39		Peptide-based, isotonic, designed for general malabsorption
Peptamen with Prebio (Nestle)	1000	Enzymatically hydrolyzed whey	40	Maltodextrin, corn starch, oligofructose	127	MCT (70%), soybean oil, soy lecithin	39		Peptide-based, isotonic formula with fiber designed for general malabsorption
Peptamen 1.5 (Nestle)	1500	Enzymatically hydrolyzed whey	67.6	Maltodextrin, corn starch	188	MCT (70%), soybean oil, soy lecithin	56		High-calorie, peptide-based, high percentage MCT oil designed for malabsorption

Peptamen AF (Nestle)	1200	Enzymatically hydrolyzed whey	75.6	Maltodextrin, corn starch, oligofructose	107	MCT, soybean oil, fish oil, soy lecithin	54.8		High-protein, peptide-based, high percentage MCT oil designed for general malabsorption and higher-calorie needs
Peptamen, Jr. (Nestle)	1000	Enzymatically hydrolyzed whey	30	Maltodextrin, cornstarch	137.6	MCT (60%), soybean, and canola oils, soy lecithin	38.4		Designed for children 1–10 y, peptide-based, 60% of fat from MCT oil
Peptamen, Jr. Fiber (Nestle)	1000	Enzymatically hydrolyzed whey	30	Maltodextrin, Cornstarch, pea fiber, oligofructose, inulin	137.6	MCT (60%), soybean, and canola oils, soy lecithin	38.4	7.2	Peptide-based complete formula with fiber and 60% of fat from MCT oil, designed for children 1–10 y
Peptamen, Jr. Prebio (Nestle)	1000	Enzymatically hydrolyzed whey	30	Maltodextrin, sucrose, Cornstarch, oligofructose, inulin	137.6	MCT (60%), soybean, and canola oils, soy lecithin	38.4	3.6	Peptide-based complete formula with prebiotics and 60% of fat from MCT oil, designed for children 1–10 y
Peptamen, Jr. 1.5 (Nestle)	1500	Enzymatically hydrolyzed whey	45	Maltodextrin, Cornstarch, oligofructose	180	MCT (60%), soybean, and canola oils, soy lecithin, tuna oil	68	5.4	High-calorie, complete peptide based formula designed for children 1–13 y, 60% of fat from MCT oil, and contains fish oil
Perative (Abbott)	1300	Partially hydrolyzed Na caseinate, whey protein hydrolysate, L-arginine	66.7	Corn maltodextrin, fructo-oligosaccharides	180.3	Canola, MCT (40%), and corn oils	37.3	6.5	Higher-calorie complete tube feeding formula designed for metabolically stressed patients with wounds, burns, or a postoperative state
Polycose (Abbott)	380/100 g powder	None	0	Glucose polymers from cornstarch	94/100g	None	0		Carbohydrate calorie modular supplement, nutritionally incomplete
Promod Liquid Protein (Abbott)	100/30 mL	Hydrolyzed beef collagen, L-tryptophan	10	Glycerine	14	None	0		Protein calorie supplement, nutritionally incomplete
Promote (Abbott)	1000	Sodium caseinate, soy protein isolate	62.5	Corn maltodextrin, sucrose	130	MCT and safflower oils, soy lecithin	26		Very high-protein complete oral or tube feeding formula

Appendix N-1. (continued)
Selected Enteral Products for Special Indications[a]

Product									Comments
Promote with fiber (Abbott)	1000	Na and Ca caseinate, soy protein isolate	62.5	Corn maltodextrin, sucrose, oat and soy fiber	138.3	Soy, MCT, and safflower oils, soy lecithin	28.2	14.4	Very high-protein complete oral or tube feeding formula with fiber
Pulmocare (Abbott)	1500	Na and Ca caseinates	62.6	Sucrose, corn maltodextrin	105.7	Canola, MCT (20%), high-oleic safflower and corn oils, soy lecithin	93.3		High-calorie, high-fat, low-carbohydrate complete oral or tube feeding designed for pulmonary patients
Renalcal (Nestle)	2000	Essential and select nonessential amino acids, whey protein	34.4	Maltodextrin, corn starch	290.4	MCT (70%), canola, and corn oils, soy lecithin	82.4		Very high-calorie, low-protein for patients with renal failure designed to maintain positive nitrogen balance, added histidine, negligible electrolytes
ReSource 2.0 (Nestle)	2000	Ca and Na caseinates	84	Corn syrup, sucrose, maltodextrin	218	Canola and MCT (20%) oils	88		Very high-calorie, high-protein oral beverage, pouch pak
Suplena with Carb Steady (Abbott)	1795	Milk protein isolates, Na caseinate	45	Corn maltodextrin, isomaltulose, sucrose, glycerin, fructo-oligosaccharides	196	High-oleic safflower and soy oils	96	12.7	Very high-calorie, low-protein, complete formula for patients with renal failure
Tolerex (Nestle)	1000	Free amino acids	21	Maltodextrin, modified corn starch	230	Safflower oil	1.5		Complete, low-fat, elemental formula
TwoCal HN (Abbott)	2000	Na and Ca caseinates	83.5	Corn syrup solids, corn maltodextrin, sucrose, fructo-oligosaccharides	218.5	High-oleic safflower, MCT (19%) and canola oils, soy lecithin	90.5	5	Complete very high-calorie feeding with fructo-oligosaccharides
Vital 1.0 Cal (Abbott)	1000	Whey protein hydrolysate, partially hydrolyzed Na caseinate	40	Maltodextrin, sucrose, fructo-oligosaccharides	130	Structured lipid (interesterified canola/MCT), canola oil, MCT	38.1	4.2	Complete, peptide-based formula for patients with impaired GI tract function

Product		Protein		Carbohydrate		Fat			Description
Vital AF 1.2 Cal (Abbott)	1200	Whey protein hydrolysate, hydrolyzed Na caseinate	75	Corn maltodextrin, fructo-oligosaccharides	110.6	Structured lipid (interesterified marine oil/MCT, MCT, canola and soy oils	53.9	5.1	Higher-calorie nutritionally complete, peptide-based formula for patients with impaired GI tract function; with fish–oil based structured lipid and prebiotic
Vital 1.5 Cal (Abbott)	1500	Whey protein hydrolysate, partially hydrolyzed Na caseinate	67.5	Maltodextrin, sucrose, fructo-oligosaccharides	187	Structured lipid (interesterified canola/MCT), canola oil, MCT	57.1	6	High-calorie nutritionally complete, peptide-based formula for patients with impaired GI tract function
Vital HN (Abbott)	1000	Partially hydrolyzed protein blend (soy and collagen), whey protein concentrate, whey protein hydrolysate, free amino acids	41.7	Corn maltodextrin, sucrose	185	Safflower and MCT (45%) oils, soy lecithin	10.8		Nutritionally complete, peptide-based elemental, low-fat, low-residue formula for patients with impaired GI tract function
Vivonex Pediatric (Nestle)	800	Free amino acids	24	Maltodextrin, modified starch	130	MCT (68%) and soybean oils	24		Nutritionally complete, elemental formula for children, unflavored, may use flavor packets
Vivonex Plus (Nestle)	1000	Free amino acids	45	Maltodextrin, modified corn starch	190	Soybean oil	6.7		High-nitrogen, low-fat elemental diet; additional glutamine arginine and branched-chain amino acids
Vivonex T.E.N. (Nestle)	1000	Free amino acids	38	Maltodextrin, modified corn starch	210	Safflower oil	2.8		Free amino acids plus additional glutamine, low fat, designed for GI tract impairment

a Sources: Abbott Nutrition Division, Abbott Laboratories, Columbus, OH (www.abbottnutrition.com; information obtained via manufacturer website 8/7/11; page last updated 2011); Nutricia North America Advanced Medical Nutrition, Scientific Hospital Supplies North America, Gaithersburg, MD (http://www.shsna.com; information obtained via manufacturer website 8/7/11; page last updated 2010); Nestle Clinical Nutrition, Glendale, CA (http://www.nestle-nutrition.com; information obtained via manufacturer website 8/7/11; page last updated 2011).

APP

Appendix N-2
Enteral Products Grouped by Usage Indication

Indication	Product
Standard adult oral	Boost, Ensure, Carnation Breakfast
Standard adult tube feeding	Jevity 1 cal, Nutren 1.0, Osmolite
High-protein oral	Boost High Protein, Ensure High Protein, Ensure Muscle Health, Ensure Clinical Strength
High-protein tube feeding	FiberSource HN, Isosource HN, Jevity 1.2 cal, Osmolite 1 cal, Osmolite 1.2 cal, Promote, Nutren Replete, Vital HN
1.5 kcal/mL	Boost Plus, Ensure Plus, Carnation Breakfast Plus, Nutren 1.5, Isosource 1.5, Jevity 1.5, Osmolite 1.5
2.0 kcal/mL	Carnation Breakfast VHC, Nutren 2.0, ReSource 2.0, TwoCal HN
Standard pediatric (>1 y)	Nutren Jr., Pediasure (1.0, 1.5), Boost Kids Essentials (1.0, 1.5)
Blenderized	Compleat, Compleat Pediatric
Clear fortified liquid	Enlive, Boost Breeze
Peptide-based adult	Peptamen, Peptamen 1.5, Peptamen AF, Perative, Vital HN, Vital (1.0, 1.5)
Peptide-based pediatric	Peptide Jr., Peptamen Jr. (1.0, 1.5), Pediasure Peptide
Free amino acid adult	Tolerex, Vivonex T.E.N., Vivonex Plus
Free amino acid pediatric (>1 y)	Elecare Junior, Neocate Junior, Neocate Splash, Vivonex Pediatric
Immune enhancing	Impact (1.0, 1.5), Impact Advanced Recovery, Pivot 1.5
Wound healing	Crucial, Isosource HN, Nutren Replete, Impact (1.0, 1.5), Perative
Diabetes	Boost Glucose Control DiabetiSource AC, Glucerna, Nutren Glytrol, ReSource Diabetishield
Kidney disease	Nepro, NovaSource Renal, Renalcal, Suplena
Liver disease	NutriHep
Pulmonary disease	NovaSource Pulmonary, Nutren Pulmonary, Oxepa, Pulmocare
Inflammatory bowel disease	Optimental, Peptamen AF, Vital AF 1.2
Carbohydrate modulars	Polycose
Protein modulars	Beneprotein, Promod
Calorie enhancers	Duocal, Benecalorie
Fat modulars	MCT oil, Microlipid

Appendix N–3.
Sources of Medical Food Modules and Modified Low-Protein Foods for Treatment of Inborn Errors of Metabolism

Company	Medical Food Module	Modified Low-Protein Modules
Abbott Nutrition Metabolic Products (Inherited Metabolic Disorders) 3300 Stelzer Road Columbus, OH 43219-3034 Tel: (800) 986-8755 (for health care professionals) Web site: www.abbottnutrition.com/Therapeutic/Inherited-Metabolic-Disorders.aspx	Medical formulas for inherited disorders involving protein, fat, or carbohydrate metabolism; protein-free formula	
Applied Nutrition 10 Saddle Road Cedar Knolls, NJ 07927 Tel: (800) 605-0410 FAX: (973) 734-0029 Web site: www.medicalfood.com/products.php	Medical protein formulas for PKU, MSUD, and GA1; medical protein bars for PKU and MSUD, LNAA powder and tablets for PKU; single amino acids	Baking mixes, cereal, snacks, sweets
Cambrooke Foods, Inc. 4 Copeland Drive Ayer, MA 01432 Tel: 1-866-4-LOW-PRO (456-9776) FAX: (978) 443 1318 Web site: www.cambrookefoods.com/	Medical protein formula for PKU, ready-to-drink medical beverages for PKU and MSUD, medical protein formula with Glytactin for PKU	Baking mixes, breads, breakfast cereal, cheeses, desserts, meat alternatives, rice and pasta, snacks, seasonings, premade frozen items
Canbrands Specialty Foods PO BOX 117 Gormley, Ontario L0H1G0 Tel: (905) 888-5008 FAX: (905)888-5009 Web site: www.canbrands.ca/cart.php		Cookies, gel-desserts, egg replacer
Dietary Specialties 8 South Commons Road Waterbury, CT 06704 Tel: 1-888-640-2800 FAX: (973) 884-5907 Website: www.dietspec.com/		Baking mixes, pasta entrees, soups, pasta, rice and porridge, sauce mixes, cake mixes, peanut butter spread, egg replacer, breads, rolls, bagels, frozen premade foods
Ener-G Foods 5960 1st Avenue South Seattle, Washington 98108 Tel: (800) 331-5222 FAX: (206) 764-3398 Website: www.ener-g.com		Breads, crackers and snacks, cookies, egg replacer, baking mixes

Appendix N–3. *(continued)*

Sources of Medical Food Modules and Modified Low-Protein Foods for Treatment of Inborn Errors of Metabolism

Mead Johnson Medical Department (Products) 2400 West Lloyd Expressway Evansville, IN 47721 Tel: (812) 429-6399 Web site: www.mjn.com/app/iwp/hcp2/ content2.do?dm=mj&id=-12490&iwpst= HCP&ls=0&csred=1&r=3508098857	Medical formulas for inherited disorders involving protein, fat, or carbohydrate metabolism; protein-free formula	
Nutricia North America – United States PO Box 117 Gaithersburg, MD 20884 Tel: (800) 365-7354 FAX: (301)-795-2301 Web site: www.shsna.com/index.htm	Medical formulas for inherited disorders involving protein, fat, or carbohydrate metabolism; protein-free formula, vitamin modules; ketogenic formula	Baking mixes, pasta, and rice, cereals, crackers, drink mix, energy bars, snacks
Nutricia North America - Canada 4517 Dobrin Street St. Laurent, QC H4R 2L8 Phone: (877) 636-2283 FAX: (514) 745-6625 Web site: www.shsna.com/index.htm	Medical formulas for inherited disorders involving protein, fat, or carbohydrate metabolism; protein-free formula, vitamin modules; ketogenic formula	Baking mixes, pasta, and rice, cereals, crackers, drink mix, energy bars, snacks
Solace Nutrition 10 Alice Court Pawcatuck, CT 06379 Tel: (888)876-5223 FAX: (401) 633-6066 Web site: www.solacenutrition.com	Medical formulas for inherited disorders involving protein metabolism; supplements for mitochondria and cholesterol disorders	
Taste Connections 612 Meyer Lane #13 Redondo Beach, CA 90278 Telephone: (310) 798-1935 FAX: (310) 971-8861 Web site: www.tasteconnections.com/		Baking mixes, premade baked items, snacks
Vitaflo USA 211 N Union St Suite 100 Alexandria, VA 22314 Tel: (888)-848-2356 FAX: (631) 693-2002 Web site: www.vitaflousa.com/default.aspx	Ready-to-drink medical protein beverages for inherited disorders involving protein metabolism; formulas and supplements for fatty acid oxidation disorders, protein-free medical formulas, single amino acid and essential fatty acid supplements, energy supplements	

PKU indicates phenylketonuria; MSUD, maple syrup urine disease; GA1, glutaric acidemia type 1; LNAA, large neutral amino acids.

Appendix O

Appendix O.
Sports/Nutrition Bars

Product (weight, g) (Manufacturer)	Calories	Protein	Fat (Saturated Fat)	Fiber	Sodium	Calcium (% DV)	Iron (% DV)
Apex Fix Crisp Bars (40 g)	150	9 g	3.5 g (2 g)	3 g	120 mg	10%	10%
Atkins' Advantage (60 g) (ANI, New York, NY)	170	8 g	12 g (4.5 g)	8 g	130 mg	20%	4%
Balance (50 g) (The Balance Bar Co, Tarrytown, NY)	200	14 g	7 g (4 g)	2 g	160 mg	15%	15%
Balance Bare (50 g)	210	13 g	9 g (3.5 g)	3 g	280 mg	10%	25%
Balance Gold (50 g)	200	14 g	7 g (4 g)	2 g	160 mg	15%	15%
Balance CarbWell (50 g)	190	14 g	7 g (4 g)	1 g	190 mg	10%	25%
Burn Bar (50 g) (Unipro, Jamul, CA)	200	15 g	6 g (2.5 g)	2 g	160 mg	25%	6%
Clif (68 g) (Clif Bar Inc, Berkeley, CA)	240	9 g	7 g (4 g)	4 g	160 mg	25%	25%
Clif's Luna Bar (48 g)	190	9 g	7 g (4 g)	3 g	210 mg	35%	30%
Clif's Luna Protein (45 g)	190	12 g	9 g (4 g)	3 g	210 mg	25%	15%
Clif Mojo (45 g)	180	9 g	8 g (1.5 g)	2 g	220 mg	8%	6%
Clif Builder's (68 g)	270	20 g	8 g (4 g)	1 g	240 mg	25%	n/a
Clif Kid Zbar (36 g)	130	3 g	4 g (1.5 g)	3 g	100 mg	30%	10%
GeniSoy (61.5 g) (GeniSoy Food Co, Tulsa, OK)	240	14 g	6 g (3 g)	2 g	310 mg	11%	15%
Kashi GoLean Crunch (45 g) (Kashi Co, La Jolla, CA)	170	8 g	5 g (2.5 g)	5 g	210 mg	20%	10%
Kashi GoLean Pro + Fiber (55 g)	190	12 g	4.5 g (3.5 g)	5 g	120 mg	10%	10%
Kashi TLC Chewy Granola Bars (35 g)	140	6 g	5 g (0.5 g)	4 g	95 mg	0%	6%
Met-Rx (100 g) (Met-Rx USA, Bohemia, NY)	410	32 g	14 g (8 g)	3 g	410 mg	15%	35%
Nature's Path Organic Optimum Energy (56 g) (Nature's Path Foods, Richmond, British Columbia, Canada)	200	7 g	3 g (0 g)	5 g	115 mg	25%	15%
Odwalla (56 g) (Odwalla, Half Moon Bay, CA)	200	3 g	5 g (1 g)	4 g	125 mg	25%	6%
PowerBar Performance (65 g) (Nestlé, Glendale, CA)	230	8 g	3.5 g (0.5 g)	2 g	200 mg	25%	25%

Appendix O. *(continued)*
Sports/Nutrition Bars

PowerBar Harvest (65 g)	250	10 g	5 g (2 g)	5 g	140 mg	20%	20%
PowerBar Pria (28 g)	110	5 g	3.5 g (2.5 g)	1	90 mg	30%	20%
PowerBar Protein Plus (65 g)	300	23 g	6 g (3.5 g)	1 g	170 mg	40%	45%
Pro 42 (105 g) (ISS Research, Charlotte, NC)	430	42 g	12 g (6 g)	2 g	95 mg	35%	110%
Probar (85 g) (Probar LLC, Heber City, UT)	370	9 g	17 g (2 g)	6 g	55 mg	8%	15%
Probar Fruition (48 g)	160	3 g	2.5 g (0 g)	4 g	10 mg	4%	6%
Promax (75 g) (Promax Nutrition, Concord, CA)	280	20 g	6 g (5 g)	1 g	170 mg	25%	40%
PureFit (57 g) (PureFit Inc, Irvine, CA)	230	18 g	6 g (1 g)	3 g	190 mg	6%	15%
Solo (50 g) (Solo GI Nutrition, Edmonton, Alberta, Canada)	200	11 g	7g (3 g)	4 g	120 mg	20%	10%
Steel Bar (70 g) (American Body Building, Aurora, IL)	270	20 g	5 g (3 g)	0 g	260 mg	10%	10%
Think Energy (35 g) (Think Products, San Francisco, CA)	140	6 g	5 g (2 g)	2 g	35 mg	15%	25%
Tigers Milk (35 g) (Schiff Nutrition Group, Salt Lake City, UT)	140	6 g	5 g (2 g)	<1 g	60 mg	15%	20%
Usana (39 g) (Usana Health Sciences, Salt Lake City, UT)	160	10 g	5 g (2 g)	2 g	135 mg	4%	10%
Worldwide Sport Nutrition Bar (78 g) (Worldwide SportNutrition, Bohemia, NY)	300	31 g	10 g (4.5 g)	2 g	330 mg	35%	15%
Zone Perfect (50 g) (Abbott Nutrition, Columbus, OH)	210	15 g	6 g (4 g)	<1 g	240 mg	10%	10%
Fruitified (50 g) (Abbott Nutrition, Columbus, OH)	180	14 g	2 g (0.5 g)	3 g	140 mg	20%	10%

DV indicates daily value.

NOTE: All values may vary slightly depending on flavor.

Appendix P

APP

Appendix P.
Sodium Content of Foods, mg per Serving

500	250	200	100	50
⅛ tsp salt	½ cup regularly seasoned spinach, beets, celery, kale, or white turnips	1 slice regular bread	½ cup of the following unsalted vegetables: beet greens, frozen mixed peas and carrots, Swiss chard	½ cup of the following fresh, frozen, or canned vegetables, canned without salt: 1 artichoke (edible base and leaves), beets, carrots, celery, dandelion greens, kale, mustard greens, peas (black-eyed), spinach, succotash, turnip greens, turnip (white), lima beans
¾ tsp monosodium glutamate	1 hard roll	½ cup canned carrots or seasoned vegetables not listed elsewhere	1 oz frozen fish fillets	1 tsp or 1 packet yellow mustard
1 bouillon cube	½ cup rice or grits cooked in salted water	1 oz natural cheddar cheese	¾ cup milk (6 oz)	1 round slice kosher or dill pickle
½ cup tomato juice	2 thin slices bacon, crisp and drained	1 tbsp catsup	½ cup pasta cooked in salted water	
1 average serving ea. (½ cup) of cooked rice, spaghetti, noodles, hominy, seasoned with salt		5 saltine crackers	1 oz tuna, drained (not rinsed)	
½ cup drained sauerkraut		1 oz plain potato chips	1 packet of BBQ sauce	
1 average frankfurter (1½ oz)				
1 oz turkey luncheon meat				
1 oz salami				
3 oz canned sardines or salmon				
3 oz shrimp (fresh) cooked in salted water				
1 tsp soy sauce				
1 oz plain salted pretzels				

From US Department of Agriculture, Agricultural Research Service. USDA National Nutrient Database for Standard Reference, Release 23. 2010. Available at: http://www.ars.usda.gov/ba/bhnrc/ndl. Accessed January 31, 2013

To help follow a lower-sodium diet, avoid foods with visible salt, such as potato chips, pretzels, or salted nuts.

Appendix Q

Appendix Q.
Saturated and Polyunsaturated Fat and Cholesterol Content of Common Foods[a]

Foods	Quantity	Saturated Fat, g	Polyunsaturated Fat, g	Cholesterol, mg	kcal
Almonds (roasted, salted, shelled)	12	1.1	3.7	0	169
Bacon (cured, cooked)	2 slices	2.1	0.7	18	84
Beef, lean	3 oz	4.3	0.4	90	215
Bread, white	1 slice	0.2	0.4	0	75
Butter	1 tbsp	7.3	0.4	31	102

Cheese
  Cheddar
  Cottage, creamed
  Cream or spread
	
	1 oz
	½ cup
	2 tbsp
		
		6.0
		1.9
		5.6
			
			0.3
			0.1
			0.4
				
				30
				19
				32
					
					114
					110
					99

Chicken (light meat, without skin)	3.5 oz	0.4	0.4	58	114
Coconut (dried, sweetened)	¼ cup	7.3	0.1	0	116
Corn oil	1 tbsp	1.1	4.1	0	124
Canola oil	1 tbsp	1.0	3.9	0	124

Egg
  Whole
  White
  Yolk
	
	1 large
	1 large
	1 large
		
		1.6
		0
		1.6
			
			1.0
			0
			0.7
				
				186
				0
				184
					
					72
					17
					55

Fish (fillet or flounder, sole)	3 oz	0.5	0.4	48	73
Hamburger (80% lean)	3 oz	5.7	0.4	77	230
Ice cream (light) vanilla	½ cup	2.2	0.2	21	137
Lamb (lean leg)	3 oz	2.8	0.3	76	162
Lard	1 tbsp	5.0	1.4	12	115
Liver (beef)	3.5 oz	1.7	0.6	392	189

Margarine
  Regular (hydrogenated)
  Liquid oil
	
	1 tbsp
	1 tbsp
		
		2.1
		2.3
			
			3.4
			3.3
				
				...
				...
					
					100
					85

Milk
  Whole
  2%
  Skimmed
	
	1 cup
	1 cup
	1 cup
		
		4.5
		3.1
		0.1
			
			0.5
			0.2
			0
				
				24
				20
				5
					
					149
					122
					83

Olive oil	1 tbsp	1.9	1.4	0	119
Oysters (Eastern)	6 medium	0.4	0.4	34	43
Peanut oil	1 tbsp	2.3	4.3	0	119
Pork (lean)	3.5 oz	2.9	1.2	74	192
Safflower oil	1 tbsp	1.0	1.7	0	120

APP

Appendix Q. *(continued)*

Saturated and Polyunsaturated Fat and Cholesterol Content of Common Foods[a]

Foods	Quantity	Saturated Fat, g	Polyunsaturated Fat, g	Cholesterol, mg	kcal
Salmon, pink (canned)	3 ½ oz	0.8	1.3	81	135
Shrimp (canned)	3 oz	0.2	0.6	214	85
Soybean oil	1 tbsp	2.1	7.9	0	120
Sweetbreads (veal thymus)	3 oz	7.3	4.0	250	271
Tuna fish, canned in vegetable oil	3 oz	1.1	2.5	26	158
Turkey (light meat)	3 ½ oz	0.4	0.3	85	139

[a]A low-cholesterol, low-fat diet should limit cholesterol intake to 300 mg per day, have less than 35% of calories as fat, and have polyunsaturated fats at least equal to saturated fats. Monounsaturated fat, hence total fat, is not included except under kcal.

From US Department of Agriculture, Agricultural Research Service. 2010. USDA National Database for Standard Reference, Release 23. Nutrient Data Laboratory Home Page. Available at: http://www.ars.usda.gov/ba/bhnrc/ndl. Accessed January 31, 2013.

Appendix R

Appendix R.
Representative Values for Constituents of Human Milk[a]

Constituent (Per L)[b]	Early Milk	Mature Milk
Energy (kcal)		650-700
Carbohydrate		
Lactose (g)	20-30	67
Glucose (g)	0.2-1.0	0.2-0.3
Oligosaccharides (g)	22-24	12-14
Total nitrogen (g)	3.0	1.9
Nonprotein nitrogen (g)	0.5	0.45
Protein nitrogen (g)	2.5	1.45
Total protein (g)	16	9
Casein (g)	3.8	5.7
β Casein (g)	2.6	4.4
κ-Casein (g)	1.2	1.3
α-Lactalbumin (g)	3.62	3.26
Lactoferrin (g)	3.53	1.94
Albumin (g)	0.39	0.41
sIgA (g)	2.0	1.0
IgM (g)	0.12	0.2
IgG (g)	0.34	0.05
Total lipids (%)	2	3.5
Triglyceride (% total lipid)	97-98	97-98
Cholesterol[c] (% total lipids)	0.7-1.3	0.4-0.5
Phospholipids (% total lipids)	1.1	0.6-0.8
Fatty acids (weight %)	88	88
Total saturated fatty acids (%)	43-44	44-45
Palmitic acid (C16:0)		20
Monounsaturated fatty acids (%)		40
Oleic acid (C18:1 ω9)	32	31
Polyunsaturated fatty acids (%)	13	14-15
Total ω3 fatty acids (%)	1.5	1.5
Linolenic acid (C18:3 ω3)	0.7	0.9
Eicosapentaenoic acid (C22:5 ω3)	0.2	0.1
Docosahexaenoic acid (C22:6 ω3)	0.5	0.2
Total ω6 fatty acids (%)	11.6	13.06
Linoleic acid (C18:2 ω6)	8.9	11.3
Arachidonic acid (C20:4 ω6)	0.7	0.5

Appendix R. *(continued)*

Representative Values for Constituents of Human Milk[a]

Water-soluble vitamins		
Ascorbic acid (mg)		100
Thiamin (μg)	20	200
Riboflavin (μg)		400-600
Niacin (mg)	0.5	1.8-6.0
Vitamin B$_6$ (mg)		0.09-0.31
Folate (μg)		80-140
Vitamin B$_{12}$ (μg)		0.5-1.0
Pantothenic acid (mg)		2-2.5
Biotin (μg)		5-9
Fat-soluble vitamins		
Retinol (mg)	2	0.3-0.6
Carotenoids (mg)	2	0.2-0.6
Vitamin K (μg)	2-5	2-3
Vitamin D (μg)		0.33
Vitamin E (μg)	8-12	3-8
Minerals		
Calcium (mg)	250	200-250
Magnesium (mg)	30-35	30-35
Phosphorus (mg)	120-160	120-140
Sodium (mg)	300-400	120-250
Potassium (mg)	600-700	400-550
Chloride (mg)	600-800	400-450
Iron (mg)	0.5-1.0	0.3-0.9
Zinc (mg)	8-12	1-3
Copper (mg)	0.5-0.8	0.2-0.4
Manganese (μg)	5-6	3
Selenium (μg)	40	7-33
Iodine (μg)		150
Fluoride (μg)		4-15

sIgA indicates secretory immunoglobulin A; IgM, immunoglobulin M; IgG, immunoglobulin G.

[a] Adapted from Picciano MF. Representative values for constituents of human milk. *Pediatr Clin North Am.* 2001;48:263-272

[b] All values are expressed per L of milk with the exception of lipids that are expressed as a percentage on the basis of milk volume or weight of total lipids.

[c] The cholesterol content of human milk ranges from 100 to 200 mg/L in most samples of human milk after day 21 of lactation.

Index

Felodipine, grapefruit juice interactions with, 1375
Female athlete triad, 278
Fentanyl, food or nutrient interactions with, 1375
Ferritin, measurement of, 636
Fertilizer, decomposition products of, in organic food, 320–321
Fetal alcohol syndrome, failure to thrive in, 670
Fiber, 397–401
 adverse effects of, 400–401
 benefits of, 399–400
 composition of, 397–398
 crude, 398
 definition of, 397
 in diabetes mellitus, 748
 Dietary Reference Intakes of, 1355
 for eating disorder patients, 935
 in enteral formulas, 1403–1413
 health claims about, 1216, 1217
 insoluble, 398
 on nutrition claims, 1214
 recommendations for, 401–402
 soluble, 398
 standard food portions ranked by amount of, 1383–1384
 in vegetarian diets, 252
Fiberoptic endoscopic examination of swallowing, 649–650, 653–654
Fight BAC! campaign, 1242–1244
Fish
 EPA recommendations for consumption of, 1263
 mercury contamination of, 1260–1261
 toxins in, 1264–1265
Fish oils, for inflammatory bowel disease, 1046–1047
Flavin adenine dinucleotide, 519
Flavored milk, 207–208
Fluid(s). See also Water
 for eating disorder patients, 935
 for sports nutrition, 271–274
Fluid therapy
 for dehydration, 723
 for inborn errors of metabolism, 729
 for preterm infants, 86–87
Fluoride
 dietary reference intake for, 1176
 in infant formulas, 67
 supplementation with, 1172–1178
 background of, 1172–1173
 excess of, 1176–1177

schedule for, 1173–1175
 toxicity of, 1178
Fluoride varnish, 1175
Fluoxetine, food or nutrient interactions with, 1371
Flushing, 848
Folate
 action of, 523–524
 deficiency of, 524–525, 872
 in inflammatory bowel disease, 1042–1043
 in kidney disease, 1015
 health claims about, 1216
 immune system interactions with, 872
 measurement of, in nutritional status assessment, 635
 for preterm infants, 100
 supplementation with, in inflammatory bowel disease, 1043
 in vegetarian diets, 252–253
Follow-up (toddler) formulas, 77–78
Food additives/GRAS substances
 allergic reactions to, 847. See also Hypersensitivity (allergy), food
 as byproducts, 1137
 chemical information about, 539–542
 contaminants, reducing exposures to, 1275–1276
 distinguished, 537–538
 FDA regulation of, 536
 federal regulation of, 536–544
 "generally recognized as safe," 535–568
 GRAS notice submissions, 538–539, 554, 555
 for infant formulas, 540–541, 546
 human studies of, 543–544
 indirect, 1272–1276
 in infant formulas, 546–554. See also Formulas
 microbiological information about, 543
 new ingredients, 554–560
 biotechnology in development of, 560–561
 safety review of, 539–544
 stanols and their esters, 555
 sterols and their esters, 555
 sweeteners. See Sweeteners
 toxicologic information about, 542–543
Food Allergen Labeling and Consumer Protection Act, 1209–1210
Food and Drug Administration
 animal growth hormones, regulation of, 563
 bioengineered microorganisms, review of, 562–563